CONGRATULATIONS

You now have access to MERLIN for
Mosby's EMT–Intermediate Textbook, second edition

by Shade, Rothenberg, Wertz, Jones, and Collins

sign on at:

http://www.mosby.com/MERLIN/Shade

A website just for you as you learn prehospital emergency care with the new **second edition** of *Mosby's EMT–Intermediate Textbook.*

what you will receive:

Whether you're a student, an instructor, or a clinician, you'll find information just for you. Things like:

- Content Updates
- Links to Related Products
- Author Information... and more

WebLinks

plus:

An exciting program that allows you to directly access hundreds of active websites keyed specifically to the content of this book. The WebLinks are continually updated, with new ones added as they develop.

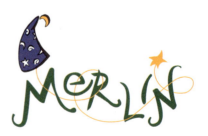

Mosby's **E**lectronic **R**esource **L**inks & **I**nformation **N**etwork

EMTINARPETSC

Mosby

An Imprint of Elsevier Science

Mosby's
EMT-INTERMEDIATE TEXTBOOK

Mosby's

edition **2**

EMT-INTERMEDIATE TEXTBOOK

BRUCE R. SHADE, EMT-P, EMS-I, AAS
Assistant Director of Public Safety
City of Cleveland, Cleveland, Ohio
Adjunct Faculty, Cuyahoga Community College, Cleveland, Ohio
Part-Time Firefighter/Paramedic
Willoughby, Ohio

MIKEL A. ROTHENBERG, MD
Emergency Care Educator
North Olmsted, Ohio
Professor of Emergency Medical Services
American College of Prehospital Medicine
Navarre, Florida

ELIZABETH WERTZ, RN, BSN, MPM, FACMPE, PHRN, EMT-P
Executive Director, Pediatric Alliance, PC
Immediate Past Chairperson, International PHTLS Division,
National Association of Emergency Medical Technicians
Chairperson, EMS for Children Advisory Committee,
Pennsylvania Emergency Health Services Council
Seven Fields, Pennsylvania

SHIRLEY A. JONES, MSEd, MHA, EMT-P
Emergency Medical Services Educator
Riverview Hospital
Noblesville, Indiana

THOMAS E. COLLINS, MD, FACEP, EMT-P
MetroHealth Medical Center
Department of Emergency Medicine
Cleveland, Ohio

with 900 full-color illustrations

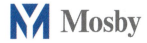

An Imprint of Elsevier Science
St. Louis   London   Philadelphia   Sydney   Toronto

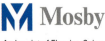
Mosby

An Imprint of Elsevier Science

Publisher: **Andrew Allen**
Editor: **Claire Merrick**
Developmental Editor: **Elaine Steinborn**
Project Manager: **John Rogers**
Project Specialist: **Kathleen L. Teal**
Designer: **Teresa Breckwoldt**

Mosby, Inc.
An Imprint of Elsevier Science
11830 Westline Industrial Drive
St. Louis, Missouri 64146

Printed in the United States of America.

International Standard Book Number: 0-323-01290-6

02   03   04   05   06/GW/RRD–W/9 8 7 6 5 4 3 2 1

PREFACE

As with the first edition the primary goal of this text is to bridge the "educational gap" between EMT–Basic training and Paramedic training according to the U.S. Department of Transportation (DOT) National Standard Curricula. The most recent changes to the EMT–Intermediate curriculum dramatically expand the role and responsibilities of the EMT–I. Today's EMT–I can perform advanced assessments, interpret ECG dysrhythmias and administer a number of essential, life saving treatments.

Some describe the new EMT–I as the Paramedic of earlier years. Having learned from the first U.S. DOT National Standard Curriculum for EMT–Paramedic, I can attest that the correlation is accurate. What does that mean for prehospital care? Without a doubt it means the delivery of better patient care. The EMT–I is now armed with the knowledge and skills to make a significant difference in patient outcome. However, along with this new role and responsibilities comes an increased burden. Doing all that may be allowed requires a higher level of competency than has ever been expected of the EMT–I. For this reason it is essential that the initial and ongoing learning experiences for the EMT–I be as productive and effective as possible.

The approach of this textbook is simple: Each objective contained in the National Standard Curriculum for the EMT–Intermediates is addressed, focusing the student on the most critical content. In addition, we have purposely exceeded the DOT objectives for EMT–Intermediate training in a number of areas to provide a more comprehensive and advanced-level textbook. We have also provided information on cutting-edge equipment and technology. By addressing a broad scope of information, *Mosby's EMT–Intermediate Textbook* offers a complete training package for a wide audience of educators and students.

Mosby's EMT–Intermediate Textbook contains 36 chapters, separated into seven divisions. The first division, PREPARATORY, addresses introductory information, including chapters on Foundations of EMT–Intermediate, Well-Being of the EMT–Intermediate, Medical-Legal Aspects, Overview of Human Systems, Emergency Pharmacology, Venous Access, and Medication Administration. Medical-Legal Aspects and Venous Access have remained separate chapters due to the importance of these two topics related to the practice of the EMT–I.

Because of its importance Division Two, AIRWAY, includes only one chapter in this new textbook. Airway Management and Ventilation are considered among the most important areas for any level of EMS provider to develop appropriate knowledge and master all the necessary skills.

Division Three, PATIENT ASSESSMENT, contains chapters on History Taking, Techniques of Physical Examination, Patient Assessment, Clinical Decision Making, Communications, and Documentation. Clinical decision making is a new and important part of patient assessment for the EMT–I and is treated as such in this textbook.

Division Four, TRAUMA, includes Trauma Systems and Mechanism of Injury, Hemorrhage and Shock, Burns, Thoracic Trauma, Head and Spinal Trauma, Abdominal Trauma, and Extremity Trauma. Although not all these topics are addressed in the most current U.S. DOT National Standard Curriculum for EMT–Intermediate, the authors felt it essential to provide readers with a more complete coverage of trauma. This was done in an effort to have this textbook serve as the single learning resource for the EMT–I student and practitioner.

Division Five, MEDICAL, includes chapters entitled Respiratory Emergencies, Cardiovascular Emergencies, Diabetic Emergencies, Allergic Reactions, Poisoning and Overdose Emergencies, Neurological Emergencies, Nontraumatic Abdominal Emergencies, Environmental Emergencies, Behavioral Emergencies, and Gynecological Emergencies.

Division Six, SPECIAL CONSIDERATIONS, includes chapters called Obstetrical Emergencies, Neonatal Resuscitation, Pediatric Emergencies, and Geriatrics.

The last section, Division Seven, ASSESSMENT-BASED MANAGEMENT, has just one chapter; Assessment-Based Management. This is a new chapter in the textbook and is designed to provide an overview of the practice of the EMT–I.

The Appendixes include a section on Medical Terminology, Advanced Airway Procedures and Administration of Thiamine and Glucagon in the Hypoglycemic Patient. These topics are not covered in the current curriculum, but were added to provide the reader with additional valuable information.

Each chapter contains a number of learning devices that have been designed to enhance the reader's comprehension and application of the material. Each chapter opens with a Case History that places the chapter content in a prehospital or clinical context. A Follow-Up to each Case History is found at the end of the chapter. Chapter Objectives appear next. Key Terms relating to the chapter are then listed. These terms also appear throughout the chapter, above the section in which they are discussed, or in the body of the text. These sections are identified by an asterisk. Each chapter concludes with a Summary, which highlights the major points discussed in the chapter.

Four types of supplemental learning material appear in the chapter text. Street Wise boxes call attention to the information that will help the EMT–Intermediate become more efficient in delivering emergency field care. Helpful Hint boxes identify background, "nice-to-know" information, giving the reader a deeper understanding of concepts and skills. Clinical Notes boxes provide the reader with background information from a clinical perspective. Student Alert boxes have been added to the second edition of this textbook to give students pointers on key areas to study in preparation for successful completion of the educational experience.

The authors and publishers are confident that both instructors and students will find that this progressive textbook facilitates an effective and enjoyable learning experience. The best of luck to you, the student, in your endeavors in advanced prehospital emergency care.

Bruce R. Shade

Mikel A. Rothenberg

Elizabeth Wertz

Shirley A. Jones

Thomas E. Collins

ACKNOWLEDGMENTS

AUTHOR ACKNOWLEDGMENTS

The first edition of this textbook came to life during a discussion Claire Merrick and I had over dinner in Bethesda, Maryland. Claire's vision and willingness to take a chance on a new market resulted in the textbook proposal moving from ideas to print on pages. The project occurred at a time when the role of the EMT–Intermediate was changing. Even though a second edition would be required in order to include all the necessary changes, Mosby took a chance and published the first edition even though the life of that printing was a short one. The second edition came about as a result of the introduction of the new U.S. DOT National Standard Curriculum for EMT–Intermediate.

As with many of these textbook projects, a lot of work goes into making words and pictures go from the authors' minds to printed pages. A number of key people made this a successful project. Claire Merrick with her "get it done or else" no nonsense approach prevented us from dawdling along, keeping this project from publishing on time. One of my strengths as an author is my determination to put only the best products out there for the reader. My worst weakness is that I beat issues to death, trying to improve them. Claire knows when to call and say, "Enough is enough." Needless to say, most of Claire's phone calls were not enjoyable ones. Claire also cut through many issues, allowing us to complete key tasks like the photo shoot for the new pictures and development of the new illustrations.

Our editor, Elaine Steinborn, was a delight to work with. Even though we nearly drove her crazy with delays (and we cannot say she didn't tell us so), last minute changes, and a host of other problems, she hung in there and delivered an outstanding textbook to production. Further, she provided emotional support along the way, helping us to see there really is a light at the end of the tunnel.

We also enjoyed the support of wonderful reviewers (listed on p. viii) who helped shape the chapters into a more readable and usable text.

Then there were the "artists." Rick Brady, a great photographer and a wonderful storyteller, created spectacular pictures and showed extraordinary patience. He even brought his whole family in to serve as models for the photo shoot. His clarity with the camera provides the reader with excellent images to better understand difficult concepts.

A refreshing and talented new artist named Jill Gregory, whom I pushed to the edge with change after change and adding new figures, did the illustrations. Much of the material I sent her were concepts that required her to use not only her artistic abilities but also her conceptual abilities. Needless to say she did a spectacular job. The second edition is one of the best-illustrated textbooks on the market.

• • •

This book is dedicated to my wife Cheri and our children, Katie and Christopher. Their sacrifice allowed me to spend the countless hours needed to bring this book to print. Throughout the years their love and support have allowed me to continue my efforts to make learning easier and more complete for out-of-hospital providers, who in turn are able to provide better patient care to those in need. My thanks and love also goes to my mother, Lucille Shade, who was an aspiring author; she encouraged me to put pen to paper. Also, to my father, Elmer Shade, Jr., who taught me the value of a hard day's work and to continually strive for what I believe.

Bruce R. Shade

• • •

To Diane, Kara, and Marc with all my love . . . without you, all my work would be in vain.

Mikel A. Rothenberg

Thanks to my parents, Helen and Bill Hodgson, for giving me the opportunity to pursue my dreams and for picking me up when the road got bumpy. To my husband, Pat, thank you for your never-ending love and support. You are truly my partner for life.

Thanks to my wonderful children: Patrick, Amanda, and Ashley. You inspire me every day. I do many of these things for you—to educate people to make a better and safer world for you. As they have grown, they have come to understand more about my dedication to writing and sharing knowledge. In fact, Ashley wants to become an illustrator (thanks to Jill Gregory for giving her encouragement!).

Patrick, I can see by your actions and the way that you treat others that you are becoming a compassionate, caring, sensitive young man. Good luck in college. Amanda, you are now my guardian angel. Even though your life was short, you taught all of us so many things. We miss you terribly every day, and we are doing our best to carry on without you. We will keep your memory alive my special daughter. Ashley, you have one of the strongest personalities I know, and you test us every day. I hope those qualities will help you change your little piece of this world.

Thank you to all of the emergency providers I have met and/or taught along the way. I truly appreciate your dedication and your willingness to make a difference. Don't ever stop your pursuit of knowledge!

And lastly, my thanks to God for giving me the ability and creativity to care for people in need and to educate others who do the same.

Elizabeth Wertz

• • •

To my father George Jones and my sister Virginia Kelleher. Thanks for all your love and support. And to Darby, Spirit, Zachary, and Chelsea.

Shirley A. Jones

• • •

The pursuit of excellent prehospital care occurs on many levels, with the ultimate driving force being the desire to provide each and every patient the exact care they require. I have been privileged throughout my adult life to work with EMS professionals who have helped instill in me the desire to use both technical and humanistic skills to care for those who are suffering.

Dr. Jonas Salk, developer of the polio vaccine, stated *"The greatest reward for doing is the opportunity to do more."* I believe this philosophy holds true for many of us in EMS.

I would like to thank my wife Katherine, whose support, dedication, and love allowed me the freedom to undertake the task of working on this book. To Katie, Tommy, Delaney Rose, and Andrew who always remind me of the important things in life. And to my parents who taught me the value of caring for others.

In addition to my parents, a special thanks to the men and women of the Pepper Pike Fire Department and Chagrin Falls Fire Department who unrelentingly encouraged and supported my desire to become a physician.

Thomas E. Collins

PUBLISHER ACKNOWLEDGMENTS

The editors wish to acknowledge and thank the many reviewers of this book, who devoted countless hours to intensive review. Their comments were invaluable in helping develop and fine-tune this manuscript.

Dennis Edgerly, EMT–P
HealthOne Hospital
Englewood, Colorado

Janet Fitts, RN, BSN, CEN, EMT-P
EMS Coordinator
East Central College
Union, Missouri

Barbara Klingensmith, MS, NREMT-P, FF
Florida State Fire College
Ocala, Florida
University of Florida
Gainesville, Florida

Jose Salazar, MPH, NREMT-P
Loudoun County Fire and Rescue
Leesburg, Virginia

William Seifarth, MS, NREMT-P
Maryland Institute for Emergency Medical Services Systems
Baltimore, Maryland

CONTENTS

Mosby's
EMT-INTERMEDIATE TEXTBOOK

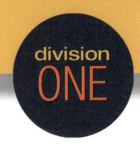

PREPARATORY

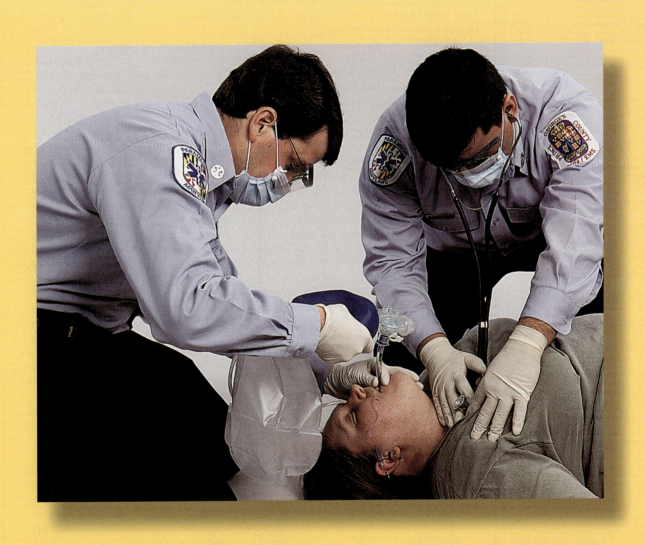

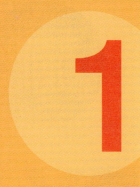

Foundations of EMT-Intermediate

Key Terms

Certification

Continuous Quality Improvement

Emergency Medical Dispatcher (EMD)

Emergency Medical Services (EMS) System

EMT–Intermediate (EMT–I)

Ethics

Health Care Professional

Licensure

Medical Direction

Profession

Professional

Professionalism

Protocols

Reciprocity

Registration

Research

Run Critiques

Standing Orders

...CASE HISTORY

Williams and Brown, EMT–Is at Station 17, report to work 5 minutes before the start of the scheduled day shift, to discover that the unit is returning from a trauma call. Their uniforms are clean, pressed, and starched, and their steel-toe leather shoes are polished. They both check the bulletin board for personnel memos and traffic notices and then sit down for a cup of coffee.

Medic 17 arrives approximately 5 minutes later; the EMT–Is begin checking the unit while the night shift crew members give their report. The crew members report that the streets department is working on a water main break at 16th and Walnut and that four ampules of naloxone and two prefilled syringes of lidocaine will expire next month. Both Williams and Brown make a note to avoid the roadwork area. While EMT–I Williams assesses all of the vehicle supplies and equipment, EMT–I Brown checks the vehicle fluid levels, radios, tires, and batteries.

A 64-year-old man awakens at 7:30 AM with a crushing chest pain. He realizes that it must be a heart attack. He and his wife were trained in CPR at the local hospital and learned to recognize the warning signs and symptoms. He also knows that it is important to act quickly. He wakes his wife and tells her to activate the EMS system by dialing 9-1-1. The emergency medical dispatcher instructs the wife to tell her husband to sit quietly until EMS arrives. The wife is also told to gather the patient's medications.

Within minutes a pumper truck, an ambulance, and a police car arrive at the home. EMT–Is Williams and Brown rush in, carrying a jump kit, oxygen, and a cardiac monitor/defibrillator. Working under established protocols, the EMT–Is place the man on oxygen and obtain a brief history of the event. As an initial assessment is performed, electrocardiogram (ECG) electrodes are applied and an intravenous (IV) line established. EMT–I Brown contacts on-line medical direction and gives the emergency department physician a brief patient report. Using telemetry, the EMT–Is transmit the ECG to the hospital for evaluation. Because the man's chest pain is still present and his vital signs are stable, the physician instructs EMT–I Brown to place a nitroglycerin tablet under the man's tongue. The man has some relief from the pain and feels confident that he is receiving good patient care. The man is gently placed on a stretcher and rolled to the ambulance for transport to the emergency department. EMT–I Williams tells the man's wife that lights and sirens are not being used in an effort to make her husband less anxious. En route to the hospital, EMT–I Brown performs an ongoing assessment of the man's pain and physical condition.

The man is delivered to the emergency department within 30 minutes of his wife's initial 9-1-1 call. The emergency department nurse and physician continue the man's care and assessment. His suspicions about a heart attack are substantiated by diagnostic tests. Thrombolytics are administered in the emergency department, and the man is transferred to the coronary intensive care unit for monitoring and recuperation. The physicians advise him that he has an excellent chance of full recovery.

CHAPTER GOAL

Upon completion of this chapter, the EMT–Intermediate will be able to understand his or her roles and responsibilities within an EMS system and how these roles and responsibilities differ from those of other levels of providers; understand the role of medical direction in the out-of-hospital environment; be able to identify the importance of primary injury prevention activities as an effective way to reduce death, disabilities, and health care costs; and value the role that ethics plays in decision making in the out-of-hospital environment.

Cognitive Objectives

As an EMT–Intermediate you should be able to do the following:

- Define the term *EMS system.*
- Define the terms *certification* and *registration.*
- Explain EMT–I licensure/certification, recertification, and reciprocity requirements.
- Evaluate the importance of maintaining your EMT–I license/certification.

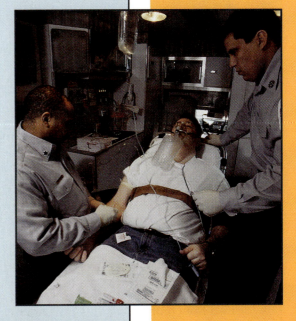

- Describe the benefits of EMT–I continuing education.
- List current state requirements for EMT–I education in your state.
- Define the terms *profession, professionalism,* and *health care professional.*
- Describe the attributes of an EMT–I as a health care professional.
- Describe how professionalism applies to an EMT–I while on and off duty.
- Describe examples of professional behaviors in the following areas: integrity, empathy, self-motivation, appearance and personal hygiene, self-confidence, communications, time management, teamwork and diplomacy, respect, patient advocacy, and careful delivery of service.
- Provide examples of activities that constitute appropriate professional behavior for an EMT–I.
- Describe the importance and benefits of quality EMS research to the future of EMS.
- Define the terms *medical direction* and *protocols.*
- Describe the role of the EMS physician in providing medical direction.
- Describe the benefits of medical direction, both on-line and off-line.
- Describe the process for the development of local policies and protocols.
- Provide examples of local protocols.
- Describe the relationship between a physician at the scene, the EMT–I at the scene, and the EMS physician providing on-line medical direction.
- Describe the components of continuous quality improvement.
- Describe the incidence, morbidity, and mortality of unintentional and alleged unintentional events in relation to injury and illness prevention.
- Identify the human, environmental, and socioeconomic impact of unintentional and alleged unintentional events in relation to injury and illness prevention.

LEARNING OBJECTIVES—cont'd

- Identify health hazards and potential crime areas within the community.
- Identify local municipal and community resources available for physical and/or socioeconomic crises.
- Identify the role of EMS in local municipal and community prevention programs.
- Identify the local prevention programs that promote safety for all age populations.
- Identify ethical responsibilities.
- Explain the premise that should underlie an EMT–I's ethical decisions in out-of-hospital care.
- Explain the relationship between the law and ethics in EMS.
- Identify the issues surrounding the use of advance directives in making an out-of-hospital resuscitation decision.

Affective Objectives

As an EMT-Intermediate you should be able to do the following:

- Defend the importance of continuing medical education and skills retention.
- Serve as a role model for others relative to professionalism in EMS.
- Exhibit professional behaviors in the following areas: integrity, empathy, self-motivation, appearance and personal hygiene, self-confidence, communications, time management, teamwork and diplomacy, respect, patient advocacy, and careful delivery of service.
- Value the need to serve as a patient advocate inclusive of those with special needs, alternative lifestyles, and cultural diversity.
- Assess personal attitudes and demeanor that may distract from professionalism.
- Value the role that family dynamics plays in the total care of patients.
- Defend the need to respect the emotional needs of dying patients and their families.
- Assess personal practices relative to the responsibility for personal safety, the safety of the crew, the patient, and bystanders.
- Advocate the need for supporting and participating in research efforts aimed at improving EMS systems.
- Advocate the need for injury prevention, including abusive situations.
- Value and defend tenets of prevention for patients and communities being served.
- Value personal commitment to the success of prevention programs.
- Advocate and practice the use of personal safety precautions in all scene situations.
- Advocate the need to show respect for the rights and feelings of patients.
- Defend personal beliefs about withholding or stopping patient care.
- Defend the value of advance medical directives.
- Assess your personal commitment to protecting patient confidentiality.
- Reinforce the patient's autonomy in the decision-making process.
- Given a scenario, defend an EMT–I's actions in a situation where a physician orders therapy that the EMT–I believes is detrimental to the patient's best interests.

Psychomotor Objectives

- None identified for this chapter.

INTRODUCTION: WHAT IS AN EMT–INTERMEDIATE?

EMT–Intermediate (EMT–I) • An emergency medical technician (EMT) who has completed training beyond the EMT–Basic level; the degree of training and skills practiced vary widely among states and EMS systems.

An **EMT–Intermediate (EMT–I)** is trained in advanced care of the acutely sick or injured. Most EMT–Is function in the prehospital care environment and serve as early links in the provision of emergency care. Some are paid, whereas others volunteer their services.

Actions taken by an EMT–I can make the difference between life and death. Proper handling and care of patients at the scene can minimize suffering, prevent further injury, and reduce recuperation time. An EMT–I is an essential component of the continuum of care and serves as a link between emergency patients and acute care resources.

Few professions offer the excitement and adventure that one experiences working as a prehospital care provider. One morning an EMT–I may be delivering a baby, that afternoon treating a patient who has abdominal pain, and the next day extricating a trauma patient from the wreckage of an overturned automobile on the freeway.

A career as an EMT–I can be exciting, but it can also challenge one's safety, composure, and humanity. Think of how disheartening it can be to perform cardiopulmonary resuscitation (CPR) for 20 minutes on a patient suffering cardiac arrest, carry him down three flights of stairs, and deliver chest compressions while off-balance in the back of a moving ambulance, only to have the patient succumb to the cardiac condition in the hospital emergency department. It can be almost as frustrating to rush to the scene of a reported serious emergency, only to find that someone has called in a false alarm or greatly exaggerated the situation to get help there sooner.

Often EMT–Is perform their duties in uncontrolled and volatile circumstances and under considerable physical and emotional stress. They often place their lives at risk to ensure the safety and well-being of the community they are sworn to serve. Long work hours, heavy workloads, lifting injuries, stress, violence, drugs, gangs, and exposure to bloodborne and airborne pathogens and hazardous materials, as well as other dangers, challenge the EMT–I's ability to remain in the field setting.

To survive as a prehospital care provider, EMT–Is must be realistic about the job. It is not all glory and excitement, nor is it mundane. With some cases it is necessary for the EMT–I to use all of the skills he or she has been trained to perform, whereas in other situations, simply holding the patient's hand or offering comfort during transport to the hospital is what is needed. To help deal with the stress inherent in the job, the EMT–I must maintain an appropriate sense of compassion and humor. Engaging in professional activities can enhance one's ability to deliver quality service.

Approach

This text presents the knowledge and skills needed by an EMT–I to function in a professional, medically appropriate, and efficient manner. Basic and advanced principles are presented, which serve as building blocks for the provision of quality patient care. This chapter describes the role of an EMT–I, what an EMS system is, and how the EMT–I works within that system. First, let us look at what an emergency medical services (EMS) system is and how an emergency call typically occurs.

Emergency Medical Services System

✂ **Emergency Medical Services (EMS) System** ● An organized approach to providing emergency care to the sick and injured.

An **emergency medical services (EMS) system** is a network of coordinated services that work as a unified whole to meet the emergency care needs of the community and to serve as a bridge between the community and the medical facilities that provide definitive health care. The primary responsibilities of an EMS system are to respond to requests for medical assistance, provide lifesaving or stabilizing treatment, and transport patients to definitive medical care. All other components of the system indirectly involved in the response, treatment, or transport of patients are considered support services. These support services are necessary to the overall operation of the EMS system.

Components of today's EMS systems, large or small, private or municipal, paid or volunteer, include some or all of the following elements as defined by the National Highway Traffic Safety Administration:
● Regulation and policy
● Resource management
● Human resources and training (including continuing education)
● Transportation
● Facilities
● Communications
● Trauma systems
● Public information and education
● Medical direction
● Evaluation

Types of Systems

EMS systems evolve as a result of geographic, political, demographic, and economic pressures that are unique to each community. Consequently, vast differences are found in EMS systems from area to area. Although many different types of EMS systems exist around the country today, no one type is superior to another. Each system offers its own unique advantages and disadvantages.

EMS systems are organized or structured in many different ways, including fire service–based, third-service, private ambulance service, hospital-based, and volunteer systems. In addition, some EMS systems are configured as public utilities or housed within law enforcement agencies.

The Emergency Call

Think back to the case history presented at the beginning of this chapter. Emergency calls, regardless of the nature, follow a similar evolution that often includes the following (Figure 1-1):
● Incident occurrence
● Recognition
● System access and dispatch
● Prehospital care
● Patient stabilization and transport
● Delivery to the hospital
● Preparation for the next event

Incident Occurrence and Recognition

The emergency call begins with the onset of illness or injury, such as the sudden onset of acute myocardial infarction, an asthma attack, a motor vehicle crash, or a

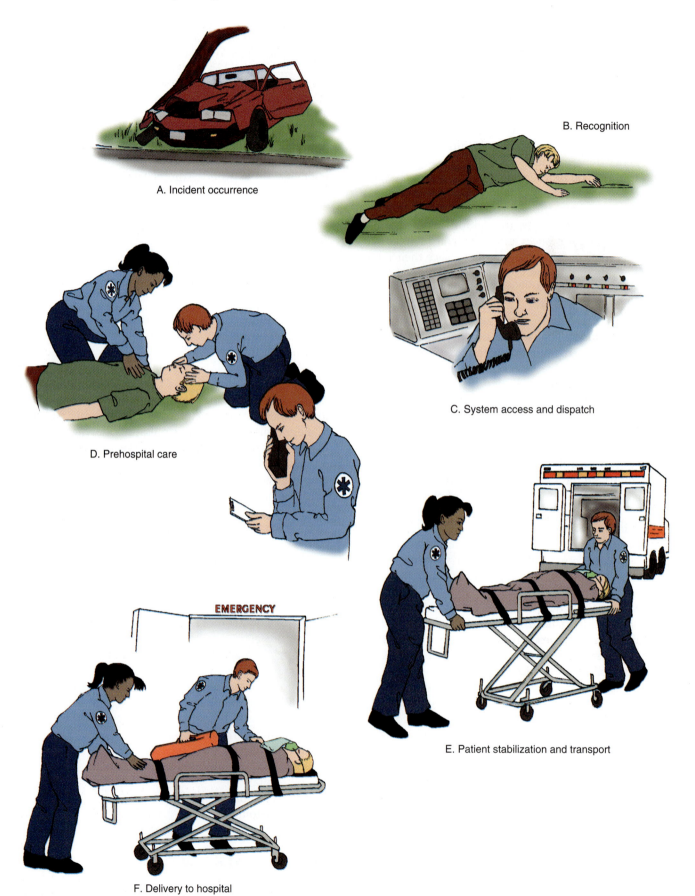

A. Incident occurrence

B. Recognition

C. System access and dispatch

D. Prehospital care

E. Patient stabilization and transport

EMERGENCY

F. Delivery to hospital

FIGURE 1-1   ▲   **Phases of emergency medical care.**

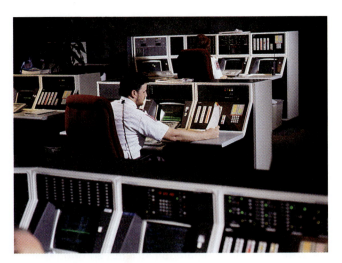

FIGURE 1-2 ▲ Emergency medical dispatchers in a computerized dispatch center.

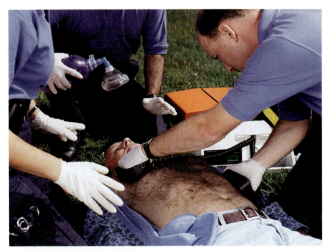

FIGURE 1-3 ▲ EMT–Is providing prehospital care.

shooting incident. The victims themselves, family members, friends, co-workers, or bystanders then recognize the incident. Once the emergency is identified, the victim may receive care from bystanders before arrival of the EMS system. Bystander care may include such procedures as the following:
- Relief of airway obstruction due to a foreign body
- CPR
- Bleeding control
- Comfort and reassurance

System Access and Dispatch

Next, a decision is made to seek medical assistance. The EMS system is then accessed, usually by phone. EMS systems receive calls for help at the dispatch center. Callers in many communities reach the EMS dispatch center by dialing 9-1-1. Other communities may access EMS via the local sheriff, police, or fire department dispatcher. In some communities people contact private ambulance services or volunteer systems directly rather than contacting a municipal service.

UNIVERSAL EMERGENCY NUMBER

The "universal" emergency phone number 9-1-1 serves much of the United States. This number eliminates the need for separate phone numbers for fire, police, and EMS systems, as well as different access numbers for each community. As a result, help can be accessed more quickly.

Emergency Medical Dispatcher ● A specially trained person who receives calls for emergency assistance and ensures proper EMS response.

Many dispatch centers are staffed with **emergency medical dispatchers (EMDs)** (Figure 1-2). The EMD's

duties go beyond answering phones and dispatching ambulances. Often the EMD also receives extensive training in computer-aided dispatch, priority dispatch, prearrival instructions, and system status management. Once the emergency call is processed, the EMD must select the most appropriate ambulance to dispatch to the scene. This decision usually is based on the distance to the call, the time of day, and the level of care needed to handle the emergency.

Prehospital Care

The treatment a patient receives before arrival at the hospital is referred to as prehospital care (Figure 1-3). Prehospital care is essentially an extension of hospital care. Prehospital care providers now deliver lifesaving treatments that were performed only by physicians just a few decades ago. Although EMTs (EMT–Basics, EMT–Intermediates, EMT–Paramedics) are delivering the care, the legal responsibility for providing advanced management skills still falls on the medical direction physician.

STREET WISE

The first rule of patient care is "Do no harm."

Stabilization and Transport

Serious and life-threatening conditions require that definitive prehospital care be provided as soon as possible. For many patients this care can be started and, to a great measure, completed in the field. However, trauma patients who require blood replacement and hemorrhage control can only be stabilized in the operating room. For these patients, resuscitation must quickly be initiated in

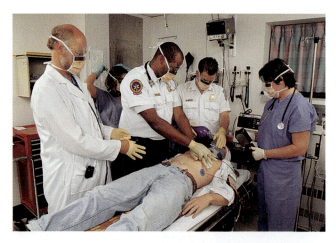

FIGURE 1-4 ▲ The EMT–Intermediate is an integral part of the professional patient care team. (From American College of Emergency Physicians; Pons PT, Cason D, chief editors: *Paramedic field care: a complaint-based approach,* St Louis, 1997, Mosby.)

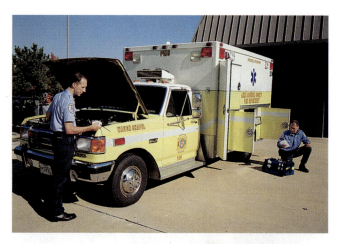

FIGURE 1-5 ▲ Preparation includes ensuring that the vehicle and equipment are in proper condition. (From American College of Emergency Physicians; Pons PT, Cason D, chief editors: *Paramedic field care: a complaint-based approach,* St Louis, 1997, Mosby.)

the field or during rapid transport to the appropriate hospital (preferably a trauma center). The ability of the EMT–I to differentiate between patients who can be stabilized at the scene and those requiring prompt transport to the hospital is critical for increasing long-term survival and reducing complications and patient disability.

In some cases patient transport to the hospital may not be necessary. The call may be a false alarm, the patient may have gone to the hospital on his or her own by the time the ambulance arrives at the scene, or the patient may refuse treatment and/or transport. Also, some EMS systems permit the EMT–I to decide when patient transport to the hospital is not warranted. Referral to another means of transport may then be provided.

Delivery to the Hospital

On arrival at the hospital, the patient receives additional treatment in the emergency department. The EMT–I must ensure that an appropriate transition from the ambulance crew to the hospital staff takes place (Figure 1-4). This includes transferring care to an individual at the same level as or higher level than the EMT–I's level of certification or licensure, informing the appropriate hospital staff of all pertinent patient information, and safely moving the patient from the ambulance cot to the emergency department bed.

Following emergency department treatment, the patient may be admitted to the hospital for further care and recuperation. After release from the hospital, the patient may need follow-up treatment and/or physical therapy as part of his or her rehabilitation.

Preparation for the Next Event

Following each emergency call, the EMT–I must restore the ambulance to its prerun condition. This includes

completing all needed documentation, replacing any medical supplies used, and cleaning the ambulance and equipment used (Figure 1-5). This must be done in a timely fashion. Quick turnarounds of the unit are necessary, since the dispatch center may be receiving additional calls for help.

EMT–INTERMEDIATE TRAINING AND CERTIFICATION

The classification of EMT–I is a little more than a few decades old. It follows the evolution of the emergency medical technician (EMT) over the past century from stretcher bearer and ambulance driver to today's health care professional.

Today's EMT–I possesses both basic skills and key advanced care skills, including additional patient assessment skills, use of advanced airway adjuncts, intravenous (IV) therapy, techniques for managing tension pneumothorax, monitoring and interpreting basic cardiac dysrhythmias, administering key life-sustaining medications, and defibrillating patients (Figure 1-6).

To practice as an EMT–I in most states, a person is required to complete a recognized EMT–I course, successfully complete a written and practical examination, and become certified or licensed. From the early 1980s through the beginning of the 1990s, the U.S. Department of Transportation (DOT) recognized three levels of EMT certification: EMT–Basic (EMT–B), EMT–Intermediate (EMT–I), and EMT–Paramedic (EMT–P). An additional level, EMT–Defibrillation, was developed by the American Heart Association in 1990 to provide for a state- or nationally-certified EMT–B who completed additional training in the use of cardiac defibrillators. In September 1993 the National EMS Education and Practice Blueprint, a consensus document, recommended that there be four lev-

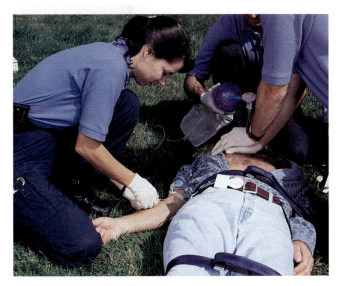

FIGURE 1-6 ▲ Intravenous therapy is an important aspect of the EMT–I's care for the patient.

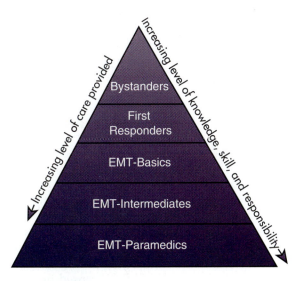

FIGURE 1-7 ▲ Pyramid of care.

els of prehospital providers: first responder, EMT–B, EMT–I, and EMT–P.

The National Standard Curriculum serves as the foundation for training of the various levels of EMTs in the United States. There is a specific curriculum for each level of EMT. The most current curriculums are the EMT–Basic: National Standard Curriculum (1994), the First Responder: National Standard Curriculum (1995), the EMT–Intermediate: National Standard Curriculum (1998), and the EMT–Paramedic: National Standard Curriculum (1999). The curriculums are developed through funding from the National Highway and Traffic Safety Administration (NHTSA). Along with the delivery of basic life support by bystanders, these four levels serve as the pyramid of care in the prehospital setting (Figure 1-7).

The current EMT–Intermediate: National Standard Curriculum was designed to address the educational needs of the traditional EMT–I and provide a solid foundation for professional practice and additional education with a heavy emphasis on clinical problem solving and decision making.

EMT–Intermediate Training

Typically, certification as an EMT–B is a prerequisite for enrollment in an EMT–I course. Proficiency in reading, writing, and math are also prerequisite skills, since documentation skills at the advanced level rely heavily on correct spelling and appropriate use of grammar, vocabulary, and syntax, whereas sufficient math skills are needed to calculate dosages for medication administration.

The EMT–I course includes didactic instruction, a skills laboratory, clinical education, and field internship (Figure 1-8).

The didactic instruction represents delivery of the knowledge or cognitive portion of the training. It is typically delivered via classroom instruction using lectures, videos, discussions, demonstrations, and simulations.

The skills laboratory is the part of the training where the EMT–I has a chance to learn and practice the needed psychomotor skills. This component is typically integrated into the curriculum in such a way as to present skills in a sequential, building fashion. The EMT–I may initially learn each skill individually and then later incorporate some or most of the learned skills into simulated patient care cases. Toward the latter part of the program, the skills laboratory may be used to present instructional scenarios to emphasize the application and integration of didactic content and skills into patient management much like the EMT–I will be expected to do in the real world.

The clinical education is an essential part of EMT–I education, since this is where the EMT–I has a chance to apply what is learned in the classroom and laboratory settings to real patient care situations. Typically, clinical education for the EMT–I student takes place in both the hospital and field settings.

An educational model, which is part of the national standard curriculum, outlines the topic areas that are included in the EMT–I training program. This revision of the curriculum includes cognitive (knowledge), psychomotor (skills), and affective (attitude) learning objectives. Learning objectives serve as a roadmap to learning.

The number of hours required for EMT–I training averages 300 to 400 total hours of instruction, including classroom time, instruction in practical skills, and clinical instruction.

Because of the advanced level of care provided, most states require the EMT–I to work under medical direction. Because advanced life support providers often treat patients understanding orders, a significant por-

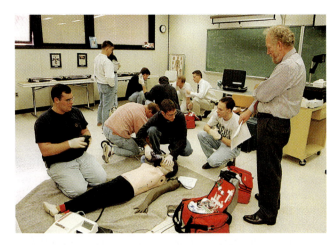

FIGURE 1-8 ▲ **An important part of the EMI course is learning and practicing new skills.**

tion of the instruction is devoted to assessment skills and dealing with as many additional potential emergency situations as possible.

The Certification Process
KNOWLEDGE AND SKILL EXAMINATIONS

At the completion of the training, the EMT–I must successfully complete written and skill examinations to demonstrate mastery of the required knowledge and skills. This is in addition to course completion and may be required by state regulations. Some states use their own testing process for EMT–Is, whereas others use the National Registry of Emergency Medical Technicians (NREMT) EMT–Intermediate Examination. Also, some states require both; the EMT–I must have national registration, as well as successfully complete a certification/licensure examination.

✖ **Registration** • Act of enrolling one's name in a "register" or book of record.

The NREMT is a private, nonprofit agency formed to provide testing and registration of EMTs on a nationwide basis. To meet the NREMT requirements for registration, the candidate must do the following:
- Successfully complete an EMT–I training program that meets DOT standards.
- Successfully pass the EMT–I written examination and practical skills testing of the NREMT.

In states in which national registration is not required, the EMT–I should view becoming nationally registered as a demonstration of commitment to excellence. To remain nationally registered, reregistration at 2-year intervals is required. Attending a structured refresher program or obtaining the required continuing education during the registration period satisfies the reregistration requirement.

✖ **Certification** • Action by which an agency or association grants recognition to an individual who has met its qualifications.

✖ **Licensure** • Process by which a government agency grants permission to an individual to engage in a given occupation on finding that the applicant has attained the minimum degree of competency necessary.

Credentialing

Following successful completion of the required training and testing, the candidate must undergo a credentialing process. The objective of credentialing is to protect the public from incompetence and provide for professional identification. **Certification** and **licensure** are common forms of credentialing used for today's prehospital care providers.

The process of credentialing varies from state to state. In some states, after meeting the necessary testing and training requirements, the process may be as simple as filling out a form that is signed by the training program medical advisor and submitted to the state EMS office. The state EMS office issues a certification card that can be carried in a wallet. In other states EMT–I certification or licensure is administered through the state department of health, board of medical examiners, or other state agency.

Meaning of EMT–Intermediate Certification

It is important to understand what certification or licensure represents. Most states or communities use certification or licensure to grant authority to an individual who has met predetermined qualifications to participate in an activity. A document is typically issued by a government or nongovernment entity that certifies fulfillment of requirements for practice in a field. There is an unfounded general belief that "licensed professionals" have greater status than those who are "certified" or "registered." A "certification" granted by a state, conferring a right to engage in a trade or profession, is in fact a "license."

Certification does not give a person the right to work as an EMT–I or to be selected for employment. Both volunteer and paid EMS systems may add other requirements, including examinations, internships, or other demonstrations of proficiency before the EMT–I is able to function in the field setting.

✖ **Reciprocity** • Mutual exchange of privileges or licenses by two certifying agencies.

Reciprocity

It is not uncommon for EMT–Is who are certified in one state to relocate to another. Rather than requiring those individuals to repeat the EMT–I training, most states have a process in place called **reciprocity** that allows the

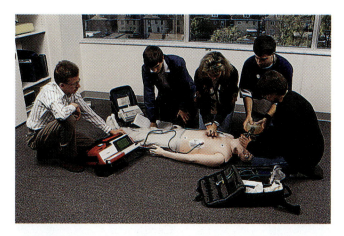

FIGURE 1-9 ▲ Continuing education activities. (Vincent Knaus from Stoy WA: *Mosby's EMT–Basic textbook,* St Louis, 1996, Mosby.)

transfer of certification or licensure. In some states reciprocity is automatic, especially if the EMT–I is nationally registered.

RECERTIFICATION AND CONTINUING EDUCATION

To maintain the right to function as an EMT–I, most states require recertification every 1 to 5 years (the average being 2 years). It is legally necessary to maintain certification or licensure as long as one practices as an EMT–I.

In some states, recertification involves participating in a refresher course, whereas in other states, EMT–Is are required to obtain a specific amount of continuing education each year. Some jurisdictions require successful completion of written and/or skills testing to become recertified as an EMT–I.

Benefits of Continuing Education

The EMT–I curriculum is designed to provide the fundamental knowledge and skills needed to serve as an entry-level EMT–I. Enrichment and continuing education are needed in some cases to bring the EMT–I to full competency. Furthermore, it is important to recognize that this curriculum does not provide a person with extensive knowledge in hazardous materials, bloodborne pathogens, emergency vehicle operations, or rescue practices in unusual environments. Another important consideration is that many of the skills and much of the knowledge learned in the EMT–I course may not be used frequently, and skill decay can occur rapidly. Continuing education helps reduce the erosion of knowledge and skills (Figure 1-9). It also keeps the EMT–I current on new procedures and treatments, allows a sharing of real-life experiences with other prehospital care providers, and encourages further professional development.

Run Critiques • Sessions in which prehospital care providers and medical direction physicians (typically in a group setting) review run reports and/or case histories to identify positive and negative aspects of care and documentation provided by EMT–Is in given cases. It allows EMT–Is to learn from others' experiences.

Continuing Education for the EMT–Intermediate

Countless continuing education opportunities are available to the EMT–I. On a local level, EMS systems, EMS associations, and hospitals often provide in-service training programs, seminars, and **run critiques.** On a state and national level a variety of conferences are held annually. These conferences expose EMT–Is to a wide range of nationally recognized experts in EMS, relaying the most current information (research updates, newest equipment, new techniques) in EMS.

Another common type of continuing education activity is the 1- or 2-day training program. A course in Prehospital Trauma Life Support (PHTLS), developed by the National Association of Emergency Medical Technicians in conjunction with the American College of Surgeons Committee on Trauma, is one example of such a program. In this course, students are exposed to basic and advanced concepts in managing trauma patients. Similar types of programs include courses in CPR, Advanced Cardiac Life Support (ACLS), Advanced Medical Life Support (AMLS), Basic Trauma Life Support (BTLS), Pediatric Life Support (PAL), and Prehospital Education for Prehospital Professionals (PEPP). Brief, information-packed courses such as these require only a modest time commitment on the EMT–I's part while providing enormous knowledge, skills learning, and remediation. Maintaining current certification in some or all of these programs may also be required for state recertification.

Alternatively, there are many excellent continuing education programs that can be conveniently reviewed while at home or on the job. These programs can be found in EMS-related textbooks, magazines, subscription videos, computer programs, and on the Internet.

EMS-Related Reading

EMS-related publishing companies have had a strong influence on the evolution of the EMS profession. A variety of EMS–related textbooks and magazines are available. EMS magazines help keep the EMT–I aware of the latest changes in a constantly evolving industry and provide excellent sources of continuing education to sharpen knowledge and skills. EMS magazines also list employment opportunities, EMS seminars, and conferences; provide details about new products and equipment; highlight tips that can be used on the job; and review various EMS–related books, videos, and computer software. An additional benefit of EMS magazines is that they provide the opportunity to write articles, communicating important information to other EMS professionals. Many offer student subscription rates.

Serving as an Instructor/Preceptor

Serving as an instructor in CPR, first aid, or EMT courses or as a preceptor in EMT–B or EMT–I field internships is another way to keep one's skills current. Teaching can serve as a source of continuing education credit. Serving as a responsible educator also establishes one as a leader and a reliable resource in the community.

PROFESSIONALISM

Professional • A person who has certain special skills and knowledge in a specific area and conforms to the standards of conduct and performance in that area. One does not need to be paid to be a professional.

Professionalism • Refers to conduct or qualities characterizing a practitioner in a particular field or occupation.

Profession • Refers to a specialized body of knowledge or skills.

Health Care Professional • Properly trained and licensed or certified provider of health care.

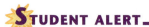
STUDENT ALERT

You should know the attributes of professionalism.

Defining Professionalism

The educational experience that one participates in to become certified should help one to become a **professional** EMT–I. **Professionalism** is necessary to promote quality patient care, instill pride in the prehospital environment, promote high standards, and earn the respect of other members of the health care team (Figure 1-10).

People who are involved in emergencies usually experience pain, fear, and great anxiety. Sick and injured patients feel vulnerable and helpless when depending on strangers for assistance. The EMT–I's professionalism can positively influence a patient's judgment of the EMS system. Patients who are made to feel at ease by the actions of caring, confident, and well-trained EMT–Is may show both psychological and physical improvement (Figure 1-11).

EMS personnel occupy positions of public trust. Society expects safety professionals to conduct themselves appropriately both on and off duty. The EMT–I is a highly visible role model. People look up to EMT–Is and trust that they will always do the right thing. Like it or not, EMT–Is are not just individual citizens. In addition to representing themselves, they also

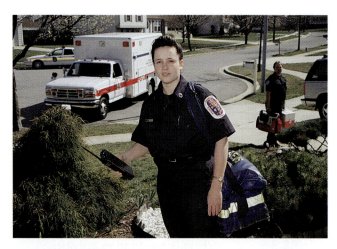
FIGURE 1-10 ▲ Professionalism is expressed in appearance and attitude. (From American College of Emergency Physicians; Pons PT, Cason D, chief editors: *Paramedic field care: a complaint-based approach,* St Louis, 1997, Mosby.)

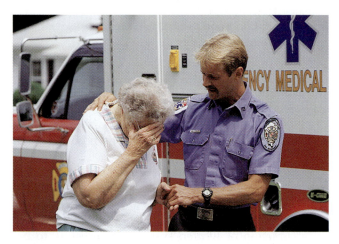
FIGURE 1-11 ▲ A gentle, appropriate touch can offer a great deal of reassurance and comfort to an ill or injured person. (From American College of Emergency Physicians; Pons PT, Cason D, chief editors: *Paramedic field care: a complaint-based approach,* St Louis, 1997, Mosby.)

represent many others, including their EMS agency; state, county, city, and/or district EMS office(s); and their peers. To a certain extent, they also represent the medical community. Unprofessional conduct, whether on or off duty, hurts the image of the EMS profession. Commitment to excellence is a daily activity that requires constant vigilance to ensure that a professional image is maintained.

Attributes of professional conduct include the following:

• *Integrity*—Having integrity is the EMT–I's single most important characteristic. The public expects EMT–Is to be honest in all of their actions. Examples of behaviors that demonstrate integrity include telling the truth, not stealing, and performing complete and accurate documentation.

- *Empathy*—Being empathetic involves identifying with and understanding the feelings, situations, and motives of others. EMT–Is must demonstrate empathy to patients, families, and other **health care professionals.** Behaviors that demonstrate empathy include showing caring and compassion for others; demonstrating an understanding of patient and family feelings; showing respect for others; exhibiting a calm, compassionate, and helpful demeanor toward those in need; and being supportive and reassuring of others.

- *A professional manner*—EMT–Is should be courteous, in control of their emotions, avoid inappropriate conversation, and appear confident. They should not eat, drink, or smoke while caring for patients.

- *Good appearance and personal hygiene*—How EMT–Is appear to others and to themselves is important. First impressions are often the longest lasting. People form an opinion about a person and his or her qualifications to do a job with their first look at the person. Being well groomed and wearing an appropriate, clean, pressed uniform (that is in good repair) projects a professional image. EMT–Is should also maintain good personal hygiene and grooming. Finally, personal protection apparel should be worn when indicated.

- *Appropriate general conduct*—EMT–Is should show interest and pride in their service. In striving to provide the best-quality patient care, they also have a responsibility to be nondiscriminatory and nonjudgmental in dealing with patients. The EMT–I should work well as a member of the prehospital team, share equally in the workload, and communicate effectively with patients, bystanders, partner(s), fellow workers, and other safety professionals. This will help the EMT–I earn the respect of others. Also, the EMT–I should instill pride in the profession and strive for high standards.

- *Being a patient advocate*—A professional places all of his or her efforts toward the patient's welfare and does not allow his or her own self-interest to come before the needs of the patient. The professional also accepts others' right to differ and does not impose his or her beliefs on others. The EMT–I must not allow personal (religious, ethical, political, social, legal) biases to affect patient care. Advocacy also means ensuring patient safety, providing reassurance, protecting patient confidentiality, and preventing patient embarrassment.

- *Treating others with respect*—EMT–Is feel and show deferential regard for others, as well as display consideration and appreciation. Being respectful and polite to others, not using derogatory or demeaning terms, and behaving in a manner to bring credit to themselves, their associations, and their profession are examples of treating others with respect. EMT–Is should call patients by their proper name (e.g., Mr. Smith), not "pops," "gramps," "bub," etc.,

and avoid making negative comments about a person's gender, race, sexual orientation, ethnicity, religion, physical appearance, profession, social status, or disability.

- *Having self-motivation/personal improvement*—A professional has an internal drive for excellence—always striving to be the best he or she can be—and enthusiastically takes advantage of learning opportunities. Attending continuing education activities, practicing skills, reading EMS-related literature, and demonstrating a commitment to continuous quality improvement are all examples of self-motivation. Also, a professional continually demonstrates self-direction, taking the initiative to complete assignments, improve and/or correct behavior that is not up to par, and take on and follow through on tasks without constant supervision. A professional is also one who accepts constructive feedback in a positive manner, looking for opportunities to make himself or herself better.

- *Self-confidence*—As a professional the EMT–I trusts or has reliance on himself or herself. EMT–Is develop an accurate assessment of their personal and professional strengths and limitations. They believe in themselves and in what they can do.

- *Maintaining good communication*—Communication is the exchange of thoughts, messages, and information. Professionals develop the ability to convey information to others verbally and in writing, as well as the ability to understand and interpret verbal and written messages. Speaking clearly, writing legibly, listening actively, and adjusting communication strategies to various situations are examples of professional behavior.

- *Exercising good time management*—Professionals organize tasks to make maximum use of time, prioritize tasks, are punctual, and complete tasks and assignments on time.

- *Employing teamwork and diplomacy*—Teamwork is the ability to work with others to achieve a common goal, whereas diplomacy is tact and skill in dealing with people. Examples of teamwork and diplomacy include placing the success of the team above self-interest, not undermining the team, helping and supporting other team members, showing respect for all team members, remaining flexible and open to change, and communicating with co-workers in an effort to resolve problems.

- *Careful delivery of service*—As a professional the EMT–I always delivers the highest quality of patient care with careful attention to detail while critically evaluating his or her performance and attitude. Examples of this include mastering and refreshing skills, performing complete equipment checks, operating the ambulance in a careful and safe manner, and following policies, procedures, and protocols, as well as the orders of superiors.

STREET WISE

To become proficient, you must be able to use all equipment and carry out procedures without having to think about them; in other words, the procedures must be "second nature." One way to accomplish this goal is to practice frequently with the equipment and rehearse all necessary skills. Handling equipment gives you a feel for each device, making it easier to use the device under less than ideal conditions, such as when the lighting is poor or you are in a hurry.

During the training program you should visit the local EMS station from time to time to observe how equipment is stored, maintained, and used. If you build a positive relationship with the crew(s), they may be willing to allow you to practice with the equipment during visits.

ROLE AND RESPONSIBILITIES OF THE EMT–INTERMEDIATE

Role

The role of an EMT–I is to provide basic and advanced care to persons experiencing medical and traumatic emergencies.

STUDENT ALERT

You should be familiar with the responsibilities of an EMT–I.

Responsibilities

The foremost responsibility of an EMT–I is to ensure his or her own safety and the safety of fellow workers. Duties typically include the following:

- Being prepared to respond to the next emergency call. This begins with being physically, mentally, and emotionally ready. Employing positive health practices, having adequate knowledge, and maintaining skills help facilitate this. The EMT–I must also ensure the availability and proper working order of appropriate equipment and supplies.
- Driving the emergency vehicle to the scene in a safe, timely, and lawful manner while exercising due regard for others.
- Assessing for and ensuring scene safety and determining the mechanism of injury (where appropriate).
- Using protective equipment in hazardous or dangerous situations, including employing body substance isolation precautions.
- Interacting with first responders who are already at the scene providing care.

- Initially controlling the scene and regulating access to potentially harmful situations. Police or other emergency personnel often assume these duties on their arrival at the scene.
- Determining the needs of those involved in the incident and communicating that information to the dispatch center, including requesting the response of and coordinating with supportive agencies as needed.
- Using basic tools and procedures to gain access to and extricate entrapped patients.
- Establishing rapport with patients and bystanders, maintaining their confidentiality, and shielding them from onlookers.
- Treating patients with the appropriate dignity, compassion, and respect.
- Rapidly assessing and managing life-threatening illnesses and injuries.
- Performing a careful patient assessment; recognizing the nature and seriousness of illnesses or injuries; prioritizing assessment, care, and transport of the patient(s); and determining the requirements for emergency medical care.
- Following given protocols to provide prompt and efficient care for illnesses or injuries.
- Assessing the effects of treatment.
- Establishing communications with medical direction, including physician consultation, when needed.
- Recognizing when the limits of field care have been reached and when prompt transportation to the appropriate medical facility is needed.
- Lifting, moving, positioning, and handling patients in such a way as to minimize discomfort and further injury, including spinal immobilization, splinting fractures, and proper lifting and carrying techniques.
- Transporting patients safely and expeditiously to an appropriate medical facility. The EMT–I must know what resources are available and be familiar with local protocols involving patient transportation. It is important to have a working knowledge of the clinical capabilities and categorizations of all hospitals in the transport area. Does each facility have an emergency department, operating suite, postanesthesia recovery room or surgical intensive care unit, and intensive care units for trauma patients? Are any of the hospitals capable of providing specialty care for trauma, pediatric, burn, cardiology, or neurology emergencies or high-risk delivery? Do any of the hospitals have acute hemodialysis, acute spinal cord/head injury management, and/or special radiological capability? What do they provide in the way of rehabilitation, clinical laboratory service, toxicology, hazardous materials/decontamination, hyperbarics, reperfusion, and psychiatric care? The EMT–I may also be responsible for making arrangements for other transportation, such as aeromedical evacuation of a critically injured motor vehicle accident victim. Local protocols should be followed in determining whether a patient will be trans-

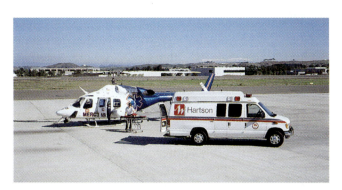

FIGURE 1-12 ▲ Helicopter and ground critical care transport units.

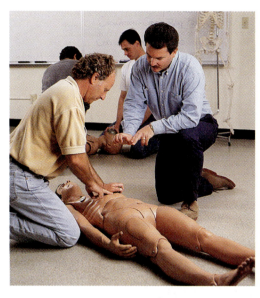

FIGURE 1-13 ▲ CPR courses prepare the public to respond appropriately in a cardiac emergency situation.

ported via ground or air. The EMT–I should also be familiar with any transfer agreements the EMS system has with hospitals and other entities (Figure 1-12).

- Communicating with medical direction when indicated for guidance on patient treatment and transfer, as well as when patient referral is warranted.
- Transferring care of patients to the emergency department staff (usually the emergency department nurse) in an orderly and efficient manner. The EMT–I must serve as the patient's advocate, providing a concise and factual briefing to the hospital staff.
- Properly completing the run sheet (run report) used by the EMS system. The EMS run report is the legal record of the events that occurred. It gives the hospital staff important information about the incident and patient history. Patient care reports must be thorough and accurate and completed in a timely manner.
- Gathering and completing needed billing information. The EMT–I should be familiar with payers and insurance systems in the community.
- Preparing for the next incident. The EMT–I is responsible for cleaning and maintaining equipment in proper working order, which ensures that quality patient care can be provided. The EMT–I must return to service as soon as possible so as to keep "downtime" to a minimum. Where appropriate, debriefing of the crew may help to glean valuable information about the emergency call, what works or does not work, and what can be done better.
- Recognizing when patient transport is not warranted and following established protocols for handling such situations.
- Keeping the emergency vehicle adequately equipped, supplied, and maintained. The EMT–I is also responsible for checking the expiration dates on IV solutions and medications, as well as testing the laryngoscopes and other such equipment for proper function.

Although primary responsibilities center on maintaining high-quality, out-of-hospital emergency care, ancillary responsibilities may involve participating in public education and health promotion programs as deemed appropriate by the community. EMT–Is serve as role models;

communities will look to them for leadership and direction in their public education and prevention activities.

Public Information and Education

The ability to recognize a serious medical emergency and activate the system may mean the difference between patient survival and death. Effective public information and education programs are needed to prepare the public to respond appropriately to medical emergencies. These programs should teach the public how to do the following:

- Recognize the signs and symptoms of serious illnesses or injuries.
- Access EMS (when, where, and how to use EMS).
- Provide lifesaving interventions such as CPR, relief of airway obstruction, and hemorrhage control (Figure 1-13).

Public information and education campaigns can also be used to reduce or prevent disease and injuries, increase compliance with treatment regimens, and reduce unnecessary use of precious EMS and non-EMS health care resources. Alternatives such as identifying less expensive transportation options and referring persons to non–hospital emergency department clinical providers and freestanding emergency clinics are effective means of reducing misuse, as well as keeping the overall cost of the system operation down. These campaigns can be developed cooperatively with health care organizations such as hospitals or other provider agencies, thereby increasing the integration of EMS into the community's health care system and public safety arena (Figure 1-14).

The EMT–I should also be an advocate for citizen involvement in the EMS system. Citizens can assist in establishing needs and parameters for system improvement, as

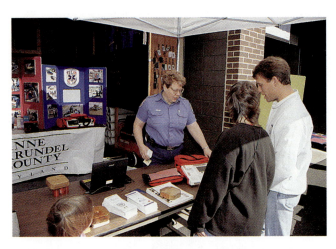

FIGURE 1-14 ▲ Educating the community about the EMS system. (From American College of Emergency Physicians; Pons PT, Cason D, chief editors: *Paramedic field care: a complaint-based approach,* St Louis, 1997, Mosby.)

well as providing an outside, objective view into quality improvement and problem resolution. This creates informed, independent advocates for the EMS system.

Marketing campaigns are an effective way of improving the image of the EMS system by increasing visibility and projecting a positive image of the EMS providers. Many systems use off-duty personnel to conduct classes or deliver speeches to schools and civic organizations. These activities can also be used to recruit future employees or volunteers into the EMS system.

EMT–Is are responsible and accountable to medical direction, the public, and their peers. The EMT–I should seek to take part in lifelong professional development and peer evaluation and assume an active role in professional and community organizations. It is also important to recognize the importance of research.

Growing Employment Opportunities

There is a wide range of jobs in which the EMT–I can practice his or her profession. Some of these jobs offer a salary, whereas others are on a volunteer basis. In addition to working in the field setting, EMT–Is are finding employment in hospital emergency departments, as well as in industrial and corporate settings. In many hospitals EMT–Is are hired to work in the emergency department. These EMT–Is typically perform nursing assistant duties, which may include obtaining patient vital signs, documenting patient information, transporting patients to the radiology department or to hospital floors, cleaning and bandaging wounds, delivering CPR, restocking supplies, splinting minor fractures, drawing blood, placing IV lines, and sometimes performing endotracheal intubation. Many EMT–Is are becoming educators and administrators in EMS systems.

Research

Until recently, treatment protocols were often drawn directly from the hospital setting. This occurred despite the marked differences between the prehospital and hospital environments. Furthermore, many protocols and procedures used today evolved without clinical evidence of their usefulness, safety, or even benefit to the patient. EMS providers must now begin to prove which patient care protocols and techniques are useful and beneficial. As changes in professional standards, training, equipment, and procedures are contemplated, they must be based on empirical data, rather than "great ideas" or "new gadget" models.

✖ **Research** • The scientific study, investigation, and experimentation conducted to establish facts and determine their significance.

Prehospital research can help eliminate much of the uncertainty associated with prehospital care. Questions such as "Why do we treat patients this way in the field?" "Does this treatment benefit many patients?" and "Does it harm some?" must be asked to continually justify EMS practices and protocols.

A number of benefits can be derived from conducting prehospital research. Most important, prehospital research has the immediate potential of saving lives or limiting morbidity by improving current and future patient care delivered in the field. Research can also prove that prehospital care makes a difference and is valuable. This is particularly important in times of recession and slow growth, when budget cuts are seen in every area of medicine and public service. Research also enhances recognition and respect for EMS professionals.

Medical Direction

✖ **Medical Direction** • Medical supervision of an EMS system and the field performance of EMTs.

Many of the services provided by an EMT–I are derived from medical practices. The care provided in the field is an extension of hospital and physician services. As such, accepted standards of medical practice must be met. Medical direction ensures that the EMT–I is providing the appropriate high-quality care. Physicians are regarded as the authorities on issues of medical care, and when properly educated and motivated, physicians are a vital component of EMS. Although the system's medical director is ultimately responsible for all of the medical care provided by his or her service, many duties may be delegated to other qualified colleagues.

✖ **Protocols** • Written instructions for the care of patients with specific conditions, illnesses, or injuries. The medical director of an EMS system is responsible for developing these protocols.

The role of the EMS physician in providing medical direction includes the following:

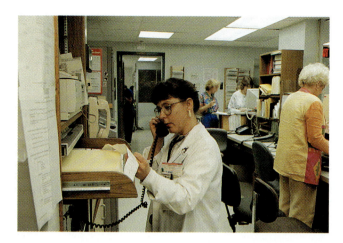

FIGURE 1-15 ▲ On-line medical direction from a physician at a hospital allows the physician to interact in the care of a patient at the scene by using information supplied by the EMS provider. (From American College of Emergency Physicians: Pons PT. Cason D, chief editors: *Paramedic field care: a complaint-based approach,* St Louis, 1997, Mosby.)

- Educating and training of EMS personnel
- Participating in the personnel selection process
- Participating in equipment selection
- Developing clinical **protocols** in cooperation with expert EMS personnel
- Participating in quality improvement and problem resolution
- Providing direct input into patient care
- Serving as an interface between the EMS system and other health care agencies
- Being an advocate for EMS within the medical community
- Serving as the "medical conscience" of the EMS system
- Being an advocate for quality patient care

STUDENT ALERT

You should know the difference between on-line and off-line medical direction and be able to define the protocols for each.

Two types of medical direction guide the EMT–I's day-to-day activities. Direct medical direction, sometimes called on-line medical direction, is care rendered under direct orders, usually over the radio or telephone (Figure 1-15). Direct medical direction is provided when the EMT–I sees a patient and contacts medical direction for instruction before rendering certain care. Direct medical direction may be supplemented by telemetry. Telemetry allows a patient's electrocardiogram (ECG) to be sent to the on-line physician for review and for help in determining appropriate treatment regimens. The hospital emergency department often provides direct medical direction. Direct medical direction may also be provided at the scene by the EMS physician. In some EMS systems the medical director responds to emergency calls.

Indirect medical direction, or off-line medical direction, includes the development of a set of written instructions, known as protocols. EMT–Is are expected to be familiar with their EMS system's protocols. When encountering a patient with a particular illness or injury, the EMT–I should initiate patient care based on the provisions of the protocol for that particular emergency.

EMS physician involvement in indirect medical direction has been divided into three phases: prospective, immediate (concurrent), and retrospective (Figure 1-16):

- *Prospective phase*—Primarily administrative in nature. Duties include training; protocol development; system design; and selection of equipment, supplies, and personnel.
- *Immediate (concurrent) phase*—Consists of both clinical and administrative responsibilities. The physician provides patient care, predominantly in the emergency department but sometimes in the field as well. The EMS physician participates in prehospital research studies. In addition, he or she performs concurrent review of the prehospital care providers' activities. This ongoing review process may take place in the field or in the emergency department. Finally, the EMS physician may give radio direction (direct medical direction).
- *Retrospective phase*—The physician reviews previous EMT–I performance, including run report review, continuous quality improvement, continuing education, and risk management, in an attempt to improve future care.

Standing Orders • EMT–I field interventions that are completed before contacting medical direction.

EMS systems usually are influenced by a combination of direct and indirect medical direction. Commonly, protocols are followed for initial care of life-threatening

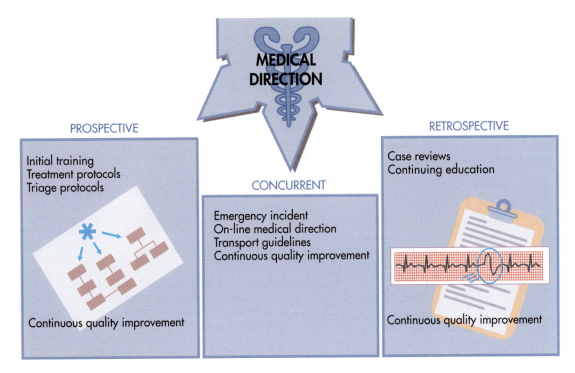

FIGURE 1-16 ▲ Types of medical direction and oversight. (From American College of Emergency Physicians; Pons PT, Cason D, chief editors: *Paramedic field care: a complaint-based approach*, St Louis, 1997, Mosby.)

problems, such as cardiac arrest, severe bleeding, major trauma, and shock. Once care has been provided to a certain point, the EMT–I is required to contact the medical director for further instructions. Portions of the protocols that are completed before the EMT–I is required to contact medical direction are referred to as **standing orders.**

All EMTs function under some sort of medical direction. In some states EMTs operate under the direction of a physician adviser. In other states the use of a medical adviser or director is only recommended, not required. Most systems, however, require active medical direction.

Medical Record Keeping

Accurate and thorough documentation of patient information and treatment is an essential ingredient in maintaining the overall quality of the EMS system. Documentation provides a record of what has taken place and conveys vital information about the patient and his or her emergency situation to other health care providers. Documentation also serves as a key element in quality improvement activities designed to make the EMS system better. This includes retrieving the run reports or electronic data, processing it to obtain the necessary information for each case, and storing it for later retrieval when indicated. Documentation is discussed in more depth in Chapter 14.

Continuous Quality Improvement

✖ **Continuous Quality Improvement** • An evaluation of services provided and the results achieved as compared with accepted standards.

The quality of an EMS system is reflected in the daily performance of its EMTs and operational efficiency. The focus of continuous quality improvement is on the EMS system and not on an individual. Ongoing quality improvement processes should be in place to monitor and evaluate the delivery of care. Continuous quality improvement is considered an essential component of modern EMS systems.

Simply stated, **continuous quality improvement** is the evaluation of EMS performance for the purpose of identifying areas of needed improvement and implementing necessary corrections. This evaluation is based on a comparison of the care delivered with the accepted standards. Management personnel and physicians responsible for system oversight most often complete these evaluations. The quality improvement process reveals problems that might not otherwise be recognized by looking at the EMS system from the surface. It can propel changes in treatment protocols and help support the EMS system to acquire additional resources at budget time. It also allows the EMS system's management and medical direction to evaluate and fix system problems in areas such as the following:

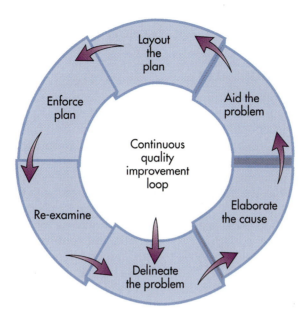

FIGURE 1-17 ▲ **Continuous quality improvement is a method of ensuring that superior medical care is provided. (From American College of Emergency Physicians; Pons PT, Cason D, chief editors:** *Paramedic field care: a complaint-based approach,* **St Louis, 1997, Mosby.)**

- Medical direction
- Financing
- Training
- Communication
- Out-of-hospital treatment and transport
- Interfacility transport
- Receiving facilities
- Agency relationships
- Specialty care units
- Dispatch
- Public information and education
- Quality improvement
- Disaster planning
- Mutual aid

A primary component of any quality improvement program is documentation. Patient care reports are checked for completeness, accuracy of charting and assessment, adherence to system treatment protocols, and patterns of error or system-related problems.

Another element used to determine levels of performance is the direct observation of patient care provided by the EMT–Is. Riding with the EMT–Is as they respond to emergency calls and provide patient care usually satisfies this evaluation.

Response time data can be used to reveal operational efficiency and can show the need for relocation of units or the acquisition of additional units. Other data that are evaluated include dispatch tapes, prehospital care data, incident reports, and emergency department and inpatient records.

Corrective action must be taken when improper care is revealed. Likewise, proper or exceptional performance must be communicated to the EMT–Is to help reinforce the behavior. Most important, quality improvement must be linked with ongoing professional education. Finally, appropriate EMS research can help enhance quality improvement efforts.

> ▶ Continuous quality improvement is a dynamic process that should involve the following steps (Figure 1-17):
> 1. Delineate system-wide problems.
> 2. Elaborate on the cause(s) of the problem.
> 3. Develop a remedy or remedies for the problem.
> 4. Lay out a plan to implement the remedy or remedies.
> 5. Enforce the plan of correction.
> 6. Reexamine the problem.

ILLNESS AND INJURY PREVENTION

Throughout your career, as you treat ill and injured patients, you may find yourself asking, "Why did this have to happen?" As an EMT–I, you are likely to respond to many tragic cases that could have been avoided. Part of the role of an EMT–I as a prehospital professional is to help reduce the incidence of injury by educating the public on illness and injury prevention, such as safe driving and accident avoidance practices.

Epidemiology
INCIDENCE, MORBIDITY, AND MORTALITY

Epidemiology is the study of the elements that influence the frequency, distribution, and causes of injury, disease, and other health-related events in a population. To help understand what epidemiology is, it is helpful to be familiar with several important concepts. Trauma is one of the most prevalent health problems that the United States faces today. Think about the following U.S. Department of Transportation facts:

- Trauma is the leading cause of death in persons ages 1 through 44.
- Trauma accounts for 80% of teenage deaths and 60% of childhood deaths.
- Fifty percent of deaths occur immediately after the trauma event.
- Injury has surpassed stroke as the third leading cause of death.
- The estimated lifetime cost of injuries is greater than $114 billion.
- For each injury resulting in death, there are an estimated 19 hospitalizations and 254 emergency department visits.

The early release of injured persons from the hospital has a host of effects on EMS services. Its implications include increased use of EMS services for supportive care and intervention.

An injury is intentional or unintentional damage to a person that is produced by acute exposure to thermal, mechanical, electrical, radiological, or chemical energy or from the lack of such essentials as heat or oxygen. Approximately 75% of all injuries are caused by mechanical or kinetic energy during events such as motor vehicle crashes, falls, and firearms being discharged. Examples of injuries that occur as a result of a lack of heat or oxygen are frostbite and drowning.

An accidental injury is referred to as unintentional. An injury that occurs because of a purposeful action to either oneself (e.g., suicide) or to another person (e.g., homicide) is called an intentional injury. Approximately one third of all deaths from injury are due to intentional injuries. A person's ability to survive an injury is influenced by factors such as physical size, age, and whether or not there is existence of underlying disease.

The years of productive life lost when an injury results in death are calculated by subtracting the age of death from 65. As an example, if a 35-year-old were to be killed in a car accident, it would be a loss of 30 years of productive life. This value can help determine the cost associated with trauma in relation to the potential earnings a person might have over his or her lifetime.

Injury risks may be defined as the real or potential hazardous situations that put individuals at risk for sustaining an injury. An example is riding a bicycle without a helmet. Falling from the bicycle can cause a head injury. This would be considered an injury risk. Injury surveillance is the ongoing systematic collection, analysis, and interpretation of injury data that are essential to the planning, implementation, and evaluation of public health practice. EMS providers serve an important role, since they are in a position to see the cause of many injuries. This information can then be reported through instruments such as the EMS run report or other documents specifically designed for this data collection. It is closely integrated with the timely dissemination of these data to those who need to know. The final link in the surveillance chain is the application of these data to prevention and control. To expand on the example of the person who received a head injury as a result of falling from a bicycle, this information could be used to develop and implement a public education program to increase the wearing of helmets while riding bicycles.

Primary injury prevention is defined as keeping an injury from ever occurring. Secondary prevention and tertiary prevention are the care and rehabilitation activities (respectively) that prevent further problems from resulting from an event that has already occurred. A teachable moment is the time after an injury has occurred when the patient and observers remain acutely aware of what has happened and may be more receptive to learning about how the event could have been prevented.

FEASIBILITY OF EMS INVOLVEMENT

More than 600,000 EMS providers in the United States are widely distributed amid the population and often reflect the composition of the community. In a rural setting the EMS provider may be the most medically educated individual. Often EMS providers are high-profile role models who are considered champions of the customer. Furthermore, EMS providers are welcome in schools and other environments and are considered authorities on injury and prevention.

ESSENTIAL LEADERSHIP ACTIVITIES

EMS organizations have an opportunity to save lives and reduce injury by establishing and maintaining prevention programs in their community. The first step to take is to lead by example. EMS management must emphasize and support the safety and wellness of its EMS providers. Policies should be put in place to promote safety throughout all aspects of work, particularly during the emergency response, while at the scene, and then during transport. EMS personnel should be provided with and required to don the proper body substance isolation (BSI) and personal protective equipment (PPE) to guard against exposure to bloodborne and airborne pathogens, as well as environmental hazards. Other topics such as proper lifting techniques; scene survival techniques (such as how to defend against violent patients or other hostile attackers); vector control; and safe response to and management of hazardous materials, temperature extremes, communicable disease, and structural risks (to name a few) should be taught and practiced. When the specific training is not available, in-house liaisons with public and private sector specialty groups can be established as a means of obtaining the needed education and training.

The next step to take is to implement the actual community-based injury prevention program. A key to the success of any prevention program is to get "buy-in" from employees at every level. EMS personnel must recognize the need and benefit of being involved in prevention activities. Education about the fundamentals of injury prevention can help to establish this understanding and appreciation. Information about prevention programs is incorporated into most of today's primary and continuing EMS education programs.

Individual EMS providers should be empowered to conduct primary injury prevention activities in their communities. There are many activities that can be done both on and off the job. It is essential that EMS managers identify and encourage interest and support. Where possible, internal budgetary support should be established to reward and/or remunerate participation. Where possible, EMS organizations should provide their EMS providers the opportunity for rotational assignments to prevention programs and salary for off-duty injury prevention activities.

RECOGNIZING THE NEED FOR OUTSIDE RESOURCES

Depending on the size of the community and its particular needs, conducting preventive education can be ex-tremely challenging, if not impractical, for the EMS system to do alone. Many EMS agencies collaborate with other groups to conduct some or all of their preventive education campaigns. Community groups such as the American Red Cross, Mothers Against Drunk Driving (MADD), and junior auxiliaries are great resources for initiating community and school programs. Hospitals (particularly trauma centers and children's hospitals) often have their own preventive education programs in which EMS agencies can partner. State highway safety offices are often able to provide funding for traffic-related projects, such as those involving child safety seats, seat belts, and drunk driving.

The financial wherewithal may not be available for EMS agencies to do all of the public education that is necessary. The good news is that financial support can often be obtained from local businesses. Large corporations will commonly donate funds or provide services in exchange for being listed as a sponsor of a given program. Advertising agencies are often willing to contribute billboard space for safety messages and public service announcements. Local television and radio stations are often willing to run public service messages at no cost. Local hospitals are frequently agreeable to including safety messages in newsletters and flyers that are distributed to a community-wide audience. Another potential source of funding for public education is local, state, and federal grant programs. In short, there are a lot of sources of financial support for community injury prevention programs.

IMPLEMENTATION OF PREVENTION STRATEGIES

In the normal course of their duties, there are many opportunities for EMT–Is to provide on-scene trauma prevention education (Figure 1-18). An example is educat-

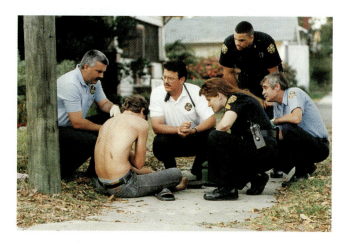

FIGURE 1-18 ▲ As part of handling emergency calls, EMT–Is should look for opportunities to provide on-scene prevention education. (From American College of Emergency Physicians; Pons PT, Cason D, chief editors: *Paramedic field care: a complaint-based approach*, St Louis, 1997, Mosby.)

ing a child about the rules for safely crossing the street following a non–life-threatening injury that occurred because the child darted across instead of looking both ways and ensuring safe passage. However, an important point to emphasize is that this education should never interfere with assessing and managing the incident or the patient's injuries.

Begin by looking at each emergency response to an injured patient and identifying whether the necessary precautions have been taken to reduce or eliminate the risk factors that are associated with that type of injury. Then identify whether there is a likelihood of possible recurrence of the given behavior. If it is unlikely that the behavior will be repeated, then the education is not needed unless it is aimed at educating others who are there with the patient.

Effective communication is an important part of the educational process. Begin by establishing rapport with the patient and family members or friends (if appropriate). A sense of timing is important; recognize whether the moment is a teachable one. In other words, is the patient receptive to the education and likely to accept and internalize it? Emotions the patient is experiencing, such as anger or fear, can interfere with his or her reception of your message. It is better to wait for the right moment to pass along the message. It is also essential to come across in as nonjudgmental and objective a manner as possible. Also, be considerate of ethnic, religious, and social diversity issues. If you offend a person in the course of delivering your message, it is unlikely that the message will be accepted and the behavior changed.

Typically, on-scene education involves telling persons how they can prevent recurrence and the need for or use of protective devices. Resources can be identified for the following:
- Safety devices
- Child-protective services
- Food, shelter, and clothing

Look for situations that are suggestive of sexual abuse, spousal abuse, or elderly abuse. These should be reported to the receiving physician at the facility where the patient is transported or to appropriate protective agencies in the community. Be sure to follow local and state policies. It may be worthwhile for EMT–Is to develop a social services resource guide for their organization to help in identifying solutions and ideas for these and other situations.

Each community needs to identify its own unique approaches to prevention. Conducting formal needs assessments will assist in identifying priorities. Consider the following types of programs:
- Flu immunizations
- Elder care clinics
- Defensive driving classes
- Workplace safety courses

- Alternative means of transportation
- After care services
- Rehabilitation
- Grief support
- Bicycle helmet programs
- Drinking-while-driving prevention programs at high schools

Also, prevention information can be listed on the local EMS agency's Internet website. The types and number of programs that can be offered are limitless. It really comes down to how much time and energy the organization can commit to preventive education programs. By collaborating with other organizations, an EMS agency can achieve a great deal more than would be possible by itself.

ETHICS AND CONFIDENTIALITY

Ethics • The discipline dealing with what is good and what is bad.

> **STUDENT ALERT**
>
> Socrates question, "How should one live?" relates to how you as an *individual* conduct yourself.

Meaning of Ethics

The word **ethics** is derived from the Greek word meaning "character" and sets standards for the rightness and wrongness of professional behavior. Whereas morals refer to social, religious, and personal standards of right and wrong, ethics relate to the rules or standards that govern the conduct of members of a particular group or profession. Ethics serve as a foundation for conduct as a practicing EMT–I. They deal with the EMT–I's relationship with his or her peers, patients, the patients' families, and society in general.

When faced with situations that call for a choice of behavior, EMT–Is must act ethically. For example, it is unethical and/or illegal to do the following:
- Make a statement to a patient about a fellow health care worker's perceived faults.
- Solicit a patient for a date.
- Give an attorney's business card to the victim of a motor vehicle accident.
- Discourage a patient from going to the hospital because he or she has no insurance.
- Fail to maintain patient confidentiality.

It is essential for EMT–Is to exemplify the principles and values of their profession. They must understand and agree to abide by both the implicit and explicit responsibilities.

EMT–Is are likely to be confronted with various ethical issues in the course of their work, such as having to decide if attempts should be made to preserve a terminally ill patient's life, meeting the needs of patients who are unable to pay, requesting medical help from others when needed, or dealing with a patient who is refusing service but who needs medical care. Because of the complexity of these issues, tomorrow's laws may decide some of today's ethical dilemmas. Sometimes, however, the EMT–I may find that a law is in conflict with what is ethically right. Obviously, this creates dilemmas that the EMT–I must work through.

Emotion should not be a factor when dealing with ethical questions. Such questions must be answered with reason and not on the basis on what other people think is right or wrong. As an individual and as a professional, you must answer these questions yourself. Maintaining your own personal code of ethics that is consistent with the professional code of ethics will help you arrive at appropriate conclusions. An important part of maintaining a personal code of ethics is to reflect on your own practice. A good rule to follow is to never do anything that is morally wrong.

When working through ethical issues, you have to ask yourself, "What is in the patient's best interest? What are the patient's rights? Does the patient understand the issues at hand? What is my professional, legal, and moral accountability?" First, determine what the patient really wants. Typically, you can use a number of sources to help you reach a conclusion. What does the patient tell you? Is there a written statement, such as an advance directive (do-not-resuscitate [DNR] order, living will, etc.), that spells out the patient's wishes? What input does the family offer? You have to use a certain amount of "good faith" in making ethical decisions. In other words, although you may not necessarily agree with the patient's wishes, it is important to respect them. By following the patient's wishes, you are showing respect for the patient. If you place the patient's well-being above all else when providing care and always do what is in the patient's best interest, there is rarely a need to worry about committing an unethical act.

There are a number of global concepts that relate to protecting patients. These include providing care that is of benefit to the patient, not doing harm, and recognizing patient autonomy. As an EMT–I you will face situations where these global concepts are in conflict with what is ethically right. An example is the patient who does not want to be resuscitated if he or she experiences cardiac arrest. Not providing care is harmful to the patient and will result in certain death. But it is the patient's wish that no resuscitative efforts be made. Thus a decision must be made regarding what is in the patient's best interest. The health care community can help establish parameters for this decision making by

taking a number of actions. These include creating treatment protocols that then serve as the norm (standard of care) for these types of cases, followed by conducting research and having prospective and retrospective reviews of decisions to help guide future decision making. Within the public arena, laws can be enacted to help protect patient rights and define the use of advance directives. These help make the patient's wishes known and reduce the potential for conflict.

Ethical Issues in Contemporary EMT–Intermediate Practice

RESUSCITATION

Probably the most challenging decisions are those surrounding resuscitation. As an EMT–I you may be confronted with a hysterical family member who, at the moment when a loved one dies, panics and insists that care be started even though a DNR order is in place. Obviously, under normal conditions, you take quick action—any delay decreases the chances of the resuscitation efforts being successful. Now you are forced to quickly decide whether to honor the patient's wishes or to follow the request of the hysterical family member. If you resuscitate the patient, he or she may experience days, weeks, or even months of additional suffering that he or she does not want. If you do not attempt resuscitation, the family member will likely be upset and may threaten litigation. Here you are forced to make an ethical decision. Begin by identifying what the patient really wants. If it is certain that the patient left clear instructions (such as an advance directive), then follow those instructions. If there is any doubt, resuscitate as you normally would. The situation gets a bit more complicated when resuscitation is started but then an advance directive is found or a family member brings it to your attention. Ethically and legally (depending on your state laws), you are obligated to stop care; however, emotionally you may want to continue. It is important to respect the patient's autonomy and stop doing that which he or she did not want. If there is any question, follow the protocols for these types of cases. It may be beneficial to contact on-line medical direction for advice.

PATIENT CONFIDENTIALITY

Confidentiality is a fundamental right. EMT–Is must hold patient care in strict confidence, as required both legally and ethically. It is unethical to divulge patients' names, details of their illness or care, or any other aspect of their care to anyone except designated EMS and law enforcement personnel. Telling friends or family about patients could result in a leak of confidential information. As an EMT–I you cannot reveal information about a patient to anyone, including the patient's own family, without the patient's permission. An exception to this rule exists if the patient is a minor or is legally certified as incompetent and you are communicating information to family members. Violation of patient confidentiality may be met with civil or administrative penalties. Sometimes EMT–Is are put into situations where they are knowledgeable of information that is required to be reported by state law. An example is neglect or abuse of children or the elderly. Here the rule of confidentiality must be breached for the public good. Each EMT–I must be knowledgeable of the requirements for reporting in his or her state.

CONSENT

Each person has a right to accept or decline medical care. This is a fundamental element of the patient-physician relationship. Although it is not as problematic when the patient asks for help, there still can be ethical dilemmas, such as "Does the patient understand the issues at hand?" or "Can the patient make an informed decision in his or her best interest?" Even more questionable is when the patient is unable to express a willingness to be treated. In patients who are unconscious, EMT–Is are obligated to initiate care based on the principle of implied consent. Here, as an EMT, you assume that if the patient were able to do so, he or she would consent to treatment. But do you really know that is what the patient wants? What happens if you bring the patient back to life but he or she spends the rest of his or her life in a coma? Have you done the patient more harm than good? These become ethical issues with which you find yourself struggling.

CARE IN FUTILE SITUATIONS

Another ethical challenge involves dealing with cases that are futile—in other words, the patient who has no chance for survival. Examples include the patient who is experiencing cardiac asystole and is unresponsive to treatment and the patient who is in cardiac arrest following blunt trauma. Neither of these patients is likely to be successfully resuscitated. To best manage these types of ethical issues, the meaning of the term *futile* must first be determined. Then who makes the decision that the situation is futile must be decided. Both of these questions must be addressed through local protocols before EMT–Is are confronted with this type of situation.

OBLIGATION TO PROVIDE CARE

Sometimes the question of whether there is an obligation to provide care creates an ethical issue. In most states the EMT–I is not legally obligated to stop at an accident scene while off duty and driving his or her own car. But the EMT–I has an ethical responsibility to stop

and help. Ethical issues also arise with patients who are not able to pay for treatment or are not in the "health plan" and in situations that involve patient "dumping" or economic triage.

CONFLICTING PHYSICIAN ORDERS

As an EMT–I, you may also find yourself dealing with ethical issues in your role as a physician extender. What should you do if the physician orders something that you believe is contraindicated or that is medically acceptable but not in the patient's best interests? How should you handle a situation where you believe the treatment is medically acceptable but morally wrong? First, the conflict may be due to miscommunication. For this reason, it is important to repeat the orders back to the physician to make sure that the orders are in fact what the physician wants to have done. If the treatment is what the physician wants done and you still believe it is inappropriate for the given situation, then you should ask the physician for an explanation. If the physician is clear on what he or she wishes done and you still believe that it inappropriate for the situation, you will need to make an ethical decision. How far are you willing to go to be a patient advocate? What are the risks associated with not following orders from a physician? Failure to follow orders will require you to defend that action and may be met with a variety of responses, including possible punitive actions. On the other hand, carrying out orders known to be contraindicated or adverse to the patient's well-being are also risky.

Code of Ethics

Many health care professions publish written codes of ethics to help guide their members who face difficult ethical decisions. A code of ethics provides a model of ideal conduct. In January 1978 the National Association of Emergency Medical Technicians issued a Code of Ethics for Emergency Medical Technicians.

The code states:

Professional status as an Emergency Medical Technician is maintained and enriched by the willingness of the individual practitioner to accept and fulfill obligations to society, other medical professionals, and the profession of Emergency Medical Technician. As an Emergency Medical Technician, I solemnly pledge myself to the following code of professional ethics:

A fundamental responsibility of the Emergency Medical Technician is to conserve life, to alleviate suffering, to promote health, to do no harm, and to encourage the quality and equal availability of emergency medical care.

The EMT Code of Ethics. Adopted by the National Association of Emergency Medical Technicians, 1978.

The Emergency Medical Technician provides services based on human need, with respect for human dignity, unrestricted by considerations of nationality, race, creed, color or status.

The Emergency Medical Technician does not use professional knowledge and skills in any enterprise detrimental to the public well-being.

The Emergency Medical Technician respects and holds in confidence all information of a confidential nature obtained in the course of professional work unless required by law to divulge such information.

The Emergency Medical Technician, as a citizen, understands and upholds the law and performs the duties of citizenship; as a professional the Emergency Medical Technician has the never-ending responsibility to work with concerned citizens and other health care professionals in promoting a high standard of emergency medical care to all people.

The Emergency Medical Technician shall maintain professional competence and demonstrate concern for the competence of other members of the Emergency Medical Services health care team.

An Emergency Medical Technician assumes responsibility in defining and upholding standards of professional practice and education.

The Emergency Medical Technician assumes responsibility for individual professional actions and judgment, both in dependent and independent emergency functions, and knows and upholds the laws that affect the practice of the Emergency Medical Technician.

An Emergency Medical Technician has the responsibility to be aware of and participate in, matters of legislation affecting the Emergency Medical Technician and the Emergency Medical Services System.

The Emergency Medical Technician adheres to standards of personal ethics that reflect credit upon the profession.

Emergency Medical Technicians, or groups of Emergency Medical Technicians, who advertise professional services, do so in conformity with the dignity of the profession.

The Emergency Medical Technician has an obligation to protect the public by not delegating to a person less qualified any service that requires the professional competence of an Emergency Medical Technician.

The Emergency Medical Technician will work harmoniously with, and sustain confidence in, Emergency Medical Technician associates, the nurse, the physician, and other members of the Emergency Medical Services health care team.

The Emergency Medical Technician refuses to participate in unethical procedures, and assumes the responsibility to expose incompetence or unethical conduct of others to the appropriate authority in a proper and professional manner.

This code stems from the premise that all EMTs should be concerned with the welfare of others. It is a professional, rather than legal, standard of behavior.

EMS ORGANIZATIONS
Benefits of Belonging

Across the country a variety of local and state EMS associations exist for the EMT–I. These organizations provide an assortment of membership benefits, including educational opportunities, newsletters, and representation on issues that affect local legislation. State associations serve not only as a clearinghouse for EMS news and training information but also as a strong, collective voice for EMT–Is when key issues are being lobbied before the state legislature.

National Association of Emergency Medical Technicians

On a national level, the EMT–I can join the National Association of Emergency Medical Technicians (NAEMT). The NAEMT was formed in 1975 by a group of nationally registered EMTs from existing state EMT organizations, national EMS leaders, and the National Registry of Emergency Medical Technicians (NREMT). The association's goals are to serve the needs of EMTs throughout the country, promote the professional status of the EMT, encourage the constant upgrading of the education and abilities of the EMT, and strive for a national standard of recognition for the skills and abilities of the EMT. The NAEMT sponsors continuing education programs on a national, regional, and local level and provides a variety of membership programs and services.

Belonging to a professional organization allows the EMT–I to be aware of the latest emergency medical technologies. It also allows communication with members from other parts of the country (or world) to share ideas with people of similar backgrounds. In addition, EMS associations that have large memberships carry a great deal of political influence. This clout enhances the prehospital care professionals' chances of obtaining favorable EMS-related positions/legislation and/or funding.

In addition to the NAEMT, key national EMS-related organizations include the following:
- American Ambulance Association (AAA)
- American College of Emergency Physicians (ACEP)
- Emergency Nurses Association (ENA)
- International Association of Firefighters (IAFF)
- National Association of EMS Educators (NAEMSE)
- National Association of Flight Paramedics (NAFP)
- National Association of EMS Physicians (NAEMSP)
- National Association of Search and Rescue (NASAR)
- National Association of State EMS Directors (NASEMSD)
- National Council of State EMS Training Coordinators (NCSEMSTC)

CASE HISTORY FOLLOW-UP ■ ■ ■

EMT–I Brown's supervisor pages him to call the station as he is waiting for his lunch order. He calls the unit from his cell phone and asks, "What's up?"

"We have a group of students from Lincoln Elementary coming in at 1:30 this afternoon. I'll place your unit on backup; I want you to come in and show them your unit and answer their questions. Okay?"

"That's great, I really enjoy the kids. I hope we don't miss anything good," Brown says. He walks back to the table and says to Williams, "We've got a show-and-tell this afternoon."

EMT–Is Williams and Brown know all of the questions and have all of the answers because they have both done public presentations for many years: "What's it like to be an EMT–I?" "What do you do when someone isn't breathing?" "What's the worst thing you've ever seen?"

Both realize they cannot tell the children about the worst thing they have ever seen, but they do enjoy recalling the story of when they delivered twin girls.

SUMMARY

Important points to remember from this chapter include the following:

- An emergency medical services (EMS) system is a network of coordinated services that work as a unified whole to meet the emergency care needs of the community and to serve as a bridge between the community and the medical facilities that provide definitive health care.
- To practice as an EMT–I in most states, a person is required to complete a recognized EMT–I course, successfully complete a written and practical examination, and become certified or licensed.
- The number of hours required for EMT–I training averages 300 to 400 total hours of instruction, including classroom time, instruction in practical skills, and clinical instruction.
- Reciprocity allows the transfer of certification or licensure from one state to another. In some states reciprocity is automatic, especially if the EMT–I is nationally registered.

- To maintain the right to function as an EMT–I, most states require recertification every 1 to 5 years (the average being 2 years).
- Continuing education is essential for helping the EMT–I reduce the erosion of knowledge and skills and to stay current on new procedures and treatment. It also encourages further professional development.
- A professional is a person who has certain special skills and knowledge in a specific area and conforms to the standards of conduct and performance in that area.
- Attributes of professional behavior include having integrity, empathy, a professional manner, good appearance and personal hygiene, and appropriate general conduct; being a patient advocate; treating others with respect; having self-motivation/personal involvement and self-confidence; maintaining good communications; exercising good time management; and employing teamwork, diplomacy, and careful delivery of service.

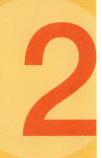

Well-Being of the EMT–Intermediate

Key Terms

Allergic Reaction

Body Substance Isolation (BSI)

Contagious

Immunization

Pathogens

Personal Protective Equipment (PPE)

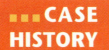

CASE HISTORY

A man is watching his grandson's Little League baseball game when he begins to experience chest pain. He does not think much about the pain until he gets home. There his wife comments on his pale, sweaty appearance. He admits that he has been having chest pain for the last hour or so. His wife immediately dials 9-1-1 and requests an ambulance.

Shortly, an ambulance and a Fire First Responder Unit arrive at the home. While they are en route, EMT–Is Randall and Emerson apply protective gloves. As soon as the ambulance comes to a stop, Randall and Emerson carry into the house the jump kit, oxygen, and a cardiac monitor/defibrillator. Following standard orders, the EMT–Is give the man oxygen, obtain a brief history of the event, perform the initial assessment, attach the electrocardiogram (ECG) electrodes and place an intravenous (IV) line. The needle used to cannulate the vein is disposed of in a "sharps" container. EMT–I Emerson then places a nitroglycerin tablet under the man's tongue. The man has some relief from the pain but still appears pale and sweaty. With assistance from the first responders, the EMT–Is place the man, who is moderately overweight, on a stretcher and roll him to the ambulance for transport to the emergency department. Several first responders assist in lifting the patient and cot into the patient module of the ambulance.

En route to the hospital, EMT–I Emerson performs an ongoing assessment of the man's pain and physical condition. The patient reminds Emerson of his father, who died of a heart attack several years ago.

CHAPTER GOAL

Upon completion of this chapter, the EMT–Intermediate will be able to understand and value the importance of personal wellness in EMS and serve as a healthy role model for peers.

Cognitive Objectives

As an EMT-Intermediate you should be able to do the following:

- Discuss the importance of universal precautions and body substance isolation practices.
- Describe the steps to take for personal protection from airborne and bloodborne pathogens.
- Explain what is meant by an exposure, and describe principles for management.

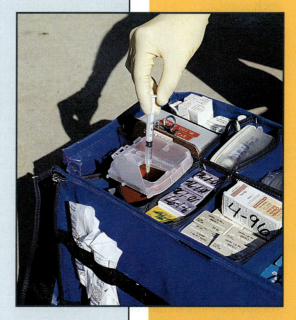

Affective Objectives

As an EMT-Intermediate you should be able to do the following:

- Advocate the benefits of working toward the goal of total personal wellness.
- Serve as a role model for other EMS providers in regard to a total-wellness lifestyle.
- Value the need to assess your own lifestyle.
- Challenge yourself regarding each wellness concept in your role as an EMT–I.
- Improve your personal physical well-being through achieving and maintaining proper body weight, regular exercise, and proper nutrition.
- Advocate and serve as a role model for other EMS providers relative to body substance isolation practices.
- Advocate and practice the use of personal safety precautions in all scene situations.

Psychomotor Objectives

As an EMT-Intermediate you should be able to do the following:

- Demonstrate the proper procedures to take for personal protection from disease.

INTRODUCTION

The job of an EMT–Intermediate (EMT–I) is a demanding one. It comes with additional responsibilities, stress, and the risk of being exposed to airborne and bloodborne pathogens. It requires physical and mental well-being. Implementing lifestyle changes can enhance personal wellness and allow the EMT–I to serve as a role model and coach for others. Personal safety is an important aspect of well-being.

PHYSICAL WELL-BEING

Factors that play a major role in maintaining physical health include good nutrition, physical fitness and weight control, adequate sleep, and prevention of disease and injury.

Good Nutrition

In the fast-paced environment in which the EMT–I works, it is easy to develop poor nutritional habits, such as eating mostly fast foods that contain high percentages of fat. Nutrition is an important part of physical well-being. Nutrients are foods that contain the elements necessary for the body to function. The six categories of nutrients are carbohydrates, fats, proteins, vitamins, minerals, and water. Food groups include sugar, fats, proteins, dairy products, vegetables, fruits, and grains. The major food groups are displayed in the Food Guide Pyramid. The base of the pyramid is made up of breads, cereals, rice, and pasta. The second level consists of vegetables and fruits. The third level consists of dairy products (milk, yogurt, and cheese). At the fourth level are meat, poultry, fish, dry beans, eggs, and nuts. The top of the pyramid is made up of fats, oils, and sweets. When planning a healthy diet, individuals should use the pyramid and eat "from the bottom up." To ensure proper nutrition, the foods closer to the base should be eaten in greater quantity, whereas the items toward the top should be consumed more in moderation (Figure 2-1). A healthy diet includes plenty of grain products, vegetables, and fruits, as well as a variety of foods that are low in fat, saturated fat, and cholesterol. A diet should also be moderate in simple sugars, salt, and sodium. Alcoholic beverages should be avoided or consumed only in moderation.

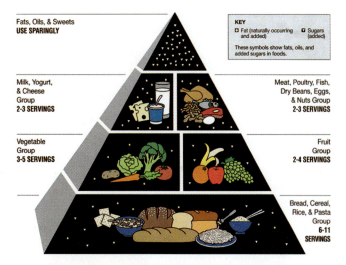

FIGURE 2-1 ▲ Food Guide Pyramid. (From US Department of Agriculture: *USDA's food guide pyramid,* USDA Human Nutrition Information Publication No. 249, Washington, DC, 1992, US Government Printing Office.)

Physical Fitness and Weight Control

As part of their day-to-day duties, EMT–Is are required to perform physically demanding tasks. For this reason, it is essential that EMT–Is be physically fit. Physical fitness can be thought of as a condition that helps one to look, feel, and do his or her best. It is individual and varies from person to person. It is influenced by age, gender, heredity, personal habits, exercise, and eating habits. Benefits of physical fitness include the following:
- Decrease in resting heart rate and blood pressure
- Increase in oxygen-carrying capacity
- Enhanced quality of life
- Increase in muscle mass and metabolism
- Increased resistance to injury
- Improved personal appearance and self-image
- Facilitated maintenance of motor skills throughout life

The demands of the job can be extremely challenging for EMT–Is who are overweight. In addition to requiring more energy, thus making the EMT–I susceptible to tiring and fatigue, excess weight can contribute to a host of injuries. Also, people who are overweight tend to be at greater risk for developing high blood pressure, diabetes mellitus, heart disease, some cancers, and other illnesses.

Although weight problems occur for many reasons, most people can control their weight through eating the right balance of foods in moderation, limiting fat consumption to no more than 65 grams (g) of fat per day in a 2000-calorie diet, and establishing and maintaining an exercise routine. Tips for controlling weight include setting realistic goals, making a commitment to change, exercising regularly, eating heathily, and then analyzing progress.

Sleep

Sleep plays an important role in being physically fit because it helps to rejuvenate a tired body. The average adult needs 7 to 8 hours of sleep each day.

When the normal and regular division between night and day is disrupted on an ongoing basis (e.g., working rotating shifts or responding to emergency calls in the early-morning hours during a 24-hour work shift), irritability, depression, and physical illness can result (Box 2-1).

Disease Prevention

EMT–Is can do a great deal to help prevent personal serious illness. As health care professionals EMT–Is have a responsibility to serve as role models in disease prevention.

CARDIOVASCULAR DISEASE

In the United States alone, cardiovascular disease accounts for more than 1 million deaths each year. For most, the risk of this disease can be reduced through

healthy living. In addition to improving cardiovascular endurance in the course of physical fitness, there are several steps that can be taken to prevent cardiovascular disease, including the following:
- Eliminating cigarette smoking
- Controlling high blood pressure
- Maintaining a favorable body fat composition through regular exercise
- Maintaining a good total cholesterol/high-density lipoprotein (HDL) ratio
- Monitoring triglyceride levels
- Reducing stress
- Having periodic risk assessments

CANCER

The term *cancer* encompasses more than 100 diseases affecting nearly all parts of the body. All can be life threatening. Cancer is caused by a change or mutation in the nucleus of a cell. Most common cancers are related to one of three environmental risk factors: smoking, sunlight, or diet.

Steps to prevent cancer include the following:
- Eliminating smoking
- Making dietary changes
- Minimizing sun exposure; using a sunscreen
- Having regular physical examinations
- Watching for the warning signs (Box 2-2)
- Conducting periodic risk assessment

BOX 2-1

GETTING YOUR Zs

Working nights, 24-hour shifts, and rotating shifts can inhibit getting enough rest. Here are some helpful tips:
- Allow some time to "unwind" and relax before trying to go to sleep.
- Consider exercise before sleeping as a way to reduce stress.
- Avoid stimulants (e.g., caffeine in coffee, soda, tea, chocolate) during the last few hours of your work shift.
- Eat simple carbohydrates (e.g., cookies or candy bar) to release serotonin (a hormone that may help induce sleep).
- Keep your sleeping area cool and dark so that your body will "think" it's nighttime.
- Make sure your family and friends know about your work shifts and your sleeping schedule to minimize interruptions.
- Try to maintain a "normal" period of dedicated sleep time each day.
- Consult a physician about your sleep difficulties when needed.

From Sanders MJ: *Mosby's paramedic textbook,* ed 2, St Louis, 2000, Mosby.

Pathogens • Microorganisms capable of causing disease in a suitable host.

INFECTIOUS DISEASE

Infectious diseases are caused by **pathogens** that include bacteria and viruses. They move from person to person in a variety of ways. Airborne pathogens are transmitted in tiny droplets that are expelled outward when a person coughs or sneezes. Other persons can then breathe in these airborne pathogens and become infected. Other pathogens are carried in a person's blood or other body fluids. When the blood or other body fluids are released from the infected person, they can access another person's body through breaks in the skin, including chapped hands, sores, and cuts, or by way of their mucous membranes (e.g., those in the mouth, eyes, or nose).

STUDENT ALERT

Whenever you come into contact with a potentially infectious body fluid, body substance, or other infectious agent, it is called an exposure.

Contagious • Refers to any disease that can be spread from person to person.

Diseases spread by pathogens can generate effects that vary from mild discomfort to the most severe effect—death. Often someone who is carrying pathogens for a disease exhibits no noticeable signs of illness (Figure 2-2). Any patient, even the young or old, may be carrying an infectious disease and be **contagious.** In the normal course of duties, the EMT–I is at risk of being exposed to infection through various means, including being splashed by blood, being stuck by a needle, or allowing blood or other body fluids to come in contact with broken or scraped skin or the mucous membranes of the eyes, nose, or mouth. Furthermore, a person can

BOX 2-2

THE SEVEN WARNING SIGNS OF CANCER (CAUTION) AS DESIGNATED BY THE AMERICAN CANCER SOCIETY

Change in bowel or bladder habits
A sore throat that does not heal
Unusual bleeding or discharge
Thickening or lump in the breast or elsewhere
Indigestion or difficulty swallowing
Obvious change in a wart or mole
Nagging cough or hoarseness

From Sanders MJ: *Mosby's paramedic textbook,* ed 2, St Louis, 2000, Mosby.

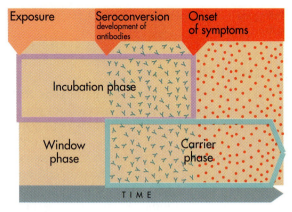

FIGURE 2-2 ▲ Stages of infection. Note that the exposed individual may be capable of spreading the disease before the onset of symptoms. (From American College of Emergency Physicians; Pons PT, Cason D, chief editors: *Paramedic field care: a complaint-based approach*, St Louis, 1997, Mosby.)

become infected through surface contamination or orally (as a result of improper hand washing).

✳ **Body Substance Isolation (BSI)** • Concept that regards all body tissues and fluids as being potentially infected. Includes bloodborne, foodborne, and airborne pathogens.

When treating any patient, it is essential to follow universal precautions and other guidelines in the workplace as established by the Centers for Disease Control and Prevention (CDC), the Occupational Safety and Health Administration (OSHA), the National Fire Protection Association (NFPA), the Federal Emergency Management Agency (FEMA), the U.S. Fire Administration (USFA), and others. These safety measures are referred to as **body substance isolation (BSI)** and offer recommendations on how a person can prevent coming into contact with blood, body substances, or any other infectious material.

The following steps should be taken to decrease the chance of being exposed to or infected by an infectious disease in the course of serving as an EMT–I:

- Follow recommended engineering and work practices.
- Maintain good personal health and hygiene habits.
- Keep your immunizations up-to-date.
- Receive periodic tuberculosis screening.
- Employ BSI/universal precautions.

Another aspect of self-protection against infectious disease is the need to remain constantly on guard. As you perform your assessment and treatment of any patient, remember that hair and clothing can hide the presence of blood or other body fluids. Moving a patient from one location to another, such as from a bed to the cot, or rolling a patient over can result in exposure to unseen body fluids, uncontrolled bleeding (worse yet—blood spurting from an arterial injury), or sharp

objects that were not initially seen. Be sure to communicate the presence of any potential hazards to your fellow providers. Just because you observe something does not mean that other emergency personnel at the scene have seen it also.

STREET WISE

Each year, in the course of inspecting or cleaning the ambulance or patient care equipment, countless EMT–Is and paramedics are stuck with contaminated needles that were not properly disposed of. Two points to remember: always make sure any needle you use is properly disposed of before leaving the ambulance, and always watch where you put your hands. If you cannot see where you are placing your hands, use a flashlight to illuminate the area.

BODY SUBSTANCE ISOLATION

The first rule to remember in body substance isolation (BSI) is to treat all blood and other body fluids as though they are infectious. This means employing proper safety measures to protect all persons, including yourself and your patients, from becoming contaminated with blood or other body fluids. Follow safe work practices, such as using disposable equipment and supplies whenever possible (particularly when performing invasive procedures), carefully placing needles and other sharp instruments in puncture-resistant containers, and laundering any reusable clothing with infection control in mind. Also, maintain good personal health and hygiene habits, such as hand washing and general cleanliness.

Hand Washing—Thorough hand washing is the most basic, effective way to prevent disease transmission. Make hand washing as soon as possible after every patient contact or after completing a decontamination procedure a normal part of your routine. This should be done even when there is no contact with body fluids or when protective gloves are worn (after removing the gloves). Waterless soaps, which are often carried on the emergency vehicle, can be used when there is no access to running water. Consider carrying your own personal waterless soap, which comes in compact and easy-to-use dispensers.

Normally, a good procedure to follow for hand washing is to first remove any rings or jewelry from your hands and arms. Then, using soap and water, lather the front and back of your hands up to 2 or 3 inches above the wrist. Vigorously rub your hands together for 10 to 15 seconds. Be sure to lather and rub between the fingers, paying at-

TABLE 2-1

U.S. Fire Administration Guidelines for Prevention of Transmission of HIV and HBV to Emergency Responders: Recommended Personal Protective Equipment for Protection Against HIV and HBV Transmission[1] in Prehospital[2] Settings

TASK OR ACTIVITY	DISPOSABLE GLOVES	GOWN	MASK[3]	PROTECTIVE EYEWEAR[3]
Bleeding control with spurting blood	Yes	Yes	Yes	Yes
Bleeding control with minimal bleeding	Yes	No	No	No
Emergency childbirth	Yes	Yes	Yes	Yes
Blood drawing	Yes[4]	No	No	No
Starting an intravenous (IV) line	Yes	No	No	No
Endotracheal intubation, esophageal obturator use	Yes	No	Yes	Yes
Oral/nasal suctioning, manually cleaning airway	Yes[5]	Yes	Yes	Yes
Handling and cleaning instruments with possible microbial contamination	Yes	Yes	Yes	Yes
Measuring blood pressure	Yes	No	No	No
Giving an injection	Yes	No	No	No
Measuring temperature	Yes	No	No	No
Rescuing from a fire[6]	Yes	No	No	No
Cleaning back of an ambulance after a medical alarm[7]	Yes	No	No	No

Modified from the CDC Guidelines, February 1989. From American College of Emergency Physicians; *Paramedic field care: a complaint-based approach,* St Louis, 1998, Mosby.

HIV, Human immunodeficiency virus; *HBV,* hepatitis B virus.

Notes for instructor:

1. The recommendations for personal protective equipment (PPE) provided in this chart are more stringent than those provided in the CDC Guidelines. The CDC Guidelines are based on application of universal precautions; this chart is based on application of body substance isolation.
2. Defined as a setting where delivery of emergency health care takes place away from a hospital or other health care facility.
3. Protective face shields can serve as both mask and eyewear to protect against blood splashes.
4. Gloves should reduce the incidence of blood contamination of hands during phlebotomy (drawing of blood samples), but they cannot prevent penetrating injuries caused by needles or other sharp instruments.
5. While not clearly necessary to prevent HIV or HBV transmission unless blood is present, gloves are recommended to prevent transmission of other agents (e.g., herpes simplex).
6. To be worn under structural firefighting gloves.
7. If other than soap and water is used, PPE recommended on the Material Safety Data Sheets (MSDS) should be worn.

tention to creases and cracks at the knuckles. Scrub under and around the fingernails with a brush. Then rinse your hands thoroughly and dry them with a paper towel. Use the paper towel to turn off the water faucet, since your contaminated hand(s) turned on the faucet.

Personal Protective Equipment (PPE) • Equipment used to protect providers from communicable disease.

Personal Protective Equipment—To achieve appropriate BSI, **personal protective equipment (PPE)** must be carried on all emergency vehicles. Recommended PPE includes protective gloves, eye protection, masks, and cover gowns (Table 2-1 above and Figure 2-3 on p. 35).

CLINICAL NOTES

Patients with spina bifida have been shown to be at risk for latex allergies.

Gloves—Latex or vinyl gloves should be used whenever there is patient contact. They provide an effective barrier against contamination from blood or other body fluids. To reduce the possibility of a delay at critical scenes while looking for and putting on gloves, many providers apply them while en route to the call.

Allergic Reaction • Hypersensitive response to an allergen to which an organism has been previously exposed and to which the organism has developed antibodies.

There are two basic types of gloves: vinyl and latex. Latex gloves come in various types, including powdered and powder free. Vinyl gloves should be used if one is allergic to latex. An indication of latex allergy is the occurrence of a rash after latex gloves are worn. Also, some patients are allergic to latex. Because of the risk for **allergic reaction,** a box of vinyl gloves or a latex allergy kit should be kept readily available in all emergency vehicles.

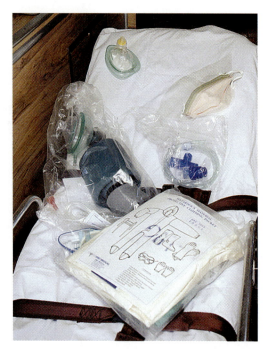

FIGURE 2-3 ▲ Personal protective equipment (PPE) is designed to protect EMS providers and patients from exposure to diseases from a variety of direct or indirect sources. (From American College of Emergency Physicians; Pons PT, Cason D, chief editors: *Paramedic field care: a complaint-based approach,* St Louis, 1997, Mosby.)

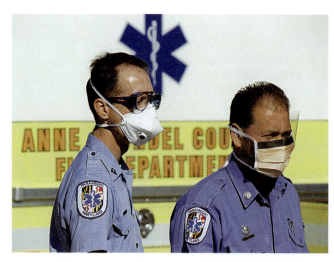

FIGURE 2-4 ▲ The face should be shielded from the danger of splashing blood or body fluids such as vomitus. (From American College of Emergency Physicians; Pons PT, Cason D, chief editors: *Paramedic field care: a complaint-based approach,* St Louis, 1997, Mosby.)

STREET WISE

Moving from performing one skill to another without changing gloves can result in accidental cross-contamination. An example is starting an intravenous (IV) line on a patient and then, while wearing the soiled gloves, using the radio or cell phone to contact medical control or write information on the run report.

If gloves become contaminated during a call, they should be replaced as soon as it is safe to do so. Also, rips or tears in vinyl or latex gloves can easily occur. For these reasons, extra gloves should be readily available. When a tear occurs and there is no contamination, remove the gloves as soon as possible, wash your hands thoroughly, and replace the gloves. If it is likely that an occupational exposure has occurred, follow your agency's exposure control policy.

Latex or vinyl gloves should never be reused. A safe way to remove gloves is to turn them inside out while pulling them off so as to avoid touching any contaminated areas. Once you remove the gloves, be sure to dispose of them properly (as described later). Also, remember to wash your hands after removing the gloves.

Since lightweight latex or vinyl gloves can tear, heavy-duty utility gloves should be worn when per-

forming cleaning or decontamination duties. Another time when a more durable glove should be worn is when patients are being extricated from an entrapment, since jagged metal or broken glass may be encountered. To ensure the necessary barrier protection, vinyl or latex gloves should be worn underneath the heavier work gloves.

Eye Protection—Eye protection should be worn whenever there is a risk of body fluids splashing into the eyes. Although goggles offer the best protection, regular prescription glasses with side shields are acceptable. Some surgical masks also have an eye shield attached (Figure 2-4). In the case of major trauma, where the exposure to a large quantity of blood is possible, a mask with eye protection is indicated. Also, eye protection should be considered when performing airway procedures such as endotracheal intubation or suctioning and when cleaning of equipment requires heavy scrubbing.

Eye protection goes beyond just the use of eyewear. Avoid allowing contaminated gloves to come into contact with your eyes, as can happen when you rub your eyes while still wearing the gloves. This can be a bit challenging when one is in the middle of treating a patient and sweat is dripping from one's brow. Using a clean 4 × 4 gauze pad is a safer alternative.

Masks—Several types of masks are available for use in the field. The basic surgical mask is designed to prevent splashed or aerosolized blood and other body fluids from coming into contact with the mouth and nose. Most of these masks are disposable and are held in place by elastic bands or ties that fit around the head. As mentioned under Eye Protection, a surgical mask with an eye shield provides more protection.

The basic surgical mask does not provide protection against airborne pathogens such as those that cause tuberculosis (TB). Patients with active TB may not even know that they have it. They can experience an assortment of signs and symptoms. The possibility of TB should be considered when encountering any patient complaining of fever, weight loss, or night sweats or who has had a continual cough. TB is not uncommon, and certain groups are considered at high risk for TB, including nursing home patients, those who are institutionalized, alcoholics, homeless persons (living in a shelter), indigent elderly persons, patients with acquired immunodeficiency syndrome (AIDS), and immigrants from countries having a high TB rate.

The release of droplets into the air that occurs with coughing can be reduced by placing a surgical mask on the patient. This should be done only if the patient's airway is patent and no breathing difficulty is noted. If a surgical mask is placed on the patient, the patient's airway and breathing must be carefully monitored. Check your local protocol for specific instructions.

Because basic surgical masks do not provide sufficient protection to providers caring for patients who may have TB, an N-95 or a high-efficiency particulate air (HEPA) respirator approved by the National Institute for Occupational Safety and Health (NIOSH) should be worn. However, because of the design of these masks, not everybody is able to wear one. EMT–Is who wear this type of mask should have a physical examination before using them in the field. In addition, fit testing should be done in advance to determine proper sizing. Both the physical examination and fit testing should be repeated periodically.

Cover Gowns—Cover gowns should be worn whenever there is the likelihood of exposure to large amounts of body fluids, such as during childbirth or when treating patients with multitrauma. Gowns provide additional protection for one's uniform but can get in the way and cause personal injury (particularly very loose fitting gowns), so care must be taken when wearing them. Overall-type coveralls with approved barrier shielding provide the best protection and are tighter fitting (Box 2-3). Be sure to follow local protocols for BSI.

Disposal of Contaminated Items—Today, to reduce the risk of disease transmission, much of the personal protective and medical equipment and supplies are designed for single use. These items should be properly disposed of after use. Disposable medical devices (other than needles or sharp objects) that become contaminated with blood or other body fluids should be

---

BOX 2-3

SIMPLIFIED FIELD SELECTION OF PERSONAL PROTECTIVE EQUIPMENT

1. If it's wet, it's infectious—use gloves.
2. If it could splash in your face, wear a full face shield or eye protection and a face mask.
3. If it could splash on your clothes, wear a gown or structural firefighting gear.
4. If the patient has a cough, place a surgical mask on the patient and a particular respirator on the crew.
5. Proper planning avoids the need for mouth-to-mouth resuscitation. Use disposable airway equipment, and carry a pocket mask.
6. When in doubt, use too much, rather than too little, personal protection equipment (PPE).
7. Always have a change of clothing available.

Modified from National Fire Academy Infection Control for Emergency Response Personnel: *The supervisor's role* (No. NFA-ICERP-IG), Emmitsburg, Md, 1992, The Academy.

---

placed in a red bag or container marked with a biohazard seal. Once the contaminated material is placed in an appropriate bag or container, it should be handled according to local protocols for disposing of biohazardous waste. Do not throw contaminated articles into a wastebasket for disposal with normal trash. Needles and other sharp objects must be disposed of in a puncture-proof container, often referred to as a "sharps" container (Figure 2-5).

Cleaning, Disinfection, and Sterilization—When nondisposable equipment is used to treat a patient or surfaces become contaminated with a patient's blood or body fluids, they must be cleaned, disinfected, or sterilized. The most basic way of removing contaminants from equipment is to clean it. Cleaning is the washing of an item with soap and water. Disinfecting includes cleaning and using a disinfectant to kill microorganisms that may be on equipment. Sterilization involves the use of chemical or physical methods to kill all of the microorganisms on an object. Cleaning and disinfecting procedures can be employed as part of one's normal duties. Sterilization is often done commercially or through the local hospital.

Following each patient encounter, clean all surfaces that came into contact with the patient. Typically, this includes patient care equipment such as backboards, ventilatory devices, oxygen administration equipment, suction equipment, splints, stretchers, and the patient compartment of the ambulance. Wash these items or surfaces down with approved soaps or disinfectants, and dispose of single-use cleaning supplies in a proper biohazard container. An effective substitute for commercial disinfectants is bleach solution diluted in water. Depending on how much organic matter is present, the

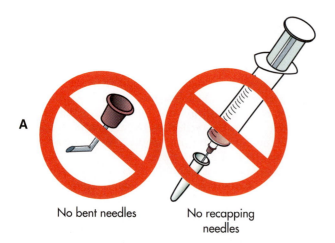

A No bent needles   No recapping needles

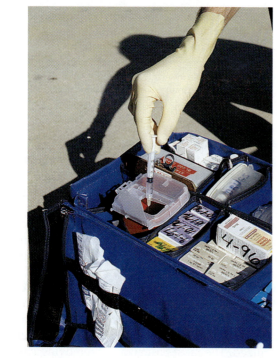

B

FIGURE 2-5 ▲ **A,** Once used, a needle should be immediately disposed of in the appropriate container, without bending or recapping. **B,** A "sharps" container that conforms to federal safety and infection control standards should be easily accessible. (From American College of Emergency Physicians; Pons PT, Cason D, chief editors: *Paramedic field care: a complaint-based approach,* St Louis, 1997, Mosby.)

recommended concentrations range from 1 part bleach to 100 parts water, to 1 part bleach to 10 parts water.

Items that are introduced into a patient's body, such as a laryngoscope blade, should be sterilized. Sterilization may be accomplished with heat, steam, radiation, or Environmental Protection Agency (EPA)–approved solutions. Contaminated equipment that requires extensive cleaning should be bagged and taken to an area specifically designated for this purpose.

Cleaning of contaminated items should never be completed in or around areas used for food preparation.

When clothing becomes contaminated, it should be bagged and cleaned according to department or agency policy. You should shower before dressing again. Many EMS systems or departments require EMS personnel to keep a spare uniform at work in the event of uniform contamination. If an occupational exposure is suspected, follow the department or agency's management procedures immediately and completely.

EXPOSURE

Even after following strict BSI techniques, the EMT–I may still be exposed to an infectious disease. It is important to know what to do in the event of an exposure. If you have been exposed to blood or any other body fluid or stuck by a needle, do the following:

- Immediately and thoroughly wash the area of contact.
- Get a medical evaluation.
- If appropriate, take the proper immunization boosters.
- Document the situation in which the exposure occurred.
- Complete any required medical follow-up.

This exposure to blood or other body fluids should be immediately reported to the receiving hospital and the designated officer in the EMS system or agency so that communications can be coordinated between the hospital and the emergency response organization. The medical facility will determine if enough information exists to identify the patient and obtain test results. The medical facility will then notify the designated officer of the findings within 48 hours of receiving the request. Check with your employer to make sure a policy is in place for this to occur in the event of an exposure.

Generally speaking, be sure to cooperate with the incident investigation and comply with all required reporting responsibilities and time frames.

✖ **Immunization** • Process of rendering a person immune or of becoming immune.

IMMUNIZATIONS/TUBERCULOSIS SCREENING

All emergency care providers should maintain **immunizations** for tetanus, diphtheria, polio, hepatitis B, MMR (measles, mumps, and rubella), and influenza. Also, they should be checked annually for TB exposure (or more frequently if a possible occupational exposure has occurred). Usually a simple skin test such as a Mantoux or purified protein derivative (PPD) test is performed. The test determines whether the provider has been exposed to TB. The department's infection control officer or physician should determine, after evaluating the potential risks to providers, how often testing should be done.

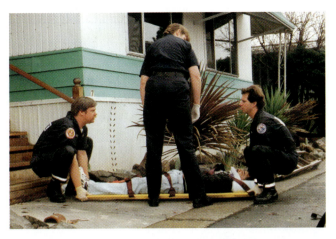

FIGURE 2-6 ▲ Use proper techniques whenever lifting and/or carrying patients. (From Sanders MJ: *Mosby's paramedic textbook,* ed 2, St Louis, 2000, Mosby.)

Injury Prevention

While working in the prehospital setting, you may find yourself in situations that can threaten your health. Every run can place you in a variety of hazardous situations. Tasks such as driving to the scene, entering a home, caring for injured patients at an accident scene, lifting stretchers, treating patients, and transporting them to the hospital all have inherent risks associated with them. You must stay alert for potential hazards. EMT–Is can minimize job-related injuries by being knowledgeable about body mechanics during lifting and moving, being alert for hostile environments, prioritizing personal safety during rescue situations, practicing safe vehicle operations, and using safety equipment and supplies.

Appropriate use of body mechanics during lifting and moving includes the following (Figure 2-6):
- Only move a patient you can safely handle.
- Look where you are walking or crawling.
- Move forward rather than backward when possible.
- Take short steps, if walking.
- Bend at your hips and knees.
- Lift with your legs, not your back.
- Keep the load close to your body.
- Keep the patient's body in-line when moving.

The most common type of run involves responding to the home of the caller, and the majority of these responses are without incident. However, what may seem to be a normal run can turn into a very dangerous, life-threatening situation for the EMT–I. Any call involving a domestic dispute, suicide attempt, severe bleeding, shooting, stabbing, or any type of violence should be approached with great caution and with the police. The police are trained to handle entering and securing these types of scenes.

Personal safety begins before responding to a call. At the start of your shift, carefully inspect the entire emergency vehicle. Check all fluid levels, and correct if low.

Examine the tires for unusual wear, damage, and proper inflation, and inspect all lights (emergency lights, as well as normal running lights) to ensure that they are working properly. Adjust the mirrors and seat position before your first call. Seat belts in the cab and patient care module must be operational and worn whenever the vehicle is in motion. Properly restrain all patients and anyone riding with the patient in the seat belts. Knowing that your emergency vehicle is in good working order can reduce anxiety and stress while responding to a call. Use emergency lights and the siren according to local procedure and state law. Typically, both must be in use when operating in the emergency mode. Proceed through all intersections, even those where you have the green light, with appropriate caution. Whenever you are operating in the emergency mode, you must exercise due regard for the safety of all others.

Have all PPE ready for use and properly stored on the emergency vehicle. Protective clothing includes turnout coat/pants, helmets, boots, gloves, eye protection, hearing protection, respiratory protection, and any other item of clothing that protects against injury, the cold, or heat. This equipment must be kept in good condition and should be inspected on a regular basis.

MENTAL WELL-BEING

Stress and Anxiety

Stress is physical or mental tension brought about by physical, chemical, or emotional factors. Stress is also brought about by the interaction of events (environmental stimuli) and the capabilities of an individual to adjust to these stimuli. People often perceive stress as generating a negative effect, such as fear, depression, or guilt. Stress can also be experienced with positive events. Anxiety is defined as uneasiness or dread about future uncertainties. Eustress is "good stress," or the response to a positive stimulus, whereas distress is "bad stress," or a negative response to an environmental stimulus. Anxiety is uneasiness or dread about future uncertainties. Being able to recognize and effectively cope with anxiety and stress associated with your job is important for career longevity in the EMS profession.

CAUSES OF STRESS

Working in EMS and stress go hand in hand. EMT–Is feel stress in many different situations. Different events trigger stress in different people. Not every person is affected by what another person considers to be stressful, but some situations cause stress in almost all EMS personnel (Box 2-4).

From Stoy WA: *Mosby's EMT–Basic textbook*, St Louis, 1996, Mosby.

BOX 2-4

SITUATIONS THAT CAUSE STRESS

- Mass casualty incident
- Infant and child trauma
- Traumatic amputation
- Infant or child abuse, elder abuse, or spouse abuse
- Death or injury of a co-worker or other public safety personnel
- Emergency response to the illness or injury of a friend or family member

---

BOX 2-5

STRESS WARNING SIGNS

- Irritability with co-workers, family, friends, or patients
- Inability to concentrate
- Physical exhaustion
- Difficulty sleeping or nightmares
- Anxiety
- Indecisiveness
- Guilt
- Loss of appetite
- Loss of interest in sexual activities
- Isolation
- Loss of interest in work
- Increased substance use or abuse (alcohol, medications, illegal drugs)
- Depression

From Stoy WA: *Mosby's EMT–Basic textbook*, St Louis, 1996, Mosby.

Other stressors at work include the following:

- The environment: heat, cold, noise
- Strain of lifting and carrying
- Fatigue
- Patient demands
- Paperwork
- Red tape
- Decision making
- Physical danger
- Communicable diseases
- Heavy workload
- Rules and regulations
- Training requirements
- Lack of advancement opportunities
- Interpersonal relationships

Not only can one expect on-the-job stress, but also stress can come from other aspects of life. Marriage, financial problems, the birth of a child, or a death in the family can be very stressful.

The business of taking care of patients in an emergency situation can be stressful. Some patients may be experiencing only a minor illness or injury (some may be experiencing no emergency at all), and it seems unnecessary to have rushed to the scene with the emergency lights and siren. Other patients may be violently injured. An EMT–I's feelings can range from anger to grief and sadness. Virtually all emergency runs involve some type of stress. EMT–Is, as well as the patients and their friends and families, will feel some of that stress. How you, as an EMT–I, interact with those involved will affect their stress, as well as your own. Watch what you say and how you say it. Avoid making comments such as "Everything will be okay" or "You have nothing to worry about." Most people can tell whether things are okay or not. A patient with burns over most of his or her body from an explosion knows that things are not going well. Tell the patient that you are there to help. Explain what you are going to do for the patient and what he or she can do to help. Not only are the words you use to help reassure the preparatory patient important, but also the way you say them will have an effect. If you do not sound sincere and look confident, the words you use will do little to reassure the patient.

SIGNS OF STRESS

Is stress real? This is a good question and one that elicits varied responses. Stress is not something that can be seen. Stress is not the difficult runs or the death of a family member. Stress is the effect that these events have on a person. The difficult run and the financial problems are examples of stressors. Stress is a physical and psychological response to any demand.

An awareness of the signs of stress, both in oneself and in co-workers, is necessary in order to know when to take steps to manage stress. Different people exhibit signs of stress in different ways (Box 2-5).

EMT–Is are faced with stressful situations everyday. Daily responsibilities call for rational, quick thinking and self-control at all times. Unfortunately, this can work against a person. Too much control and too many expectations can be hazardous to one's mental and physical health.

MANAGING STRESS

A person who chooses a career in EMS must develop an understanding of job-related stress and effective stress management. Just as everyone reacts differently to stress, so, too, are the ways to deal with it. To manage stress effectively, a person must recognize the early warning signs of anxiety. Many warning signs appear during the emergency response or within 24 hours after the event. Some may be delayed for quite some time and may not appear for months or years after the event.

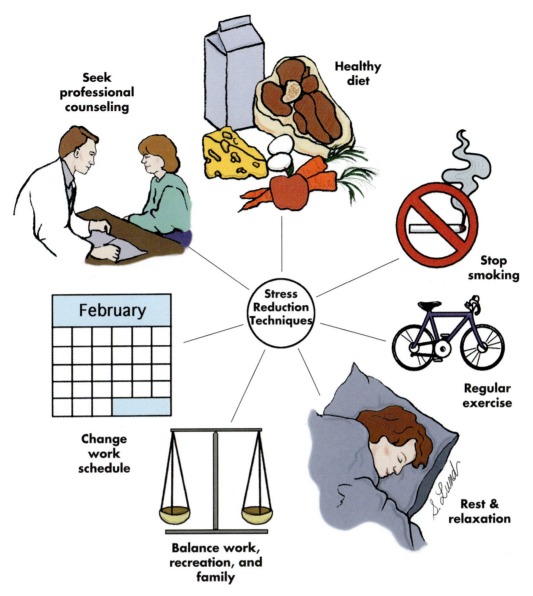

FIGURE 2-7 ▲ Stress reduction techniques. (From Stoy WA: *Mosby's EMT–Basic textbook,* St Louis, 1996, Mosby.)

Managing stress starts with being healthy. A person's ability to manage stress is directly related to his or her physical well-being. Eating right; quitting smoking; engaging in regular exercise, rest, and relaxation; balancing work and recreational activities; spending time with family and friends; changing the work schedule; and seeking professional counseling all contribute to a healthy lifestyle (Figure 2-7). These activities help prevent the EMT–I from becoming angry, isolated, strained, or even worse, relying on drugs and alcohol. Prevention is the best medicine.

Eating properly can be difficult when much of the shift is spent taking call after call. When there are just a few minutes to eat, it is easier to stop at a local fast-food restaurant for a quick meal between calls. The healthier thing to do is to bring a lunch, dinner, or snacks to work. Not only does this ensure good eating habits, it can help save a great deal of money. Also, unhealthy snacks should be replaced with fruits and vegetables, since they are healthy and help replace the vitamins and minerals a body uses under stressful situations. It is also a good idea to cut back on fats and sugars, replacing them with complex carbohydrates such as pastas, vegetables, and whole-grain foods. Sugars and caffeine provide a quick pick-me-up, but they can cause a letdown just as quickly.

Another thing EMT–Is should do is to take time for themselves. At least 30 minutes, three times a week, should be set aside for exercise. If necessary, exercise or hobby time should actually be planned on a calendar. The entire family can be involved, taking walks, riding bicycles, or participating in a sport the whole family can enjoy. Exercise can be made fun; it does not have to be a grueling, boring activity. An exercise is more likely to be continued if it is enjoyable. Setting goals while planning an exercise schedule (such as increasing cardiorespiratory endurance, increasing strength, and increasing flexibility) can help a person stay with the schedule. Before any exercise program is started, especially running or weight lifting, it should be approved by a physician to make sure it is healthy and safe.

It is also important for EMT–Is to know when to say "no"; they should not be afraid to turn down extra shifts. Working too many hours can be dangerous for both EMT–Is and their patients. As EMT–Is tire, their judgment may become clouded, they may not use proper lifting techniques, or they could fall asleep at the wheel. Just as the body needs exercise and a proper diet, it also needs sleep. EMT–Is should realize their limitations.

Also, EMT–Is must learn how to relax while at work. They may not be able to sleep, but relaxation techniques can help reduce or eliminate the effects of stress. It takes practice to relax while at work. Finding a quiet place free from distractions, listening to music, reading, meditating, or just daydreaming can all help. The EMT–I must do something to occupy his or her mind—preferably a non–EMS-related activity. Once it is determined what works for a person, it should be done on a regular basis.

HELPFUL HINT

- Deep breathing is a good stress reliever that can be incorporated into your relaxation techniques. Take a long, deep breath, and try to fill your lungs. Hold your breath for about 3 to 5 seconds, and then exhale through your mouth. Repeat this one or two times. Deep breathing can be done anywhere, virtually any time you feel uptight or stressed. Deep breathing exercises will help relax you, lower your blood pressure, and slow your pulse.

Balancing work, family, rest, and social activities can help alleviate stress. However, some situations can produce an overwhelming amount of stress. This is called critical incident stress. Understandably, a plane crash or any incident involving a large number of victims can have a devastating effect on the EMT–I. Also, a given situation may have a more profound effect on some persons than on others. A father who treats a critically injured child the same age as his own may experience profound stress. Critical incident stress needs to be managed immediately.

CRITICAL INCIDENT STRESS MANAGEMENT

Critical incident stress management (CISM) is an organized, formal, peer, and mental health support network and process. It enables emergency personnel to vent feelings and facilitates understanding of stressful situations. It is a useful method of preventing delayed reactions to stress.

The initial step is to defuse the emotions that have emerged as a product of the incident. The next step is to educate EMT–Is about stress reactions and how to manage them. The third step is to identify and extend qualified help to those who need it.

Components of CISM include preincident stress training, on-scene support to distressed personnel, individual consults, defusing services immediately after a large-scale incident, mobilization services after a large-scale incident, critical incident stress debriefing 24 to 72 hours after an event, and follow-up services. It can also include specialty debriefings for nonemergency groups in the community, support during routine discussions of an incident, and advice to command staff during a large-scale incident.

Situations in which CISM should be considered include the following:
- Line-of-duty injury or death
- Disaster
- Emergency co-worker's suicide
- Infant or child death
- Extreme threat to the emergency worker
- Prolonged incident that ends in loss or success
- Victims known to operations personnel
- Death or injury of a civilian caused by operations
- Other significant event

Two key parts of the CISM process are defusing and debriefing. Defusing is done immediately after a large-scale incident. It is an informal gathering that lasts less than an hour and occurs within 8 hours of the incident. It permits the initial release of feelings of those involved.

During the debriefing, the group of responders are brought together to form a trusting relationship. This assures everyone involved that there is a group of peers who will support each other throughout the challenging time. A debriefing team handles the debriefing. The debriefing team usually consists of peers who have been trained in the CISM process. The team is usually headed by a mental health professional. The debriefing session can last from 1 to 3 hours.

Peer support is the key idea in the CISM process. It makes sense for EMT–Is to share their feelings with those who can understand what they are feeling. EMT–Is should communicate with their partner(s), helping one another through the day. They must not be afraid to offer help.

EMT–Is must be familiar with CISD programs available in their system. If such a program does not exist, they should find out where emergency responders can go for help.

SUMMARY

Important points to remember from this chapter include the following:

- Nutrition is an important part of physical well-being. A healthy diet includes plenty of grain products, vegetables, and fruit and a variety of foods that are low in fat, saturated fat, and cholesterol. A diet also should be moderate in simple sugars, salt, and sodium.
- Because of the demands of the job, it is essential that EMT–Is be physically fit.
- Sleep helps to rejuvenate a tired body. On average, adults need 7 to 8 hours of sleep each day.
- EMT–Is have a responsibility to serve as role models in disease prevention.
- Infectious diseases are caused by pathogens that include bacteria and viruses. Any patient, even the young or old, may be carrying an infectious disease.
- To decrease the chance of being exposed to or infected by an infectious disease, the EMT–I should follow recommended engineering (i.e., puncture-resistant containers) and work practices, maintain good personal health and hygiene habits, keep immunizations up-to-date, receive periodic tuberculosis (TB) screening, and employ body substance isolation (BSI) procedures.
- Thorough hand washing is the most basic, effective way to prevent disease transmission.
- Recommended personal protective equipment (PPE) includes protective gloves, eye protection, masks, and cover gowns.
- Because of the risk for allergic reaction, a box of vinyl gloves or a latex allergy kit should be kept readily available in all emergency vehicles.
- Eye protection should be worn whenever there is a risk of body fluids splashing into one's eyes.

- Basic surgical masks are used to prevent splashed or aerosolized blood and other body fluids from coming into contact with the EMT–I's eyes, mouth, or nose.
- Disposable medical devices (other than needles or sharp objects) that become contaminated with blood or other body fluids should be placed in a red bag or container marked with a biohazard seal and then disposed of according to local policy.
- Needles and other sharp objects must be disposed of in a puncture-proof container, often referred to as a "sharps" container.
- When nondisposable equipment is used to treat a patient or surfaces become contaminated with a patient's blood or other body fluids, the equipment or surfaces must be cleaned, disinfected, or sterilized.
- It is important that the EMT–I knows the steps to follow in the event of an exposure. An exposure to blood or other body fluids should be immediately reported to the receiving hospital and the designated officer in the EMS system or agency so that communications can be coordinated between the hospital and the emergency response organization.
- All emergency care providers should maintain immunizations for tetanus, diphtheria, polio, hepatitis B, MMR (measles, mumps, and rubella), and influenza. Also, they should be checked annually for TB exposure (or more frequently if a possible occupational exposure has occurred).
- Stress is physical or mental tension brought about by physical, chemical, or emotional factors. Stress is also brought about by the interaction of events (environmental stimuli) and the capabilities of an individual to adjust to these stimuli.
- EMT–Is must be aware of the signs of stress, both in themselves and in co-workers, so that they know when to take steps to manage stress.
- A person's ability to manage stress is directly related to his or her physical well-being. Eating right; quitting smoking; engaging in regular exercise, rest, and relaxation; balancing work and recreational activities; spending time with family and friends; changing the work schedule; and seeking professional counseling all contribute to a healthy lifestyle.
- Critical incident stress management (CISM) is an organized, formal, peer, and mental health support network and process. It enables emergency personnel to vent feelings and facilitates understanding of stressful situations.

3 Medical-Legal Aspects

Key Terms

Abandonment

Assault

Battery

Consent

Do-Not-Resuscitate
(DNR) Order

Duty to Act

Expressed Consent

False Imprisonment

Good Samaritan Laws

Gross Negligence

Implied Consent

Informed Consent

Libel

Negligence

Ordinary Negligence

Scope of Practice

Slander

Standard of Care

Tort

Tort Law

...CASE HISTORY

EMT–I Reynolds is attending the annual state EMS conference and is taking a break after sitting in on a talk about medical-legal issues in EMS. She pours a soda and sits in the lobby to think about the complex issues of which the lawyer spoke.

Several groups of people are in the lobby discussing personal medical liability, assault charges stemming from invasive field interventions, and false imprisonment for using hard restraints. One group is discussing a charge against an EMT–Intermediate training institute for violating the American Disabilities Act because it failed to accommodate a hearing-impaired student.

EMT–I Reynolds wants a few quiet minutes to herself, when she overhears EMT–I Thomas, who works at her service, saying, "I heard Tom Reilly from platoon B is HIV positive."

EMT–I Reynolds stands and walks away, disgusted with Thomas's gossiping.

LEARNING OBJECTIVES

CHAPTER GOAL
Upon completion of this chapter, the EMT-Intermediate will be able to understand the legal issues that affect decisions made in the out-of-hospital environment.

Cognitive Objectives
As an EMT-Intermediate you should be able to do the following:
- Review legal and ethical responsibilities.
- Identify and explain the importance of laws pertinent to the EMT–I.
- Differentiate between licensure and certification as they apply to the EMT–I.
- List the specific problems or conditions encountered while providing care that an EMT–I is required to report, and identify in each instance to whom the report is to be made.
- Define the terms *abandonment, advance directives, assault, battery, breach of duty, confidentiality, consent (expressed, implied, informed, involuntary), do-not-resuscitate (DNR) orders, duty to act, emancipated minor, false imprisonment, immunity, liability, libel, minor, negligence, proximate cause, scope of practice, slander, standard of care,* and *tort.*
- Differentiate between the scope of practice and the standard of care for EMT–I practice.

- Discuss the concept of medical direction, including off-line medical direction and on-line medical direction, and its relationship to the standard of care of an EMT–I.
- Review the four elements that must be present to prove negligence.
- Given a scenario in which a patient is injured while an EMT–I is providing care, determine whether the four components of negligence are present.
- Given a scenario, demonstrate patient care behaviors that would protect the EMT–I from claims of negligence.
- Explain the concept of liability as it might apply to EMT–I practice, including physicians providing medical direction and EMT–I supervision of other care providers.
- Review the legal concept of immunity, including Good Samaritan statutes and governmental (civil) immunity, as it applies to the EMT–I.
- Review the importance and necessity of patient confidentiality and the standards for maintaining patient confidentiality that apply to the EMT–I.
- Review the steps to take if a patient refuses care.
- Identify the legal issues involved in the decision not to transport a patient or to reduce the level of care being provided during transport.
- Review the conditions under which the use of force, including restraint, is acceptable.
- Explain the purpose of advance directives relative to patient care and how the EMT–I should care for a patient who is covered by an advance directive.
- Discuss the responsibilities of the EMT–I in relation to resuscitation efforts for patients who are potential organ donors.
- Review the importance of providing accurate documentation (oral and written) in substantiating an incident.
- Review the characteristics of a patient care report required to make it an effective legal document.

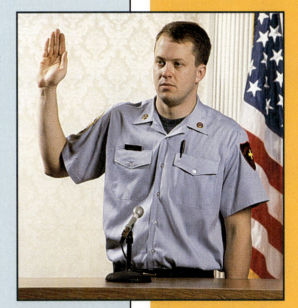

Affective Objectives
As an EMT-Intermediate you should be able to do the following:
- Assess your personal commitment to protecting patient confidentiality.
- Defend personal beliefs about withholding or stopping patient care.
- Defend the value of advance medical directives.

Psychomotor Objectives
- None identified for this chapter.

INTRODUCTION

Legal issues are an important aspect of patient care for the EMT–Intermediate (EMT–I). Understanding some basic legal concepts is helpful for the EMT–I, as is have a working knowledge of applicable state laws and regulations. The information in this chapter should not be substituted for legal advice. Laws vary widely from state to state. Consult an experienced attorney or your local EMS authority for interpretation of specific rules and regulations as they pertain to your EMS system. Remember, ignorance of the law is rarely, if ever, an acceptable excuse or defense.

ESSENTIAL PRINCIPLES

Prevention of Legal Problems

In dealing with legal issues, prevention of problems is the cardinal rule. Appropriate emergency medical care and accurate call documentation are the best protection for medical-legal questions. Successful suits against most health care providers involve failure to follow one of the following practices:

- Caring for patients as if each is a family member. Many malpractice claims against health care providers stem not from what the provider did, but how he or she did it.
- Following state and local guidelines and protocols concerning prehospital care, including appropriate use of on-line and off-line medical direction. Do not perform procedures that you are not certified to do or allowed to do within protocol guidelines. Know your department's policies and procedures, and always follow them.

Case example—Proper adherence to standard protocols is an acceptable defense against allegations of negligence. In *Fairchild v. United States,* plaintiffs claimed that medical personnel should have been sent at an earlier time to the decedent's aid. In brief, the case involved a man who was hiking through Grand Canyon National Park and became ill on the trail. Another hiker relayed the patient's signs and symptoms to a ranger. The ranger determined, on the basis of the information given him, that the decedent was suffering from heat exhaustion. The ranger instructed bystanders to give the decedent oral fluids and observe him. No ranger responded to the scene. According to the transcript, the patient was conscious and alert and had no vomiting; these findings ruled out the more serious possibility of heat stroke. Had heat stroke been present, a professional rescuer would have been sent to the scene.

The appellate court reasoned that the ranger's decision not to go to the scene was based on evidence that the decedent was suffering from heat exhaustion, not heat stroke, and that this treatment was in accordance with the accepted protocol and procedures established by the National Park Service. Thus as a matter of law, the ranger's failure to come to the scene did not constitute negligence (*Fairchild v. United States,* Case No. 93C 6953, 1996 WL 197692 [N.D. Ill., Eastern Div. Apr. 22, 1996]).

- Keeping proper, thorough, and accurate patient care documentation as required by the EMS system. It is important that handwriting be legible. Because legal proceedings can take place years after the original event, ensure that run reports can be easily read for years after an incident.

To reduce negligence claims, all EMT–Is and EMS systems should adhere to the following practices:

- Provide and use appropriate education, training, and continuing education. Remember, recertification requirements are usually only minimum standards.
- Provide appropriate medical direction, both on-line and off-line. This includes case review and continuous quality improvement programs with direct involvement by the medical director.
- Always have accurate and thorough documentation. The one most important legal defensive measure is this: "Document, document, document." Do it regularly, on a timely basis, and accurately (Figure 3-1).
- Always maintain a professional attitude and demeanor. The way the EMT–I appears to patients and to the public as a professional is often related to a person's willingness to pursue legal action. Unprofessional behavior invites more legal problems than do professional actions.

Legal Duties and Ethical Responsibilities of the EMT–Intermediate

The legal duties of the EMT–I are to the patient, the medical director, and the public. These are generally set by local, state, and federal statutes and regulations and are based on generally accepted standards.

Besides legal duties, the EMT–I carries, as a professional, ethical responsibilities. This means that one's conduct should be morally desirable. Ethical responsibilities of the EMT–I include the following:

- Responding to the physical and emotional needs of every patient with respect
- Maintaining mastery of skills
- Participating in continuing education and refresher training
- Critically reviewing performance and seeking improvement
- Reporting honestly and respecting the confidentiality of both patients and co-workers
- Working cooperatively and with respect for other emergency professionals

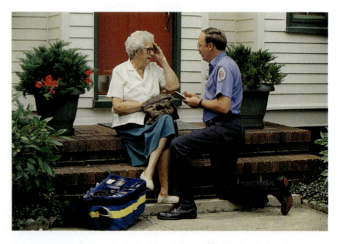

FIGURE 3-1 ▲ Documentation is an important part of the EMT–I's job. (From American College of Emergency Physicians; Pons PT, Cason D, chief editors: *Paramedic field care: a complaint-based approach,* St Louis, 1997, Mosby for ACEP.)

A recent review of EMS legal cases revealed the following:
- Most cases involved a patient care incident resulting in death or significant physical injury.
- The majority of allegations involved inadequate assessment or treatment, delay in ambulance arrival, failure of ambulance arrival, or failure to transport the patient to the hospital.
- Immunity to liability was claimed as a defense in 53% of cases and was used by both public and private EMS providers.
- The appellate court outcome was similar whether or not liability immunity was used as a defense.

Data from Morgan DL et al: Liability immunity as a legal defense for recent emergency medical services system litigation, *Prehosp Disaster Med* 10:82-91, April-June, 1995.

REVIEW OF THE LEGAL SYSTEM

Types of Law

There are five basic types of laws, all of which may apply to the EMT–I:

- *Legislative law*—Deals with laws enacted at the federal, state, or local levels by the legislative branches of government, including Congress, city councils, district boards, and state general assemblies.
- *Administrative law*—Deals with regulations developed by a government agency (e.g., the Federal Aviation Administration). Generally, the agency has the authority to enforce these specific rules, regulations, and statutes.
- *Common law*—Deals with laws that are "judge made" and based on individual legal cases. This type of law is also called case law. The word *common* refers to the fact that these laws are derived, via the courts, from society's acceptance of customs or norms over time.
- *Criminal law*—Deals with laws that prohibit the performance of any act considered damaging to the public. Violations of these laws result in crimes, and violators may be prosecuted and tried in a criminal proceeding—a trial before a judge, and sometimes a jury—in which evidence is heard and a verdict of "guilty" or "not guilty" is reached. If a guilty verdict is reached, a fine, imprisonment, or both, may result. Typical criminal acts include robbery, assault, and murder.
- *Civil (tort) law*—The area of law dealing with private complaints brought by a plaintiff against a defendant for an illegal act or wrongdoing (tort). Complaints are enforced by bringing a civil lawsuit against the defendant in which the plaintiff requests the court to award damages (usually money).

    A **tort** is the breach of a legal duty or obligation resulting in an injury, either physical, mental, or financial. **Tort law** (also called civil law) is different from criminal law. Under tort law, the plaintiff, or injured person, files a lawsuit, or legal action, against the defendant, or person accused of committing the breach of duty. If the plaintiff successfully proves that the defendant caused harm by violating a legal duty, the plaintiff may collect damages—monetary compensation awarded by the court. Injuries include medical bills, loss of employment, pain, suffering, and loss of ability to be with others (loss of consortium).

Failing to perform the job appropriately can result in civil or criminal liability. The best legal protection is provision of appropriate assessment and care coupled with accurate and complete documentation. Since laws differ from state to state and area to area, it is important to always get competent legal advice.

How Laws Affect the EMT–Intermediate

There are several specific areas of the various types of law that directly affect the EMT–I. These include laws regarding the following:

- *Scope of practice*—The range of duties and skills an EMT–I is allowed and expected to perform when necessary is referred to as the **scope of practice.** This range is usually set by state law or regulation and by local medical direction.
- *Medical direction*—Medical direction by a licensed physician is required for EMT–I practice. It may be off-line or on-line, depending on state and local requirements. Each system should have a policy to guide EMT–Is in dealing with the on-scene physician (see later discussion).
- *Medical Practice Act*—Each state has a set of laws, called the Medical Practice Act, that governs the practice of medicine within that state. These laws, although different from state to state, define limits for the scope of practice, which includes those patient assessment and treatment skills that medical direction physicians allow EMT–Is to perform. EMT–Is must be familiar with the appropriate state act that defines the scope of practice.
- *Certification*—Certification grants recognition to an individual who has met predetermined qualifications to participate in an activity (e.g., function as a cardiopulmonary resuscitation [CPR] instructor). It is usually granted by a certifying agency or professional association, not necessarily a government agency.
- *Licensure*—Licensure is the process of occupational regulation by a government agency, such as the state medical board. Licensure grants permission to an individual who meets established qualifications to engage in the profession or occupation (e.g., function as an EMT–I). Licensure, certification, or both, may be required by state or local authorities for a person to practice as an EMT–I.
- *Motor vehicle laws*—Motor vehicle codes vary considerably from state to state. Many areas, for example, require that a person possess a chauffeur's license to

drive an emergency vehicle. Thus EMT–Is must be familiar with appropriate state statutes regarding the operation of emergency vehicles, paying particular attention to sections dealing with speeding, right-of-way, and the use of lights and a siren. The motor vehicle code of each state also sets standards for equipping and operating an emergency vehicle, such as an ambulance.

Case example—While operating an ambulance under emergency conditions, EMS providers have limited immunity from traffic laws. The plaintiff EMT–I was operating an EMS ambulance and, after stopping, proceeded through a red light with all warning devices activated. The ambulance was hit by another vehicle. The EMT–Is were transporting a woman with severe shortness of breath. The EMS system contended that it was operating an authorized "emergency vehicle" engaged in an "emergency operation" at the time of the accident. The appellate court agreed; since the ambulance was engaged in an emergency operation, the driver had a qualified privilege to proceed past a red light and could be held responsible for the accident only if her conduct demonstrated a reckless disregard for the safety of others (*Mulholland v. Nabisco, Inc.*, 693 NYS 2d 242 [NY App Div, 1999]).

- Mandatory reporting requirements—These vary from state to state but often include the following:
  - Child abuse and neglect; elderly abuse; spouse abuse
  - Sexual assault
  - Gunshot and stab wounds
  - Animal bites
  - Communicable diseases
    The content of the report and to whom it must be made is set by law, regulation, or policy.
    Various laws regarding protection for the EMT–I, depending on the locality, may include the following:
- Laws requiring that other health care providers and hospitals notify the EMT–I if there is evidence of exposure to a communicable disease (e.g., a patient the EMT–I transported to the hospital turns out to have bacterial meningitis)
- Immunity statutes, including governmental (civil) immunity and Good Samaritan laws
- Laws covering special crimes against an EMT–I, including assault or battery to EMT–Is while they are doing their duties and obstruction of EMT–I activity and patient care

NEGLIGENCE

Legal Accountability of the EMT–Intermediate

The EMT–I is expected to act in a reasonable and prudent manner and to provide a level of care and transportation consistent with his or her education and training. Failure to meet these expectations—negligence—can result in legal accountability and liability.

Components of Negligence

Negligence, or medical liability, is conduct that falls below the standard of care. This conduct may entail either doing something that should not have been done or failing to do something that should have been done. For example, defibrillating a responsive patient in normal sinus rhythm is doing something that should not have been done. Failure to defibrillate an arrested person in ventricular fibrillation, however, would be considered failing to do something that should have been done. In either of these two cases, the care rendered the patient would be considered negligent because it falls below the standard of care. Although the EMT–I may violate the standard of care, a legal finding of professional negligence is not as simple.

- **Negligence** • Professional conduct that falls below the standard of care; also known as medical liability.
- **Ordinary Negligence** • Acts of omission that occur in an attempt to deliver proper care.
- **Gross Negligence** • The willful and reckless giving of care that causes injury to the patient.

STREET WISE

Giving either the wrong care or substandard care is considered negligent, or below the standard of care.

For the EMT–I to be found negligent, the following four requirements must be met (Figure 3-2):
- The act or omission must have been within the EMT–I's duty to act.
- The act or omission must have been below the standard of care.
- An injury must have occurred to the patient.
- The act or omission must have been the proximate (direct) cause of injury.

DUTY TO ACT

Duty to act means that the EMT–I has an obligation to provide care. Generally, just by being dispatched and responding to a scene, the EMT–I has incurred a duty to act. This duty applies to both paid and volunteer EMS systems.

Duties include the following:
- Duty to respond and render care
- Duty to obey laws and regulations
- Duty to operate an emergency vehicle reasonably and prudently
- Duty to provide care and transportation to the expected standard
- Duty to provide care and transportation consistent with the scope of practice and local medical protocols

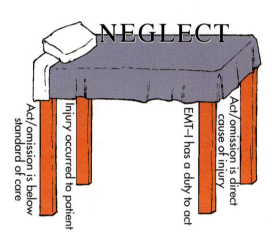

FIGURE 3-2 ▲ The four elements of negligence.

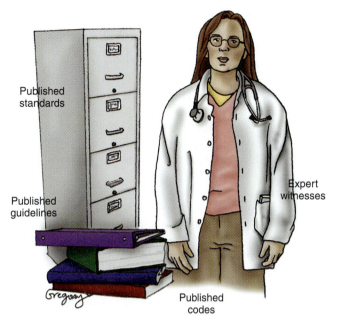

FIGURE 3-3 ▲ Elements that establish the standard of care.

- Duty to continue care and transportation through to its appropriate conclusion

ACT OR OMISSION BELOW THE STANDARD OF CARE

Practicing by the accepted standard of care involves exercising the care, skill, and judgment that would be expected under like or similar circumstances by a similarly trained, reasonable EMT–I in the location involved. The standard of care is established by court testimony and reference to published codes, standards, criteria, and guidelines applicable to the situation (Figure 3-3).

Violation of the standard of care is usually established by testimony from expert witnesses and from various rules, regulations, and protocols that may be presented. An expert witness is an individual who has special knowledge, not normally possessed by the average person, about a subject; for example, a physician may serve as an expert witness in medical negligence cases.

An act or omission below the **standard of care** may include providing improper care, performing skills the EMT–I is not certified to do, violating rules and regulations set forth by the EMT–I's EMS system, or using equipment that fails to work properly. Breach of duty may include the following:
- *Malfeasance*—Performing a wrongful or unlawful act.
- *Misfeasance*—Performing a legal act in a way that is harmful.
- *Nonfeasance*—Failure to perform a required act or duty.

Sometimes negligence may be so obvious that it does not require extensive proof. The legal term for this is *res ipsa loquitur*—literally, "the thing stands for itself." This principle suggests that the plaintiff's injury could only have been caused by the defendant's negligence. Usually the relationship must be so clear that no expert witness testimony is necessary to prove it.

Still another concept involves negligence per se—the legal assumption that negligence occurred simply by the fact that a statute was violated and injury resulted.

INJURY TO THE PATIENT

Generally, for the EMT–I to be found negligent, the injury to the patient must have resulted in damages that can be estimated in financial terms. It is not necessary, however, for the damages merely to represent absolute monetary losses. Pain, suffering, and loss of companionship are often successfully claimed as damages in professional negligence lawsuits. Direct damages are called compensatory damages and may include the following:
- Medical expenses
- Lost earnings
- Conscious pain and suffering
- Wrongful death

In some states juries are allowed to award punitive damages ("punishing damages"), which are intended to punish **gross negligence,** or willful and wanton (deliberate) misconduct. Punitive damages are usually not covered by malpractice insurance.

PROXIMATE CAUSE

Proximate cause means that something was directly responsible for damage. Within reasonable medical probability, the error of the EMT–I must be the direct cause of the patient's injuries. The patient may claim to have suffered a new injury or worsening of his or her original problem as a result of the EMT–I's negligence.

To establish proximate cause, the plaintiff must prove the following:

- The action or inaction of the EMT–I was the cause of or worsened the damage.
- The fact that the EMT–I's act or inaction would result in the damage must have been reasonably foreseeable by the EMT–I. This means that a reasonable person would recognize in advance the potential for a particular event to occur.

Proximate cause is usually established by expert witness testimony. Whether or not one is familiar with the intricacies of the legal system, three important facts bear remembering:

- Excellent patient care, appropriate use of medical direction, professional behavior, and good judgment are the best ways to avoid legal problems.
- The EMT–I should immediately consult with a supervisor if he or she receives any kind of legal notice or subpoena or is requested to sign any legal documents related to his or her work as an EMT–I.
- The EMT–I should consider consulting an attorney as well if he or she has any questions or receives a subpoena.

Defenses Against Negligence Charges

There are several potential legal defenses against allegations of professional negligence.

GOOD SAMARITAN LAWS

Good Samaritan laws may provide immunity from prosecution or civil suit for people who render care at the scene of an emergency. Most states have Good Samaritan laws in place to protect persons who provide assistance at emergency scenes. These laws may apply to laypersons or medical personnel. Good Samaritan laws vary widely from state to state in the scope of their coverage and requirements. A trial or hearing may be required to decide if the EMT–I's actions place him or her within the scope of the particular state's Good Samaritan law (Figure 3-4).

These laws typically have the following three conditions:

- The charge is not gross negligence. Good Samaritan law immunity usually covers charges of **ordinary negligence** but not charges of gross negligence (e.g., patient abandonment). Proving gross negligence may be difficult in a court of law.
- The provider must give care without charging a fee for service.
- The provider must give only care that is appropriate for his or her certification level.

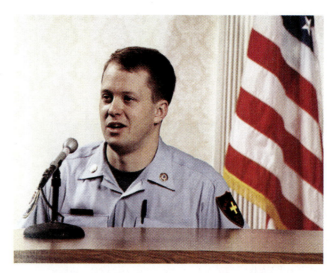

FIGURE 3-4 ▲ Testifying at trial. (From McSwain NE et al: *The basic EMT: comprehensive prehospital patient care,* St Louis, 1997, Mosby.)

! HELPFUL HINT

- Remember that Good Samaritan laws do not prevent anyone from initiating a lawsuit. They may, however, allow an EMT–I to successfully defend himself or herself by claiming immunity. Good Samaritan laws have not been well tested in the courts. Therefore many attorneys caution their EMS clients not to rely heavily on these laws for protection. These laws do *not* prevent an EMT–I from being sued. In the United States anyone is free to sue anyone for any reason.

Many questions remain to be answered regarding Good Samaritan laws. These include concerns as to vagueness in the laws and the true definition of "fee for service" (i.e., career versus volunteer EMT) prehospital care.

GOVERNMENTAL (CIVIL) IMMUNITY

Governmental (civil) immunity means that an EMS service may be protected from a charge of negligence because it is a designated government agency. These laws vary from area to area. Although immunity laws vary widely from state to state, some experts believe that the trend is toward limiting government agency protection. Nonetheless, as with Good Samaritan laws, EMT–Is should not rely on civil immunity statutes for protection.

Case example—A recent court decision in Maryland found that the state's Good Samaritan statute does not provide immunity to a paramedic employed by a municipal fire department that bills the patient for its services, regardless of the "token" amount of the bill (*Chase v. Mayor and City Council of Baltimore,* 126 Md App 427, 730 A 2d 239 [Md Sp App, 1999]).

GROSS NEGLIGENCE SUPERSEDES IMMUNITY

Litigation involving emergency medical services is becoming more common. Courts have upheld liability immunity in certain cases; on the other hand, gross negligence supersedes this defense and may also result in significant punitive damages.*

Case example—A child with epiglottitis was placed into a city ambulance at the office of his personal pediatrician. The paramedics offered to take the child to the nearest hospital, 6 minutes away. Instead, the physician insisted that the child be taken to a children's hospital, much farther away, and proceeded to intubate him before placing him into the ambulance. The physician signed a form releasing the city from liability. The tube plugged shortly thereafter, resulting in hypoxic brain damage to the child, who died 3 days later. The plaintiff and physician claimed that the EMS suction device was functioning improperly and that the ambulance's oxygen cylinders were empty. Because of the signed release, the city and ambulance service were found innocent. The jury reached a judgment against the physician for $2,500,000 (*Wilson v. Herman,* Docket No. L11975-89 [Middlesex County, NJ Sup Ct, 1994]; reported in *Medical Malpractice Verdicts, Settlements and Experts* 10:16, July 1994).

Case example—A woman with breathing difficulty was, according to relatives, refused transport to the hospital by the local EMS crew. Her daughter drove her there, and she died of a heart attack en route. EMS claimed that the relatives refused transport and that the woman might have died anyway, even if transported by ambulance. A confidential settlement was reached (*Jennings v. Atlanta South Ambulance, Inc.,* Case No. E01168 [Fulton County, Ga Sup Ct, 1994]; reported in *Medical Malpractice Verdicts, Settlements and Experts* 10:17-18, July 1994).

Case example—A 38-year-old woman visiting on business developed severe abdominal pain. She was 3 months' pregnant. She was seen at a local emergency department three different times, where a urinary tract infection and gastritis were diagnosed. An ultrasound examination was never done. Two days later, EMS was called because the patient was having severe abdominal pain. The patient was on the third floor of a walk-up building. According to reports, she was ordered by the EMS technicians to get out of bed and walk down the three flights of stairs. She tried but collapsed by the side of her bed. Reportedly, the EMS technicians refused to carry her down the stairs in a chair and left the apartment. The patient died 70 minutes later. The plaintiff argued that the technicians were negligent for leaving the patient while she was in obvious distress, as well as for failing to diagnose her ectopic pregnancy. Liability was conceded before trial. The jury reached a $41,032,000 verdict against the defendants (*Plotkin v. NYCHHC,* Case No. 16631/88 [Kings County, NY Sup Ct, 1994]; reported in *Medical Malpractice Verdicts, Settlements and Experts* 10:20, August 1994).

Case example—An Indiana appellate court has held that "a municipality that provides emergency medical services to the public may be held liable under federal civil rights laws for restricting access to lifesaving medical devices" (*Culver-Union Township Ambulance Service v. Steindler,* 611 NE 2d 698 [Ind Ct App, 1993]; reported in Bushnell K: *Medical Liability Reporter* 15:185). The plaintiffs alleged that ambulance personnel failed to adequately respond to the patient's condition and failed to promptly transport him to a medical facility. Damages were sought against the town that owned the ambulance. Although a municipality is not constitutionally required "to provide emergency medical services to the general public, the town in this case had affirmatively undertaken to render such services to the patient and allegedly had adopted a policy that unduly restricted the patient's access to lifesaving equipment."

*Data from Shanaberger CJ: Case law involving base-station contact, *Prehosp Disaster Med* 10:75-81, April-June, 1995.

GOVERNMENTAL (CIVIL) IMMUNITY

A common defense when EMS providers are named in a lawsuit is that of civil immunity. Generally, this doctrine defeats simple negligence actions. On the other hand, most states still recognize a cause of action for "willful and wanton" negligence, similar to that cited in most Good Samaritan statutes. For example, in one case the estate of a worker who had died of heat stroke after collapsing at work brought suit against EMTs who had treated him, alleging negligent care (*Brock v. Anderson Road Association,* 222 Ill Dec 451, 677 NE 2d 985 [Ill App Ct, 1997]). The circuit court dismissed the complaint, and the plaintiff appealed. The appellate court held that the immunity provision of the state's Emergency Medical Services (EMS) Systems Act applied with regard to the negligence claim. The court further opined that since there was no evidence presented that the treatment of the patient constituted willful or wanton misconduct, the circuit court's decision was affirmed. Despite several jurisdictions' similar findings, EMS providers should not *ipso facto* assume that they are immune from liability (see case example of *Carrola v. Guillen* below).

In *Hansen v. Horn Rapids ORV Park of the City of Richland* (85 Wash App 424, 932 P 2d 724 [1997]), a participant in a motorcycle race held in a city park brought suit against several parties, including the

Continued

GOVERNMENTAL (CIVIL) IMMUNITY—cont'd

city, alleging negligence of the EMTs who treated his injuries during the race. Summary judgment was granted by the superior court, and the plaintiffs appealed. The court of appeals held that none of the parties, including the city, owed a nondelegable duty to the patient to provide first aid. Thus they could not be held vicariously liable for alleged negligence of the EMTs. In a related case (*Proveaux v. Medical University of South Carolina,* 482 SE 2d 774 [SC 1997]), the Supreme Court of South Carolina held that a physician, whose salary had to be approved by a state-run medical college, was entitled to civil immunity when sued for medical malpractice.

Case example—Civil immunity does not guarantee summary judgment. Survivors of a woman treated by firefighters and paramedics sued for negligence and gross negligence. The district court denied summary judgment on the basis of civil immunity because a genuine issue of fact existed as to whether or not the EMS providers exercised civil discretion in providing care. The EMS providers appealed, and the district court decision was upheld. The patient was an elderly woman found by paramedics to be in severe respiratory distress. They moved her to the ambulance, where

they contacted medical control, requested backup, administered medications, and intubated her. She then developed cardiac arrest. They left for the hospital after a third paramedic arrived at the scene. The patient died shortly after arriving at the hospital. The entire call, from dispatch to hospital, took 24 minutes. Plaintiffs' allegations included improperly used equipment, violation of treatment and transportation protocols (including failure to promptly transport the patient to the hospital), and failure to surrender authority to an on-site physician (*Carrola v. Guillen,* 935 SW 2d 949 (Tex Ct App [1996]).

COMMENT: The basis for the court's decision in *Carrola v. Guillen* focused on the issue of medical versus governmental discretion. Government-employed medical personnel are not immune from liability if the discretion they exercise is medical and not governmental (*Kassen v. Hatley,* 887 SW 2d 4, 11 [Tex, 1994]). In other words, once a government health care provider begins to treat a patient, the duty owed to that patient is the same as that owed by any similar professional. If the government-employed health care provider is medically negligent, immunity does not necessarily apply.

STATUTE OF LIMITATIONS

The statute of limitations denotes a limited number of years following an incident during which a lawsuit may be filed. The statute period is set by law, varies from state to state, and may differ between adults and children.

CONTRIBUTORY NEGLIGENCE

Contributory negligence is a defense theory alleging that the plaintiff may have contributed to his or her own injuries. Damages awarded by the jury may be reduced or eliminated on the basis of the plaintiff's contribution to his or her own injury. Expert witness testimony is usually required to establish that the patient contributed to his or her own injuries.

Case example—EMTs are liable even if the patient is also negligent. The plaintiff had a diagnosis of hypoglycemia since the mid-1970s. While skiing, she became dizzy and nearly lost consciousness. Apparently, she had not followed her prescribed diet that day. A ski patrolman, who was also an EMT, administered intravenous (IV) glucose. Immediately, the patient experienced redness and swelling in the arm where the IV line was located. Surgery was required, and she lost partial use of the arm. The plaintiff claimed that the skiing corporation was liable for the actions of the ski patrolman, whose negligence resulted in her injuries.

An initial jury verdict found in favor of the defendant ski corporation, ruling that the plaintiff was 95% liable for her in-

juries because of failure to follow her diet. Under Colorado law, the remaining 5% of damages was not recoverable—a plaintiff seeking recovery must prove that his or her own fault is less than 50%. On rehearing, the federal district court ruled that "while Ms. Spence's neglect of her dietary regimen undoubtedly precipitated the situation requiring treatment by an EMT, there was no evidence that her hypoglycemia—or her failure to control the hypoglycemia—contributed in any way to the specific arm injury that was the basis for her damage claim." Judgment was entered for the plaintiff (*Spence v. Aspen Skiing Co.,* 820 F Supp 542, 542 [D Colo, 1993]).

COMMENT: Many courts have held that the defense of contributory negligence is inapplicable when a patient's conduct provides the occasion for medical attention, care, or treatment that later is the subject of a medical malpractice claim (*Jensen v. Archbishop Bergan Mercy Hospital,* 236 Neb 1, 459 NW 2d 178 [1990]; *Whitehead v. Linkous,* 404 So 2d 377 [Fla Dist Ct App, 1981]; *Matthews v. Williford,* 318 So 2d 480 [Fla Dist Ct App 1975]). The court in Spence found that "all patients, regardless of how they sustain an illness or injury, may reasonably expect competent treatment from those into whose hands they have placed themselves" (820 F Supp at 542).

LIABILITY INSURANCE

The sophistication of EMS has created the obligation and expectation to provide quality patient care. Many EMT–Is are not covered by Good Samaritan laws, and as a result, more EMT–Is are being named as defendants in malpractice suits. For these reasons, many EMS systems and individual EMT–Is have purchased malpractice insurance. Some larger EMS systems are self-insured, meaning they have the money available to cover possible claims without outside companies.

Although most EMS systems carry some type of insurance, this insurance may or may not provide adequate protection for the individual provider. EMTs should check with their particular EMS system to clarify the extent to which they are covered by the system's malpractice insurance. Separate (individual) malpractice insurance is recommended for career EMT–Is and those whose EMS system lacks adequate coverage. The specific dollar amounts of insurance necessary differ from area to area. Colleagues, insurance agents, attorneys, supervisors, and risk management or continuous quality improvement personnel may be able to provide suggestions regarding individual malpractice insurance.

Service-supplied malpractice insurance alone may be very limited in coverage, and it may not cover any medical care administered while the EMT–I is off duty. On the other hand, individual medical liability insurance is written for each EMT–I's specific needs. The insurer then acts as an advocate for the EMT–I, not for the EMS service.

Despite who provides malpractice coverage, the EMT–I should understand the contract and be familiar with reporting requirements. Some insurers require that the EMT–I report any incident, no matter how small, that may develop into a lawsuit. If a potential suit is not reported on a timely basis, the insurer may refuse to provide coverage if a suit actually occurs.

SPECIAL LIABILITY CONCERNS

Liability of the EMT–Intermediate Medical Director

The medical director for any EMS program is subject to liability in a variety of situations, such as the following:
- *On-line*—The medical director is responsible for providing on-line medical control—direct supervision regarding patient care—usually on either the radio or phone.
- *Off-line*—Off-line supervision is provided by use of protocols, including standing orders.
- *Indirect supervision*—The medical director is responsible for EMT–Is under his or her control. This is often called the "borrowed servant" doctrine in legal terms. Although the EMT–I may work for an ambulance service or EMS division, the medical director is still "where the buck stops." Similarly, depending on the degree of supervision and control of EMT–Basics by EMT–Is, an EMT–I may also be liable for the actions of the EMT–Basic.

Other Liability Considerations

All members of the EMS team, including the medical director, must pay careful attention to nonmedical, but related, legislation, particularly concerning the areas of civil rights, disabilities, and off-duty performance:
- *Civil rights*—Various federal, state, and local laws state that an EMS system may not discriminate in providing service to a patient because of race, color, sex, national origin, or in some cases, ability to pay. In addition, patients should be provided with appropriate care despite their disease/condition (e.g., HIV/AIDS, other communicable disease).
- *Disabilities*—Closely related to civil rights legislation is the Americans with Disabilities Act that prohibits discrimination based on a person's disability, including certain diseases such as HIV/AIDS. This law has been interpreted broadly by the courts to include patients with disabilities who allegedly were treated differently from those without disabilities. The law provides severe civil penalties for violations.
- *Off-duty EMT–I*—Laws regarding whether or not an off-duty EMT–I can perform procedures that require physician delegation vary from state to state. Check your local regulations before you are faced with the situation.

THE ANATOMY OF A MALPRACTICE SUIT

The Case

EMT–Is Jones and Smith are called to the home of Mr. Reid, an accountant age 60 years, who is in cardiac arrest. Mr. Reid's adopted son, Mr. Law, is performing one-person CPR. EMT–I Jones joins Mr. Law in performing two-person CPR while EMT–I Smith calls for advanced life support (ALS) backup. After EMT–I Smith discovers that the ambulance radio will not work, he takes the oxygen tank and bag-valve-mask equipment from the ambulance and joins EMT–I Jones. Between the EMT–Is and Mr. Law, CPR is performed for 5 minutes. Mr. Reid does not respond. At that time, EMT–I Jones notices that the oxygen tank is empty and runs back to the ambulance to get another one.

The three men again perform CPR, using a new oxygen tank, for another 5 minutes. When there is no response, EMT–Is Smith and Jones decide to transport Mr. Reid to the nearest hospital, which is 10 minutes away.

On arrival at the hospital emergency department, the emergency physician notes that Mr. Reid is in a cardiac rhythm known as ventricular fibrillation, a chaotic quivering of the heart that results in the absence of cardiac output. She administers an electrical shock, or defibrillation, to Mr. Reid, resulting in normal cardiac contraction.

After other ALS therapy, Mr. Reid's heart is again beating normally and he is breathing on his own. However, he remains unresponsive. In fact, Mr. Reid never does wake up, although his other bodily functions are normal. He requires around-the-clock care in a nursing home for the rest of his life.

The Lawsuit

Mr. Law later sues on behalf of Mr. Reid against EMT–Is Smith and Jones, the ambulance company, and the medical director of the ambulance service. He claims that the EMT–Is spent too much time performing CPR in the field. The lawsuit also questions whether EMT–Is Smith and Jones should have carried an automated external defibrillator on their unit and tried to use it on Mr. Reid. Combined with the fact that the first oxygen tank was empty and that their radio was broken, Mr. Law's attorney states that Mr. Reid's brain was deprived of sufficient oxygen to allow for him to recover responsiveness, although the heart problem was reversed at the hospital.

The suit claims the following:

- A duty to act existed because EMT–Is Smith and Jones were dispatched and responded to the call for help.
- An act below the standard of care occurred because EMT–Is Smith and Jones performed CPR for too long before taking Mr. Reid to the hospital. The suit also states that the EMT–Is should have ensured that the first oxygen tank was full before using it. The ambulance service's protocols require that oxygen tanks be checked before and after each run. A review of the checklist for that day revealed that EMT–Is Smith and Jones had failed to check their oxygen supply properly. Substandard care also may have occurred because EMT–Is Smith and Jones failed to attempt defibrillation.
- An injury occurred to the patient because Mr. Reid never regained responsiveness, although the emergency department physician could treat the heart problem. The suit claims compensable damages for the cost of nursing home care for the rest of Mr. Reid's expected life and for loss of wages because he is now unable to work as an accountant.
- The failure of EMT–Is Smith and Jones to ensure an adequate oxygen supply during CPR, to provide early defibrillation, and to transport Mr. Reid as soon as possible to the hospital directly caused the brain injuries that prevented the patient from regaining responsiveness.

What Happens When A Lawsuit Is Filed?

COMPLAINT FILING

When people believe they have been injured as a result of malpractice, they seek the advice of an attorney. After investigating the facts and agreeing that the case has merit, the attorney will file a *complaint* for the individual in the appropriate court. The complaint states the reasons for the charge of negligence and asks for damages. The person who files the complaint, along with his or her attorney, is known as the *plaintiff.*

When a complaint is received, the court issues a *subpoena* to the defendant, the individual charged with negligence. The defendant has a certain number of days to file an *answer* to the complaint with the court.

DISCOVERY

The defendant's attorney investigates the facts and prepares an answer to the complaint. Once the answer has been filed, both sides begin a process known as *discovery.* During the discovery phase, each side tries to find out as much as possible about the opposition's case. Both sides will usually have expert witnesses, who will testify in support of either the plaintiff's or the defendant's case.

DEPOSITION

Much of the discovery process consists of the taking of *depositions.* A deposition is a sworn statement, usually taken in an attorney's office. Although the setting for a deposition is informal, the testimony offered is recorded by a court reporter. Anything said in a deposition may ultimately be used in a trial, if one occurs.

The plaintiff's attorney will usually take a deposition from both the plaintiff and the defendant, trying to discover both sides of the story. Both sides will depose each other's expert witnesses. Attorneys for both sides are always present at the deposition and may cross-examine the person being questioned.

SETTLEMENT

After preliminary information is obtained through the discovery process, both sides will reevaluate their case. At this stage, the involved parties, including the malpractice insurance company, usually try to reach some type of agreement, or settlement. This process is known as a settlement conference. The court reporter is not usually present during these meetings.

TRIAL

If an out-of-court settlement is not reached, a trial date is set. A trial is the presentation of both sides of the case in a court and may take place several years after the alleged incident occurred. Usually a jury will decide whether the defendant is guilty; however, sometimes, the case is heard only by a judge. If the judge or jury finds the defendant liable, they will state what damages should be paid to the plaintiff.

APPEAL

The liable party may pay the damages after the trial or file an appeal. An appeal is a complaint filed with a higher-level court stating that something was done improperly during the trial. The side filing the appeal usually believes that an error during the trial wrongly led to a verdict against them. The appellate court will decide whether to let the decision of the lower-level court stand, change the decision, or order a new trial.

● ● ●

The lawsuit process may take years. A lawsuit may not even be filed until years after the event has occurred. The maximum period from the occurrence of an alleged injury to the ultimate filing of a lawsuit is called the *statute of limitations*. This period varies from state to state but is usually no greater than 2 or 3 years.

CONFIDENTIALITY

Confidentiality of the EMT–I–patient relationship is very important. Court cases (case law) have almost uniformly supported the patient's right to confidentiality except under very specific circumstances. All aspects of encounters with patients should be considered absolutely confidential. No information should be shared with anyone, including relatives, friends, and other "trusted" people. This confidential information includes, but is not limited to, patient history, assessment findings, and treatment rendered.

The release of information requires specific written permission from the patient or a legal guardian. Permission is not required for release of certain information under the following circumstances:

- Information is released to other providers with a need to know to provide care (e.g., other on-scene EMS providers, hospital emergency department staff, medical control personnel).
- Information is required by law.
- Information is required for third-party billing.
- Information is released in response to a proper subpoena.

Improper release of information or release of inaccurate information can result in liability. Possible charges include the following:

- *Invasion of privacy*—The release, without legal justification, of information about a patient's private life that might reasonably expose the individual to ridicule, notoriety, or embarrassment is an invasion of privacy. The fact that the information is true is not a defense.
- *Defamation*—Making an untrue statement about someone's character or reputation without legal privilege or consent of the individual is considered defamation.
- *Libel*—**Libel** is the injury of a person's character, name, or reputation by false and malicious writings. An EMT–I can be sued for writing something in a run report that could be considered harmful to a patient. Thus the written record must be accurate and confidential. Avoid slang terms; do not write, "Patient is high as a kite." Instead, write, "Patient appears to be intoxicated." Avoid labels when describing behavior; do not write, "Patient walked like a drunken slob." Instead, write, "Patient's gait was unsteady."
- *Slander*—**Slander** is the utterance of false statements that defame and damage another's reputation. Limit oral reporting to appropriate personnel. Again, avoid slang terms; describe the patient's behavior rather than giving an "editorial" opinion of his or her condition. An EMT–I may be sued for slander if he or she says something false or malicious about a patient that injures a patient's character, name, or reputation.

PATIENT TRANSFER LAWS: EMTALA/COBRA

EMT–Is are often involved in transferring patients between health care facilities (hospital to hospital, hospital to nursing home, etc.). Emergency department physicians and hospitals are now subject to the provisions of the Consolidated Omnibus Budget Reconciliation Act of 1985 (COBRA), which has been renamed the Emergency Medical Treatment and Active Labor Act (EMTALA) (42 USC § 1392dd). EMTALA specifies several responsibilities of the emergency department that must be met before transferring a patient.

Significance of EMTALA for EMT–Intermediates

Because EMT–Is perform many patient transfers, it is essential to be aware of EMTALA's patient transfer provisions. These provisions are meant to prevent unstable emergency patients from being transferred between care facilities solely for economic reasons. The transfer of any patient should satisfy EMTALA requirements. If the patient's condition deteriorates in transit, it may be because he or she was not adequately stabilized before transfer.

In addition, EMTALA provisions apply to hospital-owned ambulance services. Once the patient is within the ambulance, he or she is legally considered to have "come to the hospital." Therefore the EMT–I and the hospital are potentially liable under EMTALA if a patient is not appropriately transported to the hospital (State Operations Manual Transmittal No. 2 [May 1998]: Responsibilities of hospitals in emergency cases; added to CCH website July 16, 1998; http://www.acep.org/policy/hcfa9807.htm).

Provisions of EMTALA

Failure to properly transfer a patient subjects the hospital and physician to significant penalties. These penalties include a fine of up to $50,000 per violation and the loss of the hospital's Medicare privileges. The provisions of EMTALA are as follows:

- All persons who present to an emergency department must undergo a medical screening examination, which may be performed by either a nurse or a physician. The purpose of this examination is to determine whether the patient is suffering from an emergency medical condition or is in active labor.
- All persons who present to an emergency department must be treated alike, regardless of their ability to pay for services.
- Unstable patients (or those in active labor) are not to be transferred unless the patient or representative so requests, or if appropriate treatment facilities are not available at the initial institution.
- Before transfer, all patients must first be stabilized unless the risk of waiting to attempt stabilization outweighs the potential benefit of transferring the patient to a more specialized facility.
- The treatment given at the transferring facility must be documented.

CONSENT ISSUES

Consent means agreement for approval. Responsive and mentally competent adult patients have the right to accept or refuse any examination, care, or transportation offered by the EMT–I. The EMT–I who performs any of these actions without appropriate patient consent risks legal action.

Competent patients may accept or refuse care. Conscious, competent patients have the right to decide what medical care and transportation to accept. The patient must be of legal age, which varies from state to state, and must be able to make a reasoned decision. To make a reasoned or informed decision, the patient must be made aware of and show understanding of the following:

- Nature of the illness or injury
- Treatment recommended
- Risks and dangers of treatment
- Alternative treatment possible and the risks
- Dangers of refusing treatment (including transport)

Remember, a conscious, competent patient can also revoke consent anytime during care and transport.

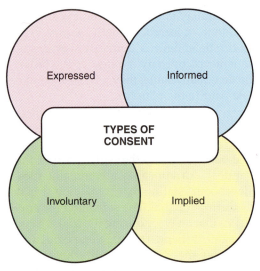

FIGURE 3-5   ▲   Types of consent.

Types of Consent

There are four general types of consent (Figure 3-5):

- *Expressed consent*—**Expressed consent** is given when the patient provides verbal or written consent for the EMT–I to examine, care for, and transport the patient to an appropriate medical facility. Expressed consent may be withdrawn anytime by the patient. Consent also can be expressed by gestures. A patient's presentation of an injury to the EMT–I usually expresses consent.
- *Informed consent*—**Informed consent** means that the patient consents to care only after receiving all the information necessary to understand his or her condition, the risks and benefits of care, and the risks and benefits of refusal of care. Similarly, a patient armed with the same information may make an informed refusal of care. In either case the patient must be given the following information so that he or she may make an informed decision:
  - The EMT–I's assessment of the situation based on his or her field impression
  - What care is being considered and why
  - An explanation of the benefits and risks (including potential side effects) of accepting or refusing examination, care, or transportation

  The degree to which the EMT–I must explain things to a patient varies, especially in an urgent situation. In nonurgent situations, and especially when a competent patient wishes to refuse care, all of the information previously mentioned should be explained to the patient and the event documented carefully.

- *Implied consent*—**Implied consent** means that the EMT–I assumes that a patient who is severely ill or injured would want care if he or she were able to respond. Legally, one is asking the question, "What would a responsible person want done under similar circumstances?" In these instances it is implied that a patient who is severely ill or injured would want care. Implied consent is effective only until the patient no longer requires emergency care or regains competence to make decisions.

- *Involuntary consent*—Treatment is allowed in certain situations granted by authority of law, whether the patient voluntarily agrees or not. Most commonly, involuntary consent involves patients held for mental health evaluation or as directed by law enforcement personnel who have the patient under arrest.

Special Consent Situations

Often consent is straightforward and the EMT–I simply proceeds with treatment. At times, however, special consent situations arise that may be problematic. These include the following:

- *Minors*—Persons younger than 18 years of age are minors in most states and cannot legally consent to or refuse medical care. Emancipated minors have been legally freed of the need for parental consent; most often this occurs if a minor becomes married. Emancipated minors can give their own consent. Emancipation may also include minors who are parents or in the armed services. Some state laws also cover an individual who is living independently and is self-supporting (e.g., a college student not living at home or receiving financial aid from parents).

  Unemancipated minors are not able to give or withhold consent; consent of a parent, legal guardian, or court-appointed custodian is usually required. The emergency doctrine applies to minors when a parent or guardian cannot be contacted. Most states also do not require parental consent for treatment of sexually transmitted diseases, pregnancy, or pregnancy-related conditions in minors.

- *Mentally incompetent adults*—A patient who has been legally determined mentally incompetent cannot give actual consent for care. In these cases consent is usually given by a legal guardian. It may be very difficult to decide competency in the out-of-hospital setting. Often others who are present at the scene, such as caretakers or friends, can be helpful. If the legally responsible party is not available, the patient can receive care under the implied consent (emergency doctrine) standard.

  Ambiguous legal issues may develop when a patient who is temporarily unable to make rational decisions refuses care. If the patient is experiencing alcohol or substance intoxication, emotional (psychiatric) problems, or certain medical conditions, he or she may be temporarily unable to make rational decisions. Usually this patient can be treated under the implied consent standard. It is always better to err on the side of caring for patients who may be mentally incompetent, regardless of cause. Serious medical problems, such as poisoning and hypothermia, may produce symptoms similar to those of intoxication. A patient who may appear to be intoxicated may actually have a serious medical problem that if left untreated may result in serious harm to the patient.

  Some states have laws that permit police officers, mental health professionals, or physicians to place apparently mentally incompetent persons into custody for their own protection. It is essential that EMT–Is be aware of local laws that make provisions for mentally incompetent persons to be treated when no one is available to give consent for them.

- *Prisoners or persons under arrest*—The court or police who have custody may authorize emergency treatment. This care is usually limited to care needed to save life or limb.

Refusal of Care or Transport

Perhaps one of the most stressful situations for the EMT–I is the patient who needs care but refuses it. Responsive adult patients have the absolute right to refuse examination, care, and transportation by EMS providers.

An EMT–I dealing with this situation should attempt to convince the patient to allow care. Often a careful explanation of the possible consequences of refusing care may change the patient's mind. Occasionally a family member, friend, or medical direction physician can help in convincing the patient to consent. In a situation in which a patient refuses care, it is important to do the following:

- Explain the consequences of the refusal of care to the patient and remember that, like consent, refusal should be based on an informed decision.
- Be certain that the patient is competent to understand the consequences of refusal. If you do not believe that the patient is mentally competent to refuse care, consider use of any local laws that permit persons to be taken into custody for their own protection.
- Always respect the patient's beliefs. If all reasonable methods to encourage consent fail, you may not legally be able to provide care. Patients may refuse care for many reasons, including religious beliefs, denial of the severity of their symptoms, or simply because of their priorities. You should not view this as a personal rejection. No matter how frustrating the situation might be, all EMS providers must maintain a high standard of professionalism.
- Accurately and thoroughly document the patient's refusal of care. Obtain a written refusal from the patient on a standardized form (Figure 3-6), and when possible, have the refusal witnessed by a family member, police officer, or firefighter. If a patient refuses to sign the form, record the details in narrative

REFUSAL OF SERVICES

I hereby refuse the emergency medical services and/or transportation offered and advised by the above named service provider and its emergency personnel,_____ hospital, and the emergency medical and nursing personnel from said hospital giving directions to the service provider. I understand that my refusal may jeopardize the health of the patient, and hereby release the above named parties from any and all claims of liability in connection with my refusal.

Signature of Patient or Legally Authorized Representative

Signature of EMT/Field RN

Witness   Date

FIGURE 3-6 ▲ A "release from liability" form.

fashion on the run report. Attempt to ensure patient understanding before allowing the patient to sign a refusal-of-care form.

Obtaining a signed refusal form may not completely clear the EMT–I from responsibility. A patient could later claim that stress, injury, or other factors led to the uninformed signing of the refusal form. Therefore the patient's refusal of care should always be documented on the run report sheet as well. In addition to vital signs and other pertinent physical observations, carefully note the patient's mental condition and establish that the patient appeared mentally competent at the time to decide to refuse care. It is also important to document that the patient received an explanation of the consequences of refusing treatment and understood or acknowledged these consequences.

❗ HELPFUL HINT

- Follow these general rules when dealing with the issue of consent:
  - When in doubt, care for the patient.
  - Obtain police assistance, particularly if a patient may be emotionally disturbed or is making an obviously irrational decision because of an altered level of awareness.
  - If available, use the EMS communications system to obtain physician direction. Some EMS systems require that an EMT–I contact medical direction before accepting a patient's refusal of care. Sometimes the physician can talk the patient into accepting needed care.

EMS-Initiated Transport Refusal

Under certain circumstances, use of the EMS system may not be the best or most appropriate choice of resources. Some EMS systems have a provider-initiated transport refusal protocol under which the EMT–I evaluates the patient and refers him or her to alternative sources of care. This decision must involve medical direction and varies, depending on the particular circum-

stances. As usual, thorough documentation is essential. Similar principles and requirements apply if, for any reason, the level of care during transportation must be downgraded.

▶ Some EMS systems will allow patients to refuse transport to the hospital after on-scene evaluation. In one large study, paramedics routinely provided a verbal explanation of the risks of refusing transport, as well as written instructions. When interviewed later, however, only 55% of patients recalled receiving written instructions and only 22% remembered being verbally advised of the risks. Over one fourth of the patients did not, in retrospect, fully understand their condition or the circumstances surrounding the original 9-1-1 call. A significant number (18%) stated that they would not take an ambulance if the same incident were to recur. Most people accessed health care after refusing ambulance transport; 6% were admitted to the hospital. These findings suggest that patients' abilities to make an informed decision are limited during an acute emergency.

Data from Schmidt TA et al: Do patients refusing transport remember descriptions of risks after initial advanced life support assessment? *Acad Emerg Med* 5:796-801, 1998.

Legal Complications Related to Consent

Various legal complications may arise that relate to consent issues. It is necessary to be aware of the following complications beforehand and prevent them from arising. Some of these "tricks and traps" may lead to charges that if accepted by a jury may result in punitive damages in a lawsuit.

- *Abandonment*—Patient **abandonment** means stopping care when it is still needed and desired by the patient and without ensuring that appropriate care continues to be provided by another qualified provider. It may occur in the field or when a patient is delivered to the emergency department without appropriate EMS-to-hospital communication.

- *False imprisonment*—**False imprisonment** is the intentional and unjustifiable detention of a person against his or her will. Depending on the locality, it may be either a civil or a criminal violation. When this charge is made, the case often involves a patient with psychiatric problems, a patient who has abused alcohol or drugs, or a suicidal patient. Depending on state or local laws, the patient's circumstances may justify the detention. Expressed consent to the detention should be obtained if possible. If the EMT–I is unable to obtain consent and detention is medically necessary, he or she must be certain to document carefully the need for as well as the method of detention. Local law enforcement officials may provide assistance under these circumstances.

- *Assault*—**Assault** involves threatening, attempting, or causing fear of offensive physical contact with a patient or other individual (e.g., threatening to restrain a patient unless he or she quiets down). Again, depending on the locality, it may be either a civil or a criminal violation.

- *Battery*—**Battery** is the unlawful touching of another person without consent (e.g., drawing a patient's blood without permission). Depending on the locality, it may be either a civil or a criminal violation.

  Charges against EMT–Is for assault and/or battery are extremely unusual. When they are made, it is usually because the patient claims that he or she did not give consent for a procedure, such as spinal immobilization or starting an IV line. The best way to avoid accusations of assault and/or battery is to obtain expressed consent from the patient (Figure 3-7).

- *Use of force*—Despite potential risks of assault, battery, or false-imprisonment charges, the EMT–Intermediate is justified in the use of force under certain circumstances. Typically, force may become necessary in order to provide appropriate care for unruly or violent patients. Note that people may be uncooperative because of a medical condition (e.g., hypoxia, hypoglycemia), just as they may be unruly because of intoxication or mental disturbances.

  The use of patient restraints must be done according to strict system protocols. At times, involvement of law enforcement personnel is helpful. Generally, use only the force considered "reasonable" to prevent harm to the patient or others. Force must never be used as a punishment to a patient.

- *Transportation of patients*—Legally, most experts believe that once a patient has consented to a certain level of care, such as by an EMT–I, this level must be maintained during the remainder of the patient encounter, including during transportation. Changes in the level of personnel attending the patient to a lower level of care may result in both medical and legal complications. In addition, emergency vehi-

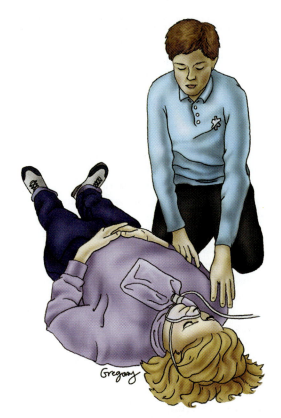

The best way to avoid accusations of assault and/or battery is to obtain expressed consent from the patient.

FIGURE 3-7 ▲ **Obtaining consent.**

cles must be operated in conformity with all applicable laws, regulations, and policies. The legal expectation is that the vehicle is operated in a manner that safeguards the patient, the crew, and the public.

RESUSCITATION ISSUES

Withholding or Stopping Resuscitation

It is well accepted that certain patients should not receive resuscitation attempts or that after a period, attempts should be stopped. To avoid potential allegations of patient abandonment and negligence, always follow a specific procedure established by local protocols. These protocols should clearly delineate the role of medical direction.

Advance Directives

Advance directives involve any of a number of written documents indicating a patient's preference for future medical treatment. These show what the patient would want or not want done under certain circumstances (e.g., terminal illness, cardiac arrest) if he or she were unable to express his or her wishes. The status of these directives depends on both state laws and local protocols.

Advance directives include the following:

- *Living will, durable power of attorney*—Certain patients do not wish to be resuscitated if they suffer a cardiac arrest. Often this desire is expressed as a written document called a living will, health care proxy, durable power of attorney for health care, or advance directive. The wording of such documents varies widely, but the intention is that the patient wishes no measures taken to resuscitate him or her in case of cardiac arrest.
- *Do-not-resuscitate (DNR) orders*—A **do-not-resuscitate (DNR) order** may be in the form of a legal document but more commonly is simply written in a letter or on a prescription pad by the patient's personal physician (Figure 3-8).

On arrival at a scene, the EMT–I may be presented with either a living will or a DNR order by a friend or family member. The legality of accepting living wills or DNR orders varies from state to state. Some states require that the EMT–I comply with the provisions in a living will or DNR order. Other states have not addressed the issue at all. It is important for the EMT–I to be familiar with the specific local legislation, policies, and protocols concerning DNR orders.

Although a lawsuit conceivably could be brought against an EMT–I for attempting to resuscitate a patient with a living will or DNR order, family members at the scene may not be in total agreement as to the best course of action. The safest course of action is to proceed with care unless it is certain that the patient's or physician's intentions are clearly and legibly documented.

If the rare instance arises in which someone physically obstructs patient care, police officers may be helpful in managing the situation. All pertinent facts must be documented concisely on the written run report.

STREET WISE

Legal authority for advance requests was granted, at least in part, by the Patient Self-Determination Act of 1990. It mandates that medical direction must establish and implement policies for dealing with advance directives. The policy should specify EMT–I care for the patient with an advance directive. It must also provide for reasonable measures of comfort to the patient and emotional support to family and loved ones.

STREET WISE

Usually CPR should be started on all patients who are without a pulse and respirations unless there is evidence of decomposition, decapitation, incineration, or massive injury incompatible with life. Do not stop CPR once it is begun unless patient care is transferred to a higher-level provider (such as the hospital emergency department) or unless instructed to do so by medical direction.

Potential Organ Donation

If a critically ill patient is identified as a potential organ donor, establish communication with medical direction as soon as possible. Based on medical direction, provide emergency care that will help maintain viable organs.

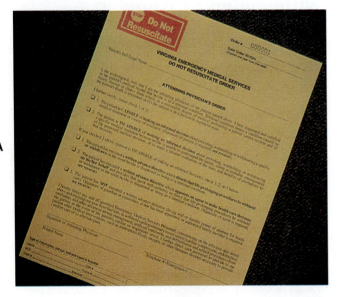

A

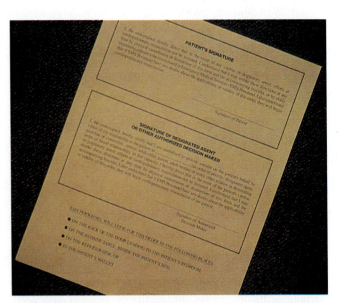

B

FIGURE 3-8 ▲ A sample do-not-resuscitate form. **A,** Front. **B,** Back.

Death in the Field

In some states EMS providers may pronounce patients dead in the field without transporting the body to a hospital. This must be done in cooperation with the local medical examiner (coroner), in conjunction with applicable laws, and according to strict protocols. Consult medical direction for guidance.

SPECIAL SITUATIONS

Situations involving child abuse, crime, motor vehicle accidents, or a physician already at the scene require special, well-defined EMS system protocols that EMT–Is must follow. The following are suggestions for dealing with these protocols.

Crime and Accident Scenes

The EMT–I's first responsibility is to maintain his or her own safety. Never enter the scene of a known violent crime until it has been secured by law enforcement personnel. Police investigation of crimes or motor vehicle accidents can be seriously hindered by emergency personnel who inadvertently disturb or destroy evidence at the scene. The role of the EMT–I is to provide good patient care and, at the same time, preserve evidence. Virtually everything at the scene may be of potential use to investigators.

At crime and accident scenes it is essential that unauthorized persons be kept off the premises. Do not touch, kick, or move anything (including vehicles or debris) unless it is absolutely necessary to provide patient care

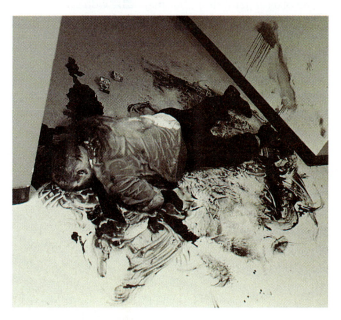

FIGURE 3-9 ▲ It is important to preserve a crime scene as much as possible when delivering patient care. (From Prehospital Trauma Life Support Committee of the National Association of Emergency Medical Technicians, in cooperation with the Committee on Trauma of the American College of Surgeons: *PHTLS: basic and advanced prehospital trauma life support,* ed 3, St Louis, 1994, Mosby.)

(Figure 3-9). If it becomes necessary to move vehicles at the scene of a motor vehicle accident, mark their original position on the pavement with a large piece of chalk or crayon. Both patient care and preservation of evidence can be accomplished, but patient care takes priority.

Make mental notes of what is observed—the position of a weapon, overturned furniture, pooled blood, or the position and location of a victim. It may be helpful to investigators if a diagram is drawn in the run report. Relay any findings to the investigating officer as soon as possible after the necessary patient care is provided.

Child Abuse

Child abuse involves the physical, sexual, or emotional maltreatment of a child. The EMT–I may be the only medical care provider who sees an abused child in both the home and the clinical context; therefore the EMT–I may be the only provider who can allow the legal system to come to the aid of such a child. It is extremely important that hospital personnel are alerted when child abuse is suspected. The EMT–I may be legally obligated to report suspected child abuse—follow all local laws and protocols. In addition, document and report any suspicious findings to the appropriate authorities. An EMT–I could be subjected to fines, imprisonment, and loss of state certification to practice for failing to report suspected child abuse.

All states have laws that protect health care professionals from liability for reporting, in good faith, suspected child abuse. It is important to note that the law does not require proof of abuse, only suspicion. On the other hand, do not speculate on the run report; state only factual information.

Having a specific protocol within an EMS system for dealing with this difficult situation is very helpful. Most important, do not delay care of the sick or injured child to pursue any suspicion of child abuse. Handle these matters after transporting the child to the hospital.

Physicians at the Scene of Patient Encounters

Occasionally a person at the scene may claim to be a physician. Usually these individuals are bona fide physicians who truly are interested in providing assistance. In rare instances EMT–Is may be confronted with a citizen who claims to be a physician but who actually is not. It is usually impossible to tell whether the person is really a physician simply because he or she claims to be one. Thus the EMT–I must follow an established protocol when dealing with a physician at the scene.

Legally, the initial responsibility for patient care rests with the on-line medical direction physician. If an on-scene physician can document his or her licensure and ability to deal with the situation, some medical direction facilities will allow him or her to take over, provided that the physician is willing to accompany the patient to the hospital. Therefore the EMT–I should contact medical direction when dealing with an on-scene physician. A physician at the scene should not be allowed to assume control of patient care against the advice of the on-line medical direction physician. If the individual continues to interfere with patient care, immediately seek police assistance.

Some EMS systems do not have the ability to contact on-line medical direction. Those systems should have written protocols for dealing with on-scene physicians. These protocols should require that if a licensed bystander physician wishes to take control, he or she *must* adhere to the following:

- Ride in the ambulance with the patient to the hospital.
- Sign all necessary care forms, including the run report.

The EMT–I must record the name, place of practice, and medical license number of the physician on the run sheet.

DOCUMENTATION

The standard rule of documentation is that "if it is not written, it was not done." Despite claims of remembering things, assume that even the best person's memory is fallible. This is particularly important, since claims may not be filed until years after an event, especially if a young child is involved. In some states the statute of limitations runs until the child achieves the legal age of majority ("legal adulthood").

Records should be maintained for a period of time that meets or exceeds any applicable statute of limitations. Many EMS systems routinely keep microfilm records for several years beyond the statute period.

Case example—In a recent court case, excellent documentation showed that despite the fact that the patient later deteriorated, she was in no acute distress at the time of the initial EMS visit. Thus there was no duty to transport her to the hospital or advise the mother of a life-threatening condition that did not exist at that time, especially when the mother stated that she did not wish the patient transported to a hospital (*Ball v. Hamilton County Emergency Medical Services*, No. 03A01-9804-CV-00139 [Tenn App, 1999]).

CASE HISTORY FOLLOW-UP ■ ■ ■

EMT–I Reynolds reports to work a few minutes early Tuesday morning after the conference, hoping to talk with EMT–I Thomas about his gossip.

"Hi, Tony. Can I have a word with you?" she asks.

"Sure, Stacy. What's up? Great conference, huh?"

"Yeah, fine, Tony. Listen, I unintentionally overheard you saying to a group of people that Tom's HIV positive."

"I didn't say that. I said I heard that he's positive," Thomas answers.

Reynolds reminds him, "Do you realize that even if he really has tested positive for HIV, it's illegal, criminally and civilly, to disclose that information? And that if he hasn't tested positive, you've committed slander?"

"Hey, we were just talking. I really wasn't thinking about it all that much. I just heard someone say it once. That's all. No big deal, right?"

EMT–I Reynolds returns, "I think it's a big deal, and I'd rather not hear anything like that said again. I'm going to mention the incident to Tom, just to let him know what's been said. I think he'll be okay to let it drop, but maybe he won't. Is everything OK on the vehicle?"

SUMMARY

Important points to remember from this chapter include the following:

- The EMT–I, like any health care professional, is subject to charges of professional negligence. Proper care of patients, adherence to established guidelines, and maintaining complete, legible documentation are key factors in avoiding legal troubles.
- Legally, the EMT–I is held to a certain standard of care. For a negligence action to be successful, it must be proved that four elements exist: a duty to act, negligent care that fell below the standard of care, damages, and the proximate cause of the damages being the EMT–I's negligence. Patient abandonment may be considered a form of negligence.
- Good Samaritan laws exist in most states, and they may or may not apply to the EMT–I. To a large extent, these laws have not been challenged in court. Thus the EMT–I is best served by assuming that Good Samaritan legislation will not necessarily provide protection against a lawsuit.
- It is advisable for individual EMT–Is to consider carrying some type of malpractice insurance, since not all jurisdictions are covered by Good Samaritan laws.
- Numerous provisions contained in the Consolidated Omnibus Budget Reconciliation Act of 1985, which was later renamed the Emergency Medical Treatment and Active Labor Act (EMTALA/COBRA), affect the transfer of patients from hospitals. These provisions were enacted to prevent the transfer of an unstable patient for purely financial reasons. Most regulations apply directly to physicians and hospitals, but the EMT–I should be aware of the major provisions of this legislation, especially regarding hospital-owned ambulance services. Good communication between all levels of emergency providers should prevent problems related to EMTALA.
- Most patients will give their consent to receive care, whether expressed or implied. A few individuals will refuse care. Keeping accurate records of any patient who refuses care may help avoid later charges of patient abandonment or negligence. When in doubt, it is generally better to attempt care of a patient rather than not to provide care. The patient should be provided, whenever possible, with adequate information to determine the benefits and risks of his or her decision.
- Encounters with patients who have living wills or physician-generated do-not-resuscitate (DNR) orders may still require the EMT–I to attempt resuscitation during cardiac arrest unless very specific requirements are met. The EMT–I should be aware of how the laws of his or her state deal with these issues.
- Crime and accident scenes require that the EMT–I pay special attention to the preservation of evidence. Police should always be present before an EMT–I attempts to enter the scene of a violent crime.
- Child abuse laws may require that all health care providers report suspected abuse to local authorities.
- Physicians who are bystanders at the scene of an emergency may be helpful or may be a hindrance to emergency care. It is ultimately the decision of the on-line medical direction physician as to whether or not the on-scene physician may assume the patient's care. Written protocols to deal with the situation are helpful. Police assistance should be enlisted if prompt cooperation is not offered by the on-scene physician.

Overview of Human Systems

4

Key Terms

Anatomical Position

Anatomy

Autonomic Nervous System

Cardiac Conduction System

Cardiac Tamponade

Cartilage

Cells

Central Nervous System

Circulatory System

Connective Tissue

Endocrine System

Gastrointestinal System

Homeostasis

Immune System

Integumentary System

Joints

Lymphatic System

Muscular System

Nervous System

Organelles

Oxygenation

Parasympathetic Nervous System

Pathophysiology

■ ■ ■ CASE HISTORY

EMT–I Jackson is precepting an EMT–I student who has just completed the anatomy and physiology portion of his class, when her unit is dispatched for a trauma call at an after-hours club. Jackson arrives on the scene in 8 minutes and is met by a police officer, who tells her that a 20-year-old has been stabbed. The suspect is in custody.

The patient is lying unconscious in a pool of blood as Jackson approaches him. Her initial assessment reveals five stab wounds: two in the chest, one in the abdomen, one in the left buttock, and one in the right thigh.

The crew ventilates the patient with 100% oxygen and a bag-valve-mask to assist his breathing and then starts two intravenous (IV) lines, per protocol. EMT–I Jackson calls medical direction to report:

"We have a male, approximately 20 years of age, with five stab wounds. He is responding to painful stimuli only. We placed an OP airway, and we're assisting ventilations with 100% O_2. We loaded the patient and began transporting immediately, starting two IVs, LR wide open en route.

"Vital signs are pulse 142 and weak; respirations 28 and labored with central cyanosis; BP is 92/68.

"The stab wounds are on the right anterior axillary line at T4, left midaxillary line at T6, left epigastric region, left midbuttock, and right anterior midthigh. The right thigh is approximately 5 cm larger than the left, and there's no response to painful stimulation of the left leg.

"We've applied a porous dressing over the open chest wound and controlled open bleeding with dry, sterile dressings over all of the other wounds. We have an ETA to your facility of approximately 12 minutes. Do you have any further orders?"

LEARNING OBJECTIVES

CHAPTER GOAL
Upon completion of this chapter, the EMT-Intermediate will understand basic anatomy and physiology and how it relates to the foundations of medicine.

Cognitive Objectives
As an EMT-Intermediate you should be able to do the following:
- Define anatomy, physiology, and pathophysiology.
- Name the levels of organization of the body from simplest to most complex, and explain each.

- Define homeostasis.
- State the anatomical terms for the parts of the body.
- Use proper terminology to describe the location of body parts with respect to one another.
- Name the body cavities and the major organs within each.
- Describe the anatomical planes.
- Identify areas of the abdomen and underlying organs.
- Define each of the cellular transport mechanisms, and give an example of the role of each in the body: diffusion, osmosis, facilitated diffusion, and active transport.
- Define the terms *metabolism*, *anabolism*, and *catabolism*.
- Describe how glucose is converted to energy during cellular respiration.
- Explain how glucose, amino acids, and fats are used for energy production.
- Describe the general characteristics of each of the four major categories of tissues.
- Name the three major layers of the skin and the tissue of which each is made.
- Describe the functions of the skeleton.
- Explain how bones are classified, and give an example of each type.
- Explain how joints are classified, and give an example of each type.
- Describe the structure and function of muscles.
- List the three types of muscles.
- State the functions of the nervous system.
- Name the divisions of the nervous system.
- Explain the structure of neurons.
- Describe the types of nerves.
- Describe the role of polarization, depolarization, and repolarization in nerve impulse transmission.
- Identify the components of the central nervous system.
- State the function of the meninges and cerebrospinal fluid.
- Identify the divisions of the autonomic nervous system, and define their functions.
- Explain how a negative feedback mechanism regulates hormonal secretion.
- State the functions of hormones.
- State the function of the hormones of the pancreas.
- Explain how insulin and glucagon work together.
- State the functions of epinephrine and norepinephrine, and explain their relationship to the sympathetic division of the autonomic nervous system.
- Describe the characteristics of blood and its composition.
- Explain the function of red blood cells, white blood cells, and platelets.
- State the importance of blood clotting.
- Describe the location of the heart.
- State the function of the pericardium.
- Name the chambers of the heart and the major vessels.
- Name the valves of the heart, and explain their functions.
- Describe coronary circulation, and explain its purpose.
- Describe the cardiac cycle.
- Explain how heart sounds are created.
- Name the parts of the cardiac conduction pathway.
- Explain the relationship between stroke volume, heart rate, and cardiac output.

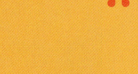

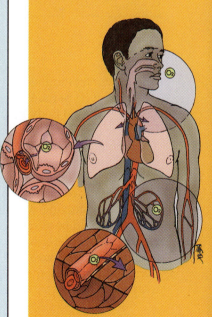

INTRODUCTION

Anatomy refers to the study of the structure of an organism and its parts. **Physiology** is the study of an organism's normal body functions, whereas **pathophysiology** is the study of disease mechanisms (Figure 4-1). Being familiar with the structure and function of the various body systems allows for better assessment of a patient's signs and symptoms. For example, if a person were to hit the breastbone (sternum) hard against the steering wheel in a motor vehicle crash, damage would be suspected not only to the bones but also to the underlying structures—the heart, lungs, and major blood vessels. Also, an understanding of normal physiology makes pathophysiology far easier to appreciate.

ORGANIZATION OF THE BODY
The Body's Building Blocks

The human body consists of increasingly sophisticated levels of organization (Figure 4-2). **Cells** are the basic building blocks of all life. In less-advanced forms, such as bacteria, the entire organism consists of a single cell. The human body contains approximately 100 trillion cells, all specialized for particular functions. Red blood cells transport oxygen, for example, and are very different from bone cells, which are designed to support weight. Cells contain various components, known as **organelles,** which carry out the processes necessary for life within each cell. An example of an organelle is the nucleus, or nerve center, of the cell (Figure 4-3).

Tissue is composed of groups of similar cells working together to accomplish a common function. There are four types of tissue: epithelial tissues, connective tissue, muscle tissue, and nerve tissue. *Organs* are composed of different types of tissue. The heart, for example, contains muscle, nerves, and connective tissue. The skin, which also is composed of many different types of tissue, is the largest organ in the body.

An *organ system,* or system, is a group of organs that have a common function and purpose. Although often found in close anatomical proximity, the organs of a system may be scattered throughout the body. Organ systems include skeletal, muscular, circulatory, respiratory,

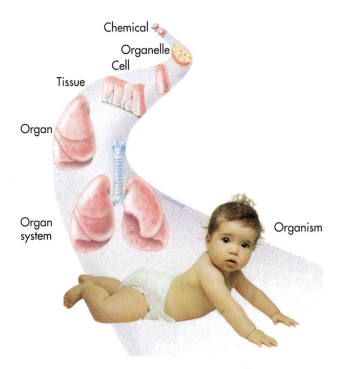

FIGURE 4-2 ▲ The levels of organization in the human body are organelle, cell, tissue, organ, organ system, and organism. (Christine Oleksyk [art], Pat Watson [photo] from Seeley R: *Essentials of anatomy and physiology,* ed 2, St Louis, 1996, Mosby.)

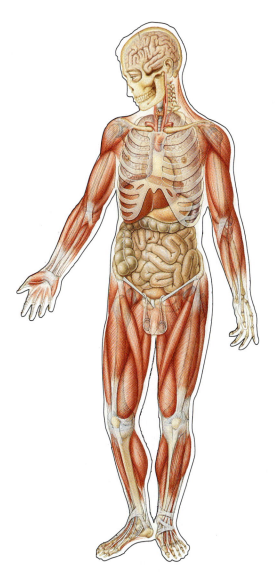

FIGURE 4-1 ▲ Anatomy refers to the study of the structure of an organism; physiology refers to the function of these structures. (From Thibodeau GA, Patton KT: *Anatomy and physiology,* ed 3, St Louis, 1996, Mosby.)

nervous, gastrointestinal, urinary, reproductive, immune, endocrine, lymphatic, integumentary, and special sensory (Figure 4-4).

Homeostasis

Homeostasis refers to the normal state of balance between all of the body's systems. Just like the system of "checks and balances" in a government, the body has internal mechanisms that regulate its functions. Some of these stimulate; others suppress—together, the "status quo" is maintained. Of course, illness or injury interferes with homeostasis. Think of the body systems as being interdependent on each other. When one dysfunctions, all the others are bound to be affected because of a disruption of homeostasis.

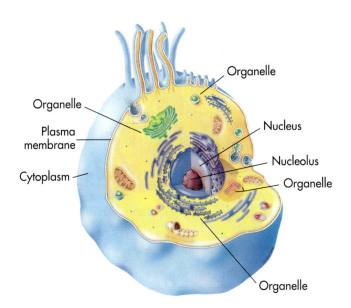

FIGURE 4-3 ▲ A typical cell in the human body. (Christine Oleksyk from Seeley R: *Essentials of anatomy and physiology,* ed 2, St Louis, 1996, Mosby.)

Organ Systems of the Body

SYSTEM	MAJOR COMPONENTS	FUNCTIONS
Integumentary	Skin, hair, nails, and sweat glands	Protects, regulates temperature, prevents water loss, and produces vitamin D precursors
Skeletal	Bones, associated cartilage, and joints	Protects, supports, and allows body movement, produces blood cells, and stores minerals
Muscular	Muscles attached to the skeleton	Produces body movement, maintains posture, and produces body heat
Nervous	Brain, spinal cord, nerves, and sensory receptors	A major regulatory system: detects sensation, controls movements, controls physiological and intellectual functions
Endocrine	Endocrine glads such as the pituitary, thyroid, and adrenal glands	A major regulatory system: participates in the regulation of metabolism, production, and many other functions
Circulatory	Heart, blood vessels, and blood	Transports nutrients, waste products, gases, and hormones throughout the body; plays a role in the immune response and the regulation of body temperature
Lymphatic	Lymph vessels, lymph nodes, and other lymph	Removes foreign substances, from the body and lymph, combats disease, maintains tissue fluid balance and absorbs fats
Respiratory	Lungs and respiratory passages	Exchanges gases (oxygen and carbon dioxide) between the blood and the air and helps regulate blood pH
Gastrointestinal	Mouth, esophagus, stomach, intestines, and accessory structures	Performs the mechanical and chemical processes of digestion, absorption of nutrients, and elimination of wastes
Urinary	Kidneys, urinary bladder, and the ducts that carry urine	Removes waste products from the circulatory system; helps regulate blood pH, ion balance, and water balance
Reproductive	Gonads, accessory structures, and genitals of males and females	Performs the processes of reproduction and controls sexual function and behaviors

FIGURE 4-4 ▲ Body systems. (Joan M. Beck from Thibodeau GA, Patton KT: *Anatomy and physiology,* ed 3, St Louis, 1996, Mosby.)

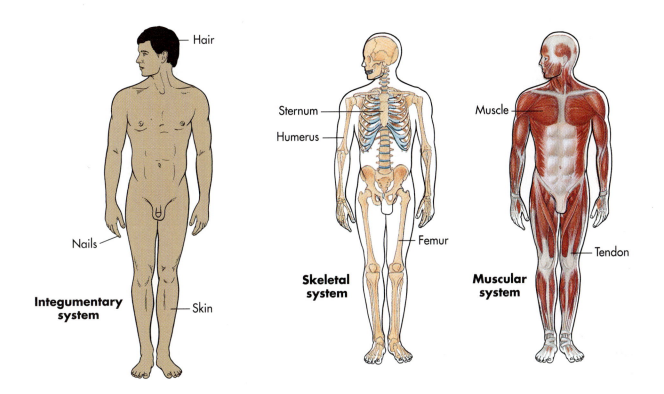

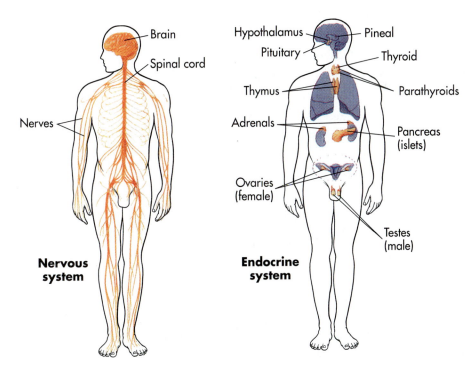

FIGURE 4-4, cont'd ▲ Body systems. (Joan M. Beck from Thibodeau GA, Patton KT: *Anatomy and physiology,* ed 3, St Louis, 1996, Mosby.)

Continued

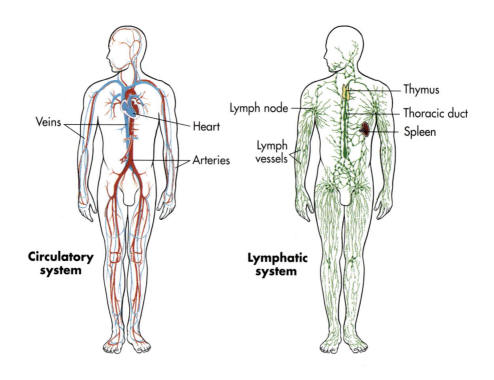

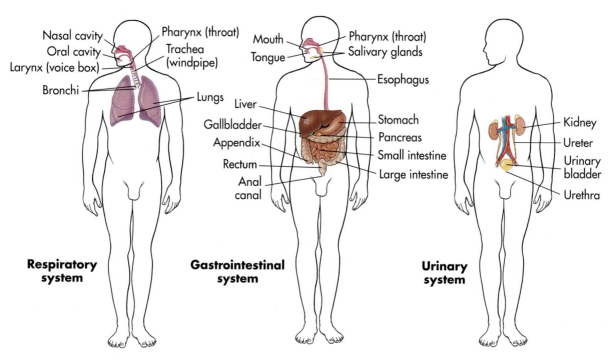

FIGURE 4-4, cont'd ▲ Body systems. (Joan M. Beck from Thibodeau GA, Patton KT: *Anatomy and physiology,* ed 3, St Louis, 1996, Mosby.)

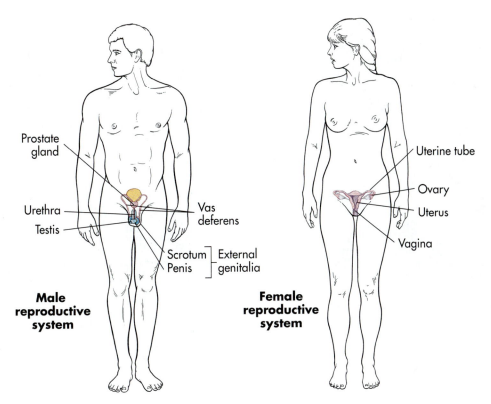

FIGURE 4-4, cont'd ▲ Body systems. (Joan M. Beck from Thibodeau GA, Patton KT: *Anatomy and physiology,* ed 3, St Louis, 1996, Mosby.)

Anatomical Terms

Just as medical terminology helps us understand the medical language, a number of terms have been devised to designate specific directions for the human body (Figure 4-5). Using standard directional terms in both written and verbal reports helps explain where the patient's symptoms and injuries are located. These terms refer to the body in the **anatomical position**—upright with eyes directed straight ahead, arms hanging by the side, feet together, and the palms of the hands facing forward (Figure 4-6).

* *Superior* means above or in a higher position. For example, the brain is superior to the heart, and the heart is superior to the intestine. The opposite term, *inferior,* means below or lower. For example, the neck is inferior to the mouth.
* *Ventral* and *anterior* mean the same thing in humans: toward the front or "belly" surface of the body. *Dorsal* and *posterior* both mean toward the back of the body.
* *Cranial* means in or near the head. *Caudal* means near the lower end of the torso (i.e., near the base of the spinal column).
* The *midline* of the body divides it into equal right and left halves. *Lateral,* as opposite to *medial,* means farther away from the midline, or toward the side.

* *Proximal* means nearest the origin of a structure. *Distal* means farthest from that point. For example, in the upper extremity (arm), the arm above the elbow is proximal to the forearm below. In the lower extremity (leg), the lower leg below the knee is distal to the thigh.

See Table 4-1 for positions, definitions, and examples of body directions.

Body Planes

For ease of description, the body is divided into imaginary planes (Figure 4-7 and Table 4-2). Understanding these terms will help in the description and documentation of patient injuries. It will also allow for better communication over the radio to the receiving hospital.

* The *frontal plane* divides the body vertically into a front and back portion. It passes through the body longitudinally from head to toe. The front portion of the body is referred to as the *ventral* or *anterior* aspect, and the back as the *dorsal* or *posterior* aspect.
* If one were to cut the body vertically into right and left portions, the imaginary cut would be referred to as the *sagittal plane.* The sagittal plane does not divide the body equally. A cut down the midline, or center, of the body separating it verti-

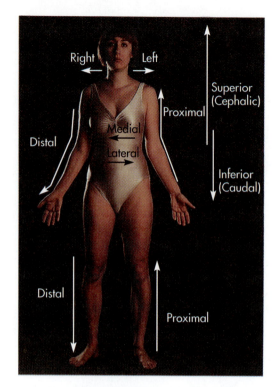

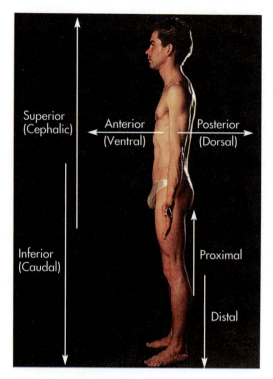

FIGURE 4-5   ▲   Directional terms for the human body. (From Seeley R: *Anatomy and physiology,* ed 3, St Louis, 1995, Mosby.)

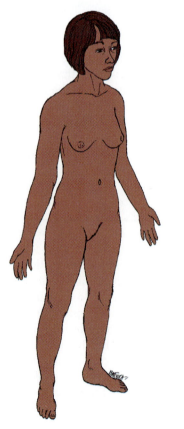

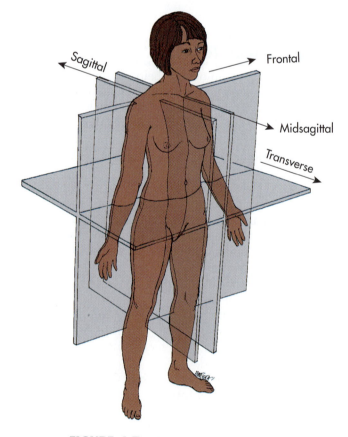

FIGURE 4-6   ▲   The anatomical position.

FIGURE 4-7   ▲   Planes of the body.

TABLE 4-1

Body Directions

POSITION	DEFINITION	EXAMPLES
Superior	Above, higher	The head is superior to the neck.
Inferior	Below, lower	The chest is inferior to the neck.
Anterior (ventral)	Toward the front	The nose is on the anterior, or ventral, surface of the head.
Posterior (dorsal)	Toward the back	The calf is on the posterior, or dorsal, surface of the leg.
Cranial	In or near the head	The brain is in the cranial cavity.
Caudal	Near the sacral region of the spinal column	The buttocks, the muscles on which a person sits, are located at the caudal end of the body.
Medial	Vertical line that passes near the midline of the body	The nose is medial to the eyes.
Lateral	Toward the side, away from the midline	The ears are lateral to the nose.
Proximal	Nearest the origin of the structure	The part of the thumb where it joins the hand is its proximal region.
Distal	Farthest from the origin of a structure	The tip of the thumb is the distal regions, compared with the part of the thumb where it joins the hand.

TABLE 4-2

Planes of the Body

POSITION	DEFINITION
Frontal	Vertical line dividing the body into a front and back portion
Sagittal	Vertical line dividing the body into right and left portions
Midsagittal	Vertical line dividing the body into right and left halves; can be thought of as the midline
Transverse	Horizontal line dividing the body into an upper and lower portion

cally into equal right and left halves is called the *midsagittal plane.*
- The *transverse plane* runs horizontally through the body perpendicular to the frontal and sagittal plane. It divides the body into an upper (superior) part and a lower (inferior) part. There could be many cross sections, each of which would be on a transverse plane.

Body Postures

Postures of the body describe the position in which the patient's body is found (Figure 4-8):
- A person in the *erect* position is standing in an upright position.
- A person in the *supine* position is lying on the dorsal surface of the body, or on the back, face up.
- A person in the *prone* position is lying on the ventral surface of the body, or on the front of the body (stomach), face down.
- A person lying in the *lateral recumbent* position is lying on the right or left side.

Body Cavities

Body cavities are hollow areas within the body that contain organs and systems (Figure 4-9):
- The hollow portion of the skull, called the *cranial cavity,* has a domed top and a base composed of several bones. The cranial cavity houses the brain and is continuous with the *spinal cavity,* also known as the *spinal* or *vertebral canal.* The spinal cavity travels through the backbone, or vertebral column, and contains the spinal cord. Organs within the cranial and spinal cavities are part of the nervous and special sensory systems.
- The *thoracic cavity (thorax),* between the base of the neck and the diaphragm, is formed by the roughly circular boundary of the rib cage. The major structures within the thoracic cavity belong to the cardiovascular and respiratory systems: the heart, major blood vessels, and lungs. The space between the lungs is known as the *mediastinum,* which contains the heart, trachea (windpipe), mainstem bronchi, part of the esophagus, and large blood vessels.
- The *abdominal cavity* is a single large cavity that extends from the diaphragm to the pelvic bones. It is bordered by the spine and the abdominal wall. The abdomen can be divided into quadrants by crossing the umbilicus (navel) with imaginary perpendicular

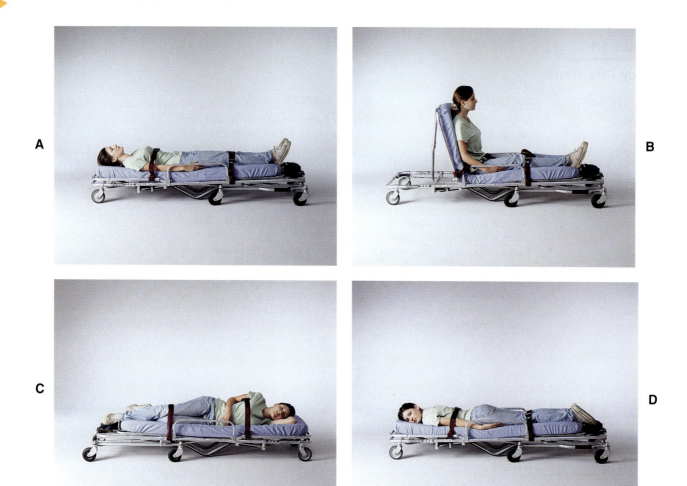

FIGURE 4-8 ▲ **A,** Patient in the supine position. **B,** Patient in the sitting position. **C,** Patient in the left lateral recumbent position. **D,** Patient in the prone position.

FIGURE 4-9 ▲ Body cavities as shown from the front (anterior) and side (lateral). (Joan M. Beck from Thibodeau GA, Patton KT: *Structure and function of the body,* ed 3, St Louis, 1992, Mosby.)

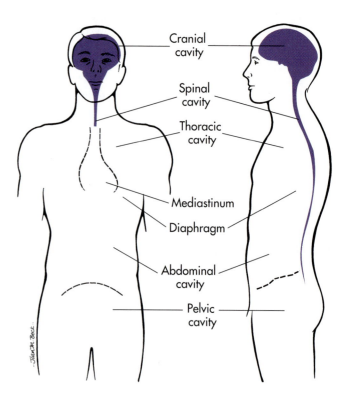

Cranial cavity

Spinal cavity

Thoracic cavity

Mediastinum

Diaphragm

Abdominal cavity

Pelvic cavity

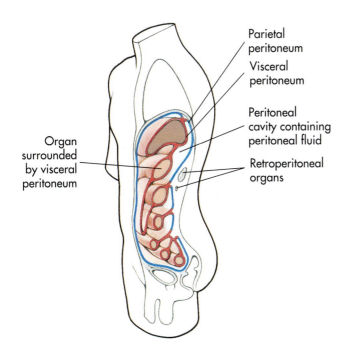

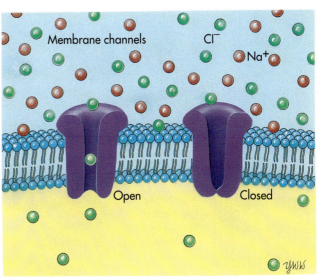

FIGURE 4-10 ▲ Lateral (side) view of the peritoneum in the human body. (Nadine Sokol from Seeley R: *Anatomy and physiology,* ed 3, St Louis, 1995, Mosby.)

FIGURE 4-11 ▲ Semipermeable cell membranes allow only certain nutrients to enter or leave the cell. (Christine Oleksyk from Thibodeau GA and Patton KT: *Anatomy and physiology,* ed 3, St Louis, 1996, Mosby.)

lines. It is important for the EMT–I to know the four quadrants and the underlying anatomy of the abdomen when assessing patients.

The abdominal cavity contains the organs of digestion and excretion, which constitute the gastrointestinal and urinary systems. The digestive organs are surrounded by the *peritoneum,* which is a double-layered smooth membrane of connective tissue. The kidneys and major blood vessels of the abdominal cavity are located in an area posterior to the digestive organs known as the *retroperitoneal space* (Figure 4-10).

• The *pelvic cavity,* making up the lower portion of the abdominal cavity, contains the organs of the gastrointestinal, reproductive, and urinary systems. The cavity is bounded by the *pelvic girdle* (pelvic bones): the *ilium, ischium, pubis, sacrum,* and *coccyx.* The strong pelvic bones provide protection for internal organs.

CELLS

Cellular Transport

Every healthy cell has an outer membrane that separates the cell contents from the fluid that surrounds it. This membrane must allow nutrients, water, and electrolytes to enter the cell and allow waste products to leave. The membrane also acts as a gatekeeper, preventing valuable proteins and electrolytes from leaving the cell while prohibiting undesirable substances from entering. The term *semipermeable* (Figure 4-11) is used to classify the cell membrane because it allows some substances to enter or

leave while restricting the passage of others. *Permeability* is the rate at which substances pass through a membrane. Smaller molecules, such as water, diffuse more easily than larger molecules, such as proteins. Other mechanisms that regulate which substances pass through the cell membrane include ion pumps (e.g., sodium pump), active transport, and diffusion.

The size and charge of molecules determine permeability. Water (H_2O) is the only substance that passes freely back and forth across the cell membrane. It is a very small molecule made up of two hydrogen atoms (H) and one oxygen ion (O). Small molecules cross the membrane much faster than larger molecules. Other substances may be too large to pass through the membrane. During the process of digestion, these substances are broken down into smaller molecules, which are allowed passage. Electrolytes, which are by their nature small, may have difficulty passing through the membrane because of their electrical charge.

Active transport processes require energy; passive transport processes do not. Several physical processes are responsible for the exchange of substances across the semipermeable membrane. These transport processes fall into two categories: passive and active. *Passive transport* processes do not require expenditure of energy, whereas *active transport* processes do. The energy required for active transport is obtained from a chemical substance called *adenosine triphosphate (ATP).* ATP is produced in the *mitochondria* (located inside each cell) from nutrients and is capable of releasing energy that enables the cell to work. Active transport breaks down ATP and

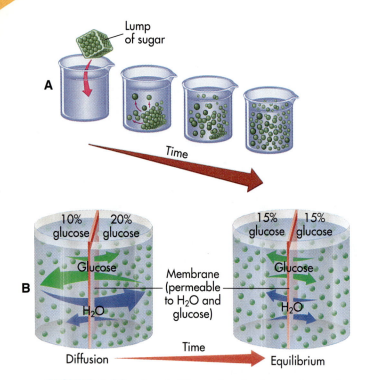

FIGURE 4-12 ▲ **A,** The molecules from a lump of sugar spread from an area of high sugar concentration in the water to areas of lower concentration, until the sugar is distributed equally throughout the container. **B,** The "membrane" allows glucose and water to pass through, creating equilibrium throughout the container. (Rolin Graphics from Thibodeau GA and Patton KT: *Anatomy and physiology,* ed 3, St Louis, 1996, Mosby.)

utilizes the resulting energy. (See later discussion on the production of ATP and cellular respiration.)

Both diffusion and facilitated diffusion are passive transport (non–energy-requiring) processes:

• *Diffusion*—Diffusion is the *continual* movement of particles from an area of higher concentration to one of lower concentration until the substances scatter themselves evenly throughout an available space (Figure 4-12). These particles are called *solutes.* When the concentration of a solute is greater on one side of a cell membrane than on the other, the solute will diffuse across the cell membrane from the area of higher concentration to the area of lower concentration. Because of the body's homeostatic mechanism, the natural tendency is to keep a balance of water and electrolytes on each side of the cell membrane. Substances that move across cell membranes by simple diffusion include oxygen, nitrogen, carbon dioxide, and electrolytes. Electrolytes, such as potassium and sodium, pass through specific channels in the membrane.

• *Facilitated diffusion*—Many molecules and ions need help diffusing across the cell membrane. In facilitated diffusion, a specialized "transport protein" with a binding site specific to one substance binds with a molecule of that substance and moves across the cell membrane. Facilitated diffusion transports molecules of a substance across a cell membrane that would otherwise be impermeable to the substance (Figure 4-13). The most important molecules moved by facilitated diffusion are glucose and the amino acids.

Despite the help of a transport protein, facilitated diffusion is still considered passive transport because the solute is moving down its concentration gradient (i.e., the molecule or ion is moving from an area of higher concentration to an area of lower concentration). Facilitated diffusion speeds the transport of a solute by providing a specific path through the cell membrane but does not alter the direction of transport.

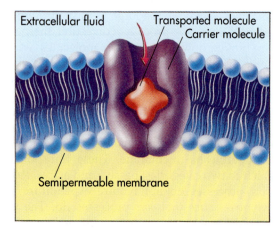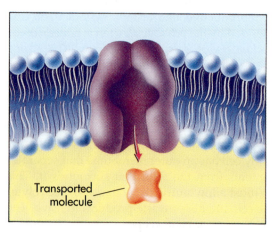

FIGURE 4-13 ▲ **A** and **B,** Carrier molecules act as facilitators to the diffusion process, escorting the transported molecule through the membrane into the cell. (Barbara Cousins from Sanders M: *Mosby's paramedic textbook,* St Louis, 1994, Mosby.)

- *Osmosis*—Osmosis is the movement of water across a semipermeable membrane (Figure 4-14). Water moves freely across the cellular membrane. Solutes such as electrolytes may or may not be able to passively pass across the cell membrane. When the concentration of a solute is higher on one side of a membrane than on the other, water will cross the membrane until the solute's concentration is equalized. The higher concentration of solute pulls fluid (water) from areas of lower concentration. For example, if there is more sodium inside a cell than outside it, water will osmose (move) into the cell. In osmosis, water (the *solvent*) moves across a semipermeable membrane from an area of lesser solute concentration to an area of greater solute concentration.

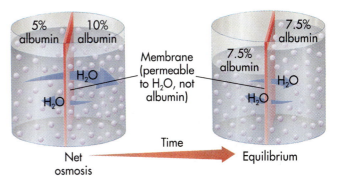

FIGURE 4-14 ▲ Osmosis is the movement of water through a semipermeable membrane. The higher concentration of solute (albumin) pulls water from areas of lower concentration, equalizing the concentration on both sides of the membrane. (David Phillip/Visuals Unlimited from Seeley R: *Essentials of anatomy and physiology,* ed 2, St Louis, 1996, Mosby.)

▶ SOLUTIONS AND OSMOTIC PRESSURE

Solutions are described by their *tonicity* (the number of particles of solute per unit volume):

- An *isotonic solution* has an osmotic pressure equal to normal body fluid, meaning that solutions are equal on both sides of the cell membrane. Examples of isotonic intravenous (IV) solutions are 0.9% normal saline and lactated Ringer's solution.

- A *hypotonic solution* has an osmotic pressure less than that of normal body fluids. When the solute concentration of a given solution is less on one side of the cell membrane than on the other, water will be drawn into the solution with a higher solute concentration. An example of a hypotonic IV solution is 5% dextrose in water (D_5W).

- A *hypertonic solution* has an osmotic pressure greater than that of normal body fluids. When the concentration of a given solute is greater on one side of the cell membrane than on the other, it draws water into the solution until the solute-to-solution ratio is equal on both sides (even though the volumes differ) (Figure 4-15). Examples of hypertonic IV solutions include 3% hypertonic saline, high-molecular-weight dextran solutions, albumin, and hetastarch.

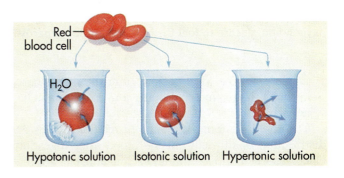

FIGURE 4-15 ▲ The effects of tonicity on a red blood cell. **A,** In a hypotonic solution, the cell swells and bursts. **B,** In an isotonic solution, the cell appears in its normal shape. **C,** In a hypertonic solution the cell shrinks. (Molly Babick/John Daugherty from Thibodeau GA and Patton KT: *Anatomy and physiology,* ed 3, St Louis, 1996, Mosby.)

moved by active transport. These include electrolytes, calcium, several different sugars, and most of the amino acids.

Cellular Metabolism and Respiration

Metabolism is the combination of all chemical processes that take place in the body resulting in growth, generation of energy, elimination of wastes, and other bodily functions. There are two steps:

- *Anabolism*—The "constructive," or building, phase, in which smaller molecules are converted to larger ones.

Active transport moves solutes against their concentration gradients, across the cell membrane from the side where they are less concentrated to the side where they are more concentrated. This transport is uphill; it reverses the tendency for substances to diffuse down their concentration gradients and therefore requires work. To pump a molecule across a membrane against its gradient, the cell must expend its own metabolic energy. Active transport is faster than diffusion. Many molecules that move via diffusion are also

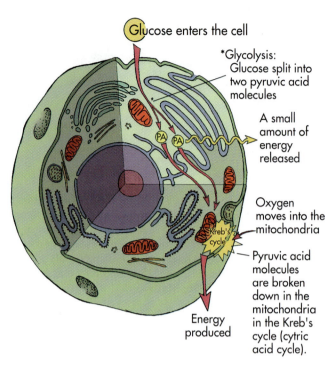

FIGURE 4-16 ▲ Aerobic metabolism occurs with oxygen and glucose to fuel the cell, and produce energy.

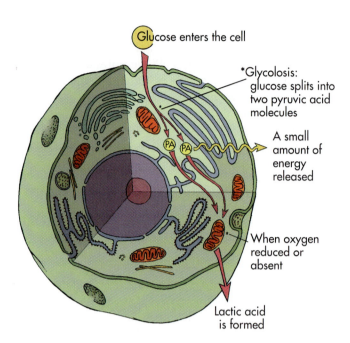

FIGURE 4-17 ▲ Anaerobic metabolism occurs without oxygen, and produces lactic acid.

- *Catabolism*—The "destructive," or breakdown, phase, in which larger molecules are converted to smaller molecules.

Usually, these terms are used in relationship to the distribution of nutrients in the blood after digestion. Once absorbed, glucose, amino acids, and fats are metabolized by the body to produce energy. Some glucose is stored in the liver as *glycogen,* which is broken down (catabolized) when necessary to raise the blood sugar (glucose) level. Through various biochemical processes, amino acids and fats are eventually used in the Krebs cycle (see below) to produce energy. Amino acids may also be converted to glucose.

Glucose is also used to generate energy via the process of *cellular respiration.* This pathway is totally different from the respiration we may think of regarding the lungs. Cellular respiration is a biochemical process resulting in the production of energy in the form of *adenosine triphosphate (ATP)* molecules. These form the "energy food" for all of the body's functions. Cellular respiration takes place in the *mitochondrion,* an intracellular organelle. Glucose is metabolized there to ATP, carbon dioxide (CO_2), and H_2O via the *Krebs cycle* and *oxidative phosphorylation.* The details of these chemical processes are not important at this point. Remember, however, that together they yield nearly 40 molecules of energy-rich ATP for each molecule of glucose metabolized, as well as CO_2 and H_2O. Another intracellular process, *glycolysis,* also contributes to ATP stores, but the majority of ATP comes from mitochondrial respiration.

These processes normally occur in the presence of oxygen and are termed normal *aerobic respiration.* When oxygen levels are lower, the above reactions do not proceed normally and the cell reverts to *anaerobic metabolism.* Less energy is produced than during aerobic respiration, and lactate acid waste products are produced (Figures 4-16 and 4-17).

TISSUES

As mentioned earlier, tissue is composed of groups of similar cells working together to accomplish a common function. There are four types of tissue (Figure 4-18):

- *Epithelial tissue* covers all external surfaces of the body and lines the hollow organs, such as the intestines, bronchi, and glands. It provides a protective barrier and aids in the absorption of food (in the intestines) and secretion of various body substances (in the sweat glands).
- **Connective tissue** binds other types of tissue together. Types of connective tissue include blood, adipose (fat) tissue, fibrous and elastic connective tissue, bone, and cartilage.
- *Muscle tissue* contracts, leading to movement of body structures. The three types of muscle tissue are skeletal muscle, cardiac muscle, and smooth muscle.
- *Nerve tissue* includes the brain, the spinal cord, and all the nerves that pass from these to various parts of the body. Nerves generate and transmit impulses throughout the body, controlling all bodily processes.

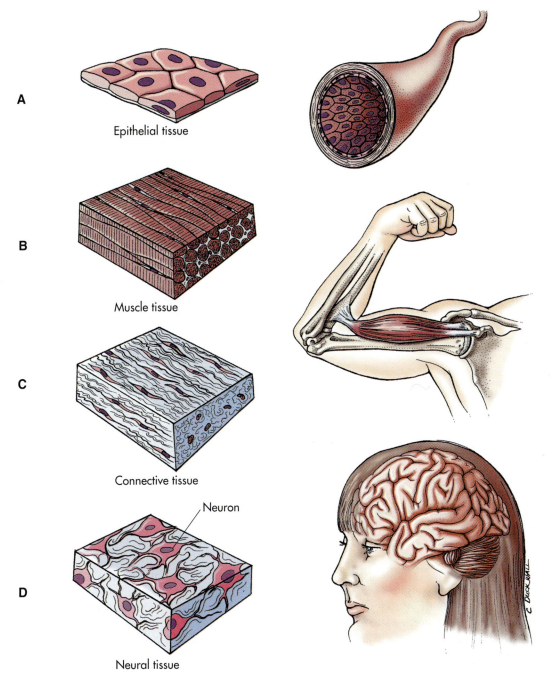

A
Epithelial tissue

B
Muscle tissue

C
Connective tissue

Neuron

D
Neural tissue

FIGURE 4-18 ▲ The four basic tissue types. **A,** Epithelial. **B,** Muscle. **C,** Connective. **D,** Neural. (From American College of Emergency Physicians; Pons PT, Cason D, chief editors: *Paramedic field care: a complaint-based approach,* St Louis, 1997, Mosby for ACEP.)

INTEGUMENTARY SYSTEM

The **integumentary system** refers to the body's external surface and includes the skin, nails, hair, sweat, and oil glands. The major functions of the integumentary system are temperature regulation, defense against disease-causing organisms, and maintenance of fluid balance.

Layers of the Integument

There are three major layers of the integument. The outermost layer is the *epidermis.* It contains no blood vessels but is rich in hair (in many locations), openings from sweat and oil glands, and nerves. Below the epidermis is the *dermis,* a thick layer that contains connective tissue, hair follicles, glands (which extend upward into the

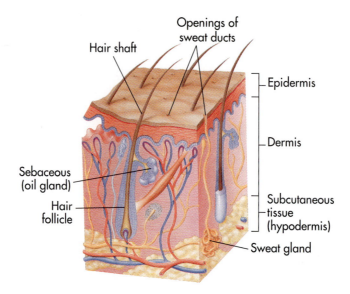

FIGURE 4-19 ▲ The integumentary system in the human body. (Rolin Graphics from Thibodeau GA, Patton KT: *Anatomy and physiology,* ed 3, St Louis, 1996, Mosby.)

epidermis), and nerve endings for temperature, touch, pain, and pressure.

Collectively, the epidermis and dermis are often called the **skin.** Below the epidermis and dermis is the *hypodermis,* usually called *subcutaneous tissue.* It attaches the skin to the underlying bone or muscle and contains much of the body's fat stores. Most nerves and blood vessels run through the dermis, extending only small branches into the epidermis (Figure 4-19).

SKELETAL SYSTEM

The **skeletal system,** composed of 206 bones, provides a framework for the human body (Figure 4-20). Bones protect internal organs and, with muscles, assist in movement. Bones also serve as a storage site for minerals, particularly calcium, and have a role in the formation of certain blood cells. Many bones have an internal cavity that contains a substance known as bone marrow. It is within the bone marrow that most of the body's red blood cells (erythrocytes) and white blood cells (leukocytes) are manufactured (Figure 4-21).

Classification of Bones

Bones are classified by their shape and size (Figure 4-22):
* *Long bones*—The relatively cylindrical bones of the arms and legs, such as the femur (thigh bone).
* *Short bones*—Smaller bones that make up the hands (carpals) and feet (tarsals).
* *Flat bones*—Regardless of size, bones that are relatively flat in three dimensions, such as the ribs.
* *Irregular bones*—Bones that have no well-defined geometrical shape, such as the vertebra.

Components of the Skeleton

The skeletal system is divided into two major components: the axial skeleton and the appendicular skeleton. The *axial skeleton* consists of the entire torso. The *appendicular skeleton* consists of the extremities (the arms and legs), as well as the *girdles,* or bony belts that attach the limbs to the body. The *shoulder girdle* attaches the upper extremity, and the *pelvic girdle* attaches the lower extremity.

AXIAL SKELETON

At the top of the axial skeleton is the *skull,* which consists of the *cranium* and the *face.* Several individual bones fuse together to make up the cranium and the face. The brain is contained within the cranium. The brain connects with the *spinal cord* through a large opening at the base of the skull called the *foramen magnum.*

The *spine,* which serves as the primary support structure of the body, consists of 33 bones called *vertebrae* and is divided into five sections. There are seven *cervical vertebrae* in the neck. The first vertebra directly beneath the skull (C1) is called the *atlas* and supports the head. The next vertebra (C2) is called the *axis.* The axis is the point at which the head turns. The remainder of the cervical vertebrae are simply numbered (C3 through C7) and have no special names. There are 12 *thoracic vertebrae* in the posterior chest, five *lumbar vertebrae* in the lower back, and five *sacral vertebrae.* The sacral vertebrae are fused into a platelike bone, the *sacrum,* which forms the posterior portion of the pelvic bone. Four *coccygeal vertebrae* are fused into the *coccyx,* or tailbone which is attached to the lower portion of the sacrum.

Attached to each thoracic vertebra is a pair of *ribs.* These 12 pairs of ribs form the *rib cage.* The upper 10 pairs

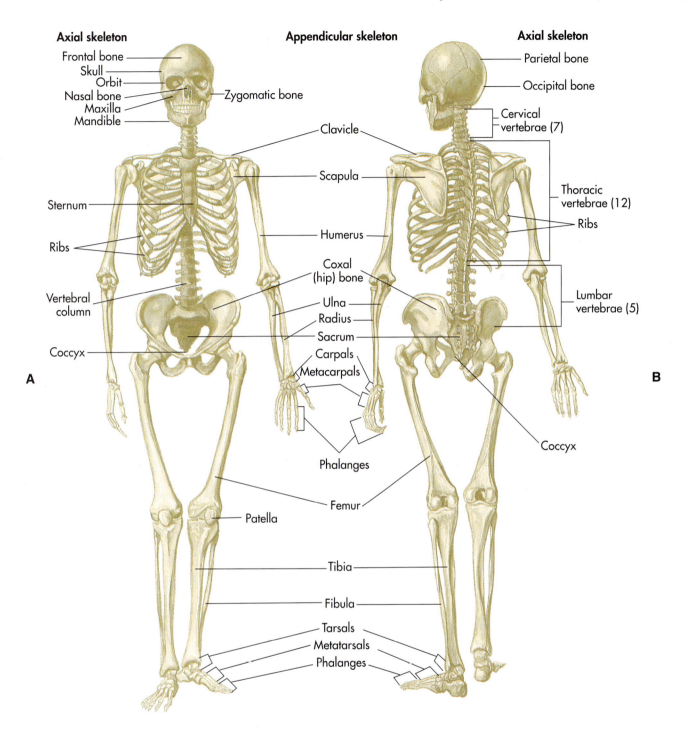

Axial skeleton

Frontal bone
Skull
Orbit
Nasal bone
Maxilla
Mandible
Zygomatic bone

Sternum
Ribs
Vertebral column
Coccyx

A

Appendicular skeleton

Clavicle
Scapula
Humerus
Coxal (hip) bone
Ulna
Radius
Sacrum
Carpals
Metacarpals
Phalanges
Femur
Patella
Tibia
Fibula
Tarsals
Metatarsals
Phalanges

Axial skeleton

Parietal bone
Occipital bone
Cervical vertebrae (7)
Thoracic vertebrae (12)
Ribs
Lumbar vertebrae (5)
Coccyx

B

FIGURE 4-20 ▲ The human skeleton. **A,** Anterior view. **B,** Posterior view. (David J. Mascaro from Thibodeau GA, Patton KT: *Anatomy and physiology,* ed 3, St Louis, 1996, Mosby.)

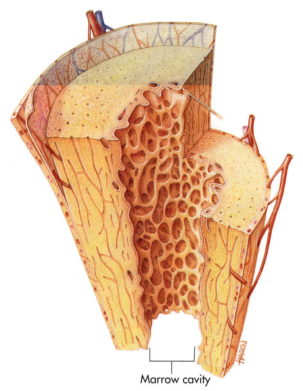

Marrow cavity

FIGURE 4-21 ▲   Bone marrow cavity. (John V. Hagen from Seeley R: *Essentials of anatomy and physiology,* ed 2, St Louis, 1996, Mosby.)

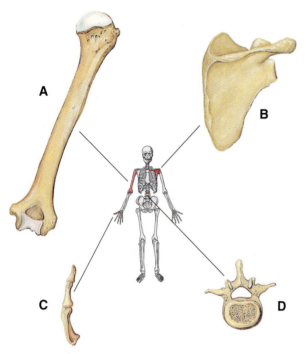

FIGURE 4-22 ▲   Types of bones. **A,** Long bone (humerus). **B,** Flat bone (scapula). **C,** Short bone (phalanx). **D,** Irregular bone (vertebra). (From Thibodeau GA, Patton KT: *Anatomy and physiology,* ed 4, St Louis, 1999, Mosby.)

attach directly to the *sternum,* or breastbone. The remaining two pair of ribs, called *floating ribs,* are held in place by cartilage.

APPENDICULAR SKELETON

The shoulder girdle attaches the upper extremity to the body and consists of the scapula (shoulder blade) posteriorly and the *clavicle* (collarbone) anteriorly. The clavicle is attached to the sternum by ligaments. The upper extremities consist of the arms, forearms, wrists, hands, and fingers.

Although the entire extremity is often called the arm, the *arm* in a purely anatomical sense actually extends only from the shoulder to the elbow. The *humerus* is the bone of the arm. The *forearm* is that portion of the upper extremity from the elbow to the wrist. Two bones make up the forearm: the *radius* and the *ulna.* The radius is the bone on the thumb side. A group of irregularly shaped bones, called the *carpals,* make up the wrist. Beyond the wrist are the *metacarpal bones,* which form the hand. Each finger is composed of a series of small bones called *phalanges.*

The pelvic girdle attaches the lower extremity to the body. It consists of a ring of bones formed by the sacrum posteriorly and the *coxae,* or *pelvic bones,* on each side. Each pelvic bone consists of three fused bones: the *ilium,* the *ischium,* and the *pubis.* The superior portion of the ilium is called the *iliac crest.* The ilium joins the sacrum to form the *sacroiliac joint.*

The lower extremities include the hips, thighs, knees, legs, ankles, feet, and toes. The *thigh* is that part of the lower extremity from the hip to the knee. The *femur* is the bone of the thigh and is the longest and strongest bone in the body. The femur articulates with the pelvic girdle at the *acetabulum;* this region is often called the *hip joint.* The *knee* is the point of articulation of the femur and the bones of the leg. It is covered with a piece of cartilage called the *patella* (kneecap).

The leg runs from the knee to the ankle and contains two bones: the *tibia* and the *fibula.* The tibia is longer and thicker than the fibula. The anterior portion of the tibia, covered only by skin, is commonly called the shin. A number of irregular bones, the *tarsals,* make up the ankle. Beyond the ankle are the *metatarsals,* which make up the foot. The toe bones, like the finger bones of the hand, are called *phalanges.*

Types of Joints

Joints occur where two or more bones meet or articulate (Figure 4-23). Movement at joints is aided by cartilage. **Cartilage** is made up of plates of shiny connective tissue that enable bones to move freely. *Ligaments* are tough white bands of tissue that bind joints together, connecting bone and cartilage (Figure 4-24).

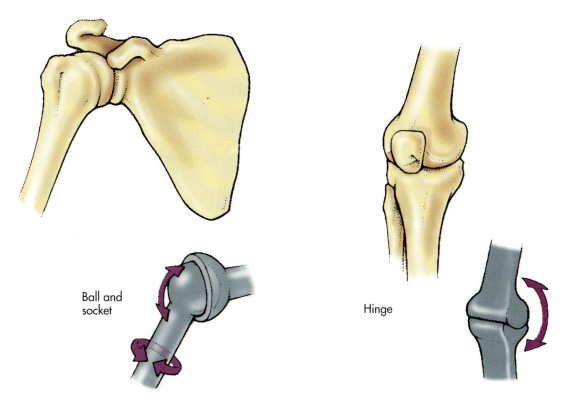

FIGURE 4-23 ▲ Examples of joints in the human body. (Duckwall Productions.)

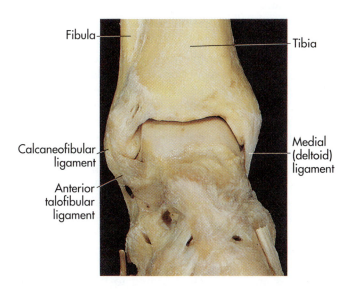

FIGURE 4-24 ▲ Ligaments bind bones and cartilage together at a joint. (Courtesy Vidic B, Suarez FR: from Thibodeau GA, Patton KT: *Anatomy and physiology*, ed 3, St Louis, 1996, Mosby.)

Tendons connect muscles to bones. There are three types of joints:

- *Immovable joints*—Joints that normally allow no motion between bones; typical immovable joints are those connecting the bones of the skull.

- *Slightly movable joints*—Joints that normally allow only a small amount of movement between bones; examples include the vertebrae and the pubic bones.
- *Freely movable joints*—Joints that allow a wide variety of movement between bones; most of the major joints of the body (e.g., shoulder, elbow, wrist, hip, knees, ankles) are freely movable.

MUSCULAR SYSTEM

The **muscular system** is composed of contractile tissues (muscle) responsible for movement. Muscles are termed either *voluntary* (under conscious control) or *involuntary* (not under conscious control). Muscle is categorized into three distinct types: skeletal, smooth, and cardiac (Figure 4-25):

- *Skeletal muscle* is voluntary and is under conscious control. There are more than 350 skeletal muscles in the body.
- *Smooth muscle* is involuntary and is not under conscious control. Examples of smooth muscle include the muscle that dilates the pupils of the eyes and the muscle of the intestinal wall. Smooth muscle works automatically; humans cannot consciously influence the contraction of involuntary muscles.
- *Cardiac* (heart) *muscle* is a special type of involuntary muscle. This type of muscle has the ability to gener-

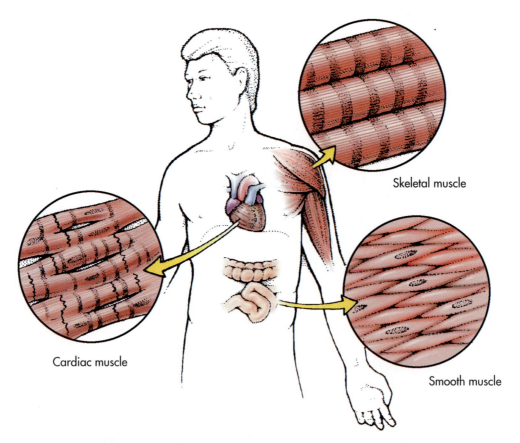

FIGURE 4-25 ▲ Examples of the three types of muscle in the human body: skeletal muscle, smooth muscle, and cardiac muscle. (Duckwall Productions.)

ate its own stimulus to contract if necessary. This property, called *intrinsic automaticity,* allows the heart to continue to pump in extreme circumstances, such as when its external nerve supply is damaged.

NERVOUS SYSTEM

The **nervous system** is an extensive network of cells that conducts information that controls and coordinates all the functions of the body. The nervous system controls two types of activities: *voluntary* (under conscious control) and *involuntary* (not under conscious control). The nervous system is divided into two parts: the central nervous system and the peripheral nervous system.

Nerve Cells, Types, and Impulses

Nerve cells are called *neurons.* Each neuron consists of three major parts (Figure 4-26):

- *Cell body*—The main part of the neuron containing the nucleus and surrounding tissues, excluding any projections such as axons or dendrites.
- *Dendrites*—A branching process that extends from the cell body of a neuron. Each neuron usually possesses several dendrites, which receive impulses conducted to the cell body.

- *Axons*—A cylinder-like extension of a neuron that carries impulses away from the cell body.

A *synapse* is the region surrounding the point of contact between two neurons or between a neuron and its *effector organ* (e.g., gland, muscle). Nerve impulses are transmitted across the synapse by the flow of chemicals, known as *neurotransmitters.* When the impulse reaches the terminal point of one neuron, the neurotransmitter is released and diffuses across the gap between cells. There it binds with a *receptor,* triggering electrical changes that either inhibit or continue the transmission of the impulse. Other substances then inactivate the neurotransmitter; collectively, these are called *inactivators* (Figure 4-27).

Nerves are classified according to the direction in which they conduct impulses. *Sensory nerves* transmit nerve impulses toward the spinal cord and the brain. *Motor nerves* transmit impulses from the brain and the spinal cord to the muscles and glands.

A *nerve impulse* is essentially the movement of sodium, potassium, and calcium ions in and out of cells, one at a time, that causes sequential changes in the electrical charge inside each cell. The resting state is called the *polarized state.* Here the concentration of potassium is higher inside the cell than outside, whereas the reverse is true for sodium and calcium. When the nerve

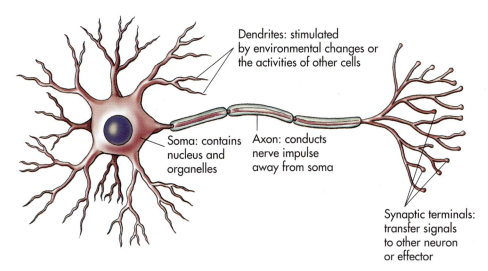

FIGURE 4-26 ▲ The neuron is the basic structural component of the nervous system. Some neurons reach several feet in length and are visible with the naked eye. (From American College of Emergency Physicians; Pons PT, Cason D, chief editors: *Paramedic field care: a complaint-based approach*, St Louis, 1997, Mosby for ACEP.)

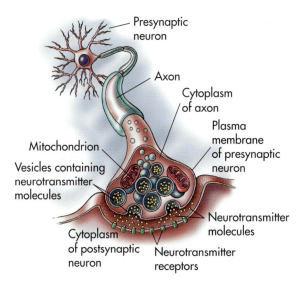

FIGURE 4-27 ▲ A synapse is formed in the space between two nerve cells, or between a nerve cell and a gland cell, muscle cell, or sensory receptor. The function of the synapse is to transmit the action potential from one cell to the other. (From American College of Emergency Physicians; Pons PT, Cason D, chief editors: *Paramedic field care: a complaint-based approach*, St Louis, 1997, Mosby for ACEP.)

impulse "hits" the next cell, it causes it to *depolarize*; sodium and calcium move inward, and potassium moves into the fluid surrounding the cell.

Depolarization occurs quickly and results in the interior of the cell becoming less negatively charged (i.e., more positive) than during the resting state. As the impulse signal moves to the next cell in line, the depolarized cell

returns back to its resting (polarized) state. Sodium and calcium flow back out, and potassium moves into the cell. This final stage is called *repolarization*. Imagine a "wave" of depolarization moving from cell to cell as the nerve impulse propagates (passes) (Figure 4-28).

Central Nervous System

The **central nervous system** consists of the brain and spinal cord. The brain, which lies in the cranial cavity, is divided into four major parts: the cerebrum, the diencephalon, the brainstem, and the cerebellum.

The *cerebrum* is the top portion of the brain and consists of the left and right hemispheres. Thinking, sensation, and voluntary movement are controlled by the cerebrum. The cerebrum is further subdivided into four lobes per hemisphere, each with different major functions as follows:

- *Frontal lobe*—Regulates higher-level thinking, such as impulse control, voluntary motor action, and personality traits.
- *Parietal lobe*—The major site for most sensory information except smell, hearing, and vision.
- *Occipital lobe*—Processing of visual information.
- *Temporal lobe*—Hearing and memory.

The *diencephalon* is the part of the brain between the brainstem and the cerebrum. Major structures include the *thalamus, hypothalamus,* and *pituitary gland.* The pituitary gland produces several proteins that control the endocrine system (see Endocrine System), as does the hypothalamus. Both the thalamus and hypothalamus are also integral in modulating pain and temperature (Figure 4-29).

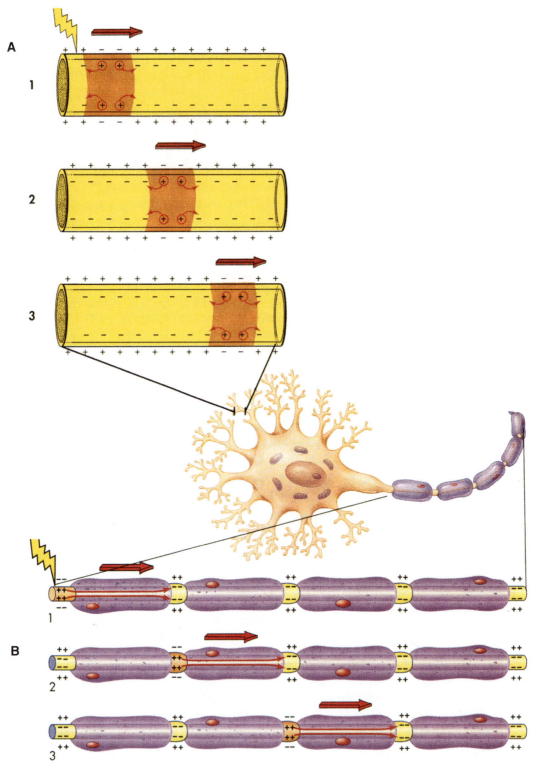

FIGURE 4-28 ▲ Conduction of nerve impulses. **A,** In an unmyelinated fiber, a nerve impulse (action potential) is a self-propagating wave of electrical disturbance. **B,** In a myelinated fiber, the action potential "jumps" around the insulating myelin in a rapid type of conduction (saltatory conduction). (From Thibodeau GA, Patton KT: *Structure and function of the body,* ed 10, St Louis, 1997, Mosby.)

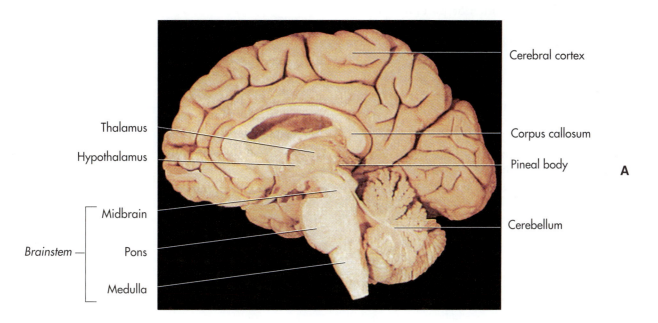

A

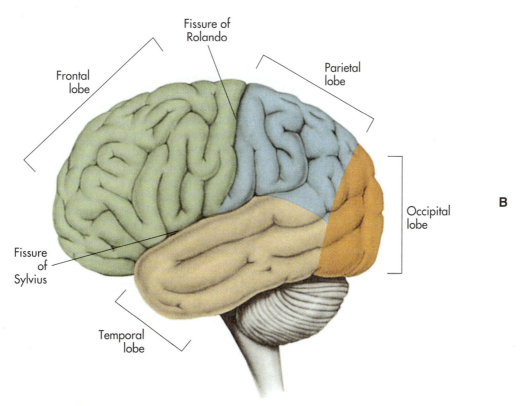

B

FIGURE 4-29 A, Section of preserved brain. **B**, Lobes of the cerebrum. (From Thibodeau GA, Patton KT: *Structure and function of the body,* ed 10, St Louis, 1997, Mosby.)

The *brainstem* consists of the medulla, pons, and midbrain. It connects the spinal cord to the remainder of the brain. This is the most inferior portion of the brain and contains important centers that control involuntary respiration, heart, and blood vessel function.

- The *midbrain* is the smallest region of the brainstem and is the point of exit of many important cranial nerves.
- The *pons* lies below the midbrain and above the medulla. It contains numerous nerve fibers, including those for sleep and respiration.
- The *medulla* connects inferiorly with the spinal cord. As well as serving as a conduction pathway for many important nerve tracts, it also coordinates heart rate, blood vessel diameter, breathing, swallowing, vomiting, and coughing.

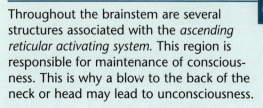

CLINICAL NOTES

Throughout the brainstem are several structures associated with the *ascending reticular activating system.* This region is responsible for maintenance of consciousness. This is why a blow to the back of the neck or head may lead to unconsciousness.

The cerebellum is located behind and below the cerebrum. Its primary function is to control the body's coordination.

CLINICAL NOTES

Abnormalities in the normal flow of cerebrospinal fluid (CSF) throughout the ventricular system may result in *hydrocephalus* (excess fluid accumulation in the brain with associated swelling). Sometimes the swelling leads to increases in pressure within the closed cranial cavity, a condition known as *increased intracranial pressure.*

SPINAL CORD

The spinal cord is a cylindrical cord of nervous tissue extending from the brainstem. It runs the length of the vertebral canal from the foramen magnum, a large opening at the base of the skull, to the level of the second lumbar vertebra. Below this level the cord divides into individual nerves known as *cauda equina.* The spinal cord receives motor nerve impulses from the brain and transmits these to the body, causing muscles to contract and movement to occur. Sensory nerve im-

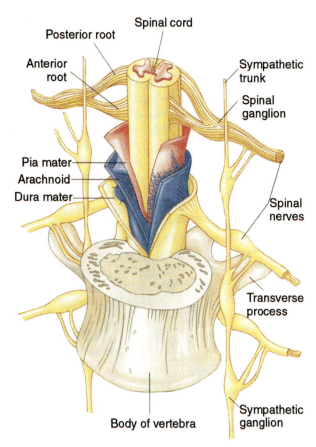

FIGURE 4-30 ▲ **The spinal cord. The meninges, spinal nerves, and sympathetic trunk are visible. (From Thibodeau GA, Patton KT:** *Structure and function of the body,* **ed 10, St Louis, 1997, Mosby.)**

pulses from the organs of special sensation are transmitted to the spinal cord and then to the brain. Both motor and sensory impulses are carried by *spinal nerves* from the spinal cord (Figure 4-30).

MENINGES AND CEREBROSPINAL FLUID

The brain and spinal cord are covered by three layers of membranes known as *meninges.* The outer layer is the *dura mater* and is the thickest. The middle layer is the *arachnoid membrane,* and the inner layer, which is closely adherent to the brain tissue, is the *pia mater. Cerebrospinal fluid (CSF),* a clear substance produced in the brain, circulates between the pia mater and the arachnoid in the *subarachnoid space.* This space is continuous from the cranial cavity to the sacrum. It fills and protects the cranial and spinal cavities, cushioning the brain and spinal cord. In the adult there is normally approximately 140 milliliters (mL) of CSF. Throughout the brain there are several hollow cavities, known as *ventricles,* that connect with the subarachnoid space and also contain CSF (Figure 4-31).

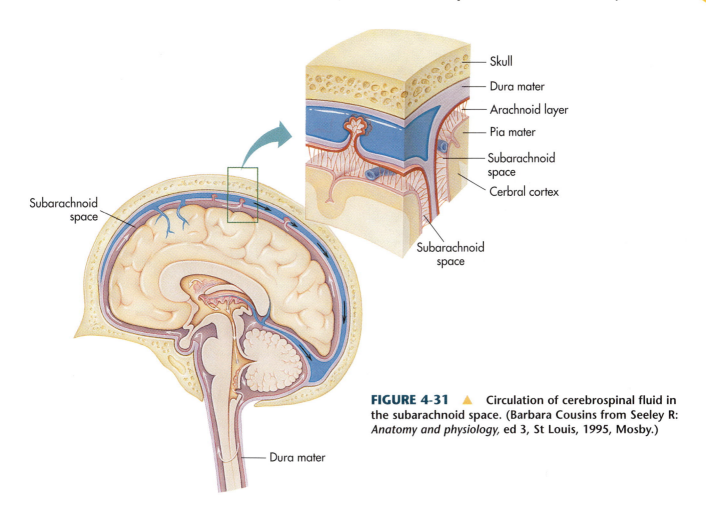

FIGURE 4-31 ▲ Circulation of cerebrospinal fluid in the subarachnoid space. (Barbara Cousins from Seeley R: *Anatomy and physiology,* ed 3, St Louis, 1995, Mosby.)

Peripheral Nervous System

The **peripheral nervous system** includes the cranial nerves, the spinal nerves, and the autonomic nervous system. There are three types of peripheral nerves:

- *Sensory nerves* transmit impulses from the organs to the spinal cord.

CLINICAL NOTES

Trauma can lead to bleeding (hematoma) within "potential spaces" formed by the meninges. Common locations are as follows (Figure 4-32):

Epidural hematoma—Bleeding in the space between the inner layer of the cranial bones and the dura.

Subdural hematoma—Bleeding in the space between the dura and the arachnoid membrane.

Subarachnoid hematoma—Bleeding in the space between the arachnoid membrane and the pia mater.

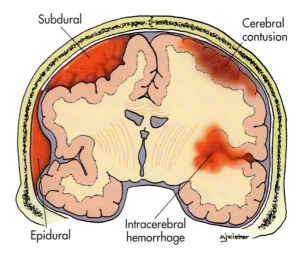

FIGURE 4-32 ▲ Types of brain injuries due to the presence of bruising or bleeding of brain tissues. **A,** Epidural hematoma. **B,** Subdural hematoma. **C,** Cerebral contusion. **D,** Intracerebral hemorrhage. (From American College of Emergency Physicians; Pons PT, Cason D, chief editors: *Paramedic field care: a complaint-based approach,* St Louis, 1997, Mosby for ACEP.)

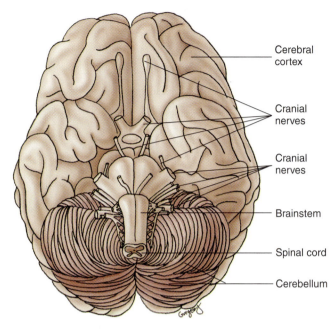

FIGURE 4-33 ▲ Cranial nerves.

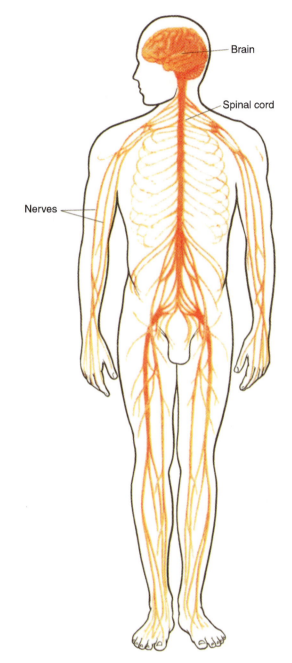

FIGURE 4-34 ▲ The nervous system. The brain and spinal cord constitute the central nervous system (CNS), and the nerves make up the peripheral nervous system (PNS). (From Thibodeau GA, Patton KT: *Structure and function of the body*, ed 10, St Louis, 1997, Mosby.)

- *Motor nerves* transmit impulses that stimulate muscle contraction and movement from the spinal cord to the muscles.
- *Mixed nerves* carry both sensory and motor messages.

Twelve pairs of *cranial nerves* extend directly from the brain. These modulate numerous functions ranging from vision to control of heart rate (Figure 4-33). Thirty-one pairs of *spinal nerves* leave the spinal cord; each pair leaves at a separate level of the vertebral column. The nerves pass from the spine via the *intervertebral foramina*. These nerves are numbered according to the regions of the vertebral column with which they are associated; there are 8 cervical pairs, 12 thoracic pairs, 5 lumbar pairs, 5 sacral pairs, and 1 coccygeal pair. The spinal nerves subdivide into numerous peripheral nerves that extend to the entire body (Figure 4-34).

AUTONOMIC NERVOUS SYSTEM

The **autonomic nervous system,** a specialized subdivision of the peripheral nervous system, regulates involuntary functions of the body (Figure 4-35). Examples of autonomic nervous system responsibilities include activity of the heart and smooth muscle. There are two divisions of the autonomic nervous system: the sympathetic and the parasympathetic nervous systems.

The **sympathetic nervous system** generates what we typically think of as the "fight or flight" response—constriction of blood vessels, elevation of the blood pressure and heart rate, and a feeling of nervousness. The **parasympathetic nervous system** works the opposite way, causing slowing of the heart rate. The parasympathetic nervous system controls intestinal activity, respiratory rate, and pupillary responses. In extreme instances, excess stimulation of the parasympathetic nervous system can lead to cardiac arrest.

Besides having opposite functions, each branch of the autonomic nervous system employs different neurotransmitters. *Norepinephrine* is the most common sympathetic neurotransmitter. It is closely related to epi-

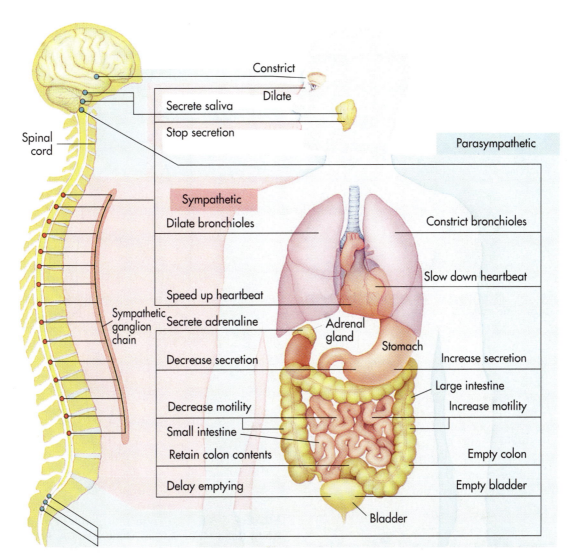

FIGURE 4-35 ▲ Organ regulation by the autonomic nervous system. The sympathetic nervous system is highlighted in red, the parasympathetic in blue. (Raychel Ciemma from Thibodeau GA, Patton KT: *Structure and function of the body,* ed 3, St Louis, 1992, Mosby.)

nephrine (adrenalin), which also functions as a sympathetic branch neurotransmitter. For this reason, the sympathetic branch is often called the "adrenergic system." Similarly, *acetylcholine* is the prime neurotransmitter in the parasympathetic branch, sometimes referred to as the "cholinergic system."

Both branches of the autonomic nervous system exert their effects by neurotransmitters that bind specific *receptors.* The two types of sympathetic receptors are important in patient care for the EMT–I and involve many of the common drugs EMT–Is use (Figure 4-36):

- *Alpha receptors*—Stimulation leads to constriction of blood vessels (vasoconstriction). This is one of the mechanisms by which drugs that raise the blood pressure (pressors, such as dopamine) work. Of course, blocking alpha receptors would lead to the opposite effect—vasodilation—and possibly hypotension.

- *Beta receptors*—These are further divided into *beta-1* and *beta-2* receptors, each with different effects. Beta-1 stimulation increases the heart rate and strength of cardiac contraction. Beta-2 stimulation leads to bronchodilation. Again, blockade of either or both receptors results in the opposite effect. Nebulized bronchodilators, such as albuterol, exert their effect primarily by stimulation of beta-2 receptors.

HELPFUL HINT

Typical sympathetic responses include tachycardia, elevated blood pressure, and a feeling of nervousness. Typical parasympathetic responses are nausea, vomiting, fainting (due to slow heart rate), and abdominal distress.

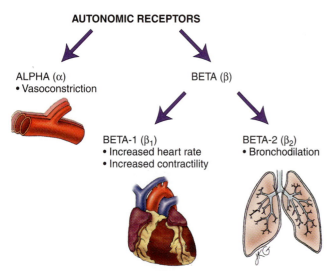

FIGURE 4-36 ▲ Receptors of the sympathetic portion of the autonomic nervous system.

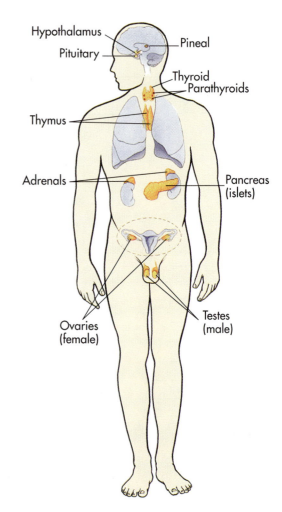

FIGURE 4-37 ▲ Endocrine glands in the human body. (Joan M. Beck from Thibodeau GA, Patton KT: *Structure and function of the body,* ed 3, St Louis, 1992, Mosby.)

ENDOCRINE SYSTEM

The **endocrine system** consists of several glands located throughout the body (Figure 4-37). These glands secrete proteins, called *hormones,* directly into the blood. Hormones regulate many body functions, such as growth, reproduction, temperature, metabolism, and blood pressure.

Regulation of Hormonal Secretion

The normal secretion of hormones is tightly regulated by a *feedback mechanism* involving the hypothalamus, the pituitary gland, the target gland, and the end-organ (the organ that the hormone affects). The steps in the process are as follows:

1. Sensors in the body alert the hypothalamus of the need to change a condition.
2. The hypothalamus releases a protein (called a "releasing factor") that travels in closely attached blood vessels to the pituitary gland.
3. The pituitary gland is stimulated to manufacture a "stimulating factor" that travels in the systemic circulation to the target gland (e.g., thyroid, adrenal, pancreas).
4. Once the target gland is stimulated by the "stimulating factor," it produces the final hormone, which is released into the blood.
5. The hormone is carried to its "target organ" and carries out the necessary task.
6. Sensors in the body then alert the hypothalamus when the necessary hormone has been produced, been released into the blood, and exerted the needed effect.

7. In response to feedback from these sensors, the hypothalamus stops producing "releasing factor" until again "informed" by the sensor mechanism that more is needed.

This process is called *negative feedback* or *feedback inhibition.* Production of the final hormone "feeds back" to the hypothalamus, causing it to cease production of further stimulating factors. In some cases the hypothalamus may also secrete inhibitory factors that terminate pituitary gland production of "stimulating factors" (Figure 4-38).

Major Endocrine Glands

The following are the major glands of the endocrine system:

- The *pituitary gland,* sometimes known as the "master gland," is located at the base of the brain in the cranial cavity. It manufactures hormones that regulate

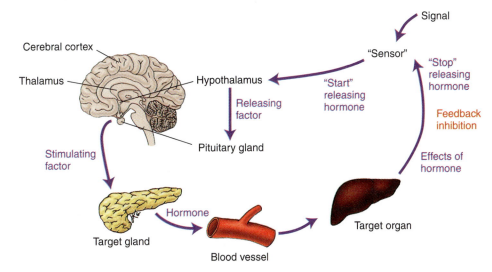

FIGURE 4-38 ▲ **Feedback inhibition.**

the function of the other endocrine glands in the body.

- The *thyroid gland* is a large gland situated at the base of the neck. It manufactures and secretes hormones that influence growth, development, metabolism, and levels of calcium in the body.

- The *parathyroid glands* are embedded in the posterior portion of the thyroid. They produce hormones that maintain normal levels of calcium in the blood.

- The *pancreas* is considered an organ of both the digestive system and the endocrine system. In addition to producing digestive enzymes, it manufactures the hormones *insulin* and *glucagon*. Both of these hormones are vital in control of the body's metabolism and blood sugar level. Lack of insulin leads to diabetes mellitus. Insulin and glucagon have opposite effects; both function to maintain a normal blood sugar level. Insulin causes the blood sugar level to decrease because it forces insulin into the cells, as if to "feed them." Glucagon, on the other hand, causes adrenergic stimulation, leading to an increase in the blood sugar level. Glucagon can also be administered clinically to raise the blood sugar level in patients with *hypoglycemia* (low blood sugar levels).

- The *adrenal glands* are located on top of each kidney. They manufacture and secrete certain sex hormones, as well as other hormones vital in maintaining the body's water and salt balance. During stress, the adrenal gland produces epinephrine and norepinephrine, which mediate the "flight or fight" response of the sympathetic nervous system mentioned previously.

- The *reproductive glands,* or *gonads,* are the *ovaries* in the woman and the *testes* in the man. These glands produce hormones responsible for the development of secondary sex characteristics (such as a deep voice and facial hair in men and breast development in women), as well as for reproduction.

BLOOD

Blood is the fluid tissue that is pumped by the heart through the arteries, veins, and capillaries. Blood consists of cells and plasma. Suspended within the pale, straw-colored plasma are several types of blood cells and dissolved chemicals, minerals, and nutrients (Figure 4-39). The average pH of the blood is 7.40 (slightly lower in venous blood than in arterial blood). Men have approximately 70 cubic centimeters (cc) of blood per kilogram (kg) of body weight, whereas women have slightly less: 65 cc/kg. In an adult man this amount equals approximately 5 or 6 liters (L) of blood.

Types of Blood Cells

There are three types of blood cells circulating in the body:

- *Red blood cells* (erythrocytes) are disk-shaped blood cells. These cells contain a protein known as *hemoglobin* that gives them their reddish color. Hemoglobin binds oxygen that is absorbed in the lungs and transports it to the tissues where it is needed.

- *White blood cells* (leukocytes) fight infection and help eliminate foreign materials from the body. There are five types of leukocytes, each of which has a role. *Neutrophils* fight bacterial infections, whereas *lymphocytes* and *monocytes* help eliminate viruses and fungal infections. *Eosinophils* and *basophils* are important in allergic reactions.

- *Platelets* are small cells in the blood that are essential for clot formation. Blood clots as a result of a series of chemical reactions. During this process,

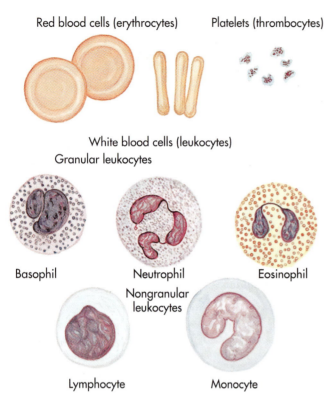

Red blood cells (erythrocytes)   Platelets (thrombocytes)

White blood cells (leukocytes)
Granular leukocytes

Basophil   Neutrophil   Eosinophil

Nongranular
leukocytes

Lymphocyte   Monocyte

FIGURE 4-39 ▲ **Erythrocytes, leukocytes, and platelets.** (Ernest W. Beck from Thibodeau GA, Patton KT: *Anatomy and physiology*, ed 3, St Louis, 1996, Mosby.)

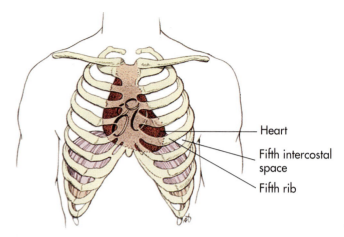

Heart

Fifth intercostal
space

Fifth rib

FIGURE 4-40 ▲ The heart is located behind the sternum (breastbone), mostly on the left side of the chest cavity. (Rusty Jones from Seeley R: *Essentials of anatomy and physiology*, ed 2, St Louis, 1996, Mosby.)

platelets aggregate together in a clump and form much of the foundation of the blood clot. The remainder of the clot consists of blood proteins, made primarily by the liver. If either part of this interdependent system fails, the patient has a problem forming a blood clot.

HEART

The **circulatory system,** sometimes referred to as the *cardiovascular system,* consists of the heart, blood, and blood vessels.

The *heart* is a muscular, cone-shaped organ, and its function is to pump blood throughout the body. It is located behind the sternum (breastbone) and is about the size of a closed fist (approximately 5 inches long, 3 inches wide, and 2 1/2 inches thick). It weighs 10 to 12 ounces in men and 8 to 10 ounces in women. Roughly two thirds of the heart lies in the left side of the chest cavity (Figure 4-40). Functionally, the heart is divided into right and left sides, which are separated by a thick wall called the *interventricular septum.* The heart muscle is referred to as the *myocardium.*

Surrounding the heart is a thick set of two pericardial membranes. Together, these membranes form the pericardial sac around the heart. The inner pericardial membrane is the *visceral pericardium,* which lies close to the outside of

the heart, or *epicardium.* The outer pericardial membrane is the *parietal pericardium.* Normally, the pericardial sac contains only a small amount of the clear *serous* ("like serum") lubricating fluid that allows the heart to contract and expand smoothly within the chest cavity.

> ● **HELPFUL HINT**
>
> • If the pericardial sac rapidly fills with fluid, such as blood, the heart is no longer able to adequately fill, and the signs and symptoms of shock result. This condition is known as **cardiac tamponade** and is a common result of penetrating chest trauma.

The normal human heart consists of two upper chambers (the *atria*) and two lower chambers (the *ventricles*). The atria receive blood returned to the heart from other parts of the body, and the ventricles pump blood out of the heart. The atria and ventricles are separated by valves that prevent backward flow of blood. Other valves are located between the ventricles and the arteries into which they pump blood (Figure 4-41).

Deoxygenated blood returns to the *right atrium* via the *superior* and *inferior vena cava,* the largest veins in the body. It passes through the *tricuspid valve* into the *right ventricle,* situated inferiorly. Blood then flows from the right ventricle through the *pulmonary (semilunar) valve* into the *main pulmonary artery.* This vessel branches, taking blood to both the left and right lungs. Blood is oxygenated in the lungs (see Respiratory System) and returned to the *left atrium* via the pulmonary veins. Blood then transverses the *mitral (bicuspid) valve* into the *left ventricle.* It is then pumped through the *aortic (semilunar) valve* into the aorta.

Normal blood flow

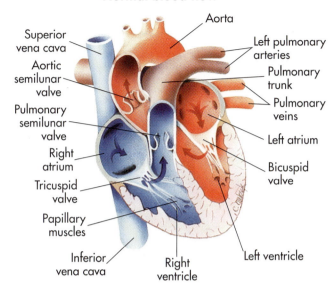

FIGURE 4-41 ▲ **Internal anatomy of the human heart. (Christine Oleksyk from Seeley R: *Anatomy and physiology*, ed 3, St Louis, 1995, Mosby.)**

Coronary Circulation

The heart receives most of its blood supply directly from the *coronary circulation.* The first branches of the aorta, immediately as the aorta leaves the heart, are the *right* and *left main coronary arteries* (Figure 4-42). These then branch into several smaller divisions, each of which supplies a particular portion of the myocardium. The major branches of the main coronary arteries are as follows:

- *Right main coronary artery*—Consists of the nodal artery (supplies the sinoatrial [SA] node), the descending right artery (supplies the anterior right ventricle), and the posterior descending artery (supplies the posterior heart wall).
- *Left main coronary artery*—Consists of the anterior descending artery (supplies the anterior wall of the left ventricle), the diagonal artery (usually supplies the lateral left ventricular wall), and the circumflex artery (usually supplies the superior left ventricle).

The blood supply to the atrioventricular (AV) node is variable. In about 60% of persons, it arises from the right side. Deoxygenated venous blood from the heart drains into five different coronary veins that empty into the right atrium via the coronary sinus.

Cardiac Cycle

The *cardiac cycle* is the repetitive pumping process of blood that begins with the onset of cardiac muscle contraction and ends with the beginning of the next con-

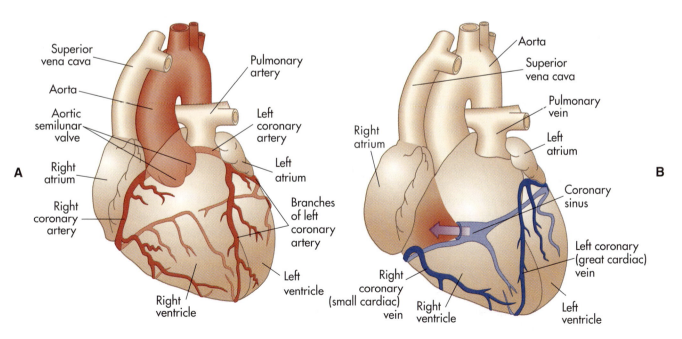

FIGURE 4-42 ▲ Coronary circulation. **A,** Coronary arteries. **B,** Coronary veins. (Network Graphics from Thibodeau GA, Patton KT: *Anatomy and physiology,* ed 3, St Louis, 1996, Mosby.)

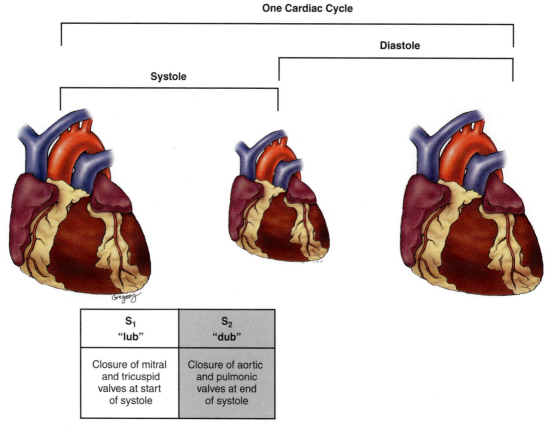

One Cardiac Cycle

Diastole

Systole

S_1 "lub"	S_2 "dub"
Closure of mitral and tricuspid valves at start of systole	Closure of aortic and pulmonic valves at end of systole

FIGURE 4-43 ▲ The normal cardiac cycle consists of two sounds, the first heart sound (S1) and the second heart sound (S2). S1 results from the closure of the mitral and tricuspid valves at the start of systole. S2 occurs when the aortic and pulmonic valves close at the end of systole.

traction. Myocardial contraction leads to pressure changes within the cardiac chambers, causing blood movement. Blood moves from areas of high pressure to areas of low pressure.

Contraction of the ventricles, with its concomitant pumping of blood into the aorta and pulmonary vessels, is known as *systole*. The *systolic blood pressure* is the pressure within the arteries during this time. *Diastole* is the relaxation phase; it is during this time that the heart receives most of its blood supply from the coronary arteries. Thus *diastolic blood pressure* not only reflects the pressure in the heart during the relaxation phase but is an indication of myocardial perfusion.

Heart Sounds

The contraction and relaxation of the heart, combined with the flow of blood, generates characteristic sounds (*heart sounds*) that can be heard with a stethoscope (*auscultation* of the heart). The normal pattern sounds much like "lub-DUB, lub-DUB, lub-DUB." The "lub" is referred to as the *first heart sound* or S_1, and the "DUB" (emphasized because it's often louder) as the *second*

heart sound (S₂). S_1 is caused by vibrations due to the sudden closure of the mitral and tricuspid valves at the start of ventricular systole. S_2 results from the closure of both the aortic and pulmonic valves at the end of ventricular systole (Figure 4-43).

There are two other heart sounds, which are not usually heard in normal individuals (Figure 4-44):

• A *third heart sound (S₃)* is a soft, low-pitched sound heard about one third of the way through diastole. Instead of hearing "lub-DUB," one hears "lub-DUB-da," with the *"da"* indicating the third heart sound. It is thought to represent the period of rapid ventricular filling due to vibrations set up by the inrush of blood. Although sometimes present in healthy young persons, most commonly an S_3 is associated with moderate to severe heart failure.

• A *fourth heart sound (S₄)* is a moderate-pitched sound occurring immediately before the normal S_1. Instead of hearing "lub-DUB," one hears *"bla'lub-DUB"* with the *"bla'"* indicating the fourth heart sound. This represents either decreased stretching (compliance) of the left ventricle or increased pressure in the atria. An S_4 is almost always abnormal.

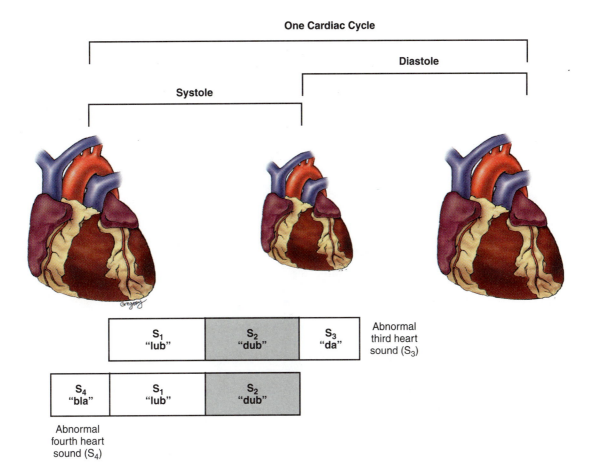

FIGURE 4-44 ▲ In addition to the normal S1 and S2, an abnormal third sound (S3) and fourth sound (S4) may sometimes be heard. These represent atrial (S3) and ventricular (S4) strain.

There are four other sounds, all abnormal, that may be heard when auscultating the heart and great vessels. Some are very easy to hear, whereas others may require years of experience.

- *Murmurs*—An abnormal "whooshing" sound indicating turbulent blood flow within the heart. If this sound is heard over a main blood vessel, it is called a bruit. Although many murmurs are "functional" (benign) and often go away, several are characteristic for heart disease.
- *Bruits*—An abnormal "whooshing" sound indicating turbulent blood flow within a blood vessel. If this sound is heard over the heart, it is called a murmur. A bruit often indicates localized atherosclerotic debris (hardening of the arteries) in a blood vessel.
- *Clicks and snaps*—Both clicks and snaps indicate abnormal cardiac valve function. They occur at different times in the cardiac cycle, depending on the disease valve. Most of these sounds, although significant, are fleeting and difficult to hear.

Cardiac Conduction Pathway

Contraction of myocardial tissue is initiated within the heart itself in a group of electrical tissues called the *sinus* or *sinoatrial (SA) node*. The electrical impulse then goes through the cardiac conduction system, which is a complex grouping of specialized tissues that forms a network of connections, much like an electrical circuit, throughout the heart (Figure 4-45). This network carries the electrical nerve impulse that causes the heart muscle to contract.

The initial electrical impulse begins high in the right atrium, in the SA node. It travels through the atria via *intraatrial pathways* to the *atrioventricular (AV) node*. The stimulus then passes into the *bundle of His*, where the conduction system divides into two portions: the *right bundle branch* and the *left bundle branch*. These fibers spread out to their respective sides of the heart. Finally, very small *Purkinje's fibers* take the current from the bundle branches to the individual myocardial cells. Normal depolarization of the myocardium progresses from atria to ventricles in an orderly fashion.

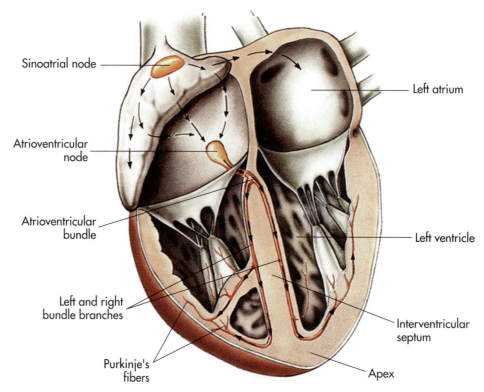

Sinoatrial node

Atrioventricular node

Atrioventricular bundle

Left and right bundle branches

Purkinje's fibers

Left atrium

Left ventricle

Interventricular septum

Apex

FIGURE 4-45 ▲ The path of electrical conduction in the heart. (Barbara Cousins from Thibodeau GA, Patton KT: *Anatomy and physiology,* ed 3, St Louis, 1996, Mosby.)

Cardiac Output

The amount of blood pumped through the circulatory system in 1 minute is referred to as the *cardiac output.* It is expressed in liters per minute. The cardiac output equals the heart rate times the *stroke volume,* or the amount of blood (volume) pumped with each heartbeat (see Figure 16-6):

Cardiac output = Stroke volume × Heart rate

Factors that influence the heart rate, the stroke volume, or both, will affect cardiac output and thus tissue oxygen delivery (perfusion).

Regulation of Heart Function

Control of the heart's rate and strength of contraction comes partially from the brain via the autonomic nervous system, from hormones of the endocrine system, and from the heart tissue. Receptors in the blood vessels, kidneys, brain, and heart constantly monitor body homeostasis. *Baroreceptors* respond to changes in pressure, usually within the heart or the main arteries. *Chemoreceptors* sense changes in the chemical composition of the blood. If abnormalities are sensed, nerve signals are transmitted to appropriate target organs, leading to release of hormones or neurotransmitters to

rectify the situation. Once conditions normalize, the receptors stop firing and the signals cease. This is very similar to the negative feedback inhibition discussed earlier under Endocrine System.

Often, stimulation of receptors leads to activation of either the parasympathetic or the sympathetic branch of the autonomic nervous system. These affect both the heart rate and the strength of heart muscle contraction *(contractility).* For example, if a patient is bleeding, baroreceptors sense an abnormally low blood volume. Although several different body responses occur at once, a major one is the release of epinephrine and norepinephrine from the adrenal glands. This causes sympathetic (adrenergic) stimulation, resulting in an increased heart rate, as well as increased contractility. On the other hand, simple fainting often results because of parasympathetic stimulation leading to a slow heart rate (bradycardia).

Another body response to volume changes involves *Starling's law of the heart.* Many years ago, the physiologist Starling noted that if a muscle is stretched a little bit before it is stimulated to contract, it contracts harder. So, if the heart is stretched, the muscle contracts harder. This is a normal defense mechanism; the amount of blood return to the right atrium varies somewhat from minute to minute, yet the normal

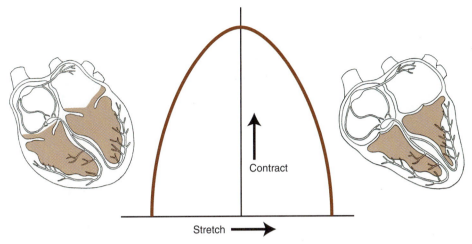

FIGURE 4-46 ▲ Starling's law of the heart. Within limits, if a muscle is stretched before it is stimulated to contract, it contracts harder.

heart continues to pump out the same percentage of blood returned. This is called the *ejection fraction.* If more blood returns to the heart, rather than having it backing up into the veins, the stretched heart pumps harder. The result is more blood is pumped with each contraction, yet the ejection fraction remains unchanged (the amount of blood pumped out increases, but so does the amount returned). It is this relationship that maintains normal cardiac output when a person changes positions, coughs, breathes, or moves (Figure 4-46).

VASCULAR SYSTEM

Arteries, Veins, and Capillaries

Arteries are blood vessels that carry blood away from the heart to the body. *Veins* transport blood from the body back to the heart (Figure 4-47). Arteries decrease in size as they move away from the heart, branching into many small *arterioles.* Arterioles then divide many times until they form *capillaries.* Capillaries are microscopic thin-walled vessels through which oxygen, carbon dioxide, and other nutrients and waste products are exchanged (Figure 4-48).

To return deoxygenated ("used") blood to the heart, groups of capillaries gradually enlarge to form *venules.* Venules then merge together, forming larger and larger veins. Eventually, the veins merge together into the immense *superior vena cava* and *inferior vena cava,* which empty into the *right atrium.*

Pathways of Circulation

Deoxygenated blood returned to the right atrium from the superior and inferior vena cava passes through the tricuspid valve into the right ventricle. From there, it is pumped through the pulmonary valve into the pulmonary artery. This is the beginning of the *pulmonary circulation,* which is designed to transport deoxygenated blood through the lungs, oxygenate it, and return it back to the left side of the heart so that the left ventricle may pump it out to the body via the *systemic circulation* (see Figure 16-8).

The main pulmonary artery branches to each lung. In the lungs the blood is oxygenated and waste products are removed. Freshly oxygenated blood is returned to the left atrium via the pulmonary veins. Blood then flows into the left ventricle, which pumps the oxygenated blood through the aorta and then to the entire body.

Blood Pressure

Blood pressure is the pressure exerted by the circulating blood on the walls of the arteries, the veins, and the chambers of the heart. The *systolic blood pressure* is the pressure within the arteries during systole, or the period of contraction. The *diastolic blood pressure* represents the pressure during cardiac relaxation. These are recorded in millimeters (mm) of mercury (Hg) and recorded as a fraction: systolic/diastolic. The normal ranges for blood pressure in adults are as follows:

- *Systolic*—100 mm Hg to 140 mm Hg
- *Diastolic*—50 mm Hg to 90 mm Hg

The blood pressure is proportional to the *cardiac output* (the amount of blood pumped by the heart each minute) times the *total peripheral resistance* (the resistance in the arterial bed) (see Figure 16-7).

Blood pressure is maintained by a complex interaction of homeostatic mechanisms (e.g., autonomic ner-

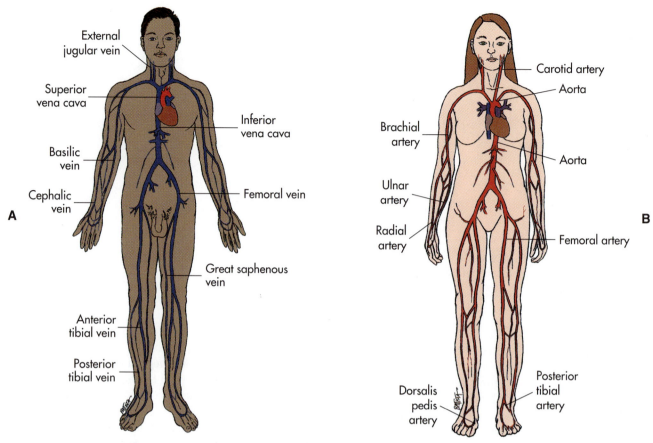

FIGURE 4-47 **A**, Major veins of the body. **B**, Major arteries of the body. (Kimberly Battista from Stoy W: *Mosby's EMT–Basic textbook,* St Louis, 1996, Mosby.)

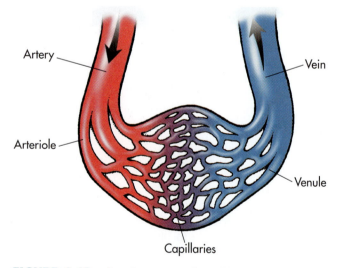

FIGURE 4-48 ▲ Oxygen, carbon dioxide, and other nutrients and waste products are exchanged through capillaries. (Duckwall Productions.)

vous system, endocrine system) that maintain normal pressure by monitoring the following:

- Blood volume
- Degree of constriction of arteries and arterioles
- Force of cardiac contraction

LYMPHATIC SYSTEM AND IMMUNITY

Lympathic System

The **lymphatic system** is a passive circulatory system that transports a plasmalike liquid called *lymph,* a thin fluid that bathes the tissues of the body (Figure 4-49). Lymph comes from excess cellular fluid and circulates through the body in thin-walled *lymph vessels,* which travel close to the major veins. Lymphatic fluid is filtered in *lymph nodes* and returns to the main circulatory system via the *thoracic duct,* which empties into the superior vena cava. The lymphatic system functions primarily to absorb fat from the intestines and to trap infection-causing organisms (such as viruses and bacteria).

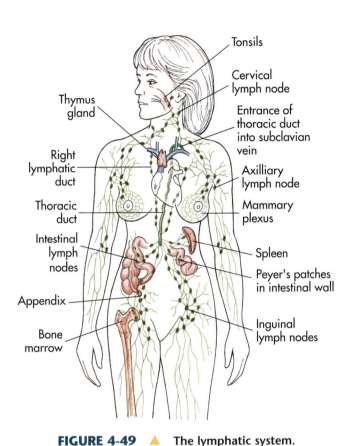

FIGURE 4-49 ▲ The lymphatic system.

Nonspecific Immunity

• Mechanical barriers (skin, secretions)
• Chemicals (histamine)
• White blood cells

Specific Immunity

• Antibody-mediated immunity
• Cell-mediated immunity

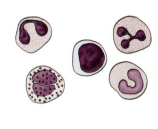
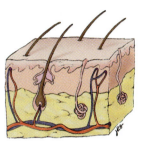

FIGURE 4-50 ▲ The immune system.

CLINICAL NOTES

The lymph nodes are the site where bacteria or viruses are trapped. They are held here until they can be destroyed by cells of the immune system. As a result, the lymph nodes or "glands" may become swollen during an infection. This swelling is an indication that the lymphatic system is properly performing its function.

Immune System

The **immune system** defends the body against bacteria, viruses, and other foreign matter. The body has two types of *immunity,* which is the ability to resist damage from foreign substances or harmful chemicals: *nonspecific immunity* and *specific immunity.* Together, nonspecific and specific immunity make up the *immune response* (Figure 4-50).

Nonspecific immunity occurs via three mechanisms:
• Mechanical barriers, such as the skin, prevent the entry of many bacteria. In addition, tears, saliva, and mucus in the respiratory tract continuously wash foreign matter away.
• Chemicals such as histamine promote inflammation in response to foreign invaders to the body.
• White blood cells (leukocytes) ingest and destroy bacterial invaders and foreign matter.

Two types of specific immunity exist:
• Foreign substances, known as *antigens,* lead to the formation of *antibodies* by the immune system. These antibodies form the basis of *antibody-mediated immunity.* When the body is exposed to a foreign antigen, the antibody attacks it and initiates a series of reactions designed to eliminate the antigen from the body.
• *Cell-mediated immunity* is achieved by the actions of *lymphocytes.* These cells seek out and destroy foreign materials, such as viruses, fungi, bacteria, and particles.

CLINICAL NOTES

Infection with the human immunodeficiency virus (HIV) leads to suppression of certain lymphocytes and a major defect in cell-mediated immunity. This is the major reason why infected persons are susceptible to serious infections.

RESPIRATORY SYSTEM

The *respiratory system* consists of the organs and structures associated with breathing and gas exchange in the body. Its function is to bring oxygen into the body and excrete carbon dioxide. By doing so, the respiratory sys-

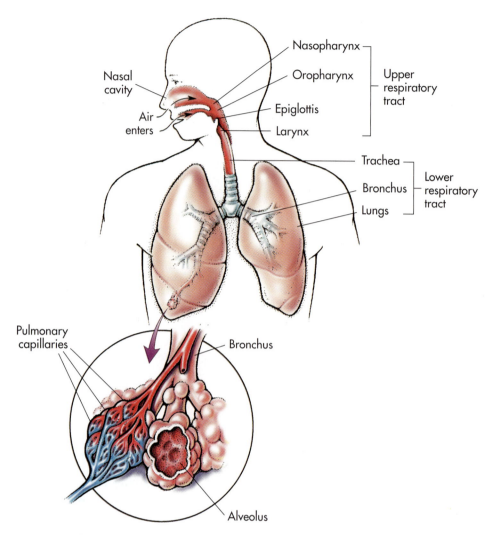

FIGURE 4-51 ▲ **The respiratory system. (Duckwall Productions.)**

tem can also exert a significant effect on acid-base and other chemical balances in the body.

The respiratory system is divided into two parts: the upper respiratory system (mouth, nasal cavity, oral cavity, larynx, and vocal cords) and the lower respiratory system (trachea, bronchi, bronchioles, and alveoli) (Figure 4-51).

Upper Respiratory System

The *upper respiratory system* consists of the mouth, nasal cavity, oral cavity, larynx, and vocal cords. Inspired air flows into the body through either the *nose* or the *mouth*. The nasal cavity is referred to as the *nasopharynx*, and the oral cavity is referred to as the *oropharynx*. These two cavities come together posteriorly to form a common cavity, the *pharynx*. Air then travels downward through the *larynx*, which contains the *vocal cords*, and into the trachea.

Lower Respiratory System

The *lower respiratory system* begins with the *trachea*, which is a tube of cartilage and other connective tissue

that extends from the larynx to the bronchi. Its purpose is to convey air to the lungs. In most adults the trachea is approximately 4 inches long. The trachea divides into the right and left *mainstem bronchi;* this region is known as the *carina.* At this point, the air enters the lungs through the *mainstem bronchi.*

The mainstem bronchi divide into *secondary bronchi,* each going to a separate *lobe* of the lung. The bronchi divide into progressively smaller branches called *bronchioles,* ending as *alveoli.* Alveoli are tiny sacs of lung tissue where gas exchange takes place. The lung contains 300 million alveoli, each about 0.33 mm in diameter. Alveoli are surrounded by capillaries. The membrane between the alveolus and the capillary is very thin, consisting of only one cell layer. Respiratory exchange between the lung and blood vessels occurs in the alveoli.

There are two *lungs:* the *right lung* and the *left lung.* The right lung has three *lobes* (upper, middle, and lower), whereas the left lung has only two (upper and lower). The lungs are covered with two connective tissue membranes known as the *pleura.* These membranes envelop each lung and line the inner borders of the rib cage, or *pleural cavity.*

Mechanics of Breathing

When a person inhales, the *diaphragm* contracts, creating a negative pressure in the chest cavity. This negative pressure "sucks" in air, expanding the lungs. Air is expired when the lung tissue collapses because of its natural elasticity, much like a balloon that has had the air suddenly released. Exhalation is a passive process and normally requires no muscular effort.

CLINICAL NOTES

The membrane closest to the lung is referred to as the *visceral pleura.* The other membrane forms the *parietal pleura.* There is a potential space between the visceral and parietal pleura, known as the *pleural space.* Normally, the two membranes are close together and a space does not exist, other than enough to contain a small amount of lubricating fluid. Under certain disease conditions or following trauma, fluid and/or air may accumulate in the pleural space, leading to respiratory problems. An abnormal collection of air in the pleural cavity is called a *pneumothorax,* and an abnormal collection of fluid is called a *pleural effusion.*

Ventilation Versus Respiration

Technically, **ventilation** refers to the movement of carbon dioxide in and out of the lungs. **Oxygenation** is a separate, but somewhat related, process. For example, a person may hyperventilate, causing a decrease in the carbon dioxide level in the blood (respiratory alkalosis) but no change in the level of oxygen. The term *respiration* refers generically to breathing. As with oxygen, people may breathe fast or slow and not necessarily significantly affect the blood concentration of carbon dioxide.

Gas Exchange in the Lungs

Oxygen is essential for the function of body processes. Inspired air contains approximately 21% oxygen. The primary waste product of the human body is carbon dioxide. Carbon dioxide is carried in the blood to the lungs. Expired air contains carbon dioxide and approximately 16% oxygen.

The primary function of the respiratory system is to provide for the exchange of gases at the alveolar-capillary membrane, the point where a single alveolus lies against a single capillary.

At the alveolar-capillary exchange surface, the alveolus and the red blood cells come very close together. Oxygen and carbon dioxide diffuse across the membrane. Oxygen moves from the alveolus to the hemoglobin molecule of the red blood cells. Carbon dioxide flows from the blood into the alveolus. When the individual exhales, carbon dioxide is breathed into the atmosphere and eliminated from the body.

CLINICAL NOTES

The large number of alveoli allow an extremely large surface area for respiratory exchange in the relatively limited space of the thoracic cavity. By wrapping the small capillaries around an enormous number of alveoli, a total surface area of more than 85 square meters (m^2) occurs. If each lung consisted of only a single sphere, like a large balloon, the surface area would be only 0.01 m^2 (1 m = 39.37 inches).

Transportation of Gases in the Blood

Oxygen is carried in the blood by *hemoglobin.* This is a complex molecule that makes up most of the red blood cell. The term *oxygen saturation,* often measured by a *pulse oximeter,* refers to the percentage of red blood cell hemoglobin that is bound to (saturated with) oxygen. Normally, this should be over 90%. The majority of carbon dioxide is transported in the form of *bicarbonate ions,* although some carbon dioxide also combines with hemoglobin (Figure 4-52).

Regulation of Respiration

The brain controls respiration. The respiratory center of the brain responds to the levels of carbon dioxide in the blood. Excess levels of carbon dioxide cause the brain to stimulate ventilation, whereas decreased levels of carbon dioxide force the brain to decrease ventilation. The brain also responds to levels of oxygen in the blood; however, the brain's response to oxygen is less predictable than its response to carbon dioxide.

DIGESTIVE SYSTEM

The *digestive system* (also called the **gastrointestinal system**) is composed of structures and organs involved in

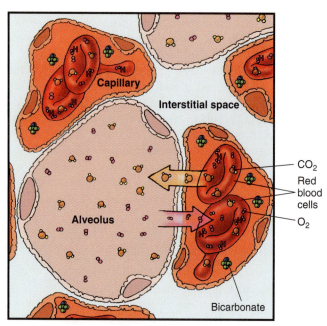

Oxygen and carbon dioxide exchange occurs in the lung between the alveoli and red blood cells in the capillaries.

FIGURE 4-52 ▲ Oxygen and carbon dioxide exchange occurs in the lung between the alveoli and red blood cells in the capillaries.

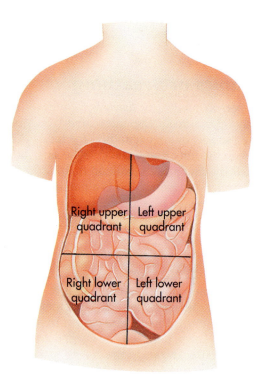

FIGURE 4-53 ▲ Organs of the abdomen.

the consumption, digestion, and elimination of food. Digestion begins in the mouth, where food is chewed by the teeth and mixed with saliva from the *salivary glands*. The partially digested food is then swallowed and travels via the *esophagus* to the *stomach*. Digestion then takes place here and in the *small intestine*. Most nutrients are absorbed in the small intestine. Water and electrolytes are absorbed and secreted in the *large intestine*.

Quadrants of the Abdomen

The abdomen is divided into imaginary *quadrants*. Because of the large number of organs in the abdomen, these quadrants enable emergency providers to distinguish the location of problems. The *umbilicus* (navel) serves as the central reference point. The diaphragm is the top of the abdominal cavity, and the pelvic bones, the bottom. The quadrants are divided by a set of imaginary perpendicular lines intersecting at the umbilicus (Figure 4-53).

The abdominal organs are identified by their location within these quadrants. Some of the organs are located in more than one quadrant. There is anatomical overlap between organs of the gastrointestinal, urinary, and reproductive systems. The major organs in each quadrant are as follows:

- *Right upper quadrant (RUQ)*—Liver, gallbladder, part of the large intestine, right kidney
- *Left upper quadrant (LUQ)*—Stomach, spleen, pancreas, part of the large intestine, left kidney

- *Right lower quadrant (RLQ)*—Appendix, part of the large intestine, right ovary, right ureter, uterus, urinary bladder
- *Left lower quadrant (LLQ)*—Part of the large intestine, left ovary, left ureter, uterus, urinary bladder

The kidneys and pancreas are not located in the abdominal cavity per se, but in an area behind the peritoneal membranes called the *retroperitoneal space*. However, injuries and illness affecting these organs often cause abdominal symptoms that are best classified by location. For this reason, these organs are included as being located within these quadrants.

Hollow Abdominal Organs

Abdominal organs are classified as hollow or solid. *Hollow organs* generally make up the digestive system, through which foodstuffs move (Figure 4-54). The *esophagus*, or swallowing tube, carries food and liquid from the pharynx to the *stomach*, an expandable organ located below the diaphragm in the left upper quadrant. Here, the food is churned and mixed with digestive juices, forming a semiliquid mass called *chyme*. Food moves through the *pyloric valve* into the *small intestine*, which is the longest part of the digestive tract and the major site of food digestion and absorption of nutrients.

The small intestine is made up of three parts: the *duodenum*, the *jejunum*, and the *ileum*. Together, the entire small intestine is often 20 feet in length. The ileum emp-

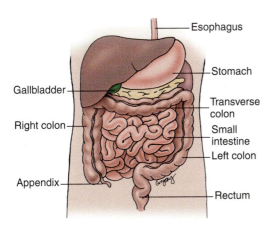

FIGURE 4-54 ▲ Hollow abdominal organs.

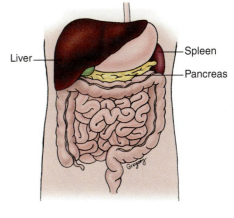

FIGURE 4-55 ▲ Solid abdominal organs.

ties into the *large intestine,* where the collection and removal of the wastes from digestion, including water, occurs. Stool is formed in the longest portion of the large intestine, the *colon.* It is stored in the *rectum* and excreted through the *anus.*

The *appendix* is a fingerlike attachment to the first part of the large intestine in the right lower quadrant. It has no known function and may become inflamed, causing *appendicitis.* The *gallbladder* is a pear-shaped organ located on the lower surface of the liver. It acts as a reservoir for *bile,* an important digestive enzyme. When a person eats fatty foods, the gallbladder contracts, releasing bile into the small intestine.

CLINICAL NOTES

Injury to a hollow organ may cause it to be punctured or to rupture. In either case, the internal contents are dumped into the abdominal cavity, which may lead to infection or irritation.

Solid Abdominal Organs

The liver, the spleen, and the pancreas are solid abdominal organs (Figure 4-55). The *liver* is a large solid organ in the right upper quadrant. It has many functions, including storage of glucose, protein synthesis, and filtering the blood of body wastes. Many drugs and chemicals also are broken down (detoxified) here. The *spleen* is a highly vascular organ located in the left upper quadrant behind the stomach. It aids in the removal of old blood cells from the circulation, as well as in fighting infection. The *pancreas* is an elongated gland located in the left upper quadrant behind the stomach. It has several functions, including the manufacture of digestive juices, as well as the hormones insulin and glucagon.

HELPFUL HINT

Injury to a solid organ may result in significant bleeding into the abdominal cavity. This injury is very serious because the patient can be in severe shock and may even bleed to death, without any signs of external bleeding.

FLUIDS AND ELECTROLYTES

Water Compartments in the Body

Water is the most abundant substance in the human body. It plays an important role in the maintenance of homeostasis and provides the cells with a life-sustaining environment. It also functions as a universal solvent for a variety of solutes. These solutes can be classified as either electrolytes or nonelectrolytes.

The average adult has a total body water content of approximately 50% to 60% of total body weight. This percentage varies depending on age and sex. In fact, a newborn's total body water content may be as high as 75% to 80% of the total body weight. Body fluid is divided into two main compartments (Figure 4-56):

- *Intracellular fluid* is found within individual cells and equals approximately 40% to 45% of total body weight. Therefore the intracellular fluid makes up approximately 75% of all body fluid.
- *Extracellular fluid* is the fluid found outside of the cell membranes. It equals approximately 15% to 20% of the total body weight, or 25% of all body fluid. Extracellular fluid is further divided into intravascular fluid and interstitial fluid:
  - *Intravascular fluid,* or *plasma*—This fluid portion of blood is noncellular and is found within the blood vessels. It equals approximately 4.5% of the total body weight.
  - *Interstitial fluid*—This fluid is located outside of the blood vessels in the spaces between the body's cells.

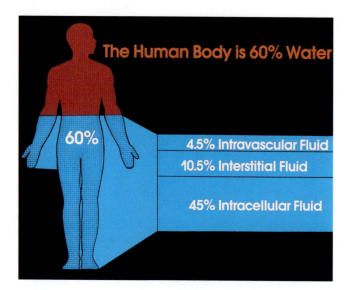

FIGURE 4-56 ▲ Body water is divided into intracellular fluid or extracellular fluid. Extracellular fluid is further divided into intravascular and interstitial fluid. (Yvonne Wylie Walston from Thibodeau GA and Patton KT: *Anatomy and physiology,* ed 3, St Louis, 1996, Mosby.)

It makes up approximately 10.5% of the total body weight. There is a delicate balance between the various fluid compartments of the body. This balance is essential in the maintenance of homeostasis.

Fluid Balance

Loss of fluid volume from any area of the body can lead to disruption of homeostasis and to shock. Normally, the total volume of water in the body, as well as its distribution in the body compartments, remains relatively constant despite wide fluctuations in the amount of water that enters and is excreted from the body on a daily basis. Water coming into the body is referred to as *intake,* whereas water excreted from the body is referred to as *output.* To maintain relative homeostasis, intake must equal output (Figure 4-57).

Several mechanisms work to maintain a balance between input and output. For example, when the fluid volume drops, the pituitary gland secretes *antidiuretic hormone (ADH).* ADH causes the kidney tubules to reabsorb more water into the blood and excrete less urine. This action allows fluid volume in the body to build up. Thirst also regulates fluid intake. The sensation of thirst occurs when body fluids become decreased, stimulating the person to take in more fluids. Conversely, when too many fluids enter the body, thirst decreases, the kidneys are activated, and more urine is excreted, eliminating the excess fluid.

The body also maintains fluid balance by shifting water from one compartment to another. Water moves in response to osmotic forces, as well as hormonal stimuli, such as ADH. Maintaining a proper balance of

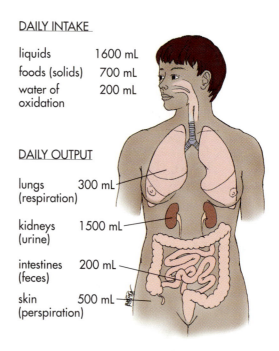

FIGURE 4-57 ▲ In order for the body to maintain relative homeostasis, daily fluid intake and output must be relatively equal. (**A,** Barbara Cousins from Thibodeau GA and Patton KT: *Anatomy and physiology,* ed 3, St Louis, 1996, Mosby. and **B,** Rolin Graphics from Thibodeau GA and Patton KT: *Anatomy and physiology,* ed 3, St Louis, 1996, Mosby.)

fluids and electrolytes within the body is necessary for life. A person may be depleted of fluids and electrolytes for several reasons, such as severe burns or severe dehydration. The patient's chances of survival may depend on how rapidly his or her internal environment is restored.

Electrolytes

Salts that break up into ions (electrically charged particles) are called electrolytes. There are two types of ions: anions and cations. *Cations* have a positive charge. Essential cations include the following (Figure 4-58):

- *Sodium (Na⁺)*—Sodium is responsible for maintaining fluid balance in the body. When sodium is eliminated from the body, water also is lost. Conversely, when sodium levels in the body rise, water is retained. Sodium is needed for the conduction of nerve impulses and for muscle contraction.
- *Potassium (K⁺)*—Potassium is required for growth and is important in the conduction of nerve impulses and muscle contraction. It also is responsible for acid-base regulation.
- *Calcium (Ca²⁺)*—Calcium is the most abundant cation in the body. It is required for blood clotting, bone growth, metabolism, normal cardiac function, and contraction of muscle.

CATIONS

ANIONS

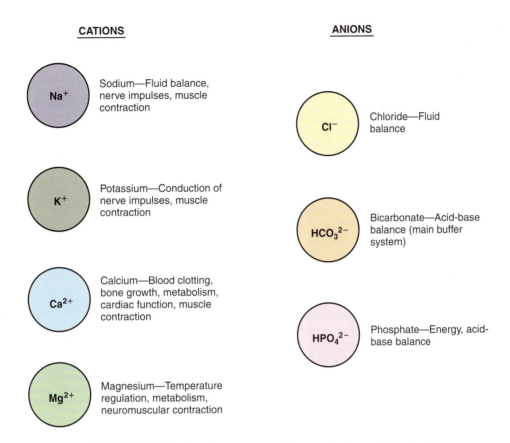

Sodium—Fluid balance, nerve impulses, muscle contraction

Potassium—Conduction of nerve impulses, muscle contraction

Calcium—Blood clotting, bone growth, metabolism, cardiac function, muscle contraction

Magnesium—Temperature regulation, metabolism, neuromuscular contraction

Chloride—Fluid balance

Bicarbonate—Acid-base balance (main buffer system)

Phosphate—Energy, acid-base balance

FIGURE 4-58 ▲ **Important cations and anions of the body.**

- *Magnesium (Mg^{2+})*—Magnesium is required for body temperature regulation, protein and carbohydrate metabolism, and neuromuscular contraction.

An *anion* has a negative charge. Essential anions include the following:

- *Chloride (Cl$^-$)*—Chloride's main function is to maintain fluid balance.
- *Bicarbonate (HCO$_3^{2-}$)*—Bicarbonate is a major buffer of the body. Its main function is to maintain acid-base balance.
- *Phosphate (HPO$_4^{2-}$)*—Phosphate helps maintain acid-base balance and is essential in providing energy for numerous biochemical reactions.

Electrolytes are measured in milliequivalents per liter (mEq/L). A milliequivalent is the concentration of electrolytes in a certain volume of solution (in this case, 1 L).

Body fluid also contains compounds with no electrical charge. These substances are called *nonelectrolytes*. Examples of nonelectrolytes include glucose, protein, urea, and similar substances.

Acid-Base Balance

Whether the blood is acidic, basic, or neutral depends on the concentration of dissolved *hydrogen (H$^+$)*. H$^+$ is an acid, so the higher the hydrogen ion (H$^+$) concentration, the more *acidic* the blood. Conversely, the lower the hydrogen ion concentration, the more *basic* (less acidic) the blood. Normal **homeostasis** functions to keep the hydrogen ion concentration within a fairly narrow range. Rather than use the term *hydrogen ion concentration*, we use *pH*, which is a mathematical expression of the same thing:

$$pH = - \text{Logarithm (base 10) [H}^+ \text{ concentration]}$$

The specifics of the math are not as important as the concept. The *lower* the hydrogen ion concentration, the *greater* the pH (more basic). Conversely, the *higher* the hydrogen ion concentration, the *lower* the pH (more acidic). The pH ranges from 0 (most acidic) to 14 (most basic), with 7.0 being neutral. The pH of pure water is 7.0, or neutral (Figure 4-59). The pH of the human body is normally slightly alkaline: approximately 7.35 to 7.45. Values higher than this indicate that the blood is *alkalotic* (too basic), whereas lower values indicate that the blood is *acidotic* (too acidic).

Chemically, an *acid* is a substance that increases the concentration of hydrogen ions in a water solution. The more hydrogen ions, the lower the pH. If the pH is below 7.0, the solution is an acid. Hydrochloric acid (HCl), the acid in the stomach, is a strong acid. A *base* is a substance that decreases the concentration of hydrogen ions. The fewer the hydrogen ions, the higher the pH. If the pH is above 7.0, the substance is a base (alkali).

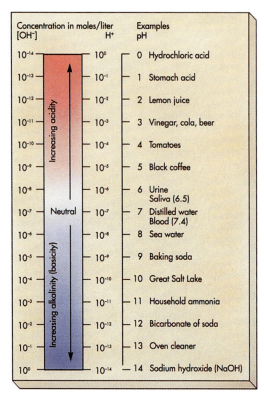

FIGURE 4-59 ▲ The pH scale. A reading of seven is considered neutral. Values less than seven are considered acidic; values higher than seven are considered basic. (From Seeley R: *Anatomy and physiology,* ed 3, St Louis, 1995, Mosby.)

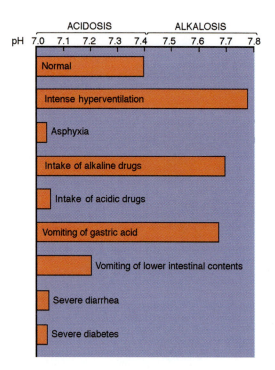

FIGURE 4-60 ▲ This graph shows the comparative pH levels in the body under various circumstances.

Acid is a normal waste product of the body's working cells. The pH in the body is a balance between the amount of acid that is produced and the amount of acid that is eliminated from the body. Body fluids must stay within this pH range to prevent serious illness. A pH above 7.45 is called *alkalosis,* whereas a pH below 7.35 is referred to as *acidosis.* Even a slight change in pH can be harmful.

BODY MECHANISMS TO MAINTAIN NORMAL ACID-BASE BALANCE

The acid-base balance of the body is highly dynamic. It varies as a result of wide fluctuations in the intake and production of acids. When changes occur in the body's acid-base balance, homeostatic mechanisms attempt to compensate. The body depends on three principal mechanisms to maintain its pH: buffer systems, the lungs, and the kidneys. These key body systems must continually readjust to maintain the acid-base balance (Figure 4-60).

Buffer System Compensation for Acid-Base Changes—A *buffer* is any substance that can reversibly bind hydrogen ions. *Buffer systems* are the fastest-acting defenses, providing almost immediate protection against changes in the hydrogen ion concentration of the extracellular fluid. Buffers act as a chemical sponge, absorbing hydrogen ions when they are in excess and donating hydrogen ions when they are depleted. The generic reaction looks like this:

$$\text{Buffer} + H^+ \leftarrow \text{H-buffer}$$

Free hydrogen ions (acid) bind with the buffer to form a weak acid (H-buffer). When the hydrogen ion concentration increases, the reaction is forced to the right and more hydrogen ions bind to the buffer, as long as available buffer is present. When the hydrogen ion concentration decreases, the reaction shifts toward the left and hydrogen ions are released from the buffer (Figure 4-61).

Three Buffer Systems—The proteins of the cells and plasma, as well as blood phosphate, act as weak buffers in the body. The body's major buffer system is the *bicarbonate/carbonic acid (HCO_4-H_2CO_3) buffer system.* The carbonic acid can then further break down into water (H_2O) and carbon dioxide (CO_2).

The buffer system is much more capable of dealing with acidosis than with alkalosis. Twenty buffers (bicarbonate) are available to combine with excess acid for every one buffer (carbonic acid) available to combine with excess base. This ratio is important because normal cellular metabolism produces an excess of acid. As long as the ratio is maintained, the pH is normal. When a pathological condition leads to an excess of acid or base, the buffer combines with the excess substance to

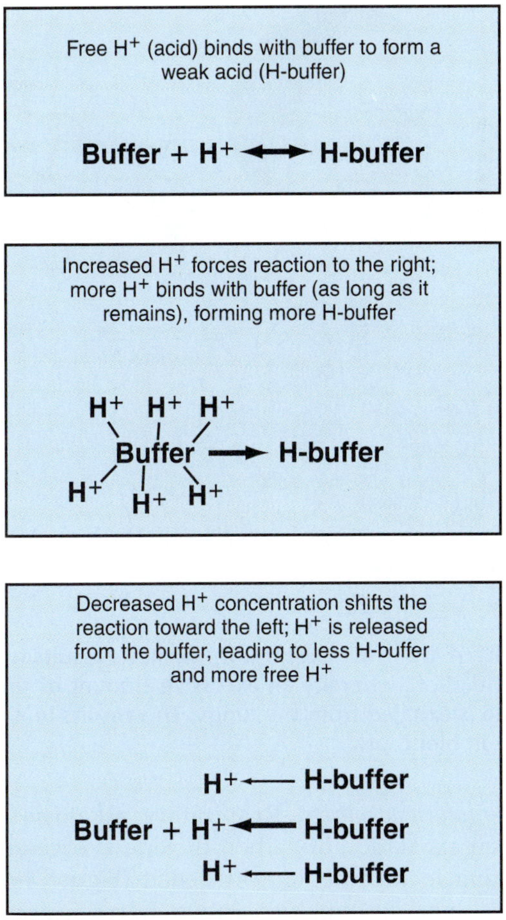

Decreased ventilation increases carbon dioxide and carbonic acid (and therefore hydrogen ions) in the blood, decreasing blood pH. The additional amount of carbonic acid may provide an additional buffering power in the face of alkalosis by lowering the pH. For example:

$$\downarrow \text{Breathing} \rightarrow \uparrow CO_2 \rightarrow \uparrow H_2CO_3 \rightarrow \uparrow H^+ \rightarrow \downarrow pH$$

Patients who are not breathing or who are breathing inadequately are likely to be acidotic because of an inadequate removal of carbon dioxide. In these cases the treatment must focus on improving ventilation.

However, patients who have metabolic acidosis (see Respiratory Versus Metabolic Processes), as in diabetic ketoacidosis, often hyperventilate to remove carbon dioxide from the bloodstream and decrease the acidosis. This situation is also true for the trauma patient. The metabolic acidosis produced by anaerobic metabolism is identified by the respiratory center in the brain. Signals are sent out to increase the respiration and eliminate more carbon dioxide.

Renal (Kidney) Compensation for Acid-Base Changes—The kidney's role in maintaining acid-base balance is complex. Very simply, the kidneys excrete hydrogen ions and form bicarbonate ions in specific amounts as indicated by the pH of the blood. When the plasma pH drops (becomes more acidic), hydrogen ions (acid) are excreted and bicarbonate ions (base) are formed and retained. Conversely, when the plasma pH rises (becomes more alkaline), hydrogen ions are retained in the body and bicarbonate ions are excreted. The kidneys are equally able to deal with alkalosis or acidosis, but there is a limitation. Because it takes at least 10 to 20 hours for kidney function to respond to an alteration in pH, the kidneys are excellent for long-term compensation but are unable to stabilize the pH in critical, rapidly developing conditions.

Respiratory Versus Metabolic Processes—Either alkalosis or acidosis can occur because of a primary respiratory or a primary metabolic abnormality. If the underlying defect is respiratory, the amount of carbon dioxide in the blood becomes either too high or too low. This causes a change in the pH quickly and in the opposite direction from the carbon dioxide change. Think of carbon dioxide as respiratory acid—blowing off more of it excretes acid and *raises* the pH; retaining it increases the blood acid level, decreasing the pH. Thus there is either a *respiratory alkalosis* or a *respiratory acidosis*. To compensate for too high or too low levels of carbon dioxide, the kidneys must excrete more or fewer hydrogen ions, depending on the level, which takes time.

On the other hand, if the primary process is metabolic, there is either too much or too little hydrogen ion concentration in the blood ("metabolic acid"), resulting in either a *metabolic acidosis* or a *metabolic alka-*

FIGURE 4-61 ▲ Acid buffering.

weaken it and produce water. For example, when a strong acid is introduced into the bloodstream, bicarbonate, a weak base, combines with it to form a weak acid, carbonic acid:

Hydrogen   Carbonic acid   Carbon dioxide

$$H^+ + HCO_3^- \leftrightarrow H_2CO_3 \leftrightarrow H_2O + CO_2$$

Bicarbonate   Water

Respiratory Compensation for Acid-Base Changes—The respiratory system plays a vital role in maintaining the acid-base balance. It regulates the concentration of carbon dioxide (and subsequently the amount of carbonic acid) in the body. For example, if excess carbon dioxide builds up, the brain detects the increase in carbon dioxide, which causes the respiratory rate to increase. As the respiratory rate increases, carbon dioxide is blown off.

Increased ventilation decreases carbon dioxide and carbonic acid (and therefore hydrogen ions) in the blood, thereby increasing the blood pH. This process helps restore normal pH in the patient who is acidotic. For example:

$$\uparrow \text{Breathing} \rightarrow \downarrow CO_2 \rightarrow \downarrow H_2CO_3 \rightarrow \downarrow H^+ \rightarrow \uparrow pH$$

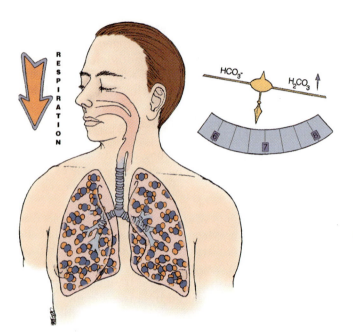

FIGURE 4-62 ▲ Respiratory acidosis occurs when carbon dioxide exhalation is decreased or inhibited, thereby creating a surplus of carbonic acid.

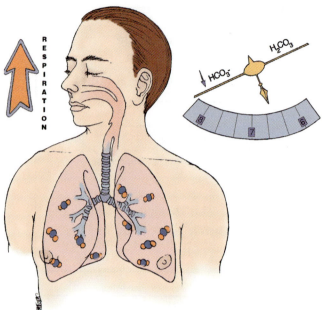

FIGURE 4-63 ▲ Respiratory alkalosis results from hyperventilation, whereby an excessive amount of carbon dioxide is exhaled from the lungs. This results in an increase in blood pH.

losis. When a metabolic problem develops, the body tends to respond quickly by changing ventilation, raising or lowering the carbon dioxide to at least partially compensate for the metabolic change. To *completely correct* metabolic changes requires that the kidneys excrete more or fewer hydrogen ions, depending on the level. This process takes hours to days to occur.

FOUR PRIMARY ACID-BASE DISORDERS

There are four primary acid-base disorders:

- *Respiratory acidosis*—**Respiratory acidosis** occurs when exhalation of carbon dioxide is inhibited (Figure 4-62). In addition to increasing the blood carbon dioxide level and decreasing the blood pH, this imbalance creates a surplus of carbonic acid. Hypoventilation (decreased respiration) is its general cause. Hypoventilation in respiratory acidosis results from problems occurring either in the respiratory center in the brain or in the lungs. Two major conditions that cause hypoventilation are central nervous system depression and obstructive lung disease. Morphine poisoning and anesthesia are examples of central nervous system depression, whereas asthma and emphysema are examples of obstructive lung diseases. Treatment is aimed at improving ventilation. Signs and symptoms of respiratory acidosis include the following:
  - Hypoventilation, seen by shallow respirations or poor exhalation
  - Disorientation and loss of mental alertness progressing to stupor, indicating central nervous system depression

- *Respiratory alkalosis*—**Respiratory alkalosis** occurs when exhalation of carbon dioxide is excessive, resulting in a carbonic acid deficit (Figure 4-63). Its root cause is hyperventilation (rapid respiration), which can be due to fever, anxiety, pain, or pulmonary infections. A hyperventilating patient blows off an increased amount of carbon dioxide, resulting in lowered carbonic acid blood levels. Therefore the blood pH is increased, and the blood carbon dioxide level is decreased. Signs and symptoms include the following:
  - Hyperventilation (deep and/or labored breathing)
  - Sensations of numbness, prickling, or tingling
  - Mental restlessness and agitation progressing to hysteria and finally unresponsiveness
- *Metabolic acidosis*—Metabolic acidosis occurs when the level of bicarbonate (a base) is low in relation to carbonic acid levels (Figure 4-64). The kidneys normally retain bicarbonate or excrete hydrogen ions in response to altered blood pH. Starvation, renal impairment, and diabetes mellitus are among the conditions that flood the plasma with acid metabolites. With renal impairment, related electrolyte imbalances may develop. Prolonged diarrhea can decrease the level of bicarbonate in the body. Treatment is aimed at eliminating carbon dioxide by ventilation. In severe cases the addition of a bicarbonate, such as sodium bicarbonate, may be required. Signs and symptoms of metabolic acidosis include the following:
  - Kussmaul breathing (deep rapid respirations), a compensatory mechanism (although absent in infants)

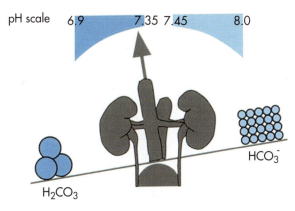

FIGURE 4-64 ▲ Metabolic acidosis occurs when the levels of bicarbonate are low in relation to carbonic acid. (From Sanders M: *Mosby's paramedic textbook,* St Louis, 1994, Mosby.)

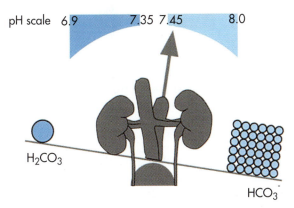

FIGURE 4-65 ▲ Metabolic alkalosis occurs when there is an excess level of bicarbonate in relation to carbonic acid. (From Sanders M: *Mosby's paramedic textbook,* St Louis, 1994, Mosby.)

- Weakness
- Disorientation
- Coma
- *Metabolic alkalosis*—Metabolic alkalosis occurs when the level of bicarbonate is high (Figure 4-65). The blood pH is increased, and the blood carbon dioxide levels are normal. Metabolic alkalosis may be due to excess intake of baking soda or other alkalis, prolonged vomiting, and other conditions that flood plasma with bicarbonate. Prolonged vomiting causes the body to lose chloride and hydrogen ions. Loss of chloride ions causes a proportionate increase of bicarbonate in the blood. Related electrolyte imbalances account for some of the clinical signs. Treatment consists of correcting the underlying cause. Signs and symptoms of metabolic alkalosis include the following:
- Slow, shallow respirations (compensatory)
- Muscular tension
- Tetany (intermittent spasms that involve the extremities)
- Mental dullness

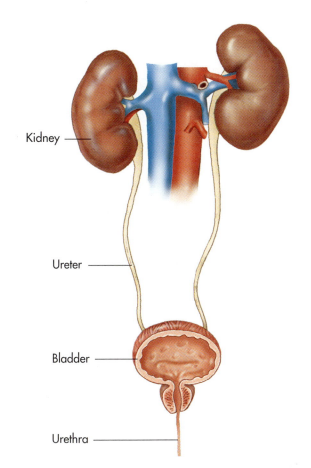

FIGURE 4-66 ▲ The urinary system. (From Sanders MJ: *Mosby's paramedic textbook,* ed 2, St Louis, 2000, Mosby.)

URINARY SYSTEM

The **urinary system** removes waste products from the blood by a complex filtration process. It also is involved in maintaining a proper balance between water and salts in the blood. The major structures of the urinary tract are anatomically intertwined with those of the digestive system. The *kidneys* are located behind the abdominal cavity, in the retroperitoneal space. These solid, bean-shaped organs filter blood and excrete body wastes in the form of urine. The kidneys also are important in the regulation of the body's fluid balance and blood pressure. The *ureters* are a pair of thick-walled hollow tubes that carry urine from the kidneys to the *urinary bladder.* The urinary bladder is a hollow, muscular sac in the midline of the lower abdominal area that stores urine until it is excreted. The *urethra* is a hollow, tubular structure that drains urine from the bladder, passing it to the outside (Figure 4-66).

REPRODUCTIVE SYSTEM

The **reproductive system** includes all of the male and female structures responsible for sexual reproduction.

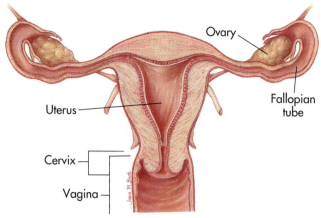

FIGURE 4-67 ▲ **Anatomy of the female reproductive system.** (Joan M. Beck from Seeley R: *Anatomy and physiology*, ed 3, St Louis, 1995, Mosby.)

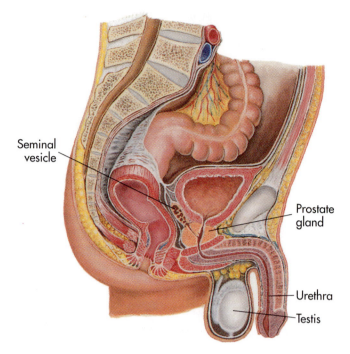

FIGURE 4-68 ▲ **Anatomy of the male reproductive system.** (George J. Wassilchenko from Thibodeau GA, Patton KT: *Structure and function of the body*, ed 3, St Louis, 1992, Mosby.)

Female Reproductive Organs

Organs of the female reproductive system include the following (Figure 4-67):

- The *uterus* is a hollow, pear-shaped organ located in the midline of the lower quadrants. It is the site of implantation, growth, and nourishment of the fetus during pregnancy.
- The *cervix* is the part of the uterus that extends into the vagina. During childbirth the baby passes through the dilated cervix into the vaginal birth canal.
- The *vagina* is the muscular tube that forms the lower part of the female reproductive tract.
- The *fallopian tubes* are two hollow tubes that extend from the uterus to the region of the ovary. These serve as a passage for movement of the ovum from the ovary and for movement of sperm from the uterus upward. The fallopian tube is where fertilization usually occurs.
- The *ovaries* are the female sex glands, and there is usually one on each side of the lower quadrants. These glands produce hormones that regulate female reproductive function and secondary sexual characteristics (breast and pubic hair development), as well as serve as the source of the *ovum*, or egg.

Male Reproductive Organs

Organs of the male reproductive system include the following (Figure 4-68):

- The *testicles*, or *testes*, are the male gonads. The testes are held in a pouch of skin known as the *scrotum*. The testes produce *sperm* and secrete male hormones, such as *testosterone*, that are responsible for secondary sexual characteristics.
- The *prostate gland* is a chestnut-shaped structure located at the base of the urethra. Together with an as-

sociated set of glands, the *seminal vesicles*, the prostate produces secretions that become part of *semen*.

- The *urethra* is a hollow, tubular structure that drains urine from the bladder. It also provides the pathway by which sperm and semen are released from the *penis*, the external male reproductive organ, during sexual intercourse.

SPECIAL SENSORY SYSTEM

The **special sensory system,** the system of the body responsible for the five senses, consists of special nerve receptors that perceive light, sound, taste, odors, and sensations from the skin or areas outside of the body.

Eyes (Vision)

The *eyes* lie within the *bony orbits* of the skull (Figure 4-69). They are held in place by loose connective tissue and several muscles. The muscles also control eye movements. The *optic nerve* enters the *globe*, or *eyeball*, posteriorly through an opening in the orbit called the *optic foramen*. The white part of the eye is called the *sclera*. The colored part of the eye is the *iris*. The iris surrounds the *pupil*, a circular opening through which light passes to the *lens*. The *cornea* is the transparent anterior portion of the eye that overlies the iris and pupil. The *anterior chamber* is the portion of the globe between the lens and the cornea. The anterior chamber is filled with a clear, watery fluid known as *aqueous humor*.

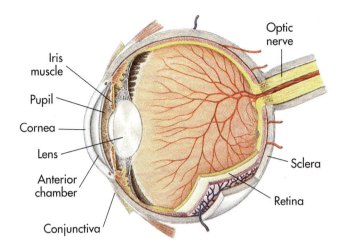

FIGURE 4-69 ▲ Horizontal section of the human eye, as viewed from above. (George J. Wassilchenko and David P. O'Connor from Thibodeau GA, Patton KT: *Structure and function of the body,* ed 3, St Louis, 1992, Mosby.)

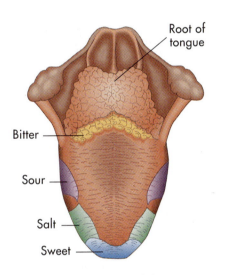

FIGURE 4-70 ▲ The surface of the tongue and the various regions sensitive to taste. (Canalith Repositioning from Thibodeau GA, Patton KT: *Anatomy and physiology,* ed 3, St Louis, 1996, Mosby.)

The *conjunctiva* is a thin, transparent membrane that covers the sclera and internal surfaces of the eyelids and stops at the iris. Tears come from the *lacrimal sacs* and pass through the *lacrimal ducts,* located on the nasal border of the eyelids. Tears are drained by ducts that lead to the nose.

The interior of the eye contains a jellylike material known as *vitreous humor.* At the rear of the interior of the globe lies the *retina.* The retina is a delicate 10-layered structure of nervous tissue that is continuous with the optic nerve. The function of the retina is to receive light, which generates nerve signals that are conducted to the brain by the optic nerve and are interpreted as vision.

Mouth and Tongue (Taste)

The mouth and tongue contain various nerves, called *taste receptors* or *taste buds,* that sense salt and sweet sensations separately. These nerves then transmit impulses back to the taste center of the brain, where they are converted into sensations perceived as taste (Figure 4-70).

Ears (Hearing)

Sound waves enter the ear through the large outside portion (the *auricle,* or *pinnae*). They travel down the ear canal to the eardrum, or *tympanic membrane.* Vibration of sound waves against the tympanic membrane sets up vibrations in three small bones on the other side, called *ossicles (malleus, incus, stapes).* Vibrations of the ossicles are converted into nerve impulses, which are transmitted to the brain via the *auditory nerve.* The brain then converts these impulses into what we experience as sound. The inner portion of the ear helps in maintaining balance (Figure 4-71).

Nose (Smell)

Special receptors, known as *olfactory nerves,* line the nasal cavity. These receptors detect various odors and transmit the message to a large nerve at the base of the brain, the *olfactory bulb.* Sensations of smell from the olfactory bulb are then transmitted to the brain and translated into sensations of smell (Figure 4-72).

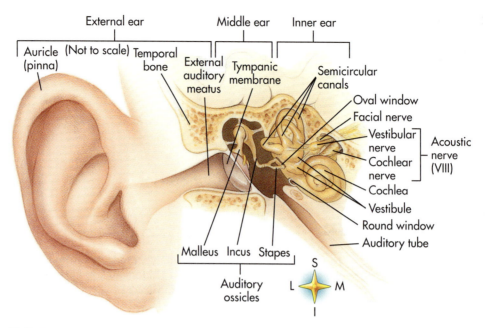

FIGURE 4-71 ▲ The ear. External, middle, and inner ears. (Anatomical structures are not drawn to scale.) (From Thibodeau GA, Patton KT: *Structure and function of the body,* ed 11, St Louis, 2000, Mosby.)

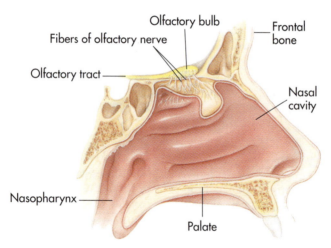

FIGURE 4-72 ▲ Sensations of smell are transmitted from the nasal cavity to the olfactory bulb in the brain. (Christine Oleksyk from Thibodeau GA, Patton KT: *Anatomy and physiology,* ed 3, St Louis, 1996, Mosby.)

EMT–I Jackson and her crew arrive at the trauma center in approximately 7 minutes. The trauma team meets them at the door and takes the patient immediately to the OR.

When EMT–I Jackson returns to the station, she asks the EMT–I student to explain the significance of the anatomical locations of the stab wounds.

"Well," he says, "nothing like putting me right on the spot. So, here goes . . .

"First, the wound at the right anterior axillary line at T4. T4 is the 'nipple line,' and an anterior axillary entry for a knife wound could cause an injury to the right lung, resulting in a pneumothorax, hemothorax, or both, as well as an abdominal injury, including a liver, gallbladder, pancreatic, or intestinal injury, or a major vessel injury in the mediastinum, including the inferior or superior vena cava. Any of these thoracic injuries could rapidly become fatal, whereas the abdominal injuries would pose a great risk for death from hemorrhage and infection.

"Second, the wound at the left midaxillary line at T6. This wound not only poses a serious risk for lung injuries but also poses an even greater risk for cardiac injury. Abdominal penetration would likely involve gastric injury, and should a major vessel have been injured in the mediastinum, it would probably have involved the descending thoracic or abdominal aorta. The patient would most likely have been dead in seconds.

"Third, the left epigastric region wound. If the knife were thrust upward, toward the head, it could have caused diaphragmatic trauma, as well as cardiac injury—and don't men often stab upward? If the knife went in perpendicular to the skin, it may have penetrated the spleen, stomach, pancreas, small intestine, or even a kidney. The patient would definitely have a hemoperitoneum. Depending on the path of the knife, the organs on the right side of the upper left abdomen could have been injured as well, including the liver or gallbladder.

"Fourth, the left midbuttock wound. This one may have injured his ischiadic or sciatic nerve, which may account for the lack of a pain response in his left leg.

"And last, the right anterior midthigh wound. This one typically wouldn't be life threatening unless it struck a major vessel and the patient was losing a significant amount of blood. However, with the 5-cm larger circumference in the right thigh, that may just be the case.

"Well, what do you think?"

EMT–I Jackson responds, "I have to admit, I'm impressed. I'll bet you pass your anatomy test."

Skin (Touch)

The sense of touch is interrelated with the function of the peripheral nervous system. Various touch receptors on the skin detect when and what we touch. Similar receptors also detect heat, cold, and pain. These impulses are transmitted to the spinal cord and then to the brain, where they are brought into conscious reality.

SUMMARY

Important points to remember from this chapter include the following:

- Anatomy is the study of body structures. Physiology is the study of the normal function of these structures, whereas pathophysiology evaluates abnormal function.
- All of the body's systems work together to maintain a state of normal function, known as homeostasis. When one system is altered, the others are necessarily affected.
- An important component of immunity is the integumentary system, consisting of the skin, nails, hair, and sweat and oil glands. This system provides the body's external covering and provides for temperature regulation and protection.
- The various organ systems of the body provide support (skeletal system), movement (muscular system), and overall control of body functions (nervous system).
- The immune system defends the body against invasion by organisms and foreign substances.
- The respiratory system facilitates intake and absorption of oxygen into the blood, which is then delivered to the tissues by the circulatory system.
- Food and water are absorbed by the digestive and lymphatic systems, whereas the endocrine system produces hormones that aid in the metabolism of food, as well as in other chemical processes.
- Body wastes are excreted by combined actions of the urinary (urine), gastrointestinal (stool), and respiratory (carbon dioxide) systems.
- Special sensory systems allow for the senses of vision, taste, hearing, smell, and touch.

5

Emergency Pharmacology

...CASE HISTORY It is 11:00 Thursday morning when EMT–Is Maloney and Rice receive a call to the local elementary school for a patient "with a history of asthma who is having trouble breathing." They arrive in approximately 4 minutes and find the patient, Rosy, age 8, sitting upright and struggling to breathe. She has inspiratory wheezes and diminished breath sounds in all of her lung fields.

EMT–I Maloney takes Rosy's pulse with her gloved hand and checks her blood pressure and pulse oximetry reading as her partner applies 100% oxygen via a nonrebreather mask. The school nurse says to the EMT–Is, "Rosy has used her inhaler about four times since she came in here today, but she hasn't been getting better. It usually works faster than this."

EMT–I Maloney prepares a nebulizer dose of albuterol while her partner takes off his gloves and calls medical direction for orders. The medical direction physician confirms the order, and EMT–I Maloney proceeds with treatment.

LEARNING OBJECTIVES

CHAPTER GOAL
Upon completion of this chapter, the EMT-Intermediate will be able to understand the basic principles of pharmacology and develop a drug profile for common emergency medications.

Cognitive Objectives
As an EMT-Intermediate you should be able to do the following:

- Differentiate among the chemical, generic (nonproprietary), trade (proprietary), and official names of a drug.
- Describe historical trends in pharmacology.
- Describe the five schedules of drugs established by the Drug Enforcement Administration.
- List the five main sources of drug products.
- Describe how drugs are classified.
- List the authoritative sources for drug products.
- Discuss special considerations in drug treatment with regard to pregnant, pediatric, and geriatric patients.

- Discuss the EMT–I's responsibilities and scope of management pertinent to the administration of medications.
- Identify the specific anatomy and physiology pertinent to pharmacology.
- List and describe general properties of drugs.
- List and describe liquid and solid drug forms.
- List and differentiate routes of drug administration.
- Differentiate between enteral and parenteral routes of drug administration.
- Describe mechanisms of drug interactions.
- List and differentiate the phases of drug activity, including the pharmaceutical, pharmacokinetic, and pharmacodynamic phases.
- Describe pharmacokinetics, pharmacodynamics, theories of drug action, drug-response relationships, factors altering drug responses, predictable drug responses, iatrogenic drug responses, and unpredictable adverse drug responses.
- Differentiate among drug interactions.
- Discuss procedures and measures to ensure security of controlled substances that an EMT–I may administer.
- Discuss considerations for storing drugs.
- List the components of a drug profile.
- List and describe drugs that an EMT–I may administer in a pharmacological management plan according to local protocol.
- Integrate pathophysiological principles of pharmacology with patient assessment.
- Synthesize patient history information and assessment findings to form a field impression.
- Synthesize a field impression and implement a pharmacological management plan.

Affective Objectives
As an EMT-Intermediate you should be able to do the following:
- Defend medication administration by an EMT–I to effect a positive therapeutic outcome.

Psychomotor Objectives
- None identified for this chapter.

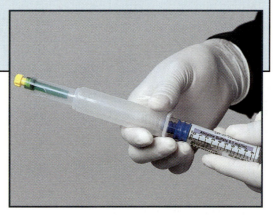

INTRODUCTION

Quick decisions on the part of the EMT–Intermediate (EMT–I) can mean the difference between life and death, especially when administering drugs. A tremendous professional and legal responsibility is involved in carrying, preparing, and administering drugs. If the wrong drug or the incorrect dose of the appropriate drug is given, the results can be fatal.

EMT–Is may administer certain emergency drugs via local protocol or standing orders, with or without contacting medical direction. This chapter includes information on certain emergency drugs and their uses, range of dosages, methods of administration, and side effects. Administration of drugs is an exacting science and can be harmful to the patient when errors are made. It is important for the EMT–I to understand the safety precautions and legal aspects of drug administration.

Continued on p. 116

PHARMACOLOGY AND DRUG NOMENCLATURE

A **drug** is any substance that, when taken into the body, changes one or more of the body's functions (Figure 5-1). For example, a particular drug may raise or lower blood pressure or increase or decrease the heart rate. Drugs are most commonly used in medicine to treat or prevent disease. Drugs are available in many forms and are administered in a variety of ways. **Pharmacology** is the term given to the study of drugs and their actions, dosages, and side effects. Pharmaceutical companies are required to list, in the drug inserts, the chemical compounds, actions, dosages, side effects, indications, and contraindications of the drugs they manufacture.

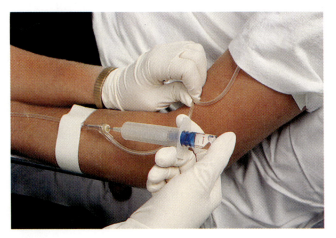

FIGURE 5-1 ▲ **Drugs introduced into the body change one or more of the body's functions. (From American College of Emergency Physicians; Pons PT, Cason D, chief editors: *Paramedic field care: a complaint-based approach,* St Louis, 1997, Mosby for ACEP.)**

> ! **HELPFUL HINT**
>
> • The written direction for the preparation and administration of a drug is called a prescription. In the United States, drugs are usually dispensed on the order of a physician. In some states specially qualified nurse practitioners or physician assistants also may prescribe drugs.

A drug may have as many as four names: chemical, generic, official, and trade. The **chemical name** is the first name given to any drug. It gives the exact description of the chemical structure of the drug. The **generic,** or nonproprietary, **name** is assigned to a drug before it becomes officially listed. It is usually the name suggested by the first manufacturer and is approved by the Food and Drug Administration (FDA). It is usually a simple form of the chemical name of the drug. The **official name** is the name under which the drug is listed in one of the official publications (e.g., the *United States Pharmacopeia* [USP]). When the drug is available for commercial distribution by the original manufacturer, a trade name (also called the brand name or proprietary name) is given. The **trade,** or proprietary, **name** is registered by the U.S. Patent Office and has the official mark of the U.S. Patent Office after its name. For 17 years the original manufacturer of the drug has the exclusive rights to production of the drug. After that time other companies may combine the same chemicals and produce their own generic equivalent of the drug. Each company that markets the drug then assigns its own trade name to its generic equivalent (Table 5-1).

DRUG LEGISLATION

Before 1906 there was little regulation of the use of drugs in the United States. In 1906 the **Pure Food and Drug Act** was passed. It was amended in 1938. The original law was enacted to prevent the manufacture and trafficking of mislabeled, poisonous, or harmful food and drugs. The amended law, called the **Federal Food, Drug, and Cosmetic Act,** required that the safety of a drug be proved before it could be distributed to the public. It also required that labels be used to list the possible habit-forming properties and side effects of drugs.

The **Harrison Narcotic Act of 1914** was the first federal legislation designed to stop drug addiction or dependence. It established federal control over the importation, manufacture, and sale of opium and coca plants and all of their compounds and derivatives. This law has been revised many times to include new and synthetic forms of potentially addictive drugs.

In 1956 the **Narcotic Control Act** was passed to amend the Harrison Act and increase penalties for the law's violation. This act also made the possession of heroin and marijuana illegal. The Bureau of Narcotics and Dangerous Drugs was an agency of the Department of Justice, which kept a registry of physicians who were permitted to give out or prescribe controlled substances.

In 1970 the **Controlled Substances Act,** which regulates the manufacture and distribution of drugs whose use may result in dependency, was passed. It went into effect on May 1, 1971. This act requires that anyone who manufactures, prescribes, administers, or dispenses such controlled substances must register annually with the U.S. Attorney General under the Drug Enforcement Administration. The following five schedules of controlled substances were established by the Drug Enforcement Administration and may be revised annually:

- *Schedule I*—Drugs that have the highest potential for abuse and have no currently accepted medical use in the United States. There is a lack of accepted safety for use of these drugs or substances even under medical supervision. Examples include heroin, marijuana, lysergic acid diethylamide (LSD), peyote, and mescaline.
- *Schedule II*—Drugs that have a high potential for abuse. These drugs have a current accepted medicinal use in the United States, but with severe restrictions. Abuse of a Schedule II drug can lead to either psychological or physiological dependence. A Schedule II drug requires a written prescription that must be filled within 72 hours of when it was written. A Schedule II drug cannot be refilled or called into the pharmacy by a medical office. Examples include morphine, codeine, secobarbital (Seconal), cocaine, amphetamines, hydromorphone (Dilaudid), and methylphenidate (Ritalin).
- *Schedule III*—Drugs that have a limited potential for psychological or physiological dependence. The prescription may be called in to the pharmacist by the physician and refilled up to five times in a 6-month period. Schedule III drugs have a limited amount of opium, codeine, or morphine. Examples include paregoric, acetaminophen with codeine (Tylenol with Codeine), and aspirin combined with caffeine and butalbital (Fiorinal).
- *Schedule IV*—Drugs that have a lower potential for abuse than those in Schedules II and III. Schedule IV drugs can be called in to the pharmacist by the medical office and may be refilled up to five times in a 6-month period. Examples include chlordiazepoxide (Librium), diazepam (Valium), propoxyphene (Darvon), and phenobarbital.
- *Schedule V*—Drugs that have a lower potential for abuse than those in Schedules I, II, III, and IV. These drugs are used for relief of coughs or diarrhea and contain limited amounts of certain narcotics. Examples include difenoxin/atropine sulfate diphenoxylate/atropine (Lomotil), brompheniramine (Dimetane Expectorant-DC), and guaifenesin (Robitussin-DAC).

REGULATING AGENCIES

Because the administration of drugs in the United States is controlled by law, several agencies have a role in monitoring and enforcing drug legislation. The **Federal Trade Commission** regulates drug advertising. The **Food and Drug Administration (FDA)** was established to review drug applications and petitions for food addi-

TABLE 5-1

Drug Names

Chemical name	2-(diethylamino)-N-(2, 6-dimethylphenyl) -,monohydrochloride
Generic name	Lidocaine hydrochloride
Trade name	Xylocaine
Chemical name	Glycerol trinitrate
Generic name	Nitroglycerin
Trade name	Nitro-Bid
Chemical name	7-Chloro-1, 3-dihydro-1-methyl-5-phenyl-2H-1, 4-benzodiazepine-2-one
Generic name	Diazepam
Trade name	Valium

tives; inspect factories where drugs, cosmetics, and foods are made; and remove unsafe drugs from the market. The FDA also ensures that the labels on food, drugs, and cosmetics are correct.

In 1970 the **Drug Enforcement Administration (DEA)** was established to oversee the control of dangerous drugs. The DEA is concerned with controlled substances only and enforces laws against the manufacture, sale, and use of illegal drugs. The DEA is also responsible for revising the list of drugs included in the schedules of controlled substances. The **Public Health Service** of the U.S. Department of Health and Human Services inspects and licenses establishments that manufacture drugs.

SOURCES OF DRUGS

At the beginning of the twentieth century, most illnesses were treated by drugs manufactured solely from plant, animal, and mineral substances. Many "secret" elixirs sold to the public and allegedly effective against a wide variety of ailments were little more than alcohol or illicit drugs. As medical science began to understand the exact mechanism of disease, researchers worked to develop more drugs to combat illnesses. Tremendous progress has been made in the development of drugs. New technologies now permit the synthetic manufacture of drugs previously unheard of. Most drugs may be derived from five different sources:

* *Plants*—Most parts of plants, including leaves, flowers, seeds, and roots, have at one time been used as drugs. For example, digitalis, a drug used to treat heart failure, is derived from the leaves of the purple foxglove flower. Morphine and opiates (opium products) are derived from the poppy plant. A further breakdown of plants includes the following:
  * *Alkaloids*—This is one of a large group of nitrogenous substances found in plants that are usually bitter; many are pharmacologically active. Examples are atropine and morphine.
  * *Glycosides*—This is a compound that contains a carbohydrate molecule (sugar) that can be found in plants. Digitalis, for example, is a cardiac glycoside that increases the force of contraction of cardiac muscle and is also used as an *antiarrhythmic*.
  * *Gums*—An excretion from various plants from which certain drugs are derived. For example, xanthan is a high-molecular-weight polysaccharide gum that when processed is used as a suspending agent in pharmaceutical preparations.
  * *Oils*—Plant oils may be used in various pharmacological preparations. For example, eucalyptus oil is a volatile oil distilled with steam from the fresh leaf of *Eucalyptus globulus* and is used as a flavor in pharmaceutical preparations and as an expectorant and local antiseptic with mild anesthetic effect.

* *Animals and humans*—Many different parts of animals have been used as drug sources, including proteins and enzymes. Substances such as epinephrine and insulin are derived from animals.
* *Minerals or mineral products*—Inorganic materials used as drugs are usually the refined forms of minerals, such as iodine, calcium, iron, and Epsom salts.
* *Synthetic sources*—Most drugs used today are manufactured in a pharmaceutical laboratory, even if they were originally available in one of the previously mentioned forms.
* *Microorganisms*—Some drugs such as penicillin and streptomycin are actually from a microorganism source.

DRUG CLASSIFICATION

Drugs can be classified into three categories:
* *Body system*—One way drugs are classified is by identifying what body system they affect. Since the vast majority of emergency drugs are used in the treatment of cardiac emergencies, they would be classified as affecting the cardiovascular system. Other drugs might impact the skeletal system or the respiratory system. Knowing which body system a drug affects helps the EMT–I understand how the body will react to a particular drug.
* *Class of agent*—The class of agent identifies how drugs affect a particular body system. For instance, drugs that are available for the control of seizure disorders are classified as anticonvulsants. Drugs that inhibit or block acetylcholine are referred to as anticholinergics. And, as discussed earlier, cardiac glycosides are naturally occurring plant substances that have characteristic effects on the heart.
* *Mechanism of action*—The mechanism of action refers to how the drug works physiologically. For instance, lidocaine decreases ventricular automaticity and excitability and raises the fibrillation threshold. It decreases conduction in ischemic cardiac tissue without adversely affecting normal conduction.

SOURCES OF DRUG INFORMATION

There are several references of drug information. The *Physicians' Desk Reference* (PDR) is widely used as a reference for drugs in current use. It contains such information as each drug's indications, therapeutic effects, dosages, administration, warnings, contraindications, precautions, side effects, and drug interactions. It also in-

HELPFUL HINT
The *Physicians' Desk Reference* (PDR) is written to be used by physicians but is readily available to the general public in offices, libraries, and bookstores.

cludes photographs of various drugs. The information is essentially the same as that included in the package insert required by the FDA in prescription medications.

Some other sources of drug information include the following:

- **American Hospital Formulary Service**—This service is distributed to practicing physicians and contains concise information that is arranged according to drug classifications.
- *Compendium of Drug Therapy*—This is published annually and is distributed to practicing physicians. It includes photographs of the drugs and phone numbers of major pharmaceutical companies and poison control centers. It also includes copies of some package inserts.
- **American Medical Association Drug Evaluation**—Drugs are evaluated according to the American Medical Association's standards.
- **Drug Inserts**—These are found in all drug packages. They supply detailed information about the drug. Many drug inserts contain the same information that is contained in the PDR.

STANDARDIZATION OF DRUGS

All drugs sold in the United States must meet and maintain high standards for therapeutic results, patient safety, and packaging safety. To meet these standards, drugs must go through strict and accurate testing, which may take several years to complete. There are several techniques available for measuring a drug's strength and purity. Two such methods are the assay and bioassay methods. An assay is an analysis or examination of a drug. A bioassay determines the strength or biological activity of a drug by noting its effect on a live animal or an isolated organ preparation, as compared with the effect of a standard preparation. The FDA is responsible for final approval of all drugs.

The **United States Pharmacopeia** (USP) consists of two volumes of drug standards for the health care provider. It defines drugs with respect to sources, chemistry, physical properties, tests to identify, storage, and dosage. It also provides directions for compounding and general use. The USP does not contain photographs of the drugs and, unlike the PDR, which is sometimes distributed to physicians at no charge, must be purchased.

SPECIAL CONSIDERATIONS IN DRUG THERAPY

Pregnant Patients

The EMT–I should always determine whether the patient is pregnant when administering drugs to a woman of childbearing age (Figure 5-2). The expected benefits should be weighed against the possible risks to the fe-

tus. Drugs that are ingested, inhaled, or absorbed by the mother have the potential to harm the fetus by crossing the placenta or through lactation. Examples of emergency drugs that rapidly cross the placenta are lidocaine, propranolol, and diazepam.

During pregnancy the metabolism in the liver is delayed and the rate of drug excretion may be increased because of the increased cardiac output.

The FDA has established a scale, with categories A, B, C, D, and X, to indicate drugs that may have documented problems in animals or humans during pregnancy. Despite this, the EMT–I should be aware that there are still many drugs whose effects are unknown during pregnancy.

Pediatric Patients

Drug dosage is based on a child's weight or body surface area rather than age (Figure 5-3), so it is important to determine the body weight of a child as soon as possible. Parents are usually the most reliable and quickest sources of such information.

Infants have immature livers and kidneys, so it is difficult for them to metabolize and eliminate the same dosages of drugs as adults. Thus in the very young, dosages of some medication must be altered to avoid adverse or toxic reactions.

Volume overload, especially in the small child, is another serious problem. The rate of fluid administration must be carefully monitored.

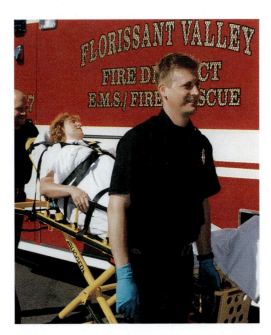

FIGURE 5-2 ▲ Drugs that are ingested, inhaled, or absorbed by the mother have the potential to harm the fetus by crossing the placenta or through lactation. (From Sanders MJ: *Mosby's paramedic textbook*, ed 2, St Louis, 2000, Mosby.)

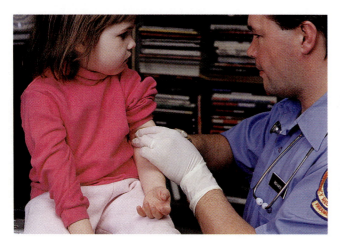
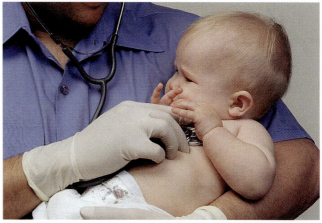

FIGURE 5-3 ▲ The drug dosage for pediatric patients is based on a child's weight or body surface area. (From American College of Emergency Physicians; Pons PT, Cason D, chief editors: *Paramedic field care: a complaint-based approach*, St Louis, 1997, Mosby for ACEP.)

Geriatric Patients

Drug-induced illness is common in elderly people. Elderly patients may take more medications, have more illnesses, and have more adverse effects from drugs than younger patients. Because of the potential contribution of polypharmacy to the clinical situation, an accurate history of specific drug use is essential and must be collected from patients, family, friends, pharmacies, and physicians (Figure 5-4).

The absorption of a drug is affected by gastric pH, motility, and ingestion of a fatty meal. The distribution of a drug is affected significantly by changes in the percentage of body fat. As people age, a change in body composition results in an increase in the percentage of body fat, a decrease in lean body mass, and a decrease in total body water. Drugs such as acetaminophen, morphine, and meperidine, which are adjusted according to body weight, appear in significantly higher concentration in a 70-year-old patient than in a 30-year-old patient. This concentration can be important if the drug has a narrow therapeutic range.

Most drugs are eliminated through the kidneys or metabolized by the liver. As a person ages, both of these systems experience changes, and these changes ultimately affect drug clearance. Drugs such as digoxin and lithium, which have a narrow therapeutic index, must be administered in decreased dosages as the patient ages, because renal function and renal blood flow both decrease with age. Blood flow through the liver also declines with age, particularly in the presence of congestive heart failure. The liver also decreases in size. Therefore several important factors of drug metabolism and clearance in the elderly patient should be considered.

SCOPE OF MANAGEMENT

One important responsibility of an EMT–I is to be able to administer medications. The basic principle of medicine is "First, do no harm." Most experienced practitioners are reluctant to administer a medication to a patient unless it is clearly needed. The medications used in prehospital care are some of the most potent available, and administration routes often leave no room for error (Figure 5-5).

An EMT–I is held responsible for safe and therapeutically effective drug administration. To provide safe, effective care that has a positive effect on patient outcome, the EMT–I must have an excellent working knowledge of both general pharmacological principles and drugs used in the prehospital environment. In addition, EMT–Is are personally responsible—legally, morally, and ethically—for each drug they administer.

The EMT–I must also be familiar with common home medications. Besides allowing for anticipation of possible drug interactions, knowledge about a patient's current medications can provide information about the patient's medical history.

Proper procedures in using drug therapy include the following:
- Use correct precautions and techniques.
- Observe and document the effects of drugs.
- Keep your knowledge base current with changes and trends in pharmacology.
- Establish and maintain professional relationships.
- Understand pharmacology.
- Perform evaluations to identify drug indications and contraindications.
- Seek drug reference literature.
- Take a drug history from the patient, including prescribed medications (name, strength, daily dosage),

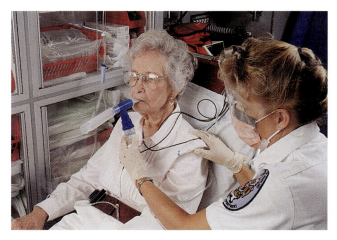

FIGURE 5-4 ▲ Drug metabolism and clearance in the elderly patient should be considered before administration of medications. (From American College of Emergency Physicians; Pons PT, Cason D, chief editors: *Paramedic field care: a complaint-based approach,* St Louis, 1997, Mosby for ACEP.)

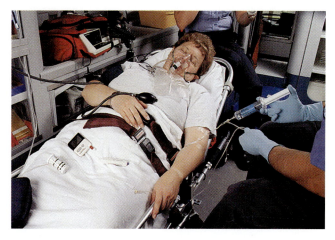

FIGURE 5-5 ▲ It is important for EMT–Is to understand all of the emergency drugs in their protocol, including the drugs' indications, range of dosages, methods of administration, side effects, and safety precautions for their use. (From American College of Emergency Physicians; Pons PT, Cason D, chief editors: *Paramedic field care: a complaint-based approach,* St Louis, 1997, Mosby for ACEP.)

over-the counter medications, vitamins, herbal preparations, and drug reactions.
● Consult with medical control.

NERVOUS SYSTEM COMPONENTS

As previously discussed (see Chapter 4), the nervous system includes the brain and spinal cord, as well as other nerves of the body. The nervous system maintains and controls all body functions by voluntary and autonomic (involuntary) responses. The two large divisions of the nervous system are the central nervous system, which consists of the brain and spinal cord, and the peripheral nervous system, which consists of motor and sensory nerves that carry information to and from the central nervous system (this system includes the somatic nervous system, which conveys information from the central nervous system to the skeletal muscles, and the **autonomic nervous system,** which regulates the internal environment of the body). The somatic nervous system produces movement only in skeletal muscle tissue. It is under conscious control and therefore voluntary. The autonomic nervous system consists of specialized peripheral nerves that control activities automatically. The autonomic nervous system is further subdivided into the sympathetic and parasympathetic nervous systems. The sympathetic part of the autonomic nervous system tends to act as an accelerator of body functions, and the parasympathetic part acts as a balance for the body.

Autonomic Nervous System

Many of the drugs used in the field of emergency medical services affect tissues and organs that receive their nerve impulses from the autonomic nervous system. This discussion of the autonomic nervous system will help explain the effects of various drugs on the human body (Figure 5-6).

The nervous system is divided into two basic components: the voluntary and the involuntary (autonomic) systems. The voluntary system is under the control of conscious thought and controls voluntary movement. The involuntary, or autonomic, nervous system controls "vegetative" functions of life by affecting vital organ functions.

The autonomic system is further broken down into two divisions, which tend to act in a reciprocal manner. Most organs are dominated by one component or the other. The two divisions are the sympathetic and the parasympathetic (Figure 5-7 and Table 5-2).

SYMPATHETIC DIVISION

The **sympathetic division** (sometimes called the *adrenergic division*) originates in the brain. Messages are sent out to the organs by two "sympathetic chains" that leave the spinal cord at approximately the first thoracic vertebra and end at approximately the second lumbar vertebra.

> ● **HELPFUL HINT**
> ● The term *adrenergic* comes from "adrenalin," a synonym for epinephrine.

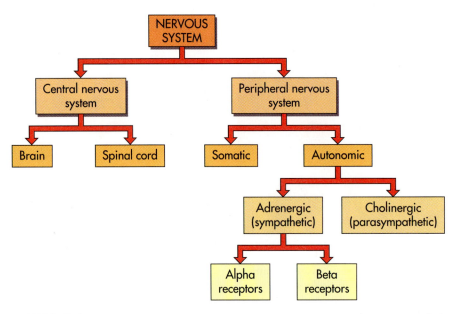

FIGURE 5-6 ▲ Overview of the nervous system. (From Sanders MJ: *Mosby's paramedic textbook,* ed 2, St Louis, 2000, Mosby.)

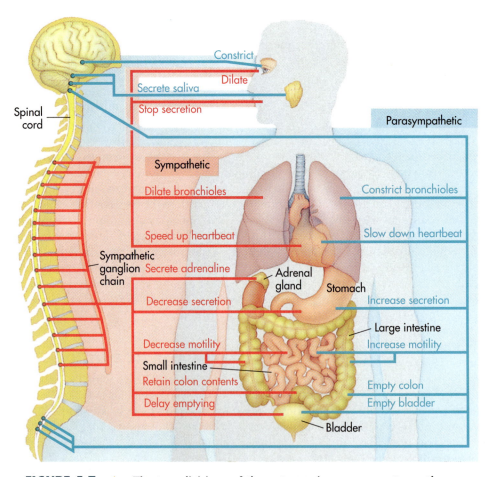

FIGURE 5-7 ▲ The two divisions of the autonomic nervous system—the sympathetic and the parasympathetic—allow for involuntary control of body systems and function in maintaining homeostasis or balance. The parasympathetic fibers are highlighted with blue, and the sympathetic fibers are highlighted with red. (From Thibodeau GA, Patton KT: *Structure and function of the body,* ed 11, St Louis, 2000, Mosby.)

TABLE 5-2

Autonomic Innervation of Target Tissues

ORGAN	EFFECT OF SYMPATHETIC STIMULATION	EFFECT OF PARASYMPATHETIC STIMULATION
Heart		
Muscle	Increased rate and force*	Slowed rate†
Coronary arteries	Dilation*‡, constriction*§	Dilation†
Systemic blood vessels		
Abdomen	Constriction§	None
Skin	Constriction§	None
Muscle	Dilation*‡, constriction§	None
Lungs		
Bronchi	Dilation*	Constriction†
Skeletal muscles	Breakdown of glycogen to glucose*	None
Metabolism	Increase of up to 100%§	None
Glands		
Adrenal glands	Release of epinephrine and norepinephrine†	None
Salivary glands	Constriction of blood vessels and slight production of thick, viscous secretion§	Dilation of blood vessels and thin, copious secretion†
Gastric glands	Inhibition§	Stimulation†
Pancreas	Inhibition§	Stimulation†
Lacrimal glands	None	Secretion†
Sweat glands		
Merocrine glands	Copious, watery secretion†	None
Apocrine glands	Thick, organic secretion†	None
Gut		
Wall	Decreased tone*	Increased mobility†
Sphincter	Increased tone	Decreased tone†
Gallbladder and bile ducts	Relaxation*	Contraction†
Urinary Bladder		
Wall	Relaxation*	Contraction†
Sphincter	Contraction§	Relaxation†
Eye		
Ciliary muscle	Relaxation for far vision*	Contraction for near vision†
Pupil	Dilation§	Constriction†
Arrector pili muscle	Contraction§	None
Blood	Increased coagulation§	None
Sex organs	Ejaculation§	Erection†

*Mediated by beta receptors.
†Mediated by cholinergic receptors.
‡Normally, there is increased blood flow through the coronary arteries as a result of sympathetic stimulation of the heart because of increased demand by cardiac tissue for oxygen. In experiments that isolate the coronary arteries, however, sympathetic nerve stimulation, acting through alpha receptors, causes vasoconstriction. The beta receptors are relatively insensitive to sympathetic nerve stimulation but can be activated by drugs.
§Mediated by alpha receptors.

The primary effect of sympathetic stimulation is an increased heart rate, bronchiole dilation, and increased metabolism and strength. These responses prepare the body for **fight or flight** when in a dangerous situation. When the sympathetic division is stimulated, impulses are transmitted electrically along the nerve fibers until they reach a synapse, or nerve junction. At this point, the transfer of the impulse across the synapse is carried by a chemical neurotransmitter called norepinephrine. This transfer also occurs at the organ to be affected.

Norepinephrine is stored and manufactured at the presynaptic neuron. When an impulse crosses, norepinephrine is secreted into the synapse. Then it is free to act on the organ or postsynaptic neuron. The effect of norepinephrine lasts only a few seconds. Any remaining norepinephrine is either absorbed by the presynaptic neuron or destroyed by an enzyme known as monoamine oxidase. In addition, whenever the sympathetic division is stimulated, epinephrine is released from the adrenal medulla, causing a more prolonged response.

Sympathetic Receptors—The two different types of receptors in the sympathetic division are the alpha (α)–adrenergic and beta (β)–adrenergic receptors. Alpha receptors are separated into alpha-1 (α_1) and alpha-2 (α_2) receptors, and beta receptors are separated into beta-1 (β_1) and beta-2 (β_2) receptors.

When α-adrenergic receptors are stimulated, vasoconstriction results. The effect of an alpha agonist on any organ depends on the type and quantity of receptors. The heart is not directly affected by alpha agonists because it has few α-adrenergic receptors.

When β_1-adrenergic receptors are stimulated, they cause an increase in the heart's contractility and force (inotropic effect), rate and automaticity (chronotropic effect), and conduction of impulses (dromotropic effect). They also cause slight vasodilation in skeletal muscle. Stimulation of β_2-adrenergic receptors results in bronchodilation.

Drugs that are sympathetic division agonists usually are described by their effect on α-adrenergic and β-adrenergic receptors. For example, a group of drugs commonly used in the treatment of asthma because of their bronchodilation effects are called beta-2 agonists. Specific examples include metaproterenol and albuterol.

Drugs That Affect the Sympathetic Division—Several drugs encountered in prehospital care are sympathetic agonists or activators. Although a few are pure alpha or beta, most have both alpha and beta effects, usually with one or the other being predominant. Some drugs, such as dopamine, have dose-related effects and may act as alpha or beta receptors depending on the dosages given. Some drugs are even selective in a beta category, affecting β_2-adrenergic receptors only.

Another commonly encountered class of drugs is the beta blockers, which are prescribed for hypertension, angina, and dysrhythmias because of their beta antagonistic actions. They occupy β-adrenergic receptors and prevent agonists, such as some of those previously discussed, from activating receptors. One of the most common beta blockers is propranolol.

PARASYMPATHETIC DIVISION

The **parasympathetic division** of the autonomic nervous system (also called the cholinergic division, derived from "acetylcholine") originates in the brain and sends messages to affect organs innervated by the cranial nerves. Pairs of cranial nerves exit directly from the brain and travel to organs without using the spinal cord as a conduit. The tenth cranial nerves, or vagus nerves, are the primary nerves of the parasympathetic division and account for approximately 75% of actions caused by parasympathetic stimulation, which affects the heart, stomach, and gastrointestinal tract.

Parasympathetic stimulation also causes increased activity in the gut for digestion. Its effects on the lungs are slight, causing only minimal bronchoconstriction. Blood vessels are not affected by parasympathetic stimulation.

When the parasympathetic division is stimulated, impulses travel along the cranial nerves. At neuron synapses and at the junction between the nerve and effector organs, the primary neurotransmitter substance is acetylcholine.

Drugs That Affect the Parasympathetic Division—Acetylcholine crosses the synapse to reach a postsynaptic neuron or effector organ. It then occupies receptor sites and is broken down by the enzyme cholinesterase. This action lasts only a few seconds at most. Cholinesterase breaks acetylcholine into acetic acid and choline. Choline is then transported back and reused in the manufacture of new acetylcholine.

Atropine, a drug commonly used in prehospital care for cardiovascular conditions, is an acetylcholine antagonist or blocker. It occupies receptor sites and prevents a parasympathetic response. It increases the heart rate by raising the discharge rate of the sinoatrial node and increases conduction through the atrioventricular node.

It is not possible to administer acetylcholine as a drug because it is broken down by cholinesterase in the blood and at synapses before it can occupy receptors. Some drugs mimic its actions, however, and can cause parasympathetic stimulation. Muscarine, a poison found in mushrooms, and pilocarpine, a drug used to treat glaucoma, are examples of these drugs.

Other drugs inhibit the breakdown of acetylcholine by cholinesterase, potentiating the parasympathetic response. Poisons such as organophosphates are such inhibitors. Accidental exposure to these poisons results in severe parasympathetic overstimulation. This condition is counteracted by using atropine as an antagonist to acetylcholine. Other drugs such as physostigmine, neostigmine, and edrophonium are also cholinesterase inhibitors. All of these drugs can be counteracted by the administration of atropine.

GENERAL PROPERTIES OF DRUGS

Drugs are commonly categorized by their effects on body function. All drugs cause cellular change, which is their **drug action,** and a degree of physiological change, which is their **drug effect.** Drug actions are achieved by a physiochemical interaction between the drug and certain tissue components in the body (usually receptors), and in general they exert multiple actions rather than a single effect. Drugs do not confer any new functions on a tissue or organ; they only modify existing functions (Figure 5-8). Drugs that interact with receptors are as follows:

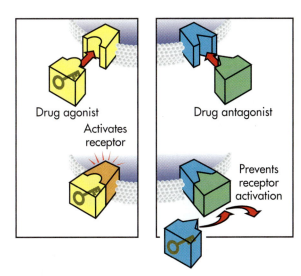

FIGURE 5-8 ▲ **Both a drug agonist and a drug antagonist must fit into a specific receptor site found on the membrane of the target cell to exhibit an effect. An "agonist" promotes an action, and an "antagonist" prevents an action. (From American College of Emergency Physicians; Pons PT, Cason D, chief editors:** *Paramedic field care: a complaint-based approach,* **St Louis, 1997, Mosby for ACEP.)**

- **Agonists**—Drugs that interact with a receptor to stimulate a response.
- **Antagonists**—Drugs that attach to a receptor prevent a response.
- **Partial agonists**—Drugs that interact with a receptor to stimulate a response but inhibit other responses.

Once administered, drugs go through four stages: absorption, distribution, metabolism, and excretion. These stages are described under Pharmacokinetics.

DRUG FORMS

Because of the EMT–I's mission of acute care and resuscitation in the prehospital setting, most drugs, to be effective, must be administered quickly and show actions rapidly. Therefore most of the medications used are injected and are usually in liquid form. The drug forms described in Tables 5-3 and 5-4 give a perspective on common drug preparations.

ROUTES FOR DRUG ADMINISTRATION

There are many routes by which a drug can be administered. The route of administration is crucial in determining the suitability of a drug, since it affects the rate at which the onset of action occurs and may affect the therapeutic response that results (Figure 5-9). Drugs are

given for either local or systemic effects. Sometimes a given route is selected because of cost, safety, or the speed with which the drug will be absorbed into the system. Certain drugs:
- May be administered by only one route
- May be toxic if given by a particular route
- May not be effective if given by a certain route
- May be given for either their local or systemic effects
- Can be absorbed only by a certain route

In the prehospital setting, the intravenous (IV) route is the most commonly used because it results in the quickest actions, but it also can be the most hazardous. The intramuscular route is commonly used in a nonemergency setting in the hospital because the muscles are highly vascular and absorption is fairly rapid. However, incorrect placement of the needle during an intramuscular injection could cause the medication to be delivered intravenously, cause nerve damage, or cause the penetration of blood vessels, resulting in the formation of a hematoma.

☀STUDENT ALERT_____
You must use aseptic techniques whenever administering medications.

Many drugs are available in unit-dose packages that contain the amount of the drug for a single dose, in the proper form for administration. Unit-dose packages are labeled with the trade name, generic name, precautions, instructions for storage, and an expiration date. The three general routes of drug administration are enteral, parenteral, and inhalation or endotracheal.

Enteral Route

The drugs given by the **enteral** route are administered along any portion of the gastrointestinal tract. These include the sublingual, buccal, oral, rectal, and nasogastric routes:
- **Sublingual**—The drug is placed under the patient's tongue and must not be swallowed. The drug is dissolved by the saliva in the mouth and is absorbed into the bloodstream through the vascular oral mucosa. The number of drugs administered sublingually is limited. Nitroglycerin is the most frequently prescribed sublingual drug and is used to treat angina pectoris. To administer the drug, the EMT–I places the tablet under the patient's tongue, where it is dissolved. The patient should avoid drinking fluids while the drug is being absorbed. Swallowing the drug may diminish or delay the effects.

TABLE 5-3

Solid Forms of Drugs

FORM	DESCRIPTION
Capsule	A powdered or granulated drug enclosed in a gelatin capsule designed to dissolve quickly in the stomach
Cream	A nongreasy, semisolid preparation used on the skin
Enteric (coated) tablet	A compressed dry form of a drug coated to withstand the stomach acidity and dissolve in the intestines (These tablets may be drugs that would be destroyed by the stomach enzymes or might be damaging to the stomach lining. They are never to be crushed or broken.)
Lozenge	A firm, compressed form of a drug, usually for a local effect in the mouth or throat (Patients should be cautioned to let lozenges dissolve slowly and avoid drinking any fluids for a period of time after using the lozenge.)
Ointment	A semisolid preparation of one or more drugs for prolonged contact with the skin; intended to be difficult to wash off
Pill	One or more drugs mixed with a cohesive material in an oval, round, or flattened shape
Powder	A drug ground into fine powder
Suppository	One or more drugs mixed in a firm base that dissolves gradually at body temperature; shaped for insertion into the body
Time-release capsule	A gelatin capsule filled with forms of the drug that will dissolve over a period of time rather than all at once
Tablet	A powdered drug compressed into a hard, small disk; may be found in many colors for easy identification; will usually dissolve high in the gastrointestinal tract; may be broken into halves or quarters only if it has been scored for that purpose

TABLE 5-4

Liquid Forms of Drugs

FORM	DESCRIPTION
Aqueous solution	One or more drugs dissolved in water
Liniment	An oily liquid used on the skin
Lotion	An emollient liquid that may be used on irritated or inflamed skin with a minimum of rubbing
Aerosol spray or foam	A liquid, powder, or foam deposited in a thin layer on the skin by air pressure
Elixir	A drug dissolved in alcohol and added flavoring; less sweet than syrups and usually preferred by adults; should not be used for patients with alcoholism or diabetes
Emulsion	A drug combined with water and oil; must be thoroughly shaken to disperse the medication evenly
Extract	A very concentrated form of drug made from vegetables or animals; may be administered as drops and usually given in a liquid to disguise the very strong taste
Fluid extract	An alcohol solution of a drug from a vegetable source; most concentrated of all fluid preparations
Paste	A drug suspended in a thin gelatin or paste base
Spirit	A concentrated alcohol solution of a volatile substance
Suspension	Finely ground drug that is dissolved in a liquid, such as water; must be shaken well before administering
Syrup	A very sweet form of medication because of a high sugar content; frequently used for children's medications and usually flavored to disguise unpleasant-tasting drugs
Tincture	An alcohol or water and alcohol solution prepared from drugs derived from plants

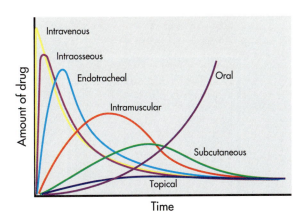

FIGURE 5-9 ▲ **The amount of time it takes to absorb a drug into the bloodstream depends on the route of administration. The chemical makeup of a drug or potential reactions with the body may determine which route is used. The route selected will be the safest and fastest. (From American College of Emergency Physicians; Pons PT, Cason D, chief editors:** *Paramedic field care: a complaint-based approach,* **St Louis, 1997, Mosby for ACEP.)**

- **Buccal**—This type of drug is dissolved between the cheek and the gum. It is absorbed across the mucous membrane of the mouth. It is a convenient, nonsterile procedure. It is not useful for drugs that taste bad and may cause an irritation to the oral mucosa.
- **Oral**—In this case the drug is swallowed and is absorbed from the stomach or small intestine. It is a convenient, nonsterile procedure. The patient must be conscious.
- **Rectal**—The drug is inserted into the rectum. It is absorbed through the mucous membranes of the rectum. It may be used in an unconscious or vomiting patient.
- **Nasogastric**—Drugs must be in a liquid form. Drugs are absorbed from the stomach or small intestine.

Parenteral Route

Giving drugs along the **parenteral** route includes using any medication route other than the alimentary canal. These are the intravenous, subcutaneous, intramuscular, transdermal, intraosseous, intrathecal, pulmonary, intralingual, intradermal, umbilical, and nasal routes:

- **Intravenous (IV)**—Injection of a sterile solution of a drug into the body by venipuncture. This method allows for an infusion of larger amounts of the drug. IV drugs have the quickest action because they enter the bloodstream immediately. Only drugs intended for IV administration should be given by this route.
- **Subcutaneous**—Injection into the fatty layer of tissue below the skin by positioning the needle and syringe at a 45-degree angle to the skin. The subcutaneous route is chosen for the drugs that should not be ab-

sorbed as rapidly as through the intramuscular or IV route. The best sites for subcutaneous injection are areas where the skin is loose and easily pinched, such as the upper arms and thighs. By this method of injection, a drug is absorbed into the body in a slow but steady rate.

- **Intramuscular**—Injection of small quantities of a drug into a muscle. Absorption is limited by the type of drug and circulation to the muscle used for injection. If a drug is injected into poorly perfused muscle, absorption is limited. Although it is possible to give some emergency drugs by this route, it is generally avoided in favor of routes that have more predictable absorption.
- **Transdermal**—Delivery of a drug to the body by absorption through the skin. Delivery is slow and maintains a steady, stable level of the drug. Dermal patches are placed on the skin, usually on the chest, upper arm, or behind the ear. Antiangina medications placed anywhere on the chest wall are very effective by this route.
- **Intraosseous**—Administration of medication directly into the bone marrow of a long bone. This technique provides rapid vascular access in the critically injured infant or child. It is not considered a replacement for IV access but is reserved for critical emergencies.
- **Intrathecal**—Injection of a drug through the theca of the spinal cord into the subarachnoid space.
- **Pulmonary**—Introduction of a drug through the pulmonary system. This may be by injecting a drug through the endotracheal tube, or the drug may be an aerosol form that the patient inhales.
- **Intralingual**—Injection of a drug within the tongue.
- **Intradermal**—Injection of a drug within the dermis.
- **Umbilical**—Injection of a drug through the umbilical cord.
- **Nasal**—Injection of a drug or substance into the nasal mucosa.

Inhalation and Endotracheal Routes

Because of the large surface area of the alveoli and vast blood supply of the pulmonary capillary beds that return blood to the left side of the heart, drugs administered through the trachea are rapidly absorbed and delivered to the heart or brachial tree for distribution. In some cases the bronchial tree itself is the target for drug effects. Bronchodilators, such as metaproterenol, are inhaled into the bronchial tree for relief of bronchospasm and act directly on the smooth muscle with only a small amount entering the circulatory system.

Several different drugs may be administered down the endotracheal tube, but it is important to deliver them in sufficient volume to ensure that they do not merely adhere to the inside of the tube. They are to be given at 2 to 2.5 times the recommended IV dose and followed with a saline flush to remove the drug from the endotracheal (ET) tube and ensure pulmonary delivery. If peripheral IV access is impossible, four drugs can be administered through the endotracheal tube. A helpful mnemonic to remember the drugs that can be given by this route is LEAN:

- **L** —Lidocaine
- **E** —Epinephrine
- **A**—Atropine
- **N**—Narcan (naloxone)

MECHANISMS OF DRUG ACTION

To create a drug action, drugs must move from their point of entry into the body to the tissues with which they react. An action of a drug administered for a **local effect** is limited to the area where it is administered. An example is lidocaine (Xylocaine) 2% jelly, which acts as a local anesthetic agent for skin disorders. A drug administered for a **systemic effect** (pertaining to the whole body rather than to one of its parts) is absorbed into the blood and then carried to the organ or tissue on which it will act. A systemic effect can be produced by administering drugs orally, sublingually, rectally, parenterally, or by inhalation. In addition, there are topical drugs that will produce a systemic effect, such as drugs that are applied to the mucous membranes in the vagina, eyes, or nose. Because mucous membranes are bathed in watery solutions and are very vascular, they are more permeable than the skin.

The **therapeutic effect** of a drug is the drug's desired effect and the reason the drug is prescribed. For example, the therapeutic effect of morphine is the relief of pain. To produce the optimal or desired therapeutic effect, a drug must reach appropriate concentrations at its site of action. The magnitude of the drug response depends on the dosage and time course of the drug in the body (Figure 5-10).

PHARMACOKINETICS

The movement of drugs in the body as they are absorbed, distributed, metabolized, and excreted is the study of **pharmacokinetics** (Figure 5-11). Drugs undergo numerous changes during their movement from the administration site to the point at which they are inactivated and excreted. To understand how a drug produces its effects, it is important to understand what happens during this process. These processes involve passive and active transport across tissue cells.

Absorption

Most drugs must be absorbed into the circulatory system for distribution and subsequent action. **Absorption** usually takes place in the mouth, dermal layers of the skin,

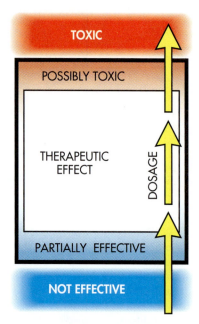

FIGURE 5-10 ▲   The therapeutic window is the balance between the desired therapeutic effect, partially effective or ineffective levels (underdosage), and toxicity (overdosage). Some drugs, such as phenytoin or theophylline, have a very narrow range of therapeutic effect, which means that they lead very easily to accidental or intentional overdose. (From American College of Emergency Physicians; Pons PT, Cason D, chief editors: *Paramedic field care: a complaint-based approach,* St Louis, 1997, Mosby for ACEP.)

subcutaneous tissue, blood vessels in the muscles, lining of the stomach and small intestines, or rectum. The following are the principal factors that affect absorption:

- *Nature of the absorbing surface*—The gradient that forces the drug across a membrane and the surface area it is exposed to both determine the ability of a drug to move across a membrane. Since osmotic force is a form of passive transport (movement from higher to lower concentrations), transport is faster if the drug passes through a single layer of cells than if it passes through multiple layers. The greater the surface area (as in the small intestine), the greater the absorption.
- *Blood flow to the site of administration*—Blood flow to the area of administration affects the speed with which the drug may move across a gradient. High blood flow rapidly removes the drug, and a high-pressure gradient is maintained. If the blood flow through the area is slow, tissue concentrations of the drug are high, thus slowing movement across the membrane surfaces.
- *Solubility of the drug*—The more soluble a drug, the easier it will pass across a surface.
- *pH*—The pH of both the drug and the body environment are factors in determining absorption.
- *Drug concentration*—Often drugs are given in a large concentration, called a loading dose, to get an imme-

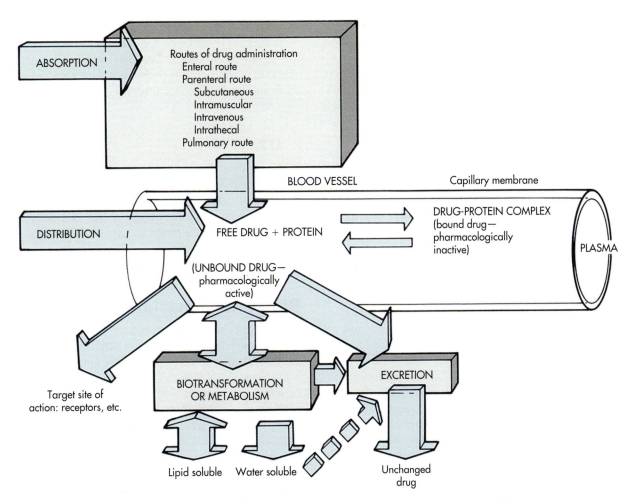

FIGURE 5-11 ▲ Pharmacokinetics: the absorption, distribution, metabolism, and excretion of a drug through the body. (From Sanders MJ: *Mosby's paramedic textbook,* ed 2, St Louis, 2000, Mosby.)

diate effect. The theory is that the drug will not be readily eliminated from the system. Drugs may also be given as a maintenance dose (a smaller dose given over a period of time) to continue the desired effect.

- *Dosage form*—The form the drug takes will have an affect on absorption. Drugs in a liquid form will be more readily absorbed than the same drugs in tablet form.
- *Routes of drug administration*—The route of administration may deposit a drug at various sites, influencing the rate of absorption. For example, in an intramuscular injection, absorption is limited by the type of drug and the circulation to the muscle used for injection. On the other hand, drugs given by the oral route are absorbed through the lining of the gastrointestinal tract. The IV route bypasses the absorption process because the drug is injected directly into the bloodstream.
- *Bioavailability*—The fraction of drug administered that reaches the central circulation is its bioavailability. Bioavailability for a drug administered intravenously is 100%.

There are three mechanisms involved in absorption:
- *Diffusion*—The constant movement of molecules from an area of higher to an area of lower concentration.
- *Osmosis*—The physical property that allows water to proceed from one side of a membrane to another.
- *Filtration*—The movement through a pressure gradient of a liquid that prevents some or all of the substances in the liquid from passing through.

Distribution

Distribution involves the transport of an absorbed drug to its target site. Some drugs that are highly water soluble are freely distributed in the vascular system and may flow easily into other body compartments where there is body water. Other drugs become bound to serum proteins in the blood and are not immediately available to act as "free" drugs on various receptors. The serum proteins are often called inert binding sites. Inert binding can also take place outside the vascular compartment, such as in body fat. This binding does not bring about any type of physiological response, and bound drugs are not available for diffusion between body compartments (Figure 5-12).

Some drugs have affinities for the same proteins and may compete with each other for free and bound status. For example, drug X is 98% bound, and drug Y, which has the same affinity, is administered. Drug Y may displace drug X and cause large percentages of the drug to become free and act on receptors. This type of action results in synergistic drug actions, in which the combined effects are much greater than if each were given individually. It also plays a part in potentiation, in which the administration of one drug enhances the effects of another. In some cases these types of effects can result in drug toxicity.

The body has certain protective mechanisms known as physiological barriers. One example is the blood-brain barrier. It prevents many drugs from leaving the blood and crossing the cerebrospinal fluid into the brain. The blood-brain barrier is highly selective, and not all drugs are allowed to cross it. In general, most drugs pass into the brain more slowly than into other tissues.

At one time it was thought that the placenta provided a protective barrier to the fetus, but this theory is now known to be untrue. Except for some vitamins and minerals, no drugs are approved "warning free" for use in the pregnant mother. With the exception of a few drugs with large molecules, almost all drugs are capable of crossing the placenta. Risks associated with drug therapy are clearly related to the stage of fetal development. The most vulnerable time for drug-induced birth defects is the first trimester, when fetal organs are developing. During the third trimester any drugs taken may have a residual effect on the fetus. At birth, the baby must rely on its own liver and kidneys to metabolize and excrete any drugs that remain in the system while in utero. Because of the newborn's decreased ability to metabolize and excrete, toxic reactions may result.

STREET WISE

A seriously ill pregnant woman may need medications for initial resuscitation or stabilization, but these drugs may affect the fetus. The decision to administer them is clearly a difficult one that must be made in consultation with medical control.

Biotransformation

As a drug is being distributed and starts to act, some of the drug's free components are starting to undergo **biotransformation** into substances for elimination from the body. Biotransformation is a series of chemical alterations of a drug that occur within the body, as by enzymatic activity. The primary organ used for this process is the liver. When the liver is exposed to a substance, structures in the hepatic cells called microsomes begin to react by metabolizing the drug into components, or metabolites, capable of being excreted. As the liver is exposed to more of the drug, hepatic cells bolster production of microsomes to handle increased drug exposure and metabolism. This process may take days and reaches maximum production of microsomes after about 2 weeks. Thus the liver is prepared to increase metabolism and elimination of a drug to which it is often exposed. When the exposure to the drug becomes less frequent or ceases altogether, the number of microsomal structures decreases (Figure 5-13).

This process of increased metabolism may eventually lead to **drug tolerance.** As the ability of the liver to metabolize improves, less drug is available to contact receptors and a higher dosage is needed to achieve the same physiological response as previously experienced. A higher dose is then given, the liver develops more microsomes to metabolize the drug, and a vicious circle begins.

Excretion

Excretion eliminates the waste products of drug metabolism from the body. The kidneys excrete most drugs, so patients with impaired renal function may be unable to eliminate drugs from their systems. Among the other structures that eliminate drugs are the intestines, lungs, sweat glands, salivary glands, and mammary glands (Figure 5-14).

Unless the drug is excreted before a repeat dose is given, a **cumulative effect** can occur. In some instances

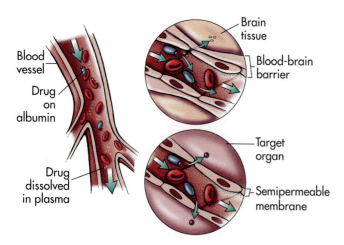

FIGURE 5-12 ▲ **Drugs being distributed to the brain and target organs via the bloodstream are dissolved in plasma or bound to proteins. The ability of a drug to cross out of the bloodstream is determined by the permeability of the membrane it is trying to cross. (From American College of Emergency Physicians; Pons PT, Cason D, chief editors:** *Paramedic field care: a complaint-based approach,* **St Louis, 1997, Mosby for ACEP.)**

the accumulation of the drug in the body may be the desired effect. However, a cumulative effect may be dangerous and result in toxic levels in the body.

PHARMACODYNAMICS

Pharmacodynamics is the study of the effects of drugs on the body. The major theory of drug action is the receptor theory, which states that drugs act by associating themselves with specific molecules, often on the cell membrane, in a manner that alters the cell's function. Receptors may be thought of as cellular "locks," with drugs being the keys. The right shape of key (the drug) with exactly the right code is inserted into the lock (receptor), and a pharmacological response occurs. Ideally, this will produce the desired therapeutic effect of the drug (Figure 5-15).

Receptors determine the quantity of drug necessary to effect a response. There are various types of receptors, such as alpha, beta, and dopaminergic. (It has been widely established that dopamine and its agonists play an important role in cardiovascular, renal, hormonal, and central nervous system regulation through stimula-

tion of α- and β-adrenergic and dopaminergic receptors.) If the drug to be administered has a tremendous affinity for the receptors (a drug's ability to bind to a receptor site), the concentration necessary to produce a response may be limited. The number of receptors in an individual patient may limit the maximal effect a drug may produce. Receptors are also responsible for selective drug action. The molecular structure of a drug determines its ability or lack of ability to bind to receptor sites. A change in a drug's structure may increase or decrease a drug's affinity to bind to receptor sites. A change in structure may also alter the drug's actions.

Agonists cause a direct change in cellular function when inserted into a receptor. Receptors may also be occupied or blocked by antagonists. An antagonist occupies a receptor site but causes no physiological response. The chemical code (key) is close enough for it to fit into the receptor (lock) but not exact enough to cause a response. Many antagonists compete for receptors and occupy sites with greater affinity than the agonist.

Drug-Response Factors

Generally, the physiological effects of a drug can be seen by monitoring the patient's condition. If the drug was given to alleviate pain, did it work? Was the blood pressure lowered when an antihypertensive drug was given? Was the dysrhythmia contained when the patient was given lidocaine? Clinically, the effects of a drug can be determined by measuring the following:

- *Plasma level profile*—A profile that is unique to each drug and that depends on the drug's rate of absorption, distribution, biotransformation, and excretion (Figure 5-16).
- *Biological half-life*—The time required for the plasma level of a drug to fall to half of a certain measured level.
- *Therapeutic threshold*—The minimum amount of drug needed in the bloodstream to cause a therapeutic effect.
- *Therapeutic index*—A quantitative measure of the relative safety of a drug; the ratio of the dose of a drug that is lethal in 50% of tested laboratory animals to the dose of the drug that is therapeutically effective in 50% of tested animals.

Factors Altering Drug Responses

A number of factors influence the actions of drugs on the body. Although genetic and psychological factors can also alter drug responses, the most common factors are listed as follows:

- *Age*—Elderly people have slower metabolic processes. Age-related kidney and liver dysfunction will extend the breakdown and excretion times in these patients. It is very important to monitor the cumulative effects of drugs in elderly patients.

  Infants and children are not simply small adults. Infants have immature livers and kidneys, so it is dif-

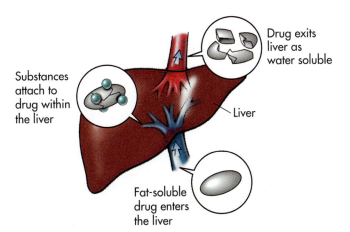

Substances attach to drug within the liver

Drug exits liver as water soluble

Liver

Fat-soluble drug enters the liver

FIGURE 5-13 ▲ The liver is the site of metabolism of most drugs. Once a drug is made water soluble by the liver, it is available for the body tissues to use or can be excreted by the kidney. (From American College of Emergency Physicians; Pons PT, Cason D, chief editors: *Paramedic field care: a complaint-based approach*, St Louis, 1997, Mosby for ACEP.)

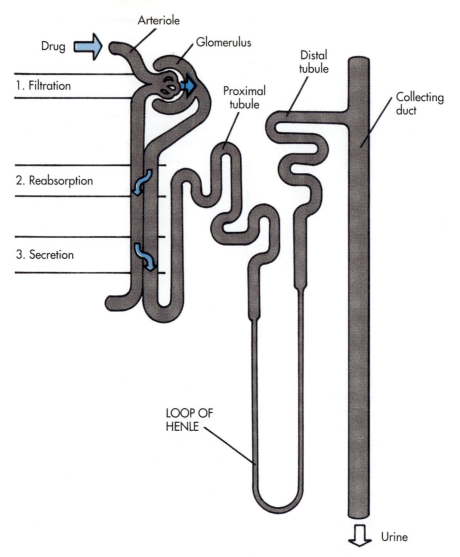

FIGURE 5-14 ▲ Drug excretion process in kidneys consists of three mechanisms: passive glomerular filtration, active tubular secretion, and partial reabsorption. (From Sanders MJ: *Mosby's paramedic textbook,* ed 2, St Louis, 2000, Mosby.)

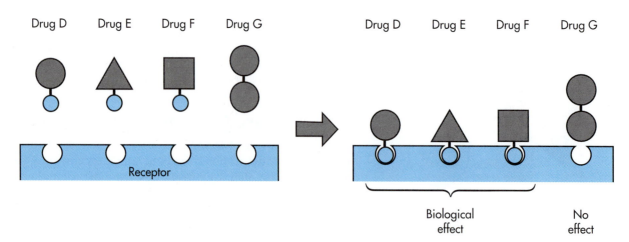

FIGURE 5-15 ▲ Lock-and-key fit between a drug and the receptors through which it acts. The site on the receptor that interacts with a drug has a definite shape. A drug that conforms to that shape can bind and produce a biological response. In this example, only the shape along the lower surface of the drug molecule is important in determining if the drug binds to the receptor. (From Sanders MJ: *Mosby's paramedic textbook,* ed 2, St Louis, 2000, Mosby.)

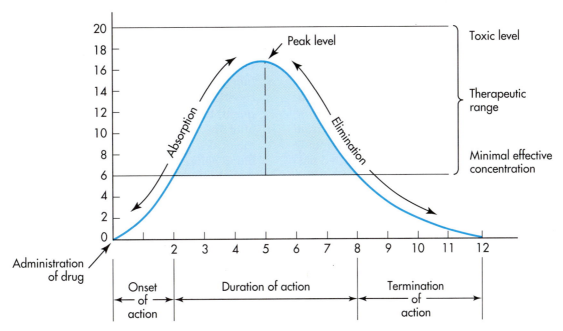

FIGURE 5-16 ▲ Plasma-level profile of a drug. (From Sanders MJ: *Mosby's paramedic textbook*, ed 2, St Louis, 2000, Mosby.)

ficult for them to metabolize and eliminate the same dosages of drugs as adults. A child's body chemistry is affected by adolescence, body proportion, and an inability to metabolize medications as effectively as adults.

- *Body mass*—Many medications have an effect on the body only within a specific concentration. To achieve a concentration of medication per unit of body water, the patient's body mass (weight) frequently serves as a guide to dosage determinations.
- *Gender*—Women and men may have different reactions to some drugs because of different body compositions and hormone levels. A woman's hematocrit (concentration of red blood cells per unit of volume) measurements are lower than a man's. Men have a lower proportion of subcutaneous fat than women. Men and women also have differences in the proportion of water volume per body weight. A woman's ability to receive medication is affected by pregnancy and considerations of the medication's effect on the unborn fetus. The use of some medications by pregnant women may cause birth defects in their children.
- *Environment and time of administration*—Fluctuations in environmental conditions such as the time of day, temperature, altitude, and noise may alter one's response to a drug.
- *Existing pathology*—If the body is compromised by a disease process, absorption, distribution, metabolism, and excretion of a drug may be altered.

Predictable Responses

All drugs have the potential for producing more than one response, desired or undesired. Drugs are given for their desired action, but some adverse drug responses are unavoidable, such as side effects. The **side effect** of a drug is any effect that is unintended. Side effects usually are predictable and may be either harmless or potentially harmful. For example, albuterol, which relaxes bronchial smooth muscle, results in bronchodilation and may have a side effect of nausea and vomiting.

Iatrogenic Responses

Administration of many drugs can lead to symptoms that mimic naturally occurring disease states. This is described as an iatrogenic drug response.

Unpredictable Responses

Some drugs produce responses that cannot be predicted on the basis of what we know about their mechanisms of action. These kinds of adverse drug responses are described as unpredictable drug responses and include the following:

- **Synergism**—Two drugs working together. One drug helps the action of the other to produce an effect that neither produces alone. For example, small doses of phenergan (a nonnarcotic antiemetic) and meperidine (Demerol) (a synthetic narcotic analgesic) are more effective for pain relief than the same dose of meperidine alone. Synergism can also have adverse effects; sedatives and barbiturates given together can cause central nervous system depression.
- **Potentiation**—One drug prolonging or multiplying the effect of another drug. For example, probenecid (Benemid) (an antigout drug) is given with penicillin (an antibiotic) to delay the excretion of penicillin and

to build up a high level of penicillin in the blood. As another example, cimetidine (Tagamet) (a gastric antisecretory) given with imipramine (Tofranil) (an antidepressant) will increase the levels of imipramine in the blood.

- **Antagonist**—A drug that prevents receptor stimulation. An antagonist drug has an affinity for a cell receptor, and by binding to it, the cell is prevented from responding. For example, naloxone is a commonly used narcotic antagonist used to treat suspected narcotic overdose and unresponsiveness with unknown etiology. Naloxone binds to the receptor sites, blocking the action of the toxic drugs. As another example, antacids taken with tetracycline (an antibiotic) prevent the absorption of tetracycline.
- **Hypersensitivity**—Also known as drug allergy. The body must build this response; the first exposure may or may not indicate that a problem is developing.
- **Idiosyncratic reaction**—An abnormal or unexpected reaction to a drug peculiar to a certain patient. This is not technically an allergy.
- **Tolerance**—An individual's capacity to endure medications. Some drugs given over a long period of time may cause the body to become resistant to their effect, requiring larger dosages to achieve the desired response. Drugs that commonly produce tolerance are opiates, barbiturates, ethyl alcohol, and tobacco.
- **Drug allergy**—A reaction occurring in a person who has been previously exposed to the drug and has developed antibodies. Drug allergies can manifest in a variety of signs and symptoms, ranging from minor to serious. The reaction can occur immediately after the patient has received the drug or may be delayed for hours or days. Signs and symptoms of a drug allergy are skin rash, fever, diarrhea, nausea, and vomiting. A life-threatening immediate reaction is called an anaphylactic reaction and results in respiratory distress, sudden severe bronchospasm, and cardiovascular collapse. In gathering the patient's history, the EMT–I must always ask about allergies of any sort, particularly allergies to drugs. If the patient is aware of existing allergies, these must be noted on the patient run report.
- **Delayed reaction** (*serum sickness*)—A hypersensitivity reaction similar to an allergy. The immune system misidentifies a protein in antiserum (a preparation of serum that has been removed from a person or animal that has already developed immunity to a particular microorganism) as a potentially harmful substance (antigen) and develops an immune response against the antiserum. Antibodies bind with the antiserum protein to create larger particles (immune complexes). The immune complexes are deposited in various tissues, causing inflammation and various other symptoms. Because it takes time for the body to produce antibodies to a new antigen, symptoms do not develop until 7 to 14 days after exposure to the antiserum. Exposure to certain medications (particularly penicillin) can cause a similar process. Unlike other drug allergies, which occur very soon after receiving the medication for the second (or subsequent) time, serum sickness can develop 7 to 14 days after the first exposure to a medication. The drug molecules probably combine with a protein in the blood before being misidentified as an antigen.

- **Anaphylactic reaction**—An acute systemic (whole body) type of allergic reaction. Anaphylaxis occurs when a person has become sensitized (i.e., the immune system has been triggered to recognize a substance as a threat to the body). On the second or subsequent exposure to the substance, an allergic reaction occurs. This reaction is sudden, severe, and involves the whole body.
- **Cross-tolerance**—Tolerance (through continued used of a drug) that increases to other drugs in the same class. For example, use of an opiate drug will cause tolerance to other opiate drugs. Heroin is a narcotic drug, and so are morphine and meperidine (Demerol). If a user develops tolerance to heroin, he or she will also show a tolerance for morphine and meperidine without using those drugs regularly.
- **Drug dependence**—A physical state where withdrawal symptoms occur when a person discontinues the use of a drug. After repeated use of a drug, the user's body becomes so accustomed to the particular drug that it can only function normally if the drug is present. Often the terms *addiction* and *dependence* are used to mean the same thing. Physical dependence is one of the factors contributing to the continued use of drugs.
- **Tachyphylaxis**—Rapid development of tolerance.
- **Cumulative effect**—Effects that take place after the primary effects are worn off but that have a permanent duration.
- **Drug toxicity**—Toxicity resulting from overdosage, ingestion of a drug intended for external use, or buildup of the drug in the blood due to impaired metabolism or excretion. Like a drug allergy, some effects are realized immediately, but others may be delayed and not be apparent for weeks or months. Most drug toxicity is avoidable if careful attention is paid to dosage and monitoring for toxicity.

DRUG INTERACTIONS

Drug interaction refers to the process that occurs when something a drug increases, decreases, or cancels the effects of the other. There are many variables that influence drug interaction, such as intestinal absorption, competition for plasma protein binding, drug metabolism or biotransformation, action at the receptor site, renal excretion, and alteration of electrolyte balance. Other variables include drug-drug interactions, drug-induced malabsorption of foods and nutrients, food-induced malabsorption of drugs, alteration of enzymes, alcohol consumption, cigarette smoking, food-initiated alteration of drug excretion, and drug incompatibilities that may occur when drugs are mixed before administration.

Some examples of drug interactions are as follows:

- Bronchodilators are used to treat the symptoms of bronchial asthma, chronic bronchitis, and emphysema. These medicines relieve wheezing, shortness of breath, and troubled breathing. They work by opening the air passages of the lungs. Foods or beverages that contain caffeine, also stimulate the central nervous system and can produce adverse effects.
- Diuretics increase the elimination of water, sodium, and chloride from the body. A commonly used diuretic is furosemide. Diuretics vary in their interactions with nutrients. Loss of potassium, calcium, and magnesium occurs with some diuretics.
- Antihypertensives relax blood vessels, increase the supply of blood and oxygen to the heart, and lessen the heart's workload. They also regulate the heartbeat. Some commonly used antihypertensives are hydralazine, methyldopa, and metoprolol. Use of sodium (salt) can diminish the effectiveness of these medications to be effective.
- Penicillins are antibiotics used for treatment of a wide variety of infections. Some commonly used penicillins are amoxicillin, ampicillin, bacampicillin, penicillin G, and penicillin V. Amoxicillin and bacampicillin may be taken with food; however, absorption of other types of penicillins is reduced when taken with food.
- Narcotic analgesics are narcotics that are used for the relief of pain. Some commonly used narcotic analgesics are meperidine and morphine. Alcohol increases the sedative effect of the medications and therefore should be avoided. Take these medications with food, because they can upset the stomach.

DRUG STORAGE AND SECURITY

Controlled substances must be locked in a secure locked box bolted to a shelf in a locked cabinet in the ambulance. The number of crew members with access to the keys or to the cabinet should be limited. Inventory forms should be kept in the cabinet with the drugs. If controlled substances are administered, records must be maintained separate from the patients' charts and must be readily available for inspection by the authorities of the Drug Enforcement Administration (DEA). Local protocols should be met when securing controlled substances. Procedures and measures to ensure the security of controlled substances are essential.

If drugs are lost or stolen, the local law enforcement agency should be notified immediately along with one's

supervisor. If drugs are expired and must be destroyed, two employees must witness the destruction of the medication and sign and date the form for destroyed substances.

When storing any drug, be aware that drug potency can be affected by temperature, light, moisture, air exposure, and shelf life. Refer to local protocols to guide the manner in which drugs are distributed, accounted for, and stored.

COMPONENTS OF A DRUG PROFILE

A drug's profile refers to its various properties. EMT–Is should become familiar with the drug profile of each medication they are required to administer. A typical drug profile includes the following information:

- *Drug names*—What are the chemical, trade, and generic names of the drug?
- *Body system*—What body system does the drug affect?
- *Class of agent*—What is the class of the drug?
- *Mechanism of action*—How does this drug work on the body?
- *Drug actions, pharmacokinetics, and indications*—Physiologically, how does this drug work? Why use this drug and not another? When should this drug be given?
- *Contraindications and side effects*—What are the **contraindications** to this drug? (When should it be avoided, and why?) Are there any adverse symptoms the patient may experience after administration?
- *Dosage*—What are the usual adult and pediatric dosages for this drug? Does the dosage vary if given by different routes?
- *Routes of administration*—By what route should this drug be given? Can it be given by other routes?
- *How supplied*—Is the drug supplied in a vial, ampule, or prefilled syringe? Always check the expiration date and concentration/dosage of the medication before it is delivered.
- *Special considerations*—Is the patient a child or older adult, or does the patient have known allergies to the medication? Always consider special needs before giving a drug.

DRUGS ADMINISTERED BY THE EMT–INTERMEDIATE

An EMT–I delivers drugs that can be given to the patient under certain conditions. The EMT–I also should be able to assist the patient in taking his or her prescribed medication. A number of medications are routinely given by the EMT–I including: delivery of the following seven medications:

- *Acetylsalicylic acid*—Acetylsalicylic acid, or aspirin, has analgesic and antirheumatic effects that are attributable to its ability to inhibit the synthesis of prostaglandins, which are important mediators of inflammation. In prehospital care, aspirin is given for its ability to inhibit platelet aggregation. Aspirin administration is strongly recommended for acute MI patients. The recommended dosage is 160 to 325 mg. The patient should be instructed to chew and swallow the aspirin. Two to four tablets of children's aspirin (80 mg each) can be used. Some side effects include stomach irritation, heartburn or indigestion, nausea or vomiting, and/or allergic reaction. Its use should be avoided in allergy due to aspirin, GI bleeding, active ulcer disease, hemorrhagic stroke, bleeding disorders, and in children with flu-like symptoms.

- *Activated charcoal*—Activated charcoal is used because it absorbs toxic substances from the gastrointestinal tract. It is used for oral poisonings and overdoses. The adult and pediatric dosages are 1 to 2 g/kg of body weight; if the charcoal is not in a premixed slurry, one part charcoal is mixed with four parts water. The solution is given to the patient orally. It is important that the patient be conscious and alert to avoid aspiration.

- *Epinephrine autoinjector*—An epinephrine autoinjector is used for severe allergic reaction. An autoinjector is a syringe with a spring-loaded needle that will release and inject the drug into the muscle. The large muscle in the thigh is the site of choice for administration.
- *Oral glucose*—This type of glucose is taken by mouth. It is indicated in a patient with a history of diabetes or in a patient with an altered level of responsiveness. The patient must be alert enough, however, to be able to take the glucose easily without aspiration.
- *Oxygen*—Oxygen is used to treat patients with conditions that cause the oxygen content to be low. These conditions may be caused by a medical or trauma condition.
- *Prescribed inhalers*—There are various types of drugs given by an inhaler device. Most commonly, the patient will present with a disease such as chronic bronchitis, emphysema, or asthma. The drug contained in the inhaler will relax bronchial muscles and make breathing easier.

Additional drugs that may be administered by the EMT–I are included in Table 5-5.

Text continued on p. 145

TABLE 5-5

Additional Drugs Used by the EMT–Intermediate

Generic name	**Adenosine**
Brand name	Adenocard
Class	Antiarrhythmic
Mechanism of action	Slows conduction time through AV node; can interrupt reentrant pathways through AV node
	Slows sinus rate
	Has direct effect on supraventricular tissue
Indications and field use	Conversion of supraventricular tachycardias, including those caused by Wolff-Parkinson-White syndrome
	Not effective in conversion of atrial fibrillation or flutter or VT
Contraindications	Sick sinus syndrome (except in patients with a functioning ventricular pacemaker); second- or third-degree AV block
Adverse reactions	Facial flushing, shortness of breath, chest pain (these occur in roughly 20% of patients; are very short-lived and well tolerated if patient is informed—before administration—of possibility of their occurrence)
Incompatibilities/drug interactions	Methylxanthines (theophylline-type drugs) prevent binding of adenosine at receptor sites; larger doses may be needed
	Dipyridamole (Persantine) causes potentiation of adenosine's effects; smaller doses may be effective
	Carbamazepine (Tegretol) may result in development of high-degree blocks
	May cause bronchoconstriction in asthmatic patients
Adult dosage	6 mg IV bolus as rapidly as possible, followed by flushing IV line; if rhythm does not convert within 2 min, repeat using 12 mg bolus; may give third dose of 12 mg 1-2 min later
Pediatric dosage	0.1 mg/kg rapid IV push (up to 6 mg); 0.2 mg/kg for second dose; maximum single dose 12 mg
Routes of administration	Rapid IV push (over 1-2 sec)
Onset of action	Seconds

AV, Atrioventricular; *CNS,* central nervous system; *COPD,* chronic obstructive pulmonary disease; *ET,* endotracheal; *GI,* gastrointestinal; *IM,* intramuscular; *IO,* intraosseous; *IV,* intravenous; *MAO,* monoamine oxidase; *PEA,* pulseless electrical activity; *SQ,* subcutaneous; *VF,* ventricular fibrillation; *VT,* ventricular tachycardia

TABLE 5-5

Additional Drugs Used by the EMT–Intermediate—cont'd

Adenosine—cont'd

Peak effects	Seconds
Duration of action	10-12 sec
Dosage forms/packaging	6 mg/2 mL vials (3 mg/mL)
Special considerations	Short half-life (<10 sec) limits side effects but may permit dysrhythmia to recur in some patients

Generic name	**Albuterol sulfate**
Brand name	Proventil, Ventolin
Class	Sympathomimetic
Mechanism of action	Relaxes bronchial smooth muscle, resulting in bronchodilation
Indications and field use	Bronchospasm from emphysema, asthma, or allergic reaction
Contraindications	Synergistic with other sympathomimetics
	Use with caution in patients with diabetes, hypertension, hyperthyroidism, and cerebrovascular disease
Adverse reactions	Excessive use may cause dysrhythmias, tachycardia, tremors, nervousness, nausea, and vomiting
Incompatibilities/drug interactions	Cyclic antidepressants, MAO inhibitors
Adult dosage	2.5 mg; dilute 0.5 mL of 0.5% solution for inhalation with 3 mL normal saline; administer in nebulizer over 5-15 min
	1-2 inhalations (90 µg each) with metered-dose inhaler; may be repeated every 15 min as needed
Pediatric dosage	Age younger than 12 yr: 0.03 mL/kg of 0.5% solution up to 1.0 mL over 5-10 min; age older than 12 yr: use full adult dose
Routes of administration	Nebulized inhaler, also in metered-dose inhaler
Onset of action	5-15 min
Peak effects	30 min-2 hr
Duration of action	3-4 hr
Dosage forms/packaging	Aerosol inhaler: 90 µg/metered spray, 100 µg/metered spray
	Solution for inhalation: 0.083% or 0.5%

Generic name	**Atropine sulfate**
Brand name	None
Class	Parasympatholytic
Mechanism of action	Inhibits acetylcholine in smooth muscle and glands, blocking parasympathetic response and allowing sympathetic response to take over
	Small doses cause sedation, and high doses cause stimulation
	Systemic effects are depressed salivary and GI secretions and bronchodilation; heart rate will increase, and there will be an increase in AV conduction
Indications and field use	First drug for symptomatic bradycardia
	Second drug (after epinephrine) for asystole or bradycardic PEA
	Poisonings by certain mushrooms, insecticides, and nerve gas
Contraindications	Use with caution in presence of myocardial ischemia and hypoxia
	Use with caution in AV block at His-Purkinje level (type II AV block and third-degree AV block with new wide-QRS complexes)
	Glaucoma, myasthenia gravis
Adverse reactions	Pupil dilation; increases myocardial oxygen demand; dry mouth
Incompatibilities/drug interactions	Antihistamines, phenothiazine antipsychotics, and tricyclic antidepressants enhance effects of atropine
Adult dosage	Asystole or PEA: 1 mg IV push; repeat every 3-5 min (if asystole persists) to a maximum dose of 0.03-0.04 mg/kg
	Bradycardia: 0.5-1.0 mg IV push every 3-5 min as needed; not to exceed total dose of 0.04 mg/kg; use shorter dosing interval (3 min) and higher doses (1 mg) in severe clinical conditions
	Poisonings: Larger doses are required; usually initial dose of 2.0 mg
	ET: 1-2 mg diluted in 10 mL sterile water or normal saline

Continued

TABLE 5-5

Additional Drugs Used by the EMT–Intermediate—cont'd

	Atropine sulfate—cont'd
Pediatric dosage	0.02 mg/kg (minimum of 0.1 mg) rapid IV push
Maximum single dose	0.5 mg in child; 1.0 mg in adolescent
Routes of administration	IV, ET, IO (IM in organophosphate poisoning)
Onset of action	1 min
Peak effects	2-5 min
Duration of action	2 hr
Dosage forms/packaging	0.1 mg/mL in 10-mL prefilled syringe (total of 1 mg)
Generic name	**Dexamethasone sodium phosphate**
Brand name	Decadron
Class	Corticosteroid
Mechanism of action	Enters target cells and binds to cytoplasmic receptors, thereby initiating many complex reactions that are responsible for its antiinflammatory and immunosuppressive effects
Indications and field use	High doses are used for treatment of unresponsive shock
	Also used in short-term management of various inflammatory and allergic disorders, such as rheumatoid arthritis and status asthmaticus; cerebral edema associated with brain tumor or head injury; control of bronchial asthma requiring corticosteroids in conjunction with other therapy
Contraindications	Systemic fungal infections and hypersensitivity to any component of this product, including sulfites
Adverse reactions	Headache, muscle weakness, fluid and electrolyte disturbances
Incompatibilities/drug interactions	When corticosteroids are administered concomitantly with potassium-depleting diuretics, patients should be observed closely for development of hypokalemia
Adult dosage	There is a great variance in recommended doses. The usual range in emergency care is 4-24 mg IV
Pediatric dosage	0.25-0.5 mg/kg dose IV/IO
Routes of administration	IV, IM
Onset of action	Rapid onset
Peak effects	None
Duration of action	Short duration
Dosage forms/packaging	4 mg/mL; available in 1-mL, 5-mL, and 25-mL vials
Generic name	**Dextrose 50% solution**
Brand name	None
Class	Hyperglycemic
Mechanism of action	Increases blood glucose (sugar) levels
Indications and field use	Hypoglycemia, coma of unknown origin, altered level of responsiveness, seizure of unknown origin
Contraindications	Intracranial hemorrhage, cerebovascular accident, delirium tremens
Adverse reactions	If IV fluid is not infusing properly in vein or infiltrates, necrosis of tissue surrounding IV site could occur
Incompatibilities/drug interactions	None
Adult dosage	25-50 g IV bolus (50-100 mL of 50% solution)
Pediatric dosage	25% dextrose at 0.5-1.0 g/kg IV bolus
	50% solution may be diluted 1:1 with normal saline or sterile water
Routes of administration	IV bolus
Onset of action	Immediate
Peak effects	Variable
Duration of action	Variable
Dosage forms/packaging	Prefilled syringe, 25 g in 50 mL
Special considerations	Draw blood sugar to confirm hypoglycemia before administering medication

AV, Atrioventricular; *CNS,* central nervous system; *COPD,* chronic obstructive pulmonary disease; *ET,* endotracheal; *GI,* gastrointestinal; *IM,* intramuscular; *IO,* intraosseous; *IV,* intravenous; *MAO,* monoamine oxidase; *PEA,* pulseless electrical activity; *SQ,* subcutaneous; *VF,* ventricular fibrillation; *VT,* ventricular tachycardia

TABLE 5-5

Additional Drugs Used by the EMT–Intermediate—cont'd

Generic name	**Diazepam**
Brand name	Valium
Class	Benzodiazepine
Mechanism of action	Affects multiple levels of CNS to decrease seizures by increasing seizure threshold
	Amnesic, sedative
Indications and field use	Grand mal seizures, especially status epilepticus
	Acute anxiety states
	Transient analgesia/amnesia for medical procedures (e.g., fracture reduction, cardioversion)
	Delirium tremens
Contraindications	Hypersensitivity, glaucoma
Adverse reactions	Thrombosis and phlebitis
	Bradycardia, hypotension, cardiovascular collapse
	Respiratory arrest, especially with elevated blood alcohol levels
	Burning proximal to IV injection site
Incompatibilities/drug interactions	Incompatible with most drugs
	Must be given close to hub of needle—can precipitate or bind with tubing
Adult dosage	5-10 mg slow IV push; can repeat at 10- to 15-min intervals; administer no faster than 5 mg/min (maximum dose 30 mg)
Pediatric dosage	For status epilepticus give 0.05-0.3 mg/kg/dose IV over 2-3 min (or until seizure activity subsides); may repeat every 30 min to maximum total dose of 5-10 mg
Routes of administration	Slow IV push; may be taken orally for anxiety
Onset of action	Minutes
Peak effects	Minutes
Duration of action	20-50 min
Dosage forms/packaging	10 mg/5 mL prefilled syringes
Generic name	**Epinephrine**
Brand name	Adrenalin
Class	Sympathomimetic
Mechanism of action	Direct-acting alpha and beta agonist:
	Alpha-1: Bronchial, skin, renal, and visceral arteriolar constriction
	Beta-1: Positive inotropic and chronotropic actions; increases automaticity
	Beta-2: Bronchial smooth muscle relaxation and dilation of skeletal vasculature
Indications and field use	Cardiac arrest: VF, pulseless VT, asystole, PEA
	Symptomatic bradycardia: After atropine and transcutaneous pacing
	Acute bronchospasm: Anaphylaxis, bronchiolitis, asthma, COPD
Contraindications	Pulmonary edema, hypothermia, hypertension
	Remember, however, there are no contraindications for use of epinephrine in cardiac arrest
Adverse reactions	Ventricular dysrhythmias, precipitation of angina or myocardial infarction, tachycardia, anxiety, hypertension, headache
Incompatibilities/drug interactions	Potentiates other sympathomimetics
	Alkaline solutions
	Patients taking MAO inhibitors, antihistamines, and tricyclic antidepressants may have heightened effects
	These interactions, although important, should not prevent use of epinephrine in cardiac arrest

Continued

TABLE 5-5

Additional Drugs Used by the EMT–Intermediate—cont'd

	Epinephrine—cont'd
Adult dosage	Cardiac arrest: First dose: 1 mg IV push (10 mL of a 1:10,000 solution); may repeat every 3-5 min ET: 2.0-2.5 mg diluted in 10 mL normal saline Profound bradycardia: 2-10 µg/min (add 1 mg to 250 mL normal saline or 5% dextrose in water to produce a concentration of 4 µg/mL) Acute bronchospasm: 0.3-0.5 mg (0.3-0.5 mL of a 1:1000 solution); may be repeated as needed and ordered SQ

Pediatric dosage	Bradycardia: IV/IO: 0.01 mg/kg (1:10,000, 0.1 mL/kg); ET: 0.1 mg/kg (1:1000, 0.1 mL/kg)
	Asystolic or pulseless arrest:
	    First dose: IV/IO: 0.01 mg/kg (1:10,000, 0.1 mL/kg); ET: 0.1 mg/kg (1:1000, 0.1 mL/kg); IV/IO doses as high as 0.2 mg/kg of 1:1000 may be effective
	    Subsequent doses: IV/IO/ET: 0.1 mg/kg (1:1000, 0.1 mL/kg); repeat every 3-5 min; IV/IO doses as high as 0.2 mg/kg (0.2 mL/kg of 1:1000 solution) may be effective
	Acute bronchospasm: Give 0.01 mg/kg (0.01 mL/kg of 1:1000 solution) SQ (maximum of 0.35 mg/dose)

Routes of administration	Cardiac: IV push, IV infusion, ET, IO Acute bronchospasm: SQ, IV, ET
Onset of action	Immediate
Peak effects	Minutes
Duration of action	Several minutes
Dosage forms/packaging	Prefilled: 0.1 mg/mL, 10-mL syringe, 1:10,000 solution Glass ampules: 1 mg/mL, 1:1000 solution Multidose 30-mL vial: 1 mg/mL
Generic name	**Furosemide**
Brand name	Lasix
Class	Loop diuretic
Mechanism of action	Potent diuretic—inhibits electrolyte reabsorption in ascending loop of Henle and promotes excretion of sodium, potassium, chloride Vasodilation, which increases venous capacitance and decreases afterload
Indications and field use	Pulmonary edema; congestive heart failure
Contraindications	Anuria, hypovolemia Hypotension (relative contraindication)
Adverse reactions	May exacerbate hypovolemia; hyperglycemia (due to hemoconcentration); hypokalemia; may decrease response to pressors
Incompatibilities/drug interactions	Acidic drugs Epinephrine, norepinephrine, isoproterenol, dopamine, dobutamine
Adult dosage	0.5-1 mg/kg (usually 20-80 mg) IV, given over 1-2 min
Pediatric dosage	1 mg/kg
Routes of administration	Slow IV push
Onset of action	5 min
Peak effects	20-60 min
Duration of action	Variable
Dosage forms/packaging	100 mg/5 mL, 20 mg/2 mL, 40 mg/4 mL vials
Special considerations	Ototoxicity and resulting deafness can occur with rapid administration
Generic name	**Isoetharine**
Brand name	Bronkosol, Bronkometer
Class	Sympathomimetic
Mechanism of action	Beta-2 agonist—relaxes smooth muscle of bronchioles, vasculature, uterus
Indications and field use	Acute bronchial asthma, bronchospasm

AV, Atrioventricular; *CNS*, central nervous system; *COPD*, chronic obstructive pulmonary disease; *ET*, endotracheal; *GI*, gastrointestinal; *IM*, intramuscular; *IO*, intraosseous; *IV*, intravenous; *MAO*, monoamine oxidase; *PEA*, pulseless electrical activity; *SQ*, subcutaneous; *VF*, ventricular fibrillation; *VT*, ventricular tachycardia

TABLE 5-5

Additional Drugs Used by the EMT–Intermediate—cont'd

Isoetharine—cont'd

Contraindications	Use with caution in patients with diabetes, hyperthyroidism, cardio-vascular and cerebrovascular disease
Adverse reactions	Dose-related tachycardia, palpitations, tremors, nervousness, peripheral vasodilation, nausea, transient hyperglycemia, life-threatening dysrhythmias; multiple successive doses can cause paradoxical bronchoconstriction
	Use with caution in patients with hyperthyroidism, diabetes, cerebrovascular disorders
Incompatibilities/drug interactions	Additive adverse effects with other beta agonists
Adult dosage	1-2 inhalations with metered-dose inhaler
Pediatric dosage	Not recommended in children under 12 yr of age
Routes of administration	Nebulized, metered-dose inhaler
Onset of action	Immediate
Peak effects	5-15 min
Duration of action	1-4 hr
Dosage forms/packaging	Metered-dose inhaler, 2-mL unit-dose of 1% solution
Special considerations	Not applicable

Generic name	**Lidocaine hydrochloride**
Brand name	Xylocaine
Class	Antiarrhythmic
Mechanism of action	Increases VF threshold
	Decreases phase 4 diastolic depolarization
	Suppresses premature ventricular ectopy
Indications and field use	Cardiac arrest from VF/VT
	Stable VT may be used following successful conversion (return of a spontaneous perfusing rhythm) from VF/VT
Contraindications	Prophylactic use in acute myocardial infarction patients not recommended
	Reduce maintenance dose (not loading dose) in patients with impaired liver function and left ventricular dysfunction
Adverse reactions	Drowsiness, confusion, fatigue, respiratory depression and arrest, cardiovascular collapse, tremors, twitching
Incompatibilities/drug interactions	None known
Adult dosage	Cardiac arrest:
	Bolus of 1.0 to 1.5 mg/kg IV; if refractory VT/VF, an additional bolus of 0.5 to 0.75 mg/kg can be given over 3 to 5 min; total dose should not exceed 3 mg/kg; the more aggressive dosing (1.5 mg/kg) is recommended in cardiac arrest due to VF or pulseless VT after failure of defibrillation and epinephrine
	ET: Use 2-2.5 times IV dose to obtain equivalent blood levels compared with IV administration
	Nonarrested patient: Stable VT and significant ventricular ectopy: 1.0-1.5 mg/kg IV push; repeat at 0.5-0.75 mg/kg IV every 5-10 min; maximum total: 3 mg/kg Maintenance infusion: On return of spontaneous circulation, start continuous infusion at 1-4 mg/min
Pediatric dosage	1 mg/kg
	Maintenance infusion: 20-50 µg/kg/min; infusion should contain 120 mg lidocaine in 100 mL 5% dextrose in water administered at rate of 1-2.5 mL/kg/hr
Routes of administration	IV bolus, followed by IV infusion; may be given ET
Onset of action	1-5 min
Peak effects	5-10 min
Duration of action	Bolus only, 20 min
Dosage forms/packaging	Prefilled syringes: 5 mg/mL, 10 mg/mL, 15 mg/mL, 20 mg/mL
	Vials: 40 mg/mL, 100 mg/mL, 200 mg/mL

Continued

TABLE 5-5

Additional Drugs Used by the EMT–Intermediate—cont'd

Generic name	**Metaproterenol sulfate**
Brand name	Alupent, Metaprel
Class	Sympathomimetic
Mechanism of action	Beta-2 agonist—acts directly on bronchial smooth muscle
Indications and field use	Bronchospasm of COPD and asthma
Contraindications	Diabetes, hyperthyroidism, and cerebrovascular or cardiovascular disorders
Adverse reactions	Dose-related tachycardia, palpitations, nervousness, peripheral vasodilation; with excessive use—lethal dysrhythmias, paradoxical bronchospasm
Incompatibilities/drug interactions	Beta blockers, MAO inhibitors, tricyclic antidepressants; potentiates other beta agonists
Adult dosage	2.5 mL of 0.4% or 0.6% unit dose (10 or 15 mg of drug, respectively) in nebulizer over 10-15 min
Pediatric dosage	6-12 years-0.1 ml (range is 0.1-0.2 ml) of 5% solution (diluted in saline solution to a total volume of 3 ml) administered by nebulizer
Routes of administration	Nebulized, metered-dose inhaler
Onset of action	1 min
Peak effects	1 hr
Duration of action	1-5 hr with single dose; up to 2.5 hr with repeated doses
Dosage forms/packaging	Vial with measuring dropper; used with nebulizer and oxygen metered-dose inhaler
Special considerations	Use caution when administering epinephrine with metaproterenol sulfate
	Antagonist—propranolol
Generic name	**Methylprednisolone sodium succinate**
Brand name	Solu-Medrol
Class	Corticosteroid
Mechanism of action	Enters target cells and binds to cytoplasmic receptors, thereby initiating many complex reactions that are responsible for its antiinflammatory and immunosuppressive effects
Indications and field use	Adjunct in treatment of bronchodilator, unresponsive asthma, hypovolemic shock (controversial), anaphylaxis, esophageal and airway burns, cerebral edema, septic shock and acute spinal cord injury
Contraindications	None for single dose
Adverse reactions	None from single dose; side effects result from long-term, repeated doses
Incompatibilities/drug interactions	None
Adult dosage	For status asthmaticus 10-250 mg given IV. Other medical emergencies may require a different dose
Pediatric dosage	For status asthmaticus 0.5-2 mg/kg given IV. Other medical emergencies may require a different dose
Routes of administration	IV bolus
Onset of action	Hours
Peak effects	8 hr
Duration of action	18-36 hr
Dosage forms/packaging	Mix-a-vials with 40, 125, 500, and 1000 mg or 20 mg/mL vials
Special considerations	Not applicable
Generic name	**Morphine sulfate**
Brand name	None
Class	Narcotic
Mechanism of action	Alleviates pain by acting on sensory cortex of frontal lobes and diencephalon
	Depresses fear and anxiety centers
	Depresses brainstem respiratory centers—decreases responsiveness to changes in $PaCO_2$; also depresses pons and medulla centers of respiratory rhythmicity
	Elevates pain threshold

AV, Atrioventricular; *CNS,* central nervous system; *COPD,* chronic obstructive pulmonary disease; *ET,* endotracheal; *GI,* gastrointestinal; *IM,* intramuscular; *IO,* intraosseous; *IV,* intravenous; *MAO,* monoamine oxidase; *PEA,* pulseless electrical activity; *SQ,* subcutaneous; *VF,* ventricular fibrillation; *VT,* ventricular tachycardia

TABLE 5-5

Additional Drugs Used by the EMT–Intermediate—cont'd

	Morphine sulfate—cont'd
	Increases venous capacitance (venous pooling) and vasodilates arterioles, reducing afterload
	Direct stimulus on chemoreceptor trigger zone in medulla, causing emesis
	Suppresses adrenergic tone
	Decreases GI motility
Indications and field use	Analgesia, especially in patients with burns, myocardial infarction, or renal colic
	Pulmonary edema
Contraindications	Respiratory depression—use with caution in patients with emphysema
	Head injuries, elevated intracranial pressure, asthma
	Use with caution in patients with liver or renal disease
Adverse reactions	Excess sedation; GI spasm; vomiting; bradycardia or tachycardia; orthostatic hypotension; respiratory depression or arrest; seizures
Incompatibilities/drug interactions	Heparin, meperidine
	Phenothiazines (potentiates sedative effect)
Adult dosage	2-4 mg slow IV push (over 1 to 5 minutes), repeat every 5 to 30 minutes as required; patient response is variable—use lowest effective dose
Pediatric dosage	0.1-0.2 mg/kg
Routes of administration	Usually given IV in field
Onset of action	Immediate
Peak effects	20 min
Duration of action	2-4 hr
Dosage forms/packaging	10 mg/mL and 15 mg/mL prefilled syringes or vials
Special considerations	Schedule II narcotic
	Beware of allergies—watch for wheals or urticaria proximal to IV site, and discontinue drug if noted
	Correct hypotension before administration
	Maximum respiratory depression 7-10 min after administration; can be reversed with naloxone
Generic name	**Naloxone**
Brand name	Narcan
Class	Narcotic antagonist
Mechanism of action	Competitive inhibition at narcotic receptor sites
	Reverses respiratory depression secondary to depressant drugs
Indications and field use	Antidote for narcotics, Lomotil, Talwin, Darvon
	Given for acutely depressed levels of responsiveness of unknown cause (differentiates narcotic-induced coma from other causes)
Contraindications	None
Adverse reactions	Acutely precipitates withdrawal symptoms, especially in neonates (nausea, vomiting, diaphoresis, increased heart rate, falling blood pressure, tremors)
	Be prepared for combative patient after administration
Incompatibilities/drug interactions	None significant
Adult dosage	Initial dose of 0.4-2 mg IV push every 2 minutes up to a total of 10 mg over short time (<10 minutes)
	If necessary, dose may be repeated in 2- to 3-min intervals to a maximum of 10 mg
	For ET administration, double dosage and dilute medication with normal saline to a volume of 3-5 mL and follow with several positive-pressure ventilations
Pediatric dosage	If 5 yr of age or younger or less than or equal to 20 kg: 0.1 mg/kg
	If older than 5 years of age or greater than 20 kg: 2.0 mg
Routes of administration	IV, ET
Onset of action	IV, within 2 min
Peak effects	Variable
Duration of action	Approximately 45 min
Dosage forms/packaging	Vials: 0.4 mg/mL (1 mL, 10 mL); 1 mg/mL (2 mL)

Continued

TABLE 5-5

Additional Drugs Used by the EMT–Intermediate—cont'd

Generic name	**Nitroglycerin**
Brand name	Nitrostat, Tridil
Class	Vasodilator
Mechanism of action	Coronary artery vasodilation
	Reduces workload on heart by causing blood pooling and peripheral vasodilation
	Smooth muscle relaxant acting on vascular, uterine, bronchial, and intestinal smooth muscle
Indications and field use	Angina pectoris, congestive heart failure, severe hypertension
Contraindications	Hypovolemia, hypotension, increased intracranial pressure, severe hepatic or renal disease
Adverse reactions	Hypotension, bradycardia, headache
Incompatibilities/drug interactions	IV: All other drugs
Adult dosage	Sublingually: Initial dose of 0.3-0.4 mg, may be repeated at 5-min intervals to a total dose of three tablets if discomfort is unrelieved
	IV: Bolus of 12.5-25 µg may be administered before initiation of continuous nitroglycerin infusion at a rate of 10-20 µg/min; infusion should be increased by 5 or 10 µg/min until desired hemodynamic or clinical response is achieved; must be mixed in glass bottles using special non-PVC tubing
Pediatric dosage	Not used
Routes of administration	IV, sublingual, topical/transdermal, aerosol
Onset of action	Immediate
Peak effects	5-10 min
Duration of action	1-10 min
Dosage forms/packaging	Tablets: 0.3 mg, 0.4 mg, or 0.6 mg
	IV: 50 mg/10 mL ampules
Generic name	**Terbutaline sulfate**
Brand name	Bricanyl, Brethine
Class	Sympathomimetic
Mechanism of action	Beta-2 agonist—has an affinity for beta-2 receptors of bronchial, vascular, and uterine smooth muscle; at increased doses, beta-1 effects may occur
Indications and field use	Bronchospasm (more prevalent in patients over age 40 yr or with coronary artery disease); used in-hospital to stop preterm labor
Contraindications	Use with caution in patients taking other sympathomimetics
Adverse reactions	Tachycardia, tremors, palpitations, nervousness, dizziness—usually dose related; tachycardia may persist as a result of beta-1 stimulus or peripheral vasodilation
Incompatibilities/drug interactions	Alkaline solutions
	Degrades when exposed to light for long periods of time
Adult dosage	0.25 mg SQ; repeat in 15-20 min
	2 inhalations separated by 60-sec interval with metered-dose inhaler
Pediatric dosage	Not recommended for patients under 12 yr of age
Routes of administration	SQ
Onset of action	15 min
Peak effects	30-60 min
Duration of action	90 min-4 hr
Dosage forms/packaging	1 mg/mL; 1-mL, 2-mL ampules
Special considerations	Use with caution in patients with cardiac disease, dysrhythmias, hypertension, diabetes, and hyperthyroidism
	Also available in oral tablets and syrup for at-home use

AV, Atrioventricular; *CNS,* central nervous system; *COPD,* chronic obstructive pulmonary disease; *ET,* endotracheal; *GI,* gastrointestinal; *IM,* intramuscular; *IO,* intraosseous; *IV,* intravenous; *MAO,* monoamine oxidase; *PEA,* pulseless electrical activity; *SQ,* subcutaneous; *VF,* ventricular fibrillation; *VT,* ventricular tachycardia

As EMT–I Maloney is administering the albuterol via inhalation and preparing the stair-chair stretcher for the patient, the school nurse collapses at her desk. EMT–I Maloney and her partner rush to the nurse to find her face flushed and diaphoretic. Her pulse is 130, and she is developing stridorous respirations.

EMT–I Maloney is puzzled for a moment, thinking the only other time she ever saw a patient "crash" like this was when a patient had an anaphylactic reaction after a bee sting.

EMT–I Maloney takes the oxygen from Rosy and immediately begins to assist ventilations on the school nurse. Her partner prepares to start an IV infusion of normal saline as EMT–I Maloney takes off her gloves and contacts medical direction for orders.

The medical direction physician asks EMT–I Maloney what she thinks is going on, and the only thing she can think to say is that it looks a lot like an anaphylactic reaction she saw once. "Is the patient allergic to anything?" the medical direction physician asks.

EMT–I Maloney goes across the hallway to the office and asks, "Is the school nurse allergic to anything?"

"Only latex," the secretary responds.

EMT–I Maloney runs back across the hall and checks the box of gloves in the nurse's office. They are hypoallergenic, nonlatex gloves.

"Doctor, she's only allergic to latex as far as we can find out, but she doesn't have latex gloves in the office."

"Are one of you wearing latex?" he asks.

"Sure, we both had on latex gloves, but we didn't touch her," EMT–I Maloney answers.

"Did one of you take your gloves off?" he asks. "Yes, my partner did, to call you and set up the stretcher," she says.

"Administer 0.3 cc of epinephrine 1:1000 subcutaneously stat," he orders.

EMT–I Maloney repeats the order back to him and administers the injection. In a few minutes the nurse is regaining responsiveness and breathing on her own easily. Rosy is doing well also, and she stares wide-eyed at her nurse.

Then EMT–I Maloney realizes that when her partner "snapped" off his gloves, he created a mist of cornstarch powder, which carried small latex particles into the air.

SUMMARY

Important points to remember from this chapter include the following:
- A drug is any substance that when taken into the body, changes one or more of the body's functions. Drugs may have as many as four names, including the chemical, generic, official, and trade names. Drugs may have natural sources, such as plants, minerals, or animals, or they may be synthesized in the laboratory.
- Consumers in the United States are protected by several regulations regarding drugs. All drugs sold in the United States must meet and maintain high standards for therapeutic results, patient safety, and packaging safety. To meet these standards, drugs must go through strict and accurate testing, which may take several years to complete. The Food and Drug Administration (FDA) is responsible for final approval of all drugs. There are several references for drug information. The *Physicians'*

Desk Reference (PDR) is widely used as a reference for drugs in current use.
- Liquid drugs administered into the body by subcutaneous, intramuscular, or intravenous (IV) routes are called parenteral drugs. Drugs administered through the parenteral route are packaged in several ways, including prefilled syringes, ampules, and vials. The routes used by the EMT–I to administer drugs include sublingual, IV, subcutaneous, inhalation, endotracheal, and transdermal.
- Administering drugs carries with it a tremendous responsibility. The EMT–I must be knowledgeable in the actions, indications, dosages, administration procedures, and side effects of the various drugs he or she may be called on to deliver. If the wrong drug or the incorrect dosage is given, the results can be fatal. EMT–Is may administer certain emergency drugs via local protocol or standing orders, with or without contacting medical direction.

6

Venous Access

Key Terms

Flexion

Half-life

HBV

HIV

Hypertonic Solution

Hypotonic Solution

Intraosseous

Ipsilateral

Isotonic Solution

Large-Bore Catheter

Needle

Sclerotic

TKO Rate

Wide-Open Rate

...■ CASE HISTORY

EMT–I Davis is on duty with Medic 6 when a call comes in for a patient who is bleeding. As EMT–I Davis and his partner, EMT–I Cooper, approach the scene (a high-rise apartment building), the dispatcher contacts them with additional information. "The patient is an 83-year-old female who's having dark stools and coffee-grounds vomiting and is cool and clammy."

A home health care nurse meets them at the door. "Hello, I'm Mrs. Brownwell," she says. "The patient's name is Helen Greenley. Her neighbors got concerned about her when she didn't show up for bingo today." She points to a large "coffee-grounds" stain on the bedding and says, "It looks like she's lost a lot of blood."

As EMT–I Davis begins his initial assessment, he notes that the patient is pale and diaphoretic. Her pulse is 142 and thready, and her respirations are 20. He measures her blood pressure at 94/72. He leans toward the patient's ear and asks, "Mrs. Greenley, are you okay?" She responds by saying, "I don't feel so well."

EMT–I Davis places her on the pulse oximeter and applies a non-rebreather mask supplied with 15 L of oxygen per minute. His partner, EMT–I Cooper, places the electrocardiogram (ECG) electrodes on the patient's chest. Her pulse oximetry reading is 90%, and the ECG shows sinus tachycardia. EMT–I Davis says to the patient, "I'm going to start an IV, Mrs. Greenley," as he places a tourniquet around her left forearm and lowers it over the side of the bed. EMT–I Cooper prepares a 1000-mL bag of normal saline with a macrodrip administration set for EMT–I Davis.

EMT–I Davis palpates a vein on the back of the patient's forearm with his gloved hand and feels confident that he will be able to get it on the first attempt. He prepares the site with povidone-iodine, then wipes it with an alcohol swab. EMT–I Cooper tears five pieces of tape to secure the intravenous (IV) line. EMT–I Davis holds Mrs. Greenley's skin taut with his thumb as he inserts the 18-gauge needle. He has the bevel pointed up as he penetrates the skin and then directs the needle into the vein. As the needle enters the vein, he sees a small amount of blood flash back into the clear plastic catheter cap. He advances the catheter and withdraws the needle.

EMT–I Cooper holds a red, puncture-proof container to his partner's side, and EMT–I Davis immediately drops the catheter stylet into it. Next, he draws a 3-mL sample of blood using a 5-mL syringe and a red-top tube.

EMT–I Davis connects the administration set and opens the flow control valve. The IV is not running. He checks the insertion site for infiltration, but there is no swelling in the surrounding tissue. He rotates the cannula and pulls it back approximately $\frac{1}{16}$ of an inch, but it still does not run. EMT-I Cooper quietly leans over and pulls the tourniquet strap loose, and the IV fluid begins to flow freely. EMT-I Davis is embarrassed to have made one of the most common and fundamental mistakes of IV therapy.

CHAPTER GOAL

Upon completion of this chapter the EMT-Intermediate will be able to understand the basic principles of venous access and IV therapy as well as relate the importance of employing appropriate Body Substance Isolation Precautions when employing these precautions.

Cognitive Objectives

As an EMT-Intermediate you should be able to do the following:

- Describe the indications, equipment needed, techniques used, precautions, and general principles of:
  - Peripheral venous cannulation
  - Obtaining a blood sample
  - External jugular cannulation
- Describe disposal of contaminated items and "sharps."

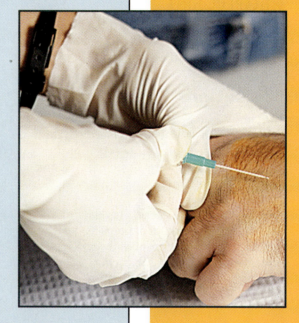

Affective Objectives

As an EMT-Intermediate you should be able to do the following:

- Comply with universal precautions and body substance isolation.

Psychomotor Objectives

As an EMT-Intermediate you should be able to do the following:

- Perfect the technique for disposal of contaminated items and "sharps."
- Demonstrate cannulation of peripheral veins.
- Demonstrate the preparation and techniques for obtaining a blood sample.
- Demonstrate cannulation of the external jugular vein.

INTRODUCTION

Intravenous (IV) cannulation is the placement of a catheter into a vein. It is used to administer blood, fluids, or medications directly into the circulatory system. It can also be used to obtain blood samples from the vein for laboratory determinations. Because IV fluids are drugs, on-line medical direction or standing orders are typically required for the EMT–I to administer IV fluids.

Large-Bore Catheter • A catheter with a large interior diameter (14 to 16 gauge).

Indications

IV therapy is an important tool in the management of the seriously ill or injured patient. Some indications for its use include cardiac disease, hypoglycemia, seizures, and shock. As an example, in hypovolemic shock, IV lines are used to counter blood loss by introducing fluid into the circulatory system. This fluid acts to restore the circulatory volume until the body is able to manufacture enough blood to regain control of the circulatory system. In medical emergencies such as heart problems, IV lines are used to establish a route for medication administration. Generally, the IV route is used to administer drugs in the prehospital setting. Giving the drug intravenously places it directly into the bloodstream, resulting in a quicker onset of action than is achieved through any other medication administration route.

Finally, an IV line can be placed as a precautionary measure in patients who are in stable condition but in whom deterioration may occur. This treatment may be for the purpose of medication access, volume replacement, or both.

> **HELPFUL HINT**
>
> - It is much easier to successfully cannulate a vein before a patient experiences circulatory collapse and venous shutdown than it is to do it afterward.

Precautions

IV therapy is an invasive vascular procedure that carries a number of risks, including bleeding, infiltration, and infection. Because performing venipuncture can be very difficult in some patients, it requires maintenance of ongoing skill proficiency. Probably the most challenging part of carrying out IV therapy is performing the venipuncture itself. Steady hands and a keen eye are needed, along with a lot of practice. Being highly skilled in this area pays off, especially in terms of successful placement and patient satisfaction.

Sclerotic • Hardened or thickened tissues.

Contraindications

Cannulation of a particular site is contraindicated in **sclerotic** veins and burned extremities. Another consideration is that attempts at IV therapy should not significantly delay transporting critically ill or injured patients to the hospital.

> **STREET WISE**
>
> When treating a critically ill or injured patient, avoid spending too much time on the scene trying to start an IV line. Rather, start the IV line(s) en route to the hospital.

Body Substance Isolation Precautions

Because performing IV therapy exposes the EMT–I to blood, body substance isolation (BSI) precautions must be followed. Regard all blood and body substances as being potentially infected with hepatitis B virus (**HBV**) or human immunodeficiency virus (**HIV**). Wear gloves whenever working with IV equipment. After each use, dispose of the gloves in an appropriate waste recepta-

cle. Wash hands before and after working with IV equipment and immediately on coming into contact with blood or other body fluids. If there is any possibility of blood or body fluid splashing, wear additional barrier protection such as a gown, mask, and eye protection. Give particular attention to the proper handling and disposal of needles and sharp instruments, as well as the use of barriers. All once-used needles must be placed in a puncture-resistant ("sharps") container as quickly as possible. For the most part, needle-stick injuries can be avoided by not bending, breaking, or recapping needles; separating them from the syringe; or manipulating them by hand. Another level of protection recommended by the Centers for Disease Control and Prevention is immunization with the HBV vaccine.

EQUIPMENT

The following equipment and supplies are needed to establish and maintain an IV line (Figure 6-1):
- IV solution
- Administration set
- Extension set
- Needles/catheters (assorted sizes)
- Protective gloves, gown, and goggles
- Tourniquet (venous constricting band)
- Tape
- Antibiotic swabs/ointment
- Gauze dressings (2 × 2s, 4 × 4s)
- 10- to 35-mL syringes
- Vacutainer holder with multisample IV Luer-lock adapter
- Assorted blood collection tubes
- Padded armboards

Intravenous Solutions

IV solutions are the fluids that are administered into the venous circulation (Table 6-1). They come in four different types: crystalloids, colloids, blood, and oxygen-carrying fluids.

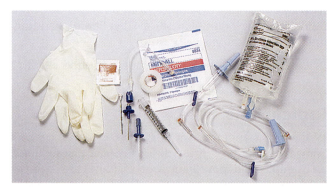

FIGURE 6-1 ▲ Equipment and supplies used to establish and maintain an IV line.

SOLUTIONS AND OSMOTIC PRESSURE

Solutions are described by their tonicity (the number of particles of solute per unit volume). An **isotonic solution** has an osmotic pressure equal to normal body fluid, meaning that solutions are equal on both sides of the cell membrane. Examples of isotonic IV solutions are 0.9% normal saline and lactated Ringer's solution. A **hypotonic solution** has an osmotic pressure less than that of normal body fluids. When the solute concentration of a given solution is less on one side of the cell membrane than on the other, water will be drawn into the solution with a higher solute concentration. A **hypertonic solution** has an osmotic pressure greater than that of normal body fluids. When the concentration of a given solute is greater on one side of the cell membrane than on the other, it draws water into the solution until the solute-to-solution ratio is equal on both sides (even though the volumes differ).

TABLE 6-1

Characteristics of Different Intravenous Solutions

SOLUTIONS	INDICATIONS	ADVANTAGES	DISADVANTAGES	CONSIDERATIONS
5% Dextrose in water (D_5W) Hypotonic sugar solution	To maintain water balance and supply calories necessary for cell metabolism	Is inexpensive and readily available	Causes red blood cell clumping, so it cannot be given with blood Is incompatible with some medications May cause water intoxication, hyponatremia, or hyperglycemia	Not the solution of choice for shock Use only to establish an emergency IV line for drug administration
0.9% Sodium chloride solution (normal saline) Isotonic crystalloid solution	For initial fluid and electrolyte (Na^+, Cl^-) replacement in all types of hypovolemia Cardiac arrest	May be used as an emergency plasma expander while whole blood is being typed and cross-matched Is readily available and inexpensive	May cause diuresis, hypernatremia, hypokalemia, and acid-base imbalance (following large infusions)	Use cautiously if patient has congestive heart failure (CHF) or renal dysfunction Monitor patient for signs of pulmonary edema or fluid overload
Lactated Ringer's solution Isotonic crystalloid solution	For initial fluid replacement in all types of hypovolemia Cardiac arrest	Closely resembles blood plasma Contains electrolyte content needed for adequate kidney function Rarely causes adverse reactions Is inexpensive and readily available Releases buffer when metabolized	May lead to volume overload, CHF, or pulmonary edema	Use with caution in patients with pulmonary edema and impaired lactate metabolism states (liver disease, anoxia) May induce hypothermia with multiple infusions

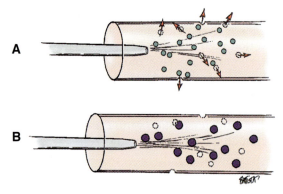

FIGURE 6-2 ▲ **A,** Crystalloid solutions move quickly across cell membranes. **B,** Colloid solutions do not move across cell membranes quickly; therefore they remain in the intravascular space for longer periods of time.

STUDENT ALERT

You should know the difference between crystalloids and colloids and be familiar with the characteristics of the IV fluids commonly used in the field setting.

CRYSTALLOIDS

Dissolving crystals such as salts and sugars in water creates crystalloid solutions. They contain no proteins or other high-molecular-weight solutes. When introduced into the circulatory system, the dissolved ions cross the cell membrane quickly, followed by the IV solution (Figure 6-2, *A*). For this reason, crystalloid solutions remain in the intravascular space for only a short time before diffusing across the capillary walls into the tissues. Because of this action, it is necessary to administer 3 L of IV crystalloid solution for every 1 L of blood lost (3:1 ratio) when treating patients who have experienced hypovolemic shock. Normal saline and lactated Ringer's solution are examples of crystalloids.

Normal Saline and Lactated Ringer's Solution— The recommended IV solutions for use in the prehospital setting are normal saline (0.9%) and lactated Ringer's solution. Both are crystalloid isotonic solutions.

HELPFUL HINT

In addition to its volume replacement benefit, lactated Ringer's solution, when metabolized by the liver, releases bicarbonate, which is a buffer.

One liter of lactated Ringer's solution contains 130 mEq of sodium (Na^+), 4 mEq of potassium (K^+), 3 mEq of calcium (Ca^{2+}), 109 mEq of chloride ions (Cl^-), and 28 mEq of lactate. One liter of normal saline contains 154 mEq of sodium ions (Na^+) and 154 mEq of chloride ions (Cl^-).

Five Percent Dextrose in Water—Five percent dextrose in water (D_5W) is a glucose solution that is isotonic in the container but hypotonic after it enters the circulatory system. The reason for this change is that glucose quickly moves from the circulation, leaving free water. In the past, D_5W was a mainstay in the management of medical emergencies. However, the American Heart Association Advanced Cardiac Life Support Guidelines for cardiac arrest no longer list D_5W as the preferred solution. This is because patients who survive are reported to have poor neurological outcomes when they have increased glucose levels. Local EMS protocols will dictate whether or not D_5W is used.

CLINICAL NOTES

Numerous other crystalloid solutions are also available. These include lesser or greater percentages of D_5W, normal saline or mixtures of lactated Ringer's solution, normal saline or half-strength normal saline, and D_5W. The following are examples of hypertonic solutions:
- 5% dextrose in 0.9% saline
- 5% dextrose in 0.45% saline (half-normal saline)
- 5% dextrose in lactated Ringer's solution
- 3% sodium chloride
- 7.5% sodium chloride
- 10% dextrose in water

The following are examples of hypotonic solutions:
- 0.45% saline (half-normal saline)
- 0.33% sodium chloride
- 2.5% dextrose in water

Half-Life • The time required by the body, tissue, or organ to metabolize or inactivate half of the substance taken in.

COLLOIDS

Colloids contain large molecules, such as protein, that do not readily pass through the capillary membrane (Figure 6-2, *B*). Therefore colloid solutions remain in the intravascular space for extended periods of time. In addition, the presence of the large molecules in colloids results in an osmotic pressure that is greater than the osmotic pressure of interstitial and intracellular fluid. This difference in pressure pulls fluid from the interstitial and intracellular spaces into the intravascular space. For this reason, colloids are often referred to as volume expanders. Plasma substitutes, plasma, packed red blood cells, and whole blood are examples of colloids. However, because colloids are expensive, have a short **half-life,** and often require refrigeration, they are not commonly used in the prehospital setting.

The following common colloids are blood derivatives:

- *Plasma protein fraction (Plasmanate)*—Plasmanate consists mostly of the protein human albumin along with a small amount of globulin and gamma globulin suspended in a saline solvent. Because of its high protein content, Plasmanate remains in the intravascular compartment, raises serum osmolarity, and pulls fluid into the vascular space from the extravascular space. It can be infused immediately without typing and crossmatching.
- *Salt-poor albumin*—This solution contains only the protein human albumin suspended in a saline solvent.

The following are artificial colloids:

- *Dextran*—Dextran consists of high-molecular-weight glucose (sugar) polymers that remain in the bloodstream because of their large size. Dextran replicates the osmotic properties of albumin, so it increases the intravascular volume. Allergic reaction is a possible side effect. Also, dextran decreases platelet adhesiveness and dilutes clotting factors, increasing the risk of bleeding.
- *Hetastarch (Hespan)*—Hetastarch is a (hydroxyethyl) starch-containing colloid with osmotic properties similar to those of albumin. Its effects can last up to 36 hours. An important benefit of hetastarch is that it does not seem to share the side effects that are seen with dextran.

CLINICAL NOTES

Unlike other blood products, a benefit of plasma substitutes is they do not carry the risk of hepatitis.

BLOOD SUBSTITUTES

A drawback to IV solutions used in the prehospital setting is that they lack the ability to carry oxygen. As discussed earlier, whole blood or blood product administration is not practical in the field. Currently under development are a number of artificial solutions that can carry oxygen and off-load it at the cellular level. Although their use remains experimental, they hold great promise for future prehospital use.

Intravenous Solution Containers

IV solutions used in the prehospital setting are typically contained in a clear plastic or vinyl bag that collapses as it empties. The size of the IV bag varies depending on its use, holding anywhere from 25 to 3000 mL of fluid. Smaller bags (100 to 250 mL) are used in the management of medical emergencies and drug administration, whereas larger bags (1000 mL) are used in the management of trauma emergencies or when the patient has experienced volume loss (Figure 6-3). Some EMS systems use IV bags of just one size.

The IV bag has two ports at the bottom of the bag: one port has a rubber stopper for the infusion of medications; the other has a plastic tab that is removed in order to insert the spiked piercing end of the IV administration set tubing into the bag. Along with a host of other information, the IV bag is labeled with the name of the solution, its contents, and an expiration date. Make sure the IV solution is the right one and that it is not expired. Just as with medications, discard any IV solution that is beyond the expiration date.

Administration Set

The administration set is the clear plastic tubing that connects the IV bag to the catheter (Figure 6-4). It allows for easy viewing in case of air bubbles or precipitation of certain medications administered through the tubing. Basic IV administration sets range from 70 to 110 inches in length. There are five primary components of IV tubing with which the EMT–I must be familiar:

- Piercing spike
- Drip chamber
- Flow clamp
- Drug administration port
- Connector end

PIERCING SPIKE

The piercing spike is the sharp, pointed end of the administration set that is inserted into the tubing insertion port of the IV bag. It comes packaged with a protective cap to prevent it from being contaminated before use (Figure 6-5).

DRIP CHAMBER

The drip chamber is the clear, cylindrical portion of the tubing where the drops passing through the adminis-

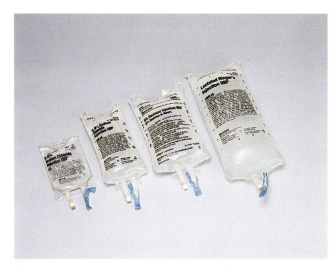

FIGURE 6-3 ▲ Various sizes of IV therapy bags.

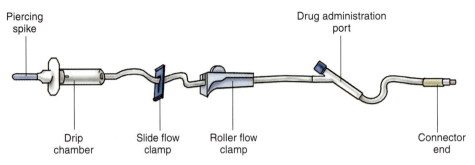

FIGURE 6-4 ▲ **An administration set.**

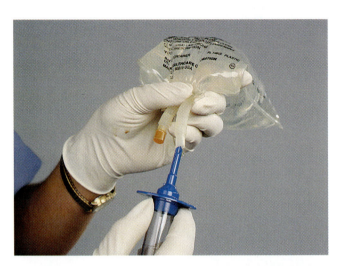

FIGURE 6-5 ▲ **Inserting piercing spike into port of IV bag. (From American College of Emergency Physicians; Pons PT, Cason D, chief editors: *Paramedic field care: a complaint-based approach*, St Louis, 1997, Mosby for ACEP.)**

❗ HELPFUL HINT

The piercing spike must be kept sterile. You can do this by uncovering the piercing spike only to insert it into the IV solution bag. Do this just before insertion. This precaution helps you avoid touching something and contaminating it. If the piercing spike becomes contaminated, discard the administration set and restart the procedure with a new one.

CLINICAL NOTES

Never use your teeth to remove a protective cap from either end of an IV administrative set, the IV bag, the IV cannulation device, or any needle that will be used on a patient.

tration set can be viewed and counted. It is located near the piercing end of the IV tubing where it connects with the IV bag. The number of drops needed to deliver 1 mL of solution is referred to as the drop factor. There are

two types of administration sets commonly used in the prehospital setting: the microdrip (mini) and the macrodrip (regular).

The top portion of the drip chamber is called the drop orifice. The drop orifice of the microdrip consists of a tiny metal barrel projecting down from the top of the drip chamber. The barrel controls fluid flow through the drip chamber. With the microdrip administration set (Figure 6-6, *A*), a smaller amount of fluid is delivered with each drop, with 60 drops being equal to 1 mL of IV solution. The microdrip delivers fluid in very precise amounts, making it useful in children and adults who require minimal fluid and when medications are administered via an IV infusion.

The macrodrip is used when a large amount of fluid is needed (Figure 6-6, *B*). With this type of drip chamber, the drop orifice consists of a large opening that allows for a bigger drop size. Depending on the manufacturer, the drop size varies with different types of administration sets. Typically, a macrodrip delivers 10, 15, or 20 drops/mL. For this reason, it is important to read the box or protective wrap in which the administration set is contained.

⭐ STUDENT ALERT

You should be familiar with the characteristics of the macrodrip and microdrip administration sets.

CLINICAL NOTES

A different type of IV administration set, the SELEC-3 from Biomedix, allows the option of three different drop volumes all in one device (Figure 6-7). By simply turning the selector top, you can choose between 10, 15, or 60 drops/mL at any time without breaking the line. This feature allows a quick response to a patient's changing needs. It also reduces inventory costs and the risk of contamination and ensures that the right administration set is always available.

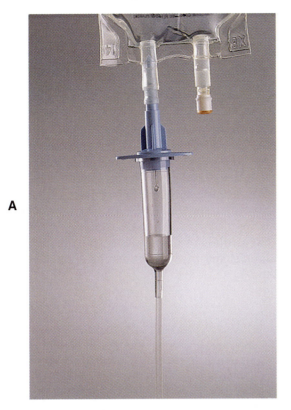
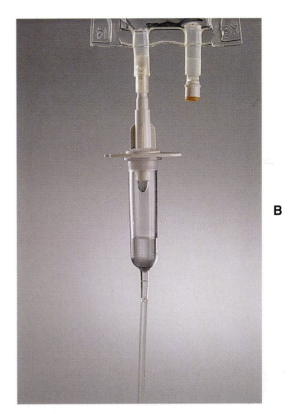

FIGURE 6-6 ▲ **A,** A microdrip chamber delivers fluids in very precise amounts. **B,** A macrodrip chamber allows for a larger drop size.

FLOW CLAMP

Below the drip chamber is the flow clamp. It has a plastic housing with a roller-type clamp that is used to control the amount of IV fluid the patient receives. The flow rate through the IV administration set can be increased or decreased, or the IV infusion turned on or off, by moving the roller up or down (moving the roller up or toward the IV bag increases the flow rate, and moving the roller down or toward the patient slows the flow rate). A second type, the slide flow clamp, moves horizontally to start or stop the flow but does not allow fine adjustments and thus cannot regulate the flow rate (Figure 6-8).

✖ **TKO Rate** • "To keep open" rate of infusing the IV solution. It is also referred to as KVO ("keep vein open"). It is equal to approximately 8 to 15 drops/min.

In the field setting, there are typically two rates for administering IV fluids. In medical emergencies in which IV lines are placed as a precautionary measure or for the purpose of administering medications, the flow is usually maintained at a **TKO rate.** In trauma or other situations in which IV fluids are being used to replace circulatory volume, the flow rate is based on the patient's response to the IV infusion.

Responses include improvement in the patient's:
● Pulse
● Blood pressure
● Capillary refill (in children younger than 6 years of age)
● Cerebral function

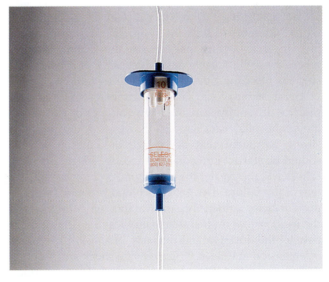

FIGURE 6-7 ▲ SELEC-3 administration set.

✖ **Wide-Open Rate** • No restriction of fluid flow from the IV bag to the patient.

There is a changing philosophy in how volume replacement should be delivered to trauma patients. Until recently, the standard of care in severely hypovolemic patients has been to infuse one to two IV lines, using large-bore catheters and macrodrip administration sets, and deliver the infusion at a **wide-open rate.** Now there

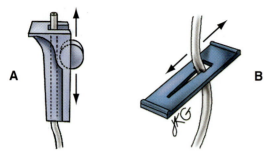

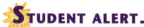

FIGURE 6-8 ▲ **A,** Roller flow clamp. **B,** Slide flow clamp.

STUDENT ALERT

You should know the IV flow rates for various medical and traumatic conditions.

are reports that using large amounts of IV fluids where there is uncontrolled bleeding (such as in penetrating trauma) may increase internal bleeding and lead to more deaths. This occurs because of a rise in blood pressure that can lead to more bleeding. Furthermore, infusing large amounts of IV fluid dilutes the clotting effect of the blood, allowing more bleeding to occur. Another problem is that traditional IV solutions used in the field setting do not have the capability to carry oxygen and are not a substitute for red blood cells. To make matters worse, attempts to start the IV line(s) may result in delays in transporting patients to the trauma facility, where they will receive definitive care that is needed to stop the bleeding, such as surgical intervention.

These factors would seem to warrant discontinuing the practice of rapidly infusing large volumes of IV fluid in the prehospital care setting. However, there is still a strong argument that aggressive fluid administration should be started immediately, since the longer a patient is in shock, the greater the risk is for developing multisystem organ failure. The patient's blood pressure is an important factor influencing survival following trauma(with the incidence of multisystem complications appearing to parallel the duration and intensity of shock. Unresolved hypotension may lead to irreversible shock and death of the organs. An additional concern is that if rapid surgical intervention does not take place, nonresuscitated patients may bleed to death while awaiting surgery.

At the present time, there does not appear to be a clear, absolute rule on how fast IV solutions should be infused as part of treating hypovolemic shock. When the patient has evidence of shock and *has external bleeding that is uncontrolled,* gain IV access en route but give only enough normal saline or lactated Ringer's solution to maintain a blood pressure high enough for adequate peripheral perfusion. Maintaining peripheral perfusion is defined as producing a peripheral pulse, maintaining the level of

consciousness, and maintaining an adequate blood pressure. A blood pressure may be considered adequate when the systolic pressure is in the range of 90 to 100 mm Hg.

When the patient has uncontrolled internal bleeding and surgical intervention is necessary, prompt transport to an appropriate facility is what is needed. Local protocol will dictate the amount and rate of IV infusion. In patients experiencing deep shock (having a blood pressure of less than 50 mm Hg), rapid fluid administration may be indicated to maintain some degree of circulation. The profound lack of circulation in this extreme shock may override concerns of increased hemorrhage secondary to rapid fluid administration. However, given the controversy of this approach, local protocols should guide such therapy.

Regardless of the flow rate, the amount of IV fluid administered in the field setting should be limited to 2 to 3 L.

CLINICAL NOTES

When treating the patient with severe blood loss and infusing IV solutions rapidly, you can increase the flow rate three to four times the normal amount by wrapping a blood pressure cuff around the IV bag and inflating it to 300 mm Hg.

DRUG ADMINISTRATION PORTS

Drug administration ports are located below the drip chamber. They are closer to the distal end of the administration set tubing. These ports consist of a self-sealing rubber stopper and a Y-shaped inlet (Figure 6-9). Medication boluses or an infusion of medication can be delivered through these ports. It is best to use the medication port that is closer to the patient.

CONNECTOR END

The connector end is the part of the IV administration set that is inserted into the hub of the IV catheter. Like the spiked piercing end, it is packaged with a protective cap to keep it from being contaminated before use. It is usually not necessary to remove the distal protective cap to drain the administration set of air, so it can be kept in place until it is time to connect it to the IV catheter. Although the design of the connectors may vary by manufacturer, the dimensions are standard and should attach to any IV catheter hub or extension set.

Three types of connectors are most often seen. The simplest connector is the slip tip. It is a male end that has a small circumference at the tip. The circumference size gradually increases as it moves back toward the tubing. To connect it, push it straight into the catheter hub (or other device). To disconnect it, rotate it a quarter of a turn and pull backward on the connector while

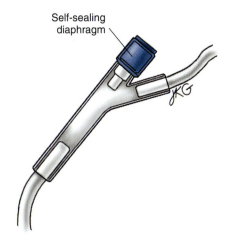

FIGURE 6-9 ▲ Drug administration port.

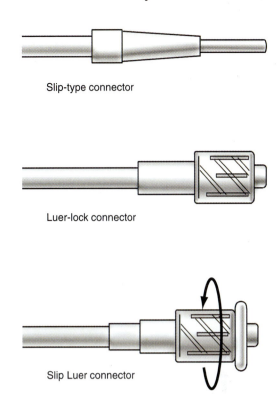

FIGURE 6-10 ▲ Three common types of connector ends.

using the other hand to hold the catheter in position. One disadvantage of the slip tip is that it can leak. Another type of connector is the Luer-lock connector. Similar to the slip tip, it has a male connector that inserts into the female end of the catheter hub. However, around the end of this connector is a threaded lip that is screwed into the hub. This connector usually prevents leakage, but because it takes more time to secure, blood can leak out of the catheter hub. The last connector is the slip Luer. It has a longer male connector than the plain Luer-lock connector. The threaded Luer lip on this device turns freely, allowing one to quickly make the connection with the slip tip and then secure the connection with the Luer-lock (Figure 6-10).

> ❗ **HELPFUL HINT**
>
> ● To reduce the amount of IV fluid needed to clear the air from the tubing, slide the flow control valve toward the spiked end of the tubing until it comes to rest against the drip chamber. Then open the control valve to flush the air out of the tubing.

Specialty Intravenous Tubing
BLOOD TUBING

Some EMS systems use IV blood tubing instead of macrodrip tubing in patients with hypovolemia. This use reduces the amount of tubing changeover required at the hospital when the patient is switched from a crystalloid solution to blood. Also, EMTs who work in an aeromedical, critical care transport or emergency department setting may be expected to set up blood tubing.

IV blood tubing has a larger internal diameter and special blood filter. It usually has a drip factor of 10 drops/mL. The filter prevents clots and other debris that have formed in the blood bag from entering the patient's circulatory system when whole blood or blood components are administered. Otherwise these clots or debris could enter and travel through the circulatory system as an embolus. This embolus could then become lodged in a blood vessel somewhere along the circulatory system, blocking blood flow past the point of occlusion. This would then result in ischemia and death of the tissue normally supplied with nutrients and oxygen by that branch of the circulatory system.

Two types of blood tubing are available: Y-tubing and straight tubing. Y tubing has two piercing spikes, one for infusing blood and the other for infusing normal saline solution. Having two piercing spikes allows normal saline to be infused as a diluent to the transfusion. It also allows immediate administration of IV fluid if the blood supply is depleted or must be stopped, as occurs in the case of a patient experiencing a transfusion reaction. Straight blood tubing is equipped with just one reservoir. For this reason, only blood is attached to the tubing. A secondary line of normal saline can be piggybacked into the tubing through a medication administration port close to the needle adapter (Figure 6-11).

> **CLINICAL NOTES**
>
> Typically, blood is delivered with normal saline. This is because the calcium chloride in IV solutions such as lactated Ringer's solution increases the potential for blood clotting.

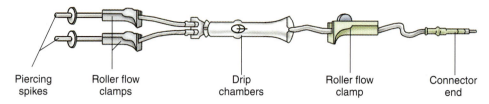

Piercing spikes   Roller flow clamps   Drip chambers   Roller flow clamp   Connector end

FIGURE 6-11 ▲ IV blood tubing.

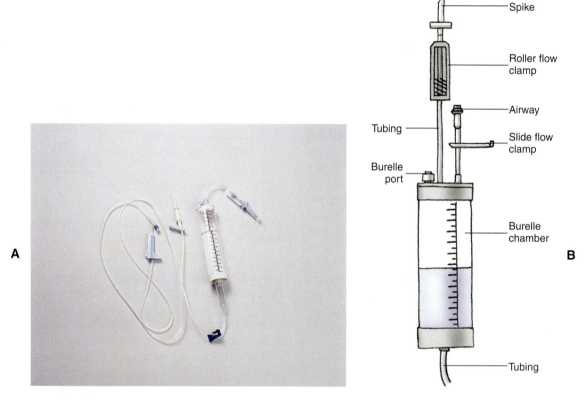

FIGURE 6-12 ▲ **A**, Volutrol chamber IV tubing is commonly used when specific amounts of fluid are to be administered. **B**, Volume control chamber IV tubing.

VOLUME CONTROL

Another type of administration set, the volume control set, is used when specific amounts of fluids are to be administered (Figure 6-12). Most commonly, this tubing is used for infant and pediatric infusions, as well as for patients who suffer from renal failure or who cannot tolerate fluid overload. Another use of the volume control administration set is to administer medications in very precise amounts.

Also referred to as burette sets, Buretrols, Volutrols, Solutols, or Metrisets, volume control sets are available with or without an in-line filter. At the proximal end of the administration set is a piercing spike that is inserted into the administration set port of the IV bag. Between the piercing spike and the fluid chamber is a flow control valve that regulates the flow of fluid into the chamber. On the top of the fluid chamber are an air vent and a self-sealing medication injection port. The main part of the vol-

ume control administration set is a fluid chamber that holds between 100 and 150 mL of fluid. The fluid chamber is calibrated in 1.0-mL increments, usually written on the side of the reservoir, to allow small, precise delivery of fluids. Below the chamber is a microdrip or macrodrip chamber. There is another flow control valve located below the drip chamber that regulates the rate at which fluid is delivered. The fluid chamber is used to measure the amount of fluid, and the drip chamber is used to ensure an accurate delivery rate. At the distal end is a connector that fits into the hub of an IV catheter or extension set.

When opened, the air vent on top of the burette chamber permits air to be displaced or replaced as fluid comes into or exits the fluid chamber. To administer a medication using this device, the drug is added to a specific amount of IV fluid by injecting it through the medication administration port after filling the chamber to the necessary level.

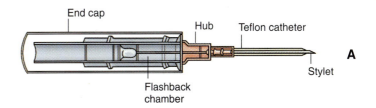

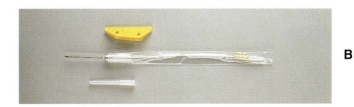

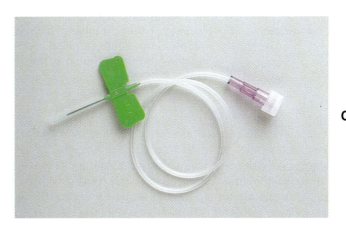

Extension Set

Extra tubing may be used to lengthen the administration set, making it easier to move the patient without disrupting the IV site. However, consider the following words of caution. More IV tubing may actually slow the IV flow rate, making its use questionable when fluid resuscitation is needed. Also, the extra tubing may get caught under the stretcher when the patient is being removed from the ambulance.

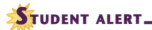 **Needle** • A sharp, stainless steel hollow tube that is used to penetrate the skin and blood vessel.

Needle/Catheter

The catheter is the tube that remains in the vein to allow the administration of IV fluids or medications. The **needle** is used to facilitate passage of the catheter through the skin and into the vein. It has a beveled tip that makes penetration of the skin and vein easier and less painful. The three basic types of IV catheters are plastic catheters inserted over a hollow needle (Angiocath, Quickcath, Jelco, etc.) (Figure 6-13, *A*), plastic catheters inserted through a hollow needle or over a guidewire (Intracath) (Figure 6-13, *B*), and hollow needles (butterfly type) (Figure 6-13, *C*). Plastic catheters are generally preferred over hollow needles in advanced life support.

STUDENT ALERT
You should know the difference between the various types of IV needle/catheters.

FIGURE 6-13 ▲ **A,** An over-the-needle catheter. **B,** A through-the-needle catheter. **C,** A hollow needle (butterfly type).

OVER-THE-NEEDLE CATHETERS

The over-the-needle catheter typically consists of a flexible plastic outer catheter and a hollow inner needle that extends just beyond the catheter. The distal end of the needle is sharp and beveled, permitting easy penetration of the skin and vein. At the proximal end of the needle is a flashback chamber that allows one to see blood return when the vein is penetrated. The needle is pulled out after insertion in the vein, leaving the catheter in place. The proximal end of the catheter has a hub where the IV tubing is attached (once the needle has been removed).

Because of their flexibility, most commonly, over-the-needle catheters are used in the prehospital setting; they can be better anchored and permit freer movement of the patient. In addition, the puncture site in the vein is the same size as the plastic catheter; therefore there is less chance for bleeding around the venipuncture site. Two other benefits of this device are that infiltration occurs less frequently than with steel needle venipuncture devices, and an armboard usually is not necessary after insertion. Because the device has both a catheter and needle, it is more difficult to insert than winged steel needles.

Over-the-needle catheters used to cannulate peripheral veins are commonly available in lengths of 1 to 2 inches (2.5 to 5 cm), with gauges ranging in size from 14 to 26.

INTRAVENOUS CATHETER SIZE

The outside diameter of the venipuncture device is called its gauge. The larger the gauge number, the smaller the diameter of the shaft (e.g., a 22-gauge catheter is small, whereas a 14-gauge catheter is large). A large-diameter (14-gauge) catheter provides much greater fluid flow than does a small-diameter (22-gauge) catheter. Catheters used for prehospital care come in a variety of sizes, which are listed in Table 6-2.

STUDENT ALERT
You should know the sizes of the IV catheters that are used for the various conditions.

Choosing the best size over-the-needle catheter for the patient is not always easy, but as a rule, except for when volume replacement is needed, smaller-sized devices are

TABLE 6-2

Different-Sized Venipuncture Devices

GAUGE	INDICATIONS FOR USE	CONSIDERATIONS
14 to 16	Adolescents and adults Volume replacement, as in trauma When viscous medications, such as 50% dextrose, are to be administered	Painful insertion Requires a large vein
18	Older children, adolescents, and adults Administration of blood and blood components and other viscous infusions	Painful insertion Requires a large vein
20	Older children, adolescents, average-sized adult patients Suitable for most IV infusions	Commonly used
22	Infants, toddlers, children, adolescents, adults (especially elderly) Suitable for most IV infusions	Used for fragile and/or small veins Slower rates must be maintained More difficult to insert through tough skin
24 to 26	Neonates, infants, toddlers, children, adolescents, adults (especially elderly) Suitable for most IV infusions, but flow rates are slower	For extremely small veins (e.g., small veins of the fingers or veins of the inner arm in elderly patients) May be difficult to insert into tough skin

better. A small needle/catheter causes less injury to the vein. It also allows greater blood flow around the tip, reducing the risk of clotting. Using a catheter that is too big for the vein invites complications. Also, some elderly patients' veins cannot accommodate a large-bore catheter. **Large-bore catheters** (14- to 16-gauge) should be used for patients in shock, cardiac arrest, or other life-threatening emergencies in which rapid fluid replacement is required. At a minimum, an 18-gauge catheter should be used in those patients requiring blood. Another time to use a larger catheter is when administering viscous medications such as 50% dextrose. When employing a large-sized catheter, be sure to choose a large enough vein to accommodate it. The other variable to consider when selecting an IV catheter is its length. The longer the catheter, the slower the flow rate. The flow rate through a 14-gauge, 5-cm catheter (approximately 125 mL/min) is twice the flow rate of a 16-gauge, 20-cm catheter. For cannulation of a peripheral vein, a needle and catheter length of 1.5 to 2 inches (5 cm) is adequate. Some over-the-needle catheters are supplied with an attached syringe (Figure 6-14). The syringe permits an easy check of blood return once the needle is inside the vein and prevents air from entering the vessel on insertion.

Other Supplies and Materials

A variety of other supplies are needed to establish and maintain an IV line. Without exception, latex or rubber protective gloves should be worn when attempting venipuncture. A tourniquet (venous constrictive band), when applied proximal to the IV venipuncture site before cannulation, delays venous return and distends the vein,

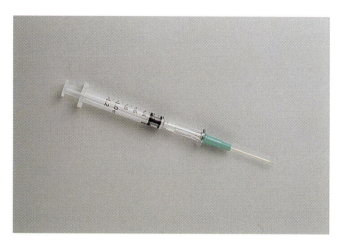

FIGURE 6-14 ▲ An IV catheter supplied with an attached syringe.

making it easier to locate and cannulate. The ideal tourniquet is easily tied, does not roll into a thin band, stays relatively flat, and releases easily. Penrose drain tubing commonly is used as a tourniquet in the prehospital setting. Also, there are a variety of tourniquets commercially available. Some are equipped with a catch mechanism to anchor them. Others have a wide, flat rubber band that is secured with Velcro. Povidone-iodine or alcohol preparations are used to cleanse the IV site before venipuncture, reducing the risk of infection. Sterile dressings are applied over the IV site to keep it clean. Adhesive tape is applied over the administration set tubing, sterile dressing, and IV catheter to hold them in place. Armboards stabilize the IV site, preventing the patient from dislodging or causing the catheter to become kinked or posi-

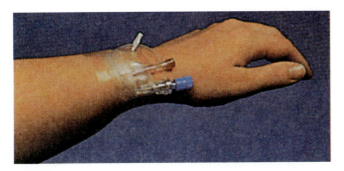

FIGURE 6-15 ▲ Intermittent infusion device in place. (From Sanders MJ: *Mosby's paramedic textbook,* ed 2, St Louis, 2000, Mosby.)

tioned against a valve in the vein. A 10- or 35-mL syringe or a Vacutainer holder with a multisample IV Luer-lock adapter fitted to it, as well as assorted blood collection tubes, are used to collect blood samples.

INTERMITTENT INFUSION DEVICE

Another popular device used in the field and hospital settings is the intermittent infusion device (Figure 6-15). It effectively eliminates the need for an IV bag and an administration set. Consisting of short tubing with a clamp, a proximal medication port, and a distal slip or Luer-lock connector, it is attached to the hub of an IV cannula that has been placed in a peripheral vein. It keeps the access device sterile and prevents blood from leaking from an open end. Alternatively, any IV cannulation device that has a catheter such as winged-tipped catheter or over-the-needle catheter device can be converted to an intermittent infusion device by way of a simple adapter plug with a latex cap that is affixed to its proximal end.

The intermittent infusion device is commonly called a heparin (or saline) lock because a heparin (or saline) flush is injected into the cap to keep blood from backing up into the venipuncture device and clotting. Two types of male adapter plugs, the long male adapter and the short male Luer-lock, are available to convert a winged needle set or over-the-needle catheter into an intermittent infusion device. Like an administration set medication injection port, the intermittent injection cap is self-sealing after the needle is removed. Some are designed to work with needleless injection systems. Although the distal end of this device is a universal size and fits the hub of a standard IV catheter, a Luer-lock tip is typically used to prevent accidental loosening.

The intermittent infusion device is particularly useful when the patient requires constant venous access but not continuous infusion. The benefits of using this device are that it creates a route for administering medications without requiring a continuous infusion of IV fluids, which can be harmful to patients experiencing circulatory overload; decreases the risk of electrolyte derangement; reduces cost (because the administration set and IV solution are not used); makes it easier to move the patient (because there is no IV bag and administration set); decreases the possibility of an IV line being accidentally pulled out; increases patient comfort and mobility; and preserves veins by reducing the need for repeated venipuncture (for withdrawing blood samples, etc).

After it is in place, the device should be flushed with saline or heparin before or after medication administration or at least once a day. A heparin flush should not be used if the patient is sensitive to heparin, has a clotting disorder, or has uncontrolled bleeding.

INTRAVENOUS SOLUTION WARMING DEVICES

Typically, IV fluids are stored in cabinets or jump kits in the EMS unit. When used, these fluids tend to be the same temperature as the air where the vehicle is parked. Thus the temperature of IV fluids can vary a lot depending on the locale, as well as the conditions under which the ambulance is stored in-between calls. The infusion of IV solutions that are less than normal body temperature can lead to the development of hypothermia in certain patients. This includes the elderly, children, the frail, and those suffering from trauma, shock, fever, or similar conditions.

Appliances are now on hand to warm IV fluids. Some are designed to fit into the cabinetry that is located in the patient module of the ambulance. Others are portable warming sacks. In-line IV fluid heaters are also available. These devices are designed to maintain the IV fluid temperature at a normal body temperature of 98° F and to prevent overheating.

One device, the Hot Sack, holds up to two 1-L IV bags, warming them to body temperature in about 1 hour (provided they are at room temperature) with even heating and no hot spots. The Hot Sack runs off of 12 volts from any vehicle. When it is not powered, it loses only 1° F in 10 minutes at 15° F outside temperature. Outside flaps in the bottom of the bag allow fluids to be administered without removing the IV bags from the Hot Sack. An optional insulated sleeve for the administrative set tubing is also available.

CLINICAL NOTES

Even IV bags at room temperature (i.e., 70° F) are colder than body temperature. Rapid infusion of a lot of fluid can lead to hypothermia.

SITES FOR PERIPHERAL VENOUS CANNULATION

Structure of Veins

Veins have three layers: the tunica intima (inner layer), tunica media (middle layer), and tunica externa (outer layer). The tunica intima is an inner elastic endothelial lining made up of layers of smooth, flat cells that allow blood cells and platelets to flow smoothly through the blood vessels. Unnecessary movement of the venipuncture device can scratch or roughen this inner surface, causing thrombus formation. Semilunar valves, designed to prevent backflow and ensure the flow of blood toward the heart, are located in this layer of the vein. These valves are found in many veins and are especially common in those of the extremities. The tunica media consists of muscular and elastic tissue. Vasoconstrictor and vasodilator nerve fibers located in this layer stimulate the vein to contract and relax. They are responsible for venous spasm that can occur as a result of anxiety or receiving IV fluids that are too cold. The tunica externa consists of connective tissue that surrounds and supports the vessel, holding it together.

Difference Between Arteries and Veins

Before choosing a vein as an IV site, make sure the blood vessel is actually a vein in order to avoid inadvertent arterial puncture (Figure 6-16). Table 6-3 shows the main characteristics of veins and arteries.

The Skin

The skin is made up of two layers: the epidermis and the dermis (Figure 6-17). The epidermis is the outermost layer. It forms a protective covering for the dermis and varies in thickness in different parts of the body. The thinnest areas of skin are on the inner surface of the limbs. The thickness of the dermis also varies with age. Elderly patients often have such thin skin on the dorsum of the hand that it does not adequately support the vein for venipuncture.

The dermis, or underlayer, is highly vascular and sensitive, containing many capillaries and thousands of nerve fibers, including those that react to temperature, touch, pressure, and pain. The number of nerve fibers varies in different areas of the body, with some areas being highly sensitive and others being only mildly sensitive. The insertion of a needle may cause great pain in one area but little pain in another.

Sites Used in Routine Situations

In noncritical patients the distal veins on the dorsum of the hands and arms often are used as IV sites. Using these veins permits the patient to freely move his or her arm. Also, the technique is relatively easy to master, and using one of these locations as the IV site does not interfere with other life-sustaining measures such as airway management (Figure 6-18). In addition, if a problem develops with more distal veins, another site higher up on the arm can be selected. The disadvantage of the more distal veins is that they are sometimes fragile and diffi-

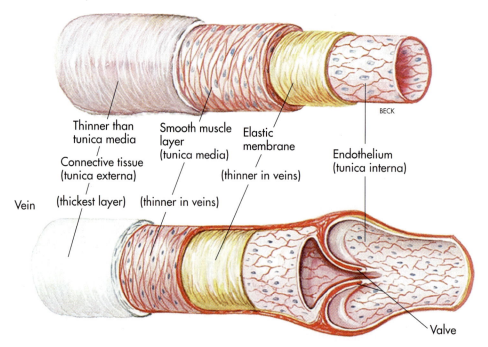

Muscular artery

Thinner than tunica media

Smooth muscle layer (tunica media)

Elastic membrane

Endothelium (tunica interna)

Connective tissue (tunica externa)

(thinner in veins)

BECK

Vein

(thickest layer)

(thinner in veins)

Valve

FIGURE 6-16 ▲ The characteristic differences between veins and arteries. (Ernest W. Beck from Thibodeau GA, Patton KT: *The human body in health and disease*, St Louis, 1992, Mosby.)

cult to cannulate. Also, in states of decreased cardiac output, medications administered through these vessels take longer to reach the central circulation. Furthermore, irritating solutions administered through these veins may cause pain and phlebitis. For a summary of IV site locations, advantages, disadvantages, and considerations for use, see Table 6-4. If available, use a vein with the following characteristics (Figure 6-19):

- Is fairly straight
- Is easily accessible
- Is well fixed, not rolling
- Feels springy when palpated

Sclerotic veins, veins near joints (where immobilization will be difficult), areas where an arterial pulse is palpable close to the vein, or veins near injured areas and edematous (swollen) extremities should be avoided as sites of IV

TABLE 6-3

Differences Between Arteries and Veins

CHARACTERISTICS	VEINS	ARTERIES
Location in the body	Superficial veins lie just under the skin and drain the skin and superficial fascia Deep veins accompany the principal arteries and take the name of the artery with which they travel	Arteries run deep and usually are surrounded by muscle, which provides them the protection they need as part of the high-pressure portion of the vascular system Occasionally an artery is superficially located; this is an aberrant artery
Color of blood	Dark red because of decreased oxygen concentration	Bright red because of usually high concentration of oxygen
Pulsation	Absent	Present
Valves	Present; they keep blood flowing toward the heart, counteracting muscular pressure that would make the blood back up Valves often cause a noticeable bulge in the vein when a tourniquet is applied	Not present; arteries are under constant pressure because the heart pumps blood through them
Direction of flow	Toward the heart	Away from the heart

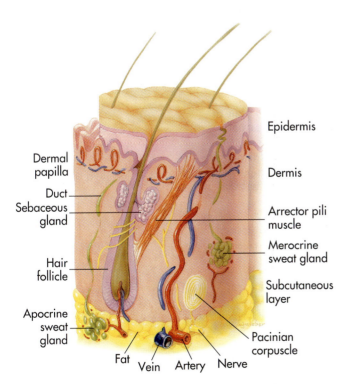

FIGURE 6-17 ▲ The skin. (From Sanders MJ: *Mosby's paramedic textbook,* ed 2, St Louis, 2000, Mosby.)

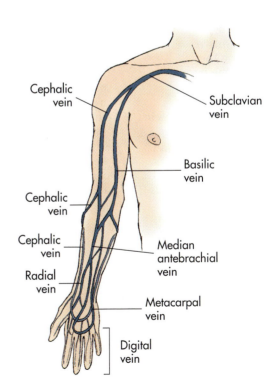

FIGURE 6-18 ▲ Venous anatomy of the arm.

TABLE 6-4

Intravenous Site Locations: Advantages, Disadvantages, and Considerations for Use

SITE	ADVANTAGES	DISADVANTAGES	CONSIDERATIONS
Digital veins Run along the lateral and dorsal portions of the fingers and are joined to each other by communicating branches	Can be used when other sites are not available	Uncomfortable for patient Infiltrate easily Cannot be used if dorsum hand veins are already being used	In some patients the veins are prominent enough to hold a 21-gauge scalp needle Adequate immobilization of the fingers with tape can keep the needle from puncturing the posterior wall of the vein
Metacarpal veins Located on the dorsum of the hand, formed by the union of the digital veins between the knuckles	Position of these veins makes them well suited for IV use Easily accessible Lie flat between the joints and metacarpal bones (the bones themselves provide a natural splint) in the large child and adult Allow the EMT–I to initiate successive venipuncture above the previous puncture site	Wrist movement is limited unless a short catheter is used Insertion is more painful because of increased nerve endings in the hands Site becomes phlebitic more easily Veins do not always dilate sufficiently to allow for successful venipuncture; when hypovolemia occurs, the peripheral veins collapse more readily than the large veins	Occasionally use of the metacarpal veins in the elderly is a poor choice because thin skin and a lack of supportive tissue in this area make securing the catheter difficult, and small, thin veins may allow extravasation of blood on venipuncture
Cephalic vein Has its source in the radial part of the dorsal venous network formed by the metacarpal veins Runs along the radial side of the forearm and upper arm	Large vein is excellent for venipuncture Readily accepts large-bore needles Does not impair mobility Its position on the forearm creates a natural splint for the needle and adapter	Proximity to the elbow may decrease joint movement Vein tends to roll during insertion	May be necessary to shave patient's arm if excessive hair makes taping the catheter and tubing in place difficult
Accessory cephalic vein Originates from either a plexus on the back of the forearm or metacarpal veins of the thumb (dorsal venous network) Sometimes arises from the portion of the cephalic vein just above the wrist and flows back into the main cephalic vein at some higher point; runs along the radial bone, ascending the arm and joining the cephalic vein below the elbow	Large vein is excellent for venipuncture Readily accepts large-bore needles Does not impair mobility	Is sometimes difficult to position the catheter flush with the skin Usually uncomfortable because the venipuncture device is at the bend of the wrist Its position on the forearm creates a natural splint for the needle and adapter	

TABLE 6-4

Intravenous Site Locations: Advantages, Disadvantages, and Considerations for Use—cont'd

SITE	ADVANTAGES	DISADVANTAGES	CONSIDERATIONS
Median antebrachial vein Arises from the palm and runs along the ulnar side of the forearm	Vein holds winged needles well in this area	Many nerve endings may cause painful venipuncture or suffer infiltration damage Infiltration occurs easily in this area	A last resort when no other means are available
Basilic vein Has its origin in the ulnar part of the dorsal venous network and ascends along the ulnar side of the forearm and upper arm; diverges toward the anterior surface of the arm just below the elbow, where it meets the median cubital vein	Can take a large-gauge needle easily Straight, strong position vein suitable for large-gauge venipuncture devices	Patient must be in an uncomfortable position during insertion Penetration of the dermal layer of the skin, where nerve endings are located, causes pain Vein tends to roll during insertion	This vein is often overlooked because of its inconspicuous position on the ulnar border of the hand and forearm; when other veins have been exhausted, this vein may still be available Vein can be brought into view by flexing the elbow and bending the arm up
Antecubital veins Located in the antecubital fossa (median cephalic is located on the radial side, median basilic is on the ulnar side, and median cubital arises in front of the elbow joint)	Readily accessible Large veins facilitate placement of large catheter Often visible or palpable in children when other veins will not dilate May be used numerous times without damage to the vein, provided good technique and sharp needles are used Because of muscular and connective tissue supporting them, they have little tendency to roll	Difficult to splint the area with an armboard Median vein crosses in front of the brachial artery, increasing risk of accidental puncture of the artery Veins may be small and scarred if blood has been drawn frequently from this site May be uncomfortable for patient because the arm must be kept straight (otherwise the catheter could kink or slide in and out of the vein, damaging it)	Location is over an area of joint flexion where any movement can dislodge the catheter and cause infiltration or result in mechanical phlebitis If these large veins are impaired or damaged, thrombophlebitis may occur, which then limits use of many available hand veins
Great saphenous vein Located at the internal malleolus	Large vein excellent for venipuncture	Circulation of the lower leg may be impaired Walking is difficult with the catheter in place Increased risk of deep vein thrombosis	
Dorsal venous network Located on the dorsal portion of the foot	Suitable for infants and toddlers	Veins may be difficult to see or find if edema is present Walking is difficult with the device in place Increased risk of deep vein thrombosis	

Continued

TABLE 6-4

Intravenous Site Locations: Advantages, Disadvantages, and Considerations for Use—cont'd

SITE	ADVANTAGES	DISADVANTAGES	CONSIDERATIONS
External jugular vein Runs from behind the angle of the jaw downward superficially across the sternocleidomastoid muscle (lateral portion of the neck) to pierce the fascia above the middle third of the clavicle; joins the subclavian vein just behind the clavicle	Easy to cannulate Is considered a peripheral vein Provides rapid access to the central circulation	Difficult to keep the dressing in place IV may be easily dislodged and positional with head movement	May not be readily accessible during arrest situation because of EMT-Is working to manage patient's airway

FIGURE 6-19 ▲ The ideal vein for delivering IV therapy is fairly straight, easily accessible, well fixed, and feels springy when palpated.

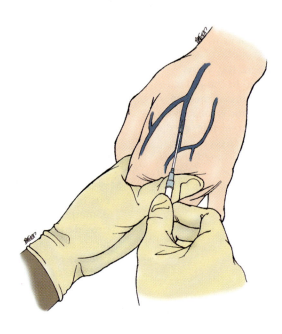

cannulation. Circulatory problems in an extremity such as dialysis fistula (arteriovenous shunt), a history of mastectomy, or an arm being treated for thrombosis or cellulitis also should prompt the selection of another extremity. If possible, the patient's nondominant hand should be used, leaving the hand used for writing free.

Sites Used in Cardiac Arrest

In cardiac arrest, the preferred sites for IV cannulation are the peripheral veins of the antecubital fossa (the area anterior to and below the elbow) because they are among the largest, most visible, and accessible veins in the arm. The more distal veins are the least preferred IV sites because blood flow from distal extremities is markedly diminished during circulatory collapse and distal peripheral veins may be difficult or impossible to cannulate.

 Intraosseous • Within or into a bone.

CLINICAL NOTES

Check your local protocol to determine if you are permitted to cannulate the external jugular vein in your community.

Other Sites

Other sites that may be used for IV cannulation include the external jugular vein, peripheral leg veins, and **intraosseous** sites. The external jugular vein is a fairly large vein that lies superficially along the side of the neck. It extends from the angle of the mandible (below the ear) and runs downward until it pierces the deep fascia of the neck just above the middle of the clavicle and ends in the subclavian vein (Figure 6-20, A). This vein is clearly visible in the adult but is difficult to cannulate in the pediatric patient because of the short neck on a child (for this reason, it is usually not attempted). A disadvantage to using the external jugular vein as an IV site is that the catheter and tubing are hard to tape down and can be displaced with movement of the patient's head. The veins of the

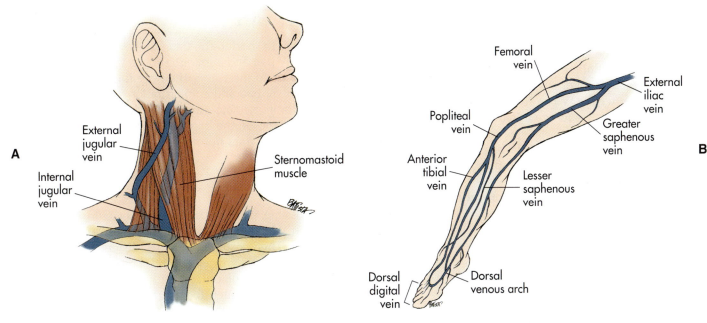

FIGURE 6-20 ▲ **A**, The jugular vein. **B**, The saphenous vein and other venous anatomy of the leg.

lower leg (Figure 6-20, *B*) should be used as a last resort in adults, because use of these veins places the patient at risk for thrombus formation. If the saphenous vein of the leg is used, it should be entered at its most distal point. Sites for IV cannulation in pediatric patients, including intraosseous cannulation, are described in Chapter 34.

PERFORMING INTRAVENOUS CANNULATION

The procedure for performing IV cannulation is as follows:
1. Explain the need for IV cannulation and describe the procedure to the patient. Determine if the patient has any allergies (especially to iodine if using iodine pads to cleanse the skin). Keep in mind that the patient may be apprehensive about the procedure and concerned that his or her condition may have worsened. This anxiety can lead to a vasomotor response that can produce syncope or venous constriction. Also, children may have completely unrealistic fears, such as being poisoned or that the IV line will never be removed. Hints for preparing the patient for venipuncture include asking the patient if he or she has ever had an IV infusion before and being supportive if the patient is fearful. You should explain to the patient:
   - Why the IV line is needed
   - That "IV" means inside the vein and that a plastic catheter will be placed there
   - That fluids containing certain nutrients or medications will flow from a bag through a length of

tubing and then through the catheter into the patient's vein
   - That he or she will experience transient pain as the needle goes in but that the discomfort will stop once the catheter is in place
   - How the patient can help by holding still when the needle is inserted and not withdrawing if there is pain
   - That the IV fluids may feel cold at first, but that the sensation should last only a few minutes
   - How this therapy will limit his or her activities
   Instruct the patient to report to you any discomfort after the IV therapy is initiated. Sometimes patients are the first to notice infiltration of the IV fluid.
2. Next, select the IV fluid to be used, and check to make sure it is:
   - The proper solution
   - Clean, without particulate matter
   - Not outdated
   - Not leaking
3. Select an appropriately sized catheter (14 to 16 gauge for trauma, volume replacement, or cardiac arrest; 18 to 20 gauge for medical conditions).

HELPFUL HINT

Displaying a confident, understanding attitude goes a long way toward helping patients feel more at ease during IV cannulation. Also, encouraging the patient to use stress reduction techniques such as deep, slow breathing can help to reduce anxiety.

4. Select the proper administration set (macrodrip for trauma, microdrip for medical conditions and drug administration).
5. Prepare the IV bag and administration set using an aseptic technique to prevent contamination, which can cause local or systemic infection.
   - Remove the IV bag from its protective envelope, and gently squeeze it to detect any punctures or leakages.
   - Steady the port of the IV bag with one hand, and remove the protective cap by pulling smoothly to the right.
   - Remove the administration set from its protective wrapping or box.
   - Slide the flow control valve close to the drip chamber.
   - Close off the flow control valve.
   - Remove the protective cap from the spiked piercing end of the administration set.
   - Invert the IV bag.
   - Using sterile technique, insert the spiked piercing end of the administration set into the tubing insertion port of the IV bag. Use one quick, smooth motion (Figure 6-21, *A*). Be careful not to puncture the side of the tubing insertion port with the tip of the spiked piercing end.
   - Turn the IV bag right side up, and squeeze the drip chamber two or three times to fill it halfway (Figure 6-21, *B*).
   - Open the control valve to flush the IV solution through the entire tubing. This should force all the air out of the tubing and prevent the accidental passing of an air embolism into the patient's circulatory system.
6. Cut or tear several pieces of tape of different lengths.
7. Employ body substance isolation precautions (at a minimum, apply gloves).

8. If possible, place the patient into a comfortable position with the selected extremity lower than the heart. This positioning helps distend the distal veins. Remove any jewelry from the arm where the IV line will be placed.
9. Apply a tourniquet. To tie it, follow these steps:
   - Place the tourniquet under the patient's arm, about 6 inches above the venipuncture site. Position it so that it is in the middle of the arm with an equal distance from either end to the patient's arm (Figure 6-21, *C*).
   - Bring the ends of the tourniquet together, placing one on top of the other (Figure 6-21, *D*).
   - Holding one end on top of the other, lift and stretch the tourniquet and tuck the top tail under the bottom tail. Do not allow the tourniquet to loosen (Figure 6-21, *E*).
   - Tie the tourniquet smoothly and snugly, being careful not to pinch the patient's skin or pull arm hair.

   To reduce the risk of pain and discomfort when using a tourniquet, avoid keeping it in place for more than 2 minutes. Also, the tourniquet should be kept as flat as possible. It should be snug but not uncomfortably tight. A tourniquet that is too tight impedes arterial, as well as venous, blood flow. Palpate the patient's radial pulse. If it cannot be felt, the tourniquet is too tight and must be loosened. Also, the tourniquet should be loosened and retightened if the patient complains of severe tightness.

   A tourniquet that is applied too tightly or kept in place too long may cause increased bruising, especially in the elderly patient whose veins are fragile. Therefore the tourniquet should be released as soon as the venipuncture device has been placed into the vein and blood samples have been drawn (if applicable).
10. Select a suitable vein by palpation and sight. Avoid areas of the veins where a valve is situated. If the vein rolls or feels hard or ropelike, select another vein. Veins can be distended for easier cannulation by:
   - Having the patient open and close his or her fist tightly five or six times
   - Flicking the skin over the vein with one or two sharp snaps of the fingers

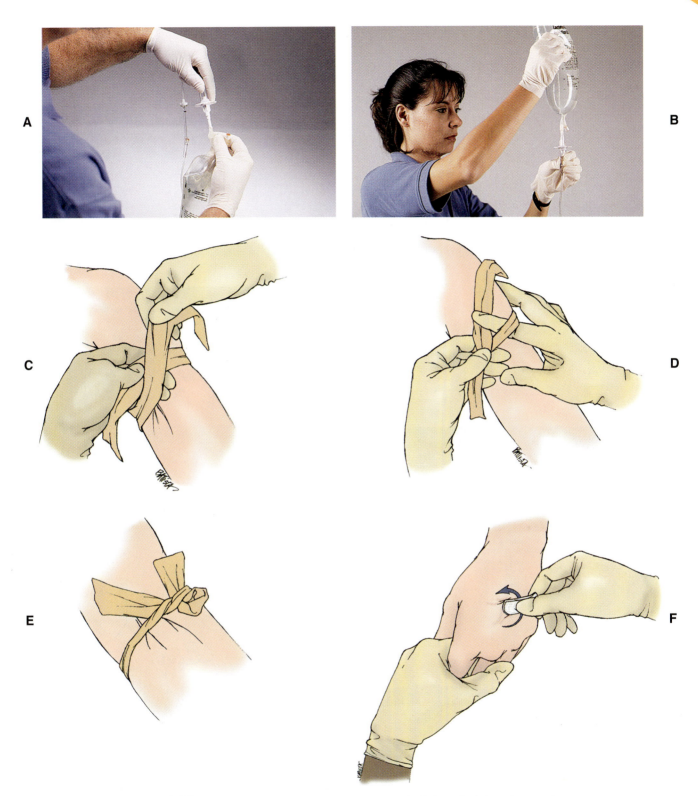

FIGURE 6-21 ▲ **A,** Insert the spiked piercing end of the administration set into the tubing of the IV bag. **B,** Squeeze the drip chamber to fill it half-way. **C,** Place the tourniquet 6 inches above the venipuncture site. **D,** Make a slip knot with the tourniquet. **E,** Complete band placement. **F,** Use povidone-iodine or an alcohol wipe to cleanse the site. *Continued*

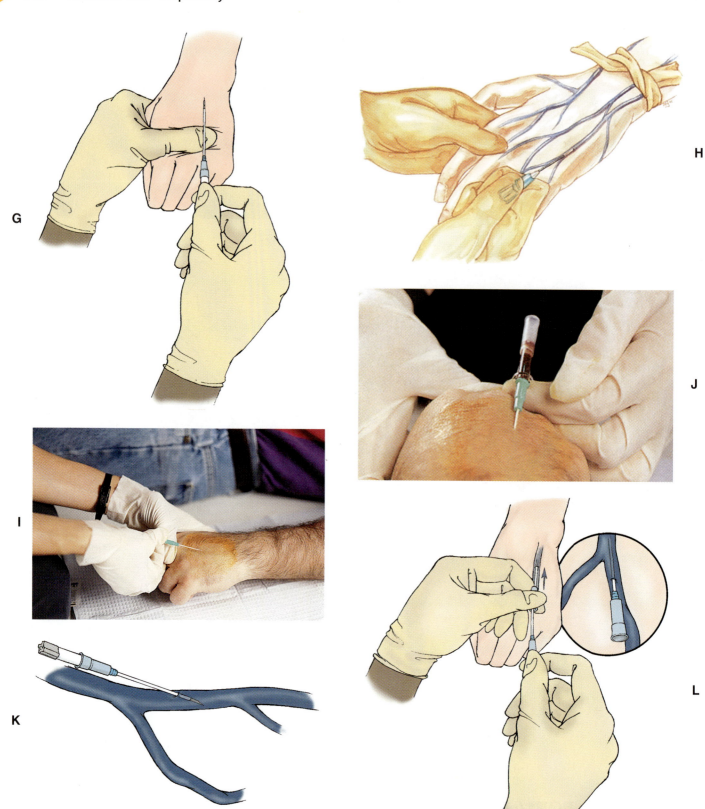

FIGURE 6-21—cont'd ▲ **G,** Pull the skin taut; the bevel of the needle should be facing up when penetrating the skin. **H,** If possible, penetrate the vein at its juncture with another vein. **I,** Penetrate the skin, and enter the vein from either the top or the side. **J,** Watch for blood in the flashback chamber. **K,** Advance the needle until the tip of the catheter is securely in the vein. **L,** Slide the catheter into the vein until the hub rests against the skin.

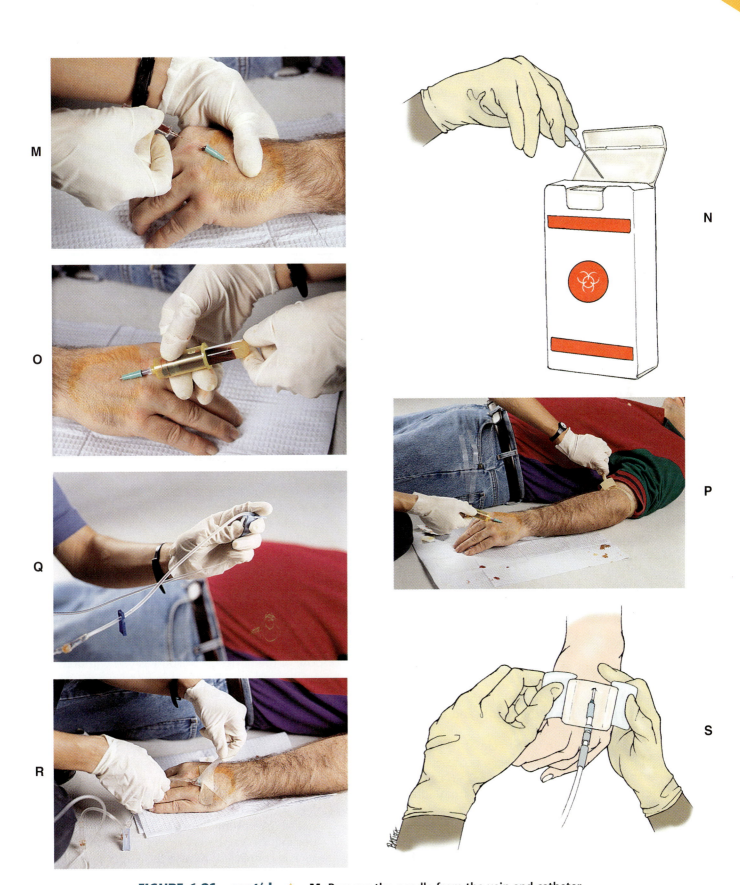

FIGURE 6-21—cont'd ▲ **M,** Remove the needle from the vein and catheter.
N, Proper disposal of the used needle. **O,** An EMT–I drawing a sample of blood.
P, Release the tourniquet. **Q,** Connect the IV tubing to the catheter. **R,** Secure the
catheter and tubing in place with tape. **S,** A commercial device used to secure the
catheter.

- Rubbing or stroking the skin upward toward the tourniquet

If a suitable vein cannot be found, or if the vein still feels small and uniform, release the tourniquet and apply it closer to the IV site. If that fails to resolve the problem, apply the tourniquet to the other arm.

11. Cleanse the site thoroughly with povidone-iodine or an alcohol wipe, using a firm circular motion (Figure 6-21, *F*). The area should be allowed to dry before penetrating the skin. It may be necessary to shave the hair around the selected insertion site to provide better adherence of the tape that is used to secure the catheter and administration set tubing.

12. Stabilize the vein by anchoring it with the thumb and stretching the skin downward. This action makes the venipuncture site taut. Stabilizing the vein helps ensure successful cannulation the first time and decreases the chance of bruising. Bruising occurs when the tip of the needle repeatedly probes a moving vein wall, nicking the vein and causing it to leak blood. When this injury occurs, the vein cannot be immediately reused, and another site must be found. This event requires the patient to endure the discomfort of another needle puncture. If the vein is in the hand, it may be helpful to have the patient flex his or her wrist.

13. Perform the venipuncture without contaminating the equipment or site.
    - Tell the patient there will be a small poke or pinch as the needle enters the skin.
    - Hold the end of the venipuncture device between the thumb and index/middle fingers—much the same as holding a pool cue. This technique allows easy visualization of the flashback chamber. Avoid touching any portion of the catheter, because a contaminated device is not usable.
    - Depending on the type of venipuncture device and manufacturer recommendations, hold the needle at a 15-degree, 30-degree, or 45-degree angle to the skin.
    - Penetrate the skin with the bevel of the needle pointed up (Figure 6-21, *G*). If significant resistance is felt, do not force the catheter. Instead, withdraw the needle and catheter together as a unit.
    - If possible, penetrate the vein at its junction or bifurcation with another vein, because it is more stable at this location (Figure 6-21, *H*).
    - Enter the vein with the needle from either the top or the side (Figure 6-21, *I*).
    - Normally, a slight "pop" or "give" is felt as the needle passes through the wall of the vein. Be careful not to enter too fast or too deeply, because the needle can go through the back wall of the vein.
    - Note when blood fills the flashback chamber of the needle (Figure 6-21, *J*).
    - Lower the venipuncture device, and advance it

another 1 to 2 cm until the tip of the catheter is well within the vein (Figure 6-21, *K*). The reason for this is that the catheter is slightly shorter than the needle. As a result, blood backflow sometimes occurs when only the needle is in the vein. Advancing the venipuncture device a bit more ensures that the catheter is correctly situated in the vein.
    - While holding the needle stable between the first and middle fingers and thumb, use the first finger and thumb of the other hand to slide the catheter into the vein until the hub is against the skin (Figure 6-21, *L*).
    - Once the catheter is within the vein, apply pressure to the vein beyond the catheter tip with the little finger to prevent blood from leaking out of the catheter hub once the needle is completely withdrawn (Figure 6-21, *M*).

14. Dispose of the needle(s) in a proper biomedical waste container (Figure 6-21, *N*).

15. Draw a blood sample (Figure 6-21, *O*). The tourniquet should be left in place while drawing blood samples.
    - Stabilize the catheter with one hand, and attach a Vacutainer holder with a multisample IV Luer-lock adapter or a syringe to the hub. Be careful not to disrupt the catheter placement while connecting the Vacutainer or syringe. Once the device is connected, release the finger pressure at the distal tip of the catheter.
    - If using a Vacutainer device, insert the blood collection tube fully into the holder and allow its internal vacuum to draw blood out of the vein. If

using a syringe, slowly withdraw the plunger to fill the syringe with blood. If blood flow into the syringe stops, it usually means that the sucking pressure of the syringe is collapsing the vein. To correct this problem, slow the rate at which the plunger is being withdrawn.

16. Once enough blood collection tubes have been filled or the syringe is completely full, release the tourniquet from the patient's arm (Figure 6-21, *P*). Next, reapply pressure to the vein beyond the catheter tip with the little finger to prevent blood from leaking out of the catheter hub once the blood-drawing device is disconnected. Disconnect the syringe or Vacutainer device from the hub of the catheter by holding the hub between the first finger and thumb and pulling the device free with the other hand.

17. Connect the IV tubing to the catheter hub. Be careful not to contaminate either the hub or the connector before insertion.

18. Open the IV flow control valve and run the IV infusion for a brief period of time to ensure that the line is patent (Figure 6-21, *Q*). To ensure proper IV flow rates, the IV container must hang at least 30 to 36 inches above the insertion site.

19. Cover the IV site with povidone-iodine ointment and a sterile dressing or a bandage.

20. Secure the catheter, administration set tubing, and sterile dressing in place with tape (Figure 6-21, *R*) or a commercial device (Figure 6-21, *S*). The tubing should be looped and secured with tape above the IV cannulation site. The loop gives the tubing more

play, making the catheter less likely to be dislodged by accidental pulls on the tubing. However, do not make the loop so small that it kinks the tubing and restricts fluid flow.

21. Adjust the appropriate flow rate for the patient's condition.

22. When using a syringe to draw blood, fill the blood collection tubes by attaching a needle to the syringe and inserting it into each blood tube to withdraw

CLINICAL NOTES

A variety of commercial transparent semi-permeable dressings are available for use in the prehospital setting. These dressings allow air to pass through them but are impervious to microorganisms. Benefits of these dressings include the following:

- They cause fewer adverse reactions than medical tape.
- The insertion site is clearly visible (allowing detection of early signs of phlebitis and swelling).
- Because the tape is waterproof, it protects the site should it become wet.
- Because the dressing adheres well to the skin, there is less chance of accidentally dislodging the venipuncture device.

STREET WISE

In some cases it is hard to get the tape to stay in place. Common problems include hairy arms and moist or wet skin. Excess hair can be shaved away from around the insertion site. However, you should take care to prevent contamination of the venipuncture site. Moist skin can be dried before applying tape. However, if the skin remains moist or wet, it may be necessary to wrap the tape around the entire arm and tape it to itself. Be careful not to wrap it so tight that blood flow is restricted.

Attach one piece of tape to the catheter hub and another piece to the administration set tubing, not one piece to both. This way, if the administration set is pulled on, it will only separate the connector from the IV catheter hub and not pull the catheter out. In addition, if the tubing requires changing, you will not have to waste time and energy trying to separate the two.

STREET WISE

In normal situations, you can ask a family member or bystander to hold the IV bag while you are on the scene taking care of the patient. It gives them something to do and frees you to do other tasks. When moving the patient to the ambulance, the IV bag typically is placed in an IV holder. This device is attached to the stretcher, looks like a pole, and has one to two hooks along with a Velcro strap that holds the IV bag in place. The IV holder folds down for easy storage when not in use. When carrying the patient out in a stair chair, Reeves stretcher, or backboard, you can keep the plastic IV bag running by placing the bag under the patient's shoulder. Placing the IV bag under the patient's shoulder also is useful in frigid temperatures when you need to keep the IV solution warm. In addition, the IV tubing should be kept under the blankets and close to the patient to prevent it from becoming chilled. An alternative method is to employ an intermittent infusion device.

the blood. The tubes are then labeled and stored in a safe location.

The number of attempts (or "sticks") made to place an IV line depends on local protocol. However, a good rule of thumb is to limit the number of attempts to three.

Although IV skills will improve with practice, some veins are particularly difficult to cannulate. Obese patients, patients in shock or cardiac arrest, chronic mainline drug users, elderly patients with fragile or "rolling" veins, and small children may pose a challenge. In shock and cardiac arrest, the patient's veins can constrict and disappear from sight. Do not waste time searching for a vein in one arm. If a good vein is not found easily, go to the patient's other arm or external jugular vein.

> **● HELPFUL HINT**
>
> To cannulate a rolling vein, do the following: First, pull the skin tight. However, be careful not to pull too tightly, or the vein will flatten, making cannulation difficult. Then pass the needle through the skin, pausing for a second to line up the needle in the same direction as the vein. Next, penetrate the vein from the side rather than the top. Try to insert the needle into the center of the vein to keep it from moving. Sometimes you have to "chase the vein" as it moves from side to side.
>
> To cannulate fragile veins, use a smaller needle and insert it into the vein carefully. The gentler you are, the better chance you have of successfully placing the IV cannula.

After Venipuncture is Performed

When it appears that the needle has penetrated a vein, try to confirm proper needle placement. Sometimes blood may not flow back into the flashback chamber of the needle (e.g., during severe hypovolemia). When this happens but you are sure you have correctly placed the catheter, start the IV infusion and carefully watch the site for signs of infiltration (e.g., coolness and swelling around the site). If infiltration occurs, remove and discard the catheter and place a dressing on the venipuncture site. Then, using sterile equipment, attempt venipuncture at another site. Other methods of determining proper placement of the catheter include the following:

- Lowering the IV bag below the IV site. If it is correctly positioned, blood backflow should be seen in the IV tubing.
- Palpating the vein above the IV site. It should be cool or the same temperature as the IV solution being infused.
- Palpating the tip of the catheter in the vein.
- Aspirating blood with a 10-mL syringe, then discarding the syringe in an approved container.

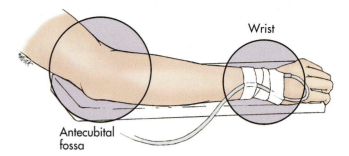

FIGURE 6-22 ▲ Common puncture sites that may require the use of an armboard.

Using an Armboard

The use of an armboard can usually be avoided simply by choosing a venipuncture site well away from any **flexion** areas. However, an armboard may be necessary when a venipuncture device is inserted near a joint or in the dorsum of the hand, or it may be used along with restraints in confused or disoriented patients (Figure 6-22).

Ask the patient to flex his or her arm, and watch the IV flow rate. If the flow stops during movement, an armboard is needed. Because armboards do not prevent rotation, they cannot always prevent infiltration. The armboard must be long enough to prevent flexion or extension at the tip of the venipuncture device. It should be covered with a soft material and applied with tape that is padded with folded gauze or tissue. Be careful when using an armboard, because one that is applied too tightly can cause nerve and tendon damage. Also, make sure the tape that keeps the venipuncture device in place is not attached to the armboard. Otherwise, any motion of the arm on the armboard can pull on and potentially displace the venipuncture device.

Regulating Fluid Flow Rates

A primary aspect of administering IV therapy is delivering accurate flow rates for the IV solutions. An infusion that runs too fast or too slow can cause the patient to suffer complications such as circulatory overload (leading to congestive heart failure and/or pulmonary edema), phlebitis, and infiltration. Some protocols call for the IV flow rate to be adjusted as ordered by medical direction. Other protocols prescribe IV solution flow rates for given conditions. When the IV flow rate is regulated with the roller clamp, the rate is usually measured in drops per minute. It is necessary to know the volume to be infused, the period of time over which the fluid is to be infused, and the number of drops per milliliter the infusion set delivers. The following formula can be used to calculate IV solution drip rates per minute.

$$\frac{\text{Volume to be infused (in milliliters)}}{\text{Time of infusion (in minutes)}} \times \text{Drip (in drops per milliliter)} = \text{Flow rate (in drops per minute)}$$

Example: You are instructed to administer 35 mL of IV fluid over 40 minutes using a microdrip administration set. The formula is 35 mL ÷ 40 minutes = 0.875 mL/min multiplied by 60 drops/mL = 52.5 drops/min (rounded to 52 drops/min) to be administered.

Once the drop rate per minute has been determined, setting the flow is easy. When the IV line has been established, the clamp is slowly opened to start fluid dripping into the drip chamber. Place your watch next to the drip chamber so that you can see both the second hand (or second indicator) and drops dripping into the chamber. Then count the drops for 1 minute (or count for 30 seconds and multiply the number by 2). Open or close the clamp as needed to adjust the drip rate. If at any time the clamp slips or the patient makes a sudden move, the drip rate may be affected. Check it periodically, using the method described previously. However, avoid spending excessive time at the scene counting for small discrepancies.

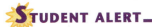

Once the flow rate has been established, be sure to check it on an ongoing basis to identify any problems with the infusion. Factors that can cause the flow rate to vary include vein spasm, vein pressure changes, patient movement, manipulations of the clamp, bent or kinked tubing, IV fluid viscosity, the height of the infusion bag, the type of administration set, and the size and position of the venous access device. Make adjustments to the flow rate as necessary to deliver the prescribed flow rate. Assess the flow rate more frequently in the following:
- Critically ill patients
- Patients whose condition can be exacerbated by fluid overload
- Pediatric patients
- Elderly patients
- Patients receiving a drug that can cause tissue damage if infiltration occurs

Documenting Intravenous Cannulation

Depending on local protocol, when an IV line is started, the following must be documented on the run report:
- Date and time of the venipuncture
- Type and amount of solution

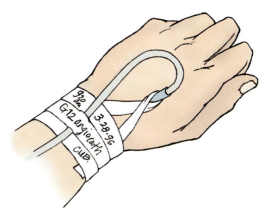

FIGURE 6-23 ▲ Document the IV cannulation by writing the necessary information on a piece of tape and applying it over the dressing.

- Type of venipuncture device used, including the length and gauge
- Venipuncture site
- Number of insertion attempts (if more than one) and the location for each
- IV flow rate
- Any adverse reactions and the actions taken to correct them
- Name or identification number of the person initiating the infusion

In addition to documenting correct IV placement, unsuccessful attempts should also be documented.

Some local protocols call for the EMT–I to document the following information directly on the tape that is used to secure the venipuncture device and administration set tubing in place:
- Date and time of insertion
- Type and gauge of needle or catheter
- Initials of the person who placed the device

To do this procedure properly, cut a piece of tape and place it on a flat surface. Write the information on it, and then apply it over the dressing. The tape should never be labeled after it has been applied over the dressing. Doing so will irritate the venipuncture site (Figure 6-23).

When the Intravenous Fluid Does Not Flow

In some cases the IV fluid does not flow as it should. Problem-solving skills can be used to determine the cause and correct the problem. The following questions should be asked (Figure 6-24):
- Was the venous tourniquet (constricting band) removed? Not releasing the tourniquet after cannulating the vein is probably the most common mistake made in both the hospital and field settings. In addition, restrictive clothing the patient is wearing or a shirtsleeve that has been pushed up too high on the arm can interfere with venous flow.

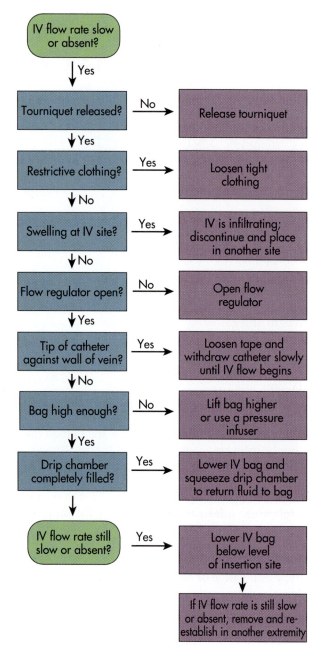

FIGURE 6-24 ▲ **A problem-solving flow chart for IV therapy.**

- Is there swelling at the cannulation site? Swelling may indicate that the catheter is displaced and there is infiltration into the tissues.
- Is the flow regulator in an open position? If it is turned off, no flow will occur. Be sure to check both the primary and secondary control valves that are part of the administration set.
- Is the tip of the catheter positioned against a valve or wall of the vein? This problem can be checked for by slightly twisting or withdrawing the catheter. It may be necessary to untape the catheter and retape it after a good flow rate has been achieved by repositioning the

catheter. In addition, a padded armboard can be used to keep the patient's hand or arm in a good position.
- Is the IV bag high enough? Sometimes when moving the patient, the cannulation site is raised higher than appropriate. This problem interferes with the gravity that is required to move IV fluid. To correct this problem, lower the extremity, raise the IV bag, or consider a pressure infuser.
- Is the drip chamber completely filled with IV solution? Inverting the bag and squeezing the drip chamber to return some of the fluid to the bag can easily correct this problem.

If the flow is still slow or absent, lower the IV bag below the level of the insertion site. If blood return is seen in the IV tubing at the connection point with the catheter, the site is patent. If problems persist, the IV line should be removed and reestablished in another extremity.

> **STUDENT ALERT**
>
> Be sure you are familiar with what to look for if the IV fluid is not flowing. Also, you should know the complications associated with IV cannulation.

Complications

All IV techniques share both local and systemic complications, including pain, catheter shear, circulatory overload, cannulation of an artery, infiltration/hematoma, local infection, pyrogenic reaction, air embolism, thrombosis, phlebitis, sepsis, and pulmonary thromboembolism. Those complications that are most likely to occur in the prehospital setting are described here.

PAIN

Pain at the puncture site is a common complication. It typically is due to penetration of the skin with the needle or extravasation of IV fluid into the tissue. Pain can lead to increased anxiety and worsening of the patient's condition. Using a smaller-gauge catheter or the sharp tip of a smaller needle to make an incision in the skin through which a larger catheter can pass more easily can reduce the pain associated with venipuncture.

CATHETER SHEAR

A catheter shear can occur when the catheter is pulled back through (through-the-needle catheter) or over (over-the-needle catheter) the needle after it has been advanced forward. Because the catheter is plastic, it can easily snag on the sharp edge of the needle and be sheared off, becoming plastic emboli. For this reason, the catheter must never be drawn back over or through the needle. The needle should always be withdrawn first and then the catheter.

CIRCULATORY OVERLOAD

Circulatory overload occurs when too much IV solution is administered or the IV solution is administered too rapidly for a given patient's condition. To prevent circulatory overload, the IV flow rate must be carefully monitored, particularly in patients prone to heart failure. All patients receiving IV fluids must be constantly watched for signs of developing congestive heart failure, in which case the IV flow rate should be significantly reduced or terminated. Signs and symptoms include headache, flushed skin, rapid pulse, increased blood pressure, rales, dyspnea, tachypnea, ing, and external jugular vein distention.

CANNULATION OF AN ARTERY

Veins tend to lie superficially, whereas arteries are found deeper in the skin. Despite this difference, an artery can be inadvertently punctured because of its close proximity to veins. Arterial puncture is characterized by the appearance of spurting bright red blood (or darker red blood in hypoxic patients). If bright red blood suddenly appears in the syringe (with over-the-needle catheters equipped with a syringe) and pushes the plunger up, the device should be completely removed. Direct pressure is then applied to the puncture site for at least 10 minutes, until the bleeding has stopped. In the patient with adequate circulatory output, the artery can be detected by checking for a pulse.

HEMATOMA OR INFILTRATION

A hematoma or infiltration at the puncture site can be caused by injury to the blood vessel, inadvertent puncture during IV cannulation, or a cannula that becomes dislodged from the vein. Fluid then accumulates in the tissues. Signs and symptoms include edema, blanching of the skin, discomfort, an infiltration site that feels cool to touch, IV fluid flowing more slowly, and an absence of blood flashback. When a hematoma or infiltration occurs at the puncture site, the catheter should be removed and the IV line reestablished at another site.

LOCAL INFECTION

A local infection can occur when appropriate cleansing techniques are not used and bacteria are introduced into the venipuncture site. Swelling and tenderness at the IV site are common signs. This infection is not seen in the prehospital setting but occurs several days following initial treatment.

AIR EMBOLISM

An air embolism occurs when air is allowed to enter the vein. It can occur during central vein cannulation, when air is not cleared from the IV administration set appropriately, or when the IV tubing becomes dislodged from the hub of the catheter. Signs and symptoms include hypotension, cyanosis, tachycardia, increased venous pressure, and loss of responsiveness.

PYROGENIC REACTION

A pyrogenic reaction occurs when foreign proteins, capable of producing fever, are present in the administration set or IV solution. It is characterized by the abrupt onset of fever (100° to 106° F), chills, backache, headache, nausea, vomiting, flushing of the face, and sudden pulse change. Cardiovascular collapse also may result. The reaction usually occurs within 30 minutes of the initiation of IV therapy. If a pyrogenic reaction is suspected, the IV line should be immediately terminated and established in the other arm, using a new administration set and solution. This complication emphasizes the need to discard any IV bag that shows leakage or cloudiness.

INTERMITTENT INFUSION DEVICE

The intermittent infusion device is used in situations where an IV route needs to be established for medication administration or repeated venous blood sampling but where continuous infusion is not required.

The following supplies and equipment are needed to place an intermittent infusion device:
- IV cannula
- One or two 3-mL syringes filled with heparin or saline flush solution and connected to a 20-gauge 1-inch needle or a needleless device
- Intermittent infusion device
- Tape or commercial securing device
- Venous blood drawing equipment
- Antiseptic swab

The following steps should be used to place an intermittent infusion device:

1. Assemble the necessary equipment.
2. Use an alcohol swab to clean the cap in the intermittent infusion device.
3. Prime the device (male adapter plug or device and tubing) with dilute heparin or saline solution (Figure 6-25, *A*).
4. Insert the IV catheter following the steps described previously (Figure 6-25, *B*).
5. Remove the needle from the over-the-needle catheter device, and properly dispose of it.
6. Obtain venous blood samples (if indicated or required by protocol).
7. Insert the distal end of the intermittent device into the hub of the IV catheter (Figure 6-25, *C*). Inject 3 to 5 mL of dilute heparin or saline solution into the lock to prevent occlusion. If resistance is felt or swelling

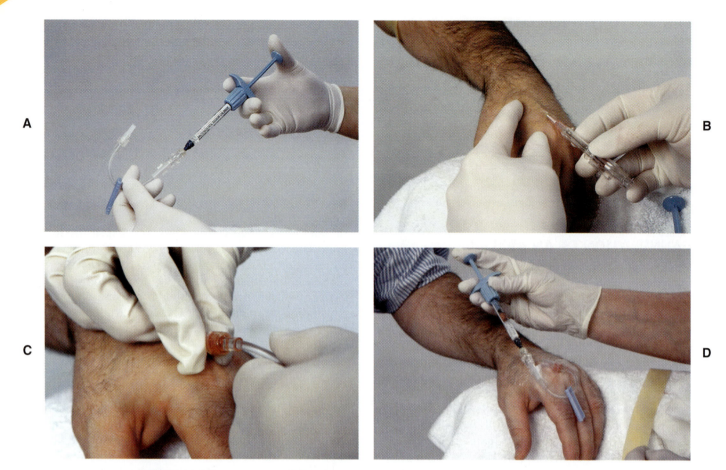

FIGURE 6-25 ▲ **A,** Priming the device with dilute heparin or saline solution. **B,** Cannulating the vein. **C,** Connecting the intermittent device to the hub of the IV catheter. **D,** Inject 3 to 5 ml of dilute heparin or saline.

occurs, restart the procedure with new equipment at another site. Cover the IV site with povidone-iodine ointment and a sterile dressing or a bandage. Secure the IV catheter and intermittent infusion device in place with tape or a commercial device.

DRAWING BLOOD

Drawing blood from a vein is done to acquire blood samples from a patient for analysis. These blood samples can reveal a great deal of information about the patient, including the blood glucose (sugar) level, hemoglobin and hematocrit levels, clotting time, presence of medications, cardiac enzyme evaluation, and more. The most commonly used venous blood assessment in the field setting is the evaluation of blood glucose levels. Information that reveals the presence of hypoglycemia will prompt the administration of 50% dextrose to resolve the glucose deficiency. Although blood samples can be drawn as a separate procedure from starting an IV, it is more practical to draw them immediately after placing the venipuncture device (but before attaching the administration tubing). This method reduces the number of painful sticks to which the pa-

tient is subjected. However, when the quality of the patient's veins is extremely fragile and drawing blood may jeopardize the IV line, blood should be drawn from another vein using a needle and syringe or a Vacutainer device.

Blood-Drawing Equipment

A variety of sizes and types of blood tubes are available to collect and store blood samples (Figure 6-26). The rubber caps on the tubes come in several colors and patterns, denoting the specific tests that are conducted with the blood that is stored in them. Most commonly used in the field setting are the red, purple, green-blue, and gray tops. Some of these tubes have small amounts of liquids or agents inside the tube to prevent blood coagulation or to aid in preserving the blood in the way necessary for a particular type of test. During the manufacture of blood tubes, a vacuum is created in the tube that acts to "suck blood" into the tube. Blood tubes can be filled by drawing blood from the vein with a syringe and then using at least a 19-gauge needle to introduce the blood into the tube or using a special holder that has a multisample IV Luer-lock adapter.

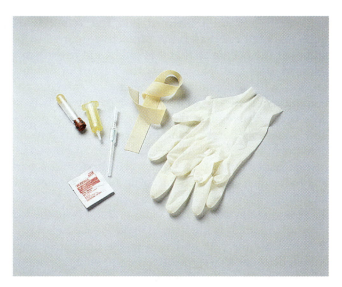

FIGURE 6-26 ▲ Equipment used to draw blood.

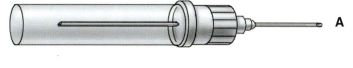

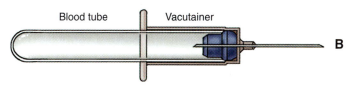

Blood tube   Vacutainer

FIGURE 6-27 ▲ **A,** Luer-lock needle. **B,** Blood collection tube fully inserted into the Vacutainer holder.

CLINICAL NOTES

The Vacutainer holder looks like the barrel of a large syringe and contains a threaded tip that is used to hold the multisample IV Luer-lock adapter or needle (Figure 6-27, *A*). On the inside end of the adapter is a needle that is used to puncture the rubber cap of the blood collection tube. The other end of the adapter attaches to the hub of the IV catheter. To draw a blood sample once the adapter is connected to the IV catheter, insert the blood collection tube (rubber cap first) into the holder and push downward with your thumb until the needle punctures the rubber cap and blood is sucked into the tube (Figure 6-27, *B*). Sometimes, using a Vacutainer device to withdraw blood in a fragile vein will cause it to collapse. If this occurs, remove the Vacutainer device and use a syringe to collect the blood sample (Figure 6-28). This way, you can control the amount of pressure used to withdraw the blood sample by applying slower, more delicate, upward pressure on the plunger of the syringe. After drawing the venous blood sample with a syringe, insert the needle of the syringe through the top of each blood tube to fill it. To prevent breaking up the blood cells (hemolyzing them), use at least a 19-gauge needle and fill each tube slowly.

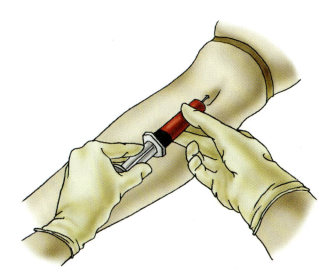

FIGURE 6-28 ▲ Using a syringe to draw a blood sample.

drawn and by whom, and any other information that may be useful, such as: "drawn before the administration of 50% dextrose." During transportation of the patient to the hospital, the filled blood collection tubes can be stored in a plastic "zip-lock" bag to prevent contaminating EMS personnel should one or more of the blood collection tubes be accidentally broken.

When blood is being drawn, each tube should be filled completely. However, small samples can be used to perform most tests if that is all that can be drawn at the time. Once the blood is obtained, the outside of the tube should be labeled with the patient's name, date, time

CLINICAL NOTES

If drawing blood for legal evaluations, such as testing persons suspected of driving while intoxicated (DWI) or under the influence (DUI), do not use an alcohol wipe to clean the skin.

CHANGING AN INTRAVENOUS BAG

Sometimes it is necessary to change an IV bag. Typically, this occurs when the bag is nearly empty of solution and the EMT–I is directed to continue the IV infusion after the bag is empty. Another situation is when the tubing or IV bag fails. Sterile procedures must be used when changing the solution bag. Any equipment that becomes contaminated must be discarded.

The following steps are used to change the IV solution bag:

1. Prepare the new IV solution bag by removing the protective cover from the IV tubing port.
2. Occlude the flow of solution from the depleted bag by moving the roller clamp on the IV administration tubing.
3. Remove the spike from the depleted IV bag. Be careful not to drop or contaminate the spike in any way.
4. Insert the spike into the new IV bag. Ensure that the drip chamber is filled appropriately.
5. Open the roller clamp to the appropriate flow rate.

If air becomes entrained within the administration tubing during this process, cleanse the medication administration port below the trapped air and insert a hypodermic needle and syringe. Pull the plunger back to aspirate the trapped air into the syringe. After the air has been removed, adjust the IV flow rate as needed.

DISCONTINUING THE INTRAVENOUS LINE

Occasionally, it may be necessary to discontinue an IV line in the prehospital setting. To perform this task, protective gloves, a sterile gauze pad, and an adhesive bandage are needed. Begin by closing the flow control valve completely. Then, while taking care not to disturb the catheter, carefully untape and remove the dressing. Next, gently hold a 2 × 2 sterile gauze dressing just above the site to stabilize the tissue while withdrawing the catheter. Remove the catheter by pulling straight back until it is completely out of the vein. To prevent blood loss, immediately cover the IV site with the 2 × 2 sterile dressing and hold it against the puncture site until the bleeding has stopped. Last, tape the dressing in place or cover it with an adhesive bandage.

USING INTRAVENOUS PROTECTIVE DEVICES

Devices are now available to help reduce the risk of accidental needle-stick injuries. One such device, the ProtectIV, works by sliding a protective guard over and completely encasing its introducer needle as the catheter is advanced forward into the vein (Figure 6-29, *A*). With one hand, the protective guard can be slid over the needle so that it is safely and irreversibly encased after use. This avoids the hazard of moving around with a contaminated needle or carrying the contaminated needle to a "sharps" container. It is as easy to use as a regular over-the-needle catheter device and comes in all of the standard sizes. Also, its translucent hub allows easy blood visualization. A porous insert provides consistently quick flashback and a barrier to flashback blood contact. The steps for its use are as follows:

1. Hold the device from the sides and not from the top and bottom. It is grooved to make it easy to hold.
2. Penetrate the skin and vein in the normal manner (Figure 6-29, *B*).
3. Once you have advanced the needle far enough into the vein, hold the device steady while you use the plastic tab that extends upward to advance the catheter into the vein. At the same time, the plastic guard of the device slides over the needle (Figure 6-29, *C*) until it is completely encased. Once it reaches the end, you will feel it "click" into place.
4. Next, while holding the plastic piece steady, twist the catheter hub to the right and pull back on the plastic piece to release the catheter hub from it (Figure 6-29, *D*). You will need to position your little finger over the distal end of the catheter to tourniquet it to prevent blood from leaking out of the catheter.
5. Connect the IV administration set tubing to the catheter hub in the normal manner, and secure the catheter and IV tubing in place.
6. Dispose of the needle in an appropriate "sharps" container.

PREPARING VOLUME CONTROL SETUPS

As discussed earlier, volume control setups allow precise amounts of IV solution to be administered to patients. This is particularly beneficial in the treatment of pediatric and geriatric patients, where controlled infusion rates are critical, as well as when administering certain dosages of medications over a specific amount of time.

The following steps should be taken to set up a volume control administration set:

1. Begin by closing the upper and lower flow clamps.
2. Insert the piercing spike into the IV bag access port.
3. Open the air vent.
4. Open the upper flow control clamp, and squeeze and release the fluid chamber to fill it with approximately 30 mL of fluid.
5. Squeeze and release the drip chamber to fill it half full.
6. Open the bottom flow regulator to flush the tubing of air.

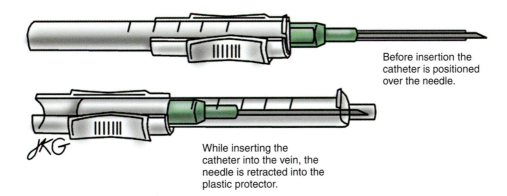

Before insertion the catheter is positioned over the needle.

While inserting the catheter into the vein, the needle is retracted into the plastic protector.

A

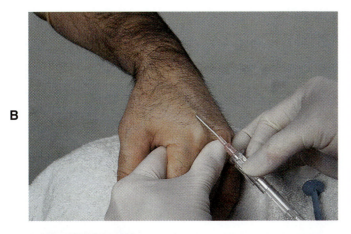

B

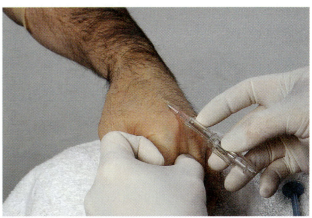

C

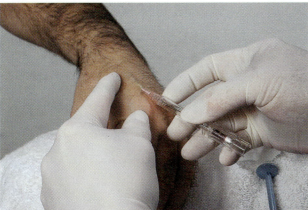

D

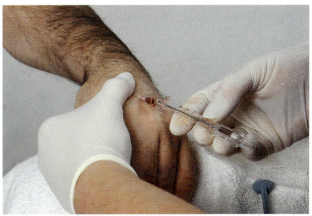

E

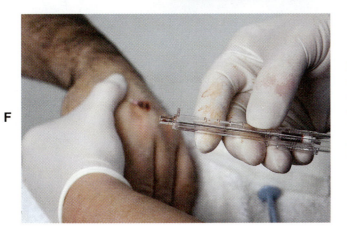

F

FIGURE 6-29 ▲ **A**, ProtectIV device. **B**, Penetrating the skin and vein with the over-the-needle catheter device. **C**, Sliding the catheter forward into the vein while withdrawing the needle. **D**, Once the plastic guard reaches the end it clicks into place. **E**, Separating the plastic guard from the catheter hub. **F**, Needle fully retracted within the protective sheath.

7. When all of the air is flushed, close the lower flow regulator.

8. Open the upper control valve to fill the fluid chamber with the desired amount of IV solution (Figure 6-30, *A*). Then close the upper control valve.

9. After the vein has been cannulated and the needle removed, insert the connector end of the administration set into the hub of the IV catheter.

10. Tape the dressing, catheter, and administration set tubing in place.

11. Open the bottom flow clamp until the desired drip rate is reached (Figure 6-30, *B*). Leave the airway valve open so that air replaces the fluid that is being infused into the patient.

The fluid chamber can be refilled if it becomes depleted and the infusion is to be continued. Start by opening the top flow regulator and allowing the needed amount of IV fluid to flow into the chamber. Then close the top flow regulator, and control the flow rate through the lower control valve.

This type of administration set can also be used to deliver a continuous flow of IV fluid. First, fill the fluid chamber with at least 30 mL of IV fluid. Next, close the air vent while leaving the top flow regulator open. The infusion rate is then controlled with the lower flow regulator.

EXTERNAL JUGULAR VEIN CANNULATION

✖ **Ipsilateral** • On the same side of the body.

As identified earlier, the external jugular vein is a fairly large peripheral vein. For this reason, EMT–Is are often permitted to cannulate this site to treat a wide range of medical emergencies.

The external jugular vein offers a number of benefits. First, it is fairly easy to cannulate. Second, because it lies so close to the subclavian vein, fluids and medications administered from this site quickly reach the central circulation and the heart.

The external jugular vein also carries with it several disadvantages. First, it is hard to access when other providers are managing the patient's airway at the same time as cannulation is being attempted. Second, because the vein lies close to the surface of the skin, it can move or "roll" when an attempt is being made to penetrate the vein. Also, the external jugular vein can be positional, with even slight movement of the head adversely affecting fluid flow through the vein. Finally, cannulation of this site can be extremely painful, so its use should be limited to patients who have decreased or total loss of consciousness.

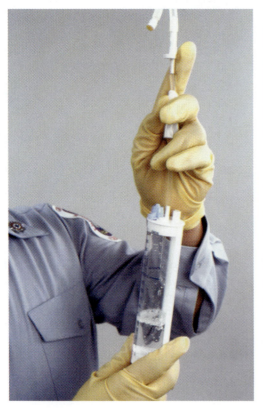
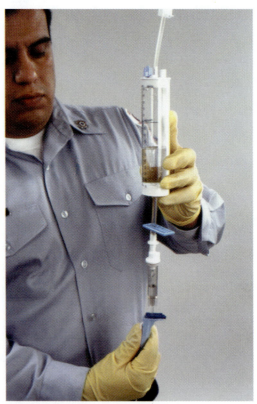

A
B

FIGURE 6-30 ▲ **A,** Open the upper control valve. **B,** Open the bottom flow clamp.

Cannulation of the external jugular vein brings with it the same complications seen with starting an IV infusion in any other vein. This includes a hematoma and/or infiltration of IV fluid into the tissues at the insertion site; cellulitis; infection; phlebitis; or an air, blood, or catheter fragment embolism. In addition, because of its close proximity to the thoracic cavity, there is a risk of puncturing the thoracic cavity and giving the patient a pneumothorax. Also, the external jugular vein is located close to several large vascular and nervous system structures that can be damaged by accidental misplacement. Finally, great caution must be exercised when cannulating the external jugular vein in trauma patients who are likely to have cervical spine injuries. The patient's neck should never be rotated or extended to make it easier to access the vein. If access cannot be obtained with the patient's head in a neutral/midline position, another IV access site should be used.

Cannulating the external jugular vein requires essentially the same equipment as is used to place an IV line in any other peripheral location. One additional item sometimes used is a 10-mL syringe that contains a few milliliters of saline. Since one of the rescuer's fingers is used to tourniquet the vein at the point when the vein meets the clavicle, a constricting band is not needed.

The procedure for cannulating the external jugular vein is as follows (Figure 6-31):

1. Place the patient into a supine, head-down position to fill the vein.
2. Turn the patient's head away from you.
3. Locate the vein, and cleanse the overlying skin with alcohol or povidone-iodine.
4. Hold the vein in place by applying pressure with your thumb on the vein above the point of entry (at the angle of the jaw).
5. Align the venipuncture device in the direction of the vein with the point aimed toward the **ipsilateral** nipple.
6. Tourniquet the vein by applying light pressure with one finger above the clavicle (where the vein meets).
7. Make the venipuncture midway between the angle of the jaw and the midclavicular line. Remember, the vein is very superficial.
8. Puncture the skin with the bevel of the needle pointed upward, approximately 0.5 to 1.0 cm from the vein.
9. Enter the vein from the top or side. If using a syringe attached to an over-the-needle catheter device, withdraw the plunger of the syringe while entering the vein. Stop withdrawing the plunger when blood flows freely into the syringe.
10. Note the return of blood, and advance the catheter.
11. While holding the catheter steady, withdraw the needle and attach the administration set tubing to the catheter hub.
12. Cover the site with povidone-iodine and a sterile dressing.
13. Secure the catheter and tubing in place.

ELDERLY PATIENTS

Elderly patients have more prominent veins and less resistant skin, which makes venipuncture easier (Figure 6-32). However, because the tissues are looser, it is more difficult to stabilize the vein. Because the veins are more fragile, the venipuncture must be done carefully and efficiently to avoid excessive bruising. It also is necessary to remove the tourniquet quickly after venipuncture, because increased vascular pressure can cause bleeding through the vein wall around the insertion site. Usually, smaller, shorter venipuncture devices work best with an elderly patient's fragile veins.

SEIZING OR MOVING PATIENTS, OR PATIENTS IN TRANSPORT

Sometimes it is necessary to place an IV line in patients who are moving or experiencing seizures or while transporting a patient to the hospital. Without a doubt it

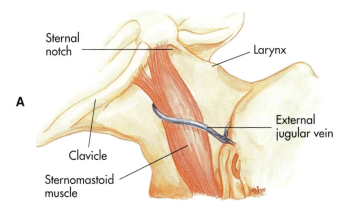
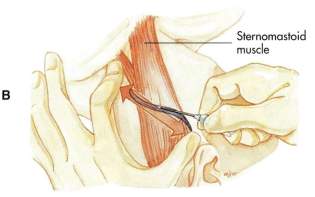

FIGURE 6-31 ▲ **A,** Anatomy of the area surrounding the external jugular vein. **B,** Proper IV cannulation of the external jugular vein. (Mark J. Weiber from Sanders MJ: *Mosby's paramedic textbook,* St Louis, 1994, Mosby.)

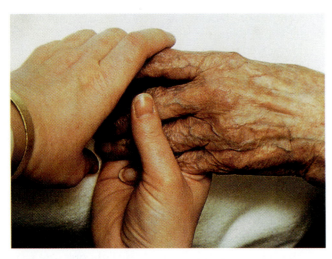

FIGURE 6-32 ▲ The skin of a geriatric patient will necessitate extra care during IV cannulation.

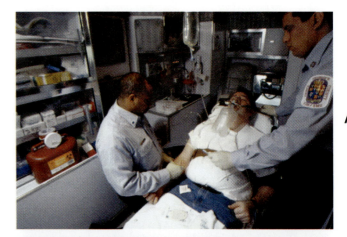

A

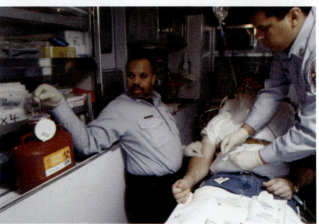

B

is more difficult to start an IV infusion when the patient is not still or is in the back of a moving ambulance; however, it can be done.

First, try to steady the extremity that will be cannulated by holding it as still as possible. If your partner or an assistant is available, have him or her hold the extremity while you perform the cannulation. Look for the biggest vein available; do not use smaller veins, since you are more likely to pass through the vein with the needle if there is sudden movement. Try to penetrate the skin and vein during a period when there is less movement. You may need to wait for a few minutes until the time is right. Hold your little and ring fingers against the patient's extremity to steady the catheter and needle during the insertion. Once you are in the vein, slide the catheter in as quickly and smoothly as possible. Once the catheter is in place, do not let go of it, since patient movement can quickly dislodge it. Immediately place one strip of tape vertically or horizontally over the hub of the catheter to hold it in place. Do not worry about using a crossover taping technique with the initial piece of tape, since all you are trying to do is keep it from be-

FIGURE 6-33 ▲ **A,** Starting an IV line in the back of the ambulance. **B,** Placing the IV needle into the "sharps" container.

coming dislodged from the vein. Then the next pieces of tape can be placed in the normal manner. Use extra tape to secure the cannula in place. Sometimes the extremity should be immobilized with an armboard or splint to prevent accidental displacement of the cannula. Wrapping the administration set tubing and extremity proximal to the cannulation site with gauze dressing can also help prevent accidental displacement (Figure 6-33).

CASE HISTORY FOLLOW-UP ■ ■ ■

EMT–I Davis makes certain that the IV line is secure by placing a 0.5-inch strip of tape under the cannula and crossing it over into a V shape to keep it from pulling out. He then loops the line and secures it with the pieces of tape.

After securing the line, EMT–I Davis places the patient's hand and wrist on a padded splint and secures them with roller gauze. He is careful not to wrap the gauze too tightly. He opens a Betadine packet and squeezes the contents onto the insertion site and then covers the site with a small gauze pad and tape.

Mrs. Greenley is beginning to talk and have meaningful movements with her hands when the ambulance arrives at the emergency department and after only 250 mL of normal saline has been administered.

SUMMARY

Important points to remember from this chapter include the following:

- Intravenous (IV) cannulation is the placement of a catheter into a vein for the purpose of administering blood, fluids, or medications into the circulatory system and/or obtaining venous blood specimens.
- Although its use is beneficial in a wide variety of situations, placement of an IV line should not significantly delay transporting critically ill or injured patients to the hospital.
- The recommended IV solutions for use in the prehospital setting are normal saline (0.9%) and lactated Ringer's solution.
  - Both are isotonic crystalloid solutions.
  - Crystalloid solutions quickly diffuse out of the circulatory system; therefore at least 3 L of IV solution must be administered for every 1 L of blood lost.

- The two most common types of administration sets are the microdrip (delivering 60 drops/mL) and the macrodrip (delivering 10 to 20 drops/mL).
- Most commonly, plastic over-the-needle catheters are used in the prehospital setting because they can be better anchored and permit freer movement of the patient.
- In noncritical patients the distal veins of the dorsal aspect of the hand and arms are preferred IV sites. The veins on the back of the hand allow the patient to freely move his or her hand, the technique is relatively easy to master, and it does not interfere with other life-sustaining measures such as airway management.
- During cardiac arrest, the preferred sites for IV placement are the veins of the antecubital fossa, because they are among the largest in the arm.
- There are some patients in whom cannulating a vein is particularly difficult, including obese persons, patients in shock or cardiac arrest, chronic mainline drug users, elderly patients with fragile or "rolling" veins, and small children.
- When the equipment is being selected for IV therapy, the IV fluid must be checked to ensure that it is not outdated, that it is clear, and that the bag has no leaks.
- When setting up the administration set, cannulating the vein, and attaching the IV solution to the catheter, the EMT–I must be sure to continually employ infection control procedures. Needles should always be discarded appropriately in a "sharps" container.
- The EMT–I must remember to release the tourniquet once the IV tubing is connected to the catheter.
- Once the IV is successfully established, the EMT–I must continually monitor the patient for signs of improvement and also for signs of circulatory overload.
- All IV techniques share a number of complications, including pain, catheter shear, circulatory overload, cannulation of an artery, infiltration/hematoma, local infection, and air embolism.

7 Medication Administration

▪▪▪ CASE HISTORY

A call came in at 2:45 PM stating that a patient was having chest pain. EMT–Is Zachary and Darby were on duty and took the run. When they arrived at 3220 Sharon Street, they saw a man about in his seventies lying on the ground near a riding lawn mower. When the ambulance crew approached Darby asked the man his name. He said his name was Mr. Jones and that he had been having chest pain. When Darby asked Mr. Jones if he had a history of heart problems, Mr. Jones said, "Yes, I am taking nitroglycerine for angina." At that point, Mr. Jones pulled out a bottle of nitroglycerin tablets from his pocket. As Darby was performing his patient assessment, he noticed Mr. Jones was sweating profusely. Mr. Jones also complained of dizziness and fatigue. As the story unfolded, Mr. Jones said he had been out in the yard for about an hour, against his wife's wishes, attempting to mow the lawn. He said he had been thirsty but did not go in the house for water for fear his wife would not let him back out in the yard.

Zachary put Mr. Jones on 15 L of oxygen by mask. Darby took the vital signs; blood pressure (BP) of 130/90, heart rate (HR) of 100, respirations of 18. After completing the history and physical examination, Darby determined that the man should take one nitroglycerin by sublingual route. The crew immediately got Mr. Jones in the ambulance and turned the air conditioning up to high. A fluid infusion of 0.9% sodium chloride (NaCl) was infused rapidly at 150 mL/hr to maintain vital signs. As the ambulance reached the hospital, Mr. Jones said his chest pain had stopped.

LEARNING OBJECTIVES

CHAPTER GOAL

Upon completion of this chapter, the EMT–Intermediate will be able to use the appropriate techniques to administer medication to a patient.

Cognitive Objectives

As an EMT–Intermediate you should be able to do the following:

- Review mathematical principles.
- Review mathematical equivalents.
- Differentiate temperature readings between the centigrade and Fahrenheit scales.
- Discuss formulas as a basis for performing drug calculations.
- Discuss applying basic principles of mathematics to the calculation of problems associated with medication dosages.
- Discuss legal aspects affecting medication administration.

- Discuss the "six rights" of drug administration and correlate these with the principles of medication administration.
- Discuss medical asepsis and the differences between clean and sterile techniques.
- Describe use of antiseptics and disinfectants.
- Describe the use of universal precautions and body substance isolation (BSI) precautions when administering a medication.

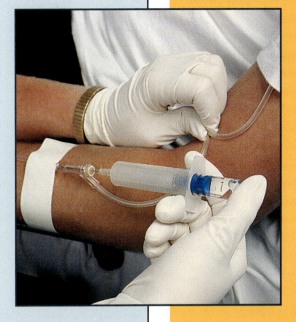

- Describe the indications, necessary equipment, required techniques, precautions, and general principles of administering medications by the inhalation route.
- Differentiate among the different dosage forms of oral medications.
- Describe the necessary equipment and general principles of administering oral medications.
- Describe the indications, necessary equipment, required techniques, precautions, and general principles of intravenous medication administration.
- Describe the indications, necessary equipment, required techniques, precautions, and general principles of rectal medication administration.
- Differentiate among the different parenteral routes of medication administration.
- Describe the necessary equipment, required techniques, complications, and general principles for the preparation and administration of parenteral medications.
- Differentiate among the various percutaneous routes of medication administration.
- Synthesize a pharmacological management plan including medication administration.
- Integrate pathophysiological principles of medication administration with patient management.

Affective Objectives
As an EMT–Intermediate you should be able to do the following:
- Comply with EMT–Intermediate standards of medication administration.
- Comply with universal precautions and BSI procedures.
- Defend a pharmacological management plan for medication administration.
- Serve as a model for medical asepsis.
- Serve as a model for advocacy while performing medication administration.
- Serve as a model for disposing of contaminated items and "sharps."

Psychomotor Objectives
As an EMT-Intermediate you should be able to do the following:
- Use universal precautions and BSI procedures during medication administration.
- Demonstrate clean technique during medication administration.
- Demonstrate administration of medications by the inhalation route.
- Demonstrate administration of oral medications.
- Demonstrate administration of medications by the gastric tube.
- Demonstrate rectal administration of medications.
- Demonstrate preparation and administration of parenteral medications.
- Perfect disposal of contaminated items and "sharps."

INTRODUCTION

With the ability to administer medications, the EMT–Intermediate (EMT–I) acquires tremendous potential for positively affecting a patient's outcome. An accurate dosage of the appropriate drug, administered at a precise rate by the correct route, can relieve pain, terminate lethal arrhythmias, or ease dyspnea. However, if the EMT–I's knowledge of that drug is incomplete, the patient may experience disastrous consequences. Death may result from administering the wrong drug, from giving it too rapidly or too slowly or by the wrong route, by giving too much or too little of it, or from not anticipating adverse drug reactions.

It is also extremely important for the EMT–I to have knowledge of basic mathematical principles to ensure that correct drug dosages are given. In addition to giving the correct drug in the correct dose, the EMT–I must be able to choose the best way to administer the drug. Drugs, depending on how they are administered, can either act on the body quickly or slowly.

SYSTEMS FOR MEASURING DRUGS

The EMT–I needs to know not only about individual drugs but also about how to administer them in the correct amount. To master this knowledge, it is necessary to understand the units of drug measurement.

The two systems for measuring drug dosage are the metric and apothecary systems. Although the apothecary system is also discussed here, the primary system of measuring drug dosages is the metric system.

Although many drugs are supplied in various dosages and packaged in unit packs of the dosages most often ordered, occasionally, the EMT–I may be required to calculate a dosage by using mathematical equations. It is necessary to master the elements of the metric system before calculations can be attempted.

Metric System

The **metric system** is used throughout the world. Because the system is based on multiples of 10, decimals are often used, but never fractions. In the metric system, the base unit of length is the meter (m), the base unit of weight is the gram (g), and the base unit of volume is the liter (L). Prefixes show which fraction of the base is being used. Prefixes often used are as follows:

micro- = (0.000001)
milli- = (0.001)
centi- = (0.01)
kilo- = (1000.0)
Symbols for the metric system are as follows:

gram = g
liter = L
kilogram = kg

milliliter = mL
milligram = mg
cubic centimeter = cc
microgram = μg
Metric units and equivalents are as follows:

1 L = 1000 mL
1 mL = 1 cc
1 g = 1000 mg
1 mg = 1000 μg
1 cc = 1 mL
1 μg = 0.001 mg
1 mg = 0.001 g

Apothecary System

The **apothecary system** is used less often today and is gradually being replaced by the metric system. The liquid measurements include the minim, fluid dram, fluid ounce, pint, quart, and gallon. The system for measuring solid weights includes the grain, dram, ounce, and pound. Roman numerals may be used for smaller numbers, such as gr V or gtt II. Fractions may be used when necessary but never decimals.

Symbols for the apothecary system are as follows:

grain = gr
dram = dr
minim = m, min
drop (s) = gtt (s)
ounce = oz
pint = pt
quart = qt
Apothecary units and equivalents are as follows:

60 grains = 1 dr
1 dr = 1 tsp
8 dr = 1 fluid ounce
60 gtt = 1 teaspoon (tsp)
3 tsp = 1 tablespoon (tbsp)

Pound-to-Kilogram Conversions

In apothecary terms, 1 **kilogram** (kg) is equal to roughly 2.2 pounds (lb). This conversion needs to be made often because many drugs are given according to the patient's body weight in kilograms. To make the conversion to kilograms, simply divide the weight in pounds by 2.2.

$$\text{Weight in kilograms} = \frac{\text{Weight in pounds}}{2.2}$$

A quick way to make pound-to-kilogram conversions is to calculate half the body weight in pounds and then deduct 10%, as follows:

EXAMPLE: 140-lb woman

$$50\% \text{ of } 140 \text{ lb} = 70 \text{ lb}$$

$$10\% \text{ of } 70 = 7$$

$$70 - 7 = 63 \text{ kg}$$

Centigrade and Fahrenheit Scales

Two of the most commonly used temperature scales are the centigrade and Fahrenheit scales. On the **centigrade scale** (also known internationally as *Celsius scale* after Anders Celsius, a Swedish astronomer who first devised it), zero is the freezing point of water and plus 100 is its boiling point. On the **Fahrenheit scale,** the temperature of the freezing point of water is plus 32 degrees, and its boiling point is 212 degrees.

Now let us compare these scales. A Fahrenheit degree represents five ninths of the change in the heat intensity indicated by a degree on the centigrade scale. Temperature on either of the two scales can be converted to the other by the following formulas:

$$\text{Degrees C} = \frac{5}{9}(^\circ F - 32)$$

$$\text{Degrees F} = (\frac{9}{5} {}^\circ C) + 32$$

Note that when converting Fahrenheit to centigrade, you should first subtract the 32 and then multiply by ⁵⁄₉. When converting centigrade to Fahrenheit, you should first multiply by ⁹⁄₅ and then add the 32.

REVIEW OF BASIC ARITHMETIC

The EMT–I must have a working knowledge of basic arithmetic to give correct drug dosages and to solve drug equations. The following is a review of basic arithmetic including converting fractions to decimals and adding, subtracting, multiplying, and dividing decimals. Also included is a section on how to round off decimals. For help or a review of addition, subtraction, and division please refer to a basic math book.

Decimals

As previously mentioned the metric system is based on the decimal system that uses multiples of ten. **Decimals** consist of a whole number, which is the number before (to the left of) the decimal point and decimal fractions, which are the numbers after (to the right of) the decimal point.

A decimal is a fraction whose denominator is a power of 10 expressed by placing a point to the left of the numerator. Recall the following:

$$\frac{2}{10} = \frac{\text{numerator}}{\text{denominator}}$$

EXAMPLES:

$$\frac{2}{10} = 0.2$$

$$\frac{25}{100} = 0.25$$

$$\frac{2}{100} = 0.02$$

$$\frac{3}{100} = 0.03$$

Changing Fractions to Decimals

To change fractions to decimals, divide the numerator by the denominator. Place a decimal point the same number of places to the right as the numerator.

EXAMPLES:

$$\frac{1}{4} = 0.25$$

$$\frac{3}{8} = 0.375$$

$$\frac{2}{3} = 0.6666$$

$$\frac{1}{12} = 0.08333$$

Adding Decimals

To add decimals, align all the decimal points in a column and then add all the numbers. The decimal point will stay in the same place after all the numbers are added.

EXAMPLES:

2.33	1.50	3.20
1.25	3.00	+2.00
3.22	+1.55	5.20
+1.23	6.05	
8.03		

Subtracting Decimals

To subtract decimals, align the decimal points in a column and then subtract the numbers. The decimal point will stay in the same place after the numbers are subtracted.

2.33	1.55	4.23
−0.44	−1.33	−2.33
1.89	0.22	1.90

Multiplying Decimals

Multiply decimals the same as whole numbers. After multiplying the numbers, perform the following:
1. Count the number of decimal places in the multiplier and the multiplicand.
2. Count that number from right to left in the product and place the decimal point.

EXAMPLES:

1.45 (multiplicand)	2.33
×0.33 (multiplier)	×0.04
435	932
+435	+000
0.4785 (product)	000
	0.0932

Dividing Decimals

To divide decimals, conduct the following:
1. Convert the divisor to a whole number by moving the decimal point to the right.
2. Move the decimal point in the dividend the same number of places to the right as in the divisor.
3. Divide.
4. Place the decimal point in the answer (quotient) directly above the decimal point in the dividend.
5. Carry out the answer to three decimal places before rounding off to two places.
   EXAMPLE:

$$.75\overline{)95800} = .75\overline{)95.800} = 1.27$$

$$\begin{array}{r} 1.277 \\ \hline 75. \\ 208 \\ 150 \\ 580 \\ 525 \\ 550 \end{array}$$

Rounding Off Decimals

To round off a decimal, first determine how many significant digits are required after the decimal point. Then look at the number to the right of the last number wanted. For example, to round off 4.113 to two digits to the right of the decimal point, look at the number 3. If 3 (in this example) is 5 or greater, the preceding point is rounded up to the next digit. If it is less than 5, the preceding digit is left as it is. The last decimal place is then dropped from the number. In this example, 4.113 would be rounded off to 4.11.
   EXAMPLES:
2.247   is rounded to 2.25
3.144   is rounded to 3.14
5.26   is rounded to 5.3
7.24   is rounded to 7.2
3.24   is rounded to 3.2

Percentages

Percent means per one hundred. Ten percent is just another way of saying "ten out of one hundred," or ten hundreths.

DETERMINING PERCENTAGE

Do the following steps to determine the percentage of one number compared to another. For example, what percent of 87 is 68?
* Divide the first number by the second:

$$68 \div 87 = 0.7816$$

* Multiply the answer by 100 (move decimal point two places to the right):

$$0.7816 \times 100 = 78.16$$

* Round to the desired precision:

$$78.16 \text{ rounded off} = 78$$

* Follow the answer with the percent (%) sign: 68 is 78% of 87

FINDING THE PERCENT OF A NUMBER

To determine the percent of a number, do the following steps:
* Multiply the number by the percent:

$$87 \times 68 = 5916$$

* Divide the answer by 100 (move decimal point two places to the left):

$$5916 \times 100 = 59.16$$

* Round to the desired precision:

$$59.16 \text{ rounded off} = 59$$

CONVERTING A FRACTION TO A PERCENT

Do the following steps to convert a fraction to a percent. For example, convert ⅘ into a percent:
* Divide the numerator of the fraction by the denominator:

$$4 \div 5 = 0.80$$

* Multiply by 100 (move the decimal point two places to the right):

$$0.80 \times 100 = 80$$

* Round the answer
* Follow the answer with the percent (%) sign: 80%

CONVERTING A PERCENT TO A FRACTION

Do the following steps to convert a percent to a fraction. For example, convert 83% to a fraction:
* Remove the percent sign
* Make a fraction with the percent as the numerator and 100 as the denominator. For example, convert $^{83}/_{100}$ into a percent.
* Reduce the fraction if needed

CONVERTING A DECIMAL TO A PERCENT

Do the following steps to convert a decimal to a percent. For example, convert 0.83 to a percent:
* Multiply the decimal by 100:

$$0.83 \times 100 = 83$$

* Add a percent sign (%) after the answer: 83%

CONVERTING A PERCENT TO A DECIMAL

Do the following step to convert a percent to a decimal. For example, convert 83% to a decimal:

- Divide the percent by 100:

$$83 \div 100 = 0.83$$

Proportions

A proportion is a statement that two ratios are equal. It can be written in two ways:

- As two equal fractions:

$$\frac{a}{b} = \frac{c}{d}$$

or

- Using a colon:

$$a : b = c : d$$

The following proportion is read as "twenty is to twenty-five as four is to five."

$$\frac{20}{25} = \frac{4}{5}$$

In problems involving proportions, we can use cross products to test whether two ratios are equal and form a proportion. To find the cross products of a proportion, we multiply the outer terms, called the extremes, and the middle terms, called the means.

Here, 20 and 5 are the extremes, and 25 and 4 are the means. Since the cross products are both equal to one hundred, we know that these ratios are equal and that this is a true proportion.

Roman Numerals

The set of roman numerals are I, V, X, L, C, D, and M. They are defined as follows:

- I means 1, II means 2, III means 3
- V means 5
- X means 10
- L means 50
- C means 100
- D means 500
- M means 1000

DRUG DOSAGE CALCULATIONS

Many of the drugs used in the field are premixed and premeasured, ready to deliver to the average adult patient. This convenience decreases both preparation time and likelihood of error. However, when giving certain drugs and drug infusions, calculation of volume or rate of delivery is often necessary. The EMT–I should use extreme caution when administering drugs, since errors in calculation could prove fatal to the patient.

Converting Units of Measure

In the metric system, it is sometimes necessary to convert measurements to the same unit of measure. For example, the physician may order 0.5 g of a drug, and the

drug container label reads 500 mg. To convert within the metric system the following rules are used:

1. To change grams to milligrams multiply grams by 1000 or move the decimal point three places to the right, as follows:

$$5 \text{ g} = ? \text{ mg}$$
$$5 \times 1000 = 5000 \text{ mg}$$
$$2 \text{ g} = ? \text{ mg}$$
$$2 \times 1000 = 2000 \text{ mg}$$

2. To change milligrams to grams divide the milligrams by 1000 or move the decimal point three places to the left, as follows:

$$100 \text{ mg} = ? \text{ g}$$
$$\frac{100}{1000} = 0.1 \text{ g}$$
$$500 \text{ mg} = ? \text{ g}$$
$$\frac{500}{1000} = 0.5 \text{ g}$$

3. To change milligrams to micrograms (μg) multiply the milligrams by 1000 or move the decimal point three places to the right, as follows:

$$5 \text{ mg} = ? \text{ μg}$$
$$5 \times 1000 = 5000 \text{ μg}$$
$$8 \text{ mg} = ? \text{ μg}$$
$$8 \times 1000 = 8000 \text{ μg}$$

4. To change micrograms to milligrams divide the micrograms by 1000 or move the decimal point three places to the left, as follows:

$$3000 \text{ μg} = ? \text{ mg}$$
$$\frac{3000}{1000} = 3 \text{ mg}$$
$$2000 \text{ μg} = ? \text{ mg}$$
$$\frac{2000}{1000} = 2 \text{ mg}$$

5. To change liters to milliliters multiply the liters by 1000 or move the decimal point three places to the right, as follows:

$$5 \text{ L} = ? \text{ mL}$$
$$5 \times 1000 = 5000 \text{ mL}$$
$$1 \text{ L} = ? \text{ mL}$$
$$1 \times 1000 = 1000 \text{ mL}$$

6. To change milliliters to liters divide the milliliters by 1000 or move the decimal point three places to the left, as follows:

$$500 \text{ mL} = ? \text{ L}$$
$$\frac{500}{1000} = 0.5 \text{ L}$$
$$1500 \text{ mL} = ? \text{ L}$$
$$\frac{1500}{1000} = 1.5 \text{ L}$$

No conversion is necessary when changing milliliters to cubic centimeters, because they are approximately the same, as indicated in the following:

EXAMPLES:

$$1 \text{ mL} = 1 \text{ cc}$$
$$3 \text{ mL} = 3 \text{ cc}$$
$$5 \text{ mL} = 5 \text{ cc}$$

Calculation of Volume

Most calculations are based on the following volume calculation formula:

$$\text{Volume to administer} = \frac{\text{Dose desired} \times \text{Volume on hand}}{\text{Dose on hand}}$$

The dose desired equals the amount of drug ordered (usually in mg). The volume on hand equals the quantity of fluid in the drug container (usually expressed in mL). The dose on hand equals the total amount of drug present in the drug container (usually expressed in mg).

EXAMPLE 1:

Give atropine, 0.5 mg, from a prefilled syringe that contains 1 mg in 10 mL of fluid:

$$\text{Volume} = \frac{0.5 \text{ mg} \times 10 \text{ mL}}{1 \text{ mg}} = \frac{5 = 5 \text{ mL}}{1}$$

A slight variation is to calculate the drug present per mL of solution:

$$\frac{1 \text{ mg}}{10 \text{ mL}} = 0.1 \text{ mg/mL}$$

Then insert this value into the previous formula:

$$\text{Volume} = \frac{0.5 \text{ mg} \times 1 \text{ mL} = 5 \text{ mL}}{0.1 \text{ mg}}$$

HELPFUL HINT

- All units in the dividend must be the same as the units in the divisor, so it may sometimes be necessary, for example, to convert 1 g to 1000 mg in order to calculate the dosage.

EXAMPLE 2:

An adult patient weighs 260 pounds and is in a coma due to a narcotic overdose. The physician orders an initial dose of naloxone at 1.5 mg intravenous (IV) push. The EMT–I has a 5-mL glass ampule containing 2.0 mg. How many mL would the EMT–I give this patient?

Calculate the volume of the dose by using the volume calculation formula:

$$\text{Volume to administer} = \frac{\text{Dose desired} \times \text{Volume on hand}}{\text{Dose on hand}}$$

$$X = \frac{1.50 \text{ mg} \times 5 \text{ mL}}{2.0 \text{ mg}}$$
$$X = 3.75 \text{ mL}$$

Calculation of Volume Based on Weight

Some drug dosages are based on the patient's weight. Normally, body weight is expressed in pounds and must be converted to kilograms.

EXAMPLE 1:

An adult patient weighs 176 pounds and is in cardiac arrest from ventricular fibrillation. At some point during the code, the physician orders an initial dose of lidocaine at 1.5 mg/kg IV push. The EMT–I has a prefilled 5-mL syringe with 20 mg/mL. How many mL would the EMT–I give this patient?

Step 1: Calculate the patient's weight in kilograms. The symbol "X" indicates for what is being solved. (NOTE: 1 kg = 2.2 lb)

$$X = 1 \text{ kg}$$
$$176 \text{ lb} \div 2.2 \text{ lb}$$
$$2.2 \text{ X} = 176$$
$$X = 80 \text{ kg}$$

Step 2: Calculate the mass (in this case, mg) of the dose.

$$\frac{X}{80 \text{ kg}} = \frac{1.5 \text{ mg}}{1 \text{ kg}}$$
$$X = 1.5 \times 80$$
$$X = 120 \text{ mg}$$

Step 3: Calculate the volume of the dose by using the volume calculation formula:

$$\text{Volume to administer} = \frac{\text{Dose desired} \times \text{Volume on hand}}{\text{Dose on hand}}$$

$$X = \frac{120 \text{ mg} \times 5 \text{ mL}}{100 \text{ mg}}$$
$$X = 6 \text{ mL}$$

Step 4: Administer 6 mL of lidocaine to the patient.

EXAMPLE 2:

A pediatric patient weighs 66 lb and is in acute bronchospasm. The physician orders an initial dose of epinephrine, 1:1000 solution at 0.01 mg/kg subcutaneously. The EMT–I has a 1-mL glass ampule containing 1 mg/mL of the 1:1000 solution. How many mL would the EMT–I give this patient?

Step 1: Calculate the patient's weight in kilograms. The symbol "X" indicates for what is being solved. (NOTE: 1 kg = 2.2 lb)

$$\frac{X}{66 \text{ lb}} = \frac{1 \text{ kg}}{2.2 \text{ lb}}$$
$$2.2 \text{ X} = 66$$
$$X = 30 \text{ kg}$$

Step 2: Calculate the mass (in this case, mg) of the dose.

$$\frac{X}{30 \text{ mg}} = \frac{0.01 \text{ mg}}{1 \text{ kg}}$$
$$X = 0.01 \times 30$$
$$X = 0.30 \text{ mg}$$

Step 3: Calculate the volume of the dose by using the volume calculation formula.

$$\text{Volume to administer} = \frac{\text{Dose desired} \times \text{Volume on hand}}{\text{Dose on hand}}$$

$$X = \frac{0.30 \text{ mg} \times 1 \text{ mL}}{1 \text{mg}}$$
$$X = 0.30 \text{ mL}$$

Step 4: Administer 0.30 mL of epinephrine to the patient.

DRUG ADMINISTRATION

Protection From Contaminants

As an EMT–I you will come in contact with patients who have a wide range of illnesses. It is imperative that you use proper protective measures to prevent acquisition of disease. These protective measures illustrate the use of body substance isolation precautions, proper hand washing, and cleaning and disposal of contaminated articles.

Body Substance Isolation

Body substance isolation (BSI) was discussed in Chapter 2—Well-Being. The correct approach to a patient requires the use of gloves. Protective eyewear and masks should be worn to prevent exposure of the EMT–I's mouth, nose, and eyes to blood droplets or other body fluids. Gowns are indicated when splashes of blood or body fluids may occur.

Hand Washing

Effective hand washing is equally as important as BSI when rendering patient care. Hand washing should be practiced before and after each patient contact and before performing any invasive procedure, such as starting an IV line or passing an endotracheal tube. Hand washing should also be performed after removing gloves, since gloves may not be a 100% effective barrier.

In the field, the use of alcohol-based hand-washing products is recommended. For alcohol to be effective in degerming, the proteinaceous (gross) matter must first be removed. Alcohol cannot penetrate through protein to kill bacteria or viruses. In the hospital the EMT–I should use the following steps for proper hand washing:

- Use the soap that is recommended in the hospital. It is the mechanical action and friction used, not the specific soap, that is important.
- Using friction, create a lather and wash for at least 15 seconds.
- Rinse hands and dry with a paper towel.
- Use the paper towel to turn off the water.

Medical Asepsis

Medical asepsis is the term used to describe those practices used to prevent the transfer of pathogenic organisms from person to person, place to place, or person to place. Medical aseptic practices are routinely used in direct patient care areas, as well as in other service areas in the health care environment. These practices interrupt a chain of events necessary for the continuation of an infectious process.

Sterilization

Certain emergency medical service (EMS) equipment may require sterilization. **Sterilization** refers to the complete destruction of all living organisms, including bacterial spores and viruses. The word *sterile* means free from or the absence of all living organisms. Any item to be sterilized must be thoroughly cleaned mechanically or by hand, using soap or detergent and water. When cleaning by hand, apply friction to the item by using a brush. After cleaning, thoroughly rinse the item with clean, running water before sterilization.

The appropriate sterilization method is determined according to how the item will be used, the material of which the item is made, and the sterilization methods available. Physical methods of sterilization comprise moist heat and dry heat. Chemical methods include gas and liquid solutions.

> **HELPFUL HINT**
>
> - Antiseptics are substances that destroy, or stop the growth of, germs on living tissue. Antiseptics are applied to skin and mucous membranes to prevent infections.

> **HELPFUL HINT**
>
> - Disinfectants are chemicals that destroy germs on nonliving objects.

Cleaning A Blood Spill

Blood presents the greatest risk for carrying infection caused by hepatitis B or HIV. Therefore it is important to clean all blood-contaminated areas after completion of a call. The following procedure is recommended:

1. Put on gloves (heavy-duty rubber).
2. Clean area with soap and water.
3. Soak area with a hospital approved disinfectant agent or a bleach and water solution. Bleach and water mixed at approximately 1½ cup bleach per 1 gallon water (1 to 10 solution) is effective and nontoxic.
4. Do not apply a bleach-water solution at 1:10 ratio to delicate stainless steel items (e.g., surgical instruments); this strength results in pitting of the surface and permanent damage to the item.

Handling and Disposal of Needles and Other Sharp Instruments

Extreme care should be taken when handling needles, scalpels, lancets, and other sharp instruments or devices; when handling sharp instruments after procedures; when cleaning used instruments; and when disposing of used needles. The Centers for Disease Control and Prevention (CDC) recommend that needles not be recapped after use. The recapping procedure often results in needle stick injuries. Needles should not be cut or bent for disposal. Place used disposable syringes and needles, scalpel blades, lancets, and other sharp items into a puncture resistant container right after their use. This equipment needs to be disposed of as infectious waste, rather than as regular trash.

Guidelines For Administering Drugs

Risks are associated in the administration of most drugs, whether in the hospital or in the more uncontrolled prehospital environment. To make risk versus benefit decisions in the field, the EMT–I must have an understanding of pathophysiology and pharmacology. This provides the background information to communicate pertinent information so that patients may be managed appropriately. Even in systems with stringent medical control, many situations occur when the EMT–I must rely on a personal knowledge base to make informed, rational decisions about management options.

Dispensing drugs by standing orders or by a direct order from a physician places tremendous responsibility on an EMT–I. If the EMT–I's knowledge of a drug is incomplete or the wrong dosage or drug is given, the patient may experience disastrous consequences. Poor documentation can be another fatal error for the EMT–I. It is imperative that a proper run report be completed. The report should include the type, dosage, and time each medication was administered. It should also report the effect that the drug had on the patient. For example, did the drug ease the patient's chest pain or make it easier for the patient to breathe?

Human error and mistakes in judgment are inevitable components of life. The point at which these meet and become actionable negligence is not always clear and is often left to the determination of a jury. EMT–I's are urged to take stock of their individual capabilities and weaknesses and be willing to confront them, before a claim arises.

Safe and Effective Medication Administration

Safe and effective medication administration in prehospital care can be summarized by the following "six rights" of drug administration:

1. "Right" patient
   Verify that this is the right patient. In a multiple casualty incident check triage tag or armband.
2. "Right" drug
   Know the indications and contraindications of the drug.
   Check the label for drug name, concentration, and expiration.
3. "Right" dose
   Be knowledgeable of the proper dosages of a drug. Verify the dose.
   Perform correct drug calculations.
   Double-check your drug calculations.
4. "Right" route
   Know what medications can be given by which routes.
   Determine how quickly or slowly the drug needs to be given for effective patient outcome.
5. "Right" time
   Know the time intervals for repeat doses.
6. "Right" documentation
   Prepare proper documentation for controlled substances.
   Record drug dosages and time given on the run report.

> **HELPFUL HINT**
>
> - If there is ever any doubt about the six rights of medication administration, check again or have someone else check.

To ensure safety when administering drugs, the EMT–I should do the following:

1. Know the policies of the medical director regarding the administration of drugs.
2. Know the local protocols or standing orders.
3. Give only the drugs that the medical director or protocols have ordered.
4. Check with the medical director or medical direction if there is any doubt about a drug.
5. Do not talk while drawing up and administering a drug. It is important to remain attentive during this task.
6. Read drug labels carefully. Make sure the drug and concentration are correct. Check the expiration date.
7. If the order is received over the radio, repeat the instructions back to medical direction.
8. Know the drugs. Be alert for color changes, precipitation, odor, or any indication that the drug has changed its properties.
9. Make sure to ask about any allergies that the patient may have to the drug. If the patient is unresponsive, attempt to elicit information from family members or friends.
10. Stay with the patient while the drug is being taken or administered. Watch for any reaction and record the patient's response.

11. Check the strength of the medication (e.g., 250 mg versus 500 mg) and the route of administration.
12. If using a syringe, measure the amount exactly; make sure there are no bubbles in the liquid.
13. Never return a drug to its container.
14. Have "sharps" containers as close to the area of use as possible.
15. Never recap, bend, or break a used needle.
16. Wear gloves for all procedures that might result in contact with blood or body fluids.

MEDICATION ERRORS

Common causes of medication errors can involve the following:

- Giving the wrong drug
- An error in drug calculations
- Drugs administered through the wrong route
- Giving the drug to the wrong patient

If an incident involving a medication error occurs, the EMT–I should do the following:

- Accept professional responsibility.
- Immediately advise medical direction or the supervisor.
- Assess and carefully monitor the patient for effects of the drug.
- Document the medication error as required by local and state drug administration policies and those of the medical direction institution.
- Modify personal practice to avoid a similar error in the future.
- Follow EMS procedures for documentation and quality improvement activities.

Equipment Used For Injections
NEEDLES AND SYRINGES

A variety of needles and syringes are used for injections. The 3-mL hypodermic syringe is the most common type used for injections. The syringe consists of a plunger, body or barrel, flange, and tip. The other types of syringes used for parenteral administration are tuberculin and insulin. Needle lengths vary from ⅜ to 1 inch or ½ inches for standard injections. *Gauge* refers to the diameter of the needle lumen. Needle gauge varies from 18 (large) to 27 (small); the higher the number, the smaller the gauge (Figure 7-1).

Most companies prepackage hypodermic syringes in color-coded envelopes with the needle attached. Separate needles and syringes may be purchased as needed. This type of syringe may be used for either subcutaneous or intramuscular (IM) injections. It is necessary to choose the package with a needle length and appropriate for the route of the injection and medication to be given. For example, an IM injection requires a needle length of at least 1 inch. The needle will vary from 20- to 25-gauge, again depending on the drug to be administered. Some drugs, such as penicillin, cannot be drawn into a syringe using a small-gauge needle.

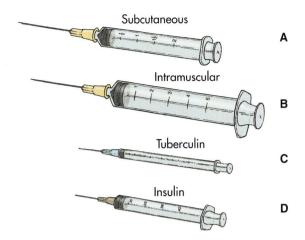

FIGURE 7-1 ▲ **Various types of syringes. A,** A subcutaneous syringe. **B,** An IM (or IV syringe). **C,** A tuberculin syringe. **D,** An insulin syringe.

Subcutaneous injections generally are given using a short, small-gauge needle—that is, 25-gauge, ⅝ inch or 23-gauge, ½ inch.

All hypodermic syringes are marked with 10 calibrations/mL on one side of the syringe. Each small line represents 0.1 (one tenth) mL. The other side of the syringe is marked in minims.

The tuberculin (TB) syringe is narrow and has a total capacity of 1 mL. There are 100 calibration lines marking the capacity. Each line represents 0.01 mL. Every tenth line is longer than the others to indicate 0.1 mL. TB syringes are used for newborn and pediatric doses and for intradermal (e.g., TB) skin tests.

The insulin syringe is used strictly for administering insulin to diabetics. It has a total capacity of 1 mL. The 1 mL volume is marked as 100 units (U), indicating the strength of 100 U of insulin per mL when full. Each group of 10 U is divided by five small lines. Each line represents

---

CLINICAL NOTES

In an effort to reduce the potential for accidental needle sticks a number of innovative products are now available. Syringes equipped with automated retraction needles work much like a standard syringe except that after injecting medication into an IV port or directly into a patient, continued pressure on the plunger activates a spring-driven retraction feature that automatically withdraws the needle and secures it with the barrel of the syringe. The contaminated needle never comes into contact with the EMT–I. Needleless IV tubings and connectors have built-in puncturing devices made of plastic that are sharp enough to pierce the rubber medication port on IV tubing or have locking ports with blunt ends or no puncturing device at all.

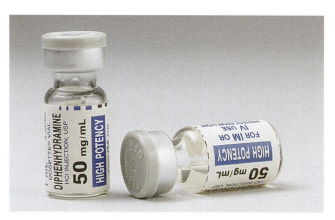

FIGURE 7-2 ▲ Vials have a self-sealing rubber stopper in the top.

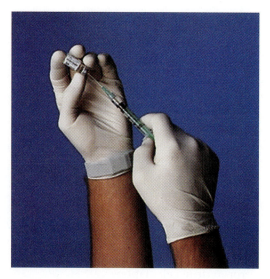

FIGURE 7-3 ▲ Withdrawing medication from vial. (From Sanders M: *Mosby's paramedic textbook,* St Louis, 1994, Mosby.)

2 U. A smaller insulin syringe with a capacity of 0.5 mL can be used when less than 50 U of insulin is ordered. The smaller insulin syringe has 50 small calibration lines, each representing 1 U of insulin. Most of the insulin used today is U-100, meaning that there are 100 units of insulin in each mL. It is important to remember that the insulin syringe must be marked U-100 to match the insulin used.

Prefilled syringes contain a premeasured amount of a medication in a disposable cartridge with a needle attached. The prefilled cartridge and needle are placed in a holder.

Drug Packaging and Preparation

Most of the drugs that the EMT–I will use are given by injection and are in liquid form. Liquid drugs administered into the body by subcutaneous, IM, or IV routes are called *parenteral drugs.* Drugs administered through the parenteral route are packaged in several ways, including vials, ampules, and prefilled syringes.

VIALS

Vials are glass or plastic containers that have a self-sealing rubber stopper in the top, from which multiple doses may be drawn (Figure 7-2). The contents of vials may be in solution, powder, or crystal form, which require reconstitution with a specific diluent, usually sterile water or saline. Vials are packaged in either single- or multidose amounts. When using a vial, the EMT–I should take the following steps:

1. Confirm the drug type, concentration, and dose.
2. Check for cloudiness and the expiration date.
3. Clean the rubber stopper with alcohol.
4. Determine the volume of drug to be withdrawn and draw that amount of air into the syringe.
5. Invert the vial, insert the needle through the rubber stopper and inject the air into the vial.

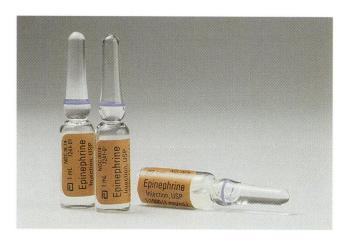

FIGURE 7-4 ▲ Ampules are breakable glass containers from which drugs are drawn into the syringe.

6. Withdraw the desired amount of solution (Figure 7-3). Remove the needle from the vial.
7. Invert the syringe and expel any trapped air.
8. Reconfirm the drug type, concentration, and dose.
9. Recap the needle, being careful not to contaminate it.

AMPULES

Ampules are breakable glass containers from which drugs must be drawn with a syringe (Figure 7-4). They are intended for single dose use. Ampules must be broken at the neck to aspirate the solution into the syringe. Once the ampule is opened, all contents from it must be either used or discarded; it must not be saved for later use, because there is no way to maintain the sterility of the solution.

Glass ampules are typical containers for inexpensive single-dose packaging. When using an ampule, the EMT–I should take the following steps:

1. Confirm the drug type, concentration, and dose.
2. Check for cloudiness and the expiration date.

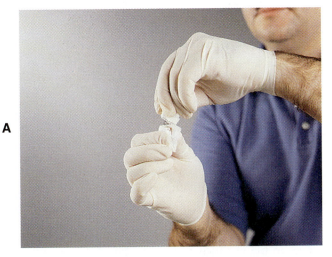
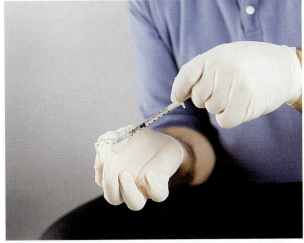

FIGURE 7-5 ▲ **A,** Break the glass top. **B,** Draw solution into the syringe and invert the needle.

3. Shake the ampule or tap the stem and top to shift the fluid to the bottom.
4. Place a gauze square or alcohol wipe over the bottle's neck and snap the top off (Figure 7-5, *A*).
5. Insert the needle into the solution without touching the sides.
6. Draw the solution into the syringe (Figure 7-5, *B*).
7. Invert the syringe (needle pointing up) and tap the syringe barrel to get the air bubbles to the top.
8. Push on the plunger to expel any trapped air.
9. Draw in more medication and repeat the procedure if necessary to have the correct amount of medication in the syringe.
10. Recap the needle, being careful not to contaminate it.

Some medications (e.g., glucagon) are packaged in a vial that contains the diluent and powder in two compartments (Mix-o-Vial). The vials are joined at the neck. Other medications are dry powders that must be reconstituted before administration. The manufacturer's instructions must be followed. Use the correct amount of the diluent prescribed for this purpose. Always mix the diluent and powder in the closed vial before withdrawing the dose.

To mix a medication from a Mix-o-Vial, the EMT–I should take the following steps:

1. Begin by confirming the labels.
2. Squeeze the vials together to break the seal.
3. Agitate or shake to mix completely.
4. With a syringe and needle and using the procedures described above, withdraw the appropriate volume of medication.

To reconstitute a medication from a Mix-o-Vial, the EMT–I should take the following steps:

1. Begin by confirming the labels.
2. Cleanse the top of the vial.
3. With a syringe and needle and using the procedures described earlier, remove all the solution from the vial containing the mixing solution.

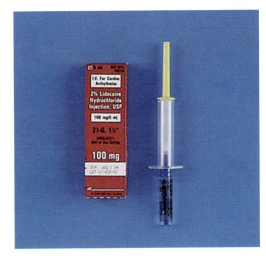

FIGURE 7-6 ▲ A prefilled syringe for medication injection. (From Sanders M: *Mosby's paramedic textbook,* St Louis, 1994, Mosby.)

4. With an alcohol wipe cleanse the top of the vial containing the powered drug and inject the solution.
5. Agitate the vial to ensure complete mixture.
6. Determine how much of the newly mixed medication is to be administered.
7. Prepare a new syringe and hypodermic needle.
8. Cleanse the rubber stopper of the vial.
9. Draw up the amount of air that is equal to the volume of medication to be withdrawn.
10. Insert the needle into the rubber stopper and inject the air.
11. Withdraw the correct volume of medication.

PREFILLED SYRINGES

Prefilled syringes are used for administration of IV, IM, or subcutaneous drugs (Figure 7-6). They are usually packaged in tamper-proof containers, and the drug solution component and syringe often must be assembled. They are intended for single-dose use. Prefilled syringes are a convenient form of packaging for emergency drugs. When using a prefilled syringe, the EMT–I should take the following steps:

1. Confirm the drug type, concentration, and dose (Figure 7-7, *A*).
2. Check for cloudiness and the expiration date (Figure 7-7, *B*).
3. If assembly is required, pop the caps off the syringe and drug cartridge and screw them together (Figure 7-7, *C* and *D*).
4. Invert the syringe and expel any excess air (Figure 7-7, *E* to *G*).
5. Reconfirm the drug type, concentration, and dose.
6. Administer the drug by the desired route.

The EMT–I also may be called on to administer medications via tablet form, such as nitroglycerin, administered sublingually; or bronchodilators, administered by aerosol or through a nebulizer mask. The different forms in which drugs may be found are listed in Chapter 5.

Administration of Drugs

To administer drugs via various routes, specific procedures must be used.

Enteral Routes of Medication Administration

Enteral administration refers to drugs that are absorbed through the gastrointestinal tract. These methods include oral and rectal administration.

ORAL ADMINISTRATION

The oral route is used for absorption of drugs through the lining of the gastrointestinal tract. The oral route is generally the most popular method of drug administration for nonemergency situations because it is a convenient, inexpensive route. Most drugs are efficiently absorbed from the gastrointestinal tract in normal circumstances. The large surface area, mixing of contents, and differences in pH enhance absorption. Some drugs, however, cannot be given orally because acids and enzymes of the gastrointestinal tract inactivate them before being absorbed. Others are so irritating to the gastrointestinal tract that they should only be taken with a meal.

To administer a medication through the oral route, the EMT–I should do the following:

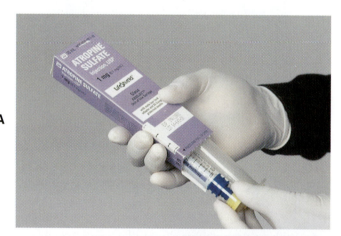

A

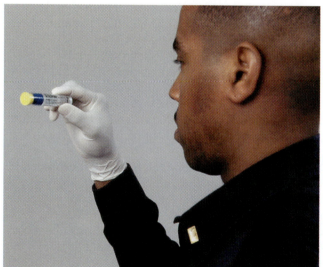

B

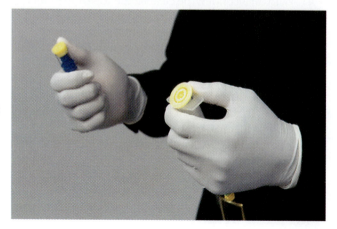

C

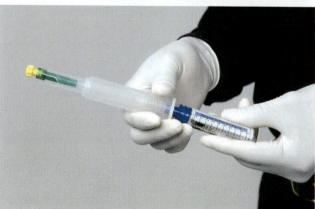

D

FIGURE 7-7 ▲ **A** to **D**, Steps in using prefilled syringes.

1. Identify the need for medication based on patient history and presenting signs and symptoms.
2. Contact medical direction for permission to administer medication or follow off-line standing orders.
3. Confirm the order, repeating to medical direction the name of the medication, dosage, and route.
4. Write down the order.
5. Reassure the patient and check for allergies.
6. Select the appropriate medication container, checking the name, dosage, and expiration date.
7. Uncap the container and remove the indicated number of tablets or in the case of a liquid, pour liquid into a calibrated cup.
8. Give the patient a glass of water and direct the patient to swallow the tablet. In the case of a liquid, direct the patient to swallow the liquid.

9. Confirm the medication administration with medical direction, record the administration time, and watch for patient response to the medication administration.

RECTAL ADMINISTRATION

The rectal route is another form of gastrointestinal administration that may have more predictable absorption than the oral route. Drugs administered rectally may have a local or systemic action and are usually in the forms of suppositories or solutions instilled through the enema procedure. Antiemetics (drugs for control of nausea and vomiting) and local analgesics (pain relievers) are commonly administered using this route. Few emergency drugs are manufactured in the form of suppositories.

To administer a medication by the rectal route, the EMT–I should do the following:

1. Perform BSI precautions.
2. Identify the need for medication based on patient history and presenting signs and symptoms.
3. Contact medical direction for permission to administer medication or follow off-line standing orders. If orders are obtained from medical direction, repeat orders back to the medical direction physician and write down the information on the run sheet.
4. Reassure the patient and check for allergies.
5. Assemble equipment: sterile gloves, suppository, lubricant, and gauze pad.
6. Open suppository package (usually foil) and drop onto a clean surface (nonsterile gauze).
7. With gloved hands, dip fingers of one hand lightly in lubricant. Pick up the suppository, holding blunted end.

E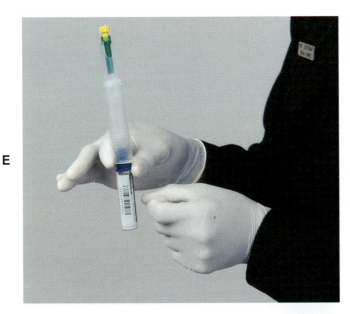

F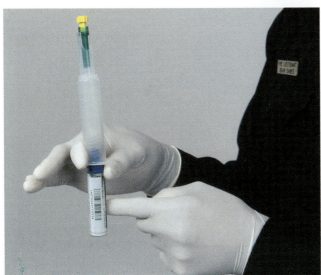

G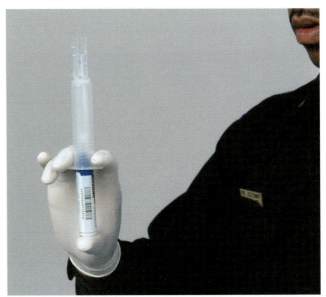

FIGURE 7-7, cont'd ▲ **E** to **G**, Steps in using prefilled syringes.

8. With one hand separate the buttocks exposing the anus. Ask the patient to breath slowly through the mouth. Insert the suppository, tapered end first. Insert about 1 to 1½ inches until it passes through the internal anal sphincter.
9. Following insertion, hold the buttocks closed. Instruct the patient not to bear down.
10. With gauze pad, dry the anal area and then dispose of the pad.

Percutaneous Routes of Medication Administration

Percutaneous administration refers to those drugs that are absorbed through the mucous membranes or skin. These include sublingual, endotracheal, and inhaled drugs.

SUBLINGUAL ADMINISTRATION

Some drugs, such as nitroglycerin, are placed in the mouth under the tongue, and this is called *sublingual administration.* Nitroglycerin passes directly through the oral mucosa into the bloodstream.

To administer a medication through the sublingual route, the EMT–I should do the following:
1. Identify the need for medication based on patient history and presenting signs and symptoms.
2. Contact medical direction for permission to administer medication or follow off-line standing orders.
3. Confirm the order, repeating to medical direction the name of the medication, dosage, and route.
4. Write down the order.
5. Reassure the patient and check for allergies.
6. Select the appropriate medication container, checking the name, dosage, and expiration date.
7. Uncap the container and remove the indicated number of tablets.

8. Direct the patient to place the tablet underneath the tongue so that it does not get swallowed or chewed (Figure 7-8, *A*).
9. Confirm the medication administration with medical direction, record the administration time, and watch for patient response to the medication administration (Figure 7-8, *B*).

ENDOTRACHEAL ADMINISTRATION

Because of the large surface area of the alveoli and vast blood supply of the pulmonary capillary beds that return blood to the left heart, drugs administered through the trachea are rapidly absorbed and delivered to the heart for distribution.

To administer a medication through the endotracheal tube, the EMT–I should do the following:
1. Ensure adequate oxygenation and ventilation of the patient.
2. Prepare the medication per medical direction.
3. Preoxygenate the patient's lungs (Figure 7-9, *A*).
4. Remove the ventilatory device from the endotracheal tube and inject the medication through a catheter deep into the tube (Figure 7-9, *B*).
5. Reconnect the ventilatory device and resume assisted breathing with several large ventilations to help enhance absorption of the medication.
6. Confirm the medication administration with medical direction, record the administration time, and watch and record patient response to the medication administration (for both desired and adverse effects).
7. Dispose of the needle/syringe in the appropriate "sharps" container. Do not recap the needle.
8. Monitor the patient for the desired therapeutic effect and any possible undesired side effects.

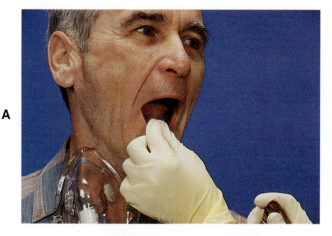

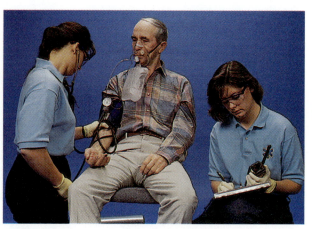

A   B

FIGURE 7-8 ▲ **A,** Have the patient place the tablet underneath the tongue.
B, Record the administration time and reconfirm the medication administration with medical direction. (Vincent Knaus from Stoy W: *Mosby's EMT–Basic textbook,* St Louis, 1996, Mosby.)

CLINICAL NOTES

Endotracheal tubes with separate injection ports are commercially available.

HELPFUL HINT

● If cardiopulmonary resuscitation is being delivered at the time of endotracheal medication administration, the EMT–I should stop chest compressions momentarily during endotracheal drug injection until several ventilations are given. Otherwise, the drug may be forced back up and out of the endotracheal tube.

AEROSOL ADMINISTRATION

Some medications can be delivered through use of a nebulizer and allow drugs to act directly on the structures of the lung or be absorbed into the systemic circulation. The proper use of a nebulizer depends on good technique. For patients older than 5 years of age, a mouthpiece is more effective than a mask. Use a mask for very young children.

To administer a medication by aerosol, the EMT–I should do the following:

1. Perform BSI precautions.
2. Identify the need for medication based on patient history and presenting signs and symptoms.
3. Contact medical direction for permission to administer medication or follow off-line standing orders. If orders are obtained from medical direction, repeat orders back to the medical direction physician and write down the information on the run sheet.
4. Reassure the patient and check for allergies. Checking for allergies to medications helps eliminate an anaphylactic reaction.

5. Explain reason for the procedure. This explanation helps calm the patient and improves the patient's cooperation with the procedure.
6. Mix the prescribed drug (using aseptic technique) with a specified amount of normal saline and pour it into the nebulizer (Figure 7-10, *A*). Some medications are available in a packaged unit dose and contain a fixed amount of diluent (usually 0.9% normal saline).
7. Attach the nebulizer to a T-piece and mouthpiece (Figure 7-10, *B*) and connect it to the oxygen regulator with oxygen connecting tubing. Alternatively, a nebulizer face mask may be used instead of a mouthpiece.
8. Adjust the oxygen flowmeter to 4 to 6 L/min to produce a steady, visible mist.
9. When the mist is visible, treatment should be started.
10. Instruct the patient to inhale slowly and deeply through the mouth and to hold the breaths 3 to 5 seconds before exhaling (Figure 7-10, *C*). Inhalation and exhalation should be continued until the aerosol canister is depleted of the medication.
11. Confirm the medication administration with medical direction, record the administration time, and watch for patient response to the medication administration (for both desired and adverse effects).
12. If changes in heart rate or dysrhythmias are noted, nebulization should be stopped and medical direction contacted for further orders.

HELPFUL HINT

● If an aerosol mask is used, the flow rate of oxygen should be maintained at 6 to 10 L/min to prevent potential buildup of exhaled carbon dioxide in the mask.

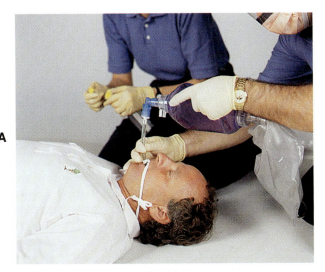

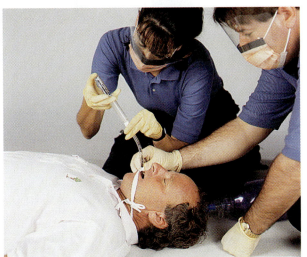

FIGURE 7-9 ▲ Endotracheal administration. **A,** Preoxygenate the patient. **B,** Inject the medication through a catheter into the endotracheal tube.

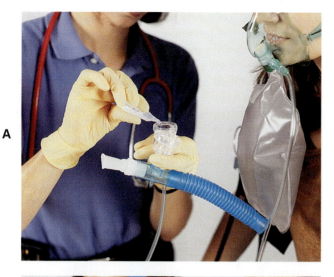

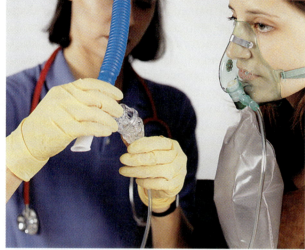

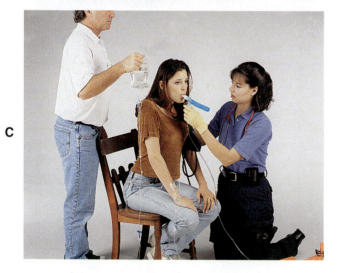

FIGURE 7-10 ▲ Aerosol administration. **A,** Mix the drug with an appropriate amount of normal saline. **B,** Connect the nebulizer to a T-piece and mouthpiece and connect to an oxygen regulator. **C,** Have the patient inhale the aerosol slowly, exhaling after 3 to 5 seconds.

An alternative form of inhalation administration is with the use of a metered dose inhaler. Metered dose inhalers (MDIs) contain a canister of liquid medication that does not require dilution or mixing. The canister fits into a mouthpiece device; when squeezed, the inhaler delivers a measured amount of medication, called a metered dose. A spacing device acts as a holding area for medication and attaches to the mouthpiece portion of the canister.

To administer a medication by an MDI, the EMT–I should do the following:

1. Perform BSI precautions.
2. Identify the need for medication based on patient history and presenting signs and symptoms.
3. Contact medical direction for permission to administer medication or follow off-line standing orders. If orders are obtained from medical direction, repeat orders back to the medical direction physician and write down the information on the run sheet.
4. Reassure the patient and check for allergies. Checking for allergies to medications helps eliminate an anaphylactic reaction.
5. Explain reason for the procedure. This explanation helps calm the patient and improves the patient's cooperation with the procedure.
6. Remove the mouthpiece and protective cap from the canister (the drug container).
7. Carefully snap off the cap and turn the mouthpiece sideways.
8. Insert the canister stem into the hole inside the mouthpiece.
9. Shake the canister and mouthpiece well.
10. Invert the MDI and hold it close to the patient's mouth advising the patient to exhale, pushing as much air from the lungs as possible.
11. Place the mouthpiece in the patient's mouth and instructing the patient to close the lips loosely around it with the tongue underneath the mouthpiece. As the patient inhales deeply over 5 seconds, press down on the canister quickly and then release it.
12. Have the patient to hold a breath for 5 to 10 seconds before exhaling.
13. Repeat the procedure in 5 to 10 minutes.

Parenteral Routes of Medication Administration

Parenteral administration is the administration of any drug by the nongastrointestinal route. It is the most

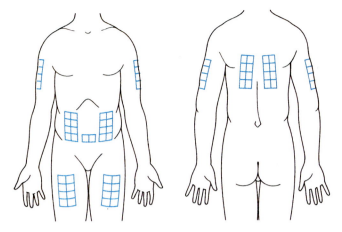

FIGURE 7-11 ▲ Commonly used subcutaneous injection sites. (From Clark JBF: *Pharmacological basis of nursing*, ed 4, St. Louis, 1993, Mosby.)

common route of medication administration that the EMT–I uses and normally involves the drug being administered by injection. Methods include subcutaneous, IM, intradermal, and IV.

SUBCUTANEOUS ADMINISTRATION

Subcutaneous administration involves the injection of a drug into the fatty tissue beneath the skin. Volumes of a drug are usually limited to quantities less than 1 mL, injected by using a 24- to 26-gauge, ½- to 1-inch needle. Subcutaneous injections are performed when the drug to be given requires a slow but steady absorption into the blood. It places the drug under the skin but above the muscle. It also avoids tendons, nerves, and blood vessels. This route is common for 1:1000 epinephrine.

Common sites for subcutaneous injections include (Figure 7-11):
- Upper lateral-posterior arm
- Abdomen
- Mid-back above the scapula
- Mid-anterior thigh

❗ HELPFUL HINT

The subcutaneous route is used for vaccines, insulin, heparin, epinephrine, and for the administration of some narcotics.

To administer a medication through the subcutaneous route, the EMT–I should do the following:
1. Perform BSI precautions.
2. Identify the need for medication based on patient history and presenting signs and symptoms.
3. Contact medical direction for permission to administer medication or follow off-line standing orders. If orders are obtained from medical direction, re-

peat orders back to the medical direction physician and write down the information on the run sheet.
4. Reassure the patient and check for allergies. Checking for allergies to medications helps eliminate an anaphylactic reaction.
5. Explain reason for the procedure and advise the patient of possible discomfort. This explanation helps calm the patient and improves the patient's cooperation with the procedure.
6. Assemble and check equipment: medication, 3-mL syringe, 25-gauge needle, antiseptic swabs, and gloves.
7. Expose and cleanse the area to be used for medication administration with the antiseptic swab (Figure 7-12, *A*). Usually the lateral aspect of either an upper arm or thigh is selected.
8. To make sure the needle does not go in too deeply, pinch the skin and dart the needle in rapidly at a 45-degree angle (Figure 7-12 *B, C*).
9. Pull back on the syringe plunger to aspirate for blood (Figure 7-12, *D*). If blood is seen in the syringe, withdraw the needle and apply firm pressure over the site with a sterile dressing. Select another site for administering the medication.
10. Inject the medication and remove the needle from the skin.
11. Apply circular pressure to the injection site to disperse the medication throughout the tissue (Figure 7-12, *E*).
12. Dispose of the needle/syringe in an appropriate "sharps" container (Figure 7-12, *F*). Do not recap the needle.
13. Store any unused medication appropriately.
14. Confirm the medication administration with medical direction, record the administration time, and watch for patient response to the medication administration (for both desired and adverse effects).

INTRAMUSCULAR ADMINISTRATION

IM administration involves the injection of small quantities of a drug into the muscle. The volume of drug administered intramuscularly is limited to quantities less than 5 mL; additional volume is unlikely to be absorbed and may cause tissue irritation. IM injection is associated with greater hazards than subcutaneous injection because of increased potential for damage to nerves.

Common sites for IM injection are as follows:
- *Deltoid muscle*—The deltoid muscle site for IM injection is located by palpating the lower edge of the acromion process. At the midpoint, in line with axilla on the lateral aspect of the upper arm, a triangle is formed (Figure 7-13).
- *Dorsogluteal*—The dorsogluteal site for administering an IM injection is found by dividing the buttock into four quadrants. The injection is given in the upper outer quadrant (Figure 7-14).

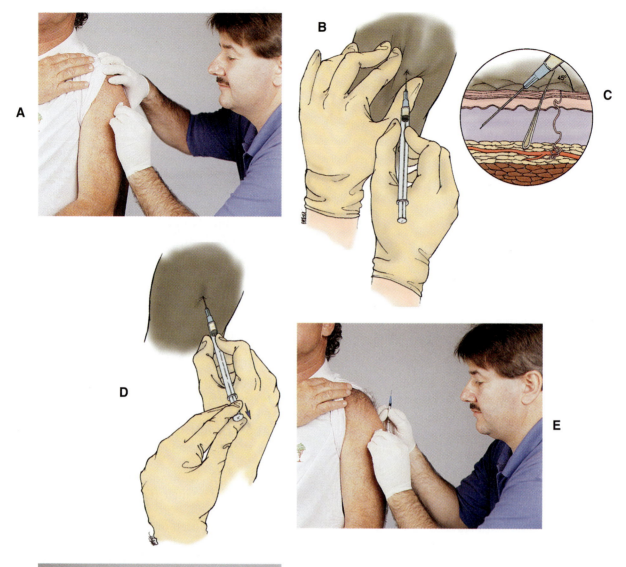

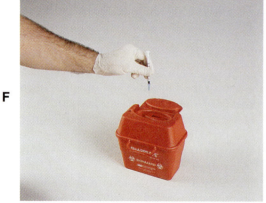

FIGURE 7-12 ▲ Subcutaneous administration. **A,** Cleanse the area. **B,** Pinch the skin and inject the needle at a 45-degree angle to the skin. **C,** A cross-section view of the skin showing proper subcutaneous injection. **D,** Aspirate for blood. **E,** Apply pressure to the injection area to disperse the medication. **F,** Dispose of all used sharp objects in a proper waste container.

• *Vastus lateralis*—Dividing the thigh into thirds horizontally and vertically identifies the *vastus lateralis* site for IM injections. The injection is given in the outer middle third (Figure 7-15).

To administer a medication through the IM route, the EMT–I should do the following:

1. Perform BSI precautions.

2. Identify the need for medication based on patient history and presenting signs and symptoms.

3. Contact medical direction for permission to administer medication or follow off-line standing orders. If orders are obtained from medical direction, repeat orders back to the medical direction physician and write down the information on the run sheet.

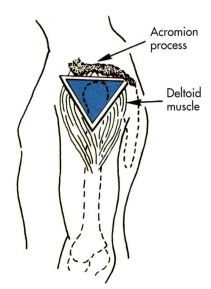

FIGURE 7-13 ▲ Deltoid muscle injection site roughly forms an inverted triangle, with the acromion process as the base. The muscle may be visible in well-developed patients. (From Clark JBF: *Pharmacological basis of nursing,* ed 4, St Louis, 1993, Mosby.)

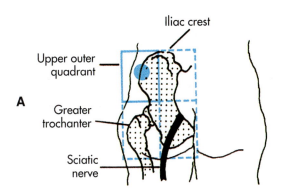

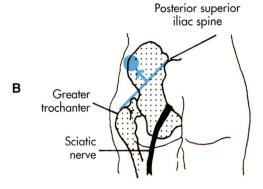

FIGURE 7-14 ▲ Two accepted methods for defining the dorsogluteal injection site. **A,** The patient's buttocks can be divided on one side into imaginary quadrants. The center of the upper outer quadrant should be used as the injection site. **B,** The paramedic locates by palpation the posterior superior iliac spine and the greater trochanter and then draws an imaginary line between the two. An injection site up and out from that line should be used. (From Clark JBF: *Pharmacological basis of nursing,* ed 4, St Louis, 1993, Mosby.)

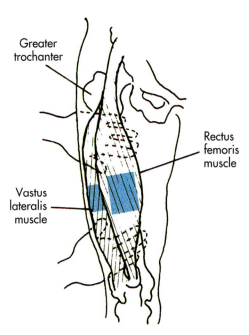

FIGURE 7-15 ▲ To define the vastus lasteralis muscle injection site and the rectus femoral muscle site, place one hand below the patient's greater trochanter and one hand above the knee. The space between the two hands defines the middle third of the underlying muscle. The rectus femoris is on the anterior thigh; the vastus lateralis is on the lateral side. (From Clark JBF: *Pharmacological basis of nursing,* ed 4, St Louis, 1993, Mosby.)

HELPFUL HINT

- The dorsogluteal site should not be used in children under 3 years of age because their muscles are underdeveloped and there is a chance of penetrating the sciatic nerve.

4. Reassure the patient and check for allergies. Checking for allergies to medications helps eliminate an anaphylactic reaction.
5. Explain reason for the procedure and advise the patient of possible discomfort. This explanation helps calm the patient and improves the patient's cooperation with the procedure.
6. Assemble and check equipment: medication, syringe, needle, antiseptic swabs, gloves.
7. Expose and cleanse the area to be used for medication administration. Use either the deltoid muscle in the shoulder or upper outer quadrant of the gluteal area.
8. To make sure the needle goes into the muscle and not the subcutaneous layer, stretch the skin over the injection site and insert the needle at a 90-degree angle to the skin (Figure 7-16).
9. Pull back on the syringe plunger to aspirate for blood. If blood is seen in the syringe, withdraw the needle and apply firm pressure over the site with a sterile dressing. Select another site for administering the medication.

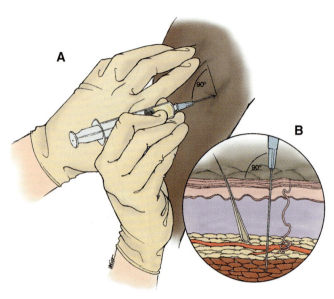

FIGURE 7-16 ▲ IM injection. **A,** For IM injections, stretch the skin across the site and inject the needle at a 90-degree angle to the skin. **B,** A cross-section view of the skin showing proper IM injection.

10. Inject the medication and remove the needle from the skin.
11. Apply circular pressure to the injection site to disperse the medication throughout the tissue.
12. Dispose of the needle/syringe in an appropriate "sharps" container. Do not recap the needle.
13. Store any unused medication appropriately.
14. Confirm the medication administration with medical direction, record the administration time, and watch for patient response to the medication administration (for both desired and adverse effects).

INTRADERMAL ADMINISTRATION

Intradermal administration involves injecting a drug directly into the skin. In the field, this route generally is limited to the administration of a local anesthetic agent to numb the skin just before performing a procedure such as establishing an IV infusion. A small amount of medication (usually less than 1 ml) is administered directly into the skin and is not intended to be absorbed into the circulatory system. The most commonly used local anesthetic is 1% lidocaine.

Various sites may be used for an intradermal injection. In all cases, avoid an area with visible superficial blood vessels. By avoiding these areas you reduce the risk of puncturing a blood vessel (see Figure 7-11).

To administer a medication through the intradermal route, the EMT–I should do the following:
1. Perform BSI precautions.
2. Identify the need for medication based on patient history and presenting signs and symptoms.

3. Contact medical direction for permission to administer medication or follow off-line standing orders. If orders are obtained from medical direction, repeat orders back to the medical direction physician and write down the information on the run sheet.
4. Reassure the patient and check for allergies. Checking for allergies to medications helps eliminate an anaphylactic reaction.
5. Explain reason for the procedure and advise the patient of possible discomfort. This explanation helps calm the patient and improves the patient's cooperation with the procedure.
6. Assemble and check equipment: medication, 3-mL syringe, 25-gauge needle, antiseptic swabs, gloves.
7. Expose and cleanse the area to be used for medication administration with an antiseptic swab.
8. Rest the patient's forearm in the palm of your hand and pull the skin tightly across the forearm with your fingers.
9. Hold the syringe parallel to the skin surface and slide the needle into the dermis.
10. Inject the medication and remove the needle from the skin.
11. Blot the area of injection while applying slight pressure.
12. Dispose of the needle/syringe in an appropriate "sharps" container. Do not recap the needle.
13. Store any unused medication appropriately.
14. Confirm the medication administration with medical direction, record the administration time, and watch for patient response to the medication administration (for both desired and adverse effects).

INTRAVENOUS ADMINISTRATION

The IV route bypasses the absorption process because the drug is injected directly into the bloodstream. Although bypassing absorption barriers has many advantages, it leaves no margin for error, making giving medications by IV administration potentially dangerous. IV injection may be delivered through a previously established IV infusion line, a heparin or saline lock, implantable port (e.g., Port-A-Cath, Hickman catheter) or directly into the vein with a sterile needle or butterfly device.

To administer a medication through an IV infusion, the EMT–I should do the following:
1. Perform BSI precautions.
2. Identify the need for medication based on patient history and presenting signs and symptoms.
3. Contact medical direction for permission to administer medication or follow off-line standing orders. If orders are obtained from medical direction, repeat orders back to the medical direction physician and write down the information on the run sheet.
4. Reassure the patient and check for allergies. Checking for allergies to medications helps eliminate an anaphylactic reaction.

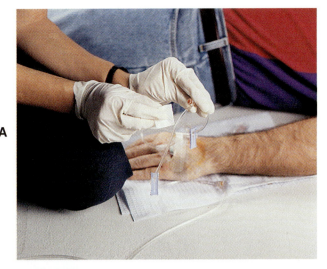

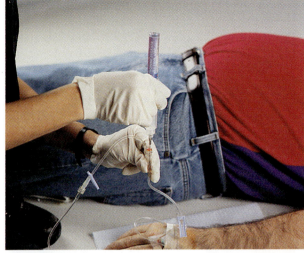

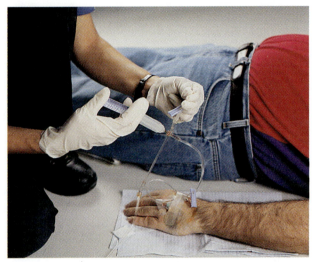

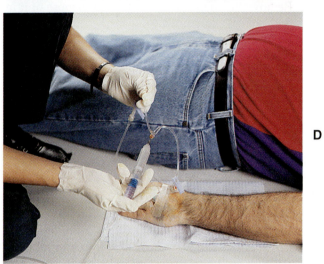

FIGURE 7-17 ▲ IV medication administration. **A,** Cleanse the medication injection site of the IV tubing. **B,** Insert the needle into the injection site. **C,** Pinch the IV tubing above the infection site to stop the flow of the IV. **D,** Administer the correct dosage.

5. Explain reason for the procedure. This explanation helps calm the patient and improves the patient's cooperation with the procedure.

6. Assemble and check equipment: medication, syringe, needle, antiseptic swabs, gloves.

7. Cleanse the medication injection site (Y-port or hub) of the IV tubing with an antiseptic swab (Figure 7-17, *A*).

8. Penetrate the injection site with the needle (Figure 7-17, *B*).

9. Stop the IV flow by pinching the IV tubing above the injection site (Figure 7-17, *C*). Closing the tubing leading to the IV bag prevents the medication from flowing up into the IV bag instead of into the patient.

10. Administer the correct dose of medication at the correct push rate (Figure 7-17, *D*).

11. Flush the IV tubing by briefly running it wide open or following the drug bolus with a 20-mL bolus of IV fluid.

12. Adjust the IV flow rate to a keep open rate.

13. Dispose of the needle/syringe in an appropriate "sharps" container. Do not recap the needle.

14. Store any unused medication appropriately.

15. Confirm the medication administration with medical direction, record the administration time, and watch for patient response to the medication administration (for both desired and adverse effects).

To administer a medication via a heparin or saline lock use the following steps:

1. Prepare one or two syringes containing 4 mL of flush solution and the medication to be administered.

2. Use an alcohol wipe to clean the cap on the heparin lock.

3. Stabilize the heparin with the thumb and index finger of one hand.

4. Insert the needle or needleless device of the syringe containing flush solution into the center of the in-

jection cap. Do not force it, if there is resistance; insert the needle or device at another angle.

5. Pull back on the plunger slightly and watch for blood return. If blood appears begin slowing injecting the flush solution. If resistance is felt, the patient complains of pain or discomfort, or if you note signs of infiltration stop immediately because the venous access device should be replaced. If none of the above signs are present you can deliver the medication.

6. Properly dispose of the hypodermic needle and syringe in the "sharps" container (if a second syringe containing flush solution has been prepared).

7. Clean the injection cap and insert the medication needle through it.

8. Deliver the medication as appropriate.

9. Remove the medication needle and dispose of it in the "sharps" container.

10. Follow the medication administration with a 2 ml saline flush from the other syringe (or the remainder of the solution if using just one flush syringe).

11. Properly dispose of the hypodermic needle and syringe. Watch the patient for response to the medication administration.

INTRAOSSEOUS ADMINISTRATION

Intraosseous administration refers to the placement of a rigid needle into a bone and the infusion of fluid and medication directly into the bone marrow. Since bone marrow is highly vascular with direct communication to the peripheral circulation, both fluids and medications may be administered effectively in this way. The administration of medication through the intraosseous route is the same as for the IV route (see Intravenous Administration), *except* that after a drug has been administered by intraosseous infusion, it must be followed by a 5-mL saline flush to make sure the drug is delivered into the systemic circulation.

CASE HISTORY FOLLOW-UP ■ ■ ■

On arrival at the hospital Mr. Jones had no chest pain and was breathing comfortably. The triage nurse checked the patient and found his BP to be 124/82 and HR to be 80. Mr. Jones was no longer sweating and thanked Darby and Zachary for their help.

As Darby and Zachary walked away, Darby said, "We could have missed that diagnosis of heat exhaustion if we had only focused on Mr. Jones's chest pain, but we caught both the angina and heat exhaustion and treated both." Zachary said, "Looks like Mr. Jones won't be mowing the lawn anymore if his wife has a say in it!"

SUMMARY

Important points for this chapter include the following:
- A basic review of arithmetic is important in beginning a study of drug administration.
- Proper drug dosages depend on correct and accurate mathematical formulas.
- Before beginning any procedure, use sterile techniques.
- Protective measures illustrate the proper use of universal precautions in the field situation.
- It is the responsibility of the EMT–I to know the proper measures for self-protection and to practice these on a routine basis.
- Health care does not offer a 100% risk-free environment, but the use of these simple measures greatly reduces the incidence of exposure in the field care environment.
- With the ability to administer medications, the EMT–I acquires tremendous potential for positively affecting a patient's outcome.
- An accurate dosage of the appropriate drug, administered at a precise rate by the correct route is an important responsibility of the EMT–I.
- Because of new drugs and techniques constantly placed on the market, maintaining current knowledge is an ongoing challenge for the EMT–I.

AIRWAY

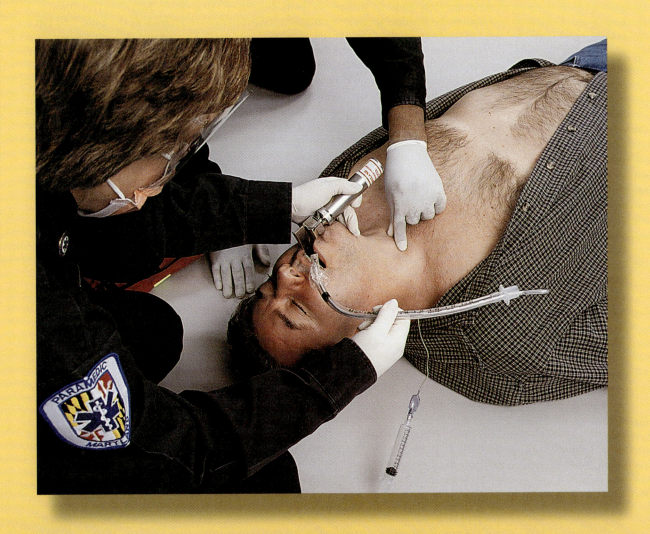

8

Airway Management

...CASE HISTORY

It is early Sunday morning (2:30 AM) when the dispatch comes in for a multiple vehicle collision on Country Meadows Road. EMT–Is Simms and Brown arrive to find a car that had crashed into a pole at high speed. EMT–I Simms gains access to the patient, a man approximately 20 years of age, through the driver's side rear window. EMT–I Simms maintains cervical spine immobilization with her gloved hands as she says, "Hi, I'm an EMT–Intermediate. Don't move. Can you hear me?" The patient doesn't answer. "Can you speak? Say something," EMT–I Simms says in a loud, firm voice. Again, there is no answer. EMT–I Simms holds the patient's head immobile and upright in straight anatomic alignment while she leans over his mouth to hear and feel if he is breathing. She can hear gurgling and stridorous respirations. They are slow and shallow. "We've got to intubate right away!" EMT–I Simms calls out to her crew. She feels the patient's carotid pulse while she holds his head immobile and notes that it is 140 and thready. Her partner, EMT–I Brown, places a nonrebreather mask on the patient with oxygen at 15 L/min and prepares to ventilate and suction. The crew extricates the patient rapidly while EMT–I Simms maintains his head alignment with her hands. A cervical spine immobilization device is applied, and the patient is secured to the backboard with padding. EMT–I Simms asks EMT–I Brown to preoxygenate and suction the patient while she prepares to place the tube. With the patient's head kept in a neutral-in-line position EMT–I Simms inserts an endotracheal tube and inflates the balloon with 5 mL of air. She then confirms placement by auscultating the epigastrium and the chest for equal bilateral breath sounds and to ensure there are no sounds of air movement in the stomach.

LEARNING OBJECTIVES ☑

CHAPTER GOAL
Upon completion of this chapter, the EMT-Intermediate will be able to establish and/or maintain a patent airway, oxygenate, and ventilate a patient.

Cognitive Objectives
As an EMT-Intermediate you should be able to do the following:
- Explain the primary objective of airway maintenance.
- Identify commonly neglected prehospital skills related to airway.
- Identify the anatomy and describe the functions of the upper and lower airway.

- Explain the differences between adult and pediatric airway anatomy.
- Define gag reflex.
- Explain the relationship between pulmonary circulation and respiration.
- List the concentration of gases that comprise atmospheric air.
- Describe the measurement of oxygen in the blood.
- Describe the measurement of carbon dioxide in the blood.
- Describe peak expiratory flow.
- List factors that cause decreased oxygen concentrations in the blood.
- List the factors that increase and decrease carbon dioxide production in the body.
- Define atelectasis.
- Define the percentage of oxygen in inspired air (FiO_2).
- Describe the voluntary and involuntary regulation of respiration.
- Describe the modified forms of respiration.
- Define normal respiratory rates and tidal volumes for the adult, child, and infant.
- List the factors that affect respiratory rate and depth.
- Define pulsus paradoxus.
- Explain the risk of infection to emergency medical service (EMS) providers associated with ventilation.
- Define and differentiate between hypoxia and hypoxemia.
- Describe causes of respiratory distress.
- Explain safety considerations of oxygen storage and delivery.
- Identify types of oxygen cylinders and pressure regulators, including a high-pressure regulator and a therapy regulator.
- List the steps for delivering oxygen from a cylinder and regulator.
- Describe the use, advantages, and disadvantages of an oxygen humidifier.
- Describe the indications, contraindications, advantages, disadvantages, complications, liter flow range, and concentration of delivered oxygen for supplemental oxygen delivery devices.
- Describe the indications, contraindications, advantages, disadvantages, complications, and technique for ventilating a patient by the following:
  - Mouth-to-mouth
  - Mouth-to-nose
  - Mouth-to-mask
  - One person bag-valve-mask device
  - Two person bag-valve-mask device
  - Three person bag-valve-mask device
  - Flow-restricted, oxygen-powered ventilation device
- Explain the advantage of the two-person method when ventilating with the bag-valve-mask device.
- Compare the ventilation techniques used for an adult patient to those used for pediatric patients.
- Describe indications, contraindications, advantages, disadvantages, complications, and technique for ventilating a patient with an automatic transport ventilator.
- Describe the Sellick (cricoid pressure) maneuver.
- Describe manual airway maneuvers.
- Describe the use of an oral and nasal airway.
- Describe the indications, contraindications, advantages, disadvantages, complications, and technique for inserting an oropharyngeal and nasopharyngeal airway

Continued

LEARNING OBJECTIVES—cont'd

- Define how to ventilate a patient with a stoma, including mouth-to-stoma and bag-valve-mask–to–stoma ventilation.
- Describe the special considerations in airway management and ventilation for the pediatric patient.
- Differentiate ET (ET) intubation from other methods of advanced airway management.
- Describe the indications, contraindications, advantages, disadvantages, and complications of ET intubation.
- Describe laryngoscopy for the removal of a foreign body airway obstruction.
- Describe the visual landmarks for direct laryngoscopy.
- Describe the use of cricoid pressure during intubation.
- Describe the methods of assessment for confirming correct placement of an ET tube.
- Describe methods for securing an ET tube.
- Describe the indications, contraindications, advantages, disadvantages, complications, equipment, and technique for extubation.
- Describe methods of ET intubation in the pediatric patient.
- Describe the indications, contraindications, advantages, disadvantages, complications, equipment, and technique for using a dual lumen airway.
- Define and explain the implications of partial airway obstruction with good and poor air exchange.
- Define complete airway obstruction.
- Describe causes of upper airway obstruction.
- Describe maneuvers used to treat complete airway obstruction.
- Explain the purpose for suctioning the upper airway.
- Identify types of suction equipment.
- Describe the indications for suctioning the upper airway.
- Identify types of suction catheters, including hard or rigid catheters and soft catheters.
- Identify techniques of suctioning the upper airway.
- Identify special considerations of suctioning the upper airway.

- Describe the indications, contraindications, advantages, disadvantages, complications, equipment, and technique of tracheobronchial suctioning in the intubated patient.
- Identify special considerations of tracheobronchial suctioning in the intubated patient.
- Define gastric distention.
- Describe the indications, contraindications, advantages, disadvantages, complications, equipment, and technique for inserting a nasogastric tube and orogastric tube.
- Identify special considerations of gastric decompression.
- Define, identify, and describe a tracheostomy, stoma, and tracheostomy tube.
- Define, identify, and describe a laryngectomy.
- Describe the special considerations in airway management and ventilation for patients with facial injuries.

Affective Objectives
As an EMT-Intermediate you should be able to do the following:
- Defend oxygenation and ventilation.
- Defend the necessity of establishing and/or maintaining patency of a patient's airway.
- Comply with standard precautions to defend against infectious and communicable diseases.

Psychomotor Objectives
As an EMT-Intermediate you should be able to do the following:
- Perform body substance isolation (BSI) precautions during basic airway management, advanced airway management, and ventilation.
- Perform pulse oximetry.
- Perform end-tidal carbon dioxide detection.
- Perform peak expiratory flow testing.
- Perform oxygen delivery from a cylinder and regulator with an oxygen delivery device.
- Perform oxygen delivery with an oxygen humidifier.
- Deliver supplemental oxygen to a breathing patient using the following devices: nasal cannula, simple face mask, partial rebreather mask, nonrebreather mask, and Venturi mask.
- Demonstrate ventilating a patient by the following techniques:
  - Mouth-to-mask ventilation

- One person bag-valve-mask device
- Two person bag-valve-mask device
- Three person bag-valve-mask device
- Flow-restricted, oxygen-powered ventilation device
- Automatic transport ventilator
- Mouth-to-stoma
- Bag-valve-mask–to–stoma ventilation
- Perform ventilation with a bag-valve-mask device.
- Perform the Sellick maneuver (cricoid pressure).
- Ventilate a pediatric patient using the one- and two-person techniques.
- Perform manual airway maneuvers, including:
  - Opening the mouth
  - Head-tilt/chin-lift maneuver
  - Jaw-thrust without head-tilt maneuver
  - Modified jaw-thrust maneuver
  - Perform manual airway maneuvers for pediatric patients, including the following:
  - Opening the mouth
  - Head-tilt/chin-lift maneuver
  - Jaw-thrust without head-tilt maneuver
  - Modified jaw-thrust maneuver
- Demonstrate insertion of an oropharyngeal airway.
- Demonstrate insertion of a nasopharyngeal airway.
- Intubate the trachea by direct orotracheal intubation.

- Perform assessment to confirm correct placement of the ET tube.
- Adequately secure an ET tube.
- Perform extubation.
- Perform ET intubation in the pediatric patient.
- Insert a dual lumen airway.
- Perform complete airway obstruction maneuvers, including the following:
  - Heimlich maneuver
  - Finger sweep
  - Chest thrusts
- Perform retrieval of foreign bodies from the upper airway using Magill forceps.
- Demonstrate suctioning the upper airway by selecting a suction device, catheter and technique.
- Perform tracheobronchial suctioning in the intubated patient by selecting a suction device, catheter and technique.
- Perform stoma suctioning.
- Demonstrate insertion of a nasogastric tube.
- Demonstrate insertion of an orogastric tube.
- Perform gastric decompression by selecting a suction device, catheter, and technique.
- Perform replacement of a tracheostomy tube through a stoma.

INTRODUCTION

A primary objective in emergency care is to ensure each patient has a patent airway and optimal ventilation. This provides for the intake of oxygen and removal of carbon dioxide. The faster care is started, the better is the patient's chance for survival. Laypersons trained in early detection and intervention in life-threatening conditions save thousands of lives each year.

✳ **Patent Airway** • An open, unblocked airway.

In the prehospital setting, emergency care professionals must be prepared to treat patients experiencing obstructed airway, aspiration, inadequate ventilation, or hypoxia. These are life-threatening conditions that require immediate intervention if the patient is to survive. Some of the procedures employed are done manually, whereas others require adjunctive equipment or ad-

vanced techniques. In contrast to the hospital environment, where care is provided in a controlled setting, managing patients in the field is often done with too few hands, little lighting, and an anxious crowd who expects the patient to be saved no matter how severe his or her condition. All these factors make the job challenging. Also at issue is that some health care providers neglect their airway skills. Basic procedures are taken for granted, and poor techniques are employed. This includes failing to create an effective seal with a bag-valve-mask device, improper positioning of the patient's head and neck, and not reassessing the patient's condition. All of these can lead to inadequate oxygenation and ventilation.

To learn these skills, understanding the normal anatomy and physiology of the respiratory system is crucial.

ANATOMY OF THE RESPIRATORY SYSTEM

The job of the respiratory system is to move air in and out of the lungs, bringing oxygen into the body and removing carbon dioxide. Oxygen is absolutely essential for human life; it is required for the conversion of essential nutrients into energy. Without it, cells of the body die. Brain death can occur within 6 to 10 minutes of the onset of cardiac arrest. Carbon dioxide is a waste product of metabolism and must be removed. For normal breathing to occur a person must have a **patent airway,** intact ventilatory musculoskeletal system, unobstructed respiratory passageways, adequate pulmonary blood flow, and appropriate neurologic stimulation.

✖ **Mucous Membrane** • A thin layer of connective tissue lining many of the body cavities through which air passes; usually contains small, mucous-secreting glands. Mucus is a thick, slippery secretion that functions as a lubricant and protects various surfaces.

CLINICAL NOTES

Inflammations of the various membranes of the body are assigned names by adding the suffix *-itis* to the anatomic name.

All of the respiratory structures leading to the microscopic alveoli (where the actual exchange of gases takes place) are lined with a highly vascular **mucous membrane.** This membrane filters the air. When inspired air finally reaches the distal passageways, it is the same temperature as the body, 100% humidified, and essentially sterile. The respiratory passageway can be thought of as having two portions, the upper and lower airways.

Upper Airway

Structures of the upper airway include the nose, mouth, pharynx, and larynx (Figure 8-1). The nose and mouth provide passageways into the respiratory system.

✖ **Maxilla** • One of a pair of large bones that form the upper jaw.

NOSE

The nose is the uppermost aspect of the airway. It consists of an external and internal portion. The external nose, or the part that protrudes from the face, is made up of a bony and cartilaginous framework covered by skin. On the front surface of the nose are two openings to the outside of the body. These openings are referred to as *nostrils* or *nares.* The union of the facial bones including the **maxilla,** frontal, nasal, ethmoid, and sphe-

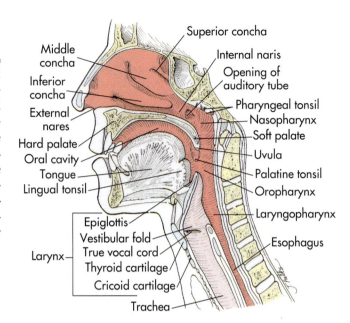

FIGURE 8-1 ▲ Anatomy of the upper airway. (Jody L. Fulks from Seeley R: *Essentials of anatomy and physiology,* ed 2, St Louis, 1996, Mosby.)

noid bones, form the walls of the nasal cavity. The roof of the nose is separated from the cranial cavity by a portion of the ethmoid bone called the *cribriform plate.* The cribriform plate has many small holes that permit branches of the olfactory nerve that are responsible for the special sense of smell to enter the cranial cavity and reach the brain. The palatine bones form the floor of the nasal cavity. This bony hard palate separates the nasal cavity from the oral cavity while a fleshy soft palate extends posteriorly from the hard palate to separate the nasopharynx from the rest of the pharynx. The orientation of the nasal floor is toward the ear. In addition to its role in respiration, the nose serves as the organ of smell (the olfactory receptors are located in its mucosa) and aids in speech.

✖ **Lateral** • To the side.

✖ **Nasal Septum** • An anatomic wall dividing the nostrils. It is made up of bone and cartilage covered by mucous membrane.

The internal nose is separated into the right and left cavity by the **nasal septum.** Each cavity has three bones, the superior, middle, and inferior turbinates (also referred to as *conchae*), which are located on their **lateral** walls. The mucous-covered turbinates are like shelves, resting parallel to the nasal floor. Their purpose is to cause turbulent airflow through the nose, forcing it to rebound in several directions during its passage. This greatly increases the surface over which air must flow as it passes through the nasal cavities. Air passing over the turbinates and through the nasal cavities is filtered, humidified, and warmed. Finer particles are trapped by the cilia of the mucous membrane and are then propelled back to the pharynx to be swallowed. Because its walls have a rich blood supply, serious bleeding can occur if the nasal passages are injured. Improper or overly aggressive placement of tubes or airways can cause significant bleeding, which may not be controlled by direct pressure. Four pairs of paranasal sinuses (cavities) drain into the nose. The cranial bones after which they are named form the frontal, maxillary, sphenoidal, and ethmoidal sinuses. These sinuses lighten the bones of the head, function as resonators for speech, trap bacteria, and serve as tributaries for fluid movement to and from the eustachian tubes, which regulate middle ear pressure, and tear ducts. The sinuses commonly become infected, and the fracture of certain sinus bones can lead to cerebrospinal fluid (CSF) leakage. On the back surface of the internal nose are two nares that serve as passageways into the nasopharynx.

Mandible • The large bone forming the lower jaw.

MOUTH

The cheeks, hard and soft palates, and tongue form the mouth, which is also referred to as the *oral cavity.* The lips are the fleshy folds that surround the opening, and the gums and teeth are located inside the mouth. The adult has 32 teeth. Although it takes significant force to dislodge any of the teeth, one or more fractured or avulsed teeth can cause airway obstruction. The hard and soft palates cover the top of the mouth, whereas the tongue, a large mass of muscle, is found on the bottom. The tongue attaches to the **mandible,** as well as to the hyoid bone through a series of muscles and ligaments. It assists with speech and swallowing of food. Because of its size and position in the airway the tongue is the most common cause of airway obstruction. The hyoid bone, shaped like a horseshoe or U is located between the chin and mandibular angle. It is unique in that it is the only bone of the axial skeleton that does not articulate with any other bone. Rather, it is suspended from the temporal bone by ligaments. The adenoids are lymph tissue located in the oropharynx and nasopharynx that filter bacteria. They often become infected and swollen.

PHARYNX

The pharynx, also called the *throat,* is a muscular conduit that extends downward from the back of the soft palate to the upper end of the esophagus. It serves as the passageway for air into the respiratory tract (anteriorly) and food and liquid into the digestive system (posteriorly). The pharynx is divided into three regions: (1) the nasopharynx (located immediately behind the nasal cavity); (2) oropharynx (located behind the mouth); and (3) laryngopharynx (the lower portion). The laryn-

gopharynx begins at the tip of the epiglottis and extends downward to where it opens posteriorly into the esophagus and anteriorly into the larynx. It is also called the *hypopharynx.*

Gag Reflex • Retching or striving to vomit; it is a normal reflex triggered by touching the soft palate or the throat.

Because the mouth and pharynx serve a dual purpose of conveying air and food and/or liquid, they are lined with sensitive nerves that activate the cough, **gag reflex,** and swallowing mechanisms to prevent the airway from being accidentally blocked or foreign matter from being drawn into the lungs.

> ### CLINICAL NOTES
>
> A cough is a forceful exhalation of a large volume of air. To initiate a cough, approximately 2.5 L of air is drawn into the respiratory passageways. Next, the glottic opening closes tightly shut to trap the air within the lungs. The abdominal and thoracic muscles then contract, pushing against the diaphragm and increasing the pressure within the tracheobronchial tree. The vocal cords suddenly open in a cough, forcing air and foreign particles out of the lungs.

Located in the front of the pharynx, just below the base of the tongue, are the epiglottis, laryngeal inlet, and mucous membrane–covered arytenoid and cricoid cartilages of the larynx. Just behind the hypopharynx are the fourth and fifth cervical vertebrae.

The epiglottis is a leaf-shaped, flexible cartilage that hangs over the larynx. It is connected to the hyoid bone and mandible by a series of ligaments and muscles. Its main function is to prevent food or liquid from entering the respiratory tree during swallowing. It also serves as an important landmark for ET intubation. Just above the epiglottis is the vallecula, the depression or "pocket" formed by the base of the tongue and the epiglottis.

> ### HELPFUL HINT
>
> • Because of their attachment to the mandible (directly and indirectly), both the tongue and epiglottis can fall back against the posterior wall of the pharynx, closing off the airway when the jaw goes slack. This problem can be corrected by using the chin-lift or jaw-thrust maneuver, which moves the mandible forward, lifting the tongue and epiglottis away from the posterior pharynx and opening the airway.

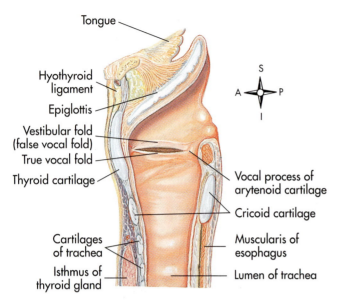

Labels on figure:
Tongue
Hyothyroid ligament
Epiglottis
Vestibular fold (false vocal fold)
True vocal fold
Thyroid cartilage
Cartilages of trachea
Isthmus of thyroid gland
Vocal process of arytenoid cartilage
Cricoid cartilage
Muscularis of esophagus
Lumen of trachea

FIGURE 8-2 ▲ Sagittal view of the larynx. (Ernest W. Beck from Thibodeau GA, Patton KT: *Anatomy and physiology*, ed 2, St Louis, 1996, Mosby.)

LARYNX

The larynx is the triangular-shaped structure that connects the pharynx with the trachea. Positioned midline in the neck, below the hyoid bone and in front of the esophagus, the larynx is made up of the thyroid cartilage, cricoid cartilage, vocal cords, and arytenoid folds. Along the lateral borders of the larynx are indentations or "hollow pockets" called *pyriform fossa.* The larynx performs several functions, including protecting the lower airway and producing voice (Figure 8-2).

The walls of the larynx consist of cartilages that prevent it from collapsing during inspiration. The main laryngeal cartilage is the thyroid cartilage. It is also referred to as the *Adam's apple* and is more prominent in men than women. The thyroid cartilage consists of two large shield-shaped pieces that form the anterior wall of the larynx and give it its V-shaped appearance. The posterior wall is open and consists of muscle. The glottic opening can be found directly behind the thyroid cartilage.

✖ **Cricothyroid Membrane** • Membrane situated between the cricoid and thyroid cartilages of the larynx.

Below the thyroid cartilage is the cricoid cartilage. It is attached to the first ring of tracheal cartilage. Unlike the thyroid and tracheal cartilages, which are open on their posterior surfaces, the cricoid cartilage is the only complete ring. It is shaped like a signet ring with the bulky portion located posteriorly. In children, the narrowest part of the laryngeal airway is the cricoid cartilage. Just behind the cricoid cartilage is the esophagus. Putting pressure on the cricoid cartilage and pushing it backward can effectively occlude the esophagus and prevent regurgitation. This procedure is referred to as the *Sellick maneuver.* Connecting the bottom border of the

thyroid cartilage with the top aspect of the cricoid cartilage is a fibrous membrane called the **cricothyroid membrane.** This is the site for surgical and alternative airway placement.

✖ **Glottis** • The slitlike opening between the vocal cords.

The cavity of the larynx extends from its triangular-shaped inlet at the epiglottis to the circular outlet at the lower border of the cricoid cartilage where it is continuous with the lumen of the trachea. At the upper end of the laryngeal cavity, extending from the anterior surface of the arytenoid cartilages to the posterior surface of the thyroid cartilage, lie the true and false vocal cords. The superior pair forms the false vocal cords (also called *vestibular folds*) and consist of elastic connective tissue covered by folds of mucous membrane. When these cords come together, they stop air from leaving the lungs (when a person holds his or her breath) and prevent foreign materials such as food or liquids from entering the airway. Below the false cords are the true vocal cords. They are cordlike structures that can vibrate to produce sound as expired air passes over them. Length and tension of the vocal cords determine the pitch of the voice. The space between the true vocal cords is referred to as the *glottic opening* or **glottis.** In the adult, the glottic opening is the narrowest portion of the upper airway (Figure 8-3, *A* and *B*). Airway patency at this level is heavily dependent on muscle tone.

Most of the larynx is richly lined with nerve endings from the vagus nerve. Due to the degree of vagal innervation, stimulation of the pharyngeal and laryngeal mucous membrane (by a laryngoscope or endotracheal [ET] tube) can cause bradycardia, hypotension, and a decreased respiratory rate.

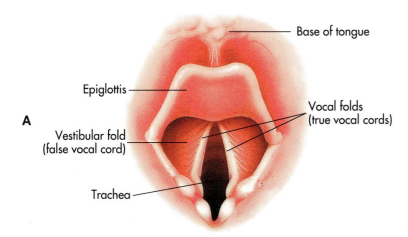

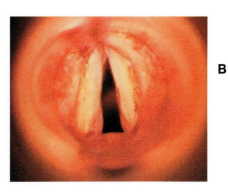

FIGURE 8-3 ▲ **A** and **B,** Vocal cords viewed from above. (**A,** From Carlyn Iverson from Seeley R: *Anatomy and physiology,* ed 3, St. Louis, 1995, Mosby. **B,** Custom Medical Stock Photography from Seeley R: *Anatomy and physiology,* ed 3, St Louis, 1995, Mosby.)

CLINICAL NOTES

The most common ailment of the larynx is inflammation, or laryngitis, and often accompanies colds, followed by a temporary diminishing or complete loss of voice. Other diseases commonly attacking the larynx include croup, diphtheria, and cancer. Laryngeal cancer is caused by cigarette smoking and by the intake of large amounts of alcohol. Persons who smoke and drink excessively run an especially high risk of developing cancer of the larynx.

A number of important structures are situated close to the larynx. The thyroid gland is located below the cricoid cartilage, lying across the trachea and up both sides. Branches of the carotid arteries cross and lie closely alongside the trachea while jugular veins branch across and lie close to the trachea.

Lower Airway

The lower airway extends from the fourth cervical vertebrae to the xyphoid process. It begins at the glottic opening and ends at the pulmonary capillary membrane. It consists of the trachea, right and left main stem bronchi, secondary bronchi, bronchioles, and alveoli.

TRACHEA

The trachea is the cylindrical tube, approximately 10- to 15-cm long, which continues from the lower rim of the larynx to the bronchi at the level of the fifth or sixth thoracic vertebra. It is situated in front of the esophagus and supported by C-shaped cartilaginous rings that extend throughout its length. These cartilages keep the tracheal walls from collapsing. The purpose of the trachea is to conduct air between the larynx and the lungs (Figure 8-4).

�֎ **Carina** • Point at which the trachea divides (bifurcates or separates into two sections) into the right and left main stem bronchi.

BRONCHIAL TREE

At the **carina,** the trachea branches into right and left main stem bronchi. There is one bronchus for each lung. The right bronchus is a more direct passageway from the trachea, because it is wider, shorter, and more vertical than the left. For this reason, aspirated foreign bodies (or incorrectly positioned ET tubes) are more likely to enter the right main stem bronchus than the left. Like the trachea, the bronchi are lined with a ciliated mucous layer and reinforced with cartilaginous rings. The main stem bronchus enters the lungs at the hilum, or root. On entering the lung, each bronchus branches into secondary bronchi, one for each lobe of the lungs (three on the right and two on the left). The secondary bronchi branch into smaller tertiary (segmental) bronchi that extend to the individual bronchopulmonary segments of each lobe. There are ten segments in the right lung and eight in the left lung. The bronchial tree continues to branch several more times. As the branches get smaller, the cartilaginous rings begin to disappear and the structures are mostly smooth muscle. The more distal por-

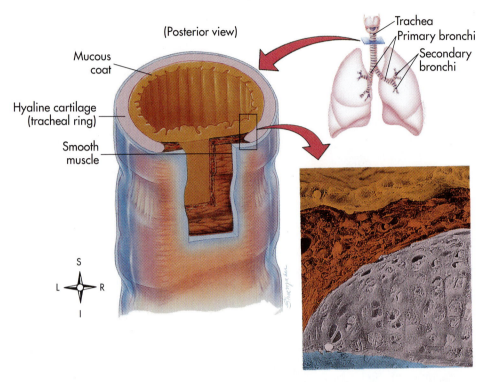

(Posterior view)

Mucous coat

Hyaline cartilage (tracheal ring)

Smooth muscle

Trachea
Primary bronchi
Secondary bronchi

S
L — R
I

FIGURE 8-4 ▲ A cross-section view of the trachea. (S. Erlandsen and J. Magney from Thibodeau GA, Patton KT: *Anatomy and physiology*, ed 3, St Louis, 1996, Mosby.)

tions are referred to as *bronchioles*. Bronchioles, in turn, branch into even smaller tubes called *terminal* and *respiratory bronchioles*, which eventually divide into microscopic branches called *alveolar ducts*. These ducts then terminate in clusters of air sacs, called *alveoli*. The continuous branching of the trachea into primary bronchi, secondary bronchi, bronchioles, and terminal bronchioles resembles a tree trunk (with its branches) and is commonly referred to as the *bronchial tree* (Figure 8-5). Beta-2 receptors of the sympathetic nervous system are also situated throughout the respiratory tree. When stimulated, they bring about bronchodilation.

Alveoli

The alveoli are hollow, grapelike structures only one or two cell layers thick (Figure 8-6). They are the most important functional units of the respiratory system because they serve as the primary site for oxygen and carbon dioxide exchange. Each alveoli lies in contact with a blood capillary, and there are millions of alveoli in each lung. The surface of the respiratory membrane inside the alveoli is covered with surfactant. This important substance decreases the surface tension of the alveoli, allowing for easier expansion and preventing collapse as air moves in and out during respiration. If surfactant is decreased or the alveoli are not inflated,

the alveoli collapse. Collapse of the alveoli is referred to as *atelectasis*.

Each microscopic alveolus is in contact with a rich capillary network arising from the pulmonary artery (Figure 8-7). The blood at the arteriole end of the pulmonary capillary is high in carbon dioxide and low in oxygen. As the blood passes through the capillaries, it comes in close proximity to outside air that has been drawn into the alveoli by inspiration. The alveoli become thinner as they expand, making diffusion of oxygen and carbon dioxide easier. Most of the carbon dioxide in the blood diffuses into the alveoli, and oxygen from the alveoli diffuses into the capillary blood. Diffusion is the process whereby particles move from an area of greater concentration to an area of lesser concentration until the distribution of particles is equal. Therefore the exchange of gases depends on differences in the concentration of gases on each side of the pulmonary membrane, which is referred to as the *diffusion gradient*.

❈ **Serous Membrane** • A two-layer epithelial membrane that lines body cavities and covers the surfaces of organs.

LUNGS

The lungs are cone-shaped, light, spongy, elastic organs; one lung is located on each side of the heart in

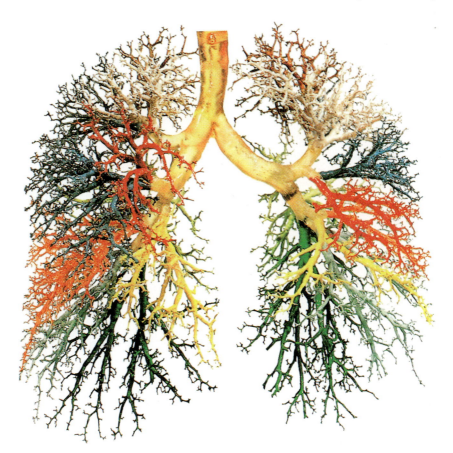

FIGURE 8-5 ▲ A plaster cast of the bronchial tree. (RMS McMinn and RT Hutchings from Thibodeau GA, Patton KT: *Anatomy and physiology,* ed 3, St Louis, 1996, Mosby.)

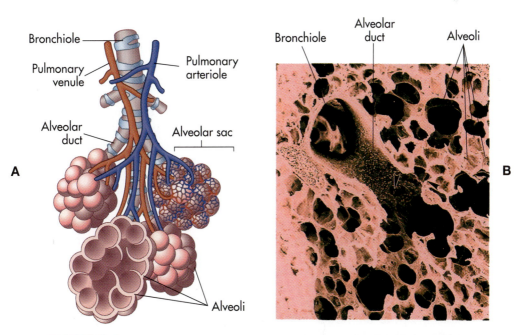

FIGURE 8-6 ▲ **A** and **B,** Anatomy of the alveoli. **A,** Terminal bronchioles branch into alveolar ducts, which terminate in alveoli. **B,** Electron micrograph scan of bronchiole, alveolar duct, and alveoli. *Arrowhead* indicates opening of alveoli into the alveolar duct. (**A,** Barbara Stackhouse from Thibodeau GA, Patton KT: *Anatomy and physiology,* ed 3, St Louis, 1996, Mosby and **B,** Joan M. Beck from Thibodeau GA, Patton KT: *Anatomy and physiology,* ed 3, St Louis, 1996, Mosby.)

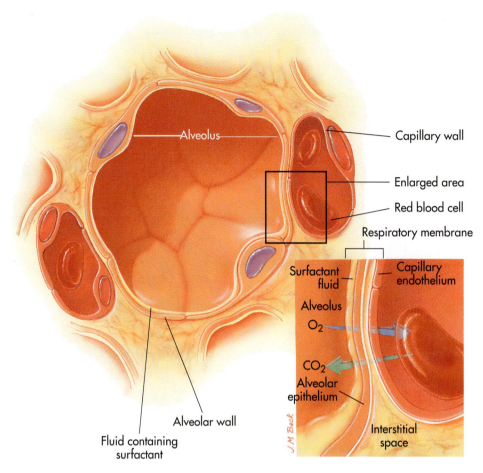

FIGURE 8-7   ▲   **The gas exchange structures of the lungs. Insert, a magnified view of the respiratory membrane. (Joan M. Beck from Thibodeau GA, Patton KT:** *Anatomy and physiology,* **ed 3, St Louis, 1996, Mosby.)**

the thoracic cavity. The lungs are large enough to fill the pleural portion of the thoracic cavity, completely extending from the diaphragm to just above the clavicles and lying against the ribs anteriorly and posteriorly. The part of the lung resting on the diaphragm is referred to as the *base;* the upper pointed portion is called the *apex.* Each lung is divided into lobes by deep, prominent fissures on the surface of the lung. The lobes are smooth and shiny on their surface. The right lung has three lobes, whereas the left has two. The primary bronchi, pulmonary blood vessels and nerves that are firmly anchored in a meshwork of dense connective tissue to form what is known as the root of the lung enter each lung through a slit on its medial surface called the *hilum* (Figure 8-8). This complex attaches to the mediastinum and fixes the positions of major nerves, vessels, and lymphatics. The lungs are freely movable except at the hilum, where root and pulmonary ligaments anchor them. The connective tissues of the root extend into the substance or parenchyma of each lung. These fibrous partitions, or trabeculae, contain elastic fibers, smooth muscles, and lymphatics. They branch repeatedly, dividing the lobes into smaller compartments; then the branches of the conducting passageways, pulmonary vessels, and nerves of the lungs follow these trabeculae to reach their peripheral destinations. The terminal partitions, or septa, divide the lung into lobules, each serviced by the tributaries of the pulmonary arteries, pulmonary veins and respiratory passageways. The connective tissues of the septa are, in turn, continuous with those of the visceral pleura. Because most of the volume of each lung consists of air-filled passageways and alveoli, the lung has a light and spongy consistency. Elastin fibers within the trabeculae, the septa, and the pleurae make the lung highly elastic and capable of tolerating great changes in volume.

Each lung is enclosed in a **serous membrane** called the *pleura.* This membrane is in the form of a sack and includes two layers: the visceral pleura and parietal pleura. The visceral layer of this membrane closely covers the lungs. The parietal layer of the pleura lines the inner surface of the chest wall, diaphragm, and mediastinum. The visceral pleura is separated from the parietal pleura by a potential space called the *pleural space,* which contains just a few drops of

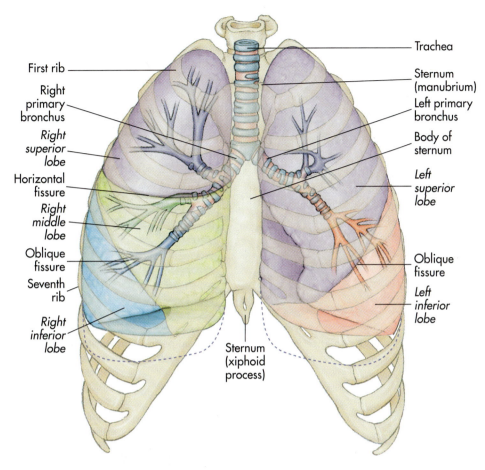

First rib

Right primary bronchus

Right superior lobe

Horizontal fissure

Right middle lobe

Oblique fissure

Seventh rib

Right inferior lobe

Trachea

Sternum (manubrium)

Left primary bronchus

Body of sternum

Left superior lobe

Oblique fissure

Left inferior lobe

Sternum (xiphoid process)

FIGURE 8-8 ▲ Lungs. (From Thibodeau GA: *Anatomy and physiology,* ed 4, St Louis, 1999, Mosby.)

pleural fluid. The fluid acts to prevent friction as the lung tissue expands and contracts in the chest cavity (Figure 8-9).

The tissues of the lungs are perfused via the bronchial arteries with oxygenated blood-containing nutrients. After the bronchial arterial blood has passed through the capillaries and collected carbon dioxide from the lung tissues, it empties into the pulmonary veins and left atrium.

Differences in the Pediatric Airway

Occlusion of the upper airway is one of the major causes of death in the prehospital setting when not appropriately managed. Therefore it is important to be aware of the significant anatomic differences between adult and pediatric airways. First, the overall size of the pediatric airway is smaller. Because of this, the airway of an infant or child is more likely to become occluded by foreign bodies, blood, vomit, loose teeth or swelling of tissue. A child less than 8 years of age has a larger tongue in comparison with the size of the mouth. A propor-

tionately smaller jaw can cause the tongue to encroach on the airway. Additionally, the child has a large, floppy, omega-shaped epiglottis, and the teeth may be absent or delicate. Due to their inability to hold the various anatomic structures clear of the airway, the weak muscles of the neck may allow obstruction to occur. The tonsils and adenoids (found in the posterior aspect of the pharynx) can also affect the patency of the airway.

The larynx lies more superior and is funnel-shaped due to narrow, undeveloped **cricoid cartilage.** The location of the vocal cords in a child is also different than in an adult. The cords of a child sit more superior and anterior on the cervical spine than those of an adult. In infants the cords are located at approximately the first (or second) cervical vertebra. As the child grows, the cords begin to move downward, closer to the level of the third vertebra. The airway of a child younger than 10 years of age is narrowest at the cricoid cartilage (Figure 8-10).

The chest wall of the child differs as well. Because the ribs and cartilage are softer, they cannot optimally contribute to lung expansion. Infants and children are more dependent on the diaphragm for breathing.

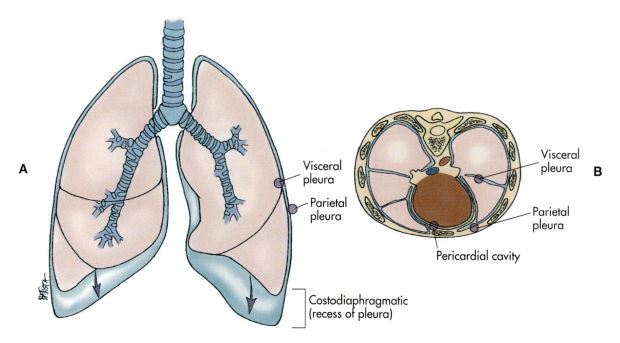

A

B

Visceral pleura

Parietal pleura

Visceral pleura

Parietal pleura

Pericardial cavity

Costodiaphragmatic (recess of pleura)

FIGURE 8-9 ▲ **A,** An anterior view of the visceral pleura and parietal pleura of the lungs. **B,** A cross-section of the visceral pleura and parietal pleura of the lungs.

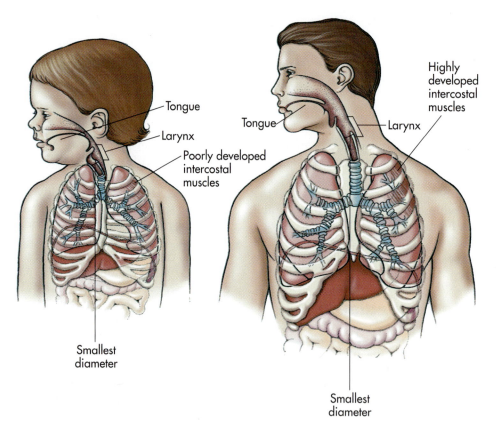

Tongue

Larynx

Poorly developed intercostal muscles

Tongue

Larynx

Highly developed intercostal muscles

Smallest diameter

Smallest diameter

FIGURE 8-10 ▲ Differences in pediatric airway. (From American College of Emergency Physicians; Pons P, Cason D, chief editors: *Paramedic field care: a complaint-based approach,* St Louis, 1997, Mosby.)

Cricoid Cartilage • The narrowest part of the child's upper airway.

PHYSIOLOGY OF THE RESPIRATORY SYSTEM

In the preceding section on anatomy of the respiratory system, the structures responsible for moving air in and out of the body were discussed. This section reviews the mechanism or process of breathing and gas exchange.

Respiration

Respiration is the exchange of gases between the body cells and the atmosphere. The major gases of respiration are oxygen and carbon dioxide. The three parts of respiration are as follows:

1. *External respiration*—This involves the exchange of gases between the circulating blood and air and is carried on by the expansion and contraction of the lungs.
2. *Internal respiration*—This involves the exchange of dissolved gases between the circulating blood and interstitial fluids in the peripheral tissues.
3. *Cellular respiration*—This is the actual use of oxygen by cells in the process of metabolism.

Respiration requires close interaction between the respiratory, central nervous, musculoskeletal, and circulatory systems. A nervous center in the brain controls the process and rate at which respiration proceeds. The regulation of respiration is largely involuntary and is controlled through chemical, physical, and nervous reflexes that monitor the body's changing carbon dioxide levels and oxygen needs.

Diaphragm • A wide, muscular partition separating the thoracic, or chest, cavity, from the abdominal cavity. It is attached to the lumbar vertebrae, lower ribs, and sternum, or breastbone. It slants upward, is higher in front than in the rear, and is dome-shaped when relaxed. Three major openings in the diaphragm allow passage of the esophagus, aorta, veins, nerves, and lymphatic and thoracic ducts.

Ventilation

The process of moving air in and out of the lungs is referred to as *ventilation*. It includes inspiration (breathing in) and expiration (breathing out). Changes in the size and gross capacity of the chest are controlled by contractions of the **diaphragm** and of the muscles between the ribs (Figure 8-11, *A*). Inspiration is initiated

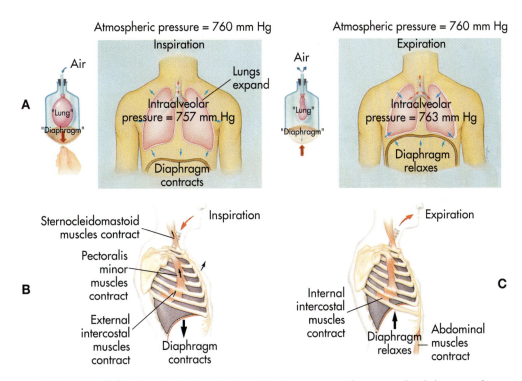

FIGURE 8-11 ▲ **A,** On inspiration, the lungs expand as a result of decreased pressure in the thoracic cavity. On expiration, the diaphragm relaxes and the lungs recoil as a result of increased pressure in the thoracic cavity. **B,** Mechanisms of inspiration. **C,** Mechanisms of expiration.

by the respiratory center in the medulla of the brain, signaling the muscles of respiration to increase the size of the chest cavity (Figure 8-11, *B*). Impulses are transmitted to the diaphragm by the phrenic nerve. The diaphragm, the major inspiratory muscle (accounting for 70% of the airflow in and out of the lungs), flattens downward against the abdominal structures. This action increases the vertical dimensions of the thoracic cavity in which the lungs are suspended, causing them to expand. The intrapulmonic pressure falls slightly below the atmospheric pressure. Normal, quiet breathing is accomplished almost entirely by this muscle. At the same time, the intercostal muscles lift the rib cage upward and outward, thus increasing the horizontal and transverse dimensions of the thoracic cavity. These actions create a potential vacuum that draws air into the enlarged lungs and fills them. The alveoli inflate and oxygen and carbon dioxide are able to diffuse across the alveolar-capillary membrane. Airway resistance must be overcome to generate flow through the airways. Changes in airway diameter affect airway resistance.

Stretch receptors in the lungs signal the respiratory center in the brain via the vagus nerve to inhibit inspiration. This is referred to as the *Hering-Breuer reflex.* Expiration occurs when the diaphragm and respiratory muscles relax and the chest cavity decreases in size (Figure 8-11, *C*). The decreasing thoracic volume increases the intrathoracic pressure, and air is forced out of the lungs. This act is passive (unless forced), and the driving force stems from the natural elasticity (recoil) of the lungs.

Minute Volume • The volume of air exchanged in 1 minute.

Respiratory Volume

Under normal circumstances, a person exchanges sufficient volumes of air to accommodate both normal and extraordinary physiologic requirements. On average, adults inhale and exhale between 500 to 800 mL of air (5 to 7 mL/kg) 12 to 20 times/min. The air inhaled and exhaled in a single respiratory cycle is referred to as the *tidal volume.* Of the 500 to 800 mL of air inhaled and exhaled, not all this air reaches the alveoli. The air remaining in the trachea and bronchi (unavailable for gas exchange) is called *dead air space,* it equals approximately 150 mL. Disease or obstruction such as chronic obstructive pulmonary disease (COPD) and atelectasis can lead to the development of additional dead space, which is referred to as *physiological dead space.* The air that reaches the alveoli for gas exchange is called *alveolar air* and equals approximately 350 mL. The air exchanged over the course of a minute is referred to as the **minute volume.** The average minute volume ranges between 6000 and 16,000 mL. These volumes of air are necessary to remove carbon dioxide and to bring in sufficient supplies of oxygen. Maximum lung capacity in the average adult male is approximately 6 L and is called the *total lung capacity.*

A number of terms are used to describe the various volumes of the lungs. Inspiratory reserve is the amount of air that can be inspired in addition to the tidal volume. Expiratory reserve is the amount of air that can be forcefully exhaled after expiring the tidal volume. Functional reserve capacity is the optimum amount of air that can be forced from the lungs in a single forced

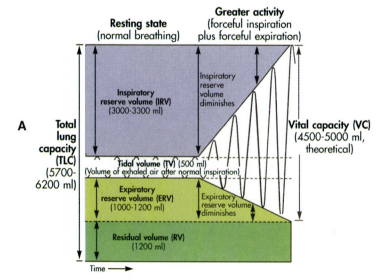

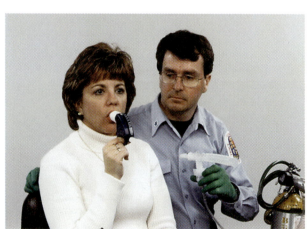

FIGURE 8-12 ▲ **A,** Ventilatory volumes. **B,** Using a peak flow meter. (**A,** From Thibodeau GA, Patton KT: *Structure and function of the body,* ed 10, St Louis, 1997, Mosby.)

expiration following optimal inspiration. The residual volume is the volume of air remaining in the lungs at the end of maximal expiration (Figure 8-12, *A*).

Various tests can be used to assess lung function including measuring the peak expiratory flow. The peak expiratory flow rate (PEFR) is the maximum, greatest expiratory flow rate in liters (L) per minute a person can deliver. It is measured by having a patient exhale forcefully into a disposable plastic chamber after taking the maximum inspiration he can. In the clinical setting the PEFR can be used to identify respiratory conditions such as asthma. Field use of PEFR allows you to evaluate the effectiveness of treatments such as bronchodilators administered to patients experiencing respiratory distress (Figure 8-12, *B*).

Exchange and Transport of Oxygen and Carbon Dioxide

✖ **Red Blood Cells (RBCs)** • Round disks that are concave on two sides and are approximately 7.5 μm in diameter. There are between 4.2 and 5.8 million RBCs.

A mature **red blood cell (RBC)** contains no nucleus. Hemoglobin, a protein in RBCs, is the most prevalent of the special blood pigments that transport oxygen from the lungs to the body cells, where it picks up carbon dioxide for transport back to the lungs to be expired. The RBCs are formed in the bone marrow. After an average life of 120 days, during which they incur substantial damage, they are broken down and removed by the spleen.

✖ **Po_2** • Abbreviation for partial pressure of oxygen.

✖ **Diffusion** • Passage of particles from an area of higher concentration to an area of lower concentration.

✖ **Fio_2** • Concentration of oxygen in inspired air.

Oxygenation

During inspiration, atmospheric air containing 21% oxygen is drawn into the respiratory passageways. The percentage of oxygen in inspired air is referred to as the **Fio_2**, which is commonly expressed as a decimal (e.g., Fio_2 = 0.95). At a 21% concentration, oxygen has a partial pressure of 160 mm Hg. By the time inspired air reaches the alveoli, a number of factors combine to reduce the **partial pressure of oxygen (Po_2)** to 104 mm Hg. The warming and humidification of the atmospheric air in the upper respiratory tract result in an increase in the partial pressure of water vapor from 5.7 mm Hg to 47 mm Hg with partial pressures of other gases declining (because the total pressure must remain at 760 mm Hg). Also, in the respiratory passageways, inspired air mixes with gas that was not exhaled on the previous exhalation (150 mL of dead space). Because dead space air contains more carbon

CLINICAL NOTES

To understand how oxygen and carbon dioxide are carried in the blood, it is helpful to comprehend partial pressures of gases. Usually, gases are found as mixtures of several gases together, like the air we breathe. Dalton's law of partial pressures states that the pressure exerted by a mixture of gases is equal to the sum of the partial pressures of each (Figure 8-13), and each gas acts as if it were present alone. The symbol used to designate partial pressure is the capital P preceding the chemical symbol for the gas. Some references still use the older symbol, a capital P and small a (Pa) to denote partial pressure. In air, the pressure of 760 mm Hg is the sum of the partial pressures of oxygen, nitrogen, carbon dioxide, water vapor, and trace gases. The partial pressure of each gas is directly related to its concentration in the total mixture. Atmospheric air contains 21% oxygen, 0.03% carbon dioxide, 78% nitrogen, and 0.97% other gases. The partial pressure of each is determined by multiplying its percentage by the sum (760 mm Hg). Atmospheric Po_2 = 21% ÷ 760 = 159.6 mm Hg (rounded off to 160 mm Hg). Partial pressure is measured in millimeters of mercury, or torr. One torr equals 1 mm Hg.

dioxide and less oxygen than inspired air, the Po_2 is reduced further. Air that finally reaches the alveoli for diffusion across the respiratory membrane registers even more partial pressure changes but still remains high in oxygen (104 mm Hg) and low in carbon dioxide. In the alveoli, this air is met by capillary venous blood oxygen that has a Po_2 of just 40 mm Hg. Oxygen diffuses in water and in a physiologic process called **diffusion**, oxygen moves across the alveolar/capillary membrane into the bloodstream until gas pressures are equal on both sides (Figure 8-14).

Oxygen is transported in arterial blood in two ways: physically, dissolved in plasma; and chemically, attached to hemoglobin. Oxygen dissolved in the plasma is referred to as the *Po_2* and oxygen bound to hemoglobin is referred to as the *Sao_2* (Figure 8-15). Although the blood is in the alveolar capillary, it absorbs enough oxygen to raise its Po_2 to 104 mm Hg. Because fluids can hold little gas in solution, just a small portion (3%) of oxygen is carried in plasma. Hemoglobin carries the majority (97%) of oxygen. When hemoglobin is in the presence of high Po_2, (e.g., in the pulmonary capillaries), oxygen binds to hemoglobin's iron molecules to form oxyhemoglobin. Hemoglobin bound to oxygen to its fullest extent (each gram of saturated hemoglobin

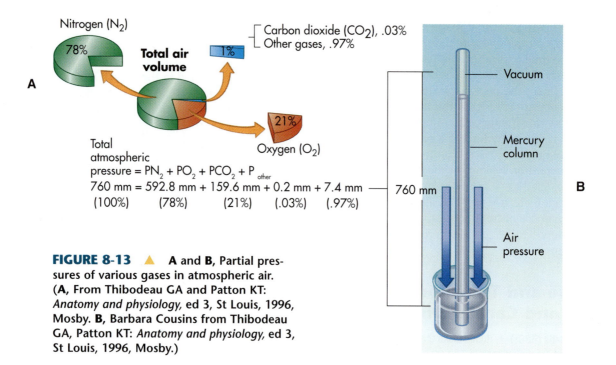

FIGURE 8-13 ▲ **A** and **B**, Partial pressures of various gases in atmospheric air. (**A**, From Thibodeau GA and Patton KT: *Anatomy and physiology*, ed 3, St Louis, 1996, Mosby. **B**, Barbara Cousins from Thibodeau GA, Patton KT: *Anatomy and physiology*, ed 3, St Louis, 1996, Mosby.)

carrying 1.34 mL of oxygen) is considered 100% saturated. Hemoglobin is close to being fully saturated at a P_{O_2} of 80 to 100 mm Hg. In this state the blood is bright red or scarlet. Oxygenated blood leaving the pulmonary capillaries has a P_{O_2} of 104 mm Hg. This blood then mixes with shunted (deoxygenated) blood. This lowers the P_{O_2} of the blood leaving the lungs through the pulmonary arteries to 95 mm Hg. This oxygen-enriched blood is then transported back to the heart via the pulmonary bloodstream where it is then pumped to the systemic capillaries. There, it comes into contact with tissues having a P_{O_2} of close to 40 mm Hg. Just like what occurred in the pulmonary capillaries, oxygen diffuses from an area of greater concentration (the bloodstream) to the area of lesser concentration (into the tissues). Oxygen then moves through the tissues to the cells where it plays an essential role in the Kreb's cycle, assisting with the production of energy. Because the cells are constantly using oxygen, a low P_{O_2} in the tissues continually exists. This condition makes for easy diffusion of oxygen from the bloodstream into the tissues. The pressure of oxygen in the blood after it has passed through the capillaries and reached the veins is lowered to 40 mm Hg. This decrease in oxygen concentration results in the blood turning bluish-red. The blood then is returned to the right side of the heart through the venous circulation. The heart then pumps this blood through the pulmonary arteries to the lungs where the cycle begins again.

✳ **P$_{CO_2}$** • Abbreviation for partial pressure of carbon dioxide.

CARBON DIOXIDE

While oxygen is moving into the tissues, carbon dioxide, a waste product of metabolism, is diffusing from the tissues (where the **partial pressure of carbon dioxide [P$_{CO_2}$]** is 50 mm Hg) into the blood (where the P_{CO_2} is 40 mm Hg). The venous blood returning to the lungs has a P_{CO_2} of 46 mm Hg. In the lungs, the carbon dioxide is removed. Once in the blood, carbon dioxide is carried to the lungs in three ways (Figure 8-16):

1. Dissolved in plasma (produces the P_{CO_2} of the blood)
2. Coupled with hemoglobin
3. Combined with water as carbonic acid and its components

Only 10% of the carbon dioxide is carried in blood plasma. Some of this 10% has a partial pressure; the rest reacts very slowly with water to form carbonic acid (H_2CO_3), which may break down further into hydrogen ions (H^+) and bicarbonate ions (HCO_3^-). Both processes are reversible. Approximately 20% of the carbon dioxide reacts somewhat faster with hemoglobin in the RBCs to form the compound carbaminohemoglobin. Approximately 70% of the carbon dioxide converts to carbonic acid in the RBCs. This process occurs in a split second due to the presence of carbonic anhydrase, a catalyzing enzyme. Just as fast, the carbonic acid

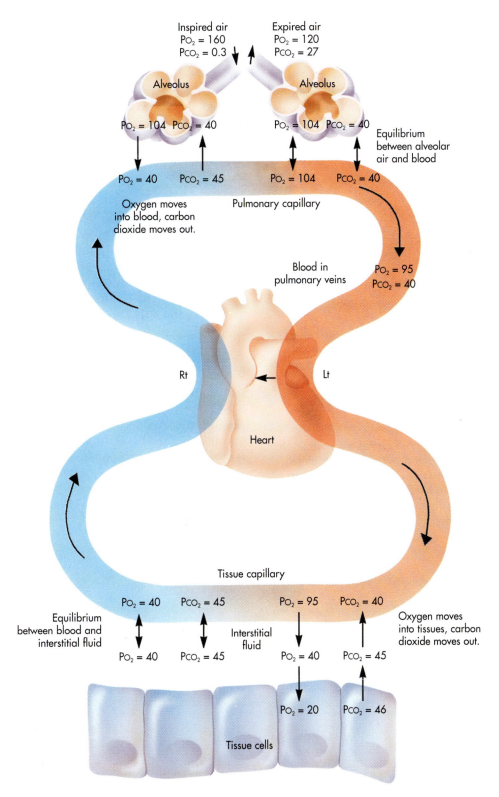

FIGURE 8-14 ▲ Oxygen and carbon dioxide diffuse across the alveolar capillaries as a result of differences in partial pressure. (Christine Oleksyk from Seeley R: *Anatomy and physiology,* ed 3, St Louis, 1995, Mosby.)

breaks down into hydrogen ions and bicarbonate ions; the hydrogen ions remain cell-bound and are neutralized by the hemoglobin, while the bicarbonate ions trade places with chloride ions in the surrounding plasma. RBCs expel excess bicarbonate yet remain electrically neutral in this process, called the *chloride shift.*

When venous blood enters the lung for gas exchange, all reversible chemical processes reverse, and carbon dioxide is once again formed. The gas diffuses into the alveoli and is expired. The exhaled air is high in carbon dioxide and low in oxygen. The amount of carbon dioxide in the body is dependent on ventilatory effectiveness. Under normal conditions, if ventilations are increased, the carbon dioxide decreases. If ventilations are decreased, the carbon dioxide will increase. In other words, carbon dioxide levels vary inversely with ventilations (Figure 8-17).

NITROGEN

Atmospheric air also contains 78% nitrogen. This creates a partial pressure of 592.8 mm Hg. Although nitrogen has no metabolic function, it is necessary for maintaining inflation of body cavities that are gas filled. The concentration of nitrogen in the alveolar gas is 74.9%. This creates a partial pressure of 569.0 mm Hg (Table 8-1).

Stimulus to Breathe
MEDULLA AND PONS

Unlike heart muscle, which contracts rhythmically even when separated from the nervous system, the respiratory muscles do not possess inherent rhythmicity. Stimuli from the brain are needed to produce the pattern of sequential inspiration-expiration. The main nervous centers for controlling the rate and depth of breathing are located in the medulla oblongata and the pons of the brainstem. Called *respiratory centers,* they

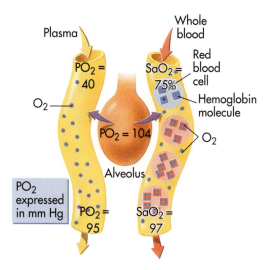

FIGURE 8-15 ▲ Hemoglobin carries approximately 97% of the oxygen in the blood while only a minimal amount is carried in the plasma. (Rolin Graphics from Thibodeau GA and Patton KT: *Anatomy and physiology,* ed 3, St Louis, 1996, Mosby.)

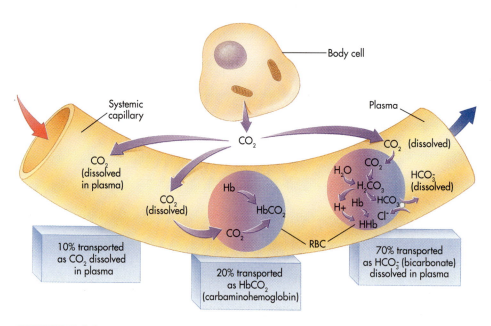

FIGURE 8-16 ▲ Carbon dioxide is transported from the body's tissues back to the lungs. Ten percent of the carbon dioxide is carried in blood plasma; twenty percent is transported in carbaminohemoglobin; seventy percent converts to bicarbonate and is transported in blood plasma. (Rolin Graphics from Thibodeau GA, Patton KT: *Anatomy and physiology,* ed 3, St Louis, 1996, Mosby.)

are comprised of scattered neurons that act as a unit to control respirations (Figure 8-18, *A*). Under resting conditions, nervous activity in the medulla produces a normal rate and depth of respirations (12 to 20 breaths per minute). The receptors of the medulla also sense the need for changing the rate and depth of respirations to maintain homeostasis. Central chemoreceptors located in the medulla are sensitive to slight changes in the concentration of carbon dioxide in the blood plasma. It is not a direct effect, because the carbon dioxide must first diffuse across the blood-brain barrier into the cerebral spinal fluid that bathes the chemosensitive area of the medulla. There, the carbon dioxide combines with water to form carbonic acid, which then dissociates into bicarbonate and hydrogen ions. The increased level of hydrogen ions stimulates the chemosensitive area, which then stimulates the respiratory center, resulting in a greater rate and depth of breathing. Consequently, carbon dioxide levels decrease as carbon dioxide is eliminated from the body. When excess carbon dioxide is present, the respiratory center stimulates the respiratory muscles to greater activity. The medulla is connected to the respiratory muscles by the vagus nerve. When the carbon dioxide concentration is low, breathing is depressed. The control centers in the medulla are in turn regulated by a number of inputs from receptors located in various areas of the body.

The pons is the apneustic center; it functions as the secondary control center for respiration if the medulla fails to initiate respiration. It also serves as the pneumotaxic center, controlling expiration.

CEREBRAL CORTEX

The cerebral cortex can influence respiration by modifying the rate at which the neurons in the medulla fire. This response allows a person to voluntarily speed up or slow down his or her breathing rate during activities such as speaking, singing, eating, or holding his or her breath during underwater swimming. However, this voluntary control has limits. Other factors such as blood carbon dioxide levels are much more powerful in controlling respirations than voluntary control. Regardless of the intent, a person will resume breathing when the body senses the need for more oxygen or if carbon dioxide levels increase to certain levels. Emotions (e.g., sobs and gasps of crying), acting through the limbic system of the brain, also can affect the respiratory center. Additionally, the activation of touch, thermal, and pain receptors also can stimulate the respiratory center, as

TABLE 8-1

CONCENTRATION OF GASES IN THE ATMOSPHERE	
Nitrogen	592.8 torr (78%)
Oxygen	159.6 torr (21%)
Carbon dioxide	0.2 torr (0.03%)
Others including water	7.4 torr (0.97%)
ALVEOLAR GAS CONCENTRATION	
Nitrogen	569.0 torr (74.9%)
Oxygen	104.0 torr (13.7%)
Carbon dioxide	40.0 torr (5.2%)
Water	47.0 torr (6.2%)

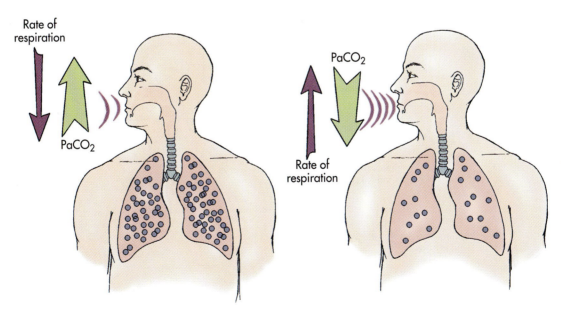

FIGURE 8-17 ▲ Carbon dioxide levels in the body are inversely proportional to ventilations. If ventilations are high, carbon dioxide levels are low. If ventilations are low, carbon dioxide levels are high.

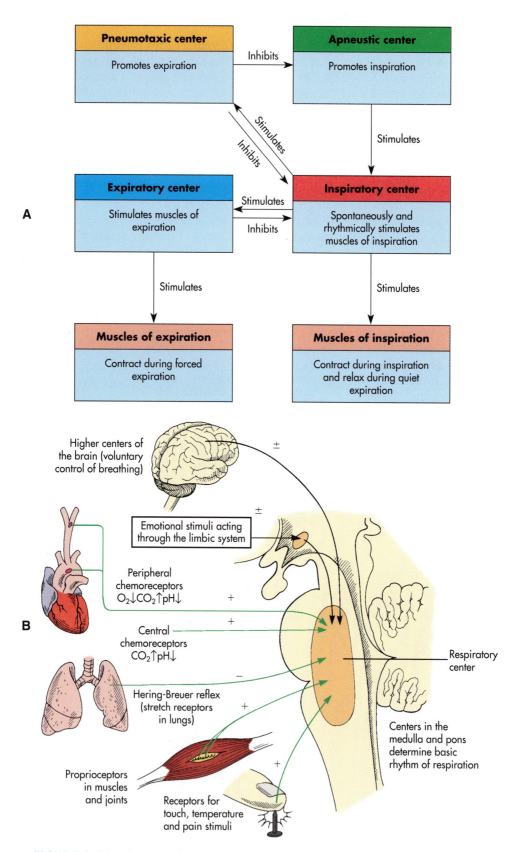

FIGURE 8-18 ▲ **A**, Respiratory centers act as a unit to control respiration. Active neurons in the respiratory center stimulate inspiration; inactive neurons cause the muscles of inspiration to relax. **B**, The regulatory mechanisms that affect the depth and rate of ventilation. (**A**, From Seeley R: *Anatomy and physiology*, ed 3, St. Louis, 1995, Mosby. **B**, Barbara Cousins from Thibodeau GA, Patton KT: *Anatomy and physiology*, ed 3, St Louis, 1996, Mosby.)

can body movements that occur during exercise. These movements stimulate proprioceptors in the joints of the limb, which in turn pass information along afferent nerve fibers to the spinal cord and brain (Figure 8-18, *B*).

PERIPHERAL CHEMORECEPTORS

Located peripherally in the aortic arch and carotid bodies are specialized receptors called *chemoreceptors.* These receptors are sensitive to increased carbon dioxide levels, increased blood acid levels, and decreased blood oxygen levels

The carotid body receptors are found at the point where the common carotid arteries divide, and the aortic bodies are small clusters of chemosensitive cells located adjacent to the aortic arch near the heart. When stimulated, these receptors send nerve impulses to the respiratory control centers in the medulla that in turn modify the respiratory rate. The peripheral chemoreceptors are sensitive to large increases in carbon dioxide and significant decreases in oxygen.

Other factors that increase or decrease respiration are as follows:

- *Body temperature*—Respirations increase with fever
- *Drug and medications*—Respirations may increase or decrease, depending on their physiologic action
- *Pain*—Increases respirations
- *Emotion*—Respirations increase
- *Hypoxia*—Respirations increase
- *Acidosis*—Respirations increase as a compensatory response to increased carbon dioxide production
- *Sleep*—Respirations decrease

PULMONARY STRETCH RECEPTORS

Specialized stretch receptors (also referred to as the *Hering-Breuer reflex*), located throughout the pulmonary airways and in the alveoli of the lungs, influence the normal pattern of breathing and act to protect the respiratory system from excessive stretching caused by harmful over inflation. When the tidal volume of air has been inspired, the lungs are expanded enough to stimulate microscopic stretch receptors. Inhibitory impulses follow afferent pathways to the medulla where the inspiratory act is curtailed. Relaxation of inspiratory muscles occurs, and expiration follows.

Modified Forms of Respiration

The body has a number of reflexes that act to protect the respiratory system, including cough, sneeze, gag reflex, sigh, and hiccough. A cough is a forceful, spastic exhalation of a large volume of air from the lungs. It aids in clearing the bronchi and bronchioles of foreign material. A sneeze is a sudden forceful exhalation from the nose that clears the nasopharynx. It is usually triggered by irritation of the nose. A hiccough is a sud-

> ### CLINICAL NOTES
>
> Individuals with chronic respiratory disease have a decreased ability to remove carbon dioxide. This condition results in a progressive increase in the carbon dioxide concentrations of the body. Over time, the respiratory centers adjust to tolerate high carbon dioxide levels. The medullary respiratory centers become dulled to these changes. The body then relies on peripheral chemoreceptors to control respirations. Respiration in these individuals is controlled by oxygen level: the rate and depth of respiration increases in response to Po_2 levels below 60 mm Hg. Because the peripheral chemoreceptors respond to low Po_2, any treatment involving high concentrations of oxygen can act to suppress the hypoxic drive thus suppressing respirations. For this reason, oxygen therapy should be administered carefully in patients who have a history of chronic respiratory disease. In those situations in which a high oxygen concentration is required (e.g., acute myocardial infarction, shock), the EMT–I should be prepared to assist the patient's breathing if respiratory depression or apnea occurs.

den inspiration caused by spasmodic contraction of the diaphragm and intermittent spastic closure of glottis. A gag reflex is a spastic pharyngeal and esophageal reflex that results from stimulus of the posterior pharynx. It may bring about nausea and vomiting. Sighing is an involuntary slow, deep breath followed by prolonged expiration. Sighing hyperinflates the lungs and opens atelectatic alveoli. A person normally sighs about once per minute.

ASSESSMENT OF THE PATIENT

The EMT–I must be skilled in assessing and managing patients who present with upper airway obstruction. Intervention in these cases may require you to employ several skills at the same time. The first step is to determine if an open airway is present. When the possibility of spinal injury exists, airway patency must be assessed and ensured in conjunction with in-line cervical spine stabilization. If airway compromise is identified, it must be resolved. Once a patent airway is ensured, respiratory effectiveness must be assessed. If the patient is not breathing adequately, assisted breathing must be provided. Following that, circulatory effectiveness must be evaluated, and measures should be taken to resolve any life-threatening deficiencies.

Body substance isolation (BSI) precautions must be employed during assessment and management of patients. At a minimum, protective rubber gloves and goggles should be worn whenever airway management is performed. If there is a chance that body fluids may be splashed or aerolyzed, wearing a mask and protective gown or overalls is pertinent. A good assessment becomes a window to the patient's condition and can make the difference between the patient surviving or not surviving. Indications of airway obstruction, hypoxia, and hypoventilation are usually evident during those first critical minutes. Intervention can resolve many life-threatening conditions.

Initial Impression

Much information is available during the approach to the patient. Is the patient responsive? Is the patient breathing? Does the patient appear to have adequate air exchange? These questions are often answered by the time the patient is reached. The absence of an open airway and/or the lack of effective breathing efforts require taking immediate steps to correct the problem (Table 8-2).

CLINICAL NOTES

The ability to breathe and the ability to protect the airway are not always the same.

Once at the patient's side, and then throughout the provision of care, the assessment should continue being made in a logical and systematic manner. Assess and ensure an open airway; also check respiratory function and evaluate circulation. The patient's level of responsiveness also should be evaluated because restlessness, agitation, disorientation, coma, and other conditions indicate decreased cerebral oxygenation. Once the initial examination is complete and the necessary intervention taken, a more thorough, focused examination can be done. However, even when the airway is initially

TABLE 8-2

Sounds and Causes of Some Common Airway Obstructions

SOUND	COMMON TYPES OF AIRWAY OBSTRUCTION
Snoring respirations	The tongue
Gurgling sounds	Accumulation of blood, vomitus, or other secretions
Stridor (a harsh, high-pitched sound heard on inhalation)	Laryngeal edema, constriction, or foreign body obstruction

patent, continuous reassessment is warranted, because airway patency may change at any time.

Indicators of respiratory function include airway patency, appearance of the neck, breathing efforts, color of the skin, breath sounds, outward signs (flaring of the nares, retraction, noisy breathing), air movement at the nose and mouth, compliance (felt during ventilatory assistance provided with a bag-valve-mask device), and the pulse rate. Devices such as the pulse oximetry unit can be used to determine the oxygen saturation. Another sign of respiratory function is silence, which indicates a complete absence of air movement.

Airway Patency

Air movement and sounds typically indicate airway patency. Sounds such as gurgling, snoring, and so on suggest obstruction of the upper airway. If an obstruction is identified, immediate steps must be taken to correct the problem.

Neck

After assessing and ensuring a patent airway, the neck should be quickly inspected for distended jugular veins, tracheal shift, or tugging. The presence of any of these indicates a likely respiratory problem.

Breathing Efforts

Observing the patient's breathing efforts helps assess the adequacy of air exchange. Air movement can be felt at the patient's nose and mouth. When an ET tube is in place, the proximal end can be checked for air movement. Normally, the chest rises and falls with each respiratory cycle. In the adult patient, the respiratory rate ranges from 12 to 20 breaths per minute. Breathing should be spontaneous and regular. Slow, fast, or irregular breathing indicates a significant problem and requires the EMT–I to intervene with assisted breathing (bag-valve-mask device, automatic ventilator, or other equipment).

Breathing at rest should be effortless. Because changes in effort may be subtle in rate and regularity, the patient must be watched carefully. Patients often compensate by preferential positioning such as upright sniffing and the semi-Fowler's position. A patient experiencing respiratory difficulty will often resist being placed in a supine position.

When assisting a patient's breathing with a ventilatory device or after placing an airway adjunct (nasopharyngeal airway, multilumen airway, ET tube) you should observe the rise and fall of the patient's chest to determine correct use and placement. When assisting a patient's breathing with the bag-valve-mask device, the effectiveness of airflow into the lungs can be gauged by noting the compliance and how quickly the bag empties. *Compliance* is defined as the stiffness or flexibility of the lung tissue. It is noted by how easily air flows into the lungs. When compliance is good, airflow occurs with a minimum amount of resistance. When compliance is poor, ventilation is harder to achieve. Compliance is poor in diseased states of the lungs, chest wall injuries, or with tension pneumothorax. Compliance also decreases when the tongue obstructs the upper airway. If poor compliance occurs during assisted breathing, look for potential causes. Is the airway open? Is the head properly extended or the jaw-thrust maneuver properly employed? Is the patient developing a tension pneumothorax? Is the ET tube occluded? Has the ET tube been inadvertently pushed into the right or left main stem bronchus? A bag that empties too quickly or "collapses" also should be regarded as ominous. It may indicate incorrect placement of the ET tube into the esophagus or a defect in the bag-valve-mask device. Devices such as the end-tidal carbon dioxide detector, esophageal detection device, and pulse oximetry device can also be used to help monitor proper placement of an ET tube or multilumen device.

Respiratory Pattern Changes

As stated earlier, breathing should be comfortable, regular, at a rate of between 12 to 20 breaths per minute, and initiated without distress. An increased respiratory rate is referred to as *tachypnea*, whereas a slower than normal rate is called *bradypnea*. A number of breathing patterns can be seen that will indicate the presence of various conditions. Cheyne-Stokes breathing is a regular pattern of gradually increasing rate and tidal volume, followed by a gradual decrease and then a short period of apnea. It is associated with brain stem insult. Kussmaul breathing is deep, gasping respirations; it is common in diabetic coma. Biot's breathing is an irregular pattern, rate, and volume with intermittent periods of apnea and is seen in increased intracranial pressure. Central neurogenic hyperventilation is a pattern of deep, rapid respirations similar to Kussmaul breathing. It is also indicative of increased intracranial pressure. Agonal breathing is a pattern of slow, shallow, irregular respirations and results from brain anoxia (Figure 8-19).

Pulsus Paradoxus

Another indicator of respiratory distress is the presence of pulsus paradoxus. This is when the systolic blood pressure drops greater than 10 mm Hg during inspiration. A change in pulse quality may also be detected. Pulsus paradoxus is seen in COPD and indicates an increase in the intrathoracic pressure. This increase in pressure within the thoracic cavity interferes with the ability of the ventricles to fill properly, leading to a decrease in blood pressure.

Pulse Oximetry

Pulse oximetry is a simple, noninvasive procedure used to determine the effectiveness of patient oxygenation (Figure 8-20). It allows for continuous monitoring, detect-

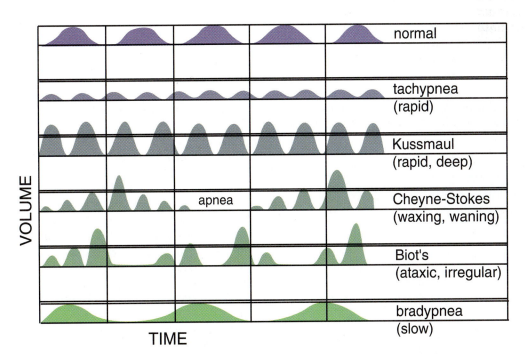

FIGURE 8-19 ▲ Normal and abnormal breathing patterns and rates. (From American College of Emergency Physicians; Pons P, Cason D, chief editors: *Paramedic field care: a complaint-based approach*, ed 1, St Louis, 1997, Mosby.)

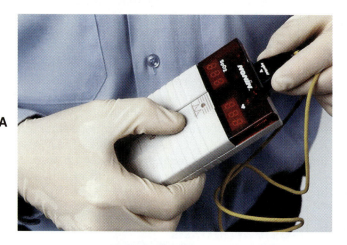

A

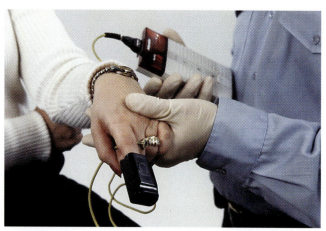

B

FIGURE 8-20 ▲ **A,** Inserting finger clip into oximeter device. **B,** Applying the finger clip and obtaining a pulse oximeter reading.

ing trends in patient's oxygenation status within 6 seconds. Pulse oximetry devices can help with the following:

- Reaffirm perceived hypoxia
- Reveal hidden hypoxia
- In conjunction with other indicators, assist in determining what oxygen adjunct should be applied and what liter flow should be administered
- Aid in monitoring clinical improvement or deterioration in acutely dyspneic patients
- In conjunction with other indicators, identify when to intubate
- Identify changes during intubation or other airway manipulations

Because normal evaluation of oxygenation is notoriously unreliable, pulse oximetry readings should be taken on all patients and recorded as part of their vital signs. Saturation readings also should be taken either before or shortly after oxygen is administered to any patient. These readings should be repeated throughout assessment, treatment, and transport of the patient.

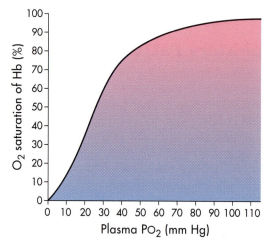

FIGURE 8-21 ▲ Oxygen-hemoglobin dissociation curve. At lower levels of O_2 saturation the levels of plasma Po_2 decrease. (From Thibodeau GA, Patton KT: *Anatomy and physiology,* ed 3, St Louis, 1996, Mosby.)

❗ HELPFUL HINT

Oxygen administration should never be delayed in the seriously ill or injured patient to obtain an initial pulse oximetry reading.

It is important to keep a patient's oxygen saturation in a normal range, because declines in saturation lead to a reduction in oxygen content, as follows:

- With 90% saturation, Po_2 drops to 60 mm Hg.
- With 75% saturation, Po_2 drops to 40 mm Hg.
- With 50% saturation, Po_2 drops to 27 mm Hg (Figure 8-21).

In addition to oxygen saturation (SaO_2), many pulse oximetry devices display a visual and audible pulse rate. However, this unit should not be used to replace palpating for a pulse or in place of the cardiac monitor when the situation dictates the use of one.

Before use, the EMT–I should test the unit on himself or herself to confirm that it is in good operating condition. To do this, turn on the unit and follow all operating recommendations set forth by the manufacturer. Make sure all the connections are secured in place properly, such as where the finger clip cable plugs into the unit (see Figure 8-21). After the unit is found to be in good operating condition, the finger clip should be placed on the patient's index finger with the outline of the finger facing up (or in some units, with the cable on the nail side of the finger). All dirt and nail polish or any obstructive covering should be removed to prevent the unit from giving a false reading. When these steps are completed, the unit will display the SaO_2 reading and typically, the patient's heart rate too.

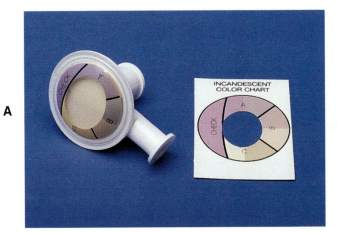 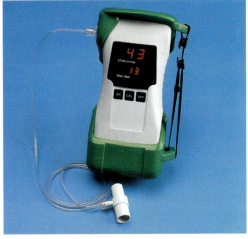

FIGURE 8-22 ▲ **A,** Colorimetric end-tidal carbon dioxide detector. **B,** Digital (or electronic) end-tidal carbon dioxide detector. (**A,** Vincent Knaus from Cummins RO, Graves J: *ACLS scenarios: core concepts for case-based learning,* St Louis, 1996, Mosby.)

Pulse oximetry should be viewed as just another tool to assist in patient monitoring. A variety of circumstances produce false readings, including the following:

- Carbon monoxide/cyanide poisoning
- Excessive ambient light on the sensor probe
- Patient movement
- Hypotension (low perfusion states)
- Hypothermia
- Use of vasoconstrictive drugs by the patient
- Nail polish
- Jaundice

Additionally, pulse oximetry cannot give information about alveolar ventilation or cellular respiration. For this reason, it is important not to accept adequate SaO_2 values while neglecting gross hypoventilation or cellular hypoxia. Another consideration is that patients with COPD may have a normally low SaO_2, so adequate histories must be obtained.

⁙ Hypoxemia • Insufficient oxygenation of the blood.

Oxygen therapy is used to treat **hypoxemia.** SaO_2 readings can help determine which oxygen adjunct should be placed on the patient, as well as the liter flow to be administered. An SaO_2 reading in the 95% to 99% range is ideal, and no supplemental oxygen is needed unless the patient's chief complaint or injury mechanism warrants it. An SaO_2 reading of 91% to 94% represents mild hypoxemia and indicates that the airway should be checked and oxygen therapy should be started at 4 to 6 L via nasal cannula. An SaO_2 reading of 85% to 90% represents moderate hypoxemia. The airway must be checked and aggressive oxygen therapy must be started at 15 L/min via nonrebreather mask. An SaO_2 reading of less than 85% indicates severe hypoxemia. In these cases, it is important to prepare to intubate or assist ventilation with a bag-valve-mask device and 100% oxygen.

CLINICAL NOTES

Pulse oximetry is a useful adjunct. However, indicators such as signs and symptoms the patient is displaying and/or the illness or injury mechanism should prompt initiation of oxygen therapy, ventilatory support, and/or intubation even in lieu of acceptable pulse oximetry readings.

☀STUDENT ALERT

End-tidal carbon dioxide devices and esophageal detector devices are now recommended tools for evaluating proper ET placement.

End-Tidal Carbon Dioxide Detectors

End-tidal carbon dioxide detectors are an effective way of verifying correct ET tube placement, as well as detecting subsequent tracheal tube displacement. These devices detect the presence of carbon dioxide in the intubated patient's expired air. End-tidal air, which closely correlates with the percentages of gases found in mixed venous blood, contains approximately 6% carbon dioxide. Particularly in patients with spontaneous circulation, a lack of carbon dioxide in the end-tidal air strongly suggests the tube has been misplaced into the esophagus.

The two types of end-tidal carbon dioxide detectors available to date are the disposable colorimetric device and the electronic monitor. Both are attached in-line between the ET tube and the ventilatory device after intubation (Figure 8-22, *A* and *B*).

The least expensive of the two devices, the disposable colorimetric device, is designed for single patient use and contains a nontoxic chemical indicator that reacts instantly to expired tracheal carbon dioxide by changing color. The reversibility of this color change allows the EMT–I to determine esophageal or tracheal intubation (after at least six breaths). The presence of a yellow color on expiration indicates correct placement in the trachea, whereas a purple color indicates improper placement in the esophagus. The color varies from expiration to inspiration as carbon dioxide levels rise and fall in a phasic manner.

The electronic device is a more expensive portable or hand-held end-tidal carbon dioxide detector, which uses an infrared analyzer to measure the percentage of carbon dioxide gas at each phase of respiration. This information is displayed on a digital readout or printout. This device can provide verification of correct ET intubation or provide continuous carbon dioxide monitoring with a cannula during transport. Newer models combine pulse oximetry, pulse rate, and respiratory rate in one unit.

Despite its usefulness, the end-tidal carbon dioxide detector sometimes produces false readings. First, carbon dioxide can inadvertently enter the stomach. It has been shown that six breaths can quickly wash out any retained carbon dioxide. Similarly, patients who ingest large amounts of carbonated liquid before arrest may produce similar false readings. Second, adequate circulation and pulmonary perfusion are required to obtain diffusion of carbon dioxide from the pulmonary capillary bed. For this reason, initial end-tidal carbon dioxide levels may be considerably lower during cardiac arrest. However, with adequate cardiopulmonary resuscitation (CPR), these levels should raise enough to allow the end-tidal carbon dioxide detector to verify proper intubation. A false reading can also be obtained in patients

with a large amount of dead space, such as in the case of a significant pulmonary embolism.

Because of the potential for inaccurate readings in some conditions, the end-tidal carbon dioxide detector should be considered as just one of many tools available for assessing correct ET tube placement and ventilatory status.

Esophageal Intubation Detectors

Another device available for verifying correct placement of an ET tube is the esophageal detector device (Figure 8-23). It comes in two types, a large syringe and a flexible bulb. Neither of these devices is a carbon dioxide detector. Rather, these simple and easy-to-use devices take advantage of the anatomic differences between the trachea and esophagus.

The syringe-type esophageal detector device resembles a large syringe with a 15-mm adapter at its distal end. After the ET tube is placed and before any ventilation attempts, the device is attached (with the compression plunger fully inserted into the syringe barrel) to the ET tube. The compression plunger is then withdrawn. If the tube is in the esophagus, its soft, unsupported walls will collapse around the end of the ET tube, preventing air from being drawn out of the device. If the ET tube is

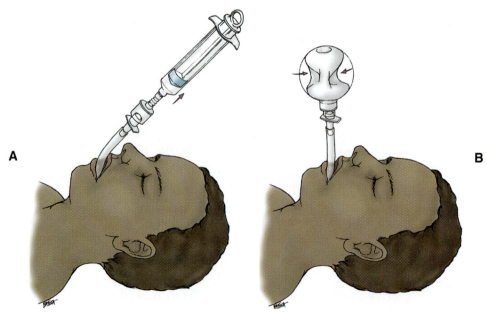

FIGURE 8-23 ▲ Esophageal intubation detector. **A,** Syringe; **B,** bulb.

in the trachea, the rigid trachea remains patent, allowing the plunger to be easily withdrawn from the device.

The bulb-type esophageal detector device works in a similar way. It is compressed before it is attached to the ET tube. As compression on the bulb is released, a vacuum is created. If the tube is in the esophagus, the bulb will not reinflate. However, if the ET tube is properly placed, the bulb will reinflate.

Benefits of these devices include that they are inexpensive; disposable; provide fast, immediate results; require no calibration; reduce the risk of ventilating the stomach; are durable; have unlimited shelf life; and are usable in low-light conditions.

Furthermore, unlike end-tidal carbon dioxide detectors, these devices are generally reliable in patients with both a perfusing and nonperfusing cardiac rhythms. However, false readings can occur with these devices in patients with morbid obesity, late pregnancy, or status asthmaticus or when there are copious tracheal secretions. In status asthmaticus the airway secretions or small airway obstruction (due to bronchospasm and so on) inhibits air aspiration from the lower airways.

Appearance of the Chest

You should note the presence of intercostal retraction or accessory muscle usage. Manifestations of respiratory compromise include the presence of nasal flaring (nostrils wide open during inspiration), tracheal tugging, retraction of the intercostal muscles, and use of the diaphragm and neck muscles to assist with inspiration.

✖ **Breath Sounds** • Sound of air passing in and out of the respiratory passageways as heard with a stethoscope.

Epigastric Sounds

Auscultation of the epigastrium should immediately follow inflation of the distal cuff of the airway device. It should be silent, with no sounds audible during ventilation (Figure 8-24).

Breath Sounds

Auscultation of the chest should immediately follow auscultation for epigastric sounds. Listening to the chest provides information about airflow into and out of the lungs. The sites usually auscultated include (1) just beneath the right and left clavicles (apexes of the lungs) and (2) the right and left lateral sides of the chest in the midaxillary line (at the level of the eighth or ninth intercostal spaces) (Figure 8-25). At each site, listen to first one side of the chest and then the other. **Breath sounds** should be equal. Additionally, six locations on the posterior chest can be auscultated. However, given that the patient is usually in a supine position during airway management, the anterior and lateral positions are most accessible. The presence of airflow with auscultation over the sternal notch reveals the correct placement of an ET tube in the trachea.

In some cases, air movement into the stomach may mimic lung sounds. Obese or barrel-chested patients are most likely to present this problem, because their breath sounds may seem distant or muffled. For this reason, it is important to ensure the presence of clear, equal, bilateral lung sounds.

Gastric Distention

It is crucial to watch for signs of gastric distention whenever providing ventilatory support. Gastric distention is suggestive of inadequate hyperextension of the head, too much pressure being generated by the ventilatory device, or improperly placed airway adjuncts.

Skin

The color and texture of the skin provide information regarding oxygenation. Early in respiratory compromise the sympathetic nervous system is stimulated in an effort to offset the lack of oxygen. This stimulation makes the skin appear pale and diaphoretic. Cyanosis is another sign of respiratory distress. When oxygen binds with hemoglobin, the blood appears bright red. Unoxygenated

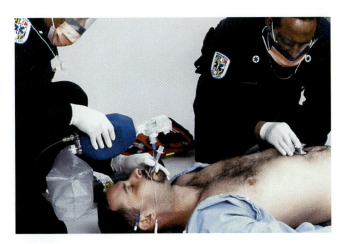

FIGURE 8-24 ▲ Auscultating the abdomen.

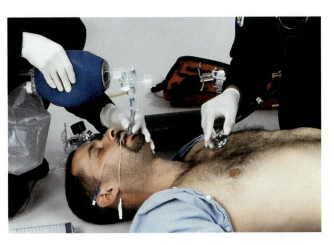

FIGURE 8-25 ▲ Auscultating the chest.

hemoglobin is blue and imparts a bluish color to the skin. However, this sign is not truly reliable because severe tissue hypoxia is possible without cyanosis. In fact, cyanosis is considered a late sign of respiratory compromise. When it does appear, cyanosis is usually seen at the lips, fingernails, and/or the skin.

✖ **Anoxia** • Lack of oxygen.

Circulatory Status

The pulse rate can also indicate respiratory compromise. Tachycardia usually accompanies hypoxemia, whereas bradycardia suggests **anoxia** with imminent cardiac arrest.

History

The history of the patient with airway obstruction or compromise may be evident, as in the case of upper airway obstruction in the responsive patient. Other causes usually are not so easily defined. When time and the patient's condition permit, appropriate questions should be asked to establish the past medical history, history of present complication, and/or the mechanism of injury.

HYPOXIA

Oxygen therapy is an essential treatment of seriously ill or injured patients. Being knowledgeable and skilled in the application of all supplemental oxygen delivery devices and the rationale for their use is important.

Pathophysiology

Oxygen plays a vital role in the body's production of energy. Without it, normal metabolism cannot occur. The movement and use of oxygen in the body is dependent on having the following:

- An adequate concentration of inspired oxygen
- Appropriate movement of oxygen across the alveolar/capillary membrane into the arterial bloodstream
- An adequate number of RBCs to carry the oxygen
- Proper tissue perfusion
- Efficient off-loading of oxygen at the tissue level

The above elements are collectively known as the *Fick Principle.*

✖ **Dysrhythmia** • A disturbance in the normal rhythm of the heart.

✖ **Hypoxia** • Reduced oxygen supply to the cells.

Hypoxia is defined as a decreased or inadequate supply of oxygen. It has several adverse effects on the body. At the cellular level, it leads to anaerobic metabolism, a physiologic process that can result in metabolic acidosis, cellular depression, and eventually, cellular death.

In the brain, it brings about swelling that results in reduced blood flow to the cerebral tissues and a worsening of the hypoxia. In the heart, it can cause cardiac **dysrhythmias** and decreased cardiac output. Hypoxia also increases myocardial and respiratory workloads because the body uses these systems to offset the hypoxia. Causes of hypoxia are listed in Box 8-1.

✖ **Kyphoscoliosis** • Lateral curvature of the spine; can interfere with normal breathing.

✖ **Fibrosis** • Abnormal formation of scar tissue in the connective tissue framework of the lungs following inflammation or pneumonia and in pulmonary tuberculosis.

Assessment

Signs of hypoxia may include changes in the patient's mental status, tachycardia, a pulse oximetry saturation reading of less than 95%, and other indications. Dyspnea and cyanosis are late signs.

BOX 8-1

CAUSES OF HYPOXIA

1. Insufficient oxygen in inspired air due to:
   - Smoke
   - Toxic gases
   - High altitude
2. Failure of the ventilatory mechanism due to:
   - Pneumothorax
   - Fractured ribs
   - Muscular paralysis
   - **Kyphoscoliosis**
3. Upper airway compromise caused by:
   - Foreign body obstruction
   - Epiglottitis
   - Croup
   - Edema of vocal cords
4. Lower airway compromise caused by:
   - Chronic bronchitis
   - Acute asthma attack
   - Tumors
   - Pneumonia
   - Pulmonary edema
   - Emphysema
   - **Fibrosis**
5. Circulatory deficiency due to:
   - Pump failure
   - Congestive heart failure
   - Congenital defects
   - Blood loss (hemorrhage)
   - Shock
   - Anemia
   - Carbon monoxide poisoning
6. Cellular deficiency as a result of:
   - Cyanide poisoning
   - Toxic shock syndrome

Treatment

Treatment of hypoxia is directed at increasing the patient's oxygen level through supplemental oxygen administration. Indications include chest pain due to myocardial ischemia, cardiorespiratory arrest, and suspected hypoxia of any cause, including major blood loss, major trauma, congestive heart failure, lung disease or injury, airway obstruction, stroke, shock, seizures, head injury, and carbon monoxide poisoning.

Supplemental oxygen raises the oxygen level by increasing the following:

- Percentage of oxygen provided to the patient (increased FiO_2 of inspired air)
- Oxygen concentration at the alveolar level
- Arterial oxygen levels
- Amount of oxygen delivered to the cells

Through these actions, supplemental oxygen decreases hypoxia and reduces the intensity of the breathing efforts and myocardial work that the body must keep up to maintain a given oxygen level. In other words, it increases the patient's ability to compensate for the hypoxia.

Oxygen Source

Oxygen used in the prehospital setting is typically stored as a compressed gas and contained in an aluminum or steel tank or cylinder. The *United States Pharmacopoeia* has color-coded cylinders containing various gases. All grades of oxygen are denoted by the colors green and white. Common sizes and volumes of the cylinders used in the prehospital setting are as follows (Figure 8-26):

D	400 L (factor: 0.16)
E	660 L (factor: 0.28)
M	3450 L (factor: 1.56)

Pressure Regulators

Depending on the surrounding temperature, the pressure in a full oxygen cylinder is approximately 2000 pounds per square inch (psi). This pressure is too high to be safely delivered to a patient. Therefore a pressure regulator is attached to the cylinder to deliver a safe working pressure of 30 to 70 psi.

With cylinders of the E size or smaller, the pressure regulator is attached to the cylinder valve assembly through use of a yoke assembly. On the inside of the yoke, a configuration of pins mate with matching holes in the valve assembly. This is referred to as a *pin-index safety system.* Since the pin position varies depending on the gas, this system keeps an oxygen delivery system from being connected to a cylinder containing another type of gas.

Cylinders greater than E have a valve assembly with a threaded outlet. The inside and outside diameters of the threaded outlets differ based on the gas in the cylinder. This keeps an oxygen regulator from being attached to a cylinder containing some other gas.

Before the pressure regulator is connected to an oxygen supply cylinder it must be cleared of any dust or dirt. Otherwise the regulator can be damaged. To perform this task, stand to the side of the main valve opening and open (crack) the cylinder valve slightly for just a brief second. This should clear any dirt or dust out of the delivery port or threaded outlet.

> **HELPFUL HINT**
>
> - Commercial companies that refill oxygen tanks typically cover the cylinder valve assembly with a protective plastic wrap or cap.

Flow Meters

A flow meter is attached to the pressure regulator to control the flow of oxygen in L/min.

Three major types of flow meters are available; the Bourdon gauge flow meter, pressure-compensated flow meter, and the constant flow selector valve. The type commonly used on portable units is the constant flow selector valve. Depending on the manufacturer it may or may not have a gauge. The adjustment of flow L/min is controlled through stepped increments (2, 4, and 6 to 15 L/min). It can be accurately used with any type of oxygen delivery device and with any size oxygen cylinder. It is rugged and functions at any angle.

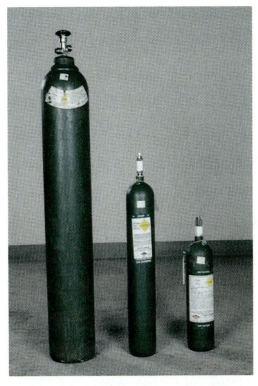

FIGURE 8-26 ▲ Oxygen tanks. (From Henry MC: *EMT prehospital care*, ed 2, St Louis, 1997, WB Saunders.)

For use in the prehospital setting, the pressure-compensated flow meter is thought to be superior to the Bourdon gauge flow meter; however, it is more fragile than the Bourdon gauge and must be operated in an upright position. For these reasons, many EMS systems use the pressure-compensated flow meter for fixed oxygen systems only. To attach a cylinder to a regulator, see Box 8-2.

STREET WISE

Safety considerations are paramount when handling oxygen cylinders. Remember, these cylinders are filled under pressure of 2000 to 2200 psi. If the neck of the cylinder is broken or the tank is punctured they can become rockets. Therefore the tank should never be left unattended and unsecured in a standing (upright) position. Also, the portable oxygen tank and regulator must be secured in place whenever transferring a patient to another location.

Oxygen cylinders should only be allowed to empty to the point where the regulator reads 200 psi. This is referred to as the safe residual pressure. To avoid accidentally running out of oxygen while treating patients, many prehospital systems maintain a policy of refilling the cylinder when it reaches 400 psi.

Oxygen delivery is measured in L/min. To estimate how long an oxygen supply will last, the following calculation can be used:

Tank life in minutes = (tank pressure in psi − 200 psi [safe residual pressure] × tank factor) ÷ L/min

An example of this calculation is as follows:

You have a D tank with 1000 psi, and you are using a nasal cannula to deliver 6 L/min. First, you subtract 200 psi (safe residual pressure) from 1000; this leaves 800 psi. Next, you multiply 800 psi by 0.16 (the tank factor); this equals 128 psi. Now you divide 128 psi by 6 L/min to yield a time of 21 minutes.

Liquid Oxygen

Because of space considerations, some EMS systems and aeromedical units use liquid oxygen. This is oxygen converted to an aqueous state. A much larger volume of oxygen can be stored in the aqueous state. To deliver the oxygen, it must be warmed. Furthermore, these oxygen units generally require upright storage and special equipment to use them.

PRECAUTIONS

Although there are no absolute contraindications to oxygen administration, it should be used with caution in patients prone to carbon dioxide retention and in premature infants. Recommended flow rates for the patient with COPD are 1 to 3 L delivered via nasal cannula or 24% to 28% via Venturi mask. If a patient develops respiratory depression, his or her breathing must be supported with a bag-valve-mask device connected to 15 L of oxygen (85% to 100%) or other ventilatory device.

Another important precaution is to avoid allowing petroleum-based substances or adhesive tape to come into contact with the valve stem of the oxygen cylinder or the oxygen regulator. These can contaminate the oxygen and contribute to spontaneous combustion when mixed with the pressurized oxygen.

Humidification

A humidifier is a nonbreakable jar of water that is attached to the flow meter. When dry oxygen coming from the oxygen cylinder passes through the water of the humidifier it is moisturized (humidified). This humidified oxygen is then delivered to the patient through an appropriate oxygen delivery device such as a nasal cannula, simple face mask, nonrebreather mask, or Venturi mask.

Oxygen that lacks this humidification can contribute to a drying out of mucous membranes of the patient's airway and respiratory tree. However, in most short-term use, oxygen dryness does not produce an adverse effect, but patients are usually more comfortable when given humidified oxygen. This is particularly true in patients who have COPD and in children.

Because of how it is used, the humidifier must be kept clean. The water reservoir is an excellent breeding ground for algae, harmful bacteria, and dangerous fungal organisms. The water in the reservoir must be replaced with sterile fresh water as often as each shift, and the reservoir should be cleaned according to manufacturer's instructions. Sterile single-patient–use humidifiers are available and preferred.

BOX 8-2

ATTACHING A CYLINDER TO A REGULATOR

The steps for delivering oxygen are as follows:
- Select an oxygen cylinder.
- Place the cylinder in an upright position and stand to one side.
- If present, remove the plastic wrapper or cap protecting the cylinder outlet.
- Crack the valve for one second to clear any dust or dirt.
- Line up the pins in the regulator yoke to the corresponding holes in the cylinder valve (smaller tanks) or the threads of the regular to the oxygen cylinder outlet (larger tanks).
- Tighten the regulator to the cylinder valve.
- Attach oxygen tubing and delivery device.

Many EMS systems no longer use humidifiers because of the lack of benefit during short transport times and the risk of infection. However, humidifiers may be beneficial during long transports and with certain pediatric patients who are experiencing inadequate breathing.

✖ **Ambient Air** • Environmental or room air.

Supplemental oxygen is administered through high-flow and low-flow systems. High-flow systems are equipped with a Venturi adapter that draws in large amounts of room air for each liter of oxygen delivered from the oxygen regulator (Figure 8-27). This action ensures delivery of precise oxygen concentrations regardless of how well the patient is breathing. In low-flow systems, oxygen travels directly from the regulator to the patient, allowing **ambient air** to be drawn into the respiratory passageways with each breath. This process dilutes the oxygen concentration from 100% (being delivered through the oxygen tubing) to a mixture of the two (100% oxygen and ambient air). The concentration delivered to the patient depends on the flow rate and type of oxygen delivery device used. With some oxygen delivery devices, the oxygen concentration varies in concert with changes in the respiratory minute volume. A patient who is breathing faster and/or deeper receives less oxygen, because he or she is taking in more ambient air, thus greatly diluting the oxygen flow of the low-flow system. Conversely, a patient whose breathing is slow and/or shallow dilutes the delivered oxygen flow with less ambient air and receives a higher concentration of oxygen. Devices that allow greater variation in the percentage of oxygen delivered to the patient are the nasal cannula and simple face mask.

Supplemental oxygen should be provided at a liter flow rate that delivers an appropriate concentration based on the patient's condition and medical history, as well as local protocols.

Oxygen Delivery Devices

The following variety of devices are used to deliver supplemental oxygen in spontaneously breathing patients:
- Nasal cannula
- Simple face mask
- Partial rebreather mask
- Nonrebreather mask
- Venturi mask

Patients needing assisted breathing usually receive high concentrations of oxygen through the device used to provide ventilatory assistance. The pocket mask, bag-valve-mask device, demand valve mask, and automatic ventilator each can provide high concentrations. Whatever oxygen administration device is used, it must be reassessed to determine the adequacy and efficiency of oxygen delivery.

NASAL CANNULA

A benefit of the nasal cannula is that it does not interfere with assessment because the patient's response to questions can be easily heard. Additionally, there is no rebreathing of expired air. The presence of nasal obstruction is the only contraindication for use of the nasal cannula.

Oxygen Concentration Delivered—The nasal cannula is a comfortable and easily tolerated device capable of delivering an oxygen concentration of 24% to 44% when supplied with flow rates of between 1 and 6 L/min. (Figure 8-28).

Precautions—The flow rate should be limited to 6 L/min. Anything greater does little to increase the inspired oxygen concentration because the anatomic

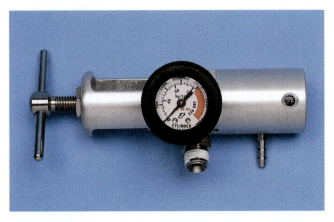

FIGURE 8-27 ▲ Oxygen regulator. (From Sanders MJ: *Mosby's paramedic textbook*, ed 2, St Louis, 2000, Mosby.)

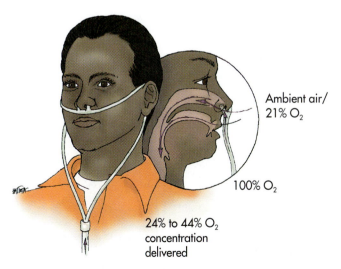

Ambient air/ 21% O₂

100% O₂

24% to 44% O₂ concentration delivered

FIGURE 8-28 ▲ A nasal cannula and the oxygen concentration delivered.

reserve (nasal cavity) is already filled. Additionally, higher flow rates dry the mucous membranes and can cause headaches. Use of the nasal cannula is recommended for patients who are as follows:

- Experiencing minor to moderate hypoxia
- Predisposed to carbon dioxide retention
- Frightened or feeling suffocated with other delivery devices
- Feeling nauseous or vomiting

Procedure—To use the nasal cannula, the following steps should be taken:

1. Explain to the patient the need for oxygen and apply the cannula.
2. Attach the nasal cannula to the oxygen.
3. Adjust the flow meter to deliver 6 L/min or less.
4. Place the two prongs of the cannula into the patient's nostrils with the tab facing up (prongs should curve upright).
5. Hook the tubing behind each ear and under the patient's chin.
6. Gently secure the cannula by sliding the adjuster upward under the patient's chin. The type that has an elastic strap fits over the ears and around the back of the head, and it is tightened by adjusting the strap on both sides simultaneously until the cannula is secure, yet comfortable.
7. Continuously monitor the oxygen level in the tank.

SIMPLE FACE MASK

Components of the simple face mask include oxygen tubing and a cone-shaped face mask that has two inlet/outlet ports (one on each side). It fits over the patient's nose, mouth, and chin. The inlet/outlet ports allow ambient air to be drawn in with each breath and carbon dioxide–filled air to escape on expiration. Oxygen is delivered to the mask through an inlet port located at its base.

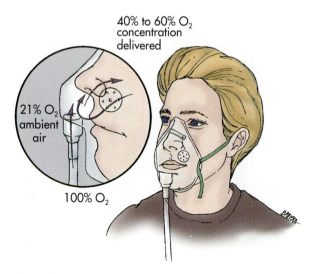

40% to 60% O_2
concentration
delivered

21% O_2
ambient
air

100% O_2

FIGURE 8-29 ▲ A simple face mask and the oxygen concentration delivered.

Oxygen Concentration Delivered—In the patient who is breathing normally, the simple face mask can deliver a concentration of 40% to 60% oxygen (Figure 8-29). Recommended flow rates used with the simple face mask range between 8 and 12 L/min. No less than 8/L should be administered through the device, because expired carbon dioxide can accumulate in the mask, resulting in hypercarbia. Flow rates of at least 8 L are needed to wash out the carbon dioxide exhaled by the patient. The simple face mask is used to provide oxygen to patients who are suffering from moderate hypoxia.

Precautions—Because the mask covers the patient's face it should be used with caution in the presence of nausea and vomiting. In the pediatric patient, flow rates of 6 to 8 L/min are generally used.

The following are some issues that accompany applying the simple face mask:

- It may feel restrictive to the patient, particularly those patients experiencing severe dyspnea.
- It is hot and confining and may irritate the skin.
- It is difficult to hear the patient speaking when the device is in place.
- It requires a tight face seal to prevent oxygen leakage.

Procedure—To use the simple mask, you should:

1. Attach the simple mask to the oxygen flow meter nipple.
2. Adjust the flow meter to deliver at least 10 to 15 L/min.
3. Apply the mask by placing it over the patient's nose, mouth, and chin.
4. Slip the loosened elastic strap over the patient's head so that it's positioned either above or below the ears.
5. Tighten the mask by adjusting the elastic strap on both sides simultaneously until the mask is secure.
6. Press the flexible metal nosepiece so that it fits the bridge of the patient's nose.
7. Continuously monitor the oxygen level in the tank.

NONREBREATHER MASK

The nonrebreather mask looks similar to the simple face mask. The difference is that, in addition to the oxygen tubing and a face mask, a reservoir bag is attached to the mask base, along with a rubber flap covering each of the air inlet/outlet ports (Figure 8-30). The reservoir collects 100% oxygen delivered through the oxygen tubing. As the patient breathes in, the 100% oxygen (contained in the reservoir) is drawn into the mask and the patient's respiratory passageways. Ambient air is kept from entering the mask during inspiration by the rubber flaps that close over the inlet/outlet ports. During expiration, the flapper valves are forced open, allowing the expired air to pass to the outside. A one-way valve positioned between the mask and reservoir keeps expired air from diluting the oxygen contained in the reservoir bag.

Oxygen Concentration Delivered—When supplied with 10 to 15 L/min, the nonrebreather mask is capable of delivering a 60% to 100% concentration of oxygen.

Precautions—Because it is a closed system that prevents breathing in of ambient air, the reservoir bag should not be allowed to totally deflate, which can cause the patient to suffocate. You should observe the reservoir bag as the patient breathes. If it collapses more than slightly during inspiration, the flow rate should be increased until only a slight deflation is seen. The reservoir bag should be kept from twisting or kinking and should be positioned outside the sheets or blankets so that it is completely free to expand. To move sufficient oxygen into the reservoir bag and remove exhaled carbon dioxide, at least 10 L of oxygen is needed. The nonrebreather mask also requires the use of a tight seal. With some patients, this tight seal may be difficult to obtain or may feel confining. Lastly, the nonrebreather mask should be employed with caution in patients who report nausea.

Use of the nonrebreather mask is recommended for the treatment of severely hypoxic patients, such as respiratory compromise, shock, acute myocardial infarction, trauma, carbon monoxide poisoning, and so forth.

Procedure—To use the nonrebreather mask, the following steps should be taken:

1. Attach the nonrebreather mask to the oxygen flow meter nipple.
2. Prefill the reservoir by using a finger to cover the exhaust portal (the connection between the mask and reservoir) (Figure 8-31).
3. Adjust the flow meter to deliver 10 to 15 L/min.
4. Apply the mask by placing it over the patient's nose, mouth, and chin.
5. Press the flexible metal nosepiece so that it fits the bridge of the patient's nose.

6. Tighten the mask by adjusting the elastic strap on both sides simultaneously until the mask is secure.
7. Make sure the one-way flaps are secure and functioning.
8. Observe the reservoir bag as the patient breathes (if it collapses more than slightly during inspiration, increase the flow rate).
9. Keep the reservoir from kinking or twisting.
10. Continuously monitor the oxygen level in the tank.

VENTURI MASK

The Venturi mask is a high-flow device that includes oxygen tubing, a face mask, and a Venturi system. As oxygen passes through the jet orifice in the mask, it draws in ambient air. The resulting mixture is delivered to the patient through the face mask. The same amount of ambient air is always entrained regardless of the rate or depth of respirations; thus fixed concentrations of oxygen (within 1%) can be provided. This mask is particularly useful with patients with COPD, with whom careful control of the inspired oxygen concentration is needed. Some Venturi masks are supplied with a dial that controls the amount of ambient air entrained, whereas others come with interchangeable caps.

Oxygen Concentration Delivered—Typically, the device delivers oxygen concentrations of 24%, 28%, 35%, or 40%. The liter flow needed depends on the oxygen concentration desired (Figure 8-32, *A* and *B*).

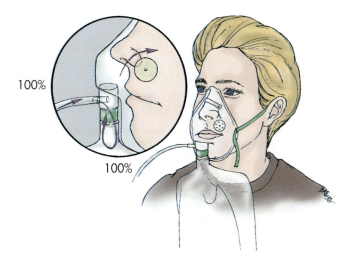

60% to 100% O_2 concentration delivered

100%

100%

FIGURE 8-30 ▲ A nonrebreather mask and the oxygen concentration delivered.

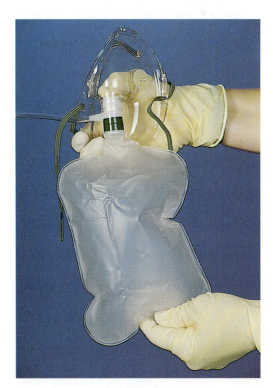

FIGURE 8-31 ▲ Inflate the reservoir bag with oxygen before placing it on the patient. (Vincent Knaus from Stoy W: *Mosby's EMT–Basic textbook,* St Louis, 1996, Mosby.)

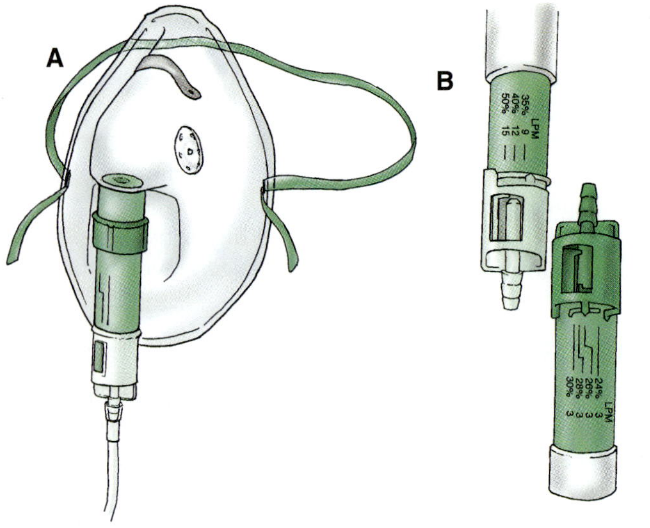

FIGURE 8-32 ▲ **A, A Venturi mask. B, Some Venturi masks are equipped with a control that regulates the amount of ambient air that can enter.**

As mentioned earlier, oxygen also can be delivered to the patient via a partial rebreather mask; bag-valve-mask device; or flow-restricted, oxygen-powered ventilation device.

Precautions—Fraction inspired oxygen concentration may be altered if the mask doesn't fit snugly, if the tubing is kinked, if the oxygen intake ports are blocked, or if less than the recommended liter flow is used.

Procedure—To use the Venturi mask, you should:

1. Attach the male adapter of the mask to the wide-bore tubing. Select the prescribed jet adapter and match the slots on the entrainment collector. Push the jet adapter onto the entrainment collector and turn it clockwise one half turn, locking it into place. Some Venturi masks have an adjustable device at the distal end of the entrainment collector that allows adjustment of the oxygen concentration. This is turned clockwise or counterclockwise to adjust the percentage delivered to the patient.
2. Attach the Venturi mask to the oxygen flow meter nipple.
3. Adjust the flow meter to deliver the required L/min.
4. Apply the mask by placing it over the patient's nose, mouth, and chin.
5. Slip the loosened elastic strap over the patient's head so that it's positioned either above or below the ears.
6. Tighten the mask by adjusting the elastic strap on both sides simultaneously until the mask is secure.
7. Press the flexible metal nosepiece so that it fits the bridge of the patient's nose.
8. Continuously monitor the oxygen level in the tank.

VENTILATION

Once a patent airway is ensured, the EMT–I then must determine if there is a need for ventilatory support.

BOX 8-3

INDICATIONS FOR HYPOVENTILATION

- Depressed respiratory function
- Drug overdose, alcohol intoxication
- Spinal injury
- Head injury
- Impaired ventilatory function
- Fractured ribs
- Flail chest
- Pneumothorax
- Chronic obstructive pulmonary disease
- Asthma
- Muscular paralysis
- Poliomyelitis

Assisted breathing must be provided to those patients who are apneic or experiencing depressed respiratory function.

Ventilation • Breathing, moving air in and out of the lungs.

Hypoventilation • A reduced rate or depth of breathing, often resulting in an abnormal rise of carbon dioxide.

Pathophysiology

As discussed earlier, adequate **ventilation** or respiratory minute volumes are needed for a sufficient intake of oxygen and removal of carbon dioxide. A decrease in either the respiratory rate or volume leads to a reduction in the respiratory minute volume. This condition is referred to as **hypoventilation.** Hypoventilation leads to the accumulation of carbon dioxide (also referred to as *hypercarbia*), development of hypoxia, and a lowered pH. Hypoventilation also can occur when the respiratory rate is so fast that the depth of breathing is reduced or when breathing is deep, but the rate is excessively slow. In both situations, too little air exchange takes place due to an overall reduction in respiratory minute volumes. Ultimately, if left uncorrected, respiratory and/or cardiac arrest can occur. A number of mechanisms can even bring about hypoventilation and are listed in Box 8-3.

Assessment

A critical component to the use of any ventilatory device is proper assessment. This assessment begins with looking at each patient during those first seconds of exposure and continuously thereafter to determine if there is sufficient air exchange. Observant evaluation of the level of responsiveness, work of breathing, respiratory rate, mucous membrane color, and pulse oximetry readings all provide critical information. If respiratory failure is imminent or present, supportive measures must be instituted. Even patients who are spontaneously breathing may require ventilatory support, because respiratory efforts that are too slow or too shallow result in hypoxia and hypercarbia and eventually lead to death. In some cases, hypoventilation is not obvious. Thus patients who have a respiratory rate outside the normal parameter (less than 12 or greater than 20 breaths per minute) may require ventilatory assistance. These patients must be closely watched and provided with ventilatory assistance as needed. Certainly, patients with respiratory rates of less than 10 or greater than 30 breaths per minute should receive ventilatory assistance.

CLINICAL NOTES

For those EMT–Is who are permitted, the use of the cardiac monitor also can provide invaluable information regarding the patient's status. However, when hypoxia is suspected, its application should not delay the administration of oxygen.

Basic Treatment

When illness or injury adversely affects a person's ability to breathe, it may be necessary to intervene and provide ventilatory support. In the prehospital setting, several procedures and devices are available for providing ventilatory assistance in the hypoventilating or apneic patient.

Assisting Breathing

To effectively assist a patient's breathing, adequate volumes of air must be delivered at a satisfactory rate. In an adult, when oxygen is not available, a tidal volume of approximately 10 mL/kilogram (kg) or 700 to 1000 milliliter (mL) delivered over 2 seconds (enough to make the chest rise clearly) is considered sufficient. When oxygen is available, a tidal volume of approximately 6 to 7 mL/kg or 400 to 600 mL given over 1 to 2 seconds until the chest rises is considered appropriate. This is true regardless of the procedure or equipment used. The following three factors challenge the ability to do this:

1. The difficulty associated with maintaining an open airway
2. Resistance to airflow
3. The need to maintain a closed ventilatory system

DIFFICULTY ASSOCIATED WITH MAINTAINING AN OPEN AIRWAY

During the act of assisting a patient's breathing, rescuers often push down on the patient's chin or face in an attempt to maintain a seal. This action forces the jaw and the tongue backward into an obstructing position, closing off the airway. When assisting a patient's breathing, you must employ a technique that ensures both an

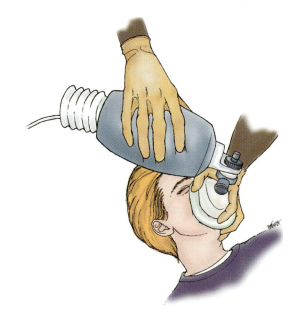

FIGURE 8-33 ▲ For effective ventilatory assistance, the EMT–I must make certain that a good seal is created and maintained, and that the lower jaw is forced forward to keep the airway open.

adequate seal and a forward disposition of the lower jaw (Figure 8-33).

RESISTANCE TO AIRFLOW

In a nonbreathing patient, frictional resistance occurs in the respiratory passageways, as does elastic resistance of the lungs and chest wall. To expand the lungs, this resistance must be overcome. It can be like blowing up a balloon—initially, it is hard to inflate the balloon, but after it begins to expand, inflation becomes much easier. Care must be taken because the high pressure required to expand the lungs can force air into the esophagus.

NEED TO MAINTAIN A CLOSED VENTILATORY SYSTEM

A closed ventilatory system must be maintained to deliver adequate volumes of air to the patient's lungs. The reason is very simple: air travels the path of least resistance. If a tight seal is not maintained between the patient's face and the mask, air can leak out. Ventilating with a bag-valve-mask device equipped with a pop-off valve can lead to the same problem when there is a great deal of airway resistance. Air tends to blow off through the valve rather than be pushed through the air passageways. Pop-off valves should be deactivated or devices equipped with them should not be used.

▶ NOTE: It is important to allow the patient to passively exhale between delivered breaths to remove carbon dioxide.

Ventilatory Assistance Procedures and Devices

Procedures and devices used to provide assisted breathing include the following:

- Mouth-to-mouth/nose breathing
- Mouth-to-mask breathing
- Bag-valve-mask device
- Flow-restricted, oxygen-powered ventilation device
- Automatic ventilator

MOUTH-TO-MOUTH/NOSE BREATHING

Mouth-to-mouth or mouth-to-nose breathing is the most basic form of ventilation. It is indicated in any apneic or inadequately breathing patient when other ventilatory devices are not available. It is a quick, effective means of assisting a patient's breathing, and when applied properly, good ventilatory volumes can be delivered because an effective seal over the patient's mouth (or nose) is easily maintained. Although this procedure requires no adjunctive equipment, use of a protective barrier is recommended. The most significant limitation of mouth-to-mouth and mouth-to-nose breathing is that it provides little oxygen (because expired air only contains 16% to 17% oxygen). Additionally, rescuers may be exposed to communicable diseases through contact with patients who have copious secretions, bleeding, or gastric regurgitation or who have a transmittable disease. When employing mouth-to-mouth or mouth-to-nose, the EMT–I should avoid overventilating the patient's lungs or breathing so quickly or deeply that he or she actually hyperventilates.

POCKET MASK

The pocket mask is a clear plastic device that covers the patient's mouth and nose, preventing contact between rescuer and patient and reducing the risk of contamination during resuscitation. Mouth-to-mask breathing has been shown to be more effective at delivering adequate tidal volumes than a bag-valve-mask device. This is because the rescuer's lungs are of greater capacity than the bag-valve-mask device. Additionally, since the pocket mask is easier to employ than a bag-valve-mask device, both hands can be used to hold the mask to the patient's face. This makes it easier to obtain an adequate face seal.

A variety of pocket masks are available; some are reusable, whereas others are disposed of after a single use. A disadvantage is that these devices are not always available. However, many are small and compact, allowing for always having one device available, whether at work or off-duty. Furthermore, they can be distributed as part of CPR training programs offered to the community. Pocket masks often are supplied with a one-way valve that keeps one from coming into contact with the patient's expired air. This valve reduces the risk of infection.

Oxygen Delivery—Many pocket masks are supplied with an inlet for delivery of supplemental oxygen to the patient. Mouth-to-mask breathing, combined with an oxygen flow rate of 10 L/min can deliver an inspired oxygen concentration of approximately 50%.

Procedure—To use the pocket mask, the following steps should be taken:

1. Perform BSI precautions.
2. Connect the oxygen tubing to the oxygen inlet of the mask.
3. Adjust the oxygen flow rate to 10 L/min or greater.
4. Attach a one-way valve to the ventilatory inlet/outlet port of the mask (Figure 8-34, *A*).
5. Kneel at the top of the patient's head and open the airway using the head-tilt procedure, provided there is no likelihood of a cervical spine injury.
6. If needed, insert an oropharyngeal airway.
7. Place the mask on the patient's face with the (a) narrow end (apex) over the bridge of the nose and (b) wide end (base) in the groove between the lower lip and chin.
8. Position both hands over the mask with the thumbs on the dome and index and middle fingers extended across the base. Press downward on the mask with the thumbs and fingers to maintain an effective seal between the patient's face and the mask.
9. Hook the ring and little fingers under the patient's jaw. Use the fingers to keep the patient's head tilted back (in nontrauma related cases) and the jaw displaced forward.
10. Take a deep breath and ventilate the patient through the one-way valve on top of the mask (Figure 8-34, *B*). Each breath should be delivered in a slow and steady manner (over at least 2 seconds). This method helps prevent gastric distention and reduces the possibility of regurgitation and aspiration.
11. Check for ventilatory effectiveness by observing chest rise and feeling for lung resistance.
12. Remove the mouth and allow the patient to passively exhale. Listen for airflow from the mask's inlet port during passive exhalation and watch the patient's chest fall.
13. When oxygen is available, ventilate the patient with a tidal volume of approximately 6 to 7 mL/kg or 400 to 600 mL over 1 to 2 seconds (until the chest rises). If oxygen is not available, a tidal volume of approximately 10 mL/kg or 700 to 1000 mL is delivered over 2 seconds (enough to make the chest rise clearly). Breaths should be delivered at a rate of at least 10 to 12 times per minute.
14. Continue the procedure until effective spontaneous breathing is restored or resuscitation efforts are ordered terminated.

BAG-VALVE-MASK DEVICE

Another tool used to provide ventilatory support is the bag-valve-mask device. It consists of a self-inflating sil-

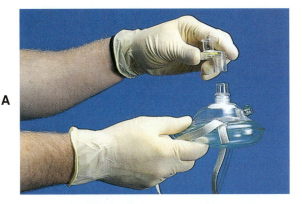
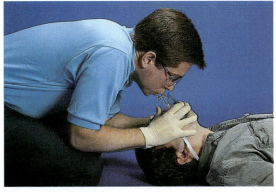

FIGURE 8-34 ▲ Mouth-to-mask ventilation with supplemental oxygen. **A,** Connect a one-way valve to the mask. **B,** After creating an appropriate seal, ventilate the patient through the one-way valve on top of the mask. (Vincent Knaus from Stoy W: *Mosby's EMT–Basic textbook,* St Louis, 1996, Mosby.)

icone or rubber bag and two valves, the nonrebreathing valve and inlet valve. Typically, the bag-valve-mask device is available in three sizes: adult (capable of storing between 1000 to 1600 mL of air), child (capable of storing 500 to 700 mL of air), and infant (capable of storing 150 to 240 mL of air). The bag-valve-mask device may be used with a mask, ET tube, esophageal obturator airway, or other airway devices. At a minimum, the bag-valve-mask device should have the following:

1. Consist of a self-inflating bag that is easy to grip and compress.
2. Be easy to clean and sterilize. With the concern over the potential transmission of infectious disease, a number of disposable units are available for use in the prehospital care setting.
3. Include a nonjam-valve system (even in the presence of large particles of vomitus).
4. Have a standard 15-mm/22-mm fitting, which allows for attachment of the device to a standard mask, ET tube, Combitube, pharyngotracheal lumen airway (PTL) or laryngeal mask airway (LMA) or tracheostomy tube.
5. Provide satisfactory performance under extremes of environmental temperatures.
6. Include a system for delivery of 85% to 100% oxygen with an oxygen reservoir and supplemental oxygen source.
7. Contain only a few parts and be easy to assemble in an emergency.

As mentioned earlier, bag-valve-mask devices used in the field setting should not be equipped with a pop-off valve. Pressures required to ventilate the patient during delivery of CPR in cardiac arrest may exceed the pop-off limit. Additionally, in patients who have poorly compliant (stiff) lungs, the tidal volume delivered may be insufficient.

The mask used with a bag-valve-mask device should be transparent, so that any vomitus or secretions around the patient's mouth can be easily seen. It should also have

an air cushion or inflatable cuff. Selecting the proper size mask is important; one that is too small or large makes it difficult to get a good seal. The mask should just cover the area between the bridge of the nose and the indentation beneath the lower lip. Ideally, the mask should only be applied for a short period, being quickly replaced by the insertion of an ET tube. ET intubation eliminates the need for a tight seal between the patient's face and a mask (the most common cause of ineffective ventilation) and protects the patient's airway from collapse.

Advantages and Disadvantages—Advantages of the bag-valve-mask device are as follows:

- It provides an immediate means of ventilatory support.
- It conveys to you a sense of compliance of the patient's lungs.
- It can be used with spontaneously breathing patients.
- It can deliver an oxygen-enriched mixture to the patient.
- It eliminates the risk of the rescuer coming into contact with a patient's blood or body fluid.
- The rescuer can ventilate for extended periods without fatigue.

Disadvantages of the bag-valve-mask device are as follows:

- It is a difficult skill to master
- It is difficult to maintain an adequate seal while delivering required volume of air
- It is sometimes difficult to deliver the required tidal volume (squeeze the bag adequately and maintain an adequate seal)
- It is difficult to ventilate a patient when cervical immobilization is in place

Indications—Indications for use of the bag-valve-mask device include patients who are apneic from any mechanism or who are experiencing unsatisfactory respiratory effort. The device is contraindicated in patients who are awake and intolerant of being ventilated.

Oxygen Delivery—When used without a supplemental oxygen source, the bag-valve-mask device only delivers 21% oxygen. When supplied with an oxygen source set at a flow rate of 15 L/min, approximately 40% to 60% oxygen is delivered. This result typically is accomplished by attaching oxygen tubing from an oxygen regulator to the oxygen inlet nipple located on the bottom or top end (depending on the manufacturer) of the bag-valve-mask device. To deliver 85% to 100% oxygen, the bag-valve-mask device must be equipped with a reservoir.

The reservoir may consist of a bag-type unit or tubing. The purpose of the reservoir is to collect a volume of 100% oxygen equal to the capacity of the bag. When the bag reexpands after having been squeezed, the 100% oxygen is drawn from the reservoir into the bag. Another device capable of delivering 85% to 100% oxygen through a bag-valve-mask device is a refill valve, or modified demand valve. It delivers 85% to 100% oxygen, depending on the capability of the device, when negative pressure from within the bag (after the bag has been squeezed and is reexpanding) triggers the refill valve to release high-flow oxygen in a sufficient volume to refill the bag. When the demand valve is attached to the reservoir port of the bag-valve-mask device, the oxygen inlet nipple must be occluded to prevent inadvertent drawing in of ambient air into the bag (Figure 8-35).

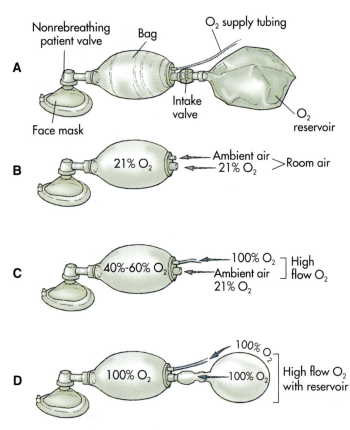

Nonrebreathing patient valve — Bag — O₂ supply tubing

A

Face mask — Intake valve — O₂ reservoir

B — 21% O₂ — Ambient air 21% O₂ — Room air

C — 40%-60% O₂ — 100% O₂ / Ambient air 21% O₂ — High flow O₂

D — 100% O₂ — 100% O₂ / 100% O₂ — High flow O₂ with reservoir

FIGURE 8-35 ▲ **A,** Components of the bag-valve-mask device. **B,** A bag-valve-mask device without a supplemental oxygen supply delivers 21% oxygen to the patient. **C,** A bag-valve-mask device with an oxygen source delivers 40% to 60% oxygen to the patient. **D,** A bag-valve-mask device equipped with a reservoir delivers nearly 100% oxygen to the patient.

✖ **Intrapulmonary Shunting** • The circulation of blood to non-ventilated alveoli, which results in the arterial blood having the same oxygen content as systemic venous blood.

In life-threatening conditions such as shock, drug overdose, and cardiac arrest, severe hypoxemia may be caused by **intrapulmonary shunting,** alveolar collapse, and decreased perfusion. For this reason the highest concentration of oxygen (as close to 100% as possible) should always be used in conjunction with providing ventilatory assistance to a patient.

Precautions—Although its use has gained widespread acceptance in the prehospital care setting, the bag-valve-mask device also has been characterized as cumbersome and difficult to use. The most common problem encountered is the inability to provide adequate ventilatory volumes to patients who are not endotracheally intubated. This situation occurs because of the difficulty providing a leak proof seal to the face while maintaining an open airway. Mask leak is a serious problem, decreasing the volume delivered to the oropharynx by as much as 40% or more. While providing ventilatory support to the patient, it is necessary to continually listen for air leaks from around the mask. Air leak indicates that a better seal needs to be established and maintained.

Poor ventilation also occurs when the bag is not squeezed completely enough to force adequate amounts of air into the patient's lungs. In patients not in cardiovascular collapse, a volume of 6 to 7 mL/kg (approximately 400 to 600 mL) over 1.5 to 2 seconds is recommended. In cardiac arrest, at least 10 to 15 mL/kg (700 to 1000 mL) of air per breath delivered over 2 seconds is needed. With four fingers on top and the thumb underneath, the bag is compressed with the right hand as completely as possible. Unfortunately, EMT–Is with smaller hands may not be able to empty the bag enough to achieve the necessary ventilatory volumes.

However, the problems of not maintaining an adequate seal, keeping an open airway, and compressing the bag sufficiently can be overcome with adequate skill practice and modifications in procedure.

When delivering assisted breathing, the resistance in the bag must be continually noted. Increased resistance (indicated by a bag that is hard to squeeze) suggests airway obstruction. A tongue that falls back against the posterior oropharynx is the most likely culprit. Unless trauma is suspected, further hyperextension of the patient's head corrects this problem. If an oropharyngeal airway has not been placed yet, it should be inserted at this point. Other possible causes include foreign body obstruction, tension pneumothorax, or severe bronchospasm. Conversely, a bag that compresses too easily indicates a leak somewhere in the system. The best indicator of effective ventilations is the rise and fall of the patient's chest.

To effectively use the bag-valve-mask device with the mask attached, the EMT–I should assume a position at the top of the patient's head. Otherwise, it is nearly impossible to maintain an effective seal between the mask and the patient's face while keeping the airway open.

Procedure—To use the bag-valve-mask device, the following steps should be taken (Figure 8-36):

1. Perform BSI precautions.
2. Unless the likelihood of trauma is present, tilt the patient's head back and mandible anteriorly using an appropriate airway maneuver.
3. If the patient is unresponsive, insert an oropharyngeal airway. If a gag reflex is present, a nasopharyngeal airway may be used.
4. Select the appropriate size mask.
5. Place mask on patient's face with narrow end (apex) over bridge of nose and wide end (base) in groove between the lower lip and chin.
6. Obtain a tight seal by applying firm downward pressure over the mask with the thumb on the dome and forefinger on the base (creating a C with the thumb and forefinger).
7. Hook the last three fingers under the jaw (these fingers form an E), and then pull the chin backward to maintain the head-tilt.
8. Squeeze the bag with one hand or between one hand and the arm, chest, or thigh (if kneeling) over 2 seconds. Compression of the bag using a smooth, steady action should be sufficient enough to produce patient chest rise. Be careful to avoid over inflating the patient's lungs. The bag should be allowed to refill completely between each compression.
9. Watch for the patient's chest to rise during ventilation and fall during passive exhalation.
10. Auscultate the chest to make sure that appropriate ventilation is occurring.
11. Connect reservoir and oxygen tubing to the oxygen inlet of the bag-valve-mask device and deliver oxygen at 12 to 15 L/min.
12. Ventilate the patient 10 to 12 times per minute or once every 4 to 5 seconds. In the patient not in cardiovascular collapse, deliver at least 6 to 7 mL/kg

of air with each breath. When delivered in conjunction with CPR, a volume of 10 mL/kg of air is needed with each breath. Slow, gentle ventilation minimizes the risk for gastric distension. Allow for adequate exhalation after each delivered breath.

13. Auscultate the chest to be sure adequate ventilation is being delivered.

Because of the problems inherent to this device, only trained and experienced personnel should use it. Additionally, because of the potential for skill degradation after only a short while, ventilating with a bag-valve-mask device should be practiced on a CPR mannequin with appropriate frequency. While delivering ventilatory support, the EMT–I must observe for gastric distension, as well as changes in the compliance of the bag, the patient's color, and level of responsiveness.

TWO-PERSON AND THREE-PERSON BAG-VALVE-MASK VENTILATION

Ventilation with a bag-valve-mask device is delivered more effectively using two EMT–Is: one holding the mask in place and maintaining an open airway and one squeezing the bag with two hands (Figure 8-37). The procedure may also be performed using three persons. Two- or three-person bag-valve-mask ventilation is especially useful for cervical spine-immobilized patients or when there is difficulty obtaining or maintaining an adequate mask seal. Advantages of the procedures are that a superior mask seal and volume delivery can be maintained. Disadvantages of the procedures include that they require additional personnel and may be difficult to perform in tight quarters such as in the back of an ambulance.

⭐STUDENT ALERT

Some guidelines no longer recommend the use of the oxygen-powered, manually triggered device. Check with your instructor to see if it will be part of your instruction. Additionally, check your local protocols to determine if its use is permitted in your EMS agency.

FLOW-RESTRICTED, OXYGEN-POWERED VENTILATION DEVICES

The flow-restricted, oxygen-powered ventilation device is a manually triggered device that delivers 100% oxygen at 40 L/min. Connected to an oxygen supply through high-pressure tubing, it is small, easy to use, and rugged, and it has an easily accessible manual control button (Figure 8-38). When the flow-restricted, oxygen-powered ventilation device is opened or activated, a steady stream of oxygen flows to the patient. Flow is limited to 30 cm of water or less to reduce the chance of gastric distension that can occur with its use.

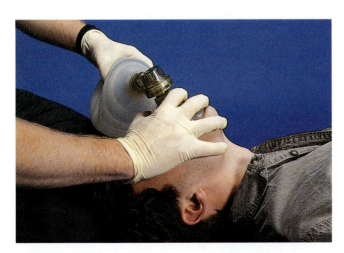

FIGURE 8-36 ▲ Bag-valve-mask ventilation procedure with one rescuer. (Vincent Knaus from Stoy W: *Mosby's EMT–basic textbook,* St Louis, 1996, Mosby.)

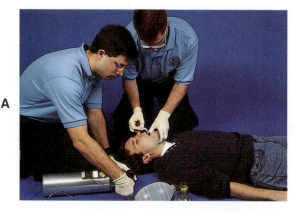
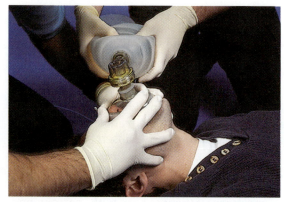

FIGURE 8-37 ▲ Bag-valve-mask ventilation procedure with two rescuers. **A,** One EMT–I opens the airway while a second EMT–I sets up the bag-valve-mask device. **B,** One EMT–I holds the mask in place while a second EMT–I ventilates. (Vincent Knaus from Stoy W: *Mosby's EMT–Basic textbook*, St Louis, 1996, Mosby.)

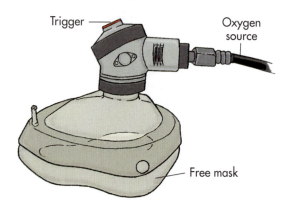

FIGURE 8-38 ▲ The flow-restricted, oxygen powered ventilation device allows a steady stream of oxygen to be delivered to the patient while the button is depressed. (Kimberly Battista from Stoy W: *Mosby's EMT–Basic textbook,* St Louis, 1996, Mosby.)

> ❗ **HELPFUL HINT**
> - The amount of pressure it takes to open the cardiac sphincter is approximately 30 cm of water.

On the delivery end, it can be attached to a face mask, Combitube airway, pharyngotracheal lumen airway, ET tube, laryngeal mask airway, or tracheostomy tube. Most of these devices contain an inspiratory release valve that also allows the flow-restricted, oxygen-powered ventilation device to be used to provide 100% oxygen to spontaneously breathing patients. The slight negative pressure created by the inspiratory effort of the patient triggers the valve from a nonflow state to a flowing state. The greater the inspiratory effort, the higher is the flow; when the inspiratory effort ceases, oxygen stops flowing.

The flow-restricted, oxygen-powered ventilation device is indicated in patients who require a high volume or high concentration of oxygen. It can be used in compliant, awake patients and with caution in unconscious patients. It is contraindicated in patients who are noncompliant or who have poor tidal volume and in small children.

Advantages and Disadvantages—Advantages of the flow-restricted, oxygen-powered ventilation device are as follows:

- It is easy to use.
- It provides high-volume or high-oxygen concentrations.
- Oxygen can be self-administered.
- Oxygen volume delivery can be regulated by inspiratory effort thus minimizing the risk of over inflation.
- Oxygen can be delivered in response to inspiratory effort—that is, there is no wasting of oxygen.

Disadvantages of the flow-restricted, oxygen-powered ventilation device are as follows:

- The device fails to provide a sense of chest compliance during ventilation; thus care must be taken not to over inflate the lungs.
- High pressures are generated by the device may cause barotrauma to lungs, resulting in pneumothorax and subcutaneous emphysema.
- It may open the esophagus causing gastric distention.
- The high oxygen flow rate quickly expends portable oxygen cylinders.

Precautions—Because the device is dependent on an oxygen source for power, another means of ventilatory support is needed if the oxygen cylinder requires changing during patient ventilation. Due to the sudden high pressure that the flow-restricted, oxygen-powered ventilation device provides, it should not be used in pediatric patients (under 16 years of age) and should be used with extreme caution in patients who are endotracheally intubated.

Procedure—To ventilate a patient with a flow-restricted, oxygen-powered ventilation device, the following steps should be taken:

1. Perform BSI precautions.
2. Assume a position at the top of the patient's head.

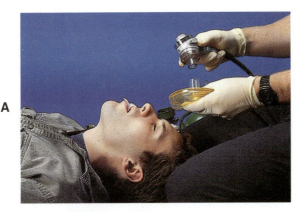
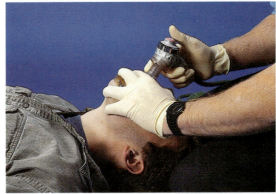

FIGURE 8-39 ▲ Ventilating a patient. **A,** Select the appropriate sized mask and attach it to the oxygen supply. **B,** Firmly hold the mask to the patient's face and deliver ventilations. (Vincent Knaus from Stoy W: *Mosby's EMT–Basic textbook,* St Louis, 1996, Mosby.)

3. Unless the likelihood of trauma is present, tilt the patient's head back and mandible anteriorly using an appropriate airway maneuver.
4. If the patient is unresponsive, insert an oropharyngeal airway. If a gag reflex is present, a nasopharyngeal airway may be used.
5. Open the regulator valve to the oxygen supply.
6. Select the proper size mask for the patient (Figure 8-39, *A*).
7. Place the mask on the patient's face with the narrow end (apex) over bridge of the nose and the wide end (base) in the groove between the lower lip and chin.
8. With both hands, firmly hold the mask to the patient's face to make a seal while maintaining an appropriate head and neck hyperextension.
9. Deliver ventilation by pushing the button of the device (Figure 8-39, *B*).
10. Watch for chest rise and auscultate the lung sounds to ensure proper ventilation.
11. As soon as the chest rises, release the pressure on the button to allow passive expiration. The flow of oxygen then ceases, and the expired air is vented out a one-way valve to the atmosphere.

AUTOMATIC TRANSPORT VENTILATORS

Automatic transport ventilators (ATVs) employed in the prehospital setting maintain the following characteristics:
- Time-cycled, constant-flow, gas-powered devices
- Lightweight, compact, and easy to use
- Designed to operate in temperature extremes from (30° F to 125° F, making them dependable in emergency situations.

These devices are indicated for situations where extended ventilation of patients is required, when a bag-valve-mask device would be used, and in cases where CPR is being delivered. Contraindications are awake patients; patients who have an obstructed airway; or

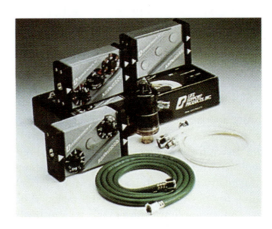

FIGURE 8-40 ▲ Automatic ventilators: Autovent 1000, 2000, and 3000. (Life Support Products, Inc.; Irvine, CA from Sanders M: *Mosby's paramedic textbook,* St Louis, 1994, Mosby.)

when there is increased airway resistance such as pneumothorax (after needle decompression), asthma, and pulmonary edema.

ATVs are equipped with a standard 15-mm inside diameter/22-mm outside diameter adapter that allows them to be attached to various airway devices and masks (Figure 8-40).

ATVs have two controls: one that regulates the ventilatory rate and one regulating tidal volume. Some devices deliver controlled ventilation only, whereas others function as intermittent mandatory ventilators, reverting to controlled mechanical ventilation in nonbreathing patients. The inspired oxygen concentration is usually fixed at 100%, but it may be adjustable depending on the device.

✖ **Adult Respiratory Distress Syndrome (ARDS)** • Pulmonary insufficiency that occurs due to a number of bodily insults. Pathologic findings include alveolar and interstitial edema due to leaking capillaries.

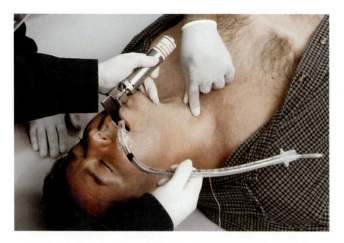

FIGURE 8-41 ▲ Cricoid pressure.

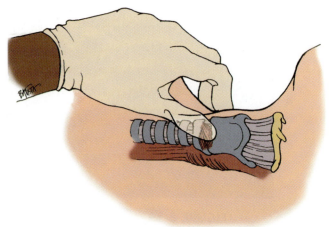

FIGURE 8-42 ▲ Cricoid pressure, known as the Sellick maneuver, prevents gastric distention and regurgitation in patients receiving artificial ventilations. (Kimberly Battista from Stoy W: *Mosby's EMT–Basic textbook,* St Louis, 1996, Mosby.)

ATVs are typically supplied with a pop-off feature that works to prevent barotrauma. The pop-off valve vents a portion of the tidal volume to the atmosphere when the preset level of airway pressure is exceeded. Unfortunately, pop-off valves can be detrimental in the presence of cardiogenic pulmonary edema, **adult respiratory distress syndrome (ARDS),** pulmonary contusion, bronchospasm, or other disorders in which high airway pressures must be exerted. To ensure proper working order, these devices must be checked regularly.

When providing ventilatory support to patients who are entracheally intubated, use of the automatic ventilator allows for performing other vital tasks. When it is used in conjunction with a face mask, proper positioning of the patient's head, as well as an effective seal between the mask and the patient's face, must be maintained.

Advantages and Disadvantages—Advantages of ATVs are as follows:
- It frees personnel to perform other tasks.
- It is lightweight, portable, durable, and mechanically simple.
- It has an adjustable tidal volume and rate.
- It adapts to portable oxygen tank.
  Disadvantages of ATVs are as follows:
- It cannot detect tube displacement.
- It does not detect increasing airway resistance.
- It is difficult to secure.
- It is dependent on oxygen tank pressure.

Cricoid Pressure

Cricoid pressure (also referred to as the *Sellick maneuver*) is a quick, effective way of preventing gastric distention and/or regurgitation in the patient who cannot protect his or her airway. It compresses the esophagus between the cricoid ring and the cervical spine. This maneuver is also invaluable when assisting a patient's breathing (e.g., with a bag-valve-mask device; flow-restricted, oxygen-powered ventilation device; and so on) and

during attempts at ET intubation. It facilitates intubation by moving the larynx posteriorly making visualization of the glottic opening and passage of the ET tube easier (Figure 8-41).

This skill is performed by applying firm pressure (about the same amount as is necessary to stop bleeding) over the cricoid cartilage and directing it posteriorly against the esophagus (Figure 8-42). This pressure closes the esophagus off to pressures as high as 100 cm H_2O.

Advantages and Disadvantages—Advantages of the Sellick manuever are as follows:
- It is noninvasive.
- It protects patient from aspiration as long as pressure is maintained.
  Disadvantages of the Sellick maneuver are as follows:
- It may lead to extreme emesis if pressure is maintained.
- A second rescuer is required for bag-valve-mask ventilation.
- Excessive pressure may obstruct the trachea in small children.

Procedure—The cricoid cartilage can be located by palpating the depression just below the thyroid cartilage. This depression is the cricothyroid membrane. The projection just below this membrane is the cricoid cartilage. Pressure is applied with the thumb and index finger of one hand to the front of the cartilage just to the sides of the midline directing it posteriorly. More pressure is required to prevent regurgitation than gastric distention. However, overzealous pressure must be avoided, since it will occlude the airway and impair tracheal intubation. This pressure is maintained until the airway is secured with an ET tube (cuff inflated) or until it is no longer needed.

Complications of the procedure include that laryngeal trauma can be produced by excessive pressure, unrelieved high gastric pressures can cause esophageal rupture, and excessive pressure can obstruct the trachea in small children. The procedure is contraindicated in patients who may have a cervical spine injury.

Artificial Ventilation of the Pediatric Patient

Pediatric patients in the prehospital setting may be in need of ventilatory assistance. Proper use of the bag-valve-mask device greatly assists in assuring the survival of the infant or child.

Providing ventilatory support in pediatric patients is challenging, since they have a flat nasal bridge that makes achieving an adequate mask seal more difficult. Furthermore, although it is important that the mask of the device is tightly secured and sealed to a patient's face, the EMT–I must be careful not to compress the mask against the face to the point where it obstructs the airway. In cases where it is difficult to obtain or maintain a seal around the patient's mouth and nose, inverting the mask on the infant or child's face may improve the situation. The proper size mask fits from the bridge of the nose to cleft of the chin. Additionally, if available, a length-based resuscitation tape such as the Broselow Tape can be used to determine the proper size mask.

The chin-lift maneuver should be performed when ventilating, as long as cervical trauma is not suspected. Care should be taken not to push too hard on the soft tissue under the chin because this may move the tongue into an obstructing position.

The ventilation rate for infants and children is at least 20 breaths per minute. It is necessary to ensure that the oxygen is attached to the bag-valve-mask device and that it is set to at least 15 L/min. It is best to use a bag-valve-mask device that provides at least 450 mL of volume and is not equipped with a pop-off valve on pediatric patients. The infant bag-valve-mask device only provides approximately 250 mL and should NOT be used in infants and neonates because it cannot give enough tidal volume and provide a long enough time for inspiration.

For children up to 8 years of age, an adult bag-valve-mask device, having a capacity of 1500 mL of air, can be used, provided care is taken to give smaller breaths. NOTE: larger breaths can cause the lungs to over inflate, and a pneumothorax may result. A host of other complications such as compromised cardiac output (due to increased intrathoracic pressure); gastric distension

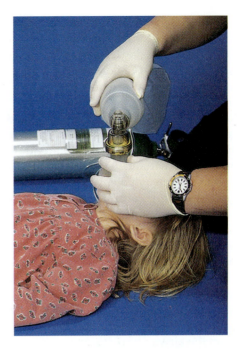

FIGURE 8-43 ▲ **Ventilating a pediatric patient with a bag-valve-mask device. (Duckwall Productions)**

leading to impaired ventilation and increased risk for regurgitation and aspiration; air leak; and air trapping can also occur with over ventilation. When airway management is performed in children over 8 years of age, an adult bag-valve-mask device should be used to provide a larger volume of ventilation. However, extreme care should be taken not to force high volumes of air into the patient's airway.

CLINICAL NOTES

Regardless of the size of the bag-valve-mask device employed, only use the force and tidal volume necessary to cause the chest to rise visibly.

Bag-valve-mask ventilation must be done with two hands: one to hold the mask on the face and maintain the head-tilt/chin-lift maneuver and one to squeeze the bag (Figure 8-43). When treating infants and toddlers, the mandible should be supported with the middle or ring finger. For older children, the fingertips of the third, fourth, and fifth fingers should be placed under the mandible to hold the jaw forward and extend the head (which accomplishes the jaw-thrust maneuver).

If there is difficulty in ventilating the child, a two-person approach should be used. One EMT–I uses both hands to maintain the airway maneuver and mask seal on the face, while the second performs the ventilation.

Maintenance of the head in a neutral, sniffing position without hyperextension is usually adequate for infants and toddlers. Hyperextension can actually occlude the infant's soft airway. Children more than 2 years of age do well with padding behind the head to displace the cervical spine anteriorly.

Obviously, if a cervical spine injury is suspected, all airway maneuvers and ventilation should be done with the head in a neutral, in-line position. A trauma jaw-thrust or chin-lift without head-tilt maneuver can be used to maintain airway patency.

The goal of the bag-valve-mask device is to achieve effective ventilation. If this goal is not achieved, the following steps should be taken:

1. Make sure the tongue is not obstructing the airway.
2. Reposition the head. Using a folded towel under the infant's or child's shoulders may help maintain the sniffing position.
3. Make sure the mask is snug against the patient's face.
4. Lift the jaw.
5. Suction the airway (if necessary).
6. Check the bag-valve-mask device for damage.
7. Provide an adequate source of oxygen.

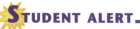

STUDENT ALERT

Placing a folded towel under infant's or child's shoulders is required for National Registry testing.

The EMT–I should watch for gastric distention, which is very common during bag-valve-mask ventilation. Appropriate suction should be readily available. If the infant or child is unresponsive, cricoid pressure (Sellick's maneuver), as described above, should be applied to minimize gastric inflation and passive regurgitation. The second EMT–I should apply this pressure with one fingertip in infants and the thumb and index finger in children. Excessive pressure should not be used because this can cause tracheal compression and obstruction in infants. Lastly, it is critical to use a child bag-valve-mask system depending on the size of the pediatric patient.

PROCEDURE

To use the bag-valve-mask device in the pediatric patient, the following steps should be taken:

1. Perform BSI precautions.
2. Position the patient properly using an appropriate airway maneuver.
3. If the patient is unresponsive, insert an oropharyngeal airway. If a gag reflex is present, a nasopharyngeal airway may be used.
4. Select the appropriate size mask.
5. Place the mask on the patient's face with narrow end (apex) over bridge of nose and wide end (base) in the groove between the lower lip and chin. Avoid compressing the patient's eyes.

6. Using one hand, place your thumb on the mask at the apex and index finger on the mask at the chin (C-grip).
7. With gentle pressure, push down on the mask to establish an adequate seal.
8. Maintain the patient's airway by lifting the bony prominence of chin with remaining fingers forming an E; avoid placing pressure on the soft area under chin.
9. Squeeze the bag with one hand. Obtain chest rise with each breath. Compression of the bag should be a smooth, steady action that avoids overinflating the patient's lungs. Begin ventilation and say, "Squeeze." Provide just enough volume to initiate chest rise; DO NOT OVERVENTILATE.
10. Allow adequate time for exhalation. Begin releasing the bag and say, "Release, release." Continue ventilations using this "squeeze, release, release" method.
11. Assess bag-valve-mask ventilation.
12. Look for adequate chest rise.
13. Listen for lung sounds at the third intercostal space and midaxillary line.
14. Assess for improvement in color and/or heart rate.
15. Apply cricoid pressure to minimize gastric inflation and passive regurgitation.
16. Locate the cricoid ring by palpating the trachea for a prominent horizontal band inferior to the thyroid cartilage and cricothyroid membrane.
17. Apply gentle downward pressure using one fingertip in infants and the thumb and index finger in children.
18. Avoid excessive pressure, as it may produce tracheal compression and obstruction in infants.

In cases of adequate ventilation, the mask seal may be best achieved with jaw displacement and the two-person bag-valve-mask technique. Although it is recognized that there may not always be an abundance of personnel at the scene, it is crucial to the child's ongoing survival to provide adequate oxygenation and ventilation. If additional personnel must be requested, it should be done so without unnecessarily delaying transport of the pediatric patient.

Ventilation of the Stoma Patient

When the patient with a stoma requires ventilatory assistance, the bystander may use the mouth-to-stoma technique, while rescue personnel generally use a bag-valve-mask device. If using the mouth-to-stoma technique, it is preferable to use a pocket mask to cover the stoma for protection from communicable disease. For either technique, the stoma site should be located and exposed it. A tight seal should be made around the stoma site and ventilation delivered as normal. Check for adequate ventilation with each breath. Be sure to seal the mouth and nose if you note air leaking from these sites (Figure 8-44).

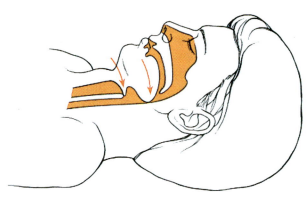

FIGURE 8-45 ▲ Unconscious patients lose muscle control, allowing the tongue to fall back against the back of the throat, causing airway obstruction. (From Henry MC: *EMT prehospital care,* ed 2, St Louis, 1997, WB Saunders.)

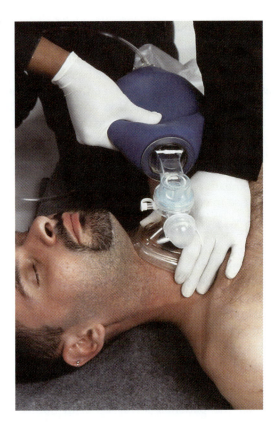

FIGURE 8-44 ▲ Ventilating a patient who has a stoma with a bag-valve-mask device.

UPPER AIRWAY PROBLEMS

Upper airway obstruction is defined as the interference of airflow through the upper airway and can represent an immediate threat to life. It may be caused by the following factors:
- The tongue
- Foreign bodies
- Vomitus
- Trauma (blood, teeth)
- Laryngeal spasm and edema

Blockage of the airway must be promptly corrected if the patient is to survive.

The Tongue
PATHOPHYSIOLOGY

The tongue is the most common cause of upper airway obstruction in the unresponsive patient (Figure 8-45). It occurs when muscle tone is depressed or absent in the supine patient. This condition allows the tongue to fall back against the soft palate and posterior pharyngeal wall infringing on the airway. To further aggravate the problem, the epiglottis can occlude the airway at the level of the larynx. With the tongue and epiglottis in obstructing positions, airflow into the respiratory system is reduced or absent. Additionally, inspiratory efforts may draw the tongue

and epiglottis into more of an obstructing position. Airway obstruction by the tongue depends on the position of the head and jaw and can occur regardless of whether the patient is in a lateral, supine, or prone position. In some cases, after a person has collapsed and before emergency care professionals have arrived on the scene, family members or bystanders may have already placed a pillow under the patient's head in an attempt to make him or her more comfortable. This movement can obstruct the airway even more. Public education efforts help tell citizens what is correct procedure in these types of emergencies.

✂ **Snoring Respiration** • Noisy, raspy breathing, usually with the mouth open.

✂ **Apnea** • Absence of breathing.

In the breathing patient, **snoring respiration** is a characteristic sign of airway obstruction caused by the tongue. In **apnea,** the initial clue to this type of obstruction is that it is difficult to ventilate the patient. After repositioning the patient's head and neck, assisted breathing should be easier to deliver.

Basic Treatment
MANUAL MANEUVERS

Treatment of this problem is directed at moving the tongue out of the way. The mandible must be lifted forward, displacing the hyoid anteriorly. This movement pulls the tongue forward and keeps the epiglottis elevated and away from the back of the throat and glottic opening. Any of the following procedures can be used to lift the mandible forward:
- Head-tilt/chin-lift maneuver
- Jaw-thrust maneuver
- Head-tilt/chin-lift and jaw-thrust without head-tilt maneuver
- Jaw-lift maneuver

In some cases such as in the spontaneously breathing patient, opening the airway with manual maneuvers may be all that is required to ensure a patent airway. These procedures are indicated in unresponsive patients who are unable to protect their own airway. Advantages to these procedures are that they require no special equipment and are safe, simple and noninvasive. A disadvantage of these procedures is that they do not protect the airway from aspiration.

Head-Tilt/Chin-Lift Maneuver—The preferred procedure for opening the airway is the head-tilt/chin-lift (Figure 8-46). This technique is considered superior to the other procedures because direct manipulation of the jaw lifts the tongue and epiglottis out of their obstructing positions. To perform the head-tilt/chin-lift maneuver, the following steps should be taken:

1. Perform BSI precautions.
2. With the patient in a supine position, move next to his or her side by the upper arm.
3. Place your uppermost hand on the patient's forehead and apply firm downward pressure with your palm to tilt the patient's head back.
4. Grasp the patient's chin with the other hand by placing your thumb on the front of the jaw and positioning your index finger under the jaw. This step should be done without putting undue pressure on the jaw.
5. Lift the jaw anteriorly to open the airway.

STREET WISE

Be careful not to compress the soft tissues underneath the patient's chin, because that can obstruct the airway. Rather, keep your fingers on the bony part of the chin.

Because this procedure causes manipulation of the head and neck, it should not be used in patients with suspected spine injury. Rather, the chin-lift or jaw-thrust without head-tilt maneuver should be used.

Jaw-Thrust Maneuver—The jaw-thrust maneuver is another useful technique for opening the airway (Figure 8-47). When employed with the head-tilt and retraction of the lower lip, it is referred to as the *triple airway maneuver*. Disadvantages of this procedure are that it is difficult to maintain if the patient becomes responsive or combative or for an extended period and it is difficult to use in conjunction with bag-valve-mask ventilation (i.e., it requires a separate rescuer to perform bag-valve-mask ventilation). To perform the jaw-thrust maneuver, the following steps should be taken:

1. Perform BSI precautions.
2. With the patient in a supine position move to the top of the patient's head.
3. Rest both your elbows on the same surface as the patient is lying.
4. Place your fingertips on each side of the patient's lower jaw, at the angles.
5. Firmly push the jaw forward while gently tilting the patient's head back.
6. Retract the patient's lower lip with both of your thumbs.

Chin-Lift and Jaw-Thrust without Head-Tilt Maneuver—In trauma patients with suspected spine injury, initial attempts at opening the airway should be done with the head kept in a neutral position. The chin-lift or jaw-thrust often can be successfully employed without the head-tilt. If the airway remains obstructed, then the head-tilt should be slowly and gently added until the airway is open.

Jaw-Lift Maneuver—The jaw-lift may also be used to open the airway in trauma patients, although it must

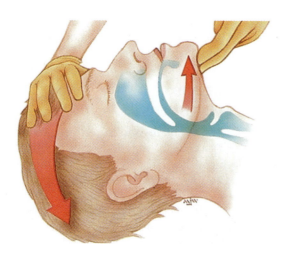

FIGURE 8-46 ▲ Head-tilt/chin-lift maneuver. (Mark J. Weiber from Sanders M: *Mosby's paramedic textbook*, St Louis, 1994, Mosby.)

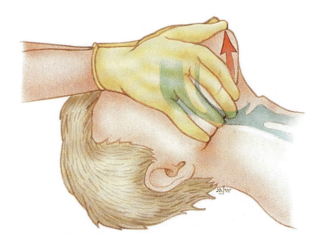

FIGURE 8-47 ▲ Jaw-thrust maneuver. (Mark J. Weiber from Sanders M: *Mosby's paramedic textbook*, St Louis, 1994, Mosby.)

be employed carefully because the thumb must be placed inside the patient's mouth. Advantages include that it can be employed in patients where cervical spinal injury is suspected and when there is a cervical collar in place. Disadvantages include that the procedure cannot be maintained if the patient becomes responsive or combative or for an extended period and it is difficult to use in conjunction with bag-valve-mask ventilation (i.e., it requires a separate rescuer to perform bag-valve-mask ventilation). To perform the jaw-lift maneuver, the following steps should be taken:

1. Perform BSI precautions.
2. With the patient in a supine position, move to the top of his or her head.
3. While keeping the patient's head in a neutral position use one hand to grasp the mandible by placing the thumb deep into the mouth, pressing downward on the tongue and positioning the index finger under the mandible.
4. Pull the jaw anteriorly to open the airway.

☀STUDENT ALERT

The term *hyperventilation* has been commonly used to describe the type of aggressive assisted breathing provided to a patient before the provision of airway management, such as ET intubation or suctioning. Hyperventilation was used to increase the patient's oxygen levels and reduce the carbon dioxide levels before the temporary cessation of ventilatory support and oxygenation and while the airway procedures were being performed. An inadvertent side effect of hyperventilation is gastric inflation. Gastric inflation can lead to serious consequences such as regurgitation, aspiration, and pneumonia. For this reason, hyperventilation has been replaced with a procedure referred to as *preoxygenation*. Preoxygenation in an adult is when oxygen is available, a tidal volume of approximately 6 to 7 mL/kg or 400 to 600 mL is given over 1 to 2 seconds until the chest rises. If oxygen is not available, a tidal volume of approximately 10 mL/kg or 700 to 1000 mL is delivered over 2 seconds (i.e., enough to make the chest rise clearly). The instructor should be consulted to determine what is considered appropriate for a specific EMT–I's learning experience. Local protocols should also be checked to identify what is considered acceptable ventilatory volumes and rates in your area.

AIRWAY ADJUNCTS

Two basic adjuncts that can be used to supplement the manual procedures previously described are the oropharyngeal airway and the nasopharyngeal airway.

However, placement of airway adjuncts should follow manual maneuvers. Potential side effects of airway devices such as activation of the gag, cough, and/or swallowing mechanisms can cause significant cardiovascular stimulation, as well as an increase in intracranial pressure.

Both the oropharyngeal and nasopharyngeal airways are designed to lift the base of the tongue forward and away from the posterior oropharynx. As their names imply, the oropharyngeal airway is inserted into the mouth, and the nasopharyngeal airway is placed into the nostril.

❗ HELPFUL HINT

- Proper head position must be maintained even when an oropharyngeal or nasopharyngeal airway is in place because these adjuncts only assist in maintaining an open airway.

Oropharyngeal Airway

The oropharyngeal airway is a plastic J-shaped device that conforms to the curvature of the palate (Figure 8-48, *A*). Once in place, it holds the base of the tongue forward, away from the posterior oropharynx, allowing air to pass around and through the tube (Figure 8-48, *B*). Oropharyngeal airways come in several sizes, ranging from No. 0 (infant) to No. 6 (large adult). The proper size must be used because an airway that is too long can press the epiglottis against the laryngeal entrance, thereby obstructing the airway. An airway that is too short fails to hold the tongue forward and may actually push it back against the posterior oropharynx.

INDICATIONS

Primary uses of the oropharyngeal airway are as follows:
- To maintain an open airway in an unresponsive, breathing patient who has no gag reflex or a patient being ventilated with a bag-valve-mask device or other positive pressure device
- As a bite block to prevent patients from biting down on and occluding an ET tube

ADVANTAGES AND DISADVANTAGES

Advantages of the oropharyngeal airway include the following:
- It can be inserted easily and quickly.
- It acts to counter obstruction by the teeth and lips.
- It facilitates suctioning of the pharynx because a large suction tube can pass on either side.

Disadvantages of the oropharyngeal airway include the following:
- It does not isolate the trachea.
- It cannot be inserted when the patient's teeth are clenched shut.

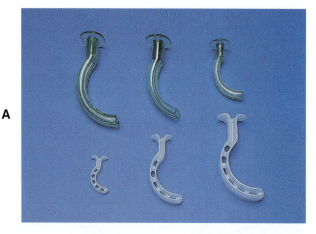
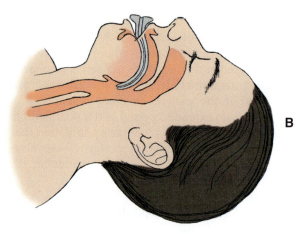

FIGURE 8-48 ▲ **A,** Oropharyngeal airways. **B,** Oropharyngeal airway in proper use. (**A,** Vincent Knaus from Stoy W: *Mosby's EMT–Basic textbook,* St Louis, 1996, Mosby. **B,** Kimberly Battista from Stoy W: *Mosby's EMT–Basic textbook,* St Louis, 1996, Mosby.)

- It can obstruct the airway if not inserted properly.
- It can easily be dislodged.
- Poor technique can produce pharyngeal or dental trauma.
- It can become occluded with emesis, blood, and so on.

CONTRAINDICATIONS

Oropharyngeal airways should not be used in patients who have a gag reflex because they can stimulate vomiting (by putting pressure on the posterior gag reflexes) or laryngospasm. Its use also should be avoided in patients who have severe maxillofacial injuries (trauma to the mandible or maxilla or significant soft-tissue damage to the tongue or pharynx).

PROCEDURE

To insert the oropharyngeal airway, the following steps should be taken:
1. Perform BSI precautions.
2. Use the head-tilt/chin-lift or jaw-thrust maneuver to open the airway. Remove any visible obstructions.
3. Ensure or maintain effective breathing and preoxygenate the patient with 100% oxygen if indicated.
4. Measure the airway to determine the appropriate size by holding it next to the patient's cheek. The proper size airway extends from the corner of the patient's mouth to the tip of the ear lobe on the same side of the face or to the angle of the lower jaw (Figure 8-49, *A*).
5. If the patient's mouth is closed, the crossfinger technique can be used to open it. This technique is performed by crossing the thumb and forefinger of one hand, placing them on the upper and lower teeth at the corner of the patient's mouth,

and then spreading the fingers apart to open the patient's jaws.
6. Move the tongue out of the way by grasping the jaw and tongue between the thumb and index finger of the left hand, lifting it anteriorly.
7. With the other hand, hold the airway at its flange end and insert it into the mouth with the curve reversed and the tip pointing toward the roof of the patient's mouth (Figure 8-49, *B*).
8. Slide in the airway along the roof of the mouth. Use caution to avoid pushing the tongue posteriorly (Figure 8-49, *C*).
9. Once the tip is past the uvula, approaching the back of the throat near the base of the tongue, rotate the airway 180 degrees until it comes to rest over the tongue (Figure 8-49, *D*). The flange of the airway should rest on the patient's lips (Figure 8-49, *E*).
10. Ventilate the patient with a bag-valve-mask device supplied with 100% oxygen (Figure 8-49, *F*) or other ventilatory device.
11. Check for proper placement of the airway by looking for chest rise. Then auscultate both sides of the chest and over the stomach with a stethoscope.

PRECAUTIONS

Care must be taken to ensure that the airway is correctly positioned because improper placement can push the tongue back against the posterior oropharynx thus obstructing the airway (Figure 8-50).

If the airway is too short or too long, it must be removed and replaced with the correct size. An indicator of improper placement is when the airway advances out of the mouth during ventilatory efforts.

An alternative method for inserting the oropharyngeal airway is to use a tongue blade to depress the

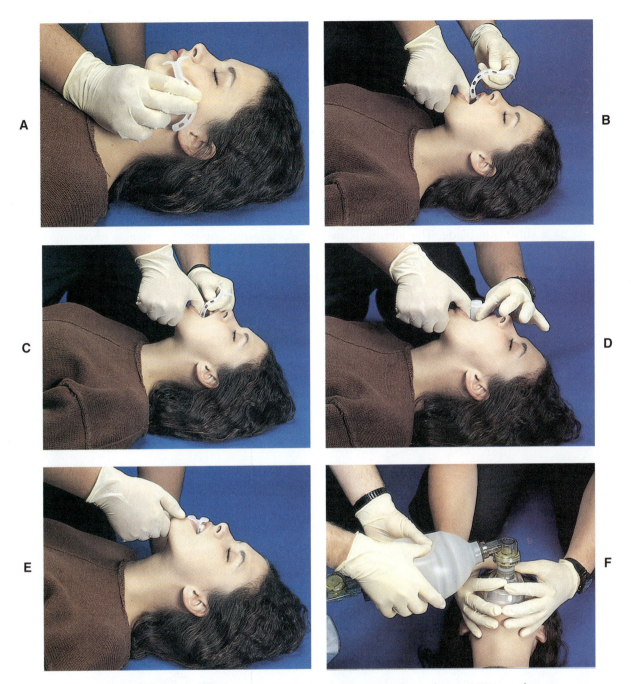

FIGURE 8-49 ▲ Inserting the oral airway (adult patient only). **A,** Measure the airway to determine the appropriate size. **B,** Open the patient's mouth and begin to insert the airway with the tip pointing toward the roof of the mouth. **C,** Slide the airway along the roof of the mouth. **D,** Rotate the airway 180 degrees. **E,** The flange of the airway should rest on the patient's lips. **F,** Ventilate the patient with 100% oxygen through a bag-valve-mask device. (Vincent Knaus from Stoy W: *Mosby's EMT–Basic textbook,* St Louis, 1996, Mosby.)

tongue while pushing the airway past it. Because its presence can stimulate vomiting or regurgitation, the airway must be immediately removed, and the EMT–I must be prepared to suction if the patient gags and/or becomes responsive.

Pediatric Oropharyngeal Airway Procedure

The best method of airway insertion is to depress the tongue with a tongue blade and insert the airway device over the blade. If a tongue blade is not available, then an alternative is to invert the airway and use the curved side as a substitute blade. The airway is inserted until the flange is against the lips and then gently rotated 180 degrees into position. The flange should be resting against the patient's lips, and extreme care must be taken to not tear any of the anatomic structures. Correct positioning of the child's head must be maintained to ensure a patent airway once the device is in place.

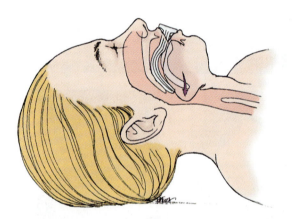

FIGURE 8-50 ▲ Improper placement of oropharyngeal airway can lead to an airway obstruction.

Nasopharyngeal Airway

The nasopharyngeal airway is a soft, uncuffed plastic tube. One end is funnel-shaped, preventing it from slipping inside the nose, whereas the other end is bevel-shaped to facilitate its passage into the nostril. It is designed to follow the natural curvature of the nasopharynx, extending from the nostril to the posterior pharynx just below the base of the tongue (also referred to as the *hypopharynx*) (Figure 8-51).

The proper size airway is slightly smaller in diameter than the opening of the patient's nostril (about the diameter of the patient's little finger) and extends from the tip of the nose to the tip of his or her earlobe. Selecting the appropriate size is important because a tube that is too short will not extend past the tongue. Conversely, a tube that is too long may pass into the esophagus, resulting in hypoventilation and gastric distention when artificial ventilation is delivered.

INDICATIONS

The nasopharyngeal airway is used to relieve soft tissue upper airway obstruction when an oropharyngeal airway is contraindicated. It can be used in patients experiencing alerted responsiveness and suppressed gag reflex.

ADVANTAGES AND DISADVANTAGES

Advantages of the nasopharyngeal airway include the following:
* It can be inserted quickly and easily.
* It bypasses the tongue.
* It may be used when a gag reflex is present.
* It can be safely placed blindly.
* It can be used in the presence of injuries to the oral cavity (trauma to the mandible, maxilla, or significant soft-tissue damage to the tongue or pharynx).

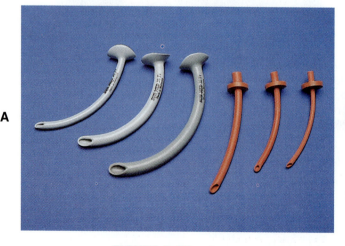

A

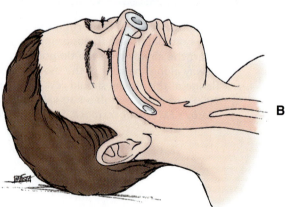

B

FIGURE 8-51 ▲ **A,** Nasopharyngeal airways. **B,** Nasopharyngeal airway in use. (**A,** Vincent Knaus from Stoy W: *Mosby's EMT–Basic textbook,* St Louis, 1996, Mosby.)

- It can be used when the patient's mouth is closed or the teeth are clenched shut.

Disadvantages of the nasopharyngeal airway include the following:

- It is smaller than the oropharyngeal airway.
- It does not isolate the trachea and therefore does not protect against aspiration.
- It is difficult to suction through.
- It can cause severe nosebleed if inserted too forcefully. This epistaxis can be difficult to control.
- It may cause pressure necrosis of the nasal mucosa.
- It may kink and clog, obstructing the airway.

CONTRAINDICATIONS

Use of the nasopharyngeal airway should be avoided in patients who have nasal obstructions or are prone to nosebleeds, or when there are indications of nasal injury. It also should be avoided in the presence of facial fractures or when skull fracture is likely because the airway can be inadvertently passed into the brain.

PROCEDURE

To insert the nasopharyngeal airway, the following steps should be taken:

1. Perform BSI precautions.
2. Open the airway manually using the head-tilt/chin-lift or jaw-thrust maneuver.
3. Ensure or maintain effective ventilatory function. If indicated, preoxygenate the patient with 100% oxygen.
4. Measure to determine the appropriate size airway for the patient (Figure 8-52, *A*).
5. Lubricate the exterior of the tube with a water-soluble gel to ease its insertion (Figure 8-52, *B*). If possible, a lidocaine gel should be used in the responsive or semiresponsive patient because its anesthetic properties make insertion more comfortable.
6. Gently push the tip of the nose upward.
7. Pass the tube into the patient's larger nostril (Figure 8-52, *C*). The curve of the airway should be upward, toward the patient's forehead and the bevel of airway toward the nasal septum.
8. Pass the airway along the floor of the nasal cavity until the flange rests firmly against the patient's nos-

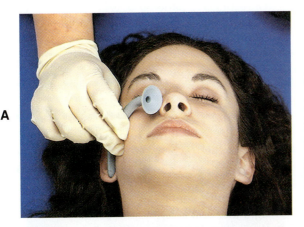
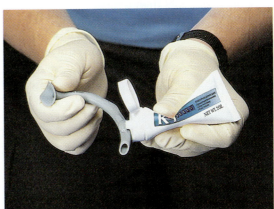
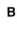
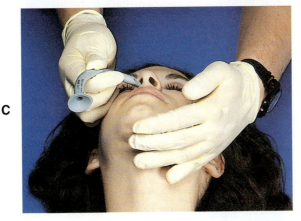
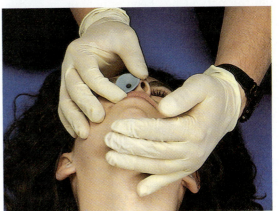

FIGURE 8-52 ▲ Inserting the nasopharyngeal airway (all ages). **A,** Measure the airway to determine the appropriate size. **B,** Lubricate the airway with a water-soluble lubricant. **C,** Insert the airway into the nostril with the bevel facing the septum. **D,** Advance the airway until the flange rests against the patient's nostril. (Vincent Knaus from Stoy W: *Mosby's EMT–Basic textbook*, St Louis, 1996, Mosby.)

tril (Figure 8-52, *D*). Avoid pushing against any resistance because it can cause tissue trauma and airway kinking. In some cases the septum may be deviated, and insertion into the one nostril cannot be accomplished, thus the other nostril must be used.

9. Verify appropriate position of the airway. Clear breath sounds, chest rise, and airflow at the proximal end of the device on expiration indicate correct placement.

10. Ventilate the patient with a bag-valve-mask device supplied with 100% oxygen or other ventilatory device (if indicated).

If resistance is met while inserting a nasopharyngeal airway, it should not be forced into the nose. Rather, the tube should be pulled out and tried in the other nostril. If resistance is such that the tube cannot be easily inserted, then a smaller-size tube may be more appropriate. If the patient gags as the last ½-inch (or so) is inserted, the airway may be too long and should be withdrawn slightly until it is tolerated.

PRECAUTIONS

Although the nasopharyngeal airway is better tolerated in semiresponsive patients than the oropharyngeal airway, its use may precipitate vomiting and laryngospasm. It also may injure the nasal mucosa causing bleeding and aspiration of clots into the trachea. Suctioning may be required to remove the secretions or blood. For these reasons, appropriate BSI precautions must be used.

ADVANCED AIRWAY MANAGEMENT

In most cases, manual airway control, ventilation, and oxygenation should precede the use of advanced airway adjuncts. This guideline is particularly important when the patient has been apneic or in cardiac arrest for several minutes before help arrives. Use of ventilatory support procedures allows you to correct profound hypoxia and hypercarbia. However, due to the high pharyngeal pressures (leading to gastric insufflation) created by most ventilatory support procedures, an advanced airway adjunct should be placed as soon as possible to prevent aspiration. The following four adjuncts to be discussed are advanced-level procedures:

1. ET tube
2. Esophageal tracheal Combitube
3. Pharyngotracheal lumen airway
4. Laryngeal mask airway

These devices offer more benefits than basic airway adjuncts; however, they also carry more risks.

Two other airway devices, the esophageal obturator airway and esophageal gastric tube airway are reviewed in Appendix A—Alternative Airway Procedures.

Endotracheal Intubation

✖ **Endotracheal** • Within or through the trachea.

✖ **Intubation** • Passing a tube into an opening of the body.

Endotracheal intubation is the insertion of an open-ended tube into the trachea to provide externally controlled breathing through a bag-valve-mask device or ventilator. It is the preferred technique for airway control in patients who are unable to maintain a patent airway in all types of medical and trauma emergencies. Due to the difficulty of the skill, the EMT–I should only perform ET intubation if he or she is trained and proficient in the procedure.

INDICATIONS

Primary uses for ET intubation are as follows:
- When ventilating an unresponsive patient through conventional methods cannot be done
- When patients cannot protect their airway (coma, respiratory and cardiac arrest)
- When prolonged artificial ventilation is needed.
- In patients experiencing or likely to experience upper airway compromise
- Unresponsive patients who lack a gag reflex
- When there is decreased tidal volume due to slow respirations
- When there is airway obstruction due to foreign bodies, trauma, or anaphylaxis

ADVANTAGES AND DISADVANTAGES

Advantages of ET intubation include the following:
- It seals the trachea, reducing the risk of aspirating blood, vomitus, and other foreign materials into the lungs.
- It facilitates ventilation and oxygenation, because a tight face seal is not required.
- It prevents gastric insufflation, because air is delivered directly into the trachea during positive-pressure ventilation.
- The direct route into the trachea allows for suctioning of the trachea and bronchi.
- It provides an effective route for administration of some medications (epinephrine, atropine, lidocaine, and naloxone). This advantage is particularly beneficial in the presence of peripheral vascular collapse such as often occurs in cardiac arrest.

DISADVANTAGES

Disdvantages of ET intubation include the following:
- ET intubation is a complicated skill requiring extensive initial and ongoing training to ensure proficiency.
- The procedure requires specialized equipment.
- The vocal cords must be visualized to place the tube (when performed orally, using a laryngoscope).

- It bypasses the physiological function of the upper airway including warming, filtering, and humidifying air.

PRECAUTIONS

Placement of the ET tube must continually be assessed; accidental displacement is a common occurrence.

CONTRAINDICATIONS

ET intubation should be avoided in patients who have epiglottitis, because insertion and manipulation of the laryngoscope into the upper airway may precipitate laryngospasm. Rather, in epiglottitis the patient's breathing should be assisted with a bag-valve-mask device until more definitive airway procedures can be performed.

COMPLICATIONS

As beneficial as ET intubation can be, there are significant and even life-threatening complications associated with this procedure, as in the following:
- Bleeding
- Laryngeal swelling
- Laryngospasm
- Vocal cord damage
- Mucosal necrosis
- Barotrauma
- Dental trauma
- Laryngeal trauma
- Misplacement into the esophagus or main stem bronchus (typically the right)

Digital Intubation • Intubation using the fingers.

ROUTES

ET intubation typically is accomplished using specialized equipment through one of two routes: orotracheal or nasotracheal. It also can be accomplished digitally (termed *digital intubation*) via the orotracheal route (see Appendix A—Alternative Airway Procedures for this information).

EQUIPMENT

The equipment and supplies used to perform ET intubation include the following:
- Laryngoscope (handle, blades, and extra batteries and bulb)
- ET tubes (various size)
- 10-mL syringe for cuff inflation and deflation
- Stylet
- Bag-valve-mask device (with supplemental oxygen and reservoir device)
- Suction equipment
- Bite block

- Magill forceps
- Tie-down tape or commercial tube holding device
- Water-soluble lubricant
- BSI supplies (gloves, mask, eyewear, or faceshield)

Laryngoscope—The laryngoscope is used to move the tongue and epiglottis out of the way. This removal allows visualization of the vocal cords and glottis, as well as placement of an ET tube. The laryngoscope consists of a handle and blade. The handle holds several batteries that serve as the energy source for the light, which is located in the distal portion of the blade. The light illuminates the airway so the upper airway structures can be seen. On the lower end of the handle is a bar where the hooked indentation of the blade is attached and locked in place (Figure 8-53).

> ### STREET WISE
> The laryngoscope also may be used in conjunction with the Magill forceps to retrieve an upper airway foreign body obstruction.

Laryngoscope blades come in a variety of sizes ranging from 0 (for the newborn) to 4 (for the large adult patient). The two types of laryngoscope blades are the curved blade (Figure 8-54, *A*), referred to as the Macintosh, and the straight blade (Figure 8-54, *B*), also referred to as the *Miller, Wisconsin,* or *Flagg.* When used properly, the tip of the curved blade is inserted into the vallecula. In this position, the tongue and epiglottis are raised out of the way when the laryngoscope handle is lifted anteriorly. Two benefits of the curved blade are that it permits more room for visualization of the glottic

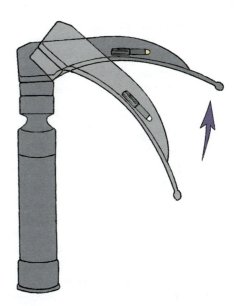

FIGURE 8-53 ▲ Lock the laryngoscope blade into the handle. (Kimberly Battista from Stoy W: *Mosby's EMT–Basic textbook,* St Louis, 1996, Mosby.)

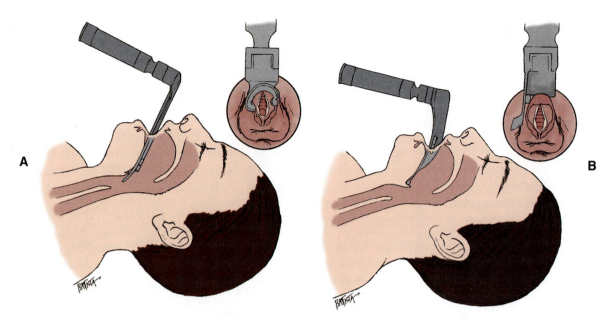

FIGURE 8-54 ▲ **A,** The Macintosh curved blade is inserted into the vallecula to raise the tongue and epiglottis out of the way. **B,** The Miller straight blade is positioned under the epiglottis to expose the glottic opening. (Kimberly Battista from Stoy W: *Mosby's EMT–Basic textbook,* St Louis, 1996, Mosby.)

opening and tube insertion and it is associated with less trauma and reflex stimulation than the straight blade, since many of the sensitive gag receptors are located on the posterior surface of the epiglottis.

In contrast, the straight blade is positioned under the epiglottis. When the handle is lifted anteriorly, the epiglottis is lifted out of the way exposing the glottic opening. The straight blade is preferred in infants because it provides greater displacement of the tongue and better visualization of the glottis, which lies higher and more anterior.

The use of one blade over the other is largely based on user preference because there are advantages to each type of blade. However, the EMT–I should be skilled in the use of both because there are cases in which one blade may be better suited for the patient than the other.

✖ **Tracheal lumen** • Cavity or channel within the trachea.

Endotracheal Tube—The ET tube is a flexible, translucent tube that is open at both ends. Its proximal end has a standard 15-mm adapter that can be connected to various devices for delivery of positive-pressure ventilation. Its distal end is beveled to facilitate placement between the vocal cords. It also has a balloon cuff that, when inflated, occludes the remainder of the **tracheal lumen.** This occlusion prevents aspiration around the tube and minimizes air leaks. Attached to the cuff is an inflating tube that has at its end a one-way inflating valve with an inlet port to accept a syringe for inflation. A pilot balloon between the one-way valve and the distal cuff reveals whether the distal cuff is in-

flated (Figure 8-55). Distal end depth centimeter (cm) markings are along the side of the ET tube for easily determining if it is placed far enough into the trachea. If the depth marking at the completion of the procedure is noted, it can be compared with the positioning of the ET tube later in the treatment and transport of the patient. If the position changes, it may indicate the tube has been advanced too far (possibly leading to main stem bronchial intubation) or has been pulled out of the trachea. The distal cuff should always be examined for leaks before placement in the trachea.

STREET WISE

Some EMT–Is tape the inflation tube to the ET tube to prevent it from being accidentally torn away from the tube.

Manufacturers commonly prewrap ET tubes in a curved position to facilitate passage into the trachea. Some ET tubes come with an O-shaped ring attachment that connects to a plastic wire running the length of the tube and ending distally. Pulling the ring bends the distal end of the tube upward. This bending helps redirect the tube, allowing easier passage into the glottic opening.

Markings on the ET tube indicate its internal diameter (ID). Tubes come in graduated sizes from 2.5 to 9.0 mm ID to lengths of 12 to 32 cm. Average sizes for

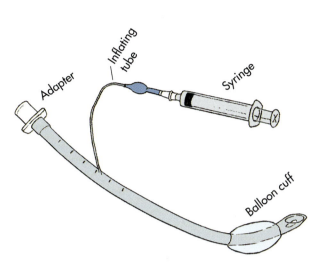

FIGURE 8-55 ▲ Components of the ET tube.

adults are 7.5 to 8.0 ID for women and 8.0 to 8.5 ID for men. When immediate placement of an ET tube is required, a 7.5 ID tube may be used for both female and male adult patients. Selection of the correct size tube is important; one that is too large can cause tracheal edema and/or damage to the vocal cords. However, a tube that is too small provides too little airflow and may lead to inadequate ventilatory volumes being delivered. Additionally, it can produce a negative pressure in the lungs, which can lead to pneumothorax and pulmonary edema. Cuffed ET tubes range in size between 5.0 and 9.0 ID.

Uncuffed ET tubes, ranging in size between 2.5 and 5.0 ID, are used for infants and children under 8 years of age because the round narrowing of their cricoid cartilage acts as a functional cuff.

Stylet—In cases where the trachea lies more anterior or the patient has a short, thick neck that makes optimal positioning of the head difficult, it may be difficult to place an ET tube. In cases like this, a semi-rigid, bendable, plastic-coated wire called a *stylet* can be used to shape the ET tube into a J or hockey-stick shape, allowing easier manipulation anteriorly. Because the stylet can cause tissue damage, it should be recessed at least one-half inch from the distal tip of the ET tube. Although a stylet is not always used, one should always be kept close at hand.

Commercial Tube-Holding Device or Tie-Down Tape—To prevent movement or accidental displacement once the tube is in place, it must be secured with a purpose-built commercial holding device or tie-down tape. Commercial tube-holding devices work quite well and are the preferred method for securing the tube in place. Tying is considered more effective than taping because tape tends to come loose when the tube or patient's face is moist.

Magill Forceps—The Magill forceps resemble a bent pair of scissors with circle-shaped tips. This device typically is used to remove foreign bodies obstructing the upper airway and to help redirect the ET tube during nasotracheal intubation.

Other Items—During intubation attempts, a suction unit should be on hand to remove secretions and foreign materials from the oropharynx. A water-soluble lubricant should be available to facilitate insertion of the ET tube. Once the ET tube is in place, an oropharyngeal airway can be used as a bite block to prevent the patient from biting and kinking the ET tube.

Use of an airway kit, or intubation wrap ensures that all the equipment and supplies needed to perform ET intubation are readily available. To eliminate potential equipment failure, the airway kit and all the equipment should be inspected at the beginning of each work shift. In volunteer settings in which specific coverage is not provided, the equipment should be checked at least once a week (Figure 8-56).

OROTRACHEAL ROUTE USING A LARYNGOSCOPE

✖ **Orotracheal** • **Through the mouth.**

Typically, the **orotracheal** route is used for ET intubation. Its prime advantage over other routes is that it allows direct observation of the ET tube as it is being passed between the vocal cords, which is an essential step for ensuring correct placement. It may be performed in

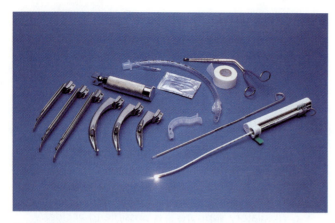

FIGURE 8-56 ▲ Equipment used in ET intubation. (Vincent Knaus from Stoy W: *Mosby's EMT–Basic textbook*, St Louis, 1996, Mosby.)

breathing and apneic patients. One disadvantage of orotracheal intubation is it requires special equipment.

To perform this procedure when no spinal injuries are suspected, the following steps should be taken:

1. Perform BSI precautions. At a minimum, gloves and goggles should be worn. A face mask and gown also should be worn when splashing is likely.
2. Use the head-tilt/chin-lift or jaw-thrust maneuver to open the patient's airway.
3. Preoxygenate with a bag-valve-mask supplied with 100% oxygen for at least 30 seconds to 1 minute to reduce carbon dioxide levels and increase oxygenation.
4. Direct a partner or first responder to provide ventilatory support of the patient (Figure 8-57, *A*, pp. 266-270).
5. Assemble and check the equipment as follows:
   - Withdraw the plunger of a 10-mL syringe to pull in 5 to 10 mL of air. Open the top part of the protective wrapper in which the ET tube is packaged. Insert the tip of the syringe into the port of the one-way inflation valve, which is connected to the distal cuff. Push the entire contents of the syringe into the distal cuff (Figure 8-57, *B*). It should be firm and have no leaks. Withdraw the air and leave the syringe connected to the inflation valve.

CLINICAL NOTES

Keep the ET tube in the protective wrapper until it is time to insert it into the trachea. This helps prevent the tube from becoming contaminated before its placement.

   - Insert the stylet and form the ET tube into the desired position. Many prefer the hockey stick position that is formed by bending the stylet and ET tube directly behind the distal balloon cuff (Figure 8-57, *C*).

STREET WISE

Use a twisting motion to properly seat the syringe. Otherwise, it may not be inserted deep enough into the one-way inflation valve to allow the introduction of air.

   - Attach the laryngoscope blade to the handle. Once it is properly seated, pull the blade up until it clicks into place and the laryngoscope bulb lights up (Figure 8-57, *D*). The bulb should appear bright white and be tightly secured in place. Note that some types of laryngoscope blades such as fiber optics do not have bulbs. Move the blade back into its unlocked position until the laryngoscope is required. This action helps conserve the life of the batteries.

STREET WISE

A yellow, flickering light provides insufficient illumination of the upper airway and suggests the batteries are weak. If the light fails to go on, you should suspect that the batteries are dead or the bulb is loose. Infrequently, the problem may lie in the contact point(s) or the wire traveling through the blade to the bulb.

✳ **Occiput** • The posterior portion of the head.

CLINICAL NOTES

It is sometimes best to remove dental appliances such as dentures and partials before intubation (unless they fit tightly).

6. Have the rescuer providing ventilatory support move out of the way (Figure 8-57, *E*). Position yourself at the patient's head.
7. Place the patient's head and neck into a "sniffing position" to align the three axes of the mouth, pharynx, and trachea. This is an optimal hyperextension of the head with elevation of the **occiput.** The sniffing position is accomplished by flexing the patient's neck forward while, at the same time, tilting the head back. Placing a rolled towel under the patient's shoulders or the occiput of the head can facilitate a sniffing position. Accomplishing this task is extremely difficult when the patient has a short, thick neck or when the patient's mobility is limited by arthritis or other such conditions. When there is

a potential for cervical spine injury, the head is firmly held in a neutral position during intubation.

8. Using the left hand, hold the laryngoscope by its handle (Figure 8-57, *F*).

9. Insert the laryngoscope blade into the right side of the patient's mouth. Using a sweeping motion, displace the tongue to the left. This action pushes the tongue out of the way allowing more room to visualize the upper airway structures and manipulate the ET tube (Figure 8-57, *G*).
10. Move the blade slightly toward the midline and advance it until the distal end is positioned at the base of tongue (Figures 8-57, *H* and *I*). Simultaneously, using the index finger of the right hand, push the lower lip away from the blade to prevent injury.
11. Visualize the tip of the epiglottis and then place the laryngoscope blade into the proper position.

12. Next, lift the laryngoscope slightly upward and forward to displace the jaw and airway structures without allowing the blade to touch the teeth (Figure 8-57, *J*). The epiglottis should come into view unless the blade has been inserted too far, in which case the blade should be withdrawn slowly until the epiglottis is seen (Figure 8-57, *K*). Conversely, if the blade is not deep enough into the airway it will need to be advanced. Placing the right thumb into the patient's mouth, grasping the chin, and lifting the jaw up while advancing the laryngoscope facilitates this advancement.

13. Suction any vomitus or secretions lying in the posterior pharynx. If suctioning fails to resolve the problem, place the patient onto his or her side to facilitate drainage of the secretions.

14. Keeping the left wrist straight, use the shoulder and arm to continue lifting the mandible and tongue at a 45-degree angle to the ground until the glottis is exposed. Often, not all the glottis can be seen, but at least the posterior third or half should be visible.

15. Grasp the ET tube in the right hand, holding it the same way a pencil is grasped (Figure 8-57, *L*). This technique permits gentle maneuvering of the tube. Hold the tube horizontal to the ground (Figure 8-57, *M*). Advance it through the right corner of the patient's mouth, directing the distal end of the tube up or down to pass it into the larynx (Figure 8-57, *N*).

16. Insert the ET tube into the glottic opening and advance it until the distal cuff disappears slightly ($\frac{1}{2}$ to 1 inch) past the vocal cords. Observe the tube as it enters the glottic opening. This is the first step in ensuring correct placement of the ET tube (Figures 8-57, *O* and *P*).
17. To prevent the tube from being accidentally displaced, hold it in place with the left hand. Do not release the ET tube before it is secured in place.
18. Inflate the distal cuff with the prefilled syringe. Use only the minimum amount of air necessary to create an effective seal (typically between 5 to 10 mL of air). This helps prevent tracheal trauma due to excessive cuff pressure. Determine how much air is needed by listening for the sound of air leaking around the tube before distal cuff inflation. The cuff should be inflated only to the point at which air leakage stops (Figure 8-57, *Q*).

Text continued on p. 270

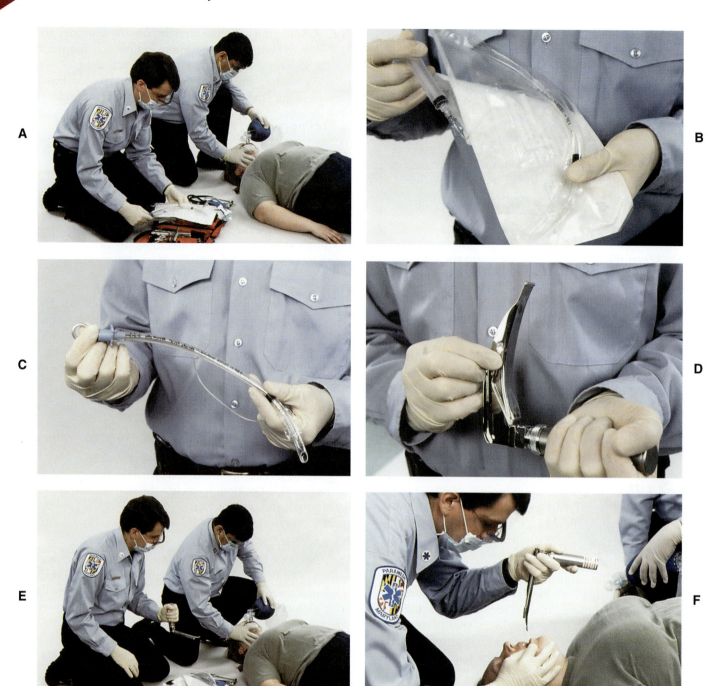

FIGURE 8-57 ▲ Orotracheal intubation using a laryngoscope. **A,** Direct a partner to provide ventilatory support. **B,** Check the distal cuff of the ET tube. **C,** Insert the stylet into the appropriate position; it must be recessed at least one-half inch from the distal tip of the ET tube) (NOTE: To make the stylet visible, this picture shows the ET tube out of the protective wrap; under normal conditions the ET tube should be kept in the protective wrapper until just before its placement. **D,** Check the bulb of the laryngoscope for brightness and tightness. **E,** Have the rescuer providing ventilatory support move out of the way. **F,** Hold the laryngoscope in left hand. (Rick Brady, Photographer.)

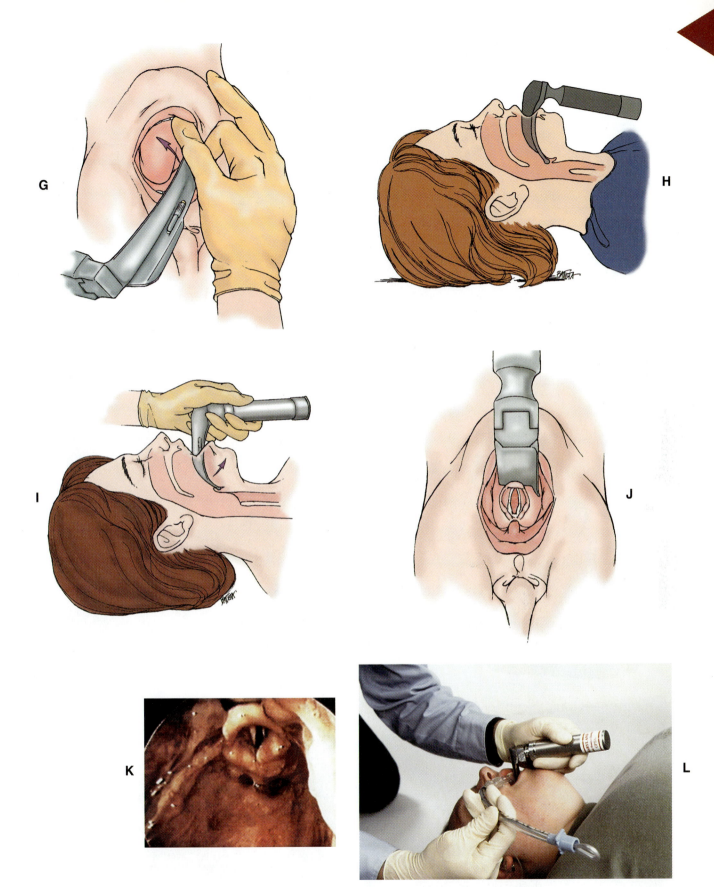

FIGURE 8-57, cont'd ▲ Orotracheal intubation using a laryngoscope.
G, Insert the laryngoscope blade into the patient's mouth and displace the tongue
to the left. **H,** Move blade toward midline and advance until distal end is positioned
at base of tongue. **I,** Lift the laryngoscope upward and forward to displace the jaw
and airway structures. **J,** An overhead view of laryngoscope placement. **K,** View of
the epiglottis and glottic opening. **L,** Grasp the ET tube in right hand. (**I,** Kimberly
Battista, Artist.)

Continued

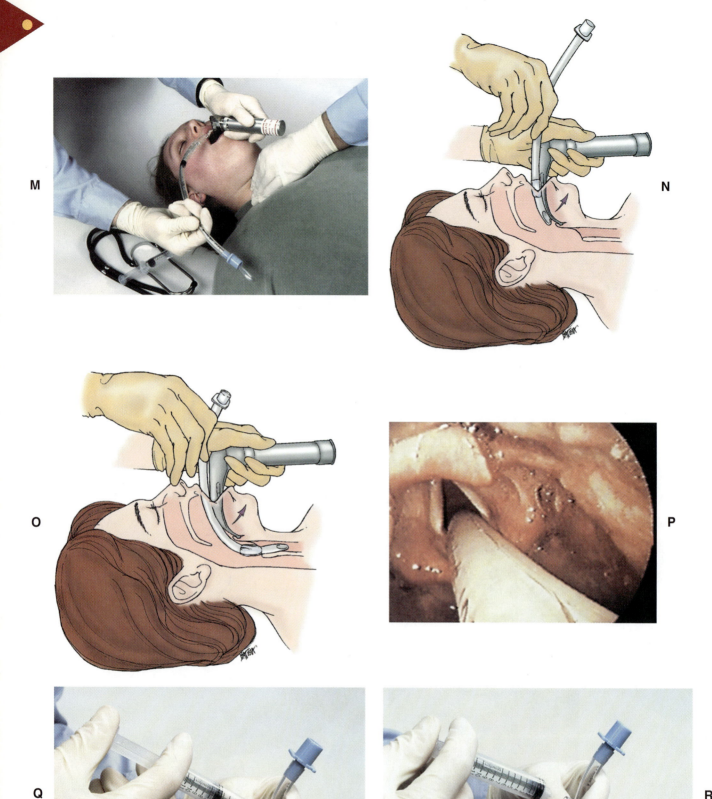

FIGURE 8-57, cont'd ▲ Orotracheal intubation using a laryngoscope.
M, Hold the ET tube horizontal to the ground. (NOTE: The other rescuer is applying cricoid pressure to make visualization of the glottic opening easier.) **N,** Advance the ET tube into the larynx. **O,** Advance the tube through the glottic opening. **P,** An ET tube passing through the glottic opening. **Q,** Inflate the distal cuff. **R,** While keeping pressure on the plunger, immediately remove the syringe.

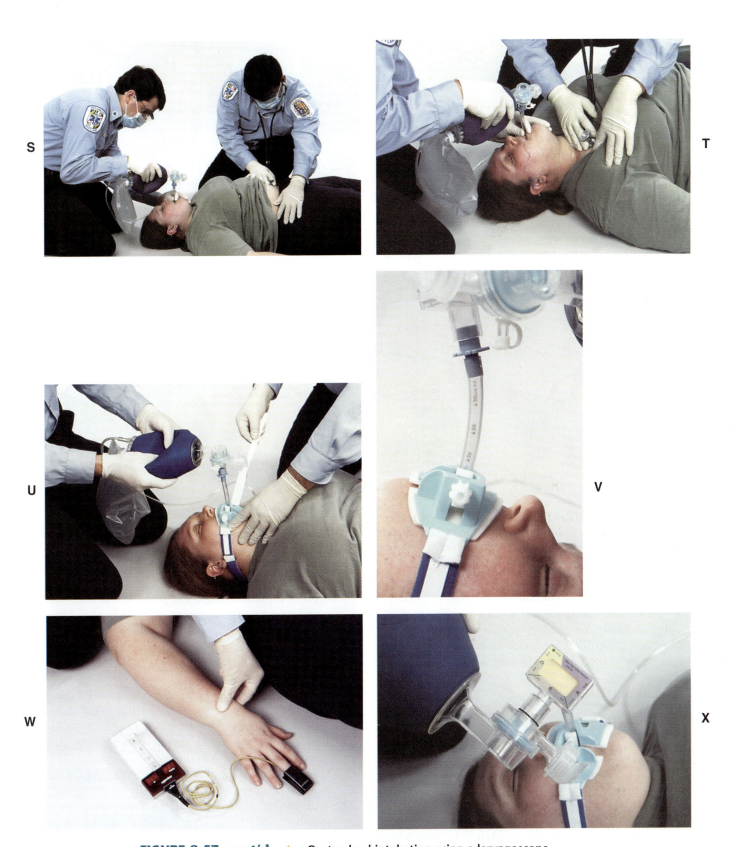

FIGURE 8-57, cont'd ▲ Orotracheal intubation using a laryngoscope.
S, Auscultate the epigastrium. **T,** Auscultate the chest. **U,** Secure the tube in place
with a commercial device. **V,** Check the tube for condensation on exhalation.
W, Apply pulse oximetry to monitor oxygen saturation. **X,** Use an end-tidal carbon
dioxide detector as a tool for assessing correct placement.   *Continued*

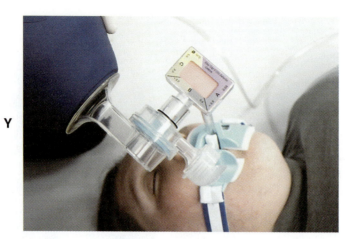

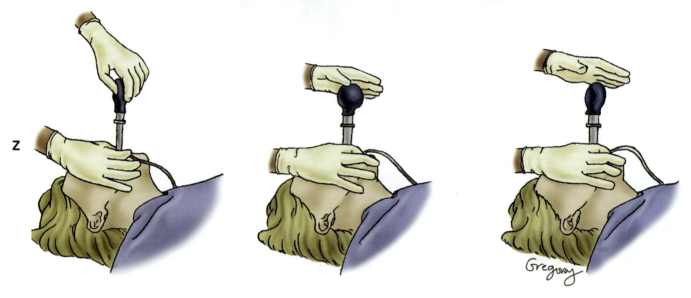

FIGURE 8-57, cont'd ▲ Orotracheal intubation using a laryngoscope. **Y,** Colormetric end-tidal carbon dioxide detectors should change colors during patient exhalation, since there is a higher presence of carbon dioxide. **Z,** Esophageal intubation detector.

19. While maintaining pressure on the plunger to keep any air from escaping and using a twisting motion, immediately remove the syringe (Figure 8-57, *R*).

20. Attach a ventilatory device to the 15- or 22-mm adapter of the tube and deliver several breaths.

> ● **HELPFUL HINT**
>
> ● When removing the syringe from the one-way inflation valve, you must be sure to maintain downward pressure on the plunger and use a reverse twisting action to prevent accidental leakage of air.

21. Recheck for proper tube placement as follows:
    - Immediately note the bag-valve-mask device compliance. Increased resistance to ventilation may be caused by esophageal placement, gastric distension, or tension pneumothorax.
    - Auscultate over the epigastrium with a stethoscope to ensure there are no sounds when ventilations are delivered (Figure 8-57, *S*).

- Next, auscultate the chest at the apices and bilateral bases for the presence of equal, bilateral lung sounds. Unequal or absent breath sounds indicate esophageal placement, right main stem placement, pneumothorax, or bronchial obstruction (Figure 8-57, *T*).
- Directly revisualize placement of the ET tube. It should rest properly between the vocal cords. Note the depth of the ET tube. In adult males the average depth is 22 cm at the teeth, and in women, it is 21 cm at the teeth.
- Palpate the distal ET cuff at the sternal notch while compressing the pilot balloon.

22. Ventilate the patient with a bag-valve-mask device supplied with 100% oxygen. When ventilating patients who are in cardiac arrest and chest compressions are being delivered, ventilate with a tidal volume of 10 to 15 mL/kg at a rate of 10 to 12 breaths per minute (1 breath every 5 to 6 seconds, each lasting 2 secconds). Insert an oropharyngeal airway to serve as a bite block. When spontaneous circulation

has been restored, continue to provide a tidal volume of 10 to 15 mL/kg (as indicated by an obvious chest rise of several centimeters). Increase the ventilation rate to 10 to 15 breaths per minute (1 breath every 4 to 5 seconds). Then aim for mild-to-moderate hyperventilation (achieved at a rate of 12 ventilations per minute at a volume of 10 to 15 mL/kg).

STUDENT ALERT

Once the ET tube is in place, there is no need to synchronize ventilation with chest compressions.

23. Secure the ET tube in place with a commercial device (Figure 8-57, *U*) or umbilical tape while continuing ventilatory support. If using umbilical tape, loop it around the ET tube at the level of the patient's teeth, securing it tightly to the tube without kinking or pinching it. Then, wrap the tape around the patient's head and tie it at the side of the neck.
24. Next, check the proximal end of the tube for breath condensation during each exhalation. Breath condensation is simply the moisture that is present in exhaled air. It should disappear each time the patient breathes in or ventilation is delivered. The absence of breath condensation during exhalation suggests improper placement of the tube (Figure 8-57, *V*).
25. A pulse oximetry unit should be applied because it provides immediate, ongoing assessment of the oxygen saturation (Figure 8-57, *W*). An end-tidal carbon dioxide detector should also be used to measure the presence of the carbon dioxide in the expired air (Figure 8-57, *X* and *Y*). Several types are available, including the colorimetric, digital, and digital/waveform units. Another device that should be used to assess correct placement is the esophageal detection device (Figure 8-57, *Z*).
26. Continue supporting the tube manually while maintaining ventilations. Regularly check to ensure proper tube position because it can be easily dislodged during resuscitation efforts, manipulation of the neck or movement of the patient. Manipulation of the neck may displace the tube up to 5 cm. During long transports in the field setting, patients are at high risk for tracheal tube displacement. For this reason a cervical collar and immobilization device should be applied to keep restless intubated patients from moving in such a way as to dislodge the ET tube.

Complications

A variety of complications can occur during ET intubation.

HYPOXIA

Hypoxia can develop before placement of the ET tube if intubation attempts are longer than appropriate or if rescue personnel fail to provide ventilatory support be-

tween procedures. For this reason, each intubation attempt should be limited to no more than 30 seconds. It is seldom absolutely necessary to place the ET tube on the first attempt. Unless placement can be easily accomplished, the first attempt may be better used to provide an initial view of the patient's anatomy. Subsequent attempts (interspersed between reoxygenation with a bag-valve-mask device and 100% oxygen) can then be used to place the tube.

INJURY TO TEETH AND TISSUE

Gently guiding the laryngoscope blade into place and not allowing it to touch the teeth can avoid injuries to the tissues or teeth. When manipulating the jaw anteriorly, it is best to employ upward traction rather than following the natural inclination to rotate and flex the wrist. From then, the left wrist should remain straight, with all lifting done from the shoulder and arm.

MISPLACEMENT OF THE TUBE

Accidental placement of the ET tube into the vallecula, pyriform sinus, esophagus, or main stem bronchus can have dire consequences.

Subcutaneous Emphysema • Presence of air beneath the skin (in the subcutaneous tissues), giving it a characteristic crackling sensation on palpation.

Vallecula and Pyriform Misplacement—Vallecula placement occurs when the tube is allowed to slip too far anteriorly and becomes lodged in the space between the epiglottis and base of the tongue. Alternatively, if the tube strays from the midline it can get hung up on either side of the epiglottis in the pyriform sinus (Figure 8-58, *A*). You can recognize this condition by the skin "bulging out" on either side of the laryngeal prominence (Adam's apple) (Figure 8-58, *B*). Forceful efforts to pass the ET tube can perforate these tissues, leading to an absence of ventilation (hypoxia, hypercarbia, death), serious bleeding, and **subcutaneous emphysema.** Vallecula misplacement can be resolved by slightly withdrawing and redirecting the tube posteriorly. Pyriform sinus misplacement can be resolved by slightly withdrawing and rotating the tube to the midline.

Endobronchial Misplacement—If the ET tube is inserted too far, it will pass into either the right or left main stem bronchus (Figure 8-59). Endobronchial intubation results in hypoxia due to one-lung ventilation. Endobronchial intubation is suspected when auscultation of the chest reveals the presence of good lung sounds on one side of the chest but diminished or absent lung sounds on the other side. Poor compliance, felt when delivering ventilations with the bag-valve-mask device; cyanosis; and other signs of hypoxia such as cardiac dysrhythmias also suggest endobronchial intubation. The pulse oximetry unit is another useful tool for detecting changes in oxygenation that can help determine that the tube has been inserted too far.

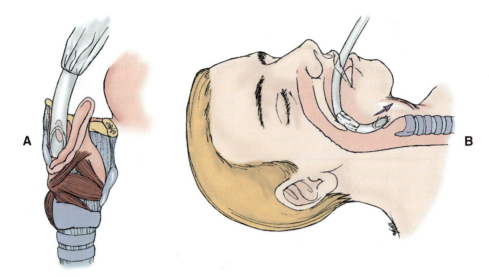

FIGURE 8-58 ▲ **A,** A misplaced ET tube in pyriform sinus. **B,** A characteristic bulge resulting from tube misplacement.

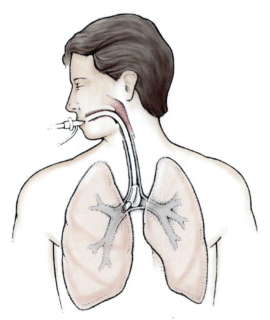

FIGURE 8-59 ▲ Misplacement of ET tube into right main stem bronchi. (Duckwall Productions)

To correct this problem, loosen or remove the securing device, deflate the distal cuff, and as ventilations continue slowly, withdraw the tube while simultaneously auscultating the left side of the chest. Stop withdrawing the tube once lung sounds heard are on the left side. Then auscultate both sides of the chest, lung sounds should be heard equally and bilaterally. Next, note the tube depth, reinflate the distal cuff, and secure the tube in place.

Some hints for preventing the tube from being inserted too far include the following:

- Advance the distal cuff past the vocal cords no more than ½ to 1 inch.

- Once in this position, continue to hold the tube in place with one hand. This prevents the tube from being accidentally inserted any further.
- Firmly secure the tube in place with umbilical tape or a commercial tube holding device to prevent it from being accidentally advanced.
- Mark the side of the ET tube at the level where it emerges from the mouth, which allows quick identification of any changes in tube placement.

✥ **Phonation** • Process of generating sounds or speech with the vocal cords.

Esophageal Intubation—Accidental misplacement of the tube into the esophagus has catastrophic results (Figure 8-60). If left uncorrected, it leads to severe hypoxia and brain death because neither assisted breathing nor oxygen are provided to the patient. Esophageal intubation can be identified by (1) an absence of chest rise and breath sounds with assisted breathing, (2) gurgling sounds heard over the epigastrium with each breath delivered, (3) an absence of breath condensation collecting inside the ET tube, (4) a persistent air leak despite inflation of the distal cuff of the ET tube, (5) cyanosis and a progressive worsening of the patient's condition, and (6) **phonation.**

As described earlier, a number of commercially available devices also can be used to indicate correct placement of the tube in the trachea. Attached to the proximal end of the tube, some devices are designed to generate a whistlelike sound with expiration when the tube is properly positioned. However, others such as the end-tidal carbon dioxide detector determine the amount of carbon dioxide present in the expired air, and the esophageal detection device is used to determine if the ET tube is situated in the trachea or esophagus.

If correct placement is uncertain, the location of the ET tube can be checked visually using a laryngoscope.

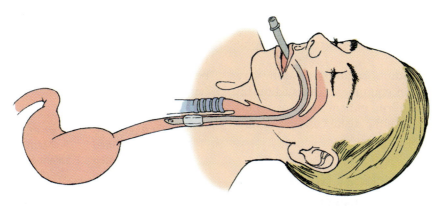

FIGURE 8-60 ▲ Misplacement of ET tube into esophagus.

If it is suspected that the tube is in the esophagus, it should be removed. When removing a misplaced ET tube, be prepared to vigorously suction the patient. The likelihood of emesis is increased, especially if gastric distension is present. Ideally, preoxygenating before attempting reintubation is best. The misplaced tube may be left in place until proper tube placement is confirmed, or it may be removed beforehand, provided diligent and vigorous suctioning is available.

CLINICAL NOTES

With some cases of esophageal intubation, vomitus will propel from the tube. This occurs due to the high gastric pressures brought about by the resuscitation efforts, particularly because several breaths usually have been delivered as a means of checking for proper tube placement. When this event occurs, the tube should be left in place, because removing it can result in vomitus traveling up into the pharynx and subsequently being aspirated into the trachea. In these cases the tube is essentially functioning as a gastric tube. You should simply displace the tube to the side of the mouth and ventilate the patient with a bag-valve-mask device until the trachea can be successfully intubated.

IDENTIFYING DIFFICULT INTUBATION

Before beginning the task of placing a definitive airway, the EMT–I should attempt to determine the likelihood of a difficult airway with an inability to ventilate. In the more controlled clinical environment, there are numer-

ous ways to assess for this potential; however, they may be difficult, if not impractical, to use in the field. Nevertheless, an attempt should be made.

The patient should be directed to open his or her mouth as wide as possible and stick out the tongue. The degree to which the EMT–I can see the pharyngeal structures is graded as classes I to IV. Class I is the best view, and class IV is the worst view. The view is indicative of how easy intubation is expected to be; however, this technique greatly varies. The actual view seen on laryngoscopy is also graded classes I to IV as to the extent the laryngeal structures that are seen. This is important to communicate to other health care professionals so that they can be alerted to the degree of ease or difficulty expected if future airway interventions are needed.

Other indicators of difficult airway and/or mask ventilation include the following:
- Short, fat neck
- Small, receding chin
- Presence of a beard
- Large tongue
- Poor mouth opening and/or neck mobility
- Facial injury with excess oral secretions
- Facial and/or neck burns
- Fractured mandible
- Laryngeal injury

Field Extubation

The need for field extubation is extremely rare. Generally, field extubating should occur only when the patient is unreasonably intolerant of the tube. Increasing sedation rather than removing the tube should address intolerance of the ET tube, as evidenced by gag reflex. The biggest concern with extubation is that patients who are awake are at high risk of laryngospasm immediately following extubation, and it is difficult to reintubate a laryngospastic patient. Extubation is indicated if the patient is able to protect and maintain an open airway, the risks for needing to reintubate are significantly reduced, and the patient is not sedated. The procedure is contraindicated if there is any risk of recurrence of respiratory failure.

To perform this procedure, begin by ensuring oxygenation, have intubation equipment and suction immediately available, confirm patient responsiveness, suction oropharynx, deflate the distal cuff and remove the tube on cough or expiration.

Pediatric Endotracheal Intubation

ET intubation may also be called for in the pediatric patient. This method provides the most effective airway control and allows direct ventilation of the lungs.

INDICATIONS

Indications for intubation of the child include the following:

- Inadequate central nervous system control of ventilation
- Functional or anatomic airway obstruction
- Excessive work of breathing leading to fatigue
- Need for high peak inspiratory pressure or positive end-expiratory pressure to maintain effective alveolar gas exchange

Begin preparing for ET intubation in the pediatric patient by selecting the appropriate equipment and supplies.

For intubation of infants and toddlers, a straight laryngoscope blade is preferred, since it provides better visualization. For older children, a curved blade (or Macintosh blade) may be more effective. Generally, the following size blades can be used for the various age groups:

0 straight	Premature infant
1 straight	Full-term infant to 1 year of age
2 straight	Two years of age to adolescent
3 straight or curved	Adolescent and above

Next, the size of the ET tube is determined. NOTE: Uncuffed tubes are used in infants and children less 8 years of age because of their "natural cuffs" at the level of the cricoid cartilage. The easiest and quickest way to determine the appropriate size ET tube is to use the external nostrils as a guide. Generally, but not always, the nares should accept the ET tube size that is to be placed into the trachea. If the tube is too small, it will not secure the airway. However, if the tube is too large, damage to the vocal cords may occur.

Several other methods may be useful when determining ET tube size for the pediatric patient. Examine the outside diameter of the patient's little finger or use the following formula for children older than 2 years of age:

$$\text{ET tube (in mm)} = (16 + \text{age in years}) \div 4$$

Using the length (height) of the infant or child is actually more accurate than using the age. Resuscitation tapes help with this method. Math is often a difficult task to perform when a child is seriously ill, and it may be necessary to use whatever method best meets his or her needs. Generally, the following size tubes are used in the various age groups:

2.5 to 3.0 uncuffed	Premature infant
3.0 to 3.5 uncuffed	Full-term infant
3.5 to 4.0 uncuffed	Infant to 1 year of age
4.0 to 5.0 uncuffed	Toddler
5.0 to 5.5 uncuffed	Preschool-age child
5.5 to 6.5 cuffed	School-age child
7.0 to 8.0 cuffed	Adolescent

PROCEDURE

To perform ET intubation in the pediatric patient, the following steps should be taken:

1. If not already done, separate the parent or guardian from the child. If possible, have someone stay with the parent to explain the procedure.
2. Manually open the airway and insert an airway adjunct such as an oropharyngeal airway if needed.
3. Preoxygenate the patient with the appropriate size bag-valve-mask device and 100% oxygen. Suction the airway as necessary.
4. Assemble the laryngoscope and blade. Check the light to make sure it works before attempting intubation.
5. Select the appropriate size tube and lubricate it with sterile water/saline or water-soluble gel. Lubricate the stylet if it is used.
6. Place the child's head in the "sniffing" position. If trauma is suspected, manually maintain a neutral position so that the head and neck are stabilized for each intubation attempt.
7. Hold the laryngoscope in the left hand, and insert it into the child's mouth from the right. Sweep the tongue to the left and move the blade into position. Because the airway is shorter and the glottis higher than an adult's, the cords will appear quickly.
8. Lift the mandible and tongue with firm, steady pressure until the glottis can be seen. Remember to keep the wrist straight and to avoid pressure on the mouth or teeth if present. If the cords are not visualized, slowly withdraw the blade and watch for the larynx to drop into view.
9. Using the right hand, introduce the ET tube to the right side of the mouth and through the glottic opening. Pass the tube through the vocal cords to about 2 to 3 cm below the vocal cords. Continue to hold the tube in place.

10. Do not let intubation attempts last more than 30 seconds. If intubation is unsuccessful, re-oxygenate the patient with a bag-valve-mask device before any subsequent attempts.

11. Once intubation is successful, ventilate the patient with a bag-valve-mask device.

12. Confirm proper tube placement as follows:
    - Observe for symmetrical chest expansion.
    - Auscultate for equal breath sounds over each lateral chest wall high in the axillae.
    - Absence of breath sounds over the abdomen.
    - Improved heart rate and color.
    - Apply the end-tidal carbon dioxide detector.

13. After confirming placement of the tube, secure it to the face while noting the placement of the distance marker at the teeth/gums. Minimize movement of the head and neck so as not to dislodge the tube. Even after the tube has been secured, continue to manually stabilize it whenever possible.

14. Continue to reassess the child to ensure proper placement of the tube throughout transport.

CONSIDERATIONS

Remember the following points when working with the airway of an infant or child:

1. Children have more soft tissue in the oropharynx and a larger tongue. Extra care must be used when inserting the laryngoscope so as not to cause injury.

2. Sweep the tongue out of the way as completely as possible to keep it from blocking your line of sight.

3. The larynx is higher in the pediatric patient than in the adult, and the epiglottis is floppy, making visualization of the cords more difficult.

4. The cricoid cartilage is the narrowest part of the upper airway, and the structures are more flexible than in an adult.

These differences may make ET intubation more challenging. Even with all these challenges, an intubation attempt should not extend beyond 30 seconds.

Throughout the intubation procedure the patient's heart rate must be monitored. Manipulation of the laryngoscope can stimulate the vagus nerve, leading to a marked decrease in the heart rate and a subsequent decrease in the blood pressure. Hypoxemia from prolonged intubation attempts can also decrease the heart rate. If there is significant decrease in the heart rate the procedure should be stopped, and high-concentration oxygen using a bag-valve-mask device should be provided. Suction equipment should be nearby, since the child's airway may become obstructed with vomitus, blood, increased saliva, or mucus. A pediatric suction catheter should be used to clear away the obstruction as quickly as possible, and providing hyperventilation with high-concentration oxygen before and after suctioning may become a priority.

MULTILUMEN AIRWAYS

The multilumen airway is designed to deliver lung ventilation when placed either in the trachea or the esophagus. Several of these devices are available including the esophageal tracheal Combitube and the pharyngotracheal lumen airway. Each of these devices is designed for blind insertion into the oropharynx and esophagus or trachea. Because serious complications with these devices can occur, the EMT–I must receive considerable training and be authorized to use them.

CLINICAL NOTES

The ET tube is the optimal adjunct to achieve adequate airway protection and ventilation during CPR.

Esophageal-Tracheal Combitube

The esophageal/tracheal dual-lumen airway, or Combitube, is a dual-lumen tube with two balloon cuffs. It is structurally and functionally similar to the pharyngotracheal lumen tube, except for a modified pharyngeal balloon and a simpler basic structure. It is an alternative device for airway control when conventional intubation measures are unsuccessful or unavailable. Two sizes are available for use: (1) a size created for patients between 4 and 5 feet tall and (2) a size created for patients more than 5 feet tall. One cuff is clear in color and located at the tip (distal cuff). The other is a larger, cream-colored cuff located near the halfway point of the tube. The blue lumen is the port used to deliver ventilations through multiple small openings in the tube between the two cuffs when the tube is placed in the esophagus. The clear lumen is the ventilation port if the tube is inserted in the trachea. When inflated, the large cream-colored cuff seals off the oropharynx and nasopharynx. The distal cuff seals off the esophagus or the trachea. A blue pilot balloon and a white pilot balloon correspond to the cream-colored and distal cuffs. Two syringes come in the kit for inflation of the cuffs (Figure 8-61, *A, B, C*).

> **HELPFUL HINT**
>
> - The Combitube airway is best described as an ET tube and a large pharyngeal tube molded into a single unit.

ADVANTAGES AND DISADVANTAGES

The advantages of the Combitube airway include the following:
- Insertion is rapid and easy.
- It is inserted blindly, requiring no special equipment or visualization of the upper airway.

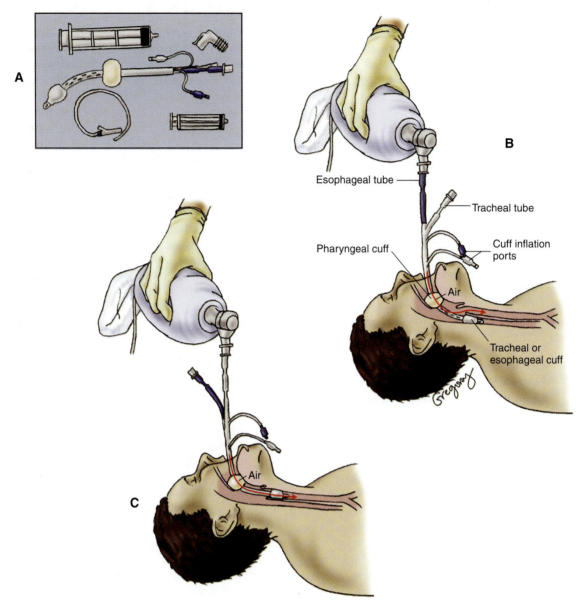

FIGURE 8-61 ▲ **A,** Combitube equipment. **B,** Combitube inserted into esophagus. **C,** Combitube inserted into trachea.

- It is inserted with the patent's head in a neutral position.
- The patient can be ventilated regardless of esophageal or tracheal tube placement.
- It has a self-adjusting, self-positioning posterior pharyngeal balloon.
- It significantly diminishes gastric distension and regurgitation.
- It is not necessary to maintain a face seal because the oropharyngeal cuff eliminates the need for a face mask.
- It can protect the trachea from upper airway bleeding or secretions if the tube is placed in the trachea.
- Allows immediate suctioning of gastric contents and decompression if the tube is placed in the esophagus.
- In an undiagnosed tracheal placement, the spontaneously breathing patient may breathe through multiple small ports in the unused lumen.

Disadvantages of the Combitube include the following:
- The trachea cannot be suctioned when the tube is in place.
- It can only be used in unconscious adults.
- It is very difficult to intubate around.

CONTRAINDICATIONS

Insertion of a Combitube should not be attempted in a responsive or semiresponsive patient who has a gag reflex. Its use also should be avoided in patients less than 4 ft tall. Additionally, it should not be used in patients who are known to have ingested a caustic substance or those who have known esophageal disease. Placement of the Combitube is not foolproof; errors can be made if assessment skills are not adequate.

The following equipment is needed for intubating a patient with the Combitube:
- Combitube kit with syringes
- Water-soluble lubricant
- Suctioning unit
- Bag-valve-device or demand valve
- Gloves
- Eye protection

PROCEDURE

To insert the Combitube, the following steps must be taken:

1. Perform BSI precautions.
2. Open the airway manually using the head-tilt/chin-lift or jaw-thrust maneuver.
3. Preoxygenate with a bag-valve-mask device supplied with 100% oxygen.
4. Ask another EMT–I to take over ventilating the patient.
5. Assemble and check the proper equipment while the patient is being preoxygenated with 100% oxygen (Figure 8-62, *A*). The Combitube must always be checked to make sure it is working properly before trying to insert it. Connect the blue-tipped syringe (drawn up with at least 100 mL of air) to the blue one-way valve tube marked *No. 1*; then connect the white-tipped syringe (drawn up with at least 15 mL of air) to the white one-way valve tube marked *No. 2*. Lubricate the tube with a water-soluble lubricant to facilitate its passage (Figure 8-62, *B*).
6. Direct the ventilator to move to the side of the patient's head and assume a position above the patient.
7. Place the patient's head into a neutral position. In an unresponsive trauma patient, the neck must be stabilized in a neutral, in-line position. The oropharyngeal airway should be removed if one has been inserted.
8. Insert the thumb of your right hand deep into the patient's mouth, grasping the tongue and lower jaw between the thumb and index finger. Lift the tongue and lower jaw anteriorly, away from the posterior pharynx.
9. Hold the Combitube so that it curves in the same direction as the natural curvature of the pharynx. Insert the tip into the mouth along the midline and advance it carefully along the tongue (Figure 8-62, *C*). Gently guide the Combitube along the base of the tongue and into the airway. Do not force the Combitube. If resistance is met, pull back and redirect the Combitube. When the Combitube is at the proper depth, the teeth or alveolar ridge will be between the heavy black lines (Figure 8-62, *D*).
10. Next, inflate the blue pilot balloon (and flesh-colored cuff) with the predrawn 100-mL blue-tipped syringe (Figure 8-62, *E*).
11. Once that cuff is inflated and the pilot balloon is tense, immediately inflate the white pilot balloon leading to the smaller distal cuff with the predrawn syringe containing 10 to 15 mL of air (Figure 8-62, *F*). The Combitube may move forward slightly, but this is normal.
12. Begin ventilation by attaching the ventilating device to the longer blue connecting tube marked *No. 1* (Figure 8-62, *G*).
13. Observe the patient's chest and listen for lung sounds. If the chest rises and falls and breath sounds are heard, the Combitube is in the esophagus (Figure 8-62, *G* and *H*). When this is the case, continue to ventilate through the blue tube.
14. If the chest does not rise and breath sounds are not heard, the Combitube is in the trachea. In this case, attach the ventilation device to the shorter clear connecting tube marked *No. 2* and ventilate the patient through it (Figure 8-62, *I*). Again, listen for breath sounds in all lung fields and in both axillae. Listen over the stomach as well.
15. Continue ventilating the patient with a bag-valve-mask device supplied with 100% oxygen or other ventilatory device.

Throughout placement of the device, the patient should be continuously monitored. Occasionally, the balloon cuffs leak or may be torn by jagged broken teeth, dentures, or bones. Thus special care must be taken when using this device, especially in the event of facial trauma. Watch for leaks by carefully squeezing the pilot balloon. The syringes can be used to keep the balloon cuffs properly inflated.

> **STREET WISE**
>
> While ventilating a deeply unresponsive patient via the blue tube (No. 1), an ET tube can be inserted around the Combitube.

Removing the Combitube—A number of factors may prompt the removal of the Combitube. Removing the device is a fairly simple procedure. First, the patient is turned on his or her side to keep the airway clear of vomitus. When ready, deflate the balloon cuffs and gently remove the tube. Because the patient may vomit when the Combitube is removed from the esophagus, a suctioning unit must be readily available.

Pharyngotracheal Lumen Airway

The pharyngotracheal lumen airway was developed to address the problems associated with the esophageal obturator airway (EOA) and esophageal gastric tube airway (EGTA). It is a two-tube, two-cuff system. The first tube is a short, wide tube with a large cuff along its lower portion. When inflated, this cuff seals off the oropharynx,

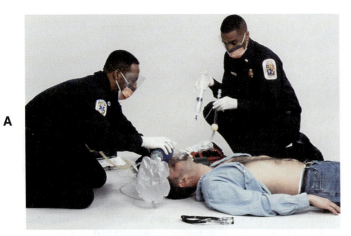

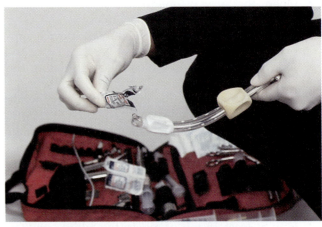

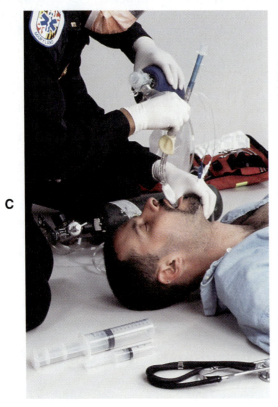

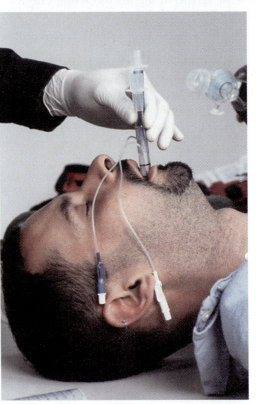

FIGURE 8-62 ▲ **A,** Assemble and check equipment. **B,** Lubricate tube. **C,** Insert Combitube into the mouth. **D,** Continue inserting tube until the teeth are situated between the heavy black lines.

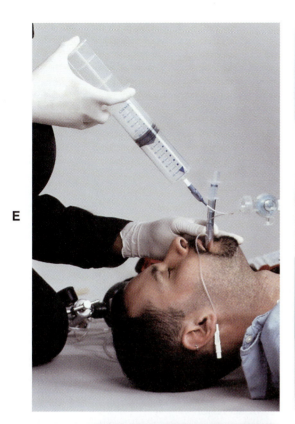

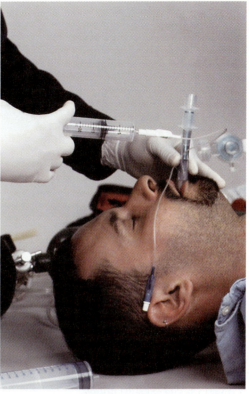

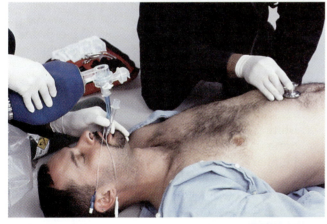

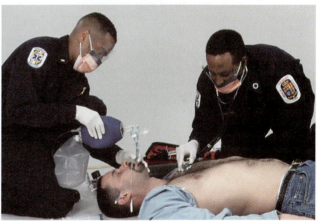

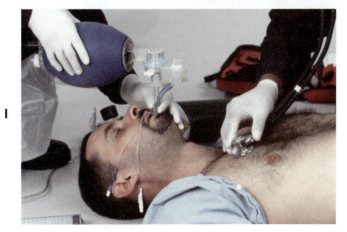

FIGURE 8-62, cont'd ▲ **E,** Inflate the blue pilot balloon. **F,** Inflate the white pilot balloon. **G,** Begin ventilating through the blue tube. **H,** While looking for chest rise and auscultating for epigastric and chest sounds. **I,** If no chest rise occurs while ventilating through the blue tube switch over to ventilating the clear

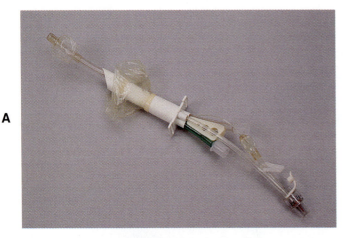

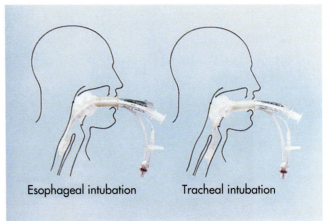

Esophageal intubation   Tracheal intubation

FIGURE 8-63 ▲ **A,** Pharyngotracheal lumen airway. **B,** Esophageal and tracheal placement of pharyngotracheal lumen airway. (**A,** From the American College of Emergency Physicians: Pons P, Cason D, chief editors: *Paramedic field care: a complaint-based approach,* St Louis, 1997, Mosby. **B,** Respironics, Inc.; Monroeville, PA from Sanders: *Mosby's paramedic textbook,* St Louis, 1994, Mosby.)

and air is introduced through the tube as its proximal end enters the pharynx. A second, longer tube travels through the first, extending past its distal end. Because of its longer length, it can be passed into either the trachea or the esophagus. At the distal end of the longer tube is a cuff that, when inflated, seals off the anatomic structure in which it is located. When the longer tube is in the esophagus, the device acts like an EOA and the patient is ventilated through the first tube. When the longer tube is in the trachea, the device acts like an ET tube and the patient is ventilated through it (Figures 8-63, *A* and *B*).

> ### 💧 HELPFUL HINT
>
> • The pharyngotracheal lumen airway is best described as an ET tube encased in a large pharyngeal tube.

Each tube has a 15-mm/22-mm connector at its proximal end for attachment of a standard ventilatory device. Housed within the second tube is a semirigid plastic stylet that allows the tube to be redirected. On one side of the cuff inflation valve is a clamp that permits deflation of the oropharyngeal cuff while keeping the other cuff inflated. The device also is equipped with an adjustable cloth neck-strap that keeps the tube in place.

ADVANTAGES AND DISADVANTAGES

Advantages of the pharyngotracheal lumen airway include the following:
- It is inserted blindly, requiring no special equipment or visualization of the upper airway.
- It can be inserted with the patent's head in a neutral position.

- It is not necessary to maintain a face seal because the oropharyngeal cuff eliminates the need for a face mask.
- It can protect the trachea from upper airway bleeding or secretions.
- When the longer tube is situated in the esophagus, the oropharynx cuff can be deflated to allow the device to be moved to the left side of the patient's mouth. This action permits ET intubation while continuing esophageal occlusion.

Disadvantages of the pharyngotracheal lumen airway include the following:
- It is sometimes difficult to identify the tube location, resulting in ventilation being delivered through the wrong tube.
- The pharyngeal or esophageal walls can be torn or ruptured during insertion.
- The device does not keep the patient from aspirating foreign materials such as blood or vomitus present in the upper airway when the longer tube is in the esophagus.
- The pharyngeal balloon can become displaced.
- It cannot be used on patients who are awake.
- It can only be used on adults.
- It can only be used orally.
- It is extremely difficult to intubate around.

CONTRAINDICATIONS

The following contraindications of the pharyngotracheal lumen airway:
- Persons less than 16 years of age
- Persons under 5 ft or more than 6 ft 7 in tall
- Ingestion of caustic substances
- A history of esophageal disease or alcoholism
- The presence of a gag reflex

PROCEDURE

To insert the pharyngotracheal lumen airway, the following steps should be taken:

1. Perform BSI precautions.
2. Open the airway manually using the head-tilt/chin-lift or jaw-thrust maneuver.
3. Preoxygenate with a bag-valve-mask device supplied with 100% oxygen.
4. Ask another EMT–I to take over ventilating the patient.
5. Assemble and check the equipment. Close the relief port with the small white cap, open the slide clamp, and blow air into the inflation valve to check the proximal and distal cuffs for proper inflation (Figure 8-64, A). Once this is done, remove the small white cap and deflate both cuffs fully. Then replace the white cap on the relief port (Figure 8-64, B).
6. Direct the ventilator to move to the side of the patient's head and kneel above the patient.
7. Place the patient's head into a neutral position. Use the tongue/jaw-lift maneuver to move the tongue out of the way.
8. Insert the device into the patient's mouth along the midline. Advance the tube until the flange rests against the patient's teeth (Figure 8-64, C).
9. Loop the white strap around the patient's head and secure it in place (Figure 8-64, D).
10. Once in place, inflate both distal cuffs simultaneously by taking a deep breath and blowing into the inflation valve (Figure 8-64, E).
11. Next, connect a ventilatory device to the green tube (oropharyngeal tube) and deliver a breath. If the chest rises, the longer tube is in the esophagus and ventilations should be continued through the green tube. A gastric tube may be inserted through the long tube into the esophagus and stomach (Figure 8-64, F and G).
12. If the patient's chest does not rise, the longer tube is in the trachea. The stylet must then be removed from the longer tube and assisted breathing provided through the tube (Figure 8-64, H).
13. Continue delivering ventilatory support with a bag-valve-mask device supplied with 100% oxygen or other ventilatory device.
14. Reassess for proper placement on an ongoing basis.

Good assessment skills are needed to properly confirm placement. Use the techniques described under ET intubation to make sure the tube is located properly.

Laryngeal Mask Airway

The laryngeal mask airway (LMA) is a device that was introduced in England in the 1980s and that is gaining popularity in the United States. The proximal end consists of a tube that looks like an ET tube. At its distal end is a silicone rubber "mask" with an inflatable outer rim.

The opening of the tube into the mask is covered by a "grille" (two vertical bars) that supports the epiglottis and keeps it from falling into the opening of the tube. An inflation line is used to inflate the mask and a pilot balloon monitors mask inflation. Once the LMA is properly positioned into a patient's hypopharynx, the cuff is inflated. This seals the larynx and situates the distal opening of the tube just above the glottis thus providing an open, secure airway. At the proximal end of the tube, a standard 15-mm adapter is attached to a bag-valve-mask device for the provision of ventilatory support.

The LMA is a more dependable method of ventilation than the face mask and provides ventilation that is equivalent to an ET tube. Although the LMA does not ensure absolute protection against aspiration, regurgitation is less likely with the LMA than with the bag-mask device (Figure 8-65, A).

The LMA comes in a variety of sizes from 1 for newborns to 4 for adults, as indicated in the following list:

Size 1	Neonates/infants up to 6.5 kg
Size 2	Infants and children up to 20 kg
Size 2½	Children between 20 to 30 kg
Size 3	Children and small adults more than 30 kg
Size 4	Normal and large adults

ADVANTAGES AND DISADVANTAGES

Advantages of the LMA include the following:
• Training in the placement and use of an LMA is simple.
• Visualization is not required for insertion and placement

Other points to remember are that it can be used when access to the patient is limited and there is a possibility of unstable neck injury. However, appropriate positioning of the patient for tracheal intubation is impossible.

Disadvantages of the LMA include the following:
• Even when successfully inserted, some patients cannot be ventilated through it. Because insertion and ventilation are not guaranteed, an alternative strategy for management of the airway must be available to the EMT–I.
• It does not isolate the trachea; therefore it does not protect the airway from regurgitation and aspiration.
• It cannot be used in patients who have a gag reflex or are semiconscious.

PROCEDURE

1. Perform BSI precautions.
2. Open the airway manually using the head-tilt/chin-lift or jaw-thrust maneuver.
3. Preoxygenate with a bag-valve-mask device supplied with 100% oxygen.
4. Ask another EMT–I to take over ventilating the patient.
5. Check for leaks by inflating the LMA mask. Remember to fully deflate the mask before insertion.

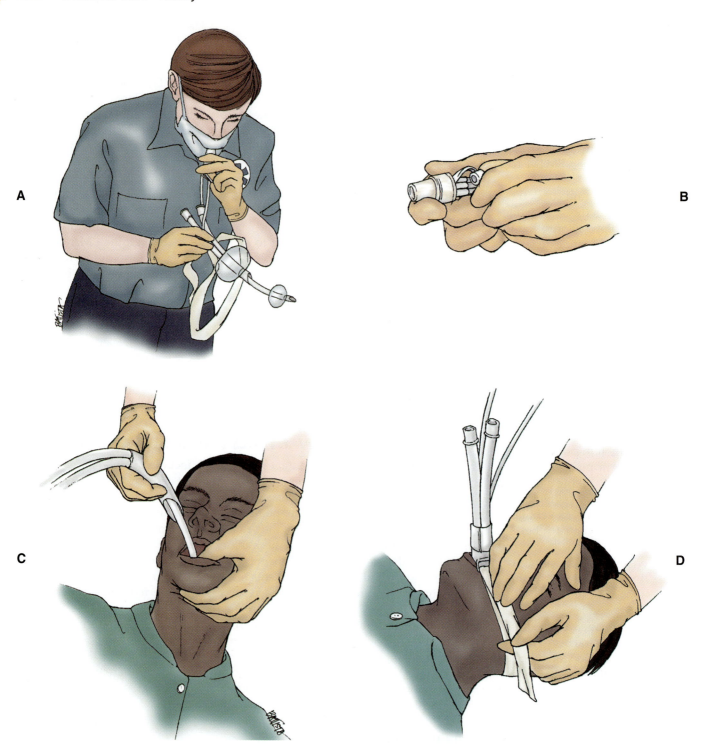

FIGURE 8-64 ▲ Ventilating a patient using a pharyngotracheal lumen airway. **A**, Check the proximal and distal cuffs for proper inflation. **B**, Replace white cap. **C**, Insert the device into the patient's mouth along the midline. **D**, Loop the white strap around the patient's head and secure the tube in place.

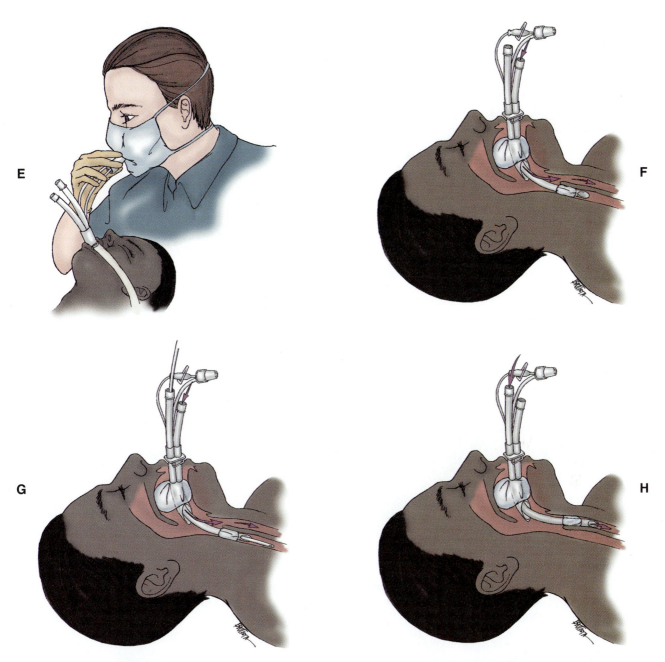

FIGURE 8-64, cont'd ▲ Ventilating a patient using a pharyngotracheal lumen airway. **E,** Inflate both distal cuffs simultaneously. **F,** Ventilate the patient through the green tube to determine if the longer tube is in the esophagus. **G,** If the longer tube is in the esophagus, a gastric tube may be inserted into the esophagus and stomach. **H,** If the longer tube is in the trachea, remove the stylet and proceed with ventilations.

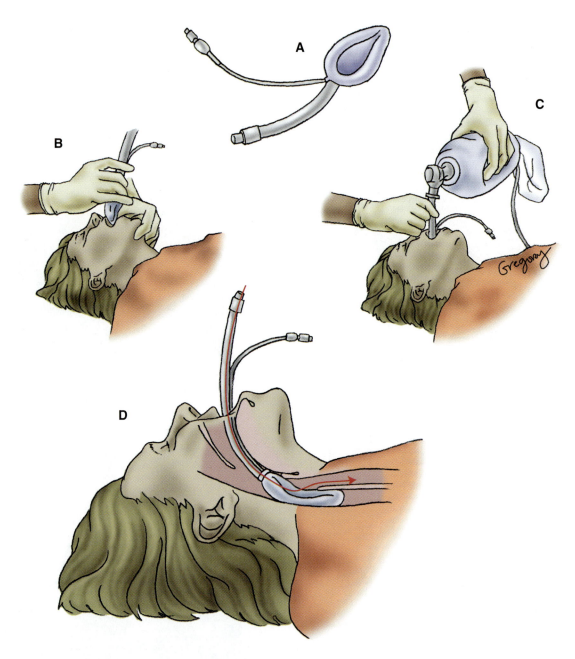

FIGURE 8-65 ▲ **A,** The laryngeal mask airway (LMA). **B,** Insert the LMA. **C,** Provide ventilatory support once the LMA is in place. **D,** Once the LMA is properly seated air has no where to go but into the trachea.

CLINICAL NOTES

Use a 20- to 50-mL syringe to deflate the cuff so it forms as a flat oval disk. Try to eliminate any wrinkles on the distal edge of the rim. A completely smooth, flat leading edge facilitates smooth insertion of the mask and avoids collision with the epiglottis. One way to correctly deflate the cuff is to press the hollow side down onto a clean flat surface, with a finger pressing the tip flat.

CLINICAL NOTES

To keep the lubricant from drying out, lubricate the mask just before insertion. Although it is important to lubricate the back of the mask thoroughly, avoid leaving globs of lubricant on the surface of the cuff or in the bowl of the mask, since this can cause blockage of the aperture or inhalation of lubricant after insertion, leading to coughing or airway obstruction.

6. Use a water-soluble lubricant to lubricate the back of the mask.

7. Direct the ventilator to move to the side of the patient's head and assume a position above the patient. Instruct to pull the lower jaw downward so that the mask is not folding over in the oral cavity as it is inserted.

8. Push the patient's head from behind using the free hand, so as to simultaneously extend the head and flex the neck. Keep this hand in this position throughout the whole insertion procedure. If necessary, use a pillow or rolled blanket to keep the neck flexed.

9. Grasp the LMA by the tube, holding it between the first finger and thumb as near as possible to the mask end. With the opening facing forward (away from self), place the extreme tip of the mask against the inner surface of the patient's upper incisor teeth (or gums). The black line on the tube should be aligned with the middle of the patient's nose.

10. Use the middle finger to push the lower jaw downward. This makes it easier to see into the mouth and verify the position of the mask. It will also enable the insertion of the index finger further into the mouth during insertion of the LMA.

11. Press the mask tip upward against the hard palate to flatten it out, simultaneously advancing it into the oral cavity. Keep it pressed upward as it is advanced and note whether it remains flattened out against the hard palate (Figure 8-65, *B*).

CLINICAL NOTES

If the mask fails to flatten out or starts to roll over as you advance it, withdraw it and start again. Check to make sure the lubricant has not dried out and the cuff is correctly deflated.

12. If the mask tip is advancing against the palate without curling over, continue inserting it. Push upward by pressing in and down with the index finger located at the junction of the mask and tube. The finger should be kept in this position while the mask is inserted into the pharynx and behind the tongue, since it provides a sense of direction as the mask tip follows the posterior pharyngeal wall downward. The mask may rarely deflect upward. If this occurs, remove and reinsert the device.

13. With one smooth motion, continue pushing with the finger (in place at the junction of the tube and mask), guiding the mask downward into position. Resistance should be felt as the mask tip comes to rest against the upper esophageal sphincter.

TABLE 8-3

Cuff Inflation Volumes

Size 1	2 to 4 mL
Size 2	Up to 10 mL
Size 2.5	Up to 15 mL
Size 3	20 mL
Size 4	30 mL

CLINICAL NOTES

If resistance is felt at this point, the mask tip has most likely folded over on itself or has impacted on an irregularity or swelling in the posterior pharynx. Force should not be used at this point, since it can cause bleeding or soreness. If tonsillar tissue is causing the obstruction, a diagonal shift in direction often allows successful insertion. Alternatively, a gloved finger inserted behind the mask to lift it forward over the obstruction may help to resolve the problem.

14. Grasp the tube firmly with the other hand and then withdraw the index finger from the pharynx. Press gently downward with the other hand to ensure the mask is fully inserted.

15. Use your prefilled syringe to inflate the cuff with the correct volume (Table 8-3). A small amount of outward movement (up to approx 1.5 cm) is normal during inflation. Expect to see a "fullness in the neck" once the mask is inflated. Usually the cuff is inflated without holding onto the tube. This allows the expanding cuff to find its correct place in the pharynx. However, in lightweight patients and some elderly patients in whom the tissues are very slack and the neck is short or at times when the mask size is too large for the patient or the cuff is overinflated, the LMA may start to slide up and out of the pharynx. When this occurs, despite using the correct size and amount of inflation, it may be necessary to hold the tube until it is secured in place.

16. Attach a ventilatory device to the 15-mm/22-mm adapter of the tube and deliver several breaths (Figure 8-65, *C* and *D*). Hold the LMA in place to prevent it from being pulled out of position by the weight of the ventilatory device.

17. Confirm tube placement by assessing for the absence of epigastric sounds and presence of bilateral breath sounds. Furthermore, an end tidal carbon dioxide detector should be used to confirm correct placement.

18. Insert an oropharyngeal airway or a bite block to prevent the patient from biting down on the tube.

19. Once proper placement is confirmed, secure the LMA in place.

20. Ventilate the patient with a bag-valve-mask device supplied with 100% oxygen or alternative ventilatory device.

COMPLICATIONS

Improper alignment of the LMA in the hypopharynx can cause airway obstruction and air escaping around the mouth, resulting from mask deflation or improper mask seal, which leads to ineffective ventilation. To optimize insertion rates and minimize complications, EMT–Is must receive adequate initial training in the use of the LMA and practice with the device regularly.

Foreign Bodies
PATHOPHYSIOLOGY

A foreign body that becomes lodged in the laryngopharynx is another cause of upper airway obstruction. In the adult, the source is usually food (particularly meat). Common factors associated with choking on food include large, poorly chewed pieces of meat; alcohol consumption; laughing, talking, or exercising while eating; or dentures. This emergency often occurs in restaurants and is mistaken for a heart attack, giving rise to the name, "cafe coronary." In children, the obstruction typically is due to food or other objects such as bubble gum, balloons, marbles, beads, coins, or small toy parts.

- **Stridor** • A high-pitched noise heard on inspiration.
- **Cyanosis** • Bluish color to the skin, seen with hypoxia.

ASSESSMENT

Airway obstruction may be partial or complete. With partial airway obstruction, air exchange may be good or poor. Good air exchange exists when the patient is able to generate an effective cough. Poor air exchange is present when the patient is unable to generate an effective cough, when **stridor** is heard during inhalation, and when there is increased breathing difficulty and **cyanosis.**

- **Retraction** • The inward movement of the soft tissues of the chest, commonly, the suprasternal notch and the intercostal spaces. Usually associated with respiratory compromise or airway obstruction.
- **Tracheal Tugging** • Condition in which the Adam's apple appears to be pulled upward on inspiration. It occurs in the presence of airway obstruction.

Airway obstruction is complete when the patient is unable to speak, breathe, or cough; airflow is not felt or heard from the nose and mouth; and spontaneous breath-

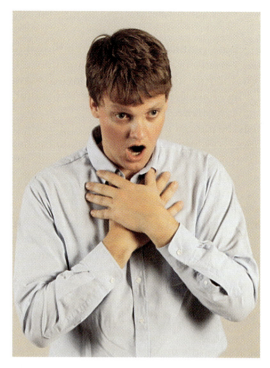

FIGURE 8-66 ▲ The typical sign that a patient is experiencing an upper airway obstruction. (American Red Cross from *First aid: responding to emergencies,* St Louis, 1991, Mosby. All rights reserved in all countries.)

ing efforts result in **retraction** of the supraclavicular and intercostal areas. **Tracheal tugging** and an absence of chest expansion also occurs. The classic sign of complete upper airway obstruction is the patient clutching his or her neck between the thumb and fingers. This gesture is referred to as the *universal distress signal* (Figure 8-66).

In complete airway obstruction, the patient becomes unresponsive quickly, and death occurs if the obstruction is unrelieved. When spontaneous breathing is absent, complete airway obstruction can be recognized by persistent difficulty that is encountered when attempting to deliver assisted breathing to the patient.

BASIC TREATMENT

With adequate air exchange, treatment is directed toward supporting and encouraging the patient to cough. Supplemental oxygen should be provided if the patient is becoming hypoxic. In poor air exchange or with complete obstruction, treatment is aimed at relieving the obstruction. This relief is accomplished by using abdominal thrusts (also referred to as the *Heimlich maneuver*).

PROCEDURE

To relieve airway obstruction in the responsive patient, the following steps should be taken:

1. Ask the victim, "Are you choking?" (Figure 8-67, *A*).

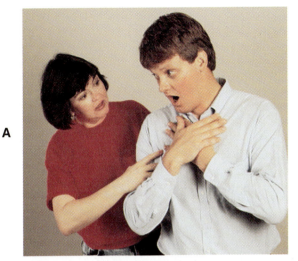

A

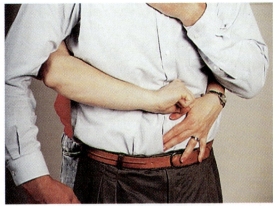

B

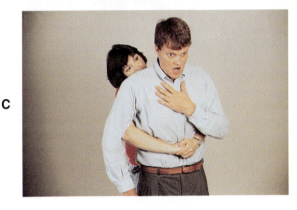

C

FIGURE 8-67 ▲ Relieving airway obstruction in conscious patients. **A,** Ask the victim, "Are you choking?" **B,** Make a fist and place the thumb side against the patient's abdomen just above the navel. **C,** Grasp the fist with the other hand and press into the victim's abdomen in an upward motion. (American Red Cross from *First aid: responding to emergencies,* St Louis, 1991, Mosby. All rights reserved in all countries.)

2. Determine if complete airway obstruction is present (as previously described).
3. Deliver abdominal thrusts.
   • Stand behind the patient and wrap the arms around the patient's abdomen.
   • Make a fist and place the thumb side against the patient's abdomen in the midline slightly above the navel but well below the xiphoid process (Figure 8-67, *B*).
   • Grasp the fist with the other hand and press into the victim's abdomen with quick upward thrusts (Figure 8-67, *C*).
4. Continue these procedures until the obstruction is dislodged or the patient becomes unresponsive.

PROCEDURE

To relieve airway obstruction in the unresponsive patient, the following steps should be taken:
1. Check for responsiveness (if in a bystander role [e.g., off duty], activate the EMS system).
2. Open the airway using the head-tilt/chin-lift maneuver.
3. Check for breathing.
4. Attempt to deliver two slow breaths.
5. Reposition the head and try to give rescue breaths again.

6. Straddle the victim's thighs and give up to five subdiaphragmatic abdominal thrusts (Figure 8-68, *A*).
7. Perform tongue/jaw-lift maneuver and finger sweep (Figs. 8-68, *B* and *C*).
8. Repeat steps until the obstruction is resolved.

DIRECT LARYNGOSCOPY

Sometimes, despite employing basic life support procedures such as the Heimlich maneuver, finger sweep, and chest thrust, the airway remains obstructed. In these cases, when the patient is unconscious and cannot be ventilated, the EMT–I can use direct laryngoscopy to remove the foreign body. Begin by inserting the laryngoscope blade into the patient's mouth as during orotracheal intubation. If the foreign body is visualized carefully, then the foreign body can be deliberately removed with the Magill forceps (Figure 8-69).

Aspiration

✖ **Regurgitation** • A passive, backward flow of gastric contents from the stomach into the oropharynx.

✖ **Aspirate** • The taking of foreign material into the lungs during inhalation.

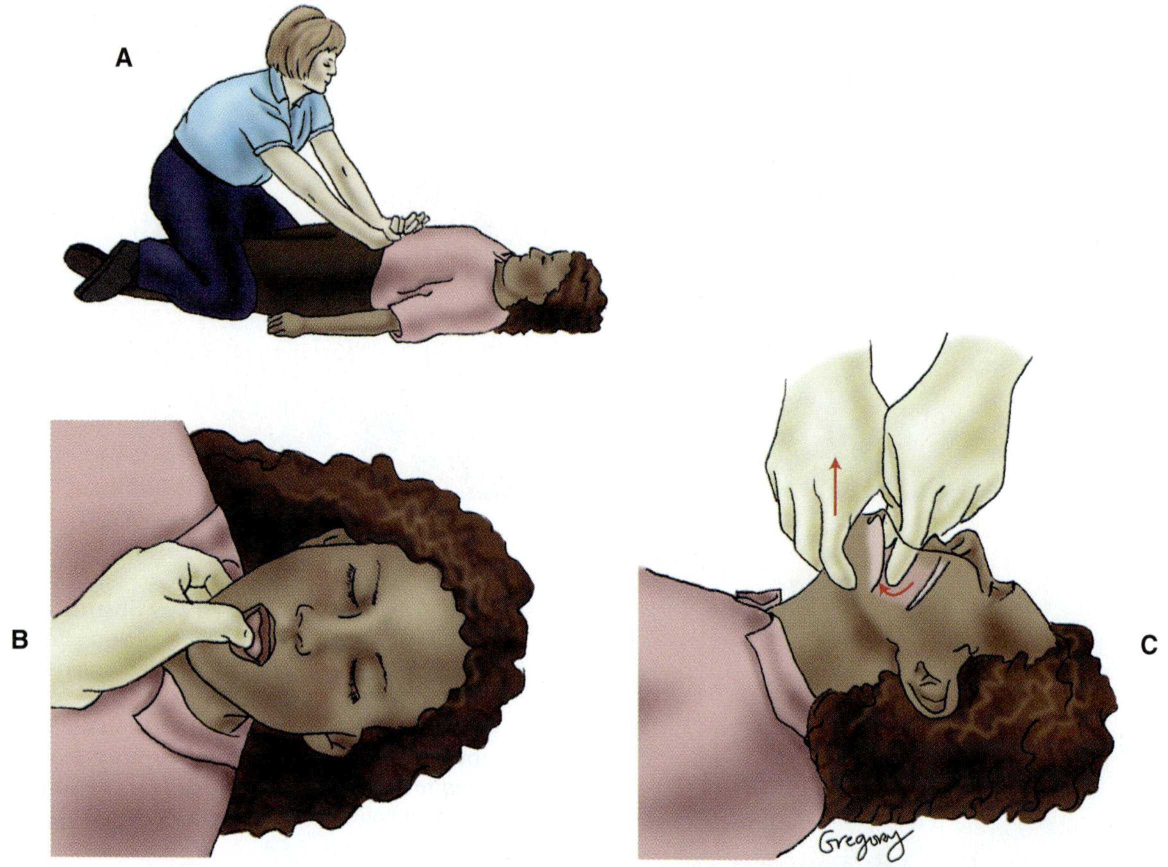

FIGURE 8-68 ▲ Relieving an airway obstruction in an unresponsive patient. **A**, Straddle the victim's thighs and give up to five abdominal thrusts. **B**, Perform tongue-jaw lift. **C**, Perform a finger sweep.

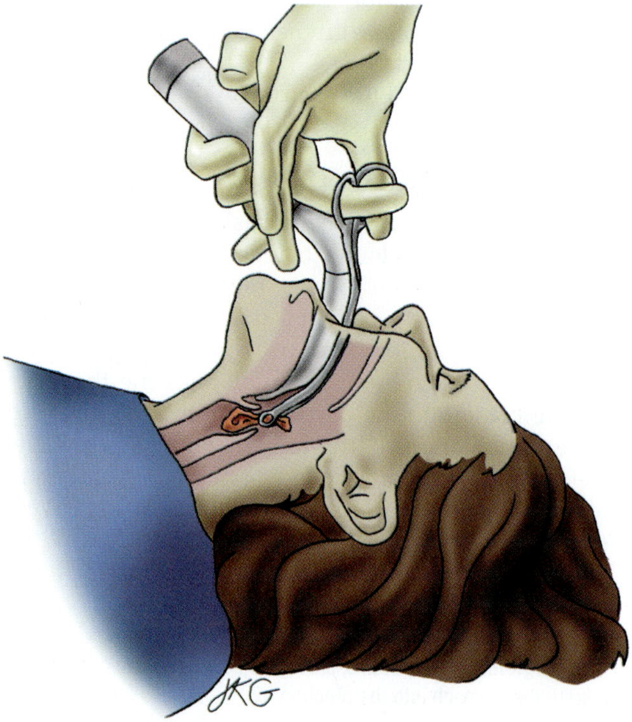

FIGURE 8-69 ▲ Using the Magill forceps to relieve an airway obstruction.

PATHOPHYSIOLOGY

Other objects including loose dentures, teeth, blood, fluids, and vomitus also can obstruct the upper airway.

Hypercarbia • Excessive partial pressure of carbon dioxide in the blood.

Vomitus, typically **regurgitation** from the stomach into the oropharynx during states of decreased responsiveness, contains partially dissolved food, protein dissolving enzymes, and hydrochloric acid. If the person **aspirates** this into the lungs, the combination can lead to increased interstitial fluid, pulmonary edema, and destruction of the alveoli. This condition seriously impairs gas exchange and leads to hypoxemia and **hypercarbia.** Furthermore, food particles can obstruct the bronchiolar airways, thus compromising airflow. Saliva, like vomitus, contains certain digestive enzymes. It too can fill the alveoli, causing similar problems. Mortality increases significantly if aspiration occurs.

ASSESSMENT

Gurgling sounds heard on inspiration and/or expiration indicates the accumulation of fluids or vomitus in the upper airway.

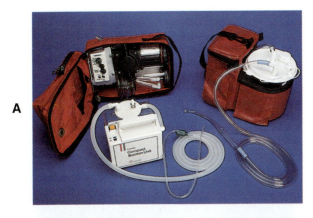

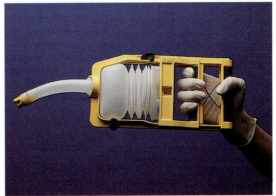

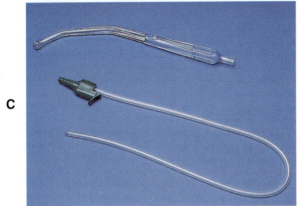

FIGURE 8-70 ▲ Types of suction units. **A,** Portable suction unit. **B,** Hand-held portable suction unit. **C,** Rigid (top) and soft (bottom) suction catheters. (From Vincent Knaus from Stoy W: *Mosby's EMT–Basic textbook,* St Louis, 1996, Mosby.)

TABLE 8-4

Comparison of Various Devices

TYPE	ADVANTAGES	DISADVANTAGES
Hand-powered	Lightweight, portable, mechanically simple, inexpensive	Limited volume, manually powered, fluid components not disposable
Oxygen-powered	Lightweight, small in size	Limited suctioning power, uses a lot of oxygen
Battery-operated	Lightweight, portable, excellent suction power, simple operation, and easy to troubleshoot most problems	More complicated mechanics, may lose battery integrity over time, some components that come into contact with fluids may not be disposable
Mounted vacuum-powered	Extremely strong vacuum, adjustable vacuum power, components that come into contact with fluids are disposable	Nonportable, cannot "field service" or substitute power source

BASIC TREATMENT

Prompt intervention with cricoid pressure, suctioning, and positioning of the patient usually can prevent aspiration.

Suctioning

Suctioning is used to remove vomitus, blood, fluids, and secretions from the airway. A variety of devices are available for the prehospital setting, including portable and stationary units (Figure 8-70, *A* to *C*). Each device is capable of generating vacuum levels of at least 300 mm

Hg when the distal end is occluded and allows a free air flow rate of at least 30 L/min when the tube is open.

Portable units allow suctioning to be done immediately rather than waiting until the patient is in the ambulance. Some are hand-, foot-, or oxygen-powered, whereas others are battery-powered. Many of today's hand-held units are capable of generating excellent suctioning pressures, and because of their small size (often weighing only 1 pound or so), they can be easily stored in an airway kit (Table 8-4).

The two most common types of suction catheters are the tonsil tip and whistle tip. The tonsil tip (also referred to as the *Yankauer suction*) is a rigid tube that has a ball-like tip with multiple holes at its distal end. Some catheters are supplied with an open tip. The tonsil-tip suction catheter is designed to remove larger particles and voluminous secretions. It can be inserted along an oropharyngeal airway or used during laryngoscopy.

The whistle-tip suction catheter is a small, easy-to-use, flexible tube that is long enough to extend into the lower respiratory tract. It can be inserted through the nares, into the oropharynx or nasopharynx, through a nasopharyngeal airway, along an oropharyngeal airway, or through an ET tube.

DISADVANTAGES

One of the disadvantages of tonsil-tip suctioning is that it is limited to suctioning of the upper airway. Additionally, vigorous insertion can cause lacerations or other injuries. As for whistle-tip suctioning, it can be ineffective in removing large volumes of secretions rapidly and is often unable to retrieve even smaller food particles.

PRECAUTIONS

Each suctioning attempt should be restricted to 15 seconds or less. This is so that during suctioning, breathing assistance is interrupted and the air the patient receives is depleted of oxygen. If possible, the patient should be ventilated with 100% oxygen both before and after each suctioning attempt. However, when fluids are present in the upper airway and assisted breathing may lead to aspiration, the airway should be cleared before ventilation is begun.

STREET WISE

Suction should not be activated during insertion of the catheter because it depletes the air of oxygen.

Once the catheter is properly positioned, suction should be applied, and the catheter withdrawn. Most suction catheters have a control opening at the proximal end that allows suction through the catheter to be started or stopped. If the suction catheter is not equipped with a control opening, one can be created by making a small slit in the catheter or suction tubing. Alternatively, turning the suction unit on and off as needed can control suction.

When fluids in the upper airway are so voluminous or thick that the tonsil-tip or whistle-tip suction catheters cannot provide adequate suctioning, the catheter should be removed and the thick-walled, wide-bore suction tubing should be used alone. Water should

be suctioned through the tubing between suctioning attempts to dilute the secretions and facilitate flow through the tubing. Any blockage of the tubing, even partial, can cut down on suction pressure and make the device less effective. It is important to keep the tubing as clean as possible.

HAZARDS

The following hazards are associated with suctioning:
- Serious cardiac dysrhythmias can occur secondary to hypoxia.
- The suction tube can stimulate the airway mucosa, causing hypertension and tachycardia or bradycardia and hypotension (vagal stimulation).
- Suctioning can stimulate the airway mucosa, triggering the patient to cough. This can result in increased intracranial pressure and reduced cerebral blood flow.

PROCEDURE

To suction the upper airway of a patient, the following steps should be taken:
1. Perform BSI precautions.
2. If possible, preoxygenate with a bag-valve-mask device supplied with 100% oxygen.
3. Determine the depth for catheter insertion by measuring from the patient's lips to the earlobe (Figure 8-71, *A*).
4. Insert the suction catheter to the proper depth (Figure 8-71, *B*).
5. Turn the suction unit on or place the thumb over suction control opening, limiting suction to 15 seconds.
6. Withdraw the catheter. When using a whistle-tip catheter, rotate it between the fingertips to keep it from adhering to the pharyngeal wall (Figure 8-71, *C*).
7. Flush out the suction catheter and tubing with saline. Then evaluate the patency of the airway and whether there is a need for additional suctioning.
8. Ventilate the patient with a bag-valve-mask device supplied with 100% oxygen or alternative ventilatory device.

ALTERNATIVE PROCEDURES

It also may be necessary to place the patient on his or her side and use the fingers to clear substances from the patient's mouth.

Tracheobronchial Suctioning

It may be necessary to suction patients through an ET or tracheostomy tube to remove mucous plugs or secretions causing respiratory compromise. Because tracheobronchial suctioning can bring about hypoxia, the patient must be preoxygenated before and after the procedure. If possible, a sterile technique should be

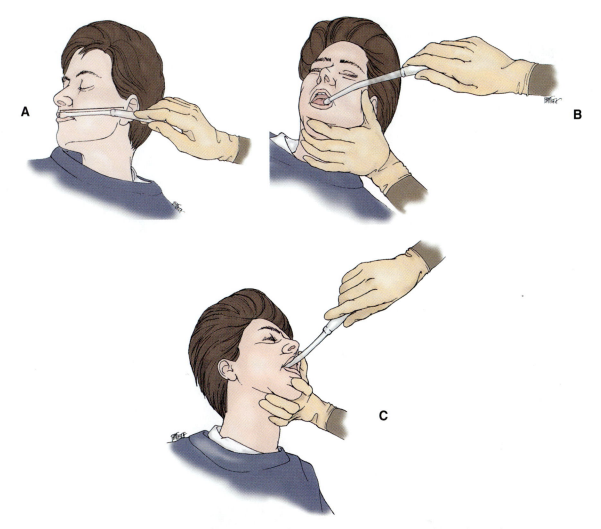

FIGURE 8-71 ▲ Suctioning a patient's airway. **A,** Measure the catheter from the tip of the patient's ear to the corner of the mouth. **B,** With suction off, insert the catheter into the patient's mouth to the proper depth. **C,** With suction on, withdraw the catheter.

used. To avoid damaging tissue, only a soft-tip catheter should be employed. It may be necessary to inject 3 to 5 mL of sterile water into the ET tube to loosen tenacious secretions. Throughout the procedure the cardiac rhythm should be monitored. If dysrhythmias or bradycardia develops the suctioning should be stopped and the patient reoxygenated.

PROCEDURE

To perform tracheobronchial suctioning, the following steps should be taken:

1. Perform BSI precautions.
2. Preoxygenate with a bag-valve-mask device supplied with 100% oxygen for approximately 5 minutes (unless the tube is completely blocked, then suctioning must begin immediately to relieve the obstruction).
3. Determine the depth for catheter insertion by measuring from the patient's lips to the earlobe.

4. Open the catheter package (if the catheter is wrapped separately) (Figure 8-72, *A*).
5. Grasp the catheter with your sterile gloved hand. Measure the catheter to determine the appropriate insertion depth. (Figure 8-72, *B*).
6. Keeping it coiled, loop it around your hand to prevent contaminating it by touching nonsterile objects.
7. Lubricate the catheter tip with a water-soluble gel or dip in sterile saline. This facilitates passage of the catheter through the ET tube.
8. Insert the suction catheter into the opening of the ET tube without touching the sides of the ET tube (Figure 8-72, *C*). Pass the tube to the proper depth (about the level of the carina or until resistance is felt) (Figure 8-72, *D* and *E*).
9. Turn the suction unit on or place the thumb over suction control opening, limiting suction to 15 seconds.
10. Withdraw the catheter rotating it between the fingertips (Figure 8-72, *F*).

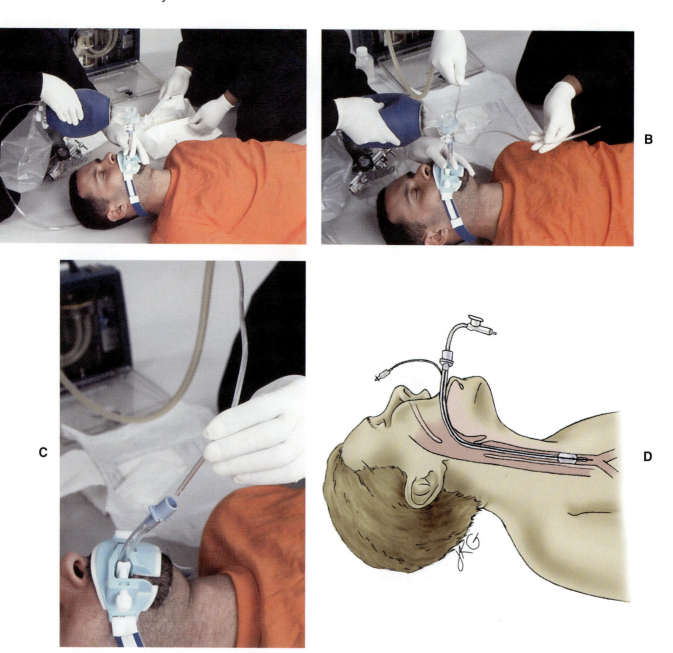

FIGURE 8-72 ▲ Performing tracheobronchial suctioning. **A,** Prepare equipment. **B,** Measure the suction catheter to determine proper insertion depth. **C,** Insert suction catheter into opening of ET tube. **D** and **E,** Pass the suction catheter to the proper depth, and withdraw the suction catheter while rotating it.

11. Flush out the suction catheter and tubing with saline and evaluate the need for additional suctioning and the patency of the airway (Figure 8-72, *G*).

12. Ventilate the patient with a bag-valve-mask device supplied with 100% oxygen or alternative ventilatory device.

To reduce the risk of contamination a fresh sterile suction catheter should be used with each suctioning attempt.

Gastric Distention

If inadequate positioning obstructs the airway or high pressures are used during ventilation, air can enter the stomach instead of the lungs. This air becomes trapped in the stomach, leading to gastric distention. As more air is introduced the abdomen becomes increasingly distended. Possible complications of this condition include decreased lung expansion due to the diaphragm pushing up against the thoracic cavity; resistance to bag-valve-mask ventilation (making it difficult to exchange

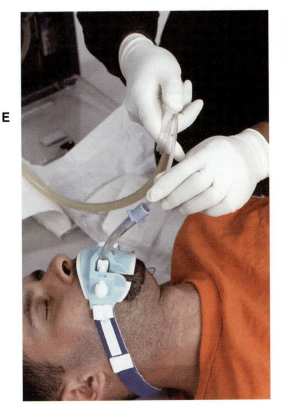

E

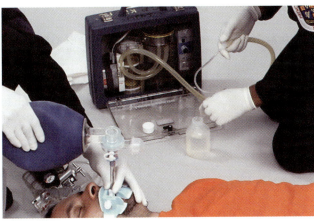

F

FIGURE 8-72, cont'd ▲ Performing tracheobronchial suctioning. **D** and **E,** Pass the suction catheter to the proper depth, and withdraw the suction catheter while rotating it. **F,** Flush the catheter and tubing with saline.

an adequate amount of air); regurgitation of the stomach contents with possible aspiration; and even gastric rupture. Gastric distension is very common when ventilating nonintubated patients. The potential for gastric distension can be reduced by increasing bag-valve-mask ventilation time for adults to 1.5 to 2 seconds and pediatric patients to 1 to 1.5 seconds.

When gastric distension occurs in the field setting and is interfering with ventilations, measures must be taken to relieve it. After placing the patient into a left lateral position (his or her side), the EMT–I should place one hand over the epigastrium, between the umbilicus and the rib cage, and slowly exert moderate pressure. A suction unit should be available to clear the upper airway in case of regurgitation (be prepared for a large volume). Relieving gastric distension is performed using extreme caution and only when absolutely necessary.

Gastric Tubes

Sometimes it is necessary to place a specialized suction tube into the stomach to relieve gastric distension and/or control emesis. It is referred to as a *gastric tube* and is indicated when a patient is likely to aspirate or there is a need for gastric lavage. Complications of this procedure include nasal, esophageal or gastric trauma from poor technique, accidental ET placement, supragastric placement, and tube obstruction. The gastric tube can be inserted through either the nasopharynx or

oropharynx. Orogastric decompression is generally preferred for unconscious patients. Orogastric decompression is contraindicated in esophageal obstruction and should be done with extreme caution in esophageal disease, esophageal trauma, and facial trauma. Nasogastric decompression is contraindicated in patients with esophageal varices, facial trauma or severe head trauma (Table 8-5).

> ### CLINICAL NOTES
>
> Nasogastric tube placement should be avoided when severe facial trauma is present, since the patient may have a fracture of the cribriform plate and the tube may be accidentally passed into the cranial cavity.

Equipment used to perform this procedure includes a nasogastric tube, 50-mL irrigation syringe, water-soluble lubricant, adhesive tape, saline for irrigation, emesis basis, and gloves.

PROCEDURE

To perform a gastric tube insertion, the following steps should be taken:
1. Assess the need for gastric tube placement.
2. Perform BSI precautions.

TABLE 8-5

Advantages and Disadvantages of Nasogastric and Orogastric Tubes

	NASOGASTRIC	OROGASTRIC
Advantages	• Tolerated by awake patients • Does not interfere with intubation • Mitigates recurrent gastric distension • Mitigates nausea • Patient can still talk	• Can use larger tubes • Can lavage more aggressively • Safe to use in facial fracture as it avoids the nasopharynx
Disadvantages	• Uncomfortable for patient • May cause patient to vomit during placement even if gag is suppressed • Interferes with bag-valve-mask seal	• May interfere with visualization during intubation • Patient may bite tube

3. Assemble the necessary equipment.
4. Prepare the patient by placing his or her head into a neutral or flexed head position.
5. Preoxygenate with a bag-valve-mask device supplied with 100% oxygen.
6. Check the nose for any deformity or obstruction that may make inserting a nasogastric tube difficult. Determine the best side for insertion (usually the patient's right nostril).
7. Determine the length of tube insertion by placing the tip of the tube at the earlobe and running the length of the tube to the nose and then the xiphoid process. Mark the point the tube should be inserted to with a piece of tape (Figure 8-73, *A* and *B*).
8. If the patient is awake, apply a local anesthetic to the nares or oropharynx. Suppress the gag reflex as well, by applying topical anesthetic to the posterior oropharynx or administering IV lidocaine. Follow local protocol.
9. Lubricate 6 to 8 inches of the nasogastric tube with viscous lidocaine (Xylocaine) or a water-soluble gel (Figure 8-73, *C*).
10. Keep an emesis basin handy in case the patient vomits.
11. Insert the tube into the nostril and advance it gently along the nasal floor or alternatively, into the oral cavity at the midline (Figure 8-73, *D*).
12. Gently advance the tube to the predetermined length (into the stomach). As the tube passes into the oropharynx, if the patient is conscious, encourage him or her to swallow or drink to facilitate passage. Do not force the tube if resistance is met. *If respiratory distress is noted, withdraw the tube immediately. This may indicate placement into the trachea or bronchus.*

HELPFUL HINT

When you feel the tube reach the nasopharyngeal junction, rotate it inward toward the other nostril. Then gently advance the tube until it is in the nasopharynx.

13. Confirm placement by the following two methods:
    • Auscultate the epigastrium for sounds (like a rush of air) while injecting 30 to 50 mL of air (Figure 8-73, *E*).
    • Aspirate gastric contents; ensure there is no reflux around the tube (Figure 8-73, *F*).
14. Tape the gastric tube in place (Figure 8-73, *G*) and connect it to low suction (if ordered).
15. Document the size of the tube inserted, degree of difficulty, tube placement checked, complications such as bleeding or vomiting, and the name of the person performing the procedure.

SPECIAL PATIENT CONSIDERATIONS

Airway Management For Patients With A Stoma

Persons with a laryngectomy (removal of the larynx) or tracheostomy (surgical opening into the trachea) breathe through an opening in the anterior neck that connects the trachea with the outside air. This opening is called a *stoma*. These patients often have tracheostomy tubes, which are made of an inner and outer cannula, in place to keep the soft tissue stoma open.

The two problems the EMT–I may see with tracheostomy patients are obstruction and stenosis.

OBSTRUCTION

A person with a laryngectomy possesses a less effective cough, making it difficult to clear secretions. If these secretions accumulate, they can form a mucous plug that can obstruct the stoma and interfere with air exchange leading to respiratory distress. The accumulated secretions can also dry, forming encrustations that can further block the airway. A tracheostomy tube typically has a fixed outer piece and an inner cannula. When mucous obstructs a double tube, the inner cannula can be

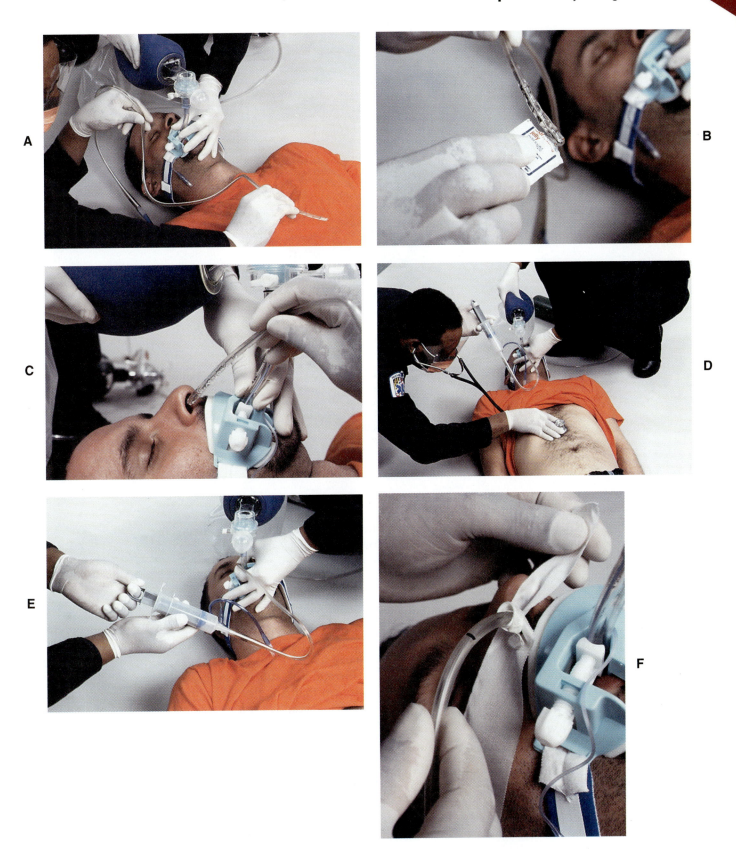

FIGURE 8-73 ▲ **A,** Place tip of tube at earlobe, then run length of tube to nose, then run length of tube from nose to xiphoid process. **B,** Lubricate tube. **C,** Insert tube into nostril. **D,** Auscultate epigastrium for sounds. **E,** Aspirate gastric contents. **F,** Tape gastric tube in place.

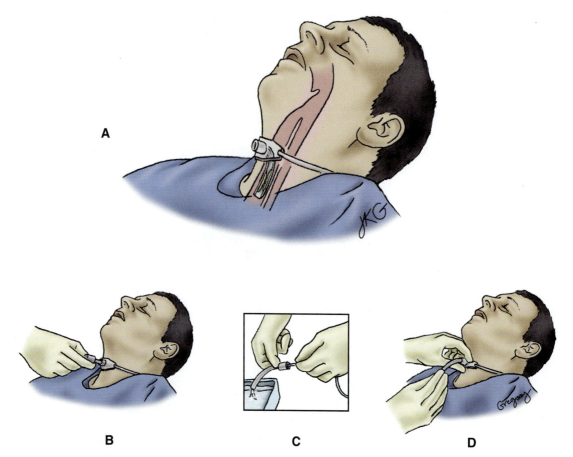

FIGURE 8-74 ▲ **A,** Obstructed tracheostomy tube. **B,** Removing inner cannula. **C,** Cleaning inner cannula. **D,** Reinserting cannula.

easily removed and cleaned with sterile water or saline, then put back (Figure 8-74, *A, B,* and *C*). Alternatively, the inner cannula can be left in place and suction used to remove the mucous. If the outer cannula must also be removed, it has to be replaced promptly because the stoma can constrict within just a few hours and prohibit replacement of the outer piece without first dilating the stoma.

STENOSIS

Tracheal stenosis is the spontaneous narrowing of the trachea at the site of the cuff. It can develop anywhere from 1 week to years after the tracheostomy tube has been placed. Any acute inflammation that leads to soft tissue swelling can reduce the diameter of the stoma and tracheal opening, producing potentially life-threatening stenosis. This stenosis can make putting the cannula back into place very difficult or impossible. If this occurs, the EMT–I must insert the largest-diameter ET tube (5.0 or greater) that will pass through the stoma before total obstruction occurs. Begin by lu-

bricating the ET tube, instruct the patient to exhale, and gently insert the tube approximately 1 to 2 cm beyond the distal cuff. Then inflate the cuff and verify comfort, patency, and correct placement. Check to ensure the tube hasn't been improperly placed into the surrounding subcutaneous tissue. This creates a false lumen that is indicated by the development of subcutaneous emphysema as well as the lack of clinical improvement in the patient.

SUCTIONING

Suctioning must be done with extreme caution if laryngeal edema is suspected, since this procedure can itself cause swelling of the soft tissue. To suction, begin by preoxygenating the patient with 100% oxygen. Inject 3 mL sterile saline through the stoma and down the trachea. Instruct the patient to exhale and then gently introduce the catheter until resistance is met. Although the patient coughs or exhales, suction the airway during withdrawal of the catheter (Figure 8-75, *A, B,* and *C*).

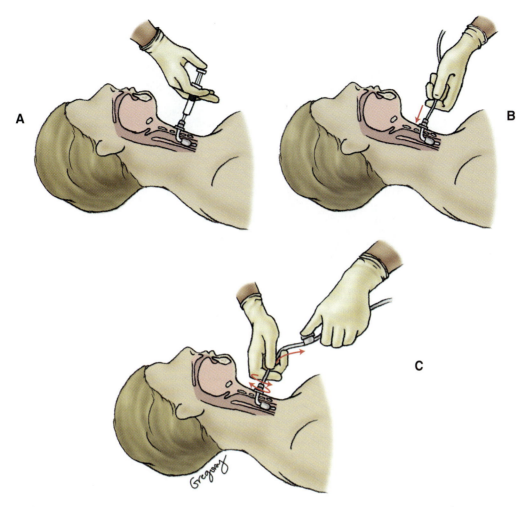

FIGURE 8-75 ▲ **A,** Instill 3 ml sterile saline. **B,** Introduce suction catheter.
C, Apply suction while withdrawing the catheter (rotating it with fingertips).

Airway Management For Patients With Facial Injuries

PATHOPHYSIOLOGY

Trauma to the head, face, or neck can lead to airway obstruction by cluttering the airway with broken teeth, facial bones, tissue, and blood. When blood is aspirated into the lungs, it can clog the bronchi and alveoli with clots that obstruct airflow. A fractured mandible, when displaced backward, can push the tongue backward with it and obstruct the airway. Direct injury to the larynx and trachea from a blunt instrument, bullet, or knife can also result in airway obstruction due to the rapid accumulation of blood in the tissues surrounding the wound or by fracturing or displacing the larynx, allowing the vocal cords to collapse into the tracheal opening. Facial injuries should lead to a high suspicion of cervical spine injury.

ASSESSMENT

As with aspiration, gurgling sounds heard on inspiration and expiration indicate the accumulation of fluids or blood in the upper airway. Stridor is indicative of upper airway obstruction due to swelling.

TREATMENT

Establishing and maintaining an open airway is a critical aspect of trauma care. Steps used to manage the trauma patient depend on the location and extent of the injuries. In-line stabilization is an important part of managing patients who sustain significant trauma. Suctioning is used to remove blood and small particles from the oropharynx and upper airway. In extreme cases, the patient's whole body should be rolled to the side while maintaining in-line support of the head to allow drainage of blood from the patient's mouth. If the trauma is limited to the mandible, insertion of a nasopharyngeal airway may be useful. Placement of an ET tube can be used to seal off the trachea, preventing aspiration.

If ET intubation is needed to manage the airway of the trauma patient special techniques must be employed to limit movement of the cervical spine during

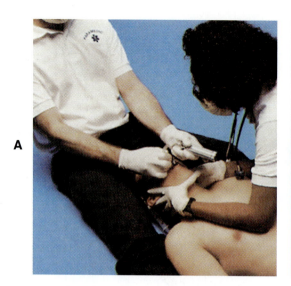
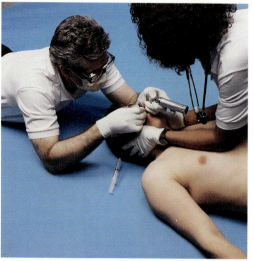

FIGURE 8-76   ▲   **A,** Intubation in a sitting position. **B,** Intubation in a prone position. (From Sanders MJ: *Mosby's paramedic textbook,* ed 2, St Louis, 2000, Mosby.)

laryngoscopy. A cervical collar alone will not provide adequate stabilization of the cervical spine.

There are several methods for performing orotracheal intubation with in-line stabilization. Most call for one team member to immobilize the head and spine while a second team member performs ET intubation. The first team member begins by facing the patient from the patient's side. Manual in-line stabilization is applied by placing the hands over the patient's ears, with the third and fourth fingers placed under the occipital skull and the thumbs on the face over the maxillary sinuses. Slight pressure is applied caudally to support and immobilize the head and neck. The second team member then intubates the patient as described earlier. Stabilization is maintained in a neutral position throughout the procedure (Figure 8-76, *A* and *B*).

If there is an inability to ventilate or perform orotracheal intubation, surgical intervention may be required.

Laryngeal Edema or Spasm

PATHOPHYSIOLOGY

Laryngeal edema and spasm also can lead to upper airway obstruction. As discussed earlier, the glottis is the narrowest part of the adult's upper airway. Edema or spasm of the vocal cords is a potentially lethal condition, because even moderate swelling can severely obstruct airflow through the glottis, resulting in asphyxia.

In adults, laryngeal edema can result from anaphylaxis, epiglottitis, and inhalation of super-heated air, smoke, or toxic substances. In children, upper airway obstruction related to laryngeal edema typically is caused by epiglottitis or croup. Epiglottitis can develop rapidly, causing the epiglottis to swell. In extreme cases, it can enlarge to the point where it obstructs the glottis and causes suffocation. With croup, there is edema of the loose tissues just below the larynx. In the smaller-diameter tracheas of children, this partial airway obstruction can cause complete airway obstruction.

ASSESSMENT

The patient with allergies may report an itching sensation in the palate, followed by the sensation of a lump in the throat. Hoarseness develops, progressing rapidly to cough and inspiratory stridor. Hives also may be present. As respiratory distress becomes more marked, retraction of the intercostal and neck muscles becomes evident on inspirations.

TREATMENT

Emergency management is aimed at reversing swelling and improving oxygenation. In the presence of allergic reaction or anaphylaxis, the administration of epinephrine can prove life saving.

CASE HISTORY FOLLOW-UP ■ ■ ■

EMT–I Simms continues to administer 100% oxygen and assist ventilations en route to the trauma center. The patient's carotid pulse grows stronger and slows from 140 to 90 per minute. His pulse oximetry reading raises from 78% to 92%, and he begins responding with purposeful movement.

In another few minutes, however, he begins to struggle against the straps, fighting EMT–I Simms' attempts to ventilate him. His face becomes flushed, and his neck muscles strain. EMT–I Simms has to extubate him.

EMT–I Simms turns on the suction and places the rigid catheter next to the patient's head as she places a 10-mL syringe in the balloon port and removes the air. She withdraws the tube.

EMT–I Simms watches the patient closely for signs of vomiting or respiratory depression as she places a nonrebreather mask on him with 15 L/min of oxygen. She notes that the patient's speech is slurred as he makes abusive comments to her and her crew. It looks as though he has a good chance of making it.

SUMMARY

Important points to remember from this chapter include the following:

- Airway management is a critical element of prehospital care.
- To be effective, airway skills must be practiced on an ongoing basis so that all necessary procedures can be performed automatically.
- Airway management centers on maintaining the respiratory system's primary function: moving air in and out of the body and supplying the bloodstream with adequate oxygen.
- To accomplish this goal, the airway must be patent, there must be adequate oxygen in the inspired air, and the respiratory minute volumes must be sufficient to remove appropriate levels of carbon dioxide.
- The airway first must be secured. Basic maneuvers such as the head-tilt/chin-lift maneuver can be used to move the tongue and epiglottis away from their obstructing positions. When a cervical spine injury is likely, the chin-lift maneuver should be employed without the head-tilt.
- A variety of procedures and devices can be used to support a patient's breathing. Of these procedures, the bag-valve-mask device offers the most advantages. However, it is difficult to use when ventilating the nonintubated patient, so its use must be practiced frequently to ensure proficiency during emergency situations.
- Inspired oxygen concentrations can be increased using a variety of delivery devices. The nonrebreather mask delivers close to 100% oxygen, making it the preferred device for severely ill or injured patients.
- ET intubation is the preferred technique for securing the airway because it prevents aspiration of foreign materials and allows for efficient delivery of assisted breathing. However, ET intubation has its hazards because accidental misplacement of the tube can result in severe hypoxia and death.
- When performing ET intubation, care must be taken to prevent injury to the teeth and tissue. Although orotracheal intubation is the most commonly used procedure, a number of alternative methods are available for use in situations when head and neck manipulation must be avoided.

PATIENT ASSESSMENT

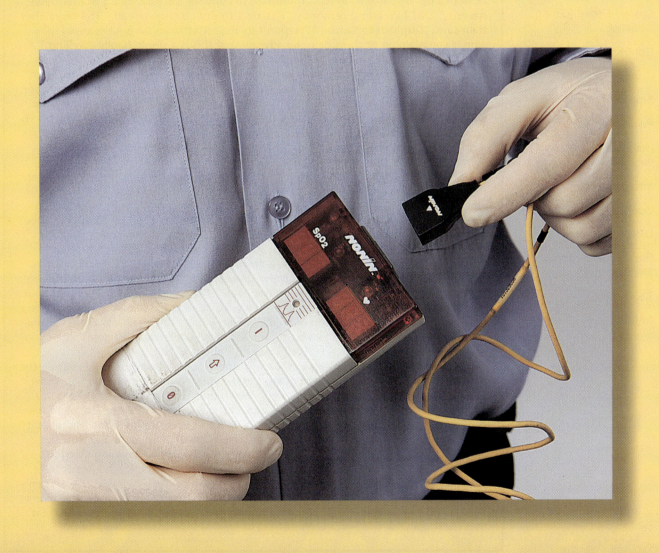

History Taking

■■■CASE HISTORY On their way back to base, EMT-Is Maloney and Woodard stop at a local fast-food restaurant; it is the first break they have had all day. Just as they place their orders, the dispatch center calls. "Dispatch to Rescue 1: prepare to copy for the 1600 block of Matthews Avenue." EMT-I Woodard responds, "Rescue 1 to dispatch: go ahead." The dispatcher then says, "Dispatch to Rescue 1: respond to 1652 Matthews for a 42-year-old man who is complaining of chest pain. Be advised that this is a single-family dwelling." As they repeat back the address to the dispatcher and start in response, Maloney tells the person at the take-out window to "put a hold on that order; we'll be back later."

As they pull up on-scene, they see an upset middle-age woman at the front door waving at them to come in. They exit the ambulance, bringing with them the jump kit, oxygen unit, drug box, and electrocardiogram (ECG) monitor/defibrillator. On entering the home they find the patient sitting on a chair in the living room. It appears he is in some discomfort, as he is clutching his chest and grimacing with pain. He seems alert and is breathing normally.

The two EMT-Is begin their assessment of the patient. EMT-I Woodard asks questions while Maloney checks for a pulse. "Sir, we are here to help you. Can you tell us why you called for the ambulance today?" The patient responds, "I've been having chest pain. . . . I didn't want to bother you, but my wife has been pestering me about getting someone over here to check me out." Woodard then asks, "What time did the pain start?" The patient answers, "It started this afternoon about 1:30 or so. . . . It was just before half-time. . .they were down by seven points. . . . I didn't tell my wife, but I've got fifty bucks riding on this game!" Next, Woodward asks, "Is there anything that seems to ease or worsen the pain?" The patient replies, "No; it's about the same as when it started." Woodard then asks, "Can you describe the pain?" The patient responds, "Well, it's kind of a dull, aching pain." "On a scale of 1 to 10, from just a little to the worst pain you have ever felt, how would rate this pain?" asks Woodard. The patient answers, "Well I'd say it's about a six."

EMT-I Maloney pulls out the stethoscope and blood pressure cuff and rolls up the patient's sleeve. He says, "Sir, I am going to take your blood pressure. Do you know what it normally is?" The patient answers, "Well, they tell me it is normally around 140 over 90 or so." His wife quickly remarks, as she hands EMT-I Woodard a half-filled medication bottle, "They have him on this high blood pressure medicine. He takes it every morning." EMT-I Woodard thanks the patient's wife, writes the name of the medication down on the run report, and then continues his questioning using the acronyms OPQRST and SAMPLE to help him recall what information he needs to gather. EMT-I Maloney finishes taking the blood pressure, then pulls out the oxygen unit, connects a nonrebreather mask to the regulator. He sets the oxygen flow rate at 15 liters (L)/min and says, "Sir, we are going to give you some oxygen to help treat that chest pain."

CHAPTER GOAL
Upon completion of this chapter, the EMT-Intermediate will be able to use the appropriate techniques to obtain a medical history from a patient.

Cognitive Objectives
As an EMT-Intermediate you should be able to do the following:

- Describe the techniques of history taking.
- Discuss the importance of using open and closed ended questions.
- Describe the use of facilitation, reflection, clarification, empathetic responses, confrontation, and interpretation.
- Differentiate between facilitation, reflection, clarification, sympathetic responses, confrontation, and interpretation.
- Describe the structure and purpose of a health history.
- Describe how to obtain a health history.
- List the components of a history of an adult patient.

Affective Objectives
As an EMT-Intermediate you should be able to do the following:

- Demonstrate the importance of empathy when obtaining a health history.
- Demonstrate the importance of confidentiality when obtaining a health history.

Psychomotor Objectives
- None identified for this chapter.

INTRODUCTION

The care health care professionals provide is directly affected by the quality of information obtained about the patient. Although data are gathered on a patient-by-patient, case-by-case basis, each part of the history has a specific purpose. Together, with the physical examination, an adequate history forms the foundation for sound patient care. The order stated here is not "set in stone," as long as all the necessary information is obtained.

Historical information often comes from a variety of *sources*. These may include the patient, family members, friends, law enforcement, and other observers. In a nonjudgmental fashion, the *reliability* of the history must be weighed; this should be conducted at the end of the evaluation and not the beginning to avoid any "first impressions" clouding an interviewer's objectivity. Many factors affect the quality of historical information; these include mental status (e.g., possible intoxication); memory; trust (e.g., in a drug overdose or crime scene injury); and motivation (e.g., Does the patient have a reason for secondary gain, such as a potential lawsuit?).

ESSENTIAL COMPONENTS OF A MEDICAL HISTORY

Regardless of the event, the history must contain certain basic information. This includes the following list:

1. *Date*—The timing of the event, accident, or injury is crucial, as is appropriate documentation, including the date of your report.
2. *Identifying data*—Age, gender, and race are all important identifiers.
3. *Chief complaint (CC)*—This is a main part of the health history and identifies, in the patient's own words, the symptoms for which the patient is seeing medical care.
4. *History of the present illness (HPI)*—This is a detailed evaluation of the CC. The HPI should provide a full, clear, and chronological account of the patient's symptoms.
5. *Past medical history (PMHx)*—This is a record of any significant past injuries, hospitalizations, operations, or diseases. Particular attention should be paid to information related to the patients' current condition (e.g., "Have you ever had chest pain like this before?").
6. *Current health status*—This section focuses on the patient's present state of health before the incident for which emergency care has been called. Factors of interest are summarized as follows:
   - *Current medications*—This includes both prescription (e.g., blood pressure medication, birth control pills) and nonprescription medications (over-the-counter [OTC] preparations, natural remedies, herbal medicines); also whether any recent changes in the patient's medications (e.g., drugs added, drugs stopped) should be confirmed.
   - *Allergies*—If patients state they are allergic to a medication, it is necessary to determine exactly what happened when they took it (e.g., Was there a rash, itching, breathing problem, shock, and so on?).
   - *Tobacco use*—Current and previous tobacco use has medical implications. Patients admitting to prior smoking need to provide the date of cessation.
   - *Alcohol, drugs, and related substances*—It may be necessary to ask specifically about which type of alcohol, since some persons actually believe beer is *not* alcohol!
   - *Diet*—Recording any recent changes, especially use of "fad diets" (e.g., liquid protein supplements), is most important.
   - *Screening tests*—There are no "routine" screening tests for all persons. Examples may include mammograms, routine chest x-rays, electrocardiograms (ECGs), or blood tests.
   - *Immunizations*—Always ask children if their "baby shots" are up-to-date. With adults, find out when a person's last tetanus shot was administered and whether he or she was vaccinated against any other infectious diseases (e.g., hepatitis).
   - *Sleep patterns*—Rather than taking a detailed sleep history, ask patients if they have trouble sleeping. If so, is it primarily in falling asleep, staying asleep (waking too early), or excessive daytime sleepiness (too tired)? Sleep disturbance may be a sign of diabetes, depression, heart failure, or many other conditions.
   - *Exercise and leisure activities*—Try to get a general sense of what else patients do besides their usual vocation (e.g., hobbies, workouts, time spent with family/friends).
   - *Environmental hazards*—Exposure to chemicals, fumes, dust, animals, radiation, or electricity may have affected the patient's complaints.
   - *Use of safety measures*—The most common safety measure about which to ask is seat belt use in motor vehicles or helmet use when operating a motorcycle. With farming accidents, determine whether safety covers (e.g., shields over power-take-off [PTO] mechanisms or grain auger bits) were in place.
   - *Family history*—Many conditions such as heart disease have a genetic pattern
   - *Home situation*—Determine if there are pets, a spouse, or significant others. This is important in domestic violence cases. Ask about general cleanliness and upkeep of home; an unkempt home may suggest that a patient is sicker than was maybe initially indicated. When taken to the hospital, some patients are more concerned for the welfare of their homes, pets, and families than for themselves.
   - *Daily life*—It may be helpful to discover what a typical "day in the life" is for the patient; even more important is how the current health problem possibly affects these activities.
   - *Important experiences*—These may include awards or other honors, as well as previous motor vehicle accidents and injuries.
   - *Religious beliefs*—In critically ill patients, it may be appropriate to ask the patient or family of a member of the clergy should be contacted.
   - *Overall outlook on life*—Find out if the patient is generally happy, sad, or relatively neutral about life.

Depending on the circumstances, obtaining all the information listed above may not be possible or even appropriate. Details are provided more for the purposes of being complete than to suggest always asking each patients each and every one of these questions. The relevant items to the patient's presenting condition should be determined. At the minimum, striving to find a history of allergies; use of medications (prescription, nonprescription, herbal, and so on); and use of drugs, alcohol, or tobacco are of the most significance importance.

TECHNIQUES OF HISTORY TAKING

Setting the Stage

ENVIRONMENT

A proper environment enhances communication between the interviewer and patient. The out-of-hospital setting does not often lend itself to an ideal history-taking atmosphere. Sometimes, placing the patient in the ambulance after a brief evaluation and continuing there is more successful. Other times, patients are more comfortable in their own homes, beds, or couches and should be interviewed there, unless medical urgency dictates otherwise.

Emergency care professionals are viewed by the patient as being in position of power and authority. During the initial interview, the patient's personal space should be respected by not getting closer than 2 to 3 feet, unless medically necessary. Typically, patients are more threatened by another person's face in close proximity to theirs than a hand or an arm. Shaking hands is a good technique to calm the patient, as well as to initially evaluate skin temperature, moisture, and strength.

DEMEANOR AND APPEARANCE

Just as an EMT-Intermediate (EMT-I) is watching the patient, the patient and bystanders are watching the EMT-I. Studies have shown that the majority of interpersonal communication occurs not by words but rather through "body language." A clean, neat, and professional appearance goes a long way. In addition, a health care professional should always treat persons with respect, regardless of the patient's presenting condition. Where possible, the patient should be referred to by name. Many individuals are offended by the use of "sir" or "madam." If you are unsure, ask patients how they are most comfortable being addressed (e.g., "What would you prefer I call you?"). Unfamiliar and potentially demeaning terms such as "Granny," "Buddy," "Bubba," "Dear," "Sweetie," or "Honey" should be avoided at all costs.

NOTE TAKING

Particularly in an uncontrolled situation, it is difficult to remember all the details. Note taking is generally well accepted by patients and essential for proper documentation. Although most patients are comfortable with note taking, if concerns arise, they should be addressed, and any reasons for taking notes should be explained to the patient (e.g., "My notes are better than my memory, and I want to make sure I give the hospital the correct information about you."). Although it requires some practice, attention should not be diverted from the patient to take notes, especially when life-threatening problems arise.

Questioning Patients

OPEN-ENDED VERSUS CLOSED-ENDED QUESTIONS

Open-ended questions should be employed whenever possible. The following are two types of medical questions:

Open-ended questions require more than a simple, often one-word answer. Examples include "Tell me about the pain" or "What things change your discomfort?"

Closed-ended, or direct, questions require a simple answer such as "yes" or "no." Examples include "Do you have pain now?" or "Does it hurt you to breathe?"

As a rule, open-ended questions tend to yield far more helpful information than closed-ended ones. Asking too many direct questions can also lead to frustration by patients, encouraging them to "close" and just say what they think you want to hear. Open-ended questions, however, allow for open discussion of many possibilities. In some cases, closed-ended questions may be better (e.g., certain nonverbal patients). Table 9-1 summarizes the differences between asking similar questions in an open-ended versus a closed-ended fashion.

CHIEF COMPLAINT

✖️ **Chief Complaint (CC)** • The main part of the health history and identifies, in the patient's own words, the symptoms for which the patient is seeing medical care.

TABLE 9-1

Open-Ended Versus Closed-Ended (Direct) Questions

OPEN-ENDED QUESTION	CLOSED-ENDED QUESTION
Describe your chest pain to me.	Does your chest hurt?
What types of things make your breathing better?	Does lying down improve you breathing?
What types of things make your pain worse?	Does it hurt when you move?
What medicines do you take?	Do you take any medications?
How much alcohol do you drink in an average week?	Do you drink alcohol?
Tell me about the timing of the pain.	When did the pain start?
What other symptoms are you feeling?	Anything else bothering you?

Several communication tricks can help obtain the most information, or **chief complaint (CC),** in a rapid, yet mutually comfortable fashion. A general, open-ended question such as "Why did you call the ambulance today?" helps get things started, followed by using the patient's lead to incorporate the following (Figures 9-1 and 9-2):

- *Facilitation*—**Facilitation** is a combination of verbal and nonverbal actions that is used to encourage the patient to say more. This includes posture, actions, or words. The most helpful is making eye contact often, but some cultures are offended by direct eye contact, especially toward members of the opposite gender. Phrases such as "Go on," "Please continue," or "I am listening" encourage the patient. Saying "I am listening" when doing something else (e.g., looking at equipment) should be avoided.

- *Reflection*—**Reflection** is repeating the patient's words (or making a summary of them) back to ensure communication. It also encourages additional responses by the patient. Done properly, reflection does not bias the story or interrupt the patient's train of thought. For example, "What I have heard so far is that you have a heaviness under your breast bone that started a half hour ago and that you have never had anything like it before, yes?"

- *Clarification*—**Clarification** requires interruption to ask additional questions to clarify points; at this stage, a few short, directed questions may be appropriate. For example, "Now, you said that breathing makes your pain worse. Is this mostly when you breath in,

when you breathe out, or all the time?" Alternatively, an open-ended question could be "Now, you said that breathing made your pain worse; when, during your breathing, is the pain made worse?"

- *Empathetic responses*—An **empathetic response** (identifying with one's feelings or symptoms) is different from sympathy (feeling sorry for someone). Although sympathy may be appropriate at some times, the point of history taking is to be professional, kind, and empathetic. Every attempt should be made to identify with what the patient is going through. Although you may have never suffered a similar condition, it is still reasonable to express to the patient things such as "You sound uncomfortable," or "I'd probably be frightened if I were in your shoes."

- *Confrontation*—**Confrontation** is more direct but potentially disruptive to a relationship with the patient. It may be extremely helpful under selected circumstances, however. For example, "I'm here to help you; if I don't know what drugs you took, I can't do you much good" or "I'm not any happier than you are that you hurt your leg; let yourself try to relax some so I can help you out better." Rarely, simply saying something like "Just do it!" is necessary for the best outcome.

- *Interpretation*—**Interpretation** requires the interviewer to synthesize what the patient has told him or her (verbally and through body language) with personal knowledge and "gut feelings." Regardless of whether the interpretation is similar to that of the patient depends on the circumstances. For example, if a patient complains of neck, upper abdomen, and left arm pain, based on answers to other questions, a possible heart attack can be suspected.

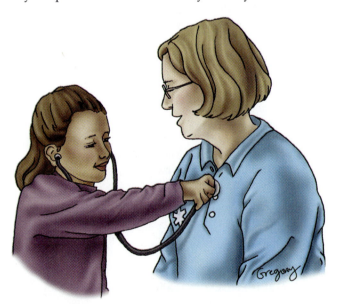

FIGURE 9-1 ▲ Facilitation is a combination of verbal and nonverbal actions that encourage the patient to say more.

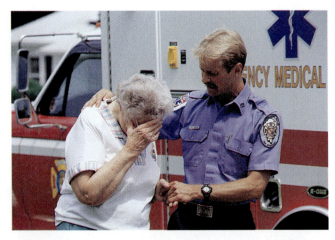

FIGURE 9-2 ▲ Empathy involves identifying with the patient's feelings or symptoms. It is very different from sympathy (feeling sorry for someone). (From American College of Emergency Physicians, Chief Editors Pons P, Cason D: Paramedic field care: a complaint-based approach, St Louis, 1998, Mosby.)

HISTORY OF THE PRESENT ILLNESS

✖ **History of the present illness (HPI)** • A detailed evaluation of the CC. The HPI should provide a full, clear, and chronological account of the patient's symptoms.

Factors that must be evaluated for any symptom to determine the **history of the present illness (HPI)** include the following:

Location: Where is it? Does it radiate (move) anywhere?

Quality: What is it like?

Quantity or severity: How bad is it? Attempt to quantify the severity of the symptom. The easiest way is to use a scale of zero (0) to ten (10), with "zero" being symptom free and "ten" being the worst pain (or other symptom) imaginable.

Duration or timing: When did it start? How long does it last?

Onset and setting: What was the patient doing when the symptoms began? Were there any emotional factors involved? Was there any exposure to an environmental agent (e.g., heat, cold, radiation, chemicals) associated with the symptoms?

Aggravating/alleviating factors: What things make the symptom better? What makes it worse?

Associated complaints: What other symptoms are present?

Although the above list incorporates some direct questions, an open-ended version should be used as much of possible during the patient interview.

The **"OPQRST"** acronym aids in remembering what you need to know about the patient's CC. It is defined as follows:

O Onset—When did the problem begin?
P Provocation—What makes the problem worse?
Q Quality—What is the problem (usually pain) like? Is it sharp, crushing, or viselike?
R Radiation—Does the pain go (move) anywhere?
S Severity—On a scale of 0 to 10 (0 being no pain and 10 being the worst pain imaginable), how bad is the pain?
T Time—Does the symptom come and go, or is it always there?

PAST MEDICAL HISTORY

✖ **Past Medical History (PMHx)** • This is a record of any significant past injuries, hospitalizations, operations, or diseases. Particular attention should be paid to information related to the patients' current condition (e.g., "Have you ever had chest pain like this before?").

To determine relevant factors in the patient's **past medical history (PMHx),** especially those that directly affect the current problem, consider the following:

- Preexisting medical problems (e.g., diabetes) or surgeries
- Medications
- Allergies
- Medical care (e.g., family physician)
- Family history
- Social history (e.g., housing environment, economic status, occupation, high-risk behavior, travel history)

CURRENT HEALTH STATUS

✖ **Current Health Status** • This is the patient's present state of health *before* the incident for which emergency care has been called.

Current health status, outlined previously under Essential Components of Medical History, can determine the use of alcohol, drugs, and other related substances. Any special diet factors of interest should also be noted.

Standardized Approach to History Taking

Over the years, several acronyms have evolved to aid in remembering what to ask during the history taking. The **"SAMPLE"** acronym is defined as follows (Figure 9-3):

S Signs and symptoms
A Allergies
M Medications
P Pertinent past medical history
L Last oral intake (fluid or solid)
E Events leading to the present situation

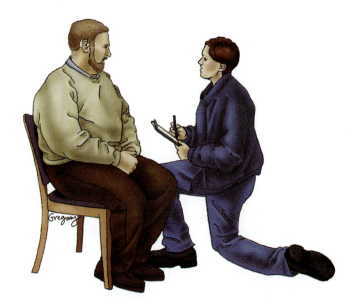

S — Signs and symptoms
A — Allergies
M — Medications
P — Pertinent past medical history
L — Last oral intake, fluid or solid
E — Events leading to the present situation

FIGURE 9-3 ▲ SAMPLE.

History Taking of Sensitive Topics

Certain topics involve both social medical issues. Because of this, many persons have difficulty talking about them. These include alcohol and drugs, physical abuse or violence, and sexual history

There is no "textbook" method for dealing with any particular patient regarding these topics. Instead, the following should be considered, to provide the best patient care possible:

- Always remain calm and professional.
- Appear completely nonjudgmental.
- Continually remind the patient that you are there to help. Don't be too reassuring, as over-assurance may hamper communication (e.g., if you say "trust me, I'm an EMT-I" too often, the patient might trust you less).

CLINICAL NOTES

A competent patient has the right to refuse to divulge information to you.

SPECIAL CHALLENGES

The Silent Patient

Despite the old saying, silence is not always "golden." Sometimes it is actually rather frustrating and confusing. At the minimum, a silent patient often makes history taking an uncomfortable experience. It does not necessarily show that the patient is hostile, problematic, or uncooperative. Patients may use silence as a way to collect their thoughts, remember details, or decide whether they trust you.

The best approach, after being certain that the patient can hear and understand you, is patience. Being alert for nonverbal clues of distress is important; these can be used as potential starting points for additional questions. Such clues include grimacing, touching or rubbing a particular area repeatedly, sweating, or crying. Sometimes a patient's silence reflects displeasure with the interviewer and possibly a lack of sensitivity. However, waiting for an answer rather than pressuring a patient to respond immediately following a question is often an effective interviewing technique.

The Talkative Patient

The opposite of the silent patient is one who talks incessantly. Under emergency circumstances, this usually reflects that the patient is nervous and scared. Sometimes, by simply acknowledging this, you help the patient relax. Faced with a limited amount of time, interviewers may become impatient. This ensures hindering the relationship with the patient. The numerous ways to cope with the talkative patient while still maintaining a professional manner and providing excellent patient care are as follows:

Lower expectations: Accept a less comprehensive history. To many, this is a last resort, because crucial information may be missed.

Give patient free reign for first few minutes of interview: Depending on the circumstances, this may not be feasible. However, remember that a patient who can verbalize extensively (1) has a patent airway and (2) is usually *not* in significant respiratory distress.

Summarize frequently: Politely interrupt and summarize, point by point, as best as possible.

Ask directed questions: Although less desirable than open-ended questions, firm direction may be exactly what is needed to maintain control over the interview.

The Patient With Multiple Symptoms

The two different scenarios that arise when dealing with patients who have multiple complaints are (1) the trauma patient with many injury-related complaints and (2) the medical patient with multiple complaints.

The crucial point for both situations is that appropriate priorities must be dealt with first. Remember that any disease or injury that threatens *airway, breathing,* or *circulation (ABC's)* must be identified rapidly and cared for immediately. The interviewer may have to direct the interview more than usual to help determine if a life-threatening problem is present.

Once you have ruled out immediate life threats, the patient should be asked to help rank his or her complaints. The following is an appropriate method to achieve this:

1. In a nonjudgmental fashion, acknowledge that many complaints are present.
2. Ask which one is the most bothersome.
3. Ask which one is the second worst, third worst, and so on.

The Anxious Patient

Everyone is usually anxious to some extent when sick or injured. Sometimes a patient speaks quickly as a response to the anxiety. Others speak much slower or even become silent (see The Silent Patient). Remember that much human communication is by nonverbal means and that close attention must be paid to these nonverbal clues. Use caution with reassurance; it is tempting to be too reassuring, which may erode a patient's trust in the interviewer.

The Angry and Hostile Patient

Anger and hostility are normal reactions to undesirable circumstances, such as illness or injury. Although the interviewer is to help, the patient may displace anger toward him or her. Mostly, this is *not* done purposefully or with negative intent. Getting angry or becoming hostile in return only escalates the situation, and no one benefits. Although history taking can be challenging at times, it is important to remain calm when responding to the patient. Of course, if there are any perceived physical dangers, obtain appropriate assistance immediately. The interviewer should not place or allow himself or herself to remain in a potentially volatile situation. This is a basic rule of scene safety regarding *any* patient encounter (see Patient Assessment, Chapter 11).

The Intoxicated Patient

Health care professionals encounter alcohol intoxication among the many patients for whom they care. The rule of scene safety discussed previously also applies. This is not the time to be judgmental; it is necessary to respect patients and not challenge them. Attempts to encourage the patient to lower his or her voice or stop cursing often simply aggravate that patient further. Many intoxicated patients also require more than the normal amount of personal space. Approaching patients like these in a small area may make them feel trapped. It is important to speak calmly and avoid sudden moves.

The Crying Patient

Crying may be due to many factors, including pain and fear. Crying is expected in many children, but it can occur in adults as well. Remember that even very small children can understand far more than they can vocalize. A gentle, calm, and professional approach is best.

At times, a patient's behavioral response seems out of proportion to the apparent degree of illness or injury. It is important to make no judgment. Remain objective and empathetic. Sometimes the best way to deal with a crying patient is simply to offer tissue paper. This simple act of kindness goes a long way to improve patient rapport.

The Depressed Patient

Depression ranges in severity from a temporary response to a situation to a severe psychiatric illness that may result in violent behavior. Signs of depression include the following:

- Sad appearance
- Crying
- Inappropriate responses, especially crying, with minimal stimuli
- Sleep disturbance
- Abnormal appetite (decreased or increased)
- Suicidal actions or gestures

Acceptance of the situation with empathy (e.g., "You sound depressed" or "You look sad") is the best communication technique. Telling the patient things like "Everything is all right" or "Things will work out" should be avoided. It is important to simply acknowledge that the patient feels bad and not press further.

The Sexually Attractive or Seductive Patient

Sometimes interviewers and patients are sexually attracted to each other. These are normal feelings but cannot interfere with the health care professional's care or behavior. If the patient becomes seductive or makes sexual advances, it should be frankly and firmly made clear that this is a professional and not personal relationship. If the patient persists, remove yourself from the situation if possible. Sometimes, having another person to "chaperone" is helpful for medical, ethical, and legal reasons.

The Patient With Confusing Behavior or History

Confusing or unusual behavior should be viewed as due to a potentially serious medical problem until proven otherwise. Hypoglycemia and hypoxia, as well as a myriad of other conditions, can mimic mental illness or dementia. A thorough history from both bystanders and the patient can assist in narrowing down the cause. It is important to remain sympathetic and professional to the patient, especially while attempting to identify the cause of the patient's behavior.

The Patient With Limited Intelligence

Many persons, even those with limited intellectual capacity, can express their basic needs, feelings, and symptoms if given a chance. The interviewer should speak clearly and in a normal tone. Although it may not always be the case, it may take more time than normal for the patient to respond to a question. Getting additional information from family or friends is always helpful. If patients are capable of communicating, the interview should be directed toward them first, ensuring patience and professionalism.

The EMT–Intermediate/Patient Language Barrier

The chances of caring for a person who does not speak English vary in different areas of the country. Spanish is the second most common language spoken by persons in the United States. Every possible step to locate a translator should be taken, including the dial-up services for language translation offered by several phone companies. It is important to be aware of local resources. In life-threatening situations, knowing a few broken words of another language is not an acceptable substitute for a translator.

The Patient With Hearing Impairment

The approach to patients with hearing impairment is similar to situations regarding a language barrier. A sign language translator should be located if the patient can sign. Patients may also be asked if they read lips. To do this, the interviewer should look them in the eyes, point to his or her mouth, and say "Do you read lips?" If the patient confirms this, it is important to speak slowly and avoid unusual terms and idiomatic language. Additionally, communication should be kept within the patient's line of vision, or all effort is lost. Another simple alternative, if the patient is able, is to communicate by writing notes.

The Patient With Sight Impairment

Many patients with sight impairment are aware of another's presence, even if they cannot visualize a person or persons. The interviewer should announce himself or herself and explain why he or she is there. Patients should be informed before they are touched, even to simply obtain vital signs.

Talking With Family and Friends

As with any patient encounter, information is confidential. When talking with family members and friends, this requirement should be maintained. However, such individuals are excellent collateral sources of data if the patient is unable to supply necessary information.

CASE HISTORY FOLLOW-UP ■ ■ ■

Assessment reveals the patient has a respiratory rate of 18; a pulse rate of 130; a blood pressure of 146/98; and cool, moist skin. Auscultation of the chest reveals clear bilateral lung sounds. The ECG monitor reveals sinus tachycardia with no ectopy and the pulse oximetry shows a SaO_2 of 94%. EMT–I Maloney examines the patient's extremities to find there is no noticeable peripheral edema.

While EMT–I Woodard writes down information on the run report, EMT–I Maloney pulls a nitroglycerin tablet out of the drug box and has the patient put it under his tongue. He then pulls out a 250 mL bag of normal saline and connects a microdrip administration set to it. An intravenous line is established and the patient is placed on the cot. He is then transferred to the back of the ambulance. On the way to the hospital, the patient tells EMT–I Woodard, "The pain in my chest doesn't seem as bad now. . . . Maybe the pain was there because my wife was nagging me so much! Hey, by the way can you find out the game score?"

SUMMARY

Important points to remember from this chapter include the following:

- History taking is an important step in the emergency care process. The better the available data, the better is the care that is given a patient.
- Essential information includes the date, identifying data, the CC, HPI, PMHx, and current health status.
- Setting the stage by maintaining a professional demeanor and appearance is important. As comfortable an environment as possible should be provided to the patient.
- Most persons do not mind if notes are taken, especially if the purpose of them is explained. Patients should always be referred to by name; it is sometimes best to ask patients how they wish to be addressed.
- Body language often sends more information than verbal clues.
- When interviewing patients, open-ended questions should be used whenever possible.
- Closed-ended (direct) questions can be used in situations in which open-ended ones fail to yield adequate information.

- Various techniques help improve the ability to communicate with a patient, including facilitation, reflection, clarification, empathetic responses, confrontation (when necessary), and interpretation.
- Both acronyms OPQRST and SAMPLE can help interviewers remember what necessary historical information should be obtained.
- Many challenging situations (e.g., silent patient, overly talkative patient, and so on) result from a person's normal responses to illness or injury—that is, anxiety and fear.
- By remaining calm and acting in a nonjudgmental fashion, an interviewer can greatly enhance the chances of communicating with the patient.
- If language barrier is presented or the patient only uses sign language, it is necessary to obtain a translator or interpreter whenever possible.
- Note writing and lip reading are potential alternative means of communication in a patient with hearing impairment.
- Treating all patients with respect and kindness, regardless of their appearances or conditions, goes a long way to enhance communication.

Techniques of Physical Examination

Key Terms

...CASE HISTORY EMT–Is Rothenberg and Collins are participating in a community blood pressure screening program being held at the township fire station, when they are dispatched to a local dinner theater for a 60-year-old man who reportedly slipped and fell on the steps outside. They arrive to find him sitting on a chair right at the entranceway to the theater. Apparently, a security guard helped him inside. The patient is awake and talking and appears to be in no distress, but the EMT–Is note that he is grimacing from pain.

They begin their assessment of the patient, Mr. Shade. EMT–I Collins asks questions while EMT–I Rothenberg feels for a radial pulse. "Sir, we are here to help you. Can you tell us what happened?"

Pointing in the direction of the steps, the patient responds, "I'd just purchased tickets for this evening's performance and I was leaving, when I twisted my ankle on the steps over there. I was just going to drive myself to the hospital, but the security guard said you guys had to see me before I leave. I think they are a bit worried I might sue."

"How long ago did it happen?" EMT–I Collins then asks.

"Oh it happened—couldn't have been more than 10 minutes ago," answers Mr. Shade.

EMT–I Collins asks, "Did you feel faint or pass out before you tripped?"

"No," replies Mr. Shade. "I just tripped. You'd think I'd learn to pick my feet up when I walk."

"Were you able to walk over to the chair by yourself, or did the security guard help you?" EMT–I Collins asks.

The patient responds, "Well, it hurt real bad when I tried to stand, so he helped me over here."

"Do you have pain anywhere else? Did you hit your head or neck when you fell?" EMT–I Collins asks.

The patient replies, "No, I just tripped and fell forward to the ground. Caught my fall with my hands out straight like this." He stretches his arms out palm side up to show his hands as he answers.

EMT–I Collins notes that the patient has swelling of his right wrist and abrasions to the palm side of both hands. He then asks, "Mr. Shade, do you feel any pain in your wrist?"

"No, not really," The patient responds.

EMT–I Rothenberg takes the patient's blood pressure while EMT–I Collins says, "Sir, I am going to take your shoe and sock off so we can take a look at your ankle and foot."

As Collins lifts the foot and ankle to remove the shoe, Mr. Shade lets out a moan and says, "Now that hurts real bad."

EMT–I Collins tells the patient as he pulls out his bandage shears, "I am going to cut your shoelace so we can get your shoe off easier."

Within a minute or so, EMT–I Collins is able to get the patient's shoe and sock off. There is obvious swelling and discoloration of the patient's ankle. EMT–I Collins then asks, "Mr. Shade, can you wiggle your toes for me?"

The patient responds by wiggling his toes. Assessment reveals normal motor, sensory, and circulatory function in all four of the patient's extremities.

LEARNING OBJECTIVES

CHAPTER GOAL
Upon completion of this chapter, the EMT–Intermediate will be able to explain the significance of physical examination findings commonly found in emergencies.

Cognitive Objectives
As an EMT–Intermediate you should be able to do the following:
- Define the terms *inspection, palpation, percussion,* and *auscultation.*
- Describe the techniques of inspection, palpation, percussion, and auscultation.
- Describe the evaluation of mental status.
- Evaluate the importance of a general survey.
- Describe the examination of the skin and nails.
- Differentiate between normal and abnormal assessment findings of the skin and nails.
- Distinguish the importance of abnormal findings of the assessment of the skin.
- Describe the examination of:
  - The head and neck
  - The eyes
  - The ears
  - The nose
  - The mouth
  - The neck
- Differentiate normal and abnormal assessment findings of:
  - The scalp
  - The skull
  - The eyes
  - The ears
  - The nose
  - The mouth
  - The neck
- Describe the survey of the thorax and respiration.
- Describe the examination of the anterior and posterior chest.
- Describe percussion of the chest.
- Differentiate the percussion sounds and their characteristics.
- Differentiate the characteristics of breath sounds.
- Differentiate normal and abnormal assessment findings of the chest examination.

Continued

Continued on p. 315

LEARNING OBJECTIVES—cont'd

- Describe the examination of:
  - The arterial pulse, including rate, rhythm, and amplitude
  - Jugular venous pressure and pulsations
  - The heart
- Distinguish normal and abnormal findings of:
  - The arterial pulses
  - Jugular venous pressure and pulsations
  - The heart
- Describe auscultation of the heart.
- Differentiate the characteristics of normal and abnormal findings associated with auscultation of the heart.
- Describe the examination of the abdomen.
- Differentiate normal and abnormal assessment findings of the abdomen.
- Describe auscultation of the abdomen.
- Distinguish normal and abnormal findings of auscultation of the abdomen.
- Describe the examination of the female external genitalia.
- Differentiate normal and abnormal assessment findings of the female external genitalia.
- Describe the examination of the male genitalia.
- Differentiate normal and abnormal findings of the male genitalia.
- Describe the examination of:
  - The musculoskeletal system
  - The peripheral vascular system
  - The nervous system
- Differentiate normal and abnormal findings of:
  - The musculoskeletal system
  - The peripheral vascular system
  - The nervous system
- Discuss the considerations of examination of an infant or child.
- Describe the general guidelines of recording examination information.

Affective Objectives
As an EMT–I intermediate you should be able to do the following:
- Demonstrate a caring attitude when performing a physical examination.

- Discuss the importance of a professional appearance and demeanor when performing a physical examination.
- Appreciate the limitations of conducting a physical examination in the out-of-hospital environment.

Psychomotor Objectives
As an EMT–I intermediate you should be able to do the following:
- Demonstrate the examination of the skin and nails.
- Demonstrate the examination of:
  - The head and neck
  - The eyes
  - The ears
  - The nose
  - The mouth
  - The neck
- Demonstrate the examination of the thorax and ventilation.
- Demonstrate the examination of the anterior and posterior chest.
- Demonstrate auscultation of the chest.
- Demonstrate percussion of the chest.
- Demonstrate the examination of the arterial pulse, including location, rate, rhythm, and amplitude.
- Demonstrate the assessment of jugular venous pressure and pulsations.
- Demonstrate the examination of the heart.
- Demonstrate the examination of the abdomen.
- Demonstrate auscultation of the abdomen.
- Demonstrate the external visual examination of the female external genitalia.
- Demonstrate the examination of the male genitalia.
- Demonstrate the examination of the peripheral vascular system.
- Demonstrate the examination of the musculoskeletal system.
- Demonstrate the examination of the nervous system.

Key Terms—cont'd

Intercostal Retractions	Obtundation	Posterior Tibial Pulse	Supraclavicular Retractions
Involuntary Guarding	Opisthotonic Posturing	Protuberant	Systole
Jaundice	Orthostasis	Pulse Oximeter	Tachycardia
Jugular Venous Pressure	Orthostatic Hypotension	Pulse Pressure	Tachypnea
Kussmaul Respirations	Pallor	Pulse Rate	Temperature
Lethargy	Palpation	Pupillary Reactivity	Tenderness
Level of Consciousness (LOC)	Paradoxical Chest Movements	Rebound Tenderness	Tenting
Lip Pursing	Paresthesias	Respiratory Rate	Tracheal Breath Sounds
Motor Tics	Peak Expiratory Flow Rate (PEFR)	Rhonchi	Tremor
Muscular Rigidity		Rigidity	Turgor
Muscle Coordination	Peak Flow Meter	Scaphoid	Vesicular Breath Sounds
Muscle Strength	Percussion	Second Heart Sound (S_2)	Vital Signs
Muscle Tone	Peritonitis	Stethoscope	Wheezes
Nasal Flaring	PERRL	Striae	
Normal Percussion Note	Pitting Edema	Stridor	
Normotension	Point of Maximum Impulse (PMI)	Stupor	
Nuchal Rigidity	Popliteal Pulse	Subcutaneous Emphysema	

OVERVIEW OF EXAMINATION TECHNIQUES AND EQUIPMENT

Examination Techniques

Any physical examination involves a combination of four different, but related, examination techniques. These are as follows:

- **Inspection**—The act of visually evaluating the patient (Figure 10-1).
- **Palpation**—The process whereby the examiner feels the texture, size, consistency, and location of certain parts of the body with the hands (Figure 10-2).
- **Percussion**—A technique involving gently striking or tapping a part of the body to evaluate the size, borders, and consistency of internal organs and to discover the presence of fluid in body cavities (Figure 10-3).
- **Auscultation**—The act of listening for sounds within the body to evaluate the condition of the heart, lungs, pleura, intestines, or other organs or to detect fetal heart sounds. Most commonly, auscultation is done with a stethoscope (Figure 10-4).

Measurement of Vital Signs

The term **vital signs** typically refers to the patient's pulse, respirations, and blood pressure. **Temperature** is also considered a vital sign, although it is less often obtained routinely in the out-of-hospital setting. The following are three important points to remember regarding vital signs:

- Vital signs are evaluated as a "set." No one vital sign will provide adequate information concerning a patient's condition.
- No one value is normal for everyone. Just as people come in all shapes and sizes, "normal" vital signs can vary within large ranges. Vital signs also vary considerably by age.
- Vital signs require continued monitoring. Besides initial readings, trends in vital signs need to be monitored to determine if the patient is getting better, worse, or staying the same. Protocols vary from system to system, but a good "rule of thumb" is to recheck vital signs every 5 to 10 minutes, or sooner if the patient's condition changes.

Height and Weight

Measurements of a patient's height and weight are important in calculation of drug doses. In the out-of-hospital setting, especially during an acute situation, exact determination of these parameters is not usually necessary—an estimate will do.

Equipment

Equipment routinely used by the EMT–Intermediate (EMT–I) in patient examination and care includes the following:

- **Stethoscope**—An instrument consisting of two earpieces connected by means of flexible tubing to a diaphragm, which is placed against the skin of the patient's chest or back to listen to (auscultate) heart and lung sounds (Figure 10-5).
- **Blood pressure cuff**—A flat, inflatable, rectangular-shaped bag attached to a pressure manometer (sometimes called a *sphygmomanometer*) wrapped around the arm or leg; the bag is inflated by squeezing a bulb, and the patient's blood pressure is measured by auscultating the pulse distal to the level of the cuff during deflation. A series of

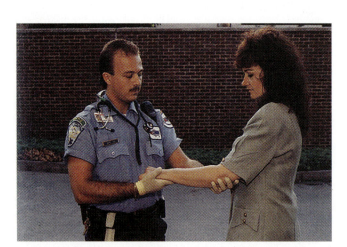

FIGURE 10-1 ▲ Visually evaluating the patient provides valuable information. (From McSwain NE, Paturas, JL: *The basic EMT: comprehensive prehospital patient care,* ed 2, St Louis, 2001, Mosby.)

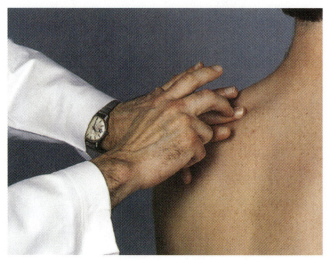

FIGURE 10-3 ▲ Percussion.

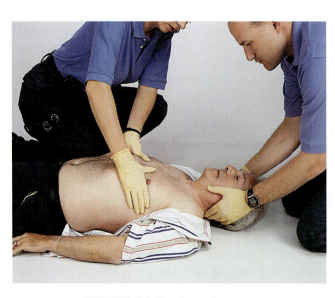

FIGURE 10-2 ▲ Palpation.

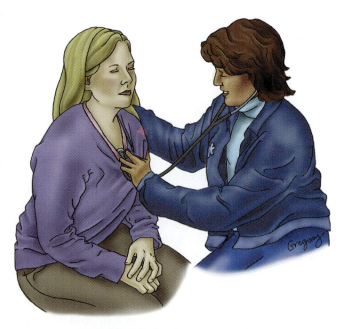

FIGURE 10-4 ▲ Auscultation.

sounds is heard, corresponding to readings on the manometer.

- *Fingerstick glucose meter*—An electronic device that determines the blood glucose (sugar) level from a drop of blood placed onto a special chemically treated dipstick. Although this measurement may also be done visually, an electronic meter is often more accurate.

- **Cardiac monitor**—An electronic device for the continuous observation of cardiac function. It may include electrocardiograph (ECG) and oscilloscope readings, recording devices, and a visual or an audible record of heart function and rhythm. An alarm system may be set to alert the EMT–I of variations from a set heart rate range (Figure 10-6).

- **Pulse oximeter**—An electronic device attached to the patient's finger, ear, or foot to determine the amount of oxygen in the blood, measured as *percent saturation of hemoglobin* (Figure 10-7). The pulse oximeter is very sensitive and will usually report changes in the arterial oxygen saturation level before the patient develops signs and symptoms of respiratory problems. Generally, a pulse oximetry reading of 95% (90% to 92% in areas of higher elevation) or better is considered as being within normal limits.

The pulse oximeter sends an infrared beam of light through the finger, toe, or earlobe. There is a direct relationship between the amount of oxygen in the blood and the ability of the blood to absorb this light (Figure 10-8). The device compares light sent into the measurement area with light coming out the other side. Using a mathematical formula, it converts this difference into oxygen saturation.

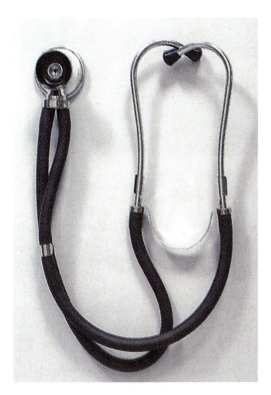

FIGURE 10-5 ▲ Acoustic stethoscope. (From Seidel HM et al: *Mosby's guide to physical examination,* ed 2, St Louis, 1991, Mosby.)

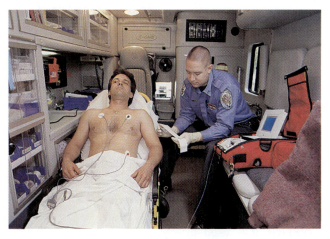

FIGURE 10-6 ▲ Monitoring a patient with three leads. (From Sanders MJ: *Mosby's paramedic textbook,* St Louis, 1994, Mosby.)

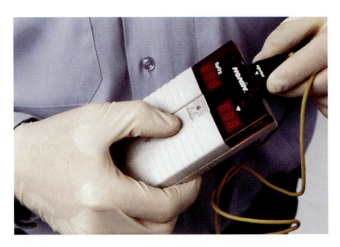

FIGURE 10-7 ▲ Pulse oximeter device.

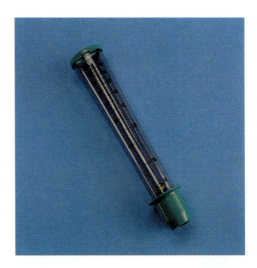

FIGURE 10-9 ▲ Peak flow meter.

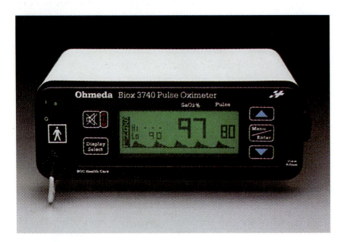

FIGURE 10-8 ▲ A pulse oximeter measures the amount of oxygen in a patient's blood using an infrared beam of light. (Courtesy Ohmeda, Louisville, Col.; from Sanders MJ: *Mosby's paramedic textbook,* St Louis, 1994, Mosby.)

Pulse oximetry is unreliable if a patient is hypothermic or hypotensive. Persons with carbon monoxide poisoning, severe vascular disease, anemia, or abnormal hemoglobin (thalassemia) may also demonstrate unreliable readings. Thus the use of oximetry is significantly limited in unstable patients and persons in cardiac arrest. Persons with cardiac ischemia may present with high pulse oximetry readings and still require oxygen.
- **Peak flow meter**—A hand-held mechanical device that measures the volume of a rapidly exhaled breath **(peak expiratory flow rate [PEFR]).** It is used primarily in the evaluation of patients with asthma, chronic obstructive lung disease, or congestive heart failure (Figure 10-9).

- **Capnometer**—An electronic device that measures how much carbon dioxide is exhaled during breathing: the *end tidal CO$_2$ (ETCO$_2$).* In the out-of-hospital setting, disposable mechanical devices are often used to detect ETCO$_2$ and help in the identification of esophageal intubation (see Figure 8-22, *A*).

GENERAL APPROACH

Establish a systematic routine to examine patients, placing special emphasis on areas suggested by the present illness and chief complaint. Depending on the situation, certain portions of the examination may be deleted if they are not related to the present problem. Remember that most patients feel vulnerable and exposed during a physical examination. Assume that there will be some apprehension and anxiety. A calm, caring, and professional manner will help allay patient anxiety.

OVERVIEW OF A COMPREHENSIVE EXAMINATION

Although not all EMT–I patient evaluations need to include a comprehensive examination, some will. The components of a complete physical examination should include the following (Figure 10-10):
- Mental status
- General survey
- Vital signs
- Skin
- HEENT (head, eyes, ears, nose, and throat)
- Neck
- Chest
- Abdomen
- Posterior body
- Extremities (peripheral pulses, musculoskeletal system)
- Neurological examination

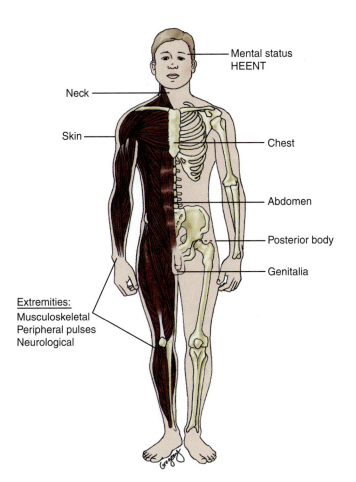

Mental status
HEENT

Neck

Skin

Chest

Abdomen

Posterior body

Genitalia

Extremities:
Musculoskeletal
Peripheral pulses
Neurological

FIGURE 10-10 ▲ **Components of the comprehensive examination.** *HEENT,* Head, eyes, ears, nose, and throat.

Mental Status

One of the best indicators of a person's condition is the mental status. A variety of conditions affect the patient's mentation, resulting in alterations from his or her normal mental state. It is important to know the patient's baseline mental status. The determination regarding a person's mental state should be based on a combination of factors: appearance and behavior, speech and language, mood, and orientation. Some patients have an altered mental status as their norm. Evaluation of these patients may be difficult.

APPEARANCE AND BEHAVIOR

Level of Consciousness—The **level of consciousness (LOC)** refers to how much awareness people have regarding their immediate surroundings. The following are the most commonly used terms related to LOC:

- Alert
- Responsive to verbal stimuli
- Responsive to painful stimuli
- Unresponsive

Descriptive terms are often applied to levels of consciousness. These include the following:

- *Normal state*—A state in which the patient is alert and responsive. The patient seems to understand questions and responds appropriately in a reasonable period.
- **Drowsiness (lethargy)**—A state in which the patient is sleepy, but otherwise normal; lethargic patients are drowsy, but they open their eyes and look at the person speaking to them, respond, and then fall back asleep.
- **Obtundation**—A reduced LOC resulting in insensitivity to unpleasant or painful stimuli; often due to an anesthetic or analgesic (pain) medication. Obtunded patients open their eyes and look at the person speaking to them, but they respond slowly and are confused.
- **Stupor**—A state of unresponsiveness where a person seems unaware of the surroundings.
- **Coma**—A state of profound unconsciousness. There are no spontaneous eye movements, and there is no response to either verbal or painful stimuli. Essentially, the patient cannot be aroused by any stimulation.

Posture and Motor Behavior—Evaluate the patient for abnormal postures and movements. Does the patient lie in bed or prefer to walk? Sometimes, posturing is purposeful (e.g., splinting to alleviate pain). Other times, nonpurposeful (not controllable by the patient) posturing occurs:

- **Decerebrate posturing**—Usually occurs in a comatose patient; the arms are extended and internally rotated while the feet are extended and in forced plantar flexion. The presence of decerebrate posturing indicates serious central nervous system pathology.
- **Decorticate posturing**—Usually occurs in a comatose patient; the upper extremities are flexed at the elbows and at the wrists; the legs may also be flexed. The presence of decorticate posturing suggests serious central nervous system pathology.
- **Opisthotonic posturing**—Acute arching of the back with the head bent back on the neck, the heels bent back on the legs, and the arms and hands flexed rigidly at the joints. Opisthotonic posturing results from severe muscle spasms, such as during a seizure or from tetanus.

As with posturing, movements may be either purposeful or nonpurposeful. Common movements that are usually not controllable by the patient include the following:

- **Rigidity**—Hardness, stiffness, or inflexibility, usually of the extremities; a sign of neurological diseases, such as Parkinson's disease.
- **Tremor**—Rhythmic, purposeless, quivering movements resulting from the involuntary alternating contraction and relaxation of opposing groups of skeletal muscles. Occurs in some elderly individuals, in cer-

tain families, and in patients with various neurological disorders, such as Parkinson's disease.

- **Motor tics**—Spasmodic muscular contraction most commonly involving the face, mouth, eyes, head, neck, or shoulders. Although these movements may appear purposeful, they are involuntary and can be consciously inhibited by the patient for only a short time. Although many tics arise from unknown causes, some medications and diseases (e.g., Tourette's syndrome) commonly cause them as well.

In addition, observe the patient for the presence of restlessness or agitation. These signs may indicate a serious underlying medical condition, such as hypoxia (lack of oxygen).

Dress, Grooming, and Personal Hygiene—At times, a patient's personal appearance may reflect his or her mental status. Patients with an altered mental status often do not pay close attention to hygiene, changing clothes, and other aspects of personal grooming. There is not necessarily, however, a relationship. Without being judgmental, observe and record any of these findings.

Facial Expression and Affect—Affect is a person's outward manifestations of emotion. Nonverbal clues make up most of human communication; watch the face carefully for expressions of anxiety, depression, anger, or happiness. Patients are said to have a **flat affect** if they appear emotionally unresponsive (e.g., no smiling or other facial expressions; quiet; give simple answers with no variation in voice tone). Persons with an altered LOC due to either psychiatric or medical problems may appear distant or act as if they are responding to imaginary people or objects. They may also act inappropriately for the situation (e.g., laughing inappropriately).

SPEECH AND LANGUAGE

As part of the mental status evaluation, assess a person's ability to speak. Observe the following:

- *Quantity*—How much does a person talk? Is it appropriate under the circumstances?
- *Rate*—A rapid speaking rate may suggest pain or anxiety; a slow rate may indicate a central nervous system problem (e.g., stroke), intoxication (drugs, alcohol), or fear. Some individuals, particularly older adults, tend to consider their words more carefully before speaking than others.
- *Loudness*—Sometimes a loud voice indicates that the patient has a hearing disorder; more commonly, it is a matter of habit and does not necessarily reflect any underlying disease or injury. Look at the entire picture before reaching conclusions.
- *Fluency*—Appropriate, fluent speech suggests a normal LOC. On the other hand, garbled speech does not necessarily indicate an alteration in the LOC. It may be due to organic causes, such as vocal cord injury or stroke.

A person's voice may change with mood, illness, or injury. Possible findings include the following:

- **Aphasia**—An abnormal neurological condition in which language function is defective or absent as a result of an injury to the cerebral cortex.
- **Dysphonia**—Difficulty in speaking; the central nervous system may be normal (e.g., hoarseness from a throat infection) or abnormal (e.g., stroke).
- **Dysarthria**—Impaired speech due to dysfunction of the tongue or other muscles essential to speech; mental function is normal.

MOOD

A person's mood may be a helpful indication of underlying illness, either physical or psychiatric. Moods range from happiness or elation (excessive happiness) to depression, anxiety, anger, or indifference. Assume that an altered mood is due to potentially treatable physical causes (e.g., intoxication, drugs, stroke, hypoglycemia) until proven otherwise. Always consider that a patient may exhibit mood instability, and preplan in your mind an avenue of escape, if necessary. Also, take any suggestion by the patient of suicide as serious—especially in teenagers and in the elderly.

ORIENTATION

The standard evaluation of a person's orientation centers around the following:

- *Time*—Date, year
- *Place*—Where are we now?
- *Person*—Who are you?

In addition, assessing a patient's remote memory (e.g., date of birth, age) and recent memory (e.g., current events) is helpful. Disorientation can occur from a variety of causes and should be considered as being due to a potentially serious medical problem until proven otherwise.

CLINICAL NOTES

We often write that a patient is "A & O × 3," meaning "alert and oriented to time, place, and person." This is appropriate in most adults; however, consider the same statement made for a 2-month-old infant: "A 2-month-old infant A & O × 3." We sometimes fall into this dangerous documentation trap. Use other terms to document the LOC in younger patients, such as "A 2-month-old infant who looks around appropriately, responds appropriately to noises and my voice, and follows me around the room with her eyes," or "A 3-year-old toddler who 'gives me five' with enthusiasm and says he is hungry enough to go out for fast food right now."

GENERAL SURVEY

- Assess the patient's level of consciousness (LOC).
- Observe the patient for signs of distress.
- Classify the patient's apparent state of health.
- Assess the skin color, and observe for obvious problems.
- Determine the patient's general weight status.
- Evaluate the patient's posture, gait, and motor activity.
- Note the patient's dress, grooming habits, and state of personal hygiene.
- Gauge whether any unusual odors of the breath are present.
- Observe the patient's facial expression.
- Obtain a set of vital signs.
- Perform additional assessment techniques as necessary.

General Survey

The **general survey** is a universal overview of the patient's general condition. It is meant to be performed in a rapid, but complete, fashion and includes many areas. Document your findings appropriately (Box 10-1).

LEVEL OF CONSCIOUSNESS

Assess the patient's level of consciousness (LOC) using the **AVPU scale:**
- **A**—Alert; the patient is alert.
- **V**—Verbal; the patient responds to verbal stimuli.
- **P**—Painful; the patient responds to painful stimuli.
- **U**—Unconscious; the patient is unconscious and does not respond.

SIGNS OF DISTRESS

Observe the patient for signs of distress. The list of possible findings is vast. Pay particular attention to those involving the ABCs (airway, breathing, and circulation). Some (noninclusive) examples are as follows:
- *Cardiorespiratory insufficiency*—Labored breathing, wheezing, cough
- *Pain*—Wincing, sweating, protectiveness (guarding) of a painful part
- *Anxiety*—Facial expression, fidgety movements; cold, moist palms

APPARENT STATE OF HEALTH

Classify the patient's apparent state of health. Possible classifications include the following:
- Acutely ill
- Chronically ill
- Frail, feeble
- Robust, vigorous

SKIN COLOR AND OBVIOUS LESIONS

Assess the skin color, and observe for obvious problems. These include abnormalities in temperature (warm, cool, hot), color (pale, cyanotic, pink), or character (dry, clammy, diaphoretic), as well as obvious lesions.

WEIGHT

Determine the patient's general weight status (e.g., emaciated, normal, obese). Also, ask if there has been a recent history of weight gain or loss.

POSTURE, GAIT, AND MOTOR ACTIVITY

Evaluate the patient's posture, gait, and motor activity. Is the patient lying quietly, or is he or she restless? Is any involuntary motor activity (e.g., tremor, tics) present? Finally, describe (if applicable) the way the patient walks:
- Is there balance?
- Is there a limp?
- Is there apparent discomfort?
- Does the patient seem to exhibit a fear of falling?
- Is the patient **ataxic** (unable to coordinate movements)?

DRESS, GROOMING, AND PERSONAL HYGIENE

Note the patient's dress, grooming habits, and state of personal hygiene. Is the dress appropriate for the temperature and current weather? Does the patient appear clean and well cared for?

ODORS OF THE BREATH

Gauge whether any unusual odors of the breath are present. These may indicate underlying conditions such as intoxication or a diabetic emergency.

FACIAL EXPRESSION

Observe the patient's facial expression. Nonverbal communication often provides more clues than verbal communication. Carefully gauge the patient's expressions at rest, during conversation, and during the examination. Look for evidence of fear, pain, or confusion.

VITAL SIGNS

Obtain a set of vital signs. These should include blood pressure, pulse, and respiratory rate. Remember to obtain sequential vital signs every 5 to 10 minutes. Changes in vital signs are often more informative than just one set.

ADDITIONAL ASSESSMENT TECHNIQUES

Perform additional assessment techniques as necessary. Depending on the circumstances, these procedures may include pulse oximetry, blood glucose monitoring, and cardiac monitoring.

> ▶ TIPS FOR EXAMINING GERIATRIC PATIENTS
> - Remember that elderly patients have decreased temperature-regulating mechanisms; they are more sensitive to cold and to changes in the temperature.
> - Preserve modesty as much as possible.
> - Remember that the elderly may have slowed physical and verbal response times.
> - Be aware that the skin normally loses its elasticity with aging and that skin turgor is routinely diminished, even in well-hydrated patients.
> - Observe the patient's surroundings carefully for clues as to the problem or for indications of abuse or neglect.
> - Be aware that depression, suicide attempts, and overdoses (deliberate and accidental) are common in the elderly.
> - Be aware that new-onset wheezing or shortness of breath is likely to be cardiac in cause.
> - Be certain that the patient is able to hear you properly. (Hearing loss can be misconstrued as an altered LOC, especially in an older person.)

Anatomical Regions

Detailed here are examination techniques, normal findings, and common abnormal findings for the major areas of the body. Although the EMT–I should be familiar with examination of each area, the actual components incorporated into the patient evaluation will depend on the circumstances. For example, an otherwise healthy patient with a simple laceration of the arm requires no more than an examination limited to the vicinity of the wound.

SKIN AND NAILS

Techniques of Examination—The skin is the largest organ in the body. It serves many vital functions and is a major component of the physical examination. During this portion of the examination, do the following (Table 10-1):

- Inspect and palpate the skin.
- Inspect the fingernails.

Characteristic Findings—In evaluating the skin and the fingernails, pay particular attention to the following areas:

- *Color*—Cyanosis and pallor (see Abnormalities) are best seen where the epidermis is thinnest (fingernails, lips, mucous membranes of the mouth, palpebral conjunctiva). In dark-skinned persons, examination of the palms and the soles may also be useful.
- *Moisture*—Is the patient diaphoretic (sweaty)? Is the skin drier than usual (scaling, cracked)?
- *Temperature*—Note changes of increased or decreased temperature to palpation both throughout the body and in localized areas.
- *Texture*—Is the skin smooth or rough? Sometimes scar tissue looks and feels leatherlike.
- *Mobility and turgor*—**Turgor** is the elasticity ("snapability") of the skin. Normally, if the skin is gently pinched up, it rapidly resumes its normal position. If it remains up ("tented"), dehydration may be present. This is called **tenting** or *decreased skin turgor.* The skin should be freely mobile (easy to move) with touch.
- *Lesions*—Lesions include scars, moles, birthmarks, wounds, and bruises.

Abnormalities—Be certain to properly document abnormalities in color, temperature, or skin and nail condition. Common abnormalities include the following:

- **Pallor**—Unnatural paleness or absence of color in the skin.
- **Cyanosis**—Bluish discoloration of the skin and mucous membranes, caused by an excess of deoxygenated hemoglobin in the blood. Cyanosis is classified as *central* or *peripheral,* depending on the cause (peripheral vascular disease versus hypoxia or cardiac problems). Central cyanosis is best seen in the lips, oral mucosa, and tongue. Cold exposure, however, can cause the lips to appear bluish. Isolated cyanosis of the nail beds, hands, or feet may be central or peripheral in origin. Anxiety and cold are common causes of peripheral cyanosis (see Figure 22-8).

TABLE 10-1

Examination of the Skin

TECHNIQUES OF EXAMINATION	NOTE THE FOLLOWING CHARACTERISTICS	DOCUMENT ABNORMALITIES
Inspect and palpate the skin	Color	Color
Inspect the fingernails	Moisture	Temperature
	Temperature	Condition
	Texture	
	Mobility and turgor	
	Lesions	

- **Jaundice**—Yellowish discoloration of the skin, mucous membranes, and sclerae of the eyes, caused by greater than normal amounts of bilirubin (a breakdown product of hemoglobin) in the blood.
- *Rashes*—General term for any type of abnormal skin eruption.
- *Bruises* (ecchymosis)—Discoloration of an area of the skin or mucous membrane caused by the leakage of blood into the subcutaneous tissues because of trauma to the underlying blood vessels or because of fragility of the vessel walls.
- *Scars*—Marks left in the skin or an internal organ by the healing of a wound, sore, or injury as a result of replacement of injured tissue by connective tissue.
- *Discoloration*—Abnormal tone or color; may be due to many causes.

HEENT (HEAD, EYES, EARS, NOSE, THROAT)

Head—Inspect and palpate the head, eyes, ears, nose, and throat area for evidence of trauma, tenderness, or deformity (Figures 10-11 to 10-13; Table 10-2). Observe the face for obvious deformities, swelling, or discoloration. Gently palpate the maxilla and mandible for possible fractures.

Eyes—Inspect and palpate the eyes, orbits, and eyelids for evidence of trauma. Pay particular attention to the position and alignment of the eyes, and to the pupils. Check the following:

- *Conjugate gaze*—The movement of each eye is controlled by the coordinated action of six muscles. These are often called the *extraocular movements (EOMs)*. **Conjugate gaze** means that the eyes move in the same direction—if a line were to be drawn from each pupil straight toward the examiner, both should

remain parallel throughout all directions of gaze. Check for proper conjugate gaze by having the patient follow your light or finger in the six cardinal directions (Figure 10-14). Injury to either the muscles or nerves of the eye will result in paralysis of one or more muscles. The result is that the eye deviates from its normal position, and the eyes no longer appear conjugate or parallel in that direction of gaze.

- *Size, shape, symmetry, and reactivity of the pupils*—Normally, both pupils should be the same size and shape and respond equally to light. Examine the pupils with a penlight, and note and compare their size and reactivity. Pupil size is classified as normal, dilated (big), constricted (small), or unequal (Figure 10-15). Unequally sized pupils in any patient with an altered LOC may be a sign of head injury or brain dysfunction.

Pupillary reactivity refers to how quickly the patient's pupils constrict when exposed to bright light. The response is classified as *reactive, slow,* or *nonreactive*. The best way to get a sense for the normal response is to practice on friends and colleagues.

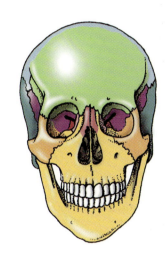
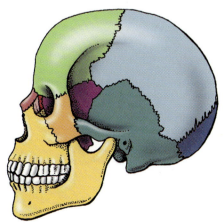

FIGURE 10-12 ▲ A normal skull, with no trauma or injury. (Duckwall Productions.)

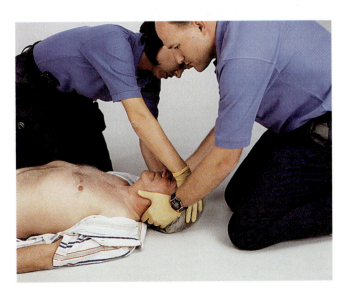

FIGURE 10-11 ▲ Assess the patient's head, checking for signs of trauma, deformity, or bleeding.

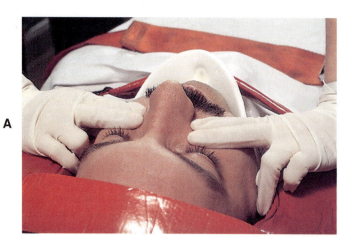

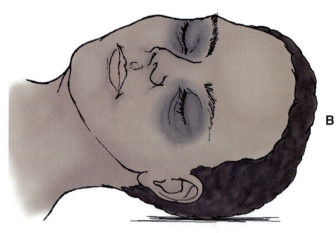

FIGURE 10-13 ▲ **A,** Palpate the area inferior to patient's eyes, checking for deformities, pain, or bruises. **B,** Raccoon eyes may indicate a skull fracture. (Vincent Knaus from Stoy W: Mosby's *EMT–Basic textbook,* St Louis, 1996, Mosby.)

TABLE 10-2

HEENT Examination

INSPECT AND PALPATE FOR TENDERNESS OR DEFORMITY	ADDITIONAL ASSESSMENT
Head	Note facial expression and contours
Scalp	Observe for asymmetry, involuntary movements, and edema
Skull	Note skin color, temperature, and condition
Face	
Eyes	Stand in front of the patient and survey the eyes
Position and alignment	Assess for conjugate gaze
Eyelids	Inspect the size, shape, symmetry, and reactivity of the pupils
Conjunctiva and sclera	Test the pupillary reactions to light (direct, consensual)
Pupils	
Ears	Inspect each auricle and surrounding tissue for deformities, drainage, tenderness, or erythema
Auricle	
Mastoid	Inspect the mastoid for discoloration and tenderness
Nose (anterior and inferior surface)	Assess for asymmetry, deformity, or foreign bodies
Mouth and pharynx	Inspect the lips; observe color, moisture, or cracking
	Note the color of the gums (normally pink)
	Inspect the teeth—any missing, discolored, loose, or abnormally positioned?
	Inspect the tongue—should appear symmetrical; note any white or reddened areas, nodules, or ulcerations
Neck	Note symmetry
	Note masses or scars
	Note any subcutaneous emphysema
	Inspect and palpate the trachea for any deviation
	Inspect for jugular venous distention
Cervical spine	Inspect
	Palpate for tenderness or deformity
	Assess for nuchal rigidity

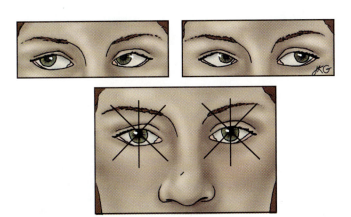

FIGURE 10-14 ▲ The six cardinal directions of gaze. Both eyes should move together in the same direction.

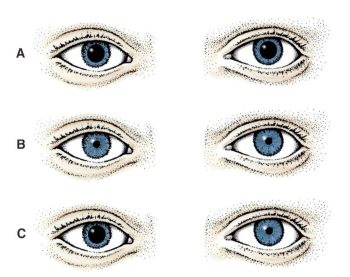

FIGURE 10-15 ▲ **A,** Dilated pupils may indicate fear, shock, or cardiac arrest. **B,** Constricted pupils may indicate shock, head injury, or poisoning. **C,** Unequal pupils may indicate head or eye trauma in a patient. (Duckwall Productions.)

To check for pupillary size and reactivity, do the following (Figure 10-16):
1. Briefly direct your light at one eye.
2. Observe for pupil constriction.
3. Remove the light, and observe for dilation.
4. Repeat for the opposite eye, and compare the responses.

HELPFUL HINT

In a brightly lit area the pupils will normally be constricted. It may be difficult to see much change when you check for reactivity. In this case, shade the eyes with your other hand.

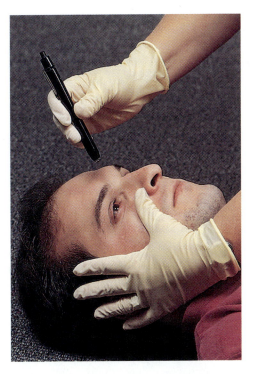

FIGURE 10-16 ▲ Check the patient's pupils for size and reactivity. (Vincent Knaus from Stoy W: *Mosby's EMT–Basic textbook,* St Louis, 1996, Mosby.)

A commonly used acronym is **PERRL,** which stands for *Pupils are Equal, Round, and React to Light.* Causes of abnormal pupillary responses include the following:
- *Dilated pupils*—Fear, shock, cardiac arrest, brain injury, drug use, blindness
- *Constricted pupils*—Head injury, bleeding in the brain, stroke, drug use, poisoning
- *Unequal pupils*—Head injury, bleeding in the brain, direct trauma to the eye, cataract surgery
- *Unresponsive pupils*—Coma, death, artificial eye, drugs

CLINICAL NOTES

Two to four percent of people have unequal pupils normally. This condition is known as anisocoria.

- *Pupillary reactions to light (direct, consensual)*—A beam of light shown into only one eye normally causes pupillary constriction in both that eye (the **direct pupillary reaction** to light) and the opposite eye (the **consensual pupillary reaction**) (Figure 10-17). Failure of this to occur indicates dysfunction of the eye, the optic nerve, or the brain.

Observe the sclera (white part of the eye) (Figure 10-18). Reddened or bloodshot sclerae may suggest alcohol consumption, drugs, or injury. Retract the lower

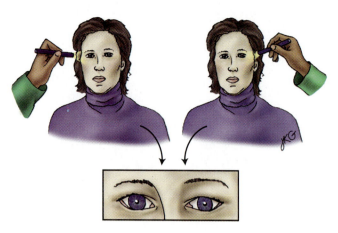

FIGURE 10-17 ▲ Direct and consensual reactions; regardless of which eye the light shines into, both pupils normally constrict equally.

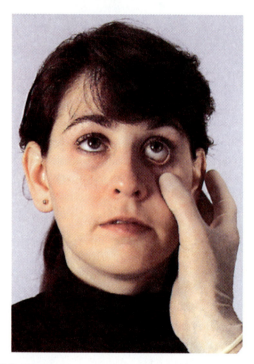

FIGURE 10-18 ▲ Inspect the cornea and sclera. (From Seidel HM et al: *Mosby's guide to physical examination,* ed 2, St Louis, 1991, Mosby.)

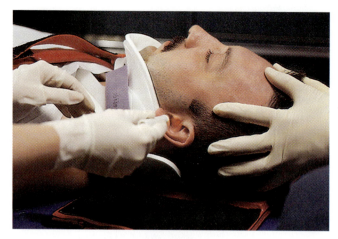

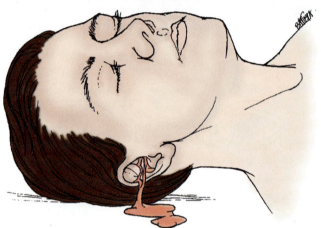

FIGURE 10-19 ▲ **A,** Inspect the patient's ears for blood or fluid. **B,** Always suspect cervical spine injury or skull fracture in a patient with blood or other fluid in the ear. (Vincent Knaus from Stoy W: *Mosby's EMT–Basic textbook,* St Louis, 1996, Mosby.)

Check the area behind the ears for discoloration. Bruising of this area is called **Battle's sign** and may suggest a basilar skull fracture (Figure 10-20). This sign usually takes time to develop and may not be visible at the scene.

CLINICAL NOTES

A drop of blood mixed with CSF will form a brown ring when placed onto a gauze pad. This is known as the "halo test," or "Bull's-eye sign." For years, this test was considered a standard way to decide whether fluid contained CSF. It has recently been questioned in the medical literature. Current trends suggest that a chemical dipstick for glucose, such as those used in blood glucose monitoring, be used instead. Follow your local protocols and medical control recommendations.

eyelids, and look at the color of the mucous membrane. A pale color may indicate poor perfusion. Palpate the orbits for fractures. Perform a brief visual acuity examination by asking the patient to count fingers. Visual acuity is a measure of the accuracy of a patient's vision. Note any blurring, double vision, or blindness.

Ears—Examine the outer ear for lacerations, bleeding, or other evidence of soft tissue trauma. Visually inspect the ear canals. Blood or clear watery fluid—cerebrospinal fluid (CSF)—in the ear may indicate a basilar skull fracture (Figure 10-19). CSF may be mixed with blood.

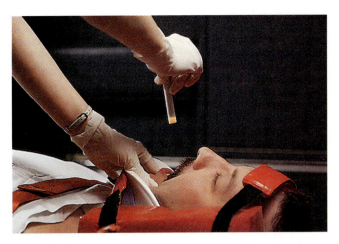

FIGURE 10-22 ▲ Inspect the patient's mouth for foreign objects and soft tissue injuries. (Vincent Knaus from Stoy W: *Mosby's EMT–Basic textbook,* St Louis, 1996, Mosby.)

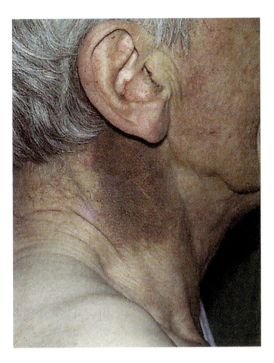

FIGURE 10-20 ▲ Battle's sign. (From Mills KLG et al: *Color atlas and text of emergencies,* ed 2, London, 1995, Mosby-Wolfe.)

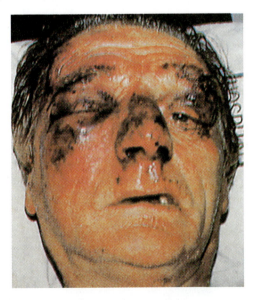

FIGURE 10-21 ▲ Observe for deformities showing a fracture or dislocated nasal cartilage. (From London PS: *A colour atlas of diagnosis after recent injury,* London, 1990, Mosby-Wolfe.)

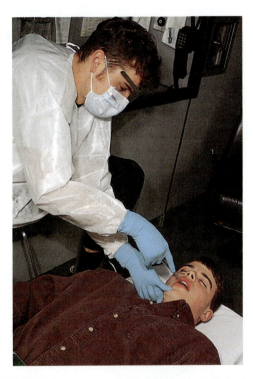

FIGURE 10-23 ▲ Suctioning is used to clear fluids from the airway. (Vincent Knaus from Stoy W: *Mosby's EMT–Basic textbook,* St Louis, 1996, Mosby.)

Nose—Observe for deformities showing a fracture or dislocated nasal cartilage (Figure 10-21). Note lacerations or other soft tissue injuries. A skull fracture may cause blood or CSF to drain into the nasopharynx, which may compromise the patient's airway.

Mouth and Throat—In the unresponsive patient, gently separate the lips and inspect the mouth for foreign material, broken teeth, or dentures. Remove den-

tures only if they are loose. Note soft tissue injuries within the mouth. Lacerations on the floor of the mouth, the inner surface of the cheek, and the base of the tongue are often overlooked (Figure 10-22).

Bleeding into the mouth can obstruct the upper airway. Suction may be required to keep the airway open and get a clear view (Figure 10-23). If the patient's airway is compromised, clear the airway and reclassify the patient as "priority" status. If you do not suspect spinal injury, position the patient to allow for drainage of blood.

While assessing the mouth, note the patient's breath odor. Alcohol ingestion usually gives off a distinct odor. A fruity odor may indicate diabetes mellitus (Chapter 24).

Neck—Assess the neck for ecchymosis, neck vein distention, open injuries, and **nuchal rigidity**—stiffness of the neck with decreased range of motion (Figures 10-24 and 10-25). This may indicate infection, such as meningitis, or may be due to muscle spasm from a whiplash type of injury. Assume that a patient with nuchal rigidity has a potentially life-threatening problem (e.g., bacterial meningitis) until proven otherwise.

Gently palpate the anterior neck for tracheal positioning (the trachea should be midline), and ask if the patient feels pain. Never palpate both sides of the neck simultaneously, since blood flow to the brain could be disrupted. Do not remove the extrication collar if it is already in place (Figure 10-26).

Ecchymosis in the neck region may signify trauma and impending airway obstruction. Normally, the neck veins are barely visible. If they are bulging outward, they are considered distended. Neck vein distention may be seen in conditions such as congestive heart failure and cardiac tamponade (Figure 10-27). Jugular vein distention (JVD) evaluation is best done with the patient sitting at a 45-degree angle.

An open wound to the anterior neck, even if it appears minor, is an emergency. If swelling develops, pressure on the trachea may obstruct the airway. If the trachea is injured, air may leak into the subcutaneous tissue, a condition known as **subcutaneous emphysema** and that feels like a crunching or crackling below the skin.

CHEST

Techniques of Examination—If it has not already been done, expose the chest and observe for symmetrical breathing, equal expansion, obvious injuries, open wounds, or scars. Observe the rate, rhythm, depth, and effort of breathing; always check for cyanosis (Figures 10-28 and 10-29; Table 10-3).

Under normal circumstances an adult breathes about 12 to 20 times per minute. Children and infants breathe faster. Adult patients whose respiratory rate is less than 10 or above 30 are often experiencing some type of compromise that requires appropriate care. The normal **respiratory rates** are as follows:
- Newborn: 40 breaths per minute
- Infant (younger than 1 year): 20 to 30 breaths per minute

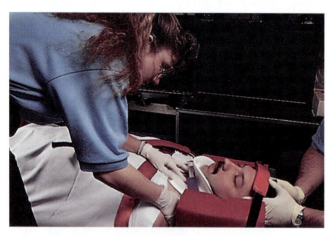

FIGURE 10-24 ▲ Carefully palpate the patient's cervical spine. (Vincent Knaus from Stoy W: *Mosby's EMT–Basic textbook,* St Louis, 1996, Mosby.)

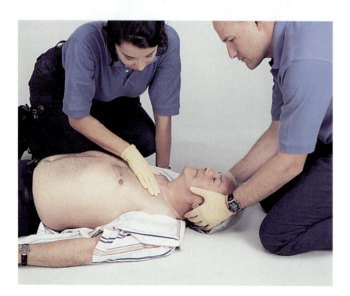

FIGURE 10-25 ▲ Assess the patient's neck for signs of trauma.

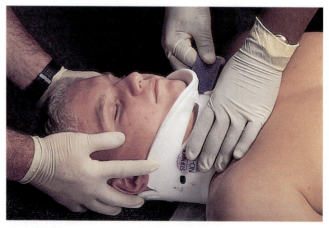

FIGURE 10-26 ▲ Apply a rigid extrication collar if a cervical spine injury is suspected. (Vincent Knaus from Stoy W: *Mosby's EMT–Basic textbook,* St Louis, 1996, Mosby.)

- Child: 18 to 26 breaths per minute
- Adult: 12 to 20 breaths per minute

Bradypnea is a respiratory rate that is too slow, and **tachypnea** is a respiratory rate that is too fast.

Some patients may try consciously to control their respiratory rates when they know they are being monitored. The following are some tips on gaining a more accurate rate:

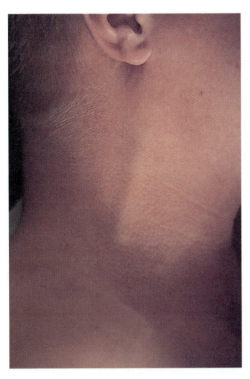

FIGURE 10-27 ▲ Distended neck veins may suggest chest injury. (Vincent Knaus from Stoy W: *Mosby's EMT–Basic textbook,* St Louis, 1996, Mosby.)

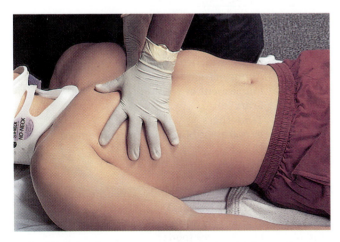

FIGURE 10-28 ▲ Assess the patient's chest, checking for paradoxical breathing or major injuries. (Vincent Knaus from Stoy W: *Mosby's EMT–Basic textbook,* St Louis, 1996, Mosby.)

- After assessing the pulse, keep your hands in place but count respirations instead.
- When counting a radial pulse, place the patient's arm across the chest; when you finish taking the pulse, count respirations (Figure 10-30).

Along with rate, assess the depth and quality of respirations. Depth is assessed by watching the rise and fall of the patient's chest while assessing respirations. Some patients are abdominal breathers whose abdomens may move more than the chest during respiration. Quality of respirations includes the adequacy of air exchange and ease of respirations. Hearing and feeling air exchange is important. Chest movement is not proof of adequate breathing.

Ease of respirations is also an important component to assess. Signs of respiratory distress include the following (see Figure 22-5):

- *Nasal flaring*—Widening of the nostrils during inspiration, known as **nasal flaring,** is more common in infants and children.
- *Paradoxical chest movements*—In **paradoxical** (asymmetrical) **chest movements,** part of the chest wall moves in a direction opposite to the rest of the chest. The most common reason for this is because part of the chest wall has been damaged. With the loss of the normal mechanical function, the injured section is unable to move in synchrony with the normal sections.
- *Use of accessory muscles*—The neck and intercostal muscles (the muscles between the ribs) participate in breathing only when respiratory difficulty is present. Thus they are considered **accessory muscles of respiration.** Their contractions can be seen as indentations between the patient's ribs and above the clavicles during inhalation. These are sometimes called **intercostal retractions** or **supraclavicular retractions.**
- *Pursed lip breathing*—Exhaling through puckered-out lips, indicating strained breathing, is known as

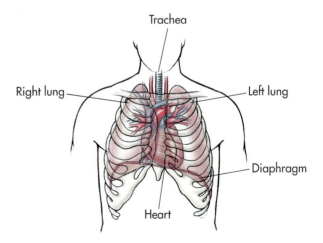

FIGURE 10-29 ▲ Normal chest structures, without trauma or injury. (Duckwall Productions.)

pursed lip breathing or **lip pursing.** Patients subconsciously breathe this way in an attempt to increase the pressure in the lungs—increased pressures cause more alveoli to remain open for a longer period, increasing the oxygen delivered to the patient (see Figure 22-10).

- *Noisy breathing*—Abnormal respiratory sounds include grunting and gurgling. **Stridor** is a high-pitched sound, usually heard on inspiration, that suggests obstruction in the airway. **Grunting** is abnormal, short and loud breaks during exhalation, which may indicate pain or severe respiratory distress, particularly in an infant or child. **Gurgling** is a bubbling sound caused by fluid in the airways, such as from heart failure, excessive oral secretions, or pneumonia.
- *Obvious difficulty* in inhalation or exhalation.
- *Cyanosis*—Bluish discoloration of the skin and lips is a late sign of respiratory difficulty (see Figure 22-8).

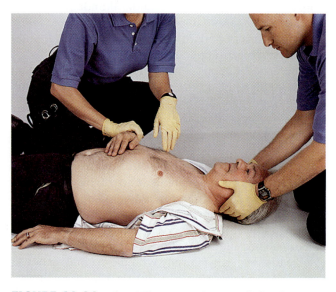

FIGURE 10-30 ▲ When counting a radial pulse, place the patient's arm across the chest; when you finish taking the pulse, count the respirations.

> ▶ The following are some common breathing patterns (see Figure 22-9):
> - **Eupnea**—Normal inhalation and exhalation.
> - **Apnea**—Absence of breathing.
> - **Bradypnea**—Slow respirations.
> - **Tachypnea**—Rapid and usually shallow respirations.
> - **Kussmaul respirations**—Rapid and deep respirations usually found in diabetic patients or others with imbalances of the acid content in their bodies.
> - **Cheyne-Stokes respirations** (pronounced "chain"-stokes)—A series of rapid then slow respirations followed by periods of apnea.

Palpate, then auscultate the chest—Palpate the chest; begin with the clavicles, and then palpate the rib cage. Note pain, tenderness, possible fractures, or subcutaneous emphysema. After palpation, auscultate the chest to verify breath sounds (Figures 10-31 and 10-32).

TABLE 10-3

Chest Examination

TECHNIQUES OF EXAMINATION	NOTE THE FOLLOWING CHARACTERISTICS	DOCUMENT ABNORMALITIES
Inspect the anterior and posterior chest	Deformities or asymmetry	Barrel chest
		Traumatic flail chest
		Open wounds
		Other evidence of trauma
		Abnormal retractions
		Impairment of respiratory movement
Palpate the anterior and posterior chest	Tenderness	Scars
	Abnormalities	Tenderness
	Respiratory expansion	Impairment of respiratory movement
Percuss in symmetrical locations	Area of abnormal percussion	Dullness
		Resonance
		Hyperresonance
Auscultate breath sounds	Normal (vesicular, bronchovesicular, bronchial, tracheal)	Discontinuous sounds (fine crackles, coarse crackles)
	Added sounds (adventitious lung sounds)	Continuous sounds (wheezes, rhonchi)
	Diminished or absent lung sounds	Effusion, consolidation

Remember, the right lung is divided into the upper, middle, and lower lobes, whereas the left lung has only two lobes: upper and lower. Try to associate the underlying lung anatomy with surface markers (Figure 10-33). Typically, lung findings are described by the region of the chest over which they are noted, *not* by the anticipated lobe of the lung.

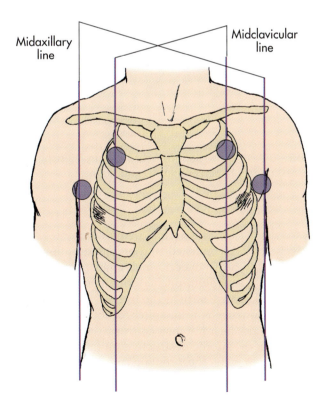

FIGURE 10-31 ▲ Ascultate the patient's lungs; listen to the flow of air in and out of the chest.

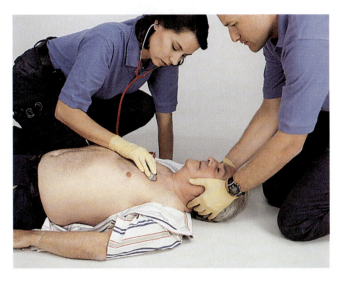

FIGURE 10-32 ▲ Proper locations for auscultating the lungs. (Kimberly Battista from Stoy W: *Mosby's EMT–Basic textbook,* St Louis, 1996, Mosby.)

As an example, a person may have abnormal lung sounds over the upper posterior aspect of the thorax. Anatomically, this could correspond to either the upper lobe or the upper portion of the lower lobe of the lung.

Examination of the Anterior and Posterior Chest—Inspect the chest for the following:
* *Deformities or asymmetry*—Check for "barrel chest deformity," traumatic flail chest, open wounds, and other evidence of trauma.
* *Impairment of respiratory movement*—Listen to the patient's breathing. Are abnormal signs present (e.g., wheezing, stridor) even without the aid of a stethoscope?
* *Abnormal retractions*—Check for inward movements of the skin between the rib interspaces during inspiration. They may also be seen in the area above the clavicles, the *supraclavicular fossa.* Although they are sometimes seen in normal thin persons, the presence of retractions, especially if the patient is short of breath, indicates increased work of breathing. Normally, diaphragmatic contraction is sufficient for adequate ventilation and oxygenation. Retractions represent contraction of the accessory muscles of respiration, such as the intercostal muscles, to help in inspiration.

Then, palpate the chest for tenderness, followed by percussion and auscultation.

Percussion of the chest helps determine whether the underlying tissues are air filled, fluid filled, or solid. It involves striking one finger against a knuckle of the other hand, which is spread over the chest. This "tapping" sends out vibrations, producing sound, much like beating on a drum (only not as strongly!) (Figure 10-34). The best way to learn is to practice. Percuss a variety of objects. When you are comfortable with the technique, practice on another person.

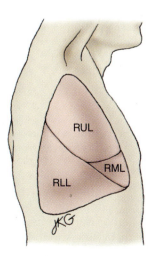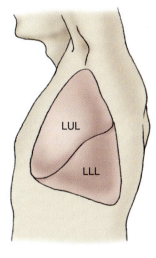

FIGURE 10-33 ▲ Try to associate the underlying lung anatomy with surface anatomy. *RUL,* Right upper lobe; *RML,* right middle lobe; *RLL,* right lower lobe; *LUL,* left upper lobe; *LLL,* left lower lobe.

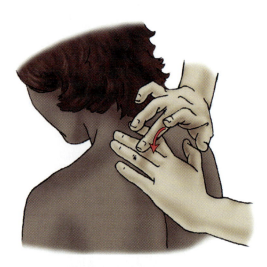

FIGURE 10-34 ▲ Technique of chest percussion involves tapping the interphalangeal joint of the nondominant hand while listening carefully to the sounds produced.

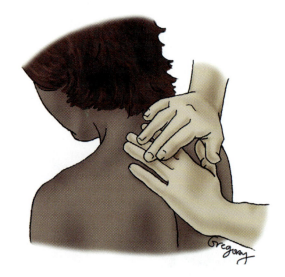

Hyperresonance over excess air (pneumothorax, COPD)

Normal percussion tone over normal lung

Dullness over solid organs and fluid-filled lungs

FIGURE 10-36 ▲ Sounds heard during chest percussion, resonance, hyperresonance, and dullness.

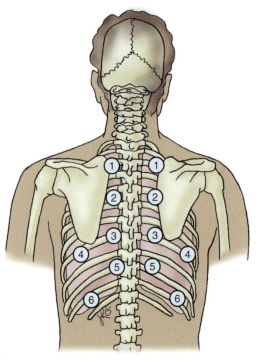

Percuss each side, alternately, from top to bottom.

FIGURE 10-35 ▲ Location for percussion and auscultation of the chest. Percuss each side, alternately, from top to bottom.

Percuss the thorax symmetrically, from top to bottom. Some prefer to do one side (left or right) in its entirety; others prefer to compare, side by side, top to bottom, as illustrated in Figure 10-35.

Sounds heard during chest percussion are classified by different terms. Sometimes, telling these apart is difficult. The most helpful rule is that the findings should be *symmetrical* on both sides of the posterior thorax. Any reproducible differences are probably abnormal (Figure 10-36).

- *Normal resonance* (the **normal percussion note**) is relatively loud, low pitched, and of long duration. This is the sound heard over normal lungs.
- **Dullness** is a medium-pitched sound normally heard over solid organs, such as the liver.
- **Hyperresonance** is a low-pitched, loud tone that is normally not heard. It may occur in the face of pneumothorax or chronic obstructive pulmonary disease (COPD) when the chest contains more air than usual.

Dullness replaces resonance when air contained in the lung is replaced with fluid or solid tissue. A similar situation occurs if the pleural space becomes filled with fluid *(pleural effusion)*. On the other hand, more air than usual, whether in the lungs (e.g., COPD) or in the pleural space (e.g., pneumothorax), makes the percussion note hyperresonant.

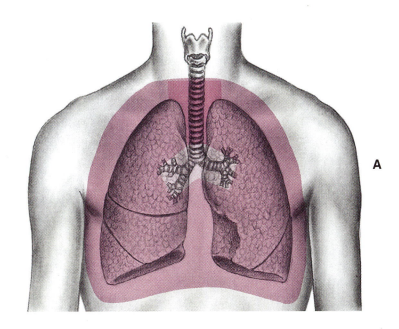

KEY:

█ Bronchovesicular
over main bronchi

█ Vesicular over lesser
bronchi, bronchioles, and lobes

█ Bronchial over trachea

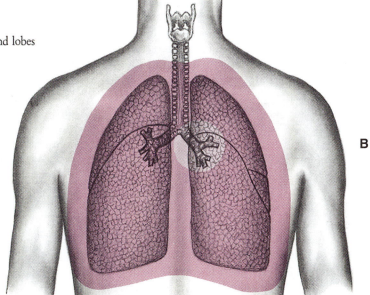

FIGURE 10-37 ▲ Expected auscultatory sounds. **A,** Anterior view. **B,** Posterior view. (From Seidel HM et al: *Mosby's guide to physical examination,* St Louis, 1987, Mosby.)

Auscultation of the chest for *normal lung sounds* (also called *breath sounds*) is vital to assess airflow through the airways. It involves listening to the sounds generated by breathing, checking for symmetry, and then determining whether additional abnormal sounds **(adventitious lung sounds)** are present. The chest should be auscultated in at least six different areas. Ascertain that breath sounds are equal on each side. If cervical spine injury is not suspected, perform both anterior and posterior auscultation.

The easiest way to understand the normal lung sounds is to practice with a partner. Four normal patterns are heard, depending on the area auscultated (Figure 10-37):

● **Vesicular breath sounds**—Normal sounds of rustling or swishing heard with the stethoscope over the lung periphery. These are usually higher pitched during inspiration and fade rapidly during expiration.
● **Bronchial breath sounds**—Normal sounds if heard over the anterior sternum; otherwise abnormal sounds heard with a stethoscope over the lungs, indicating *consolidation* (filled with fluid) or compression of a normal lung. Expiration and inspiration produce loud, high-pitched sounds with a short

silent period between the inspiratory and expiratory sounds. Expiration lasts longer.

- **Bronchovesicular breath sounds**—Sounds that are between tracheal sounds and vesicular sounds. These may be normal in the first and second interspaces anteriorly and between the scapulae, but otherwise they suggest fluid in the lungs.
- **Tracheal breath sounds**—Normal breath sounds heard during auscultation over the trachea. Inspiration and expiration are equally loud, with the expiratory sound being heard during the greater part of expiration, whereas the inspiratory sound stops abruptly at the height of inspiration, with a pause before the sound of expiration is heard.

Adventitious lung sounds are additional sounds heard during auscultation of the chest and are usually abnormal. There has been much debate over the use of terms, and experts continue to disagree. The most practical way to classify added sounds is by their duration throughout the respiratory cycle:

- *Discontinuous sounds*—These are sounds that are, by definition, not present for the entire respiratory cycle (full inspiration to full exhalation). These intermittent sounds may follow a pattern, such as being present only during inspiration, or they may occur in a random fashion. If the patient's condition is serious enough, some usually discontinuous sounds may become continuous (e.g., crackles in severe congestive heart failure).

  The general term for discontinuous sounds is **crackles.** Some use the term *rales* to indicate a similar sound, but *crackles* is a far more descriptive and understandable term. Crackles are crackling or bubbling sounds that represent fluid in the alveoli and are present in heart failure or pneumonia. Some further differentiate crackles into *fine crackles* (quieter, higher pitched) and *coarse crackles* (louder, higher pitched). One way to get an idea of the sound of crackles is to rub your hair together between the thumb and index finger close to your ear.

- *Continuous sounds*—Again, there is some overlap between continuous and noncontinuous sounds. Wheezes and rhonchi tend to be more continuous than crackles. **Wheezes** are squeaking, high-pitched sounds that may occur on either inspiration, expiration, or both. They represent spasms in the airways and are present in asthma, COPD, and heart failure. **Rhonchi** are coarser and sound like "gurgling." They are often present over the larger airways only and may be present on both inspiration and expiration. Rhonchi indicate mucus or other type of material in the larynx, trachea, or bronchi. They are often present in upper respiratory infections such as bronchitis.

As in the rest of the body, symmetry is important. Lung sounds should be relatively similar on both sides of each part of the chest. *Diminished* or *absent* lung sounds suggest either pleural effusion (fluid), consoli-

dation (fluid in the lungs for any reason), collapsed lung, or a surgically removed lung.

CARDIOVASCULAR SYSTEM

Evaluation of the cardiovascular system involves examination of four areas (Table 10-4):

- Arterial pulse
- Blood pressure
- Jugular venous pressure and pulsation
- Heart

Arterial Pulse—When assessing vital signs, the most commonly used pulses are the radial, carotid, brachial, and femoral. In the conscious patient the radial pulse is used most often. In patients with shock or poor circulation, the radial pulse may be either absent or difficult to assess. In these patients, palpate the carotid or femoral pulse.

It is important to assess for three particular characteristics during palpation of the pulse: *rate*, regularity, *(rhythm)*, and character *(amplitude)* (Figure 10-38).

The **pulse rate** (sometimes called *heart rate*) is measured as beats per minute. The normal adult pulse rate is 60 to 100 beats per minute. A heart rate that is greater than 100 beats per minute is called **tachycardia,** whereas a heart rate less than 60 beats per minute is called **bradycardia.** Athletes and patients taking certain blood pressure or cardiac medications may have a resting pulse rate as low as 40 beats per minute. This may be considered normal for these patients if the patient is not dizzy or showing other signs or symptoms of hypoperfusion.

Normal pulse ranges for various age-groups are as follows:
- Newborn to 3 years old: 100 to 160 beats per minute
- Child (3 to 8 years old): 70 to 150 beats per minute
- Older child (8 to 12 years old): 55 to 110 beats per minute
- Adolescent (12 to 18 years old): 60 to 110 beats per minute
- Adults (over 18 years old): 60 to 100 beats per minute

Also assess the *regularity* of the pulse. Normally, the pulse has very regular intervals between beats. Certain conditions such as heart disease or drugs can cause the pulse to be irregular. An irregular pulse may suggest a rhythm disturbance of the heart called a **cardiac dysrhythmia.** Some patients will complain that they feel dizzy or notice "skipped" or "extra" beats. If the patient has an irregular pulse, counting the rate for a full minute is helpful. Determine the frequency and nature, if possible, of the irregularities. For example, the pulse may skip every four beats, or pause every third beat—

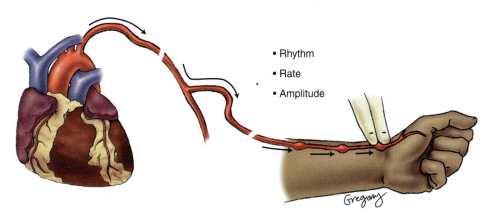

FIGURE 10-38 ▲ Characteristics to monitor in the pulse.

TABLE 10-4

Cardiovascular Examination

TECHNIQUES OF EXAMINATION	NOTE THE FOLLOWING CHARACTERISTICS	DOCUMENT ABNORMALITIES
Evaluate the arterial pulse	Rate Rhythm Amplitude	Bradycardia Tachycardia Irregular heartbeat Weak, thready, or bounding pulse
Evaluate the blood pressure	Systolic pressure Diastolic pressure Pulse pressure Orthostatic hypotension (if applicable)	Hypertension Hypotension Orthostasis
Evaluate the jugular venous pressure and pulsation	Distention If palpable (should not be)	Bulging Distention Palpable (probably is actually the carotid)
Evaluate the heart	Inspect and palpate the chest Locate the point of maximum impulse (PMI) Assess the apical pulse Listen to heart tones	Bradycardia Tachycardia Irregular heartbeat Distant or muffled heart tones

this information may be helpful in determining the cause of the problem.

If you feel an irregular pulse after repeated checks, suspect cardiac abnormalities. The combination of a rapid and irregular pulse may be dangerous because the heart's chambers do not have enough time to refill with blood between contractions. Blood that the heart pumps out during each contraction decreases significantly, resulting in a reduction in perfusion (circulation through body tissues). If allowed by your local protocols, place the patient on a cardiac monitor if you have not already done so.

Character is another important component of the pulse. Pulse character is usually described as follows:
● *Strong*—Easily palpated.
● *Weak*—Difficult to palpate.

● *Bounding*—Visible through the skin.
● *Thready*—Weak, unsteady, and usually rapid.

Weak and thready pulses are associated with shock. A bounding pulse may be caused by exercise, heat injury, stroke, or high blood pressure.

▶ NOTE: The authors assume that the reader is familiar with how to take a blood pressure, using either auscultation (stethoscope), palpation, or an automated device.

Blood Pressure—The **blood pressure** is a measurement of the force within the arteries created by the flow of blood and is measured with a *sphygmomanometer,* sometimes known as a **blood pressure cuff** or "BP cuff." Blood pressure is measured in millimeters of mercury (mm Hg). A measurement of 120 mm Hg means that there is enough pressure within the vessel to support a column of mercury 120 mm tall. Although some sphygmomanometers use mercury, air and electronic devices are becoming increasingly common.

Each contraction of the heart, or **systole,** generates a wave of pressure in the arterial tree. The peak level of this wave is known as the *systolic pressure.* The *diastolic pressure* is the low point of the wave and reflects the force maintained between beats, or **diastole,** when the heart is at rest.

Blood pressure readings are recorded as a figure that looks like a fraction (e.g., 120/80 mm Hg). The first or upper number is the systolic pressure. The second or bottom number is the diastolic pressure. Because most gauges have a scale in increments of 2 mm Hg, blood pressure is usually read as an even number. Digital units may also use odd numbers.

Like other vital signs, there is no single blood pressure that is normal for everyone. There is a wide range considered within normal limits **(normotension).** The normal systolic blood pressure range for an adult at rest is 90 to 140 mm Hg. Diastolic pressure ranges from 60 to 90 mm Hg. Blood pressure ranges may be affected by the following:

- *Age*—Blood pressure usually increases in the elderly.
- *Sex*—Females tend to have lower blood pressure.
- *Body size*—Smaller patients may normally have a lower blood pressure.

> Normotensive ranges for various age-groups are as follows:
> - Newborn (average): 70/40 mm Hg
> - Up to 1 year: 86/60 mm Hg
> - Over 2 years: See formula below
> - Adult (average): 100 to 140/50 to 90 mm Hg

> The lower limit of normal for systolic blood pressure in a child over 2 years of age may be estimated by the following formula:
>
> Systolic lower limit = 70 + (2 × Age in years)
>
> Levels below this number in a child should be considered abnormal under the appropriate circumstances (i.e., a sick patient or evidence of injury). Other signs of shock are usually present in a child long before the blood pressure drops. A decrease in blood pressure in a child is a *late* sign of shock and should indicate a need for "priority" care.

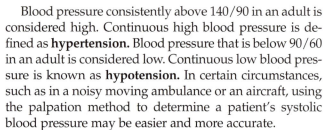

CLINICAL NOTES

Measurement of blood pressure in newborns and children younger than 3 years old is difficult in the field. Follow your local protocols.

Blood pressure consistently above 140/90 in an adult is considered high. Continuous high blood pressure is defined as **hypertension.** Blood pressure that is below 90/60 in an adult is considered low. Continuous low blood pressure is known as **hypotension.** In certain circumstances, such as in a noisy moving ambulance or an aircraft, using the palpation method to determine a patient's systolic blood pressure may be easier and more accurate.

Certain cardiovascular conditions may cause the blood pressure to be different in each of the upper extremities. If time permits, measure the blood pressure in each arm.

> ► ELECTRONIC BLOOD PRESSURE MONITORS
> Electronic blood pressure monitors are excellent for continuous monitoring of blood pressure. However, in emergencies they are not appropriate for initial measurements for the following reasons:
> - The initial readings tend to be inaccurate.
> - They take more time to put into use than manual methods.
> - As with any electronic device, they are subject to operator and equipment failure.
> You should maintain proficiency in traditional blood pressure monitoring and use a manual sphygmomanometer for the initial assessment.

> ► ERRORS IN BLOOD PRESSURE MEASUREMENT
> Errors can occur in the measurement of blood pressure. Generally, most are avoidable.
> - If the cuff size is too small, it will act as a tourniquet and the reading will be falsely high.
> - If the cuff size is too large, the reading will be falsely low.
> - Sounds may be heard incorrectly.
> - The cuff may be placed too loosely. The recorded blood pressure will not be correct, but it is impossible to predict with reliability in which direction (falsely high or low) the error will occur.

Orthostatic Hypotension—In some individuals the blood pressure drops suddenly when the person stands up. This condition is known as **orthostatic hypotension.** Orthostatic hypotension is more common in smaller females, the elderly, and patients who are dehydrated or bleeding internally. There are many causes for **orthostasis,** including volume loss for any reason, such as bleeding or diarrhea. Remember that orthostatic changes are somewhat subjective, and normal findings vary from patient to patient. Overall, "positive" findings of orthostatic change include the following (Figure 10-39):

- An increase in the pulse rate of 10 to 20 beats per minute or greater
- A decrease in the systolic blood pressure of 10 to 20 mm Hg or greater

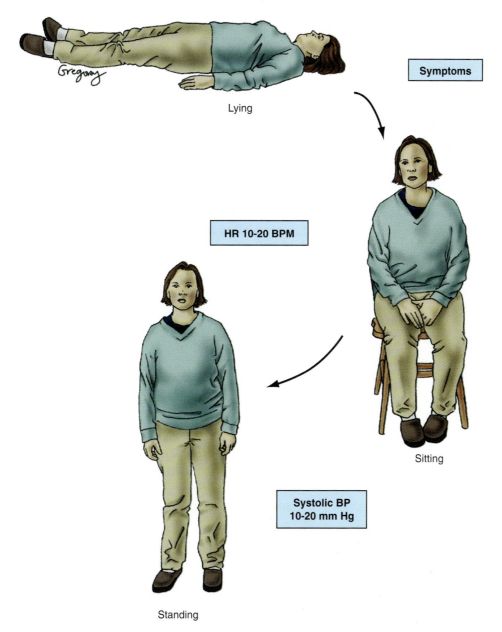

Lying

Symptoms

Sitting

HR 10-20 BPM

Systolic BP
10-20 mm Hg

Standing

FIGURE 10-39 ▲ Orthostasis.

● Symptoms in the patient (These may include weakness, dizziness, or feeling like one is going to pass out. Even if the pulse and blood pressure do not change, many experts consider a patient who develops symptoms with positional changes to have a positive test.)

When checking for orthostatic changes, take both the blood pressure and pulse with patients first lying down. Then, sit them up for 2 minutes and repeat the procedure. If the test is positive (blood pressure decreases, pulse increases, or patient is symptomatic), they are orthostatic; there is *no* need to stand them up to see "how low will it go!" If the test is negative, and you wish to continue checking, recheck the pulse and blood pressure after allowing the patient to stand for 2 minutes. The most helpful sign is if the patient develops symptoms, whether or not the pulse or blood pressure change.

▶ Often, there is no need to determine orthostatic vital signs, especially if patients are obviously unstable in the initial position you find them. Perform this part of the assessment only if you think it will contribute to your care of the patient.

Pulse Pressure—Changes in the pulse pressure are helpful in recognizing early shock. The difference between systolic blood pressure and diastolic blood pressure is the **pulse pressure.** The normal value is 40 mm Hg. During early shock, cardiac tamponade, or tension pneumothorax, the resistance to flow in the blood vessels goes up. This is reflected as an increase in diastolic blood pressure and a narrowing (decrease) in the pulse pressure. As shock progresses and the body's compensatory mechanisms fail, this finding is no longer reliable.

Jugular Venous Pressure and Pulsation— Normally, the neck veins are barely visible. Their level of distention is called the **jugular venous pressure.** If they appear to be bulging outward, they are considered distended. Neck vein distention may be seen in condi-

tions such as congestive heart failure and cardiac tamponade (see Figure 10-27). Venous pulsations are rarely palpable; if a pulse is felt, it is most likely the carotid artery. In addition, venous pulsations are eliminated by light pressure on the vein just above the sternal end of the clavicle; arterial (carotid) pulsations are not eliminated by this pressure. Finally, the level of venous pulsations changes with position, dropping as the patient becomes more upright; carotid pulsations are not changed by position.

Heart—As part of inspection and palpation of the chest, find the **point of maximum impulse (PMI)** of the heart. This is in the fifth intercostal space of the thorax, just medial to the left midclavicular line, where the *apical beat* of the heart is observed (Figure 10-40). Place the stethoscope here to obtain an *apical heart rate* and to listen for heart tones.

Normal heart tones or heart sounds are discussed in detail in Chapter 4. The contraction and relaxation of the heart, combined with the flow of blood, generates characteristic sounds (heart sounds) that can be heard with a stethoscope (auscultation of the heart). The normal pattern sounds much like "lub-DUB, lub-DUB, lub-DUB." The "lub" is called the **first heart sound (S_1),** and the "DUB" (emphasized because it is often louder) is the **second heart sound (S_2)** (Figure 10-41).

Listen over the PMI for distant or muffled heart tones. The intensity of heart tones varies from person to person. Those with hyperexpanded chests, such as in COPD, may have normally distant heart tones.

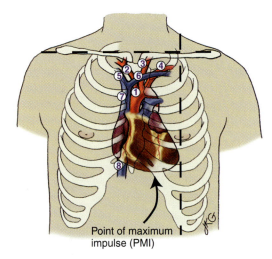

Point of maximum impulse (PMI)

FIGURE 10-40 ▲ **Point of maximum impulse.**

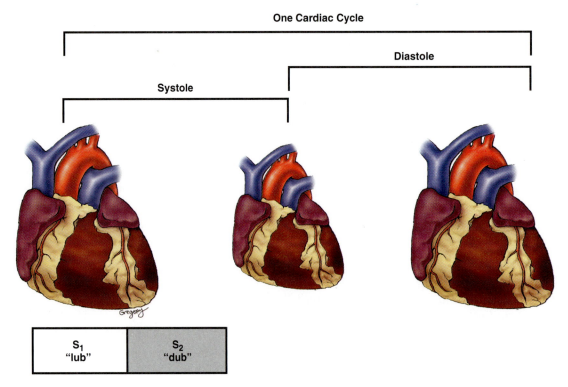

FIGURE 10-41 ▲ **One cardiac cycle.**

ABDOMEN

General Approach—Examine the abdomen with the patient in a supine position, if possible. Ask patients to point out tender areas first and examine these last. Some people are extremely sensitive to touch over the abdomen ("ticklish"). In this case, start palpation with your hand on top of the patient's (Table 10-5).

Inspect the Abdomen—Inspect the abdomen for signs of obvious injury, ecchymosis, or swelling. Note the following:

- *The skin*—Scars, **striae** ("stretch marks"), dilated veins, rashes, or lesions. Pinkish striae may be a sign of endocrine disease, whereas dilated veins, especially those that appear like a "bundle of worms" suggest severe liver disease (Figure 10-42).
- *Contour*—What is the general shape of the abdomen? It may be flat, rounded, **protuberant** (protrudes; fat tissue is the most common cause), or **scaphoid** (markedly concave or hollowed). Is it symmetrical, or is there swelling ("bulges"), either localized or diffuse? Are there bulges over the flanks? Depending on the location, abnormal abdominal bulges may indicate a hernia, mass, or fluid in the abdominal cavity (*ascites*) (Figure 10-43).
- *Pulsations*—In a thin individual the presence of normal pulsations in the upper abdominal aorta is common. Excessive pulsation or pulsations well below the epigastrium may indicate an aortic aneurysm.

Auscultate the Abdomen—In the abdominal examination, perform auscultation before palpation. Otherwise, the bowel may be jarred and alter the ability to listen to **bowel sounds** properly. Normally, the abdomen is relatively noisy; these "gurgles" represent normal peristalsis of food through the gut. Bowel sounds may be absent, increased (hyperactive), or decreased (hypoactive) (Figure 10-44):

- *Absent bowel sounds*—The total absence of bowel sounds is extremely worrisome and suggests serious intraabdominal pathology. To be certain that bowel sounds are *really* absent, most experts recommend listening for a minimum of 15 to 30 seconds in *each* of the four quadrants.
- *Decreased (hypoactive) bowel sounds*—Hypoactive bowel sounds are a very subjective finding, meaning that they are present, but not as audible as in most abdomens. There is a significant difference between the *total absence* of bowel sounds and *decreased* bowel sounds. It is for this reason that you must listen in all four quadrants, and for a period, before concluding that bowel sounds are really absent. Absent bowel sounds often indicate an acute surgical condition (e.g., peritonitis).
- *Increased (hyperactive) bowel sounds*—Hyperactive bowel sounds are far less diagnostic than are absent ones. Anxiety, diet, or hunger may cause *borborygmi*—rumbling, gurgling, and tinkling noises indicating hyperperistalsis. When the bowel sounds are *increased* or normal, listening in all four quadrants is not necessary.

Bruits may also be heard over the abdomen. These are moderate- to high-pitched "whooshing" sounds that represent turbulent blood flow in arteries. The significance of the bruit depends on its location:

- A bruit in the epigastric region, or upper quadrant—especially if present during both systole and

---

TABLE 10-5

Abdominal Examination

TECHNIQUES OF EXAMINATION	NOTE THE FOLLOWING CHARACTERISTICS	DOCUMENT ABNORMALITIES
Inspect the abdomen, including the flanks	Skin	Scars
	Contour (flat, rounded, protuberant, scaphoid [markedly concave or hollowed])	Striae ("stretch marks")
		Dilated veins
	Symmetry	Rashes and lesions
	Swelling	Bulges at the flanks
	Pulsations (aortic pulsation sometimes visible)	Abnormal bulges
		Hernias
		Distention
		Ascites
		Abnormal pulsations
Auscultate the abdomen (*before* palpation)	Bowel sounds	Absence
	Absence most important	Increased (hyperactive)
	Quantity, quality less helpful	Decreased (hypoactive)
	Bruits over arteries	
Palpate the abdomen	Light palpation	Muscle guarding
	Deep palpation	Rigidity
	Rebound tenderness (assess for peritoneal irritation)	Masses
		Tenderness, rebound

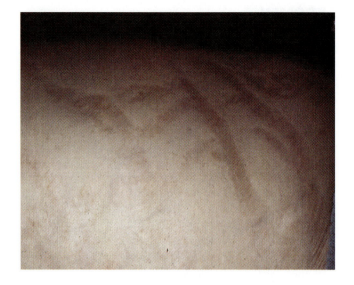

FIGURE 10-42 ▲ Striae. (From Seidel HM et al: *Mosby's guide to physical examination,* St Louis, 1991, Mosby.)

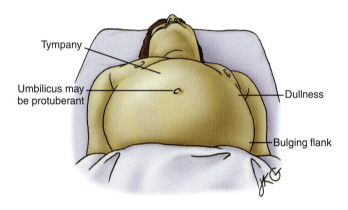

Tympany

Umbilicus may be protuberant

Dullness

Bulging flank

FIGURE 10-43 ▲ Abdominal distention.

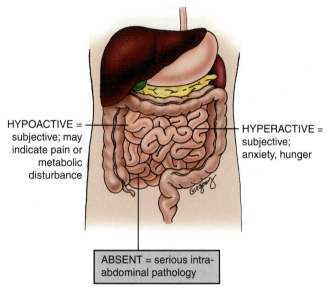

HYPOACTIVE = subjective; may indicate pain or metabolic disturbance

HYPERACTIVE = subjective; anxiety, hunger

ABSENT = serious intra-abdominal pathology

FIGURE 10-44 ▲ Auscultate bowel sounds.

diastole—suggests renal artery stenosis due to atherosclerosis. This is an uncommon but surgically treatable cause of hypertension (high blood pressure).

- A bruit over the lower abdomen or back suggests an aortic aneurysm.

- Bruits over the groin (a femoral artery) are common in systole; a murmur that persists through both systole *and* diastole may suggest potentially significant arterial occlusion.

Palpate the Abdomen—Perform palpation in two separate stages:

- *Light palpation*—Gently palpate the entire abdomen, keeping your hand and forearm horizontal to the abdomen, fingers together, and flat on the abdominal surface. Barely raise your hand off the skin when you move it around. Note **tenderness (pain with movement or palpation), guarding,** and **muscular rigidity,** as well as any masses or lesions. Observe the patient's face for any painful response or grimace (Figure 10-45). Consider what organs lie beneath the area of the abdomen being palpated (Figure 10-46).

Guarding is present when the patient moves or deliberately tenses the abdominal muscles to avoid pressure from the palpating hand. If muscular rigid-

ity (hardness or stiffness) persists despite your best efforts to calm the patient **(involuntary guarding),** it may be an indication of peritoneal irritation (peritonitis), especially if the bowel sounds are also absent. Sometimes, peritoneal irritation is so extensive that the abdominal muscles become "rock hard." This degree of spasm has been likened to feeling a hard board on the abdomen, thus the term **boardlike rigidity.** Weight lifters may have such extensive abdominal muscles that their abdomen feels this way normally.

Palpate posteriorly at the *costovertebral angle (CVA)* at the junction of the twelfth rib and the twelfth thoracic vertebra (Figure 10-47). CVA tenderness may indicate a kidney disorder.

- *Deep palpation*—Palpate the same area as with light palpation, except gently press a little harder and

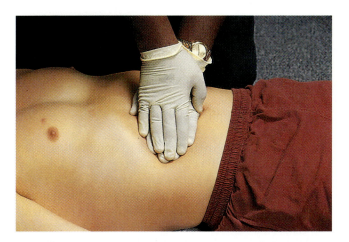

FIGURE 10-45 ▲ Palpate the patient's abdomen, checking to see if it is soft, firm, or distended. (Vincent Knaus from Stoy W: *Mosby's EMT–Basic textbook,* St Louis, 1996, Mosby.)

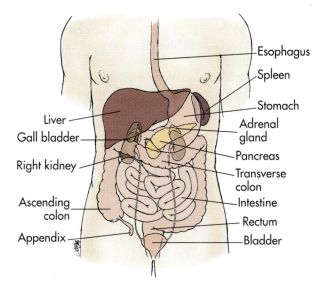

FIGURE 10-46 ▲ Organs of the normal abdominal cavity.

deeper. If the patient is tender with direct pressure, quickly withdraw your hand and see if the sudden withdrawal (which jars the peritoneal contents) worsens the pain. If the pain is worse with the sudden release of the pressure (withdrawal) than with direct pressure, the patient is said to have **rebound tenderness.** Rebound tenderness suggests peritoneal irritation **(peritonitis)** (Figure 10-48).

▶ NOTE: Findings of discoloration, rigidity, exposed intestines (evisceration), or severe pain indicate a serious problem. Classify these patients as "priority."

GENITALIA

The genital examination may be awkward or uncomfortable for both the patient and for the provider. A

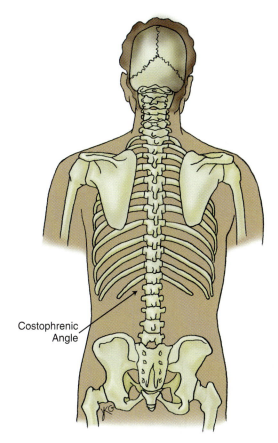

FIGURE 10-47 ▲ Costophrenic angle.

male examiner of a female patient typically has a female attendant present. This is both for patient comfort and legal protection. Some female examiners work alone with female patients, although a chaperone may be helpful, if available, for patients and examiners of both sexes.

The out-of-hospital physical examination of the genitalia is limited. In both men and women, inspect the external genitalia; carefully note any inflammation, discharge, bleeding, or swelling (Table 10-6).

EXTREMITIES

Although discussed separately here, the peripheral vascular system, as well as the nervous system, is examined at the same time as the extremities. Consider the functional implications of any illness or injury and the underlying anatomy. Assess the patient's general appearance, body proportions, and ease of movement. Be certain to note any limitations in the range of motion or any unusual increase in the mobility of a joint. Decreased range of motion is common in arthritis, inflammation, or fibrosis (excess scar tissue) (Table 10-7).

Assess for the following (Figures 10-49 and 10-50):
● *Signs of inflammation*—These include swelling, tenderness, increased heat, redness, and decreased function. Either trauma or infection can cause inflammation. Swelling may involve a joint or other structures.

- *Crepitus*—**Crepitus** is a palpable or audible crunching produced by movement of a body part.
- *Deformities*—These can be produced by anything that restricts the range of motion, including scar tissue and misalignment of bones.
- *Muscular strength*—This is described under Nervous System (p. 348).

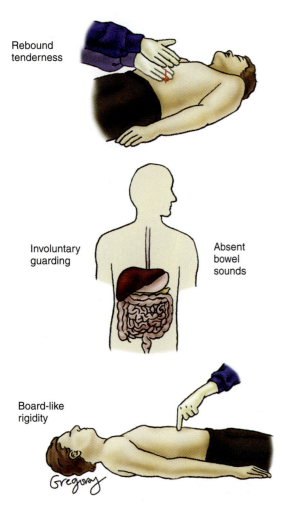

FIGURE 10-48 ▲ **Signs of peritonitis.**

- *Symmetry*—Note whether the injury or other findings are isolated to one side or if they are bilateral. Symmetrical findings are common in massive trauma (e.g., bilateral ankle fractures after a fall) and are the rule in certain medical conditions (e.g., rheumatoid arthritis).
- *Atrophy*—Loss of substance, especially muscle mass, is known as **atrophy.** This usually indicates a chronic condition.
- *Pain*—Try to localize the patient's complaint as much as possible without causing more discomfort.
- *Tenderness*—Try to localize the patient's complaint as much as possible without causing more discomfort.
- *Peripheral pulses*—This is discussed under Peripheral Vascular System (below).
- *Motor function*—This is described under Nervous System (p. 348).
- *Sensory function*—This is described under Nervous System (p. 349).

PERIPHERAL VASCULAR SYSTEM

Examination of the peripheral vascular system is integrally linked with both the neurological examination and the examination of the extremities. Usually, these are all done simultaneously (Table 10-8).

Assess the Arms—Inspect the upper extremities from fingertips to shoulders, noting the following (Figure 10-51):

- *Size, symmetry, swelling*—Normally, the upper extremities should be equally sized and symmetrical. Any localized swelling is abnormal.
- *Color of the skin and nail beds*—Look particularly for cyanosis, areas of decreased circulation (pallor), and inflammation. In some cases of chronic venous insufficiency, the skin becomes excessively pigmented ("bronze edema"). This is more common in the legs than in the upper extremity.
- *Texture of the skin*—Assess for uniformity of texture; isolated changes may indicate an underlying vascular problem. A leatherlike texture to the skin may indicate chronic venous insufficiency.

TABLE 10-6

Examination of the Genitalia

TECHNIQUES OF EXAMINATION	NOTE THE FOLLOWING CHARACTERISTICS	DOCUMENT ABNORMALITIES
Assess the external male genitalia	Inspect the external genitalia	Inflammation Discharge Bleeding Swelling
Assess the external female genitalia	Inspect the external genitalia	Inflammation Discharge Bleeding Swelling

Generally, any pulse can be classified as one of the following:

- Increased
- Normal
- Diminished
- Absent

Palpate the upper extremity pulses—radial and brachial. Compare the amplitude of each side of the body. These should be equal. Note any differences or diminished pulse strength (Figures 10-52 and 10-53).

Assess the Legs—The patient should be lying down without socks or stockings on for the most adequate examination possible. First, inspect the lower ex-

tremities from the groin and buttocks to the feet, looking for the following (Figure 10-54):

- *Size, symmetry, swelling*—Normally, the lower extremities should be equally sized and symmetrical. Any localized swelling is abnormal.
- *Rashes, scars, ulcers, wounds, or other lesions*
- *Color and texture of the skin*—Look particularly for cyanosis, areas of decreased circulation (pallor), and inflammation. In some cases of chronic venous insufficiency, the skin becomes excessively pigmented ("bronze edema"), especially in the legs. Assess for uniformity of texture; isolated changes may indicate an underlying vascular problem.

TABLE 10-7

Extremity Examination

TECHNIQUES OF EXAMINATION	NOTE THE FOLLOWING CHARACTERISTICS	DOCUMENT ABNORMALITIES
Assess the entire patient first	General appearance	
	Body proportions	
	Ease of motion	
Assess joint motions, in general	Range of motion	Limitations in range of motion
		Unusual increase in mobility of a joint
Assess the extremities	Signs of inflammation	Swelling
	Crepitus	Tenderness
	Deformities	Increased heat
	Muscle strength	Decreased function
	Symmetry	
	Atrophy	
	Pain	
	Tenderness	
	Peripheral pulses	
	Motor function	
	Sensory function	

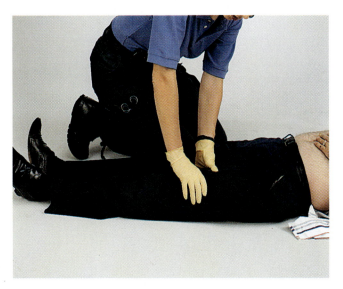

FIGURE 10-49 ▲ Palpate the patient's upper leg.

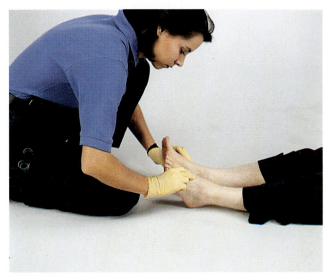

FIGURE 10-50 ▲ Palpate the patient's lower leg, checking for pulse, motor function, and sensation.

TABLE 10-8

Peripheral Vascular System Examination

TECHNIQUES OF EXAMINATION	NOTE THE FOLLOWING CHARACTERISTICS	DOCUMENT ABNORMALITIES
Assess the arms	Size, symmetry, swelling	Localized swelling
	Color of the skin and nail beds	Cyanosis, pallor, inflammation
	Texture of the skin	"Bronze edema"
	Brachial pulse	Asymmetry of pulses
	Radial pulse	Abnormal pulse strength
Assess the legs	Size, symmetry, swelling	Localized swelling
	Rashes, scars, ulcers, wounds, or other lesions	Cyanosis, pallor, inflammation "Bronze edema"
	Color and texture of the skin	Leatherlike texture of venous insufficiency
	Uniformity of texture	Edema
	Temperature	Pitting edema
Assess the lower extremity pulses	Femoral pulse	Decreased
	Popliteal pulse	Absent
	Dorsalis pedis pulse	Overly pulsatile
	Posterior tibial pulse	

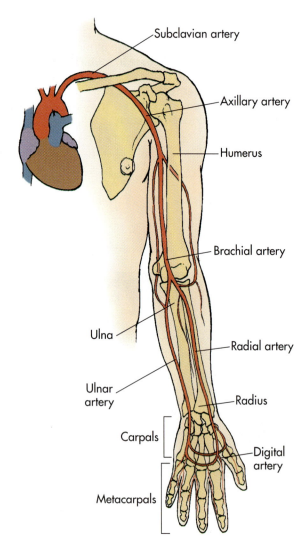

FIGURE 10-51 ▲ Structure of the normal arm.

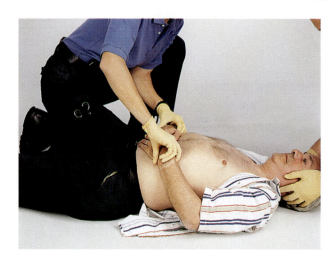

FIGURE 10-52 ▲ Check the distal pulses of the arm.

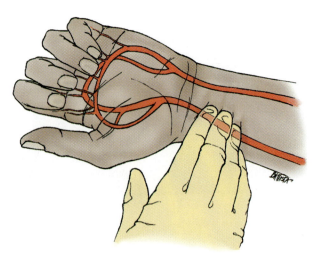

FIGURE 10-53 ▲ The radial pulse point is used most often to assess an adult patient's pulse.

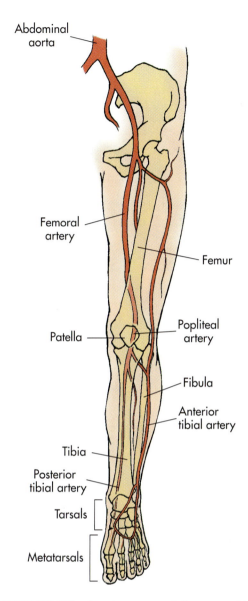

Abdominal aorta

Femoral artery

Femur

Popliteal artery

Patella

Fibula

Anterior tibial artery

Tibia

Posterior tibial artery

Tarsals

Metatarsals

FIGURE 10-54 ▲ Structure of the normal leg.

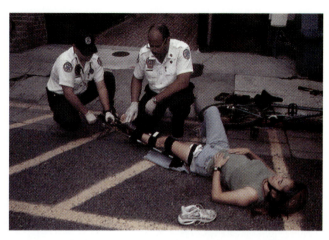

FIGURE 10-55 ▲ Pulse locations in the leg. (From McSwain NE, Paturas, JL: *The basic EMT: comprehensive prehospital patient care,* ed 2, St Louis, 2001, Mosby.)

A leatherlike texture to the skin may indicate chronic venous insufficiency.

Lower Extremity Pulses—Now, palpate the pulses to assess arterial circulation (Figure 10-55):

- **Femoral pulse**—Located in the inguinal region, about halfway between the anterior-superior iliac spine and the symphysis pubis.
- **Popliteal pulse**—Located in the popliteal fossa of the back of the knee joint. Palpating this pulse is easier if the leg is flexed first. Typically, the popliteal pulse is more difficult to find than the other lower extremity pulses. If it appears bounding or a pulsatile mass is present, the patient probably has a popliteal artery aneurysm, not a normal pulse.
- **Dorsalis pedis pulse**—Located on the dorsum of the foot, lateral to the great toe extensor tendon. This

pulse may be congenitally absent in some people or may be more lateral than usual.

- **Posterior tibial pulse**—Located posterior to the medial malleolus of the ankle.

A decreased or absent arterial pulse indicates partial or complete arterial occlusion in the proximal vessels. When an artery is blocked, all the pulses distally are usually affected. Chronic arterial insufficiency can lead to a glistening, thinned appearance of the skin.

Temperature—Note the temperature of the feet and legs. They should be equal on both sides. Bilateral cold feet are most often due to the environment, rather than to arterial disease.

Edema—Check for **edema** (swelling due to accumulation of fluid in the tissues).

Pitting edema is said to occur when pressure over an edematous area results in a depression in the skin (Figure 10-56). This usually persists for less than 5 minutes. To check for pitting edema, press firmly but gently with your thumb for at least 5 seconds:

- Over the dorsum of each foot
- Behind each medial malleolus
- Over the shins

Typically, edema (both nonpitting and pitting) is graded on a 4-point scale:

- 1+=Slight edema
- 2+=More edema
- 3+=Moderate edema
- 4+=Marked edema

▶ NOTE: This rating scale is subjective; there have been no scientific data to this point that document how to best quantitate the amount of edema. The best way to report edema is give your best estimate of how much, and whether or not it is pitting. For example: "The patient has 4+ pitting edema of both lower legs."

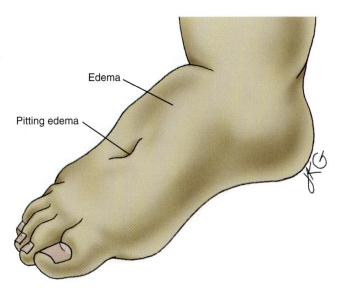

FIGURE 10-56 ▲ Pitting edema.

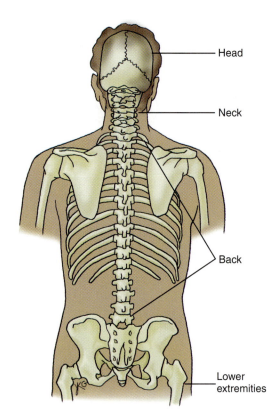

FIGURE 10-57 ▲ **Parts of the spine examination encompass the head, neck, back, and lower extremity examinations.**

SPINE

Parts of the spine examination encompass the head, neck, back, and lower extremity examinations (Figure 10-57). Specific spine-related portions of the complete patient examination are detailed here. Incorporate them into the rest of the examination. The parts of the spine that need to be examined depend on the clinical presentation. Of course, in trauma the cervical spine rates high priority (Table 10-9).

Inspect the Spine—Inspect the spine both from the side and from behind, if possible. From the side, assess that the normal cervical, thoracic, and lumbar curves are visible (Figure 10-58). From behind, an imaginary line drawn from the spinous process of T1 should run perpendicular to the ground and between the gluteal cleft (Figure 10-59). Assess for any obvious deformity, swelling, or bruising.

Palpate the Spine—Gently palpate the spine over the spinous processes. Palpate the muscles of the neck and back for symmetry, tenderness, and spasm (an area that is "harder" than the rest). Also, examine the costovertebral angle for deformities and pain. Reduce patient movement, since back injuries can be easily aggravated.

NERVOUS SYSTEM

General Approach—Many students find the nervous system and its examination very complex and somewhat threatening. Even if you are not comfortable with the official terminology for each test, if you remember the word *symmetry*, the approach becomes much easier. Just about everything that is evaluated during examination of the nervous system involves bilateral tests—strength, sensation, and reflexes. The re-

sults on one side of the body should parallel those on the other side. If there are obvious asymmetrical responses, the test result is probably abnormal. On the other hand, it is certainly possible to be "symmetrically abnormal" as well.

Volumes have been written about the neurological examination. The amount of detail required for the EMT–I varies greatly and depends on the situation. Many components of this examination are actually completed while assessing other areas of the body (e.g., arms, legs). Keeping the principle of symmetry in mind, organize your findings into three categories (Figure 10-60; Table 10-10):
- Mental status and speech
- Motor system
- Sensory system

Assess the Mental Status and Speech—Much of this portion of the examination is discussed earlier in this chapter (see p. 319) and is not repeated here. An important part of the neurological assessment is the evaluation of patient's LOC—the patient's degree of awareness of his surroundings. The LOC is the best indicator of the condition of the central nervous system. Any changes should be noted; deterioration indicates the need for urgent medical attention and reclassification as a "priority" patient.

TABLE 10-9

Spine Examination

TECHNIQUES OF EXAMINATION	NOTE THE FOLLOWING CHARACTERISTICS	DOCUMENT ABNORMALITIES
Inspect the spine	From the side: normal cervical, thoracic, lumbar curves From the back: symmetrical (line from T1 to gluteal cleft)	Deformity Asymmetry Swelling Bruising
Palpate the spine	Spinal processes Neck and back muscles Costovertebral angle	Symmetry Tenderness Spasm Deformity Pain

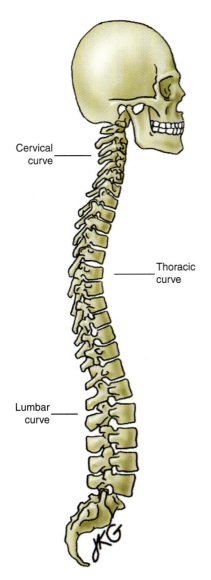

Cervical curve

Thoracic curve

Lumbar curve

FIGURE 10-58 ▲ From the side, assess that the normal cervical, thoracic, and lumbar curves are visible.

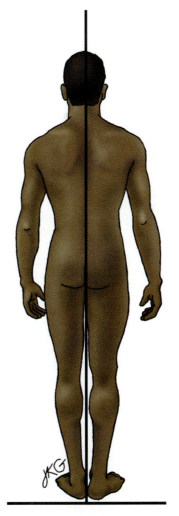

FIGURE 10-59 ▲ An imaginary line drawn from the spinous process of T1 should run perpendicular to the ground, between the gluteal cleft.

In addition to the AVPU scale, the **Glasgow Coma Scale** is a helpful guide. Although this scale has become somewhat controversial in recent medical literature, it is still widely used. The three main areas assessed are eye opening, verbal response, and motor response.

The maximum score possible is 15, and the minimum is 3. Adults scoring below 9 have a poor neurological prognosis. A separate scale has been devised for children.

Evaluate motor response on the basis of the patient's best response to either a verbal command or a painful stimulus. Six points are the maximum possible in this category. The motor response is scored as follows:

6 = Patient obeys a simple command, such as "Lift your right hand up."
5 = Patient moves a limb in an attempt to locate a painful stimulus and remove it.
4 = Patient attempts to withdraw from a painful stimulus.
3 = Patient flexes the arms and wrists in response to painful stimuli (decorticate posturing).
2 = Patient extends the arms at the elbows in response to painful stimuli (decerebrate posturing).
1 = Patient has no motor response to pain on any limb.

Evaluate verbal response on the basis of the best answer to questions of time, place, and person: "What day is this?" "What place is this?" "What is your name?" There are a maximum of 5 possible points in this category, scored as follows:

5 = Patient is oriented to time, place, and person.
4 = Patient is able to converse but is not oriented to time, place, or person.
3 = Patient speaks in only short phrases or uses words that make no sense.
2 = Patient responds with incomprehensible sounds such as moans and groans.
1 = Patient has no verbal response.

Evaluate eye opening from what stimuli, if any, are required for the patient to open his eyes without assistance. The maximum points possible in this category are 4. Eye opening is scored as follows:

4 = Patient opens his or her eyes spontaneously.
3 = Patient opens his or her eyes in response to being spoken to or shouted at.
2 = Patient opens his or her eyes only in response to pain.
1 = Patient exhibits no response.

CLINICAL NOTES

The AVPU scale evaluates what stimulus it takes to get a response. The Glasgow Coma Scale evaluates what response results from the stimulus given. Both scales are valuable.

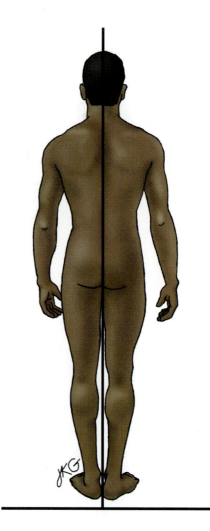

FIGURE 10-60 ▲ Use the principle of symmetry to help organize nervous system findings.

Assess the Motor System—Observe the patient's body position during movement and at rest. Are there any involuntary movements? If so, note their quality, rate, rhythm, and amplitude. Many involuntary movements (e.g., tremors, tics) vary in relation to the patient's posture, activity, emotional state, and energy level (worse with fatigue).

Muscle Tone—When a normal muscle with an intact nerve supply is relaxed voluntarily, it maintains a small amount of tension known as **muscle tone.** Check the patient's muscle tone by feeling the resistance to passive stretch. Have the patient relax as much as possible, and take each major joint through passive range of motion. "Passive" means that the examiner does all the work; the patient should not contribute any muscular effort.

Muscle Strength—Strength varies markedly among people. The dominant (right or left) side is usually somewhat stronger. Overall, test **muscle strength** by asking the patient to try to move against your resistance. Some patients are simply too weak to be tested in

TABLE 10-10

Examination of the Nervous System

TECHNIQUES OF EXAMINATION	NOTE THE FOLLOWING CHARACTERISTICS	DOCUMENT ABNORMALITIES
Assess the mental status and speech	Level of consciousness (LOC): AVPU, Glasgow Coma Scale Posture and motor behavior Dress, grooming, personal hygiene Facial expression and affect Speech and language Mood Orientation	Altered LOC Decerebrate, decorticate posturing Rigidity, tremor, tics Flat affect Aphasia, dysphonia, dysarthria Mood disturbance Disorientation to time, place, or person
Assess the motor system	Body position and movements Muscle tone Muscle strength Muscle coordination	Involuntary movements Decreased or increased tone Decreased strength (based on the "0 to 5 scale") Inability to perform rapidly alternating movements with hands
Assess the sensory system	Pain sensation Temperature sensation (may be optional) Light touch	Increased sensitivity Decreased sensitivity Asymmetry of response

this fashion. Test them against gravity alone or with gravity eliminated.

A uniformly accepted method for grading muscle strength uses a scale of 0 to 5:

- 0 = No detectable muscle contraction
- 1 = Barely detectable muscle contraction
- 2 = Active movement with gravity eliminated
- 3 = Active movement against gravity
- 4 = Active movement against gravity and some resistance
- 5 = Active movement against full resistance without fatigue (*normal*)

In a normal person, muscle strength would be rated as 5/5. In contrast, a patient who is weak might have upper extremity muscle strength of 1/5 and lower extremity muscle strength of 2/5.

Although many physical examination texts present examination of the upper extremity first, out-of-hospital teaching has always stressed attention to the *lower extremities first*, since they suffer more serious injuries (e.g., fractured femur). Follow your local protocols.

- Ask the patient to move the toes (flexion and extension) and then to press the feet against your hands (plantar flexion) and up again (dorsiflexion). Note any inability to move. If you suspect spinal or back injury, do not have patients move their feet.
- Ask the patient to move the fingers (flexion, extension, finger abduction) and then to squeeze your hands (grip). Note any loss or deficit of grip strength. If you suspect spinal or back injury, do not have patients move their arms.

Muscle Coordination—Test **muscle coordination** (the ability of groups of muscles to move as a whole) by having patients perform a series of rapidly alternating movements, such as turning their hands over repeatedly (Figure 10-61).

▶ *Paralysis* is the loss of movement, the loss of sensation, or both. Paralysis of both arms and both legs is *quadriplegia*. Paralysis of the arm and leg on one side of the body is *hemiplegia*. Paralysis of both legs is *paraplegia*.

Assess the Sensory System—Use the principle of symmetry to perform the sensory examination. Compare symmetrical areas on each side of the body. Normally, sensation of all types (e.g., pain, temperature, touch) should be equal on both sides. It is also important to compare pain, temperature, and touch in the distal and more proximal portions of *each* extremity. Explain to patients what you are going to do, then have them keep their eyes closed during the actual examination.

Pain Sensation—Pain sensation is usually tested using a clean safety pin or other sharp tool. The stimulus must be hard enough to be felt, but light enough not to cause bleeding. Practice on a partner until you are comfortable with the "right touch." Another excellent technique is to use a light pinch. In light of infection hazards and body substance isolation precautions, the pinch is the recommended technique for the EMT–I.

Temperature Sensation—Most examiners eliminate this portion of the sensory examination if pain sensation

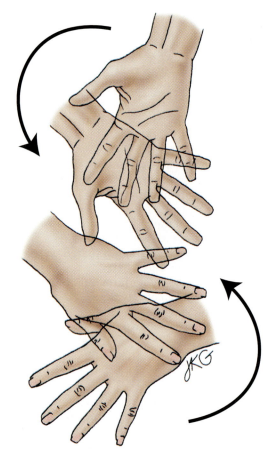

FIGURE 10-61 ▲ Rapidly alternating hand movements help evaluate the patient's coordination.

is normal. If necessary, or if there is any question about whether or not sensation is intact, check temperature sensation by using water in a small vessel or tube that is either chilled or warmed. Have the patient, again with the eyes closed, identify either "cold" or "warm" on various parts of the body.

Light Touch Sensation—Using a fine wisp of cotton, touch the skin lightly. Compare the patient's response on both sides. Note areas of decreased, as well as areas of *increased*, sensitivity to light touch.

▶ NOTE: Checking a person's response to more than one sensation is important, since pain, temperature, and light touch are all carried in different fibers of the spinal cord.

When assessing the conscious patient, ask about any numbness or tingling sensation in the arms or legs. These sensations, known as **paresthesias,** could indicate

HELPFUL HINT

- To assess equality of sensation, stroke the outside of one extremity and then the outside of the other. Ask the patient if it feels the same on both sides.

possible spinal cord damage or local circulatory problems. Care for any patient who complains of numbness or tingling in the extremities, or inequality of sensation, particularly following an injury, as though a spinal injury exists.

PHYSICAL EXAMINATION OF INFANTS AND CHILDREN

The physical examination of infants and children has many similarities to that of the adult. The priorities of airway, breathing, and circulation are unchanged. There are, however, some differences in the approach to the patient:
- Unless it is necessary to detect a life-threatening situation, perform painful or potentially distressing portions near the end of the examination.
- Assess areas where the patient complains of pain last.

Pediatric examination is detailed in Chapter 34. The material included here summarizes key information.

Anatomical Differences Between Children and Adults

Infants are individuals under the age of 1 year, whereas the term **child** refers to individuals from age 1 to 8 years. The overall size of the pediatric airway is smaller than in the adult, making an infant or child far more likely to suffer airway obstruction due to a foreign body. There are also relative size differences in the tongue and epiglottis in children younger than 8 years old. These differences, combined with the tonsils and adenoids, also affect patency of the airway.

Other major differences between pediatric and adult patients include the following (Figure 10-62):
- The internal organs of infants and children are larger in proportion to body size than in adults, and the skeleton is smaller. Since more internal organs are essentially packed into a "smaller space," there is a higher incidence of internal injuries, particularly to the liver.
- The head is relatively larger in infants, predisposing them to head injury.
- Children's bones are softer and more flexible, as a rule, than in the adult. Many bony injuries involve *bending* the bone, not *breaking* it.
- The infant and child's nervous system is not as well developed as in the adult, and their responses to stimuli may be slower or different.

Approach to the Pediatric Patient

The EMT–I is faced with unique challenges when dealing with pediatric patients. These include the following:
- Fear of strangers and of the unknown
- Presence and role of the parents
- Differences in levels of understanding

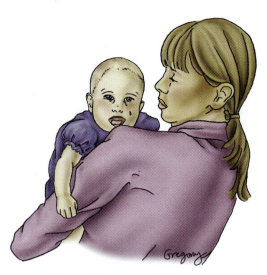

- Airway problems more likely
- More organs in smaller space
- Internal injuries (liver)
- Head larger; head injuries
- Bones bend, not break
- Response may be slower

FIGURE 10-62 ▲ **Differences in pediatric patients.**

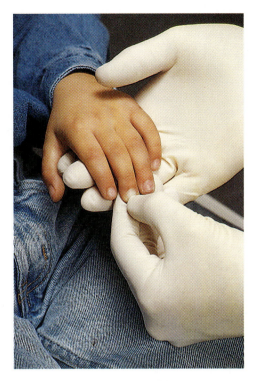

FIGURE 10-63 ▲ Capillary refill may be assessed in children under the age of 6 years. (Vincent Knaus from Stoy W: *Mosby's EMT–Basic textbook,* St Louis, 1996, Mosby.)

The Initial Evaluation

The initial examination of any pediatric patient should focus on the following:

- *Responsiveness*—Use the AVPU scale to assess the child or infant's level of responsiveness.
- *Respiratory status*—Most serious pediatric problems and cardiac arrests start with a primary respiratory event, unlike in the adult. *Prevention* of deterioration in a pediatric patient is far more likely to be successful than resuscitation once a situation has worsened. The first sign of respiratory distress in an infant is usually tachypnea.
- *Circulatory status*—A slow or irregular pulse is a poor sign. Skin color, temperature, and capillary refill should also be evaluated. Young children have poor collateral circulation, especially in a cold environment, so capillary refill may not provide an accurate assessment of perfusion (Figure 10-63).

RECORDING EXAMINATION FINDINGS

Documentation is essential for good patient care and provides a sound basis for defense of any possible licensure or negligence action. Many EMS systems have standard report forms with checkoff boxes and often space for a narrative report. Be certain that they contain the appropriate choices, and plenty of room for narrative information.

SUMMARY

Important points to remember from this chapter include the following:

- Physical examination is a multifaceted process that, along with the history, is key in the EMT–I's care for patients. The basic techniques of all examinations involve inspection (looking), palpation (touching), percussion (tapping), and auscultation (listening to). Measurement of the patient's vital signs is generally limited to the pulse rate, respiratory rate, and blood pressure in the out-of-hospital setting, although temperature may be important under many circumstances. As with any test, "normal" vital signs follow a continuous spectrum; a normal test does not necessarily mean a normal patient.
- The comprehensive examination covers the following areas:
  - Mental status

- General survey
- Vital signs
- Skin
- HEENT (head, eyes, ears, nose, and throat)
- Neck
- Chest
- Abdomen
- Posterior body
- Extremities (peripheral pulses, musculoskeletal system)

- Neurological examination
- The amount of detail necessary and which areas to cover depend on each patient's particular circumstances. Examination techniques are similar in adults, children, and infants, although there are several significant anatomical differences in younger patients that the EMT–I must be aware of. All findings should be appropriately documented, according to local protocols.

11

Patient Assessment

...CASE HISTORY It is early afternoon on a rainy, winter day. EMT–Is Smith and Jones are eating lunch at the base when the alarm sounds: "Unit three . . . Respond as backup to a motor vehicle crash with injuries . . . Intersection of Highway K and Mexico Road . . . Time out 1230." En route, the EMT–Is are advised that three cars are involved and there are multiple patients. Police are on the scene, and fire/rescue personnel have been dispatched. The air medical crew has been placed on standby. ETA is 5 minutes.

As the EMT–Is approach the crash site, they see warning lights and police blocking access to the intersection. There are cars and people everywhere, and the scene looks very busy. Two of the cars are still on the roadway, and the third car is on its side because of the impact. The EMT–Is don their protective gear and report to the command post established by the fire department.

The EMT–Is are directed to the first ambulance that arrived on the scene. In the patient compartment they find a woman holding a child in her lap, talking to a police officer. They hear her say that she and her 3-year-old child were front-seat passengers in one of the cars at the intersection, and they were able to exit the car after impact. The patients are visibly shaken but have no apparent injuries. EMT–I Smith performs a brief initial assessment on the woman and obtains an initial set of vital signs. The child is whimpering and clinging to his mother. He will not cooperate for an examination, so EMT–I Smith attempts to palpate major body regions through his winter clothing. His mother states that she thinks he is okay and is just scared from the crash. She wants him to be "checked out" at the emergency department. The police officer offers to stay with them so that EMT–I Smith can care for other patients at the scene. EMT–I Smith returns to the command post and helps EMT–I Jones and the other crews.

There are a total of seven patients, two of whom have serious injuries and are flown out to the trauma center. EMT–Is Smith and Jones transport the mother and her child and one other patient with minor injuries to a local hospital. The other crews transport the remaining patients. En route back to the base, EMT–I Smith is advised by dispatch to contact his medical direction physician. She wants to talk to him about one of the patients he transported.

▶ NOTE: The authors assume that the reader is already familiar with the basics of obtaining a history and performing a physical examination (see Chapters 9 and 10). Unless necessary for special emphasis, these details are not repeated here.

CHAPTER GOAL

Upon completion of this chapter, the EMT–Intermediate will be able to integrate the principles of history taking and techniques of physical examination to perform patient assessment on an emergency patient.

Cognitive Objectives

As an EMT–Intermediate you should be able to do the following:

- Describe and recognize common hazards found at the scene of a trauma patient and those found at the scene of a medical patient.
- Differentiate safe from unsafe scenes.
- Describe methods for making an unsafe scene safe.
- Discuss common mechanisms of injury.
- Predict patterns of injury on the basis of the mechanism of injury.
- Discuss the reasons for identifying the total number of patients at the scene.
- Explain the reasons for identifying the need for additional help or assistance.
- Summarize the reasons for forming a general impression of the patient.
- Review methods of assessing mental status and level of consciousness in the adult, child, and infant as detailed in Chapter 10.

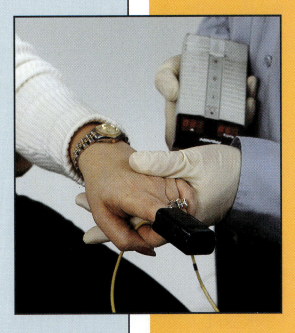

- Discuss methods of assessing the airway in the adult, child, and infant.
- State reasons for management of the cervical spine once the patient has been determined to be a trauma patient.
- Analyze a scene to determine if spinal precautions are required.
- Describe methods used for assessing if a patient is breathing.
- Differentiate between a patient with adequate breathing and one with inadequate breathing (minute ventilation).
- Distinguish between methods of assessing breathing in the adult, child, and infant.
- Compare the methods of providing airway care to the adult, child, and infant.
- Describe the methods used to locate and assess a pulse.
- Differentiate between locating and assessing a pulse in the adult, child, and infant.
- Discuss the need for assessing the patient for external bleeding.
- Describe normal and abnormal findings when assessing skin color.
- Describe normal and abnormal findings when assessing skin temperature.
- Describe normal and abnormal findings when assessing skin condition.
- Explain the reasons for prioritizing a patient for care and transport.
- Identify patients who require expeditious transport.
- Describe the evaluation of the patient's perfusion status based on findings in the initial assessment.

- Describe orthostatic vital signs, and evaluate their usefulness in assessing a patient in shock.
- Apply the techniques of physical examination to the medical patient.
- Differentiate between the assessment done for a patient who is unresponsive or has an altered mental status and the assessment done for other medical patients.
- Discuss the reasons for reconsidering the mechanism of injury.
- State the reasons for doing a rapid trauma assessment.
- Recite examples and explain why patients should receive a rapid trauma assessment.
- Apply the techniques of physical examination to the trauma patient.
- Describe the areas included in the rapid trauma assessment, and discuss what should be evaluated.
- Identify cases where the rapid assessment may be altered to provide patient care.
- Discuss the reasons for doing a focused history and physical examination.
- Describe when and why a detailed physical examination is necessary.
- Discuss the components of the detailed physical examination in relation to the techniques of examination.
- State the areas of the body evaluated during the detailed physical examination.
- Explain what additional care should be provided while doing the detailed physical examination.
- Distinguish between the detailed physical examination performed on a trauma patient and that performed on a medical patient.
- Differentiate between patients who require a detailed physical examination and those who do not.
- Discuss the reasons for repeating the initial assessment as part of the ongoing assessment.
- Describe the components of the ongoing assessment.
- Describe trending of assessment components.
- Discuss medical identification devices/systems.

Affective Objectives
As an EMT–I Intermediate you should be able to do the following:
- Explain the rationale for crew members to evaluate scene safety before entering.

- Serve as a model for others, explaining how patient situations affect your evaluation of the mechanism of injury or illness.
- Explain the importance of forming a general impression of the patient.
- Explain the value of performing an initial assessment.
- Show a caring attitude when doing an initial assessment.
- Attend to the feelings that patients with medical conditions might be experiencing.
- Value the need for maintaining a professional, caring attitude when doing a focused history and physical examination.
- Explain the rationale for the feelings that these patients might be experiencing.
- Show a caring attitude when doing a detailed physical examination.
- Explain the value of doing an ongoing assessment.
- Recognize and respect the feelings that patients might experience during assessment.
- Explain the value of trending assessment components to other health care professionals who assume care of the patient.

Psychomotor Objectives
As an EMT–I Intermediate you should be able to do the following:
- Observe various scenarios and identify hazards.
- Demonstrate the scene size-up.
- Demonstrate the techniques for assessing mental status.
- Demonstrate the techniques for assessing the airway.
- Demonstrate the techniques for determining if the patient is breathing.
- Demonstrate the techniques for determining if the patient has a pulse.
- Demonstrate the techniques for determining if the patient has external bleeding.
- Demonstrate the techniques for determining the patient's skin color, temperature, and condition.
- Demonstrate the ability to prioritize patients.
- Using the techniques of examination, demonstrate the assessment of a medical patient.
- Demonstrate the patient care skills that should be used to assist with a patient who is responsive with no known history.

INTRODUCTION

Patient assessment is a structured method of evaluating a patient's condition. An organized, well-developed patient assessment is a valuable tool for providing patient care. The patient assessment is the process of looking for, asking about, and recognizing the symptoms and signs of an abnormal condition. A *symptom* is a subjective indication of a disease or condition as perceived by the patient. For example, the patient may complain of the symptom chest pain. A *sign* is an objective finding such as a rash or a deformed arm. Patient assessment is a process that continues throughout the time spent with a patient, because a patient's condition can change quickly. Continual assessment allows the EMT–Intermediate (EMT–I) to recognize critical situations early and to influence patient outcomes positively (Figure 11-1).

Patient assessment is a team process. While an EMT–I is assessing a patient, other team members are initiating lifesaving care, gathering additional information, and ensuring that equipment is ready for use (Figure 11-2). Typically, one individual acts as team leader. This person may be assigned as part of the shift schedule or determined by the members of the crew. Designating a team leader in advance will reduce confusion at the scene. Patient assessment skills are best

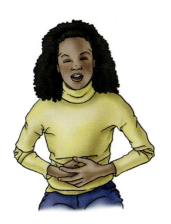 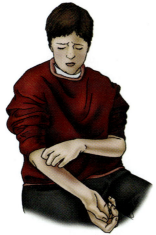

A *symptom* is a subjective indication of a condition as perceived by the patient.

A *sign* is an objective finding such as a rash or a deformed arm.

FIGURE 11-1 ▲ Signs and symptoms.

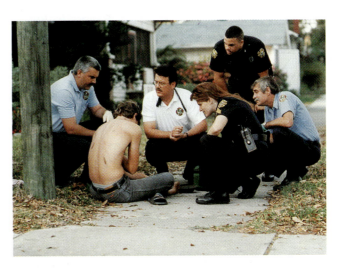

FIGURE 11-2 ▲ Patient assessment is a team process. (From American College of Emergency Physicians; Pons PT, Cason D, chief editors: *Paramedic field care: a complaint-based approach*, St Louis, 1997, Mosby for ACEP.)

mastered by practice and experience. This chapter provides direction and guidance for properly developing patient assessment skills. It is up to the individual EMT–I to put this information into daily practice and to develop proficiency.

The patient assessment and care process is discussed in six phases: scene size-up (scene assessment), initial assessment, focused history and physical examination of the medical patient, focused history and physical examination of the trauma patient, detailed physical examination, and ongoing assessment (Figure 11-3).

> Before 1994 the Department of Transportation (DOT) curriculum for basic-level out-of-hospital care providers divided patient assessment into four phases:
> - Scene assessment
> - Primary survey
> - Resuscitation
> - Secondary survey
>
>   The revised EMT–I curriculum now teaches six phases of patient assessment:
> - Scene size-up
> - Initial assessment
> - Focused history and physical examination of the medical patient
> - Focused history and physical examination of the trauma patient
> - Detailed physical examination
> - Ongoing assessment
>
>   Resuscitation is performed as necessary throughout patient assessment as soon as life-threatening problems are identified.

SCENE SIZE-UP
General Approach

The **scene size-up** (scene assessment) is an assessment of the scene and surroundings that provides valuable information to the EMT–I. Initially, potential scene hazards that may endanger the EMT–I or the patient are identified. Then the "whole picture" of the call is evaluated (Figure 11-4). Scene size-up allows the EMT–I to ensure a safe environment for rescuers and patients, anticipate potentially hazardous situations, and call for appropriate resources. For example, as the EMT–I drives up to a home, he or she notices a man on the front porch waving a butcher knife. From the immediate scene size-up, the EMT–I knows to wait for police to secure the scene.

Before any care is given to the patient, the EMT–I should begin a rapid assessment of the circumstances of the call that is based on dispatch information, previous knowledge, and on-scene observations:
- *Dispatch information*—In many areas dispatchers are trained to gather more information than just location

and possible problems (Figure 11-5). The emergency medical dispatcher (EMD) can provide information on the following:
- Scene conditions
- Number of patients
- Patient conditions
- Medical history

> ### HELPFUL HINT
> Not all dispatchers are trained as EMDs. To qualify as an EMD, a person must undergo specific training, including the use of prearrival instructions and call prioritizing.

- *Previous knowledge*—If the EMT–I is aware of a situation potentially requiring special assistance, he or she may need to direct the EMD to dispatch police or other emergency agencies immediately. Potentially hazardous situations include calls to high-risk parts of a response area (high crime or drug use areas), known unsafe situations (gang fights, shootings, stabbings), and sometimes just a "gut feeling" based on the EMD's information.
- *On-scene observations*—The following are five considerations regarding on-scene observations:
  - Is the scene safe? Is it safe for responders, the patient, and bystanders? If the scene is unsafe, the EMT–I should attempt to make it safe, if possible. Otherwise, the EMT–I should *not* enter the scene.
  - Should body substance isolation precautions be taken? In general, the answer to this question should always be *yes*.
  - Is this a medical or a trauma patient? If medical, what is the nature of the illness? If trauma, what is the mechanism of injury?
  - How many patients are involved?
  - Is additional help required? The EMT–I should recognize and request backup immediately on arrival (or en route). Canceling a request for additional help during the response is better than not having requested necessary assistance in the first place.

Body Substance Isolation Precautions

The EMT–I can be exposed to many contagious diseases during normal patient contact. Some of these diseases, such as HIV infection, hepatitis, and meningitis, can be deadly. Other diseases, such as chickenpox, influenza, and common colds, are not deadly but may cause an EMT–I to miss work or spread disease to family members and colleagues.

The use of protective equipment reduces the chances of being exposed to contagious diseases. **Body substance isolation (BSI) precautions** (formerly called

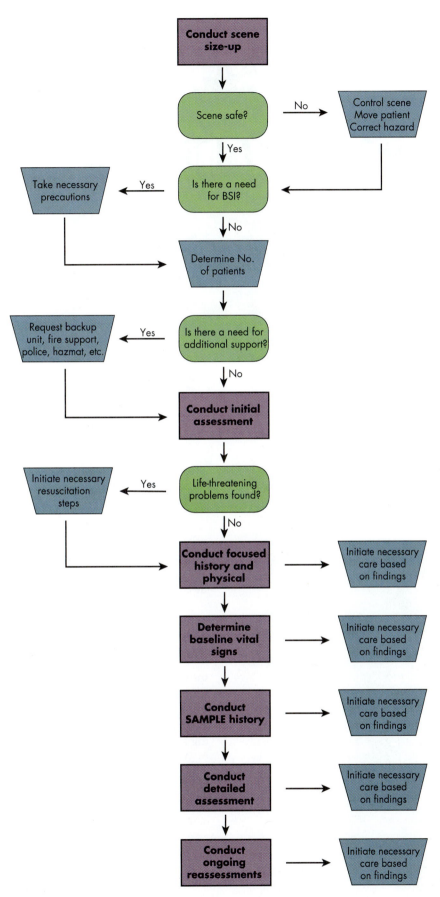

FIGURE 11-3 ▲ Algorithm demonstrating the necessary steps in patient care and assessment.

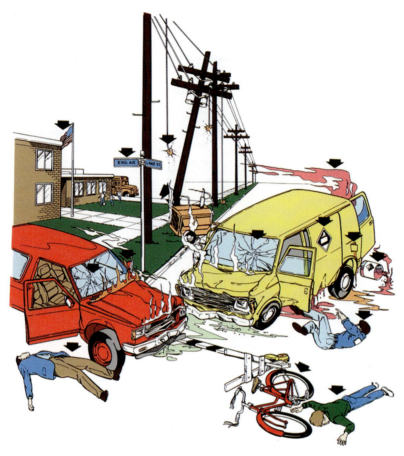

FIGURE 11-4 ▲ Many different hazards can be present at an emergency scene. (Courtesy the American Red Cross. All rights reserved in all countries. From *First aid: responding to emergencies,* St Louis, 1991, Mosby.)

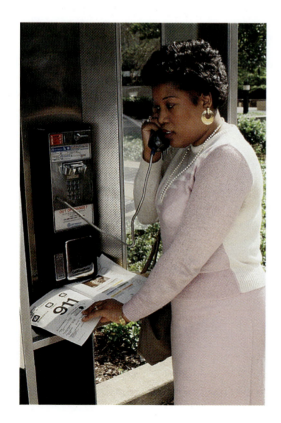

FIGURE 11-5 ▲ Gathering information from a caller. (Courtesy the American Red Cross. All rights reserved in all countries. From *First aid: responding to emergencies,* St Louis, 1991, Mosby.)

universal precautions) are a set of guidelines for health care providers that reduce exposure to contagious diseases. The Centers for Disease Control and Prevention recommends that health care providers use the following set of BSI precautions during all patient encounters:

• Wear latex or vinyl gloves when in contact with blood or other body fluids, mucous membranes, or nonintact skin of any patient or when handling items soiled with blood or body fluids. For those incidents in which large amounts of blood or body fluids are present, wear thicker gloves or use two pairs of gloves. Although medical gloves provide a good barrier, they may not provide protection from sharp objects such as wood, metal, or glass. Work-type gloves, with latex or vinyl gloves underneath, are appropriate until the hazard has been removed (Figure 11-6, *A*).

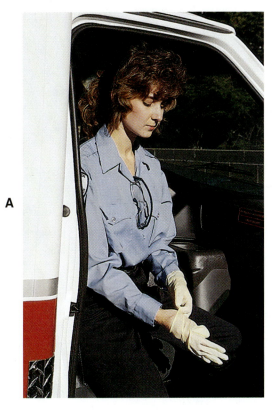

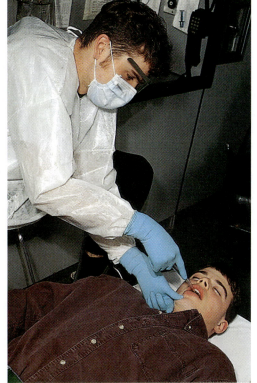

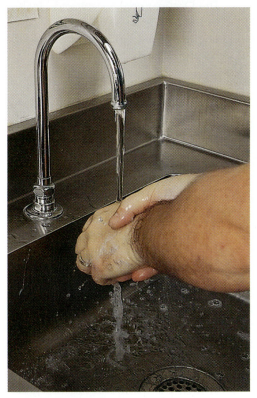

FIGURE 11-6 ▲ Body substance isolation precautions. **A,** Latex or vinyl gloves must be worn whenever there is potential for contact with blood or body fluids of any patient. **B,** Protective eyewear, a facial mask, and a gown should be worn whenever there is a potential for splash exposure to blood or other body fluids of any patient. **C,** Thorough hand washing is important. (Vincent Knaus from Stoy W: *Mosby's EMT–Basic textbook*, St Louis, 1996, Mosby.)

- Wear protective eyewear or masks whenever blood or body fluids may splash or spray near the eyes, nose, or mouth. EMT–Is are often victims of splash exposure. Blood and other body fluids splashed into the eyes can transmit certain diseases. When the potential for splash exposure is high, wear eye protection such as safety glasses. These glasses resemble regular glasses with the sides near the eyes also covered. Some health care professionals recommend that basic eye protection be worn during any incident.

- A mask provides protection against splash exposure to the mouth and nose, and against airborne pathogens. Because different manufacturing standards are used for masks that protect against body fluid exposure and those that protect against airborne disease, check the package labeling to be certain the right mask is being used. The mask works best when worn by the EMT–I, not by the patient. An antiinfection mask placed over the patient's mouth and nose may interfere with assessment of the patient's airway. However, an alert, cooperative patient with a productive cough may be asked to wear a mask (particularly if an infectious airborne disease is suspected). Follow your local protocols (Figure 11-6, *B*).

- Wash hands thoroughly if they are contaminated with blood or body fluids. Also wash hands before and after treating each patient, even if gloves have been worn.
- Avoid recapping needles; always dispose of sharp objects in medical waste containers. Many items used by EMT–Is for patient care are now disposable, such as sheets, pillowcases, airway masks, and splints. Disposable items are usually designed for single use only. Single-use items are the best way to prevent transmission of diseases, but making all equipment disposable is not practical. Equipment manufacturers may provide helpful guidelines after potential infectious disease exposure.
- Dispose of medical waste properly. Place single-use items in plastic bags, and dispose of them in the proper containers. Follow your local protocols for waste disposal.

These guidelines are not simply good protection for EMT–Is and their patients; they are the law. EMS systems and hospitals are required to ensure that protective equipment and proper medical waste disposal areas are available. The Occupational Safety and Health Administration (OSHA) and state agencies may levy significant civil penalties against EMS systems that fail to comply with these procedures.

Scene Safety

The main purpose behind scene safety is to prevent illness or injury to EMT–Is or bystanders and to prevent further illness or injury to the patient(s). Look for hazards such as collapsed structures, chemical spills, fire, weapons, and violent people. If the scene is unsafe, do *not* enter. No matter how critically ill or injured the patient is, a dead or injured EMT–I will not be of help. Instruct dispatch to notify the appropriate agencies for emergency assistance.

To assess scene safety, consider whether a hostile situation exists, or if any special equipment or personnel (e.g., fire department, hazardous materials teams) will be required:

- Consider the environment. What is the location of the emergency? Will the patient have to be moved, and if so, are there many flights of steps, narrow corridors, or nonfunctioning elevators? Is there a fire (or risk of fire)? Is the patient in the wilderness or at a great height? What is the weather like? If the patient is inside and it is snowing outside, he or she will need protection against the environment. Is there a possibility of air or fluid chemical contamination? *All* of these factors must be considered when determining whether a scene is safe.

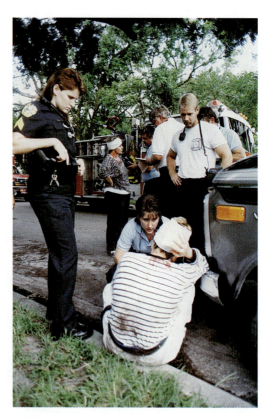

FIGURE 11-7 ▲ Enter the scene only when you know it is safe. (Craig Jackson, photographer.)

- Preserve patient modesty as much as possible during all phases of patient contact. Sometimes, hiding the patient from the view of onlookers is difficult. Usually, however, the best solution is to assess the patient in the back of the ambulance, if possible, or in another private location.
- Is the situation hostile? If a crime has occurred, have the perpetrators been captured? Is their location known? Do not assume that there is only one perpetrator. Also, note the bystanders' mood—are they hostile or supportive? If any doubts exist, do not enter (or remain on) the scene unless law enforcement assistance is present (Figure 11-7).
- Is special equipment required? At this time, decide whether self-contained breathing apparatus or protective clothing is required. Make this decision *before* entering the scene. *Do not* attempt water rescue or entry into a fire or hazardous materials incident without proper training and equipment.

Deciding not to enter an unsafe scene can be very stressful and difficult. This is a decision, however, that must occasionally be made. Remember, an injured or otherwise incapacitated EMT–I is of no benefit to a patient. Also, an injured EMT–I would increase the number of victims that must be cared for by the remaining rescue personnel. Self-protection *must* be the primary concern.

Personal Protection

Sometimes a patient or bystander may pose a threat to an EMT–I. Recognizing danger signs is important, as is following a few key rules to reduce the chance of death or injury:

- Potentially violent situations may not be obvious. If outright signs or even "gut feelings" reveal danger, do not enter until police have secured the area.
- If a patient becomes violent during the incident, move to a safe area and await police arrival.
- Take a position to avoid being cornered or injured by doors, objects, or vehicles.
- Realize that persons of both sexes and of any race, age, and economic status have the potential to injure an EMT–I. Do not let size or an initially calm disposition catch you off guard.
- Avoid being judgmental. Some patients become violent because of medical problems, medication, or simple emotional stress. Do not attribute all violent behavior to alcohol or illicit drug abuse.
- After the scene and patient are secured, provide care as needed.
- Documentation is important, especially when the care given differs from that set by protocols. If physical restraints are needed, carefully document this fact in the run report. EMS systems should have well-established protocols regulating the use of force to ease patient care (see Chapter 3).
- In some systems, body armor (bulletproof vests) is worn. The carrying of weapons is discouraged except by EMS personnel who function in law enforcement capacities. Persons untrained and unfamiliar with proper weapon use can be injured or killed with their own weapons.

Mechanism of Injury/Nature of Illness

As part of the general impression, a decision must be made as to whether the patient has been the victim of trauma or has a medical problem (Figure 11-8). Sometimes the decision is obvious, as in the case of a person struck by a moving car or a man who has collapsed with shortness of breath and no known trauma. Other times, the picture may not be quite so clear, as in the case of a person who suffers a heart attack while driving a car, causing a crash. In such situations it will be necessary to make the best decision possible on the basis of the information available at the time.

If trauma is involved, determine what happened. Did the patient fall? Was the patient stabbed? Was there a motor vehicle accident? What was the size of the knife blade? What was the caliber of the gun? How much damage was done to the car?

Obtain information from the patient, from family members, or from bystanders (including other emer-

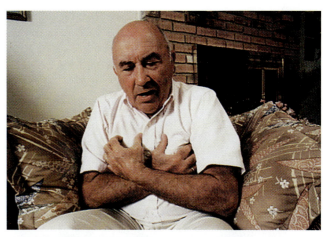

FIGURE 11-8 ▲ Emergencies can be either medical or trauma in nature. (Courtesy the American Red Cross. All rights reserved in all countries. From *First aid: responding to emergencies,* St Louis, 1991, Mosby.)

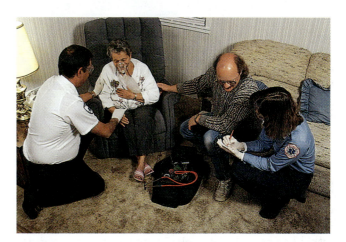

FIGURE 11-9 ▲ Talking with family members or bystanders can be an excellent way to gather information about an emergency scene. (Vincent Knaus from Stoy W: *Mosby's EMT–Basic textbook,* St Louis, 1996, Mosby.)

gency care professionals) regarding the trauma (Figure 11-9).

While assessing the mechanism of injury, determine how many patients are present and decide whether additional help will be required. Also, consider the need for spinal immobilization. If multiple patients are involved, the triage procedure should begin at this point. Since EMT–Is are less likely to call for help once they have become actively involved in patient care, obtain additional help (e.g., law enforcement, fire, rescue, advanced life support [ALS], utility services) *before* beginning care. Then begin appropriate patient triage according to protocols. If the responding crew can manage the situation, consider spinal precautions in all victims and continue care.

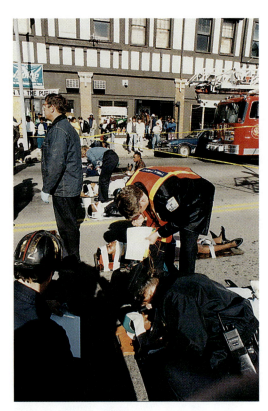

FIGURE 11-10 ▲ **Many emergency scenes involve a number of patients.**

In the medical patient, try to identify the nature of the illness. Is the patient short of breath? Does the patient have chest pain? Is the patient dizzy? The patient, family, or bystanders may provide invaluable information. While determining the nature of the medical illness, determine how many patients are present and decide whether additional help will be required. Do not assume, just because it is a "medical call," that there is only one patient. Many conditions (e.g., fume exposure, food poisoning, infectious disease) may result in multiple patients. As in a trauma scene, if multiple patients are involved, the triage procedure should begin at this point (Figure 11-10). If trauma and potential injury to the cervical spine are suspected, stabilize the patient's spine.

INITIAL ASSESSMENT

The next step in patient assessment is the **initial assessment** (formerly called the primary survey) (Figure 11-11). The initial assessment is a rapid, organized, and systematic evaluation:

- Form a general impression of the patient. This is necessary to determine the priority of care and is based on an immediate assessment of the environment and the patient's chief complaint.
- Quickly determine the nature of the illness or the mechanism of injury.

- Provide spinal stabilization if indicated.
- Identify and manage immediately any life-threatening conditions.
- Assess the patient's mental status.
- Assess the airway. Is it patent? If not, open it.
- Assess breathing. Is it present? Is it adequate?
- Assess circulation. Determine the pulse rate. At the same time, check for bleeding and evaluate the skin for color, temperature, and moisture. In children under 6 years of age, determine adequacy of capillary refill.
- Identify "priority" (unstable) patients. At this point, a decision should be made whether to begin transport or wait for paramedic backup. Follow your local protocols.

Approach the patient face-to-face, if possible. This allows for the development of rapport and also saves patients from having to turn their heads to see who is coming. Make eye contact with the patient, and introduce yourself: "I am EMT–Intermediate Smith, and we are here to help you." If spinal injuries are suspected, tell the patient not to move.

General Impression of the Patient

The EMT–I's immediate sensory assessment of the situation, combined with the patient's chief complaint, is what forms the general impression (Figure 11-12). Everything seen, heard, or smelled when approaching the patient should be noted. Is the patient comfortable, or is he or she writhing in pain? Does the patient look healthy, or does he or she look barely alive? What is the patient's chief complaint? Is there a medical problem (such as chest pain), or has trauma occurred (such as a shooting)?

Life-Threatening Problems or Injuries

Look for life-threatening problems or injuries (such as marked difficulty breathing or severe bleeding), and treat these immediately. A general impression of the patient's condition forms the basis for the rest of patient care. If the patient does not look well, treat him or her as unstable ("priority") according to local protocols. Remember, appearance is only one of many criteria used to determine the severity of a patient's condition.

STREET WISE

Not all sick patients look bad; sick appearance is only one of many criteria used to assess patients.

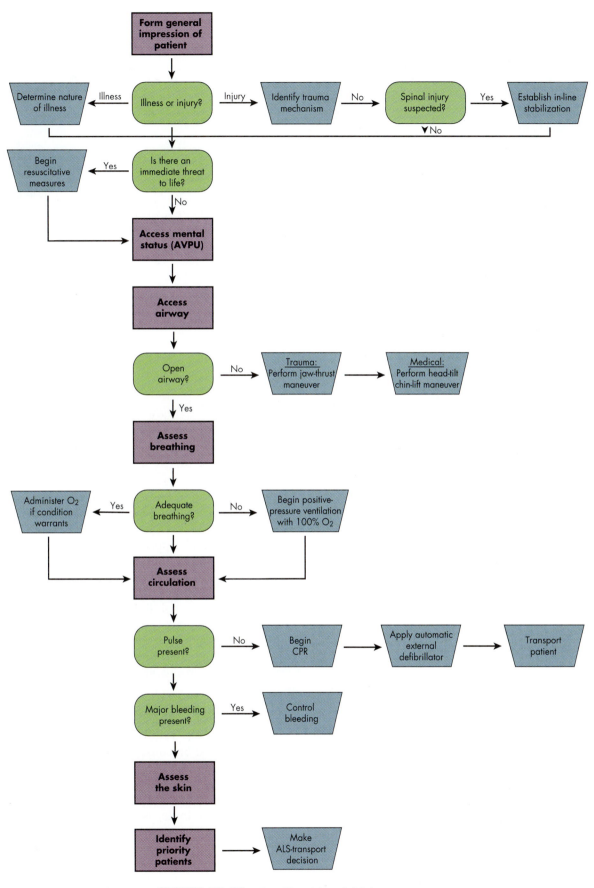

FIGURE 11-11 ▲ Algorithm, initial assessment.

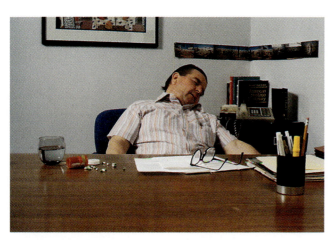

FIGURE 11-12 ▲ Form a general impression of the scene, using all of your senses to take in information. (Courtesy the American Red Cross. All rights reserved in all countries. From *First aid: responding to emergencies,* St Louis, 1991, Mosby.)

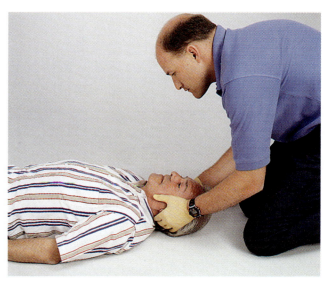

FIGURE 11-13 ▲ For patients with suspected trauma injuries, perform the jaw-thrust maneuver without hyperextension.

Assess the Patient's Mental Status

Determine the patient's level of responsiveness using the AVPU mnemonic:
- **A**—Patient is *A*wake and *A*lert.
- **V**—Patient responds to *V*erbal stimulus.
- **P**—Patient responds to *P*ainful stimulus.
- **U**—Patient is *U*nresponsive.

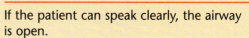

STREET WISE

An initial conversation with the patient will give a good impression of the mental status. Consider a patient who is unresponsive, especially if no gag or cough reflex is present, as "priority" status. Even a patient who responds verbally but does not follow commands appropriately should be treated as a "priority" case.

Assess the Patient's Airway Status

The patient who is responsive and can speak clearly has an open airway. In these patients the initial survey can continue. An open airway must be ensured in patients who are unresponsive.

▶ NOTE: This information is not intended to replace material taught in a standardized health care provider cardiopulmonary resuscitation (CPR) course. The authors assume that the reader has already received and is properly trained in CPR.

For semiresponsive or unresponsive medical patients, perform the head-tilt/chin-lift maneuver. If the airway is not clear, clear it. For trauma patients or those

STREET WISE

If the patient can speak clearly, the airway is open.

patients with an unknown nature of illness, stabilize the cervical spine and perform the jaw-thrust maneuver (Figure 11-13). In the case of two EMT–Is working together, one EMT–I provides airway and spine protection while the other EMT–I continues the initial survey. If a second EMT–I is not available, it is most important to maintain the airway and protect the spine. Once the jaw thrust is done, stabilize the neck until it is properly immobilized (Figures 11-14 to 11-17).

There are many forms of mechanical airway adjuncts that EMT–Is may find helpful. These adjuncts are discussed in detail in Chapter 8.

Assess the Patient's Breathing

Immediately assist ventilation of or ventilate patients with inadequate breathing. These patients include the following:
- Patients who are not breathing (respiratory arrest)
- Adult patients whose respiratory rate (number of breaths per minute) is less than 10 per minute or greater than 30 per minute
- Patients who have decreased levels of responsiveness

Quickly determine whether the patient is breathing by looking, listening, and feeling for air exchange:
- Look for rise and fall of the chest.
- Listen for air moving in and out of the patient's nose or mouth.

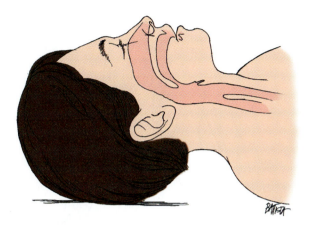

FIGURE 11-14 ▲ A normal airway—the patient is breathing adequately. (Kimberly Battista from Stoy W: *Mosby's EMT–Basic textbook,* St Louis, 1995, Mosby.)

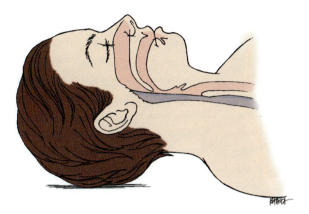

FIGURE 11-16 ▲ Fluid in the airway may obstruct a patient's respiration.

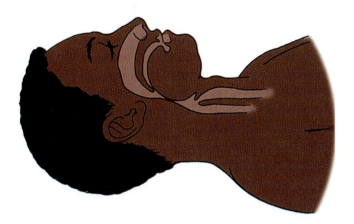

FIGURE 11-15 ▲ If the patient becomes unconscious, the tongue may slide back in the mouth, obstructing the airway. (Kimberly Battista from Stoy W: *Mosby's EMT–Basic textbook,* St Louis, 1995, Mosby.)

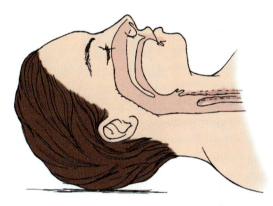

FIGURE 11-17 ▲ The airway can also become constricted, blocking the patient's ability to breathe adequately.

• Feel for exhaled air against your chin, face, or palm of your hand with the rise and fall of the patient's chest.

All three of these sensations must be present to conclude that the patient is breathing adequately. If any of these signals are absent, the patient may not be breathing enough to oxygenate the body tissues and remove carbon dioxide. Also, a patient whose rate of respiration is greater than 20 or less than 12 breaths per minute will often be unable to maintain sufficient air exchange and will become hypoxic and hypercarbic. At a minimum, these patients should receive a high concentration of supplemental oxygen.

The patient should be ventilated by either mouth to mask or by adjunct devices whenever inadequate air exchange is suspected. Always, supplemental oxygen should be used. Two initial ventilations of 1.5 to 2.0 seconds each should be given, followed by one breath every 5 seconds. Some EMS physicians recommend

▶ The specific term for the amount of air exchanged in 1 minute is *minute ventilation.* This is better determined in the pulmonary function laboratory than in the field. If a person's minute ventilation is inadequate, signs of inadequate breathing and cyanosis may be present.

ventilating the apneic or unresponsive patient every 3 to 5 seconds. Any patient with difficulty breathing should be treated as a "priority" patient.

Even if breathing is present and the patient is responsive, high-concentration oxygen (15 L/min nonrebreather mask) still may be required. All patients with a serious illness or injury should receive high-concentration oxygen. An unresponsive patient with adequate respirations should receive high-concentration oxygen.

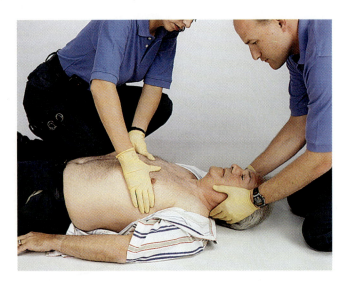

FIGURE 11-18 ▲ Palpating for equal expansion of the chest.

Also, the EMT–I should palpate the chest for equal expansion during the initial assessment of the trauma patient (Figure 11-18). This will help identify the presence of flail chest that can lead to significant interference with effective ventilation.

Assess the Patient's Circulation

The order of priorities in the circulatory assessment is as follows:
- Check for a pulse.
- Stop major bleeding if present.
- Evaluate perfusion by assessing the skin color, temperature, capillary refill, and condition.

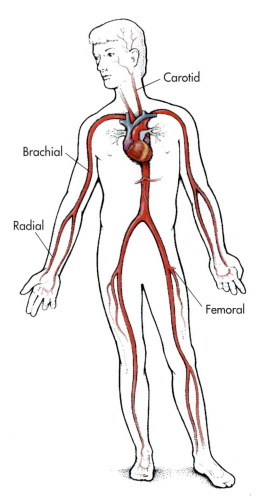

FIGURE 11-19 ▲ Check for a pulse. (Duckwall Productions.)

CHECK FOR A PULSE

If the patient is responsive, check quickly for a radial pulse. In a child under 1 year of age, palpate the brachial pulse. If no radial pulse is present, palpate the carotid pulse. If the patient is unresponsive, feel for the carotid pulse first (Figure 11-19).

If the patient is pulseless:
- *Medical patient over 12 years of age*—Start CPR and apply the automated external defibrillator (AED) or standard defibrillator.
- *Medical patient under 12 years of age*—Start CPR.
- *Trauma patient*—Start CPR.

Even if carotid and radial pulses are present, a pulse rate less than 60 beats per minute or greater than 100 beats per minute (in adult patients) should be considered potentially life threatening if combined with other pertinent findings, such as hypotension, chest pain, or severe dizziness.

The presence of certain pulses often suggests that various minimum systolic blood pressure levels are present. These numbers are only estimates, however. For example, if a radial pulse is present, the patient's systolic blood pressure is approximately 80 mm Hg.

▶ ASSESSMENT OF EFFECTIVE VENTILATION
There are several ways to decide whether the patient is receiving effective ventilatory assistance. A combination of the following indicators is usually most helpful:
- *Rise and fall of the chest wall*—The chest wall should rise with inhalation and fall with exhalation.
- *Auscultation of the lungs*—Good movement of air in all of the lung fields should be heard during inspiration.
- *Skin color*—As the patient becomes better oxygenated, his or her color should improve (i.e., the patient should "pink up").
- *Heart rate*—Typically, persons develop tachycardia and then bradycardia with respiratory compromise. A change toward normal in the heart rate should be seen with proper ventilation.
- *Pulse oximetry*—If a person is not being effectively ventilated, the pulse oximetry reading may be low.

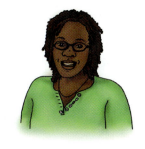

Warm, pink, dry skin is normal.

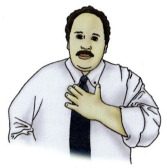

Pale, cool, and clammy skin indicates shock.

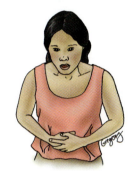

Hot, dry skin may indicate heat injury, medication overdose, or infection.

FIGURE 11-20 ▲ **Conditions indicated by skin color, temperature, and moisture.**

Knowing the following values will help with a more rapid estimate of the patient's blood pressure:
- Carotid: 60 mm Hg systolic
- Femoral: 70 mm Hg systolic
- Radial: 80 mm Hg systolic

CHECK FOR MAJOR BLEEDING

If major bleeding is present, control it using a standard measure, such as direct pressure, elevation, pressure points, bandages, or a tourniquet.

ASSESS THE SKIN TO DETERMINE PERFUSION STATUS

The color, temperature, and moisture of the patient's skin can suggest abnormal situations (Figure 11-20):
- Warm, pink, dry skin usually indicates adequate circulation. This is the normal skin condition.
- Pale, cool, and clammy skin indicates shock.
- Hot, dry skin may indicate serious medical emergencies, such as heat injury, medication overdose, or infection.

The patient's face, lips, nail beds, mouth, earlobes, and eyelids are all places where color may be assessed. In dark-skinned patients, look for color changes in the nail beds, under the tongue, and in the conjunctiva.

Some abnormal skin colors and the conditions leading to them are as follows:
- *Red*—Alcohol or cocaine ingestion, anaphylactic (allergy) shock, hyperthermia, stroke, heart attack
- *Pale*—Shock, stress, heart attack, anemia, hypothermia
- *Yellow (jaundice)*—Liver disease, gallbladder disease, kidney disease
- *Mottled red, pale, or blue*—Poor perfusion (often seen in cardiac arrest)

Another sign assessed at the time of evaluating skin color and temperature is capillary refill. Capillary refill is assessed by pressing on the patient's nail bed or palmar surface of the hands or feet. Normally, a pink color returns within 2 seconds when the pressure is released. If refill is slow or absent, the patient's circulation may be inadequate.

This test has been the subject of much controversy in recent medical literature. Some experts state that the test is questionable in adults. For example, some women and elderly patients of both sexes may have refill times of up to 10 seconds and still have adequate circulation. The 1994 DOT EMT–Basic curriculum recommends that this test be used only in children under 6 years of age (Figure 11-21). Even in young children, the test is unreliable if the patient is in a cold environment or has just come out of the cold. Local protocols and medical direction instructions will determine the use of this test.

> ### HELPFUL HINT
> - Remember the following points when removing a patient's clothing to ease examination and care:
>   - Use caution in extremely cold environments, especially when transferring the patient to metal backboards or scoop stretchers.
>   - Prevent further exposure to toxic substances that may burn or irritate the skin.
>   - In hot weather, remember that skin contact with certain surfaces (such as metal parts of a stretcher) can cause burns.

To better assess and care for the patient, it may be necessary to remove some or all clothing. The nature of the incident will dictate to what extent this must be done. Protecting the patient from embarrassment as much as possible without compromising patient care is important.

Identify "Priority" (Unstable) Patients

"Priority" patients are unstable patients who require more advanced-level care when possible. Depending on the EMT–I's location and protocols, identification of a

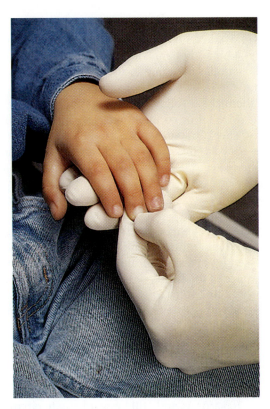

FIGURE 11-21 ▲ Assessing capillary refill. (Vincent Knaus from Stoy W: *Mosby's EMT–Basic textbook,* St Louis, 1996, Mosby.)

patient as "priority" may simply mean rapid transportation to the nearest medical facility. In certain cases, paramedic backup may be requested at the scene or en route. In some EMS systems an air medical helicopter service may be activated. Local protocols should be followed in determining whether patients are "priority" status.

The availability of care may play a role in this decision making. For instance, if paramedic care is 20 minutes away and the appropriate hospital is 5 minutes away, transporting the patient to the hospital would be more prudent. In other situations, initiating transportation and meeting the paramedic unit at a point en route may be appropriate. "Priority" does not necessarily mean a high-speed ambulance ride with lights and siren. The important factor is starting transportation or providing advanced care rapidly. Local EMS protocols and the recommendations of medical direction should always be followed.

Listing all conditions or situations that would give a patient "priority" status is impossible. Overall, erring on the side of caution is best. Some general guidelines for the identification of "priority" patients include the following:

- Poor general impression
- Altered mental status
- Unresponsive patients, especially if there is no gag reflex
- Responsive patients who are unable to follow simple commands

- Difficulty breathing
- Shock (hypoperfusion)
- Complicated childbirth
- Chest pain with suspected cardiac origin
- Hypoxia that fails to correct rapidly (within 1 to 2 minutes of field intervention)
- Multiple trauma (including severe burns)
- Severe hypertension
- Uncontrolled bleeding
- Severe pain anywhere

After "priority" patients are identified, transport can be expedited and the appropriate focused history and physical examination continued.

Lifesaving procedures are performed as the need is identified. These include techniques such as relief of airway obstruction, control of hemorrhage, artificial respiration, CPR, defibrillation of cardiac arrest victims, and initiation of shock management (e.g., administration of epinephrine in anaphylactic shock and administration of glucose [sugar] in severe hypoglycemia) (Figure 11-22).

STREET WISE

Perform resuscitation concurrently with the initial survey, "treating as you go." If an obstructed airway is detected during the initial survey, stop and take care of the problem before continuing the survey.

✖ **Focused History and Physical Examination** • An in-depth examination to determine the severity and cause of the patient's condition. It includes both a hands-on examination and a gathering of the patient's history.

FOCUSED HISTORY AND PHYSICAL EXAMINATION: MEDICAL PATIENT

The information sought during the **focused history and physical examination** is limited and is specifically related to the acute problem for which care is being provided. Only the suspected condition is evaluated. The focused history and physical examination differ for medical and trauma patients.

Responsive Medical Patient

In the responsive medical patient, obtain the history first. Ascertain the chief complaint in the patient's own words, if possible. Then assess the complaint using the **OPQRST** acronym:

- **O**—Onset; when did the problem begin?
- **P**—Provocation; what makes the problem worse?

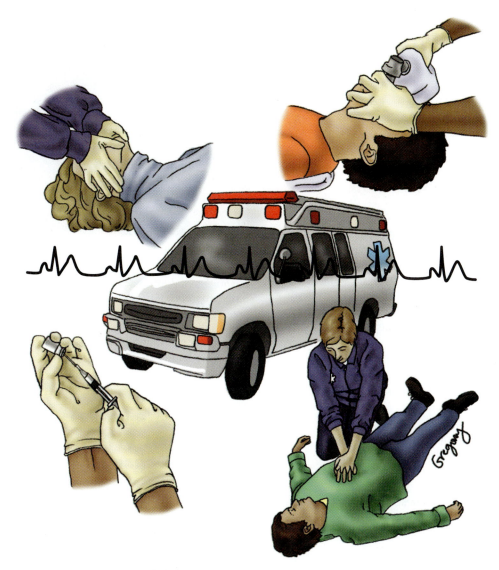

FIGURE 11-22 ▲ Lifesaving procedures.

- **Q**—Quality; what is the problem (usually pain) like? Is it sharp, crushing, viselike?
- **R**—Radiation; does the pain go (move) anywhere?
- **S**—Severity; on a scale of 0 to 10 (0 = no pain, 10 = the worst pain imaginable), how bad is the pain?
- **T**—Time; does the symptom come and go, or is it always there?

In addition, determine if there are any associated symptoms. Finally, summarize the patient's past medical history and current health status.

Once a focused history has been obtained, perform a focused physical examination, paying particular attention to the patient's chief complaint. Assess the following areas as necessary, using the techniques detailed in Chapter 10.

- Head
- Neck
- Chest
- Abdomen
- Pelvis
- Extremities
- Posterior aspect of the body

Then obtain baseline vital signs, including orthostatic measurements if indicated. Using all of the information available, provide emergency medical care. Consult local protocols and on-line medical direction as necessary.

Unresponsive Medical Patient

In the unresponsive medical patient, perform a rapid assessment. Position the patient to protect the airway, and assess the following as necessary:

- Head
- Neck
- Chest
- Abdomen
- Pelvis

- Extremities
- Posterior aspect of the body

Obtain baseline vital signs, and obtain whatever information possible from relatives and bystanders. Remember to look for medical alert tags on the patient's wrist or chest. Then provide care based on signs and symptoms.

FOCUSED HISTORY AND PHYSICAL EXAMINATION: TRAUMA PATIENT

Reconsider the Mechanism of Injury and Transport Decision

Reconsider the patient's mechanism of injury before proceeding with the history and physical examination. This helps identify "priority" patients and guide further assessment. Persons with any of the following circumstances should be considered "priority" patients until proven otherwise:

- Ejection from vehicle
- Death in same passenger compartment
- Falls greater than 20 feet
- Rollover of vehicle
- High-speed vehicle crash
- Vehicle-pedestrian crash
- Motorcycle crash
- Unresponsive or altered mental status
- Penetrations of the head, chest, or abdomen

In infants and small children the following additional factors should be considered when determining "priority" status:

- Falls greater than 10 feet
- Bicycle collisions
- Passenger in any medium-speed collision

Look for Hidden Injuries

Some of the most serious injuries are not immediately obvious, particularly the following:

- *Seat belt injuries*—If buckled, seat belts by themselves may produce potentially serious intraabdominal injuries. Do not assume that a patient has no injury just because of seat belt use.
- *Air bag injuries*—Air bags may not be effective without concomitant use of a seat belt. Recall that a patient can still hit the steering wheel after air bag deflation. Always lift the deployed air bag and look at the steering wheel for deformation after the patient has been removed. Regard any visible deformation of the steering wheel as an indicator of potentially serious internal injury and act accordingly (Figure 11-23).
- *Child safety seat injuries*—Despite many media warnings, some individuals still place small children in

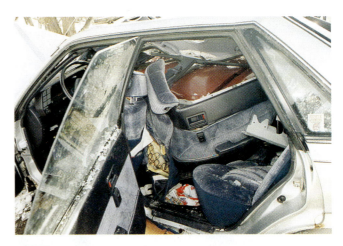

FIGURE 11-23 ▲ Deformed steering wheel. (From American College of Emergency Physicians; Pons PT, Cason D, chief editors: *Paramedic field care: a complaint-based approach*, St Louis, 1997, Mosby for ACEP.)

safety seats that are in the direct path of an expanding air bag. This trauma may cause serious injury to a small child.

Perform A Rapid Trauma Assessment If Warranted by the Mechanism of Injury

Perform a rapid trauma physical examination on patients with a significant mechanism of injury to detect life-threatening injuries. In the responsive patient, obtain historical information before and during the trauma assessment. Be certain to continue spinal stabilization and continuously reconsider your transport decision. Change to "priority" status if necessary.

Assess the patient's mental status. Then inspect and palpate, looking and feeling for signs of injury. The acronym for the rapid head-to-toe examination in a trauma patient is DCAP-BTLS. Look and feel for the following signs of injury:

- **D**—Deformity
- **C**—Contusions
- **A**—Abrasions
- **P**—Punctures/penetrations
- **B**—Burns
- **T**—Tenderness
- **L**—Lacerations
- **S**—Swelling

Use the techniques detailed in Chapter 10 to do the following:

- Assess the head and neck, and then place a cervical collar.
- Assess the chest.
- Assess the abdomen.
- Assess the pelvis.
- Assess all four extremities.

- Using spinal precautions, roll the patient over and assess the posterior body

Throughout the examination, look for medical identification devices and obtain the patient's history, including the following:
- Chief complaint
- History of present illness
- Past medical history
- Current health status

If No Significant Mechanism of Injury Exists

For patients with no significant mechanism of injury (e.g., a cut finger), do the following:
- Perform a focused history and physical examination of the injuries based on the techniques of examination discussed in Chapter 10. Limit your examination to the specific injury site.
- Assess baseline vital signs.
- Obtain a patient history, including the chief complaint, history of the present illness, past medical history, and current health status.

DETAILED PHYSICAL EXAMINATION

The **detailed assessment** (Figure 11-24) (sometimes called the secondary survey) is an organized subjective and objective examination of the patient. This examination is patient and injury specific; it gathers more detailed patient information than that provided in the initial and focused assessments. Special emphasis needs to be placed on areas suggested by the chief complaint and history.

The patient's injury or illness will indicate whether this part of the patient assessment is necessary. A patient with a simple cut finger, for example, would not require a detailed assessment. However, a victim of multiple trauma would. Identifying illness or injuries also allows EMT–Is to begin patient care, which may prevent further injury and decrease pain.

For "priority" patients, the detailed assessment (if indicated) can be performed en route to the hospital (Figure 11-25). Sometimes, the time required to care for life-threatening conditions will not allow for completion of the detailed assessment.

STREET WISE

For "priority" patients, perform the detailed assessment en route to the hospital.

After obtaining the patient history, proceed with examination of the following areas as necessary, using the techniques outlined in Chapter 10. The head-to-toe examination (secondary survey) is a thorough examination of the body to identify wounds, fractures, and other injuries or signs of illness.
- Mental status
- General survey
- Skin
- Head
- Eyes
- Ears
- Nose and sinuses
- Mouth and pharynx
- Neck
- Thorax and lungs
- Cardiovascular system
- Abdomen
- External genitalia
- Peripheral vascular system
- Musculoskeletal system
- Nervous system

Accurately record examination findings and baseline vital signs.

ONGOING ASSESSMENT

Patient assessment is an ongoing process that must be continued during definitive field management and transportation. In a stable patient the assessment is repeated every 15 minutes. In an unstable patient the assessment is repeated every 5 minutes.

Ongoing assessment includes the following parameters:
- Reassess the patient's mental status.
- Monitor the airway.
- Monitor the breathing rate and quality.
- Reassess the pulse rate and quality.
- Monitor the skin for color, temperature, and condition.
- Realign patient priorities as needed.
- Reassess vital signs.
- Repeat the focused examination regarding the complaint or injuries.
- Check the efficacy of interventions.

Definitive Field Management

Definitive field management includes the lifesaving modalities described previously and treatment of less-threatening problems to the extent possible in the field. This process includes airway maintenance and ventilation, as well as the use of intravenous (IV) fluids and the pneumatic antishock garment for shock, according to local protocols. In many patients, cardiac monitoring is appropriate. If a patient has trauma, fracture stabilization, bandaging, and immobilization to the stretcher will improve comfort and ensure a safer transport to the hospital.

If an IV line is started, drawing blood for the hospital to analyze is helpful. Local protocols also may include use of the fingerstick blood glucose (sugar) test in the field.

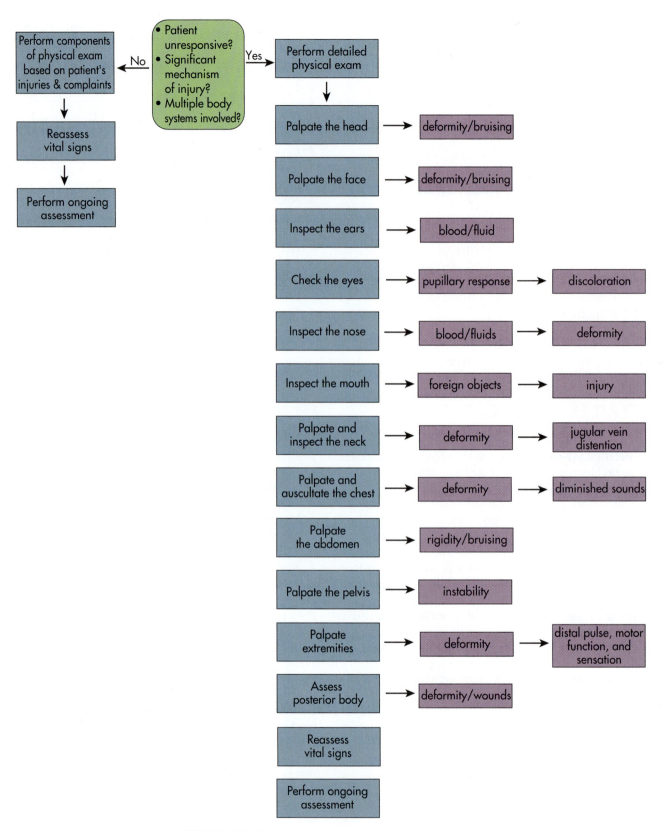

FIGURE 11-24 ▲ Algorithm, detailed examination.

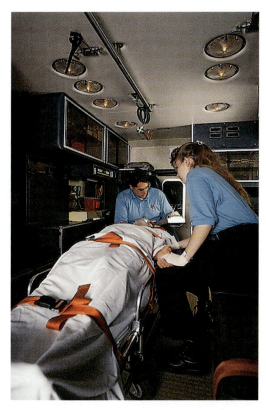

FIGURE 11-25 ▲ It may be necessary to perform the detailed assessment while en route to the receiving facility if the patient is a "priority."

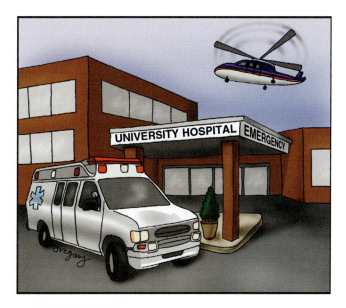

FIGURE 11-26 ▲ Direct transport to a specialty center.

Transportation

The facility to which the patient is transported depends on factors such as patient condition, available facilities, and available transport modes. It is generally accepted that patients should be directly transported to the most appropriate facility for their condition. If possible, and if allowed by local protocols, the patient's wishes to be taken to a certain hospital should be taken into consideration.

Many EMS systems now include specialty centers for the following:

- Multisystem trauma
- Acute myocardial infarction (chest pain emergency departments)
- Burns
- Spinal cord injuries
- Pediatric trauma
- Eye injuries
- Extremity reimplantation
- Neonatal emergencies
- Hyperbaric medicine
- Behavioral and psychiatric emergencies

In many EMS systems the EMT–Is determine which patients are referred to a specialty center on the basis of written protocols. Other systems require transport authorization from medical direction. Depending on the level of care available, transport time, and patient condition, some patients are directed to the closest emergency department for initial evaluation and lifesaving treatment. Usually, however, direct transport to the appropriate specialty center is best for the patient (Figure 11-26).

Different modes of transportation are available; conditions, local protocols, and medical direction will dictate which mode is used. Air medical transportation, especially EMS helicopter transport, has become a common vehicle for transporting critically ill and injured patients to the appropriate specialty center. General guidelines for when helicopter transport is *not* appropriate include the following:

- During lightning or high-wind conditions
- During heavy cloud periods (unless the helicopter can fly on instruments)
- For combative patients
- For patients contaminated by hazardous materials
- For patients whose size prohibits proper securing inside the aircraft
- When ground transport is faster, including waiting time for the helicopter to reach the scene

▶ SOME TIPS FOR TRANSPORTING GERIATRIC PATIENTS INCLUDE THE FOLLOWING:

- A geriatric patient may think he or she is being brought to the hospital to die and may resist transport.
- Explain clearly everything that is being done to the patient.
- Give these patients choices whenever possible.
- Ensure that someone will take care of the patient's possessions.
- Use family members whenever possible to help reassure the patient.

Follow the "three R's" rule of medical transportation: Get the "right person" to the "right place" in the "right amount of time."

Contacting Medical Direction

Once transport is begun, the receiving facility should be contacted, either directly or through the medical direction facility. Some EMS systems require that units also call in during the resuscitation phase of the incident. At this point, EMT–Is should take the time to provide only "need to know" information, such as the following:

- Nature of the incident
- Number of patients being transported
- Life-threatening problems
- Care being rendered
- Results of that care
- Estimated time of arrival (ETA) at the facility

If additional information is necessary to update the patient's condition, a follow-up call can be made en route. Some EMS systems require that medical direction contact be made at specific times. If a certain procedure requires permission from medical direction, more information (such as vital signs or specific injuries) may be needed before contact is made with medical direction.

The appropriate run reports need to be filled out in a clear and readable format. A well-documented report is essential for proper transfer of care to the receiving facility and for defense if patient care ever needs justification in a hearing or negligence suit.

CASE HISTORY FOLLOW-UP ■ ■ ■

EMT–I Smith is back at the base and feeling a little nervous as he places the call to the hospital. A million things are running through his mind. Did he miss a major injury to a patient? Did he leave out some important patient information? Was his radio report inaccurate? Was his paperwork not complete? He hates emergency responses like this car crash. The scenes are always busy, and so many things need to be done at once. Overlooking something important is so easy.

The medical direction physician comes to the phone. Her voice is friendly, yet she sounds concerned. She asks EMT–I Smith about his assessment of the 3-year-old child. EMT–I Smith feels sick to his stomach, and before answering the physician's question, he asks if the child is okay. The physician tells him that the boy will be fine but that he had a right midshaft femur fracture and had lost quite a bit of blood by the time he got to the emergency department. According to the mother, the child was sitting on her lap when the crash occurred and was thrown to the floorboard of the car.

EMT–I Smith mentally reviews his physical examination of the child. He remembers that the child had a lot of winter clothing on and did not want to be touched. He recalls feeling the boy's chest, abdomen, arms, and legs and thinking that his right thigh felt a little larger than the left as he palpated through the boy's clothes. If only the boy had grimaced or shown some reaction, EMT–I Smith would have removed his clothing and performed a more thorough examination.

EMT–I Smith apologizes to the physician and refrains from making excuses. She tells him not to be too hard on himself and that "we all need to learn from our mistakes." Yet EMT–I Smith knows the crucial point is that he did not do a good patient assessment. He was distracted by the scene and by the number of patients. He knows that he is ultimately responsible for this error and vows never to let this kind of thing happen again.

SUMMARY

Important points to remember from this chapter include the following:

- Patient assessment is a structured method of evaluating a patient's physical condition. The process involves six phases: scene size-up (scene assessment), initial assessment (primary survey), focused history and physical examination of the medical patient, focused history and physical examination of the trauma patient, detailed assessment (secondary survey), and ongoing assessment (which includes definitive field management and transportation).
- During the scene size-up, the EMT–I must evaluate the "whole picture" of the call. The purpose of this phase is to provide a safe environment for EMS personnel and the patient. On arrival, five critical decisions must be made:
  - Is the scene safe?
  - How many patients are involved?
  - Is additional help needed?
  - Is this a medical or a trauma patient?
  - Is there a need for body substance isolation precautions?
- The initial assessment is an organized approach to the patient that includes the following tasks:
  - Form a general impression of the patient.
  - Determine if any life-threatening conditions are present. If so, treat these immediately.
  - Evaluate the patient's level of responsiveness.
  - Assess the airway. If the patient is responsive and can speak clearly, the airway is open. Otherwise, an open airway must be ensured.
  - Assess breathing, and immediately ventilate patients with inadequate breathing.
  - Assess circulation by checking the pulses. Look for and treat bleeding, and assess the skin.
  - Identify "priority" (unstable) patients who require more advanced-level care as soon as possible.
- During the initial assessment, perform lifesaving procedures as needed if they have not already been done.

- The focused history and physical examination evaluates the patient on the basis of the suspected condition. In trauma patients the EMT–I must first reconsider the mechanism of injury and the transport decision and then perform the rapid trauma assessment. The acronym for this examination is DCAP-BTLS (see text).
- Following the rapid trauma assessment, the EMT–I should obtain baseline vital signs. These vital signs should include pulse, respirations, blood pressure, pulse oximetry, and temperature (according to local protocol). Similar information must be obtained in the medical patient.
- The detailed assessment is a more detailed examination that is patient and injury specific. The patient's illness or injury should suggest whether this part of the patient assessment needs to be done. There are three parts to the detailed assessment: the chief complaint (the main problem for which EMS was called), a detailed exploration of the chief complaint and related problems, and a head-to-toe survey as indicated by the patient's condition.
- Patient assessment is an ongoing process that is continued while the EMT–I provides definitive field management and transportation to the hospital. During this process the EMT–I reassesses the patient's mental status, airway, breathing, pulse, skin, and vital signs. Treatment priorities are modified as needed, and the focused examination repeated as necessary. The effects of any treatment provided to the patient should be continuously monitored.
- Many conditions cannot be completely managed in the field. The job of the EMT–I is to provide lifesaving care when necessary, stabilize the patient, and appropriately "package" the patient for transportation to more definitive care, usually at a hospital. Local protocols will most often determine to which medical facility the patient is taken. Medical direction and/or the receiving facility should be contacted according to local protocols. The EMT–I should be sure to document all care given on the appropriate run report in a clear and legible fashion.

12

Clinical Decision Making

...CASE HISTORY It is 5 o'clock in the morning on December 25 when EMT–Is Budin and Phillips return from their fourth call of the morning. Shortly after returning to the station, they receive a call for a 54-year-old woman experiencing shortness of breath. On arrival at the scene, they are met by a local police officer, who reports that the woman appears well and is sitting in a chair talking with her daughter. The women reports that she has noticed increasing shortness of breath for the past 72 hours but has been hesitant to call 9-1-1 because she wishes to stay with her family, who is visiting for the holidays. The patient's daughter wants the EMT–Is to make sure her mother is "okay" so they can attend church services in a few hours.

LEARNING OBJECTIVES

CHAPTER GOAL
Upon completion of this chapter, the EMT–Intermediate will be able to apply the decision-making process to form a field impression from information gathered during patient assessment.

Cognitive Objectives
As an EMT-Intermediate you should be able to do the following:
- Compare the factors influencing medical care in the out-of-hospital environment with other medical settings.
- Differentiate between critical life-threatening, potentially life-threatening, and non–life-threatening patient conditions.
- Evaluate the benefits and shortfalls of protocols, standing orders, and patient care algorithms.
- Define the components, stages, and sequences of the critical thinking process for EMT–Is.
- Apply the fundamental elements of critical thinking for EMT–Is.
- Describe the effects of the "fight or flight" response and the positive and negative effects on decision-making capabilities.
- Develop strategies for effective thinking under pressure.

- Summarize the "six R's" of putting it altogether: read the patient, read the scene, react, reevaluate, revise the management plan, and review performance.

Affective Objectives
As an EMT–Intermediate you should be able to do the following:
- Defend the position that clinical decision making is the cornerstone of effective EMT–I practice.
- Practice the facilitation behaviors when thinking under pressure.

Psychomotor Objectives
- None identified for this chapter.

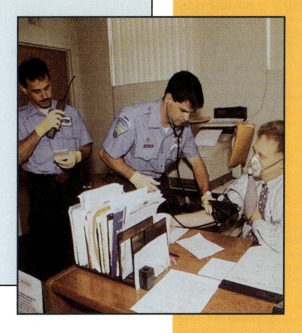

INTRODUCTION

In the practice of prehospital care, the EMT–Intermediate (EMT–I) must be able to function in a chaotic environment that at most times bombards the provider with numerous sources of information. The ability to properly gather the information, evaluate its usefulness, and use it in synthesizing a treatment plan is the cornerstone of effective EMT–I practice. The key to success involves the development of a pattern that can be used for manipulating data in different situations.

In developing management plans, the EMT–I must have a solid foundation of knowledge and facts on which the treatment decisions are made. Basing a therapy on partial assessment or neglect of key information can result in inappropriate and dangerous care.

It is easy to make a decision. The challenge is to make the best decision in a time-critical manner, often with severely limited data. The EMT–I must possess the skills to independently make patient care decisions without the benefit of numerous other professionals to help.

The ability to effectively gather information, evaluate its quality, and synthesize the information into a management plan is additionally challenged by the enormous pressure under which the EMT–I operates. Time is crucial in many injuries and illnesses. Family members may be prompting the EMT–I to hurry. The rain, cold, heat, or snow may be forcing a decision to initiate treatments immediately or wait to perform them during transport. Mass casualty incidents almost instantaneously deplete the resources of the first units to arrive and require the rationing of medical personnel and equipment.

HELPFUL HINT
- Clinical decision making is the ability to quickly integrate an enormous amount of information from multiple sources to form a correct treatment plan.

The Practice Environment

The out-of-hospital environment is a unique atmosphere in which to apply medical skills and therapies. Many of the procedures and treatments used by EMT–Is were developed to function best within a hospital setting. However, emergency departments are well lit, seldom bounce around, and are devoid of extremes of temperature and weather—the opposite of conditions that EMT–Is may face daily. A tremendous number of variables can affect almost every aspect of the emergency call, including weather, patient position, contamination, hostile animals, locked entrances, bystanders, and environmental factors.

The Spectrum of Patients

There is no clear definition of what constitutes an emergency. Every individual will have a unique interpretation of when an ambulance needs to be summoned. The EMS system provides a safety net of emergency care and typically responds to all calls for help regardless of type. Thus EMT–Is are exposed to a broad spectrum of patient illness, injury, and acuity of distress.

✚ **Major Trauma** • Injuries or mechanism that place the patient at great risk of death or disability

It is often very clear when a patient has sustained **major trauma** and incurred injuries to numerous organ systems. These high-profile victims usually generate many calls to 9-1-1, and the EMT–I should be informed by dispatch of the potential for a serious situation. Usually the mechanism of injury itself is enough to alert the provider as to the potential for serious injury. Other obvious critical life threats include penetrating trauma to the chest, abdomen, or head.

Patients with advanced forms of malignancy may appear emaciated or obtunded, or to have minimal respirations. These patients, along with those who have exacerbations of chronic diseases such as congestive heart failure or chronic obstructive pulmonary disease (COPD), can appear to be in extreme distress.

It is often said that very ill and basically healthy patients present with the clearest treatment solutions. The group in between—patients with "potentially serious" injuries or illnesses—require the greatest amount of scrutiny and evaluation. Patients with blunt trauma to the abdomen from a motor vehicle collision can initially appear well but quickly deteriorate as a result of internal bleeding due to liver or splenic lacerations. Chronic medical conditions may affect a patient's response to new illnesses or injuries. A patient with chronic congestive heart failure may have very little reserve to tolerate pulmonary insult from an acute disease such as pneumonia.

Some injuries and illnesses are quite distressful for the patient but clearly not life threatening. A fractured and deformed wrist or other fracture can be painful to the patient and distracting to the EMT–I but generally is not considered life threatening (Figure 12-1). An otherwise healthy adult with acute gastroenteritis may "feel like dying" because of the frequent episodes of forceful vomiting and diarrhea. However, this generally is a self-limited disease that responds well to diet manipulation and rehydration; it is usually not life threatening.

GUIDANCE AND AUTHORITY

✚ **Protocols/Standing Orders/Algorithms** • Well-defined practice guidelines for specific patient presentations, illnesses, or injuries. Developed with the local medical director, these often negate the need to contact on-line medical command for orders.

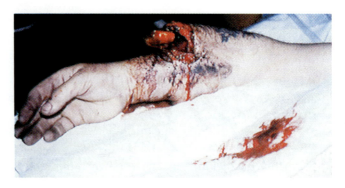

FIGURE 12-1 ▲ Open fracture. (From London PS: *A colour atlas of diagnosis after recent injury,* London, 1990, Mosby-Wolfe.)

There are an infinite variety of patient presentations to the multitude of diseases and injuries humans can endure. There is no absolute way to prepare EMT–Is for each potential patient encounter. Instead, EMS systems have evolved a framework of tools to assist in the approach, evaluation, and management of common patient problems.

Protocols, standing orders, and patient care **algorithms** essentially have the same goal of providing well-defined, structured performance guidelines. The strength of these practice parameters is a standardized approach to common presentations. Universal practice patterns lend themselves well to quality improvement initiatives and performance benchmarking.

✚ **Medical Ambiguity** • Vagueness in symptoms or complaints that limits the ability to determine a specific diagnosis.

The value of guidelines such as protocols is in the general approach to the classic presentation of common problems. Weaknesses in protocols are encountered when patients present "outside the box" of common occurrences. A patient may be focused on one aspect of an acute illness and neglect to inform the EMT–I of other important symptoms. This type of **medical ambiguity** can cause the EMT–I to misclassify the patient and begin an evaluation and treatment course that may neglect the primary derangement.

It is also a challenge when patients have multiple complaints or disease states that require the consideration of multiple protocols and algorithms. The focused nature of protocols makes integration of multiple treatment guidelines difficult and confusing. Since protocols commonly follow a step-by-step progression to direct a specific type of treatment, there are no clear points at which other protocols can, or should, be initiated.

A common pitfall in EMT–I practice is the overreliance on algorithms or protocols without an adequate understanding of the intellectual basis of the treatment plan. This is commonly referred to as "cookbook medicine." The EMT–I student should be aware that although there are common disease states and injury patterns, there is also tremendous variability in how individuals react to physiological insults and subsequent therapy. Proper understanding of anatomy, normal physiology, the pathophysiology of disease states, and the body's response to traumatic injury will allow for integration of the common treatment modalities with the unique characteristics of the patient.

❗ HELPFUL HINT

- Understanding the physiology involved in treatment protocols will provide a better understanding of which treatments to select when patients do not fit into one particular protocol.

CRITICAL THINKING: COMPONENTS, STAGES, AND SEQUENCE

The mechanism of collecting, integrating, and synthesizing information takes part largely at the subconscious level. The product of this thought process is an understanding of the patient's illness or injury and the development of a treatment plan. Reviewing these critical thinking steps will help provide an understanding of how these important diagnostic and therapeutic conclusions are made.

Concept Formation

✖ **Concept Formation** • A pattern of understanding based on the initial information gathered.

The EMT–I begins to form the first concepts **(concept formation)** the instant the call comes in over the radio, phone, or pager. The EMT–I will immediately have a first *impression* as to how the call is affecting other activities the EMT–I is involved in at the time. Additional stimuli will be encountered as information is relayed from dispatch and the EMT–I approaches the scene. The immediate patient environment will also influence the EMT–I's decision making.

Once at the patient's side, the EMT–I gathers important data during the initial assessment. These data help form the foundation for deciding how critical the patient's condition may be. The physical examination provides information concerning what body systems are injured or what abnormal functions are present.

If conscious, the patient may verbalize a chief complaint. This information helps the EMT–I determine what the patient is most concerned about but may not be specific to the actual acute problem. The history will indicate how quickly the problem developed and if the patient attempted to treat the condition personally.

General patient affect can provide clues to the patient's mental status. This is important to consider because mental status directly relates to perfusion of the central nervous system, electrolyte disturbances, intoxication, head trauma, and psychological disorders.

CLINICAL NOTES

In addition to the senses of touch, sight, smell, and hearing, there are numerous tools for collecting critical data, including sphygmomanometers, pulse oximetry, and simple blood glucose monitors. The incorrect use of all ancillary devices can produce false and misleading data. Do not use these tools on patients without clearly understanding their limitations.

Data Interpretation

✖ **Data Interpretation** • Comparison of current information with past education and experience to draw conclusions.

Data interpretation begins as soon as the EMT–I learns about the call. As patient assessment proceeds, all of the information regarding physical findings and patient symptoms are integrated into the EMT–I's knowledge of normal anatomy and human physiology. The EMT–I's attitude regarding the reliability of the data and prior experience with similar data will help determine how the information will be used.

Application of the Principle

As the data are processed, the EMT–I begins to formulate an initial impression of what disease processes or injuries are affecting the patient. This working diagnosis then guides the EMT–I toward specific treatment protocols. Initial interventions are selected on the basis of the cumulative interpretation of all the data received concerning the current patient, as well as data on similar patients who have been cared for in the past.

Evaluation

One of the most important habits an EMT–I can develop is the ability to constantly reassess the patient. Optimal care is not provided by taking a single "snapshot" of the patient and basing all ongoing treatment decisions on the data gathered during only the initial evaluation. The EMT–I should routinely reevaluate the vital signs and physical state of the patient to determine the response to therapies or progression of the physiological insult. As new information is learned, the working diagnosis may be expanded or changed. This may necessitate modifications in the current treatment protocols and planned therapies.

Reflection on Action

Another important habit, similar to constantly reassessing the patient, is to critique the actions and interventions performed on each call. Honest and in-depth reflection on the aspects of the run that were challenging will help the EMT–I prepare for the next patient with similar problems.

FUNDAMENTAL ELEMENTS OF CRITICAL THINKING

Eight elements form the foundation of critical thinking for the EMT–I:

- *Adequate fund of knowledge*—The level of understanding the EMT–I possesses regarding how injuries and diseases affect patients. This is acquired through training, continuing education, and patient encounters.
- *Focus on specific and multiple elements of data*—The ability to recognize the specific critical data that must be gathered from multiple sources to form the basis of the complete examination and treatment.
- *Information stimuli*—The ability to gather and organize the data stimuli in a pattern that leads to a general understanding of the situation.
- *Identification of and dealing with medical ambiguity*—The ability to recognize that similar problems can present with a variety of manifestations for each unique patient.
- *Differentiation between relevant and irrelevant data*—The ability to recognize important data that are being presented, along with a tremendous amount of extraneous data that are not particularly useful to the EMT–I.
- *Analysis of and comparison with similar situations*—The ability to integrate data gathered in the current situation with any previous similar situations experienced.

- *Recall of contrary situations*—The ability to recall past adverse patient encounters that may guide the current situation.
- *Articulation of assessment-based decisions and construction of arguments*—The ability to explain the reasoning behind conclusions drawn from the evaluation and treatment plans initiated.

APPLICATION OF ASSESSMENT-BASED PATIENT MANAGEMENT

Patient Acuity Spectrum

Spectrum of Acuity • The wide range of patient presentations, illnesses, or injuries. This ranges from the patient who appears totally normal, as well as the most critical patient who is close to or experiencing cardiac arrest.

Each individual has a unique definition of what actually constitutes an emergency. This leads to a wide variety of reasons why the 9-1-1 system is activated and an ambulance is dispatched. The **spectrum of acuity** is wide, and the percentage of EMS calls that are truly life-threatening emergencies is small (Figure 12-2). These involve the high-acuity patients for whom EMT–I intervention and

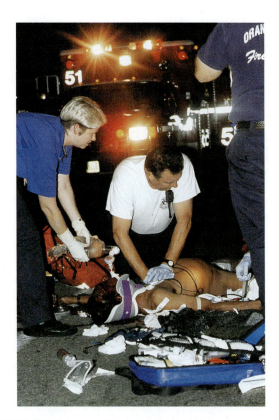

FIGURE 12-2 ▲ Life-and-death situations in EMS are infrequent when compared with the total call volume. (Craig Jackson, photographer.)

rapid transportation to the hospital are the critical factors for survival.

Ambulance calls that represent minor medical illnesses or injuries are generally straightforward and require little critical thinking on the part of the EMT–I regarding appropriate treatment. Patients who possess obvious life threats, either from illness or from trauma, often demonstrate very clear problems with very specific interventions that the EMT–I is prepared to perform. These patient presentations typically follow well-established guidelines or protocols, and little critical thinking is necessary.

The greatest challenge EMT–Is face is performing accurate assessments and interventions for patients whose conditions are neither low nor high acuity. The condition of these moderate-acuity patients can be further compromised by injuries or illnesses with progressive decompensation. EMT–I interventions play a crucial role in stabilizing this type of patient.

CLINICAL NOTES

Compared with the mildly ill or severely ill patient, the moderately ill or injured patient can be the most difficult to correctly identify and treat.

Thinking Under Pressure

One of the true attributes that separate the seasoned, veteran EMT–I from a new graduate is the ability to work under extreme pressure. In almost every environment in which EMT–Is respond, there is *someone* who is having an emergency. The scene will be emotionally charged, and patients will be frightened. Family members may express severe stress as they try to comfort loved ones during the crisis. All of these factors challenge the EMT–I to remain focused and apply skills and training to benefit the patient.

✖ "Fight or Flight" Response • The body's physiological reaction to stressful situations that involves activation of the sympathetic nervous system.

Our bodies prepare for stressful encounters. The sympathetic nervous system releases adrenaline, which is responsible for the **"fight or flight" response.** The useful aspects of this adrenaline surge are the heightened senses of vision and hearing. Muscle strength and reflexes also are increased as the body prepares for the challenge. Unfortunately, critical thinking skills may become impaired during this process, and the ability to focus on problems and perform thorough assessments can be diminished.

The key to quality performance under pressure is the development of habits of evaluation and management that can be applied to every patient encountered. These habits will naturally lead the EMT–I to perform the im-

portant aspects of care that can be easily overlooked when one is placed under stress. These habits are learned in initial EMT–I training and subsequent runs throughout the career of the EMT–I. Technical aspects of care and performing procedures should become second nature to the EMT–I and should require very little critical thinking.

Mental Checklist

The clinical decision-making habits that the EMT–I will need to develop revolve around a number of actions that will overlap throughout the patient encounter. These actions include the following:
- Stop and think.
- Scan the situation.
- Decide and act.
- Maintain clear, concise control.
- Perform regular and continual reevaluation of the patient.

Facilitating Behaviors

✖ Facilitating Behaviors • Patterns of behaviors and actions that promote efficient and appropriate patient care.

With each patient encounter, the EMT–I will gain more experience in general patient assessment and management. Certain behaviors **(facilitating behaviors)** typically facilitate efficient patient care and are important to highlight early in the training process. The first rule is to *stay calm.* Anxiety in caregivers typically provokes or worsens anxiety in the patient. A confident, steady approach to the patient imparts the feeling of trust that is critical in treating acute illness and injury. An unorganized, sloppy examination by the EMT–I will be recognized by the patient and emergency department staff and will typically result in crucial pieces of information being missed. A habit of patient assessment needs to be developed that is systematic and can be followed reflexively under stressful situations.

Anticipating potential changes in the patient's condition will enable the EMT–I to mentally prepare for ad-

STREET WISE

Patient assessments and therapies rarely occur in calm, peaceful settings. The patient, family members, or bystanders may all be very emotional. If you become angry, loud, or obviously frustrated, the anxiety of those around you may be heightened and even interfere with care. Maintaining a calm, professional demeanor will instill trust in the quality of care being provided and facilitate communications and treatment.

ditional therapies or procedures and avoid hesitation in the face of a sudden, unexpected finding.

In assessing the patient for the current acute event, two questions should be addressed:

- What is the current working diagnosis and best treatment plan?
- What additional problems could the patient potentially develop, and how should they be treated?

CLINICAL NOTES

Emergency service providers not only need to be aware of the "most common" explanations for patient complaints, but they also need to be aware of the "most life threatening." Always assume a worst-case scenario when initially evaluating a patient. When faced with multiple working diagnoses, pursue the diagnosis that carries the worst potential outcome for the patient. Always err on the side of the patient.

 Clinical decision making incorporates multiple styles of information management:
- Situation analysis
  - Reflective in nature versus impulsive action
  - Promotes a thorough assessment before initiating therapies
  - Allows prior experiences and training to influence action
- Data processing style
  - Divergent development of ideas versus convergent focused processing
  - Allows for consideration of multiple diagnoses
- Decision-making style
  - Anticipatory actions versus reactive actions
  - Allows EMT–Is to prepare for additional interventions

Each situation that the EMT–I faces requires a unique combination of all types of information management styles.

Situational Awareness

Situational Awareness • The integration of all facets of the scene and patient care, resulting in an overall picture of the current event.

It is common practice to mention "scene survey" as one of the first actions the EMT–I accomplishes on arrival. Overall **situational awareness** requires that the EMT–I constantly read the scene to gather new data and identify any potential threats (Figure 12-3). The same is true for the patient. Ongoing patient assessments allow the EMT–I to quickly detect improvement due to interven-

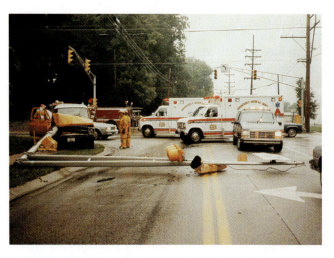

FIGURE 12-3 ▲ Every scene should be evaluated for potential dangers to the responding crew. (From American College of Emergency Physicians; Pons PT, Cason D, chief editors: *Paramedic field care: a complaint-based approach,* St Louis, 1997, Mosby for ACEP.)

tions or worsening conditions that require treatment. The assumption that the patient always has the potential to deteriorate will help motivate the EMT–I to maintain proper diligence.

Putting It All Together: "The Six R's"

How is clinical decision making applied to the patient? The mental habits that EMT–Is develop through training and experience are applied in the preparation for the run, response, initial assessment, focused examination, interventions, ongoing examination, and ongoing treatment. Clinical decision making is the cumulative effort of training and experience applied to a particular patient problem. The "six R's" include the crucial points in this process:

- Read the patient.
- Read the scene.
- React.
- Reevaluate.
- Revise the management plan.
- Review performance at the run critique.

READ THE PATIENT

Immediately on encountering the patient, the EMT–I will develop questions and begin to formulate assessments. Simple observation while approaching the patient can prompt several critical questions:

- What is the level of consciousness?
- Is the patient interacting with bystanders or family?
- Is there any obvious respiratory distress?
- Is there obvious deformity or bleeding?
- Is the skin pale or cyanotic?

Talking with the patient will allow the EMT–I to gain further insight into the current crisis. The chief complaint will reflect what the patient is most concerned about, whereas the history of the illness or injury may give clues regarding other conditions the EMS providers will need to address. Talking to the patient also provides immediate assessment of the airway and general neurological function.

Touching the patient provides general clinical information about skin texture and hydration status, temperature, and diaphoresis. Palpation of the pulse for regularity, strength, and rate will assist the EMT–I in assessing basic cardiac function. Auscultation of lung sounds helps determine the quality of ventilation and identify the physiological insults of bronchospasm and pulmonary edema. By this time, the ABCs (airway, breathing, circulation) have been performed and apparent critical life threats have been identified. Accurate vitals signs complete the initial patient assessment and help determine a level of acuity for the patient.

It is important to recognize factors that limit the EMT–I's ability to read the patient. Certainly, patients at a very young age may not be able to verbalize a chief complaint or accurately describe pain or discomfort. At the other extreme, patients who have suffered stroke, dementia, or other illnesses may not be able to effectively communicate with the EMT–I. Medications and intoxicants (drugs or alcohol) can also alter a patient's perception of pain and misdirect the provider. Recognizing these limitations will prevent the EMT–I from drawing conclusions based on insufficient or inaccurate data.

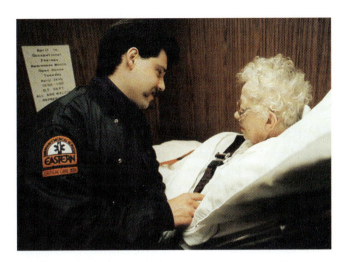

FIGURE 12-4 ▲ Elderly patients may be unable to effectively communicate relevant history or symptoms. This may deprive the EMT–I of pertinent information. (Craig Jackson, photographer.)

> **STREET WISE**
>
> A language barrier between the patient and EMS personnel can severely limit the amount of accurate information that can be gathered (Figure 12-4).

READ THE SCENE

On arrival at the scene, a survey of the immediate surroundings should be performed. This can provide information regarding the mechanism of injury, number of victims, and environmental conditions affecting the patient and social issues that may have influenced the patient's need for emergency assistance.

REACT

The hallmark of being a good EMT–I is having the ability to recognize a life-threatening emergency and react quickly. The initial assessment is designed to quickly identify critical patients and prompt the EMT–I to intervene with airway, respiratory, and cardiac support.

The reaction of the EMT–I is influenced by the most typical illness or injury pattern that fits with the patient complaints and examination. While considering the "most common" presentation, the EMT–I must be prepared to react to sudden deteriorations in the patient or to the discovery of more life-threatening conditions.

�֍ **Working Diagnosis** • The medical illness or injury that is perceived to be affecting the patient. Based on current information, the diagnosis can be modified and changed as additional information is gathered.

✖ **Reevaluation** • Ongoing assessment of the patient to determine a change in condition or response to therapy.

There will be occasions when a clear **working diagnosis** would not be apparent after the initial assessment and focused examination. In these instances, the habitual **reevaluation** of the ABCs while treating the specific signs and symptoms may be the safest treatment plan.

REEVALUATE

After the working diagnosis is established and therapy initiated, the EMT–I must routinely reevaluate the condition of the patient. Assessment for deterioration in condition and response to interventions will help the EMT–I prepare additional treatment and monitoring goals. As the critical issues are identified and addressed, a more complete secondary examination will allow the EMT–I to identify less serious or less obvious problems that may be affecting the patient.

REVISE

As patient care proceeds, the EMT–I will become more confident in assessing the patient and establishing the working diagnosis. Ongoing evaluations will also help determine trends in the patient's vital signs and overall condition. At this stage the EMT–I will have the opportunity to further revise the initial assessment and modify the planned therapies.

REVIEW

Establishing well-organized patient assessment habits will guide the EMT–I in every patient encounter. Crucial to the development of these habits is the critique of each run. Accomplished formally at "run review" training, informally during conversation about the call, or through personal reflection, the review of the call will allow the EMT–I to reinforce habits that were efficient and helpful in the patient care, while modifying or abandoning those habits that did not particularly assist in care.

STREET WISE

What if your interventions do not improve the condition of the patient?

There will be times when prehospital treatment fails to help the patient. In these situations consider the following possibilities:

- The initial working diagnosis is incorrect.
- Additional problems are contributing to the patient's condition.
- Therapeutic interventions are incorrect or inadequate.
- The patient's condition may be exceeding the limits of care that an EMT–I can provide.

CLINICAL NOTES

Remember that patient information is confidential and should only be discussed with appropriate personnel.

SUMMARY

Important points to remember from this chapter include the following:

- Critical decision making incorporates all past experiences and training into an almost subconscious process that facilitates the gathering of data, synthesis of information, and development of a working diagnosis.
- The practiced EMT–I will develop habits that allow for efficient preparation, assessment, interventions, and review that build from the experience of each call.

13 Communications

...CASE HISTORY

EMT–I Walters has just received a phone call from an attorney representing his ambulance service. It seems as though an emergency response handled by EMT–I Walters and a previous partner has become part of a lawsuit against his EMS service and his medical direction hospital. EMT–I Walters has no immediate recall of the incident because it happened several years ago. The attorney briefly describes it for him, based on the patient's hospital records.

The call occurred 2 years ago on September 5, at 0445. EMT–I Walters and his partner were dispatched to a motor vehicle crash where a driver had struck a utility post head-on. EMT–I Walters begins to remember the incident. It was a rainy morning and the end of a busy shift. He pulled up on the scene to find a group of bystanders surrounding the patient, who was lying face down on the pavement next to the car. The bystanders said that they had been with the patient at a party and were following him back to his apartment. They were concerned that he was "too drunk to drive." As EMT–I Walters secured the patient's head and neck to place him supine, he heard the group say that they pulled their friend from the car after the crash and moved him to the pavement. The patient was breathing, smelled of alcohol, and had vomitus on his face and neck. The EMT–Is maintained cervical spinal stabilization, suctioned the patient's airway, and administered high-concentration oxygen.

The patient was disoriented but could follow simple commands. He had a laceration on his forehead from striking the windshield, but there were no other obvious signs of injury. During the physical examination, EMT–I Walters noted that the patient could not move his lower extremities. He appeared to have no sensation below the level of his umbilicus, and EMT–I Walters marked the area on the patient's skin where the sensation stopped. The EMT–Is secured the patient's neck and spine to a long backboard and prepared him for transport. En route, EMT–I Walters contacted medical direction and gave the following report:

"We are en route to your facility with a 24-year-old male who was involved in a head-on collision. He was removed from the car by friends and placed prone on the pavement prior to our arrival. We immobilized his spine and placed him in a supine position. He has a laceration on his forehead from striking the windshield. He is disoriented but able to follow simple commands. He is unable to move his lower extremities and has no sensation or movement below the level of his umbilicus. Strength and motion in the upper extremities are within normal range. Vital signs are stable. Friends state that the patient has been drinking. He has vomited once. The patient's airway was suctioned, and he was placed on high-flow oxygen. He is fully immobilized on a long backboard. Our ETA is 8 minutes."

After delivering the patient to the emergency department, EMT–I Walters carefully documented the specifics of the call on the prehospital care report and returned to service. Later that week, he heard that the patient suffered a complete cord lesion and was permanently paralyzed.

CHAPTER GOAL

Upon completion of this chapter, the EMT–Intermediate will be able to follow an accepted format for the dissemination of patient information in verbal form, either in person or over the radio.

Cognitive Objectives

As an EMT–Intermediate you should be able to do the following:

- Identify the importance of communications when providing EMS.
- Identify the role of verbal, written, and electronic communications in the provision of EMS.
- Diagram a basic communication model.
- Identify the importance of proper verbal communications and terminology when communicating during an EMS event.
- List factors that impede and enhance verbal communications.
- Identify the components of the local EMS communications system and describe their function and use.
- Describe the function and use of cellular phones in EMS communications.
- Identify and differentiate among simplex, multiplex, and duplex communications systems; digital communications; and trunking.
- Describe the functions and responsibilities of the Federal Communications Commission.
- Identify the importance of proper written communications during an EMS event.
- List factors that impede and enhance effective written communications.
- Recognize the legal status of written communications related to an EMS event.
- State the importance of data collection during an EMS event.
- Identify technology used to collect and exchange patient and/or scene information electronically, including facsimiles (faxes) and computer communications.
- Recognize the legal status of patient medical information exchanged electronically.
- Describe the phases of communication necessary to complete a typical EMS event.
- Describe how the emergency medical dispatcher functions as an integral part of the EMS team. List appropriate information to be gathered by the emergency medical dispatcher.
- Identify the role of the emergency medical dispatcher in a typical EMS event.
- Identify the importance of prearrival instructions in a typical EMS event.
- Describe the purpose of verbal communication of patient information to the hospital.
- Describe information that should be included in patient assessment information that is verbally reported to medical direction.
- Organize a list of patient assessment information in the correct order for electronic transmission to medical direction according to the format used locally.

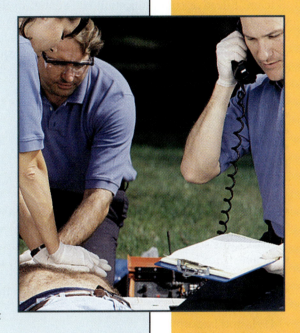

INTRODUCTION

An EMT–Intermediate (EMT–I) functions as part of the EMS team. Effective communication is essential to the smooth and efficient operation of the team. There must be a coordinated communications system that allows information to flow internally and externally in both routine and emergency modes. Communication routinely takes place between the following:

- Callers and the dispatch center
  - Requests for help
  - Verification of addresses/locations
  - Updates on patient or scene status
- The dispatch center and EMT–Is
  - Dispatch information and response to emergency calls and nonemergency calls
  - Updates to and reports from responding teams (hazards, patient information, directions for accessing the scene)
  - Requests for backup units and/or rescue, fire, or law enforcement specialty teams
  - Resolving communication difficulties between the field and the emergency department
- EMT–Is and backup units
  - Communicating equipment needs
  - Scene and patient updates
  - Advice on what routes should be used to best access the scene
- EMT–Is who are working together on the ambulance
  - Communication that ensures safety of team members when they are apart (such as the use of portable radios)
  - Communication between team members and the dispatch center in multiple-patient incidents
  - Routine conversations during the course of working together
- EMT–Is and the emergency department
  - Medical direction and advice
  - Information about patients being transported to their facility
- EMT–Is in the field and EMS system administration
  - Sending and receiving messages

- Routine activities such as sending the unit to the ambulance repair facility for vehicle maintenance
- The dispatch center and public safety units (fire, police, and other EMS units), as well as other community agencies
  - The EMS system and the public in general
  - Public relations and education
  - Media coverage
  - Evacuation information, storm or hazard warnings
- The dispatch center and disaster networks
  - Personnel, resource, and equipment needs
  - Number of patients distributed to area hospitals
- Emergency departments
  - Relaying patient information
  - Announcing bed and resource availability
  - Announcing availability of air and ground ambulance units

Communications that take place as part of providing EMS are done verbally, through written means, or electronically.

Idea • The intended meaning of the communication.

Encode • To put an idea or message into a language or code.

BASIC COMMUNICATION MODEL

Communication is the exchange of information between an individual or group and other persons. Think of the types of communication you participate in daily or that go on around you. From the routine to emergencies, communication generally follows the same basic model (Figure 13-1). First, you form an **idea** or message you wish to pass along. Then you **encode** it in a language that can be understood by the person who will receive the message or in a manner that is appropriate for the situation. This might be words, numbers, symbols, pictures, codes, signals or any number of other things.

Next, you select the medium for sending your message, such as speaking to someone face-to-face, speaking over the radio or phone, leaving a voice mail, writing a

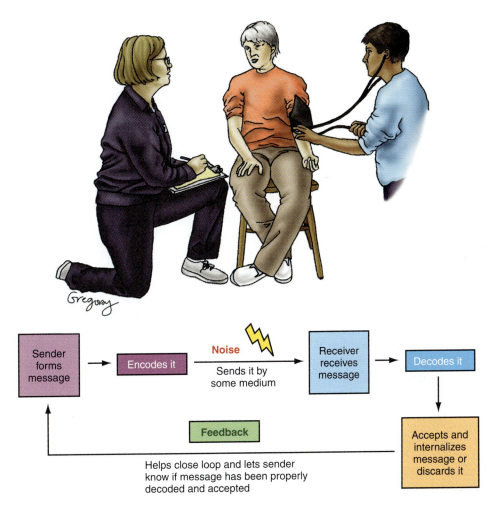

FIGURE 13-1 ▲ **Basic communication model.**

note or letter, or sending a fax or electronic mail. Pagers that have a text display are another means of getting a message to someone. Gestures and body language can also effectively communicate a message. When you think about it, there is no shortage of communication media—today's technology allows us to communicate at an unparalleled rate of speed and efficiency.

✳ **Decode** • To convert a message into understandable language.

✳ **Feedback** • Confirmation from the receiver that a message has been received and understood.

Your message then arrives at its destination, and the receiver **decodes** it into language the he or she understands. Ideally, the receiver accepts or internalizes the message. However, in some cases the message may be received and decoded but the receiver does not agree with it and fails to act on it. Last, the receiver provides **feedback** to you that the message has been received and understood. Feedback is critical to closing the communication loop or circle. Without feedback the message may remain out there and you have no idea that it has not been received, decoded, and accepted.

STREET WISE

An example of the communication model in action:

EMT–I Jones: "Mrs. Smith, we are here to help you. Why did you call for the ambulance?"

Mrs. Smith: "I called you all because I am having chest pain."

EMT–I Jones: "You say you are having chest pain?"

Mrs. Smith: "Yes. Yes, I am."

EMT–I Jones: "When did the chest pain start?"

Mrs. Smith: "Oh, it started about half an hour ago."

EMT–I Jones: "I see. The chest pain started approximately half an hour ago. What were you doing when the pain started?"

Mrs. Smith: "Well, I was watching television. My favorite soap opera had just started."

Feedback is particularly critical in emergency communications.

VERBAL COMMUNICATION

Verbal communication is a good way to exchange system and patient information with other members of the EMS team. Some communication is effective, whereas other communication fails to achieve its intent. **Semantic** (meaning of words) and technical (equipment) factors can either boost or hinder communication.

Semantics

The term *semantics* relates to the meaning of words. Words commonly used in communication mean different things to different people. Employing words or phrases that are vague or abstract invites varying interpretation. Also, technical language and medical terminology can create confusion when used in the wrong setting. One way to improve communications is to make sure they are unambiguous and to the point and that they avoid technical or semantic jargon that cannot be clearly understood by all parties.

Sometimes a code, symbol, abbreviation, or acronym used by a person or agency is unfamiliar to the receiver, thereby creating a gap in communication. It is important to use only codes with which all persons are familiar. Many EMS systems, as well as fire and police departments, have eliminated or greatly reduced their use of codes and gone to using plain English. It is also helpful to identify a standard set of appropriate abbreviations and acronyms and ensure that everyone knows them. These should include abbreviations and acronyms commonly used by the physicians, nurses, and other health care professionals in the local hospitals.

Noise • Things that interfere with receiving a message.

Noise

Although we typically think of noise as loud sounds, **noise** in the communication model is anything that interferes with communication. People have a tendency to listen to only part of the message and block out other information. It may be that the receiver is daydreaming, thinking about other things, or not in a mood to listen when the message is delivered. Also, new information may conflict with established values, beliefs, or expectations. Uncomfortable environmental conditions can also distract the receiver. He or she may be hungry, thirsty, angry, or tired and not ready to receive the message. It may be that several messages are being delivered to the receiver all at once and he or she cannot effectively decode the message. Think about emergency scenes and conditions under which the EMT–I works. Often they are extremely hectic and loud.

Perceptions and cultural differences can also interfere with the message being decoded and interpreted in the intended manner. What is considered normal in one part of the world may be offensive in another. Touching someone on the arm can be comforting, or it may be offensive.

In face-to-face communication, facial expressions and the body language of the sender can also influence how a message is received. If a person says he or she is not angry but his or her face paints a different picture, the receiver may not believe what the person says. Voice inflection, tone, pitch and the words used also play a role in verbal communication. Words that seem calming and reassuring when said in a controlled tone may seem insincere when said in an excited or loud voice.

Overcoming noise may not always be possible, particularly in emergency situations. For this reason, it is important to get feedback from the receiver to ensure that the receiver understands and accepts the message. Furthermore, look for the best time to deliver the message. If the person you are trying to communicate with is in the midst of several communications, it is better to wait until he or she is able to give his or her full attention. This may not always be possible in emergency situations, so you have to use your best judgment. If a message must be communicated promptly, first try to get the receiver's attention and then deliver the message. Follow that up by asking the receiver to repeat back the information you provided.

COMMUNICATION EQUIPMENT

The communications network that carries the emergency and routine communications must consist of reliable equipment capable of providing clear communication to all necessary agencies or systems. When setting up a communications system, the EMS service must consider the unique nature of its resources, geography, and funding. Modern EMS communications systems have specific equipment needs. The typical configuration includes telephones, radios, repeater systems, recording equipment, and pagers.

Telephones

Enhanced 9-1-1 • An emergency phone system that includes a visual display of the caller's phone number and address.

The widespread availability of the telephone makes it an excellent communication link for EMS systems. In fact, the telephone is one of the most common devices the public uses to reach the EMS system. **Enhanced 9-1-1** is the recommended phone system for EMS systems.

Dedicated Land Lines • Telephone lines with continuous direct connection from one geographical location to another.

The telephone also allows EMS systems to communicate internally, as well as externally, for routine and emergency situations. **Dedicated land lines** are often used by dispatchers to notify EMS personnel of emergency calls and are a reliable method of communicating with receiving hospitals, medical direction facilities, remote radio communication receivers, communication consoles, and police and fire dispatch centers. Dedicated land lines eliminate the need for the dispatcher to go through a switchboard, dial a phone number, or confront busy signals. Their biggest benefit is in saving time.

Cellular Phones

Cellular phones are another timesaving way for the public to access EMS systems, particularly in the case of motor vehicle crashes and other emergencies that motorists might encounter. They also are popular for use in the prehospital setting because of their ease of use and decreasing cost.

Cellular communication allows for excellent reception and better continuity in transmission than is achieved with typical radio systems. The geographical area served by a cellular telephone network is divided into regions called cells, each with its own base station and antenna that interconnects the mobile units and the telephone network. When the transmission falls out of one cell's range, it is immediately picked up by another cell. Most major metropolitan and many rural areas are now covered by cellular systems, and the network is growing.

Cellular phones can be used by EMS systems for dispatch, on-scene communications, scene-to-hospital communications, and delivery of on-line medical direction. In addition to voice communication, cellular phones allow transmittal of 12-lead electrocardiograms (ECGs), faxes, and computer data to the dispatch center and the hospital. Communications between the EMT–I and the hospital must be conducted over a telephone line that is dedicated to this purpose. Otherwise, there is a risk of getting a busy signal when attempting to establish communications with the hospital.

An advantage of cellular communications is that a person can be less formal than when talking over the radio. This promotes discussion and can reduce on-line time. It allows the physician to speak directly to the patient when necessary, such as when the patient refuses to be treated or transported to the hospital. Furthermore, the conversations conducted via cellular technology are more private and less likely to be picked by public scanners. This helps ensure patient confidentiality.

Disadvantages of cellular phones are that geography can interfere with the signal and cell sites may be unavailable or can become tied up with public communications. This can be the case during disasters, when cellular systems are tied up with a large volume of calls being made by private citizens and the news media.

Radios

Radios are the primary means of communications between the dispatch center and EMS teams. Radios allow communication between the following:
- The EMS team and the base station or communication dispatch center
- EMT–Is on the EMS team (using portable radios)
- The EMS team and other responding or on-scene units
- The EMS team and receiving hospitals or facility(ies) providing medical direction
- The EMS team and other public agencies (police and fire departments)

The radio system consists of three primary components: the base station, mobile two-way radios, and portable radios.

BASE STATION

The base station is the most powerful radio in the system, with a typical power output of 80 to 150 watts. A remote console may control it. Usually, the base station is located in a dispatch center that serves as the communications network for the EMS system. In some communities one dispatch center is responsible for all fire, police, and EMS communications. Many base stations are multiple-channel systems, but often the dispatch center communicates on only one channel at a time.

MOBILE RADIOS

Mobile two-way radios are mounted in vehicles such as ambulances, rescue units, and supervisory vehicles. With a typical power output of 20 to 50 watts, they allow communication to take place between the base station and emergency teams on the road. The characteristic transmission range is 10 to 15 miles over average terrain. This range is diminished in mountainous areas, where dense foliage is present, and in cities with large buildings. Mobile radios often have multiple channels.

PORTABLE RADIOS

Portable radios allow EMT–Is to communicate while away from the ambulance. These radios are hand-held devices with a typical power output of 1 to 5 watts. This low-power output significantly limits the range of the radios, allowing a range of only 1 to 5 miles. Like mobile radios, portable radios can be equipped with multiple channels. Some EMS systems equip each EMS team with one portable radio, whereas other systems provide a portable radio for each team member on duty.

RADIO SYSTEM CHARACTERISTICS

Each radio component serves as both a transmitter and a receiver. As such, they are referred to as transceivers.

make it ideal for use in major metropolitan operations. Frequencies in the 800-MHz range also can be tied to a computer system that can send voiceless communications to a computer in the vehicle.

Additional Communication Equipment

PAGERS

EMS agencies and fire departments are adapting existing technology to meet their internal and external communication needs. Pagers are devices that alert the user that someone is trying to contact him or her, usually by beeping or vibrating. The liquid crystal display can show short messages or telephone numbers. These messages can be sent to one or more persons at a time. Many systems require each member to wear a pager both on and off the job.

Alphanumeric pagers can be used to routinely update field personnel and administrators with vital information, including the following:

- Location of incoming emergency calls
- Significant EMS or fire calls
- Multiple-casualty incident calls
- What hospitals are on divert status
- Developing severe weather
- Existence of open shifts

REPEATER SYSTEMS

Portable radios allow EMT–Is to communicate from the patient's side or from remote locations. Unfortunately, using portable radios to communicate directly with hospitals or the dispatch center is sometimes impossible because of their short range. This drawback is due to their small size, low power output, and short antenna height. Poor output is sometimes a problem with mobile radios as well. To overcome this dilemma, some EMS systems use repeater systems to increase the range of their portable and mobile radios. Repeater systems are devices that receive transmissions from relatively low wattage transmitters on one frequency and retransmit them at a higher power on another frequency, increasing the range of the transmissions (Figure 13-3). Some repeater units are mounted on the vehicle, whereas others are mounted on towers.

RECORDING EQUIPMENT

Today, most EMS systems use recording equipment to maintain an active record of the radio and phone communications taking place within the system. Communications that take place between EMT–Is and medical direction also are recorded. Therefore keep in mind that radio and phone communications might be replayed for a variety of reasons, including

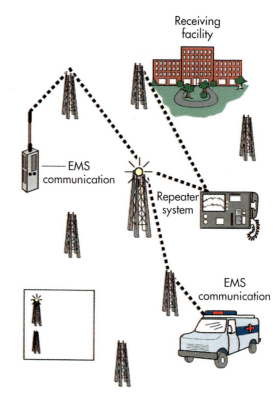

FIGURE 13-3 ▲ Repeater systems allow EMS systems to overcome poor output capabilities of portable radios. (Fox Photography.)

(but not limited to) media broadcast, educational activities, disciplinary hearings, and litigation. Professionalism in all communications within the EMS system is of paramount importance.

Rapid changes in both the communication needs of the EMS community and the available equipment require continual monitoring, upgrading, and training.

FEDERAL COMMUNICATIONS COMMISSION

The Federal Communications Commission (FCC) is the federal agency that controls and regulates all radio communications in the United States. The FCC's primary functions include licensing and allocating radio frequencies, establishing technical standards for radio equipment, and establishing and enforcing rules and regulations for radio equipment operation. The FCC is also responsible for monitoring frequencies for appropriate usage and spot-checking base stations and dispatch centers for appropriate licensing and records.

State and local governments may have additional requirements for radio operations. In some communities, regional plans are used to ensure cooperation of all radio users. In other areas there are minimum equipment standards for ambulance licensure that specify the type of radio equipment to be used.

WRITTEN COMMUNICATION

As members of the EMS team, EMT–Is routinely use written communication to convey information throughout the EMS system. This includes using forms to document the condition, as well as the cleaning and maintenance, of emergency vehicle(s) and medical equipment; recording daily checks of drug and fluid expirations; preparing incident reports that explain various occurrences during the workday; adding to call records that list or log dates, times, or other specifics of calls; and filling out information required for system administration, including training, work assignment, payroll, and benefit information.

The most important EMT–I written communication involves documenting the appropriate information regarding each emergency run. This includes the patient's condition and treatment information. Proper documentation during an EMS event provides a written, legal record of each case. It conveys important clinical information from the EMS team to the emergency department staff. Once the patient is delivered to the hospital, this documentation becomes a part of the medical record. When completing documentation, remember that all patient information is confidential and can only be shared with the nurse or physician who is continuing care of the patient in the emergency department.

Medical direction uses patient documentation to perform quality improvement audits to monitor a system's compliance with existing patient care protocols. The EMS run report tells a story as to the EMT–I's assessment and the care provided in the prehospital setting. Proper documentation shows that appropriate protocols are being followed and that the care provided meets the standard of care. Further information gleaned from quality improvement may be used to change or introduce new protocols or procedures. The EMS run report may also be used to gather important system data, such as patient billing information and data for research.

When completing written communication, keep in mind that it is an effective means of representing yourself as a professional to other health care providers.

ELECTRONIC INFORMATION GATHERING

Technology can be used to collect and exchange patient and scene information electronically. An advantage to electronic information gathering is that it can allow for real-time capturing of information. In other words, as an EMT–I is assessing a patient and entering information into a computer or wireless voice or data device, the information can be sent to the hospital, thereby allowing the receiving physician and nurses to know the condition of the patient being treated. Also, medical diagnostic technology can be integrated into the information being sent. This reduces dependence on traditional written documentation. It can also provide for advanced notification to the receiving hospital and reduce the time to in-hospital diagnosis and therapy. Electronic documentation carries with it the same responsibility of ensuring patient confidentiality. This may require additional equipment or software to prevent others from accessing patient information that is being sent electronically.

Some EMS systems no longer keep paper records, maintaining an electronic file of necessary information instead. This eliminates the need to maintain storage space for completed EMS run reports, makes it easier to look up a given EMS run, and facilitates data collection for quality improvement, research activities, and patient billing. In busy EMS systems the retrieval and utilization of paper EMS run reports can be a time-consuming process.

Biotelemetry • The process of transmitting physiological data, such as an electrocardiogram (ECG), over distance, usually by radio.

Oscilloscope • A television-like screen that displays an electrical current, such as the impulse that travels through the heart's conduction system.

Biotelemetry

Biotelemetry has been used in the prehospital setting for almost three decades. The electrical activity (voltage changes) in a patient's heart picked up by an ECG is converted into audio tones, which are transmitted to the hospital. The receiver at the hospital converts the audio signal back into measurable voltage changes, which can be traced on an **oscilloscope** and/or onto an ECG tape (Figure 13-4).

Interference • Something that prevents or inhibits clear reception.

Interference is a problem that can occur during telemetry transmission. Loose ECG electrodes, muscle tremors, 60-MHz noise, fluctuations in transmitter power, and interference of the actual radio transmission cause it.

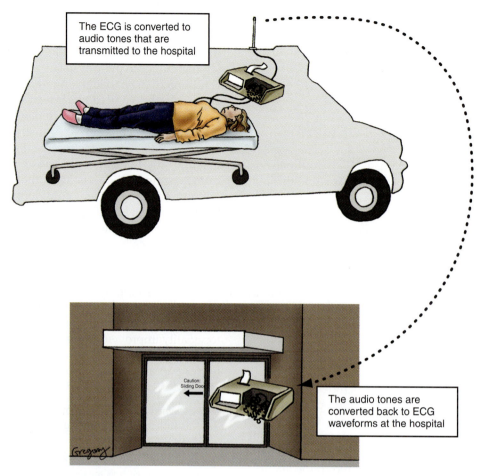

The ECG is converted to audio tones that are transmitted to the hospital

The audio tones are converted back to ECG waveforms at the hospital

FIGURE 13-4 ▲ **Biotelemetry is the transmission of a patient's ECG to the hospital.**

Computers

Computers have changed the world we live in. Although it may seem like they have been around forever, the first so-called personal computer was introduced in 1975. From the desktop, to laptop and notebook computers, to hand-held computers, these devices play a significant role in everyday life. The future is open to smaller and more powerful designs. Just as computers have become indispensable in the home, they also play an important role in the prehospital environment. Aside from their use in administrative functions, training, and computer-aided dispatch, they are also used to gather and document patient information. A benefit of entering patient information directly into the computer is that it effectively eliminates a step; with handwritten run reports the information either has to be retyped or scanned into the computer in order for it to be used for administrative or quality assurance purposes.

Once information is stored in the computer, it can be sorted by various categories. This allows the EMS system to use it for a variety of functions, including conducting quality assurance activities and researching various aspects of patient care. With information stored in the computer, the EMS system can quickly provide data and reports. Reports can be generated in a variety of formats depending on how the information is to be used.

Computers can communicate with other computers through a variety of means, including networks, cellular technology, and the Internet. E-mail is an effective means of communicating information throughout an organization, as well as to outside agencies.

Just as computers offer a number of advantages, there are some drawbacks. Computers and the software that is used are subject to the limitations of the computer and the operator. Not everyone is computer literate, and this can lead to problems getting efficient and effective use of the equipment. Furthermore, there is some loss of flexibility when a computer is being used to document the EMS event, since the computer document typically uses a prescribed format, as compared with written reports, where information can be entered in any manner that is appropriate to the situation.

Facsimiles

The facsimile, or "fax," technology that is commonplace in government, businesses, and homes throughout the world can also be used as an effective communication tool in the prehospital care setting. Fax machines scan printed information, digitize it line by line, and then transmit it over normal telephone lines to another fax machine that then decodes and prints ir. Faxes can also be generated and sent or received through computers or cellular technology.

Advantages of facsimile technology are that it provides earlier notification to the hospital of patient information and produces another piece of medical documentation. Also, it can be an effective tool for communications throughout an organization, as well as outside of it. An example is that employee work schedules can be generated at EMS headquarters and distributed to employees at remote base stations via a fax.

✖ **Encrypting** • Scrambling a message in order to prevent illicit access to the information.

A disadvantage of facsimile technology is that there must be access to a fax machine (or device such as a computer that can send or receive the fax) at both ends (sender and receiver). Using cellular technology, pen-based computers can be configured to send a copy of the run information to a fax machine while the EMT–I is en route to the hospital with the patient. However, when the EMS run report is sent via fax, steps must be in place to ensure patient confidentiality. The fax must be received in a secure location rather than one that serves as the general emergency department fax machine. This may require the hospital emergency department to maintain a dedicated phone line and fax machine for receiving EMS run reports. Furthermore, there must be a mechanism in place that permits the EMS run reports to be handled only by authorized personnel. One additional consideration is to make sure that faxes sent via cellular technology cannot be viewed or retrieved by anyone other than those who were intended to receive the fax. This requires **encrypting** the message.

TYPES OF COMMUNICATIONS

EMS communications can be broken down into three types: routine, emergency response, and patient care or medical related.

Routine Communications

Much of the communication that takes place in the EMS system is routine in nature. This communication occurs over the phone, on the ambulance radio, using portable radios, or by written or electronic means. Routine communication could include EMT–Is advising the dispatch center that they are taking time to eat lunch, are picking up supplies or equipment, or are en route to have vehicle maintenance performed. It may also include messages from the dispatch center to the crew.

Emergency Communications

Emergency communications include all exchanges of information that occur from the beginning until the end of an emergency call.

The steps in the progression of a typical EMS event include the following:
1. Incident occurrence
2. Recognition
3. System access and dispatch
4. Prehospital care
5. Patient stabilization and transport
6. Delivery to the hospital
7. Preparation for the next event

A variety of communication links in the EMS chain are necessary to accomplish these seven steps.

THE CALL FOR HELP

Communication between the person requesting help and the dispatcher typically occurs via the public telephone system, ideally 9-1-1 or some other widely publicized emergency number. In a 9-1-1 system the call for help is received at a public safety answering point (PSAP). Many 9-1-1 systems display the address and phone number of a call's origin. This is referred to as enhanced 9-1-1. If the caller is incoherent or unsure of his or her location, enhanced 9-1-1 is invaluable and potentially lifesaving. Calls for help also may come into the communications center from other emergency agencies, such as police or fire departments, via nonpublic telephone or radio. Public agencies such as school districts, regional transit authorities, or housing authorities may place calls for assistance as well.

✖ **Prearrival Medical Instructions** • The emergency medical dispatcher's instructions to the caller for appropriate emergency measures.

EMERGENCY MEDICAL DISPATCHER

The person with whom the caller comes into initial contact is typically the emergency medical dispatcher

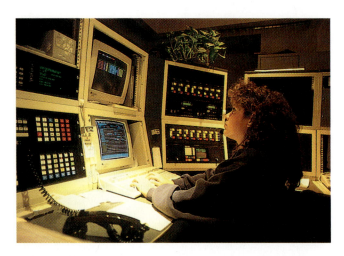

FIGURE 13-5 ▲ An emergency medical dispatcher is a critical part of the EMS chain of communication. (Fox Photography.)

(EMD). The EMD is an essential part of the EMS team and does the following (Figure 13-5):

- Obtains, in a rapid and controlled manner, as much information about the emergency from the caller as possible
- Coordinates the appropriate emergency response to the scene
- Provides **prearrival medical instructions** by telephone for the caller to follow until emergency care arrives
- Monitors and coordinates communications between EMS and other public safety personnel
- Helps to ensure the safety of the providers at the scene (calls for police, fire department, hazardous materials team, or additional EMS units, if needed)
- Assists with the resolution of communication difficulties
- Collects incident data and maintains written records
- Gathers key pieces of information from the caller, including the following:
  - Location (including the address or closest intersection) and nature of the emergency (the ambulance can be dispatched as soon as these are known)
  - Call-back number (in case of accidental telephone disconnection) and name of the caller (if applicable)
  - Specific information that will help in determining the resources needed to handle the case (e.g., seriousness of the emergency, entrapment of victim[s], fire hazards at the scene)

Once this essential information has been gathered, the EMD may find it necessary to provide prearrival telephone medical instructions to the caller. The provision of prearrival instructions may continue throughout the time the ambulance is being dispatched and responding to the scene. This instruction allows for the delivery of emergency care until the first responding unit arrives. This care may be life sustaining in critical incidents. Also, it can provide emotional support for the caller, bystanders, or even the patient. Last, the information regarding the patient's condition obtained during the provision of prearrival instructions can be provided to the responding unit(s), thus allowing them to better prepare.

Next, the EMD must make appropriate decisions regarding which response vehicles to send to a scene. As such, the EMD is responsible for the following:

- Knowing the location of all units
- Knowing the capabilities (basic or advanced life support, specialty equipment, etc.) of the various units
- Determining if any support services are necessary

INITIAL DISPATCH COMMUNICATION

The initial communication between the EMD and the EMT–Is often involves the EMD alerting the EMT–Is of an emergency call and directing them to the scene. This communication may be done through telephone notification, voice or digital radio communication, radio paging, tone alert systems, and/or mobile data terminals. Initial dispatch communication usually includes the address, age, and sex of the patient, as well as the type of emergency to which the EMT–Is are to respond. Next, the EMS team typically recites the call information back to the EMD, confirming that the information has been communicated without error. While the EMS team is en route to the scene, the dispatch center may update them with additional information regarding the scene or patient.

RUN TIMES

From the time the call is received by the unit until the unit is back in quarters, a variety of communications take place. At a minimum, the EMS team calls the dispatch center when the unit is:

- En route to the scene
- At the scene
- En route to the hospital
- Arriving at the hospital
- In service and returning to quarters
- Off the air at quarters

Some systems use mobile data terminals in the ambulance to transmit this information to the dispatch center. Sending the information may be as simple as pushing a button for each event time.

With each communication between the dispatch center and the EMT–Is, the EMD will usually announce the time. For the purpose of clarity, military time (the 24-hour clock) is used.

CALLING ON-SCENE

Next, the EMT–Is call "on-scene," advising the dispatch center of their arrival. Communications that im-

Example of on-scene radio communications:
"Rescue 1532 to dispatch, show us on-scene."
"Dispatch to Rescue 1532, you are on-scene at 1338."
"Rescue 1532 to dispatch, this is a two-car crash with four patients. Two are critically injured; the other two have minor injuries. We need two backup units for transport. We also need police out here for traffic control."
"Dispatch to Rescue 1532, that's affirmative. Rescue 1542 is en route already. We will start another unit right away."
"Dispatch to Rescue 1532, is the fire department on-scene with you?"
"Rescue 1532 to dispatch, that's affirmative; they were here when we arrived."

mediately follow this call may include a scene survey or report from the EMS team of any hazards present. In addition, assistance may be requested on the basis of the number of patients found or the severity of the patient's condition.

MEDICAL COMMUNICATIONS

If the patient's condition warrants it, the next radio communication is between the EMS team and medical direction. The EMS team contacts medical direction for advice or to pass on patient information to the receiving hospital. This communication can be done either at the scene or en route to the hospital.

CALLING EN ROUTE TO THE HOSPITAL, ON ARRIVAL, AND "RETURNING TO SERVICE"

The EMT–Is then call dispatch en route to the hospital and also on arrival at the hospital. Finally, the EMS team advises the dispatcher that they are "returning to service" when leaving the hospital.

If a call is completed without any patient being transported to the hospital, the EMS team advises the dispatcher of the reason (e.g., "The patient refused transport" or "The patient was gone on our arrival."

Medical Communications • Communications between the EMT–I and medical direction or the receiving hospital.

Medical Communications

EMT–Is can bridge the gap between the prehospital setting and the emergency department by communicating findings and treatments provided to the medical direction physician or the receiving hospital. Depending on

local, regional, or state requirements, this communication may be mandated by law or protocol. Most EMS systems have guidelines for when to communicate patient or medical information. These communications may occur via radio, cellular phone, or land line.

PURPOSE OF MEDICAL COMMUNICATIONS

One of the most important purposes of **medical communications** is to obtain orders for patient care in the field. The EMS team can also solicit advice from medical direction when they are uncertain of the course of action to take with a given patient. Medical communications also provide the hospital with information regarding the patient's condition so that the hospital can begin preparing to provide care. Communication with medical direction can also provide help in dealing with obviously ill patients who are refusing care. A medical direction physician may be able to convince the patient of his or her need for treatment and/or hospital care. Medical direction can also resolve uncertainty as to the continuation or termination of resuscitation (e.g., patients with questionable do-not-resuscitate orders) and assist in resolving difficulties with non-EMS physicians who are interfering at the scene. Finally, EMT–Is might find it useful to consult with a physician when patient transport is deemed unnecessary.

CLINICAL NOTES

How well you communicate can make the difference between whether or not you receive an order to administer a particular medication or treatment. Therefore it is essential for you to establish credibility with the medical direction physician. Start by being well organized and concise. Provide information that is pertinent, not everything in the patient's entire medical history. Before starting your radio or phone report, stop for a few seconds and relax; take a few deep breaths if necessary. This is particularly important when dealing with a taxing situation.

Oral Report • A description of the case given by the EMT–I to medical direction or the receiving hospital.

ORAL REPORT

An **oral report** should be given by the EMT–Is when communicating with the medical direction physician or the receiving hospital. The EMT–Is must paint a clear picture of what they find at the scene, remembering that they are the eyes and ears of the physician. A standard format should be employed to permit efficient use of radio time and allow the physician to quickly receive and assimilate information regarding the patient's condition (Figure 13-6). The following are useful elements of the report in the order they are given:

- Identification number and level of training of the provider
- Description of the scene
- Patient's age and sex
- Chief complaint
- Associated signs and symptoms
- Brief, pertinent history of the present illness
- Pertinent past medical history, medications, and allergies
- Physical examination findings, including the following:
  - Level of responsiveness
  - Vital signs
  - General appearance and degree of distress
  - Trauma index or Glasgow Coma Scale (if applicable)
  - Pertinent findings of the physical examination
- Treatment given so far

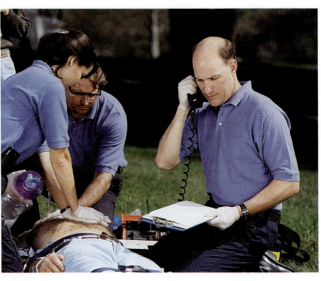

FIGURE 13-6 ▲ A standard list of patient information allows the emergency department to receive and assume care of a patient quickly. (James Silvernail from Sanders MJ: *Mosby's paramedic textbook,* St Louis, 1994, Mosby.)

- Response to treatment
- Advanced life support given on standing orders
- Orders being requested
- Name of the patient's private physician
- Estimated time of arrival at the hospital

When communicating from the field, the EMS team must provide the physician with a complete and accurate report and be prepared to provide additional information when requested.

Treatment Orders • Treatment directives given to the EMT–I by medical direction.

TREATMENT INSTRUCTIONS

Good communication skills are necessary if the patient is to receive appropriate treatment. Any **treatment orders** given by the physician should be repeated back him or her to prevent mistakes. EMT–Is should be prepared to question orders that do not seem appropriate for the patient's condition, that are unclear, or that they are not authorized to perform. Once the orders have been carried out, the patient's response to treatment should be reported back to medical direction. The patient's vital signs should be reported to the medical direction physician with each medication administration. Changes in the patient's condition should also be reported. These changes can be relayed to the hospital directly or through the communication center. The patient's privacy must be protected throughout all medical communications.

NOTIFYING THE RECEIVING HOSPITAL

Hospitals must be notified of patients they will soon receive. This notification is an important element in

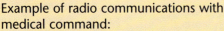

STREET WISE

Example of radio communications with medical command:

"General Hospital, this is Rescue 4, EMT–Intermediate Shade, on-line number 581. We are at the home of a 59-year-old, 80-kg responsive male who is complaining of substernal chest pain that radiates to his neck. He says it started suddenly about half an hour ago while he was watching TV. He took two nitroglycerin tablets without relief.

"He also states he is short of breath and feels nauseated. He has a past history of heart-related problems and takes nitroglycerin, Isordil, and Procardia XL. He is a patient of Dr. Marcus.

"The patient appears in moderate distress at this time. He is clutching his chest, but he is able to talk in full sentences. Vitals are as follows: he is alert and oriented; BP is 162/94; pulse is 108 and irregular; respirations are 18 and slightly labored; skin cool and moist. He has clear bilateral lung sounds, and there is no JVD [jugular venous distention] or peripheral edema. The ECG shows sinus tachycardia with frequent unifocal PVCs [premature ventricular contractions]. Pulse oximetry showed 92% on room air.

"We started him on oxygen at 15 L/min via nonrebreather mask, placed an IV of normal saline, and gave him two baby aspirin and three nitroglycerin tablets without relief. We are requesting permission to administer 1 to 3 mg of morphine sulfate IV. Our ETA to your facility is 15 minutes."

the overall provision of care. If the emergency department knows of the patient's problem before his or her arrival at the hospital, they can mobilize resources, determine bed availability, and prepare teams within the hospital to deal with the patient's condition.

COMMUNICATIONS BASICS

Echo • To immediately repeat back each radio transmission received.

Proper radio use results in efficient and effective communications. However, there is more to proper radio use than picking up the microphone and speaking. Transmissions must be clear, and content must be concise and professional (Figure 13-7). The following rules apply to using the radio:

* Before beginning to talk, always listen to the frequency to be sure no one is transmitting.
* Press the transmission button on the microphone, and wait 1 second before speaking.
* Keep the microphone approximately 2 to 3 inches from the mouth.
* Speak slowly and clearly, pronouncing each word distinctly.
* Speak in a normal pitch, keeping your voice free of emotion.
* Keep the transmission brief. If longer transmissions are needed, pause for a few seconds after every 30 seconds or so to allow other units to transmit information if needed.
* Give the name of the unit or number from which the call is originating. Next, address the unit being called (e.g., "Dispatch center to Unit 5.").
* The unit being called should signal that they are ready to receive the communication by saying, "Go ahead." A response of, "Stand by," indicates that the unit is not ready to receive the communication.
* Always get confirmation that the message was received.
* Use proper unit numbers, hospital numbers, names, and titles.
* Do not use slang or profanity over the air.
* Avoid using codes and abbreviations unless they are part of your system and everyone understands them.
* When transmitting a number that might be confused, give the number and then the individual digits.
* Receive the full message from the sender. Do not attempt to cut that person off so that you can speak.
* Do not use a person's name or divulge confidential information that is not essential to the radio report.
* Because EMT–Is rarely act alone, use "we" instead of "I."
* Avoid words that are difficult to hear, like "yes" or "no." Use "affirmative" and "negative."
* Use a standard format for transmitting information.
* Use EMS frequencies only for EMS communications.

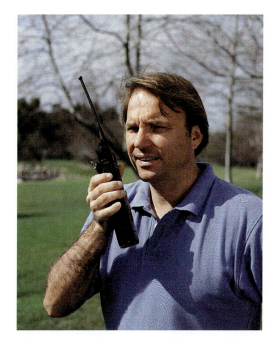

FIGURE 13-7 ▲ Clear and concise messages given over the radio allow for better communication and patient care.

* Before transmitting, reduce the background noise as much as possible by closing the window or turning the volume down on other radios.
* When the medical direction physician gives treatment orders, **echo** them to the physician.
* Hold portable radios in an upright (vertical) position to achieve maximum radio coverage.

☆TUDENT ALERT

To get the best reception with portable radios, keep the radio in a vertical, upright position.

It is important to understand that the airwaves are public and that scanners are popular. More than just the EMS community can overhear EMS communications, and inappropriate language is subject to fines and penalties by the FCC. In addition, unprofessional communication creates a bad public image. It can lead to a loss of credibility with colleagues in prehospital and hospital settings and in one's own agency.

SYSTEM MAINTENANCE

Communication equipment is costly and breakable. Dropping it, submerging it in water, or exposing it to harsh environments can cause damage. In addition, beverages spilled onto radio equipment surfaces can harm the internal parts. Careful handling is essential.

Radios must be checked on an ongoing basis to ensure that they are working properly. Only qualified individuals should repair malfunctioning radio equipment.

Portable radio batteries should be recharged according to the manufacturer's instructions. Spare batteries should always be available. Regular cleaning of radio equipment will improve its physical appearance. Exterior surfaces should be wiped with a moist cloth and mild detergent. Harsh cleaning agents should be avoided.

COMMUNICATIONS WITH THE PUBLIC

The EMS system continually interacts with the general public, which is responsible for funding the system. Public relations programs and the news media help make the public aware of the resources that the EMS system offers and helps teach the public about how and when to use the EMS system. Blood pressure screenings, demonstrations, open houses, extrication/disaster drills, short news spots, and programs on the dangers of drinking and driving all contribute to public awareness of the EMS system.

The news media also is valuable when vital information must be distributed quickly and/or to large communities. Evacuations due to weather or other disasters fall into this category.

Perhaps the least costly and most effective communication program is everyday contact with patients, family, and bystanders. Each run has the potential for wide public interaction, and serious events draw media coverage. Media involvement should be positive and productive; far-reaching damage can be inflicted to systems that disregard or antagonize these communications specialists.

Dealing With the Press (Media)

EMS systems and their personnel are being increasingly thrust into positions of interaction with the news media (Figure 13-8). These interactions can either boost public confidence or cause widespread public mistrust. In all situations, however, the patient comes first, and care cannot be delayed in favor of talking to a reporter.

Many EMS systems designate a public information officer (PIO) to design and implement public information programs and to respond to questions from the media. However, even when there is a PIO in the service, news reporters often want to get as close to the story as possible. This means they may request interviews with the EMT–Is who were on the scene or who directly experienced the topic of their story. As such, you may be called on to represent your service in a television, radio, or newspaper interview. Be sure to obtain permission from your agency before participating in an interview, because some EMS systems may prohibit such activities or require prior permission.

When giving an interview, remember the following:
- Relax and be yourself. Make your EMS system appear human.
- Know your system's policy on what kind of information can be released to the media.

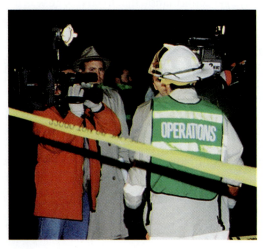

FIGURE 13-8 ▲ The news media are often found at large-scale emergency scenes. Be prepared to interact accurately and professionally.

- Use simple terms and explain information in a way that a layperson can understand. Most people will not understand work-related jargon, even though the reporter may.
- Brief yourself by reviewing the appropriate material beforehand (EMS run report, reference materials, etc.)
- Know what information is a matter of public record.
- Maintain patient confidentiality at all times.
- Speak clearly, and be brief. Answer questions directly. Do not beat around the bush. Do not give more information than you are asked for.
- Give only the facts. If you do not have an answer to a question, do not speculate or guess.
- Take a few seconds to think of the appropriate response to questions you are asked. If you are uncertain about a question, ask for clarification.
- After you answer a question, some reporters will say nothing, hoping you will feel compelled to say more. Do not volunteer information. Instead, ask for the next question.
- If a reporter says, "Would you say…," and then adds a quote for you to agree to, do not agree. Always make your own statement.
- Do not be fooled when reporters close their notebooks and say, "I know the official position, but just between us, how do you feel about it?" Nine times out of 10, they will use the quote.
- Do not respond to "what if" questions. When you guess, what you say could return to haunt you.
- Some reporters will ask you two questions at once. Answer the first question and then ask the reporter to repeat the second question.
- Always anticipate other issues for which the reporter may be looking for answers. If you are unprepared for the question, take a few seconds to think of the appropriate answer. Do not be afraid to say, "I don't know" or "I don't have any comment on that issue."

Although the EMS team's top priorities are safety and patient care, news reporters may not recognize the importance of these two duties. If a reporter is hampering your ability to provide care, suggest first that the reporter speak to someone else and then request that the reporter allow you to attend to the tasks at hand. If, after reasonable requests for cooperation, the reporter persists, get assistance from the local police. However, be certain that patient care, not your pride, is being compromised before soliciting police intervention.

Although EMS personnel cannot expect the news media to be a cheerleader for them, they can expect to be treated fairly (especially if a good relationship already exists). To establish a positive working relationship with local media, try being responsive to their needs and honest when responding to inquiries.

COMMUNICATIONS IN DISASTER SITUATIONS

Any number of problems can hinder communications during a disaster, including the following:
- Overloaded radio frequencies
- Incompatible frequencies between agencies
- Damage to the communications infrastructure
- General equipment failure

In disaster situations the EMS communications system is a key component of a meaningful and organized response (Figure 13-9). EMS services must cooperate with other agencies in establishing guidelines for radio use in mass casualty or disaster events. A disaster plan should be in place to allow communications with other agencies and hospitals, as well as emergency response and coordinating personnel. The plan must anticipate and provide for the breakdown of any component of the communications system and specify alternate means of communication. For example, during a disaster, telephone lines might not be available or may be overloaded. Guidelines must be in place for overriding the existing communications system components and restricting nonessential communications. Emergency radios should be available in the event of land line failure, and alternate radio frequencies must be designated in case the usual channels become overloaded. It is important that all responders use a common language so that all "players" can understand each other. Codes that some responders may not understand should be avoided.

In disasters and multiple-casualty incidents (MCIs) an incident command system (ICS) should be put in place as soon as possible. The ICS is a management sys-

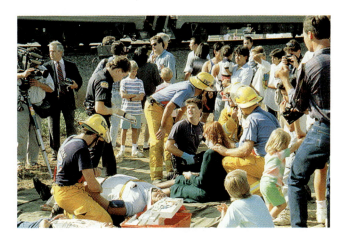

FIGURE 13-9 ▲ Communication at disaster scenes can be chaotic. (Colin C. Williams, photographer.)

tem designed to control, direct, and coordinate emergency response operations and resources.

In MCIs it is crucial that patients be dispersed to various hospitals without overloading a single emergency department. Tracking patients from the scene of the event to the destination is important. This requires a predetermined format designed to provide information on the status of victims treated in the field by EMS personnel or in designated first-aid areas. EMS personnel should design and test disaster communication procedures well in advance so that resources can be coordinated reliably under stress.

CASE HISTORY FOLLOW-UP ▪▪▪

According to the attorney, EMT–I Walters' previous partner has a different memory of the event. In fact, he remembers applying a Kendrick extrication device and removing the patient from the wrecked car. He has no recollection of the patient's paralysis. Lucky for EMT–I Walters, his partner, the EMS service, and the hospital, the patient's contention that his paralysis resulted from inappropriate handling at the scene and at the emergency department can be dispelled because of Walters' excellent documentation.

EMS communications provide for an orderly and safe emergency response, allow for state-of-the-art prehospital patient care, and may sometimes help to protect the EMT–I and other members of the health care team from litigation. Had it not been for the clear and concise radio report taped by the hospital and the carefully documented prehospital care report, this case scenario may have had a much different outcome.

SUMMARY

Important points from this chapter include the following:

- A working knowledge of EMS communications is important for all prehospital care providers.
- Access to the system begins with the citizen making the call and does not end until the patient is delivered to the hospital and the run report is completed. Effective and concise communication is required among all involved parties for the system to work.
- Modern EMS communications systems have specific equipment needs. The typical configuration includes telephones, radios, repeater systems, and recording equipment. The most powerful radio in the system is the base station, with a typical power output of 80 to 150 watts.
- The ambulance is equipped with mobile two-way radios and/or cellular phones to allow communication between the EMS team and the base station, the EMS team and other responding or on-scene units, the EMS team and the receiving hospitals or facility(ies) providing medical direction, and the EMS team and other public agencies (police and fire departments).

- Portable radios are hand-held devices with a typical power output of 1 to 5 watts. Portable radios allow communications to take place while EMT–Is are away from the ambulance.
- Poor output is sometimes a problem with mobile and portable radios. Repeater systems may be used to increase the range of these devices. Repeater systems are devices that receive transmissions from relatively low-wattage transmitters on one frequency and retransmit them at a higher power on another frequency. This increases the range of the transmissions.
- The Federal Communications Commission (FCC) is the federal agency that controls and regulates all radio communications in the United States. EMS communications can be broken down into three types: routine, emergency response, and patient care or medical related.
- Skill and knowledge on the part of all parties (EMT–Is, emergency medical dispatchers) are required to communicate well on the radio. Transmissions must be clear, and the content must be concise and professional.

14 Documentation

...CASE HISTORY

EMT–I Johnson reports to work at 7:00 AM on Monday, ready for a typical EMS week of shootings, stabbings, and heart attacks. His supervisor hands him a subpoena to appear for a deposition the coming Wednesday morning and a manila envelope with a prehospital report from the call.

EMT–I Johnson opens the envelope and begins to study the report. The call occurred just 2 weeks after he received his EMT–Intermediate certification. The report states that the call occurred on November 5, at 2035, at 425 Miami Lane. The patient was Natalie Browning, age 23 years. EMT–I Johnson wrote that her chief complaint was SOB and that she was combative and intoxicated on alcohol. He recorded that he had to restrain her with hard restraints and that her behavior was obnoxious.

LEARNING OBJECTIVES

CHAPTER GOAL

Upon completion of this chapter, the EMT-Intermediate will be able to apply the necessary knowledge and skills to properly document various types of EMS events.

Cognitive Objectives

As an EMT-Intermediate you should be able to do the following:

- Identify the general principles regarding the importance of EMS documentation and ways in which documents are used.

- Explain the role of documentation in agency reimbursement.

- Apply the principles of documentation to computer charting as access to this technology becomes available.

- Evaluate a finished document for errors and omissions.

- Identify and use medical terminology correctly.

- Recite appropriate and accurate medical abbreviations and acronyms.

- Evaluate a finished document for proper use and spelling of abbreviations and acronyms.

- Identify and eliminate extraneous or nonprofessional information.

- Analyze the documentation for accuracy and completeness, including spelling.

- Record pertinent information using a consistent narrative format.
- Describe the differences between subjective and objective elements of documentation.
- Identify and record the pertinent, reportable clinical data of each patient interaction.
- Explain how to properly record direct patient or bystander comments.
- Note and record "pertinent negative" clinical findings.
- Record all pertinent administrative information.
- Correct errors and omissions using proper procedures as defined under local protocols.
- Revise documents, when necessary, using locally approved procedures.
- Describe the potential consequences of illegible, incomplete, or inaccurate documentation.
- Evaluate the confidential nature of an EMS report.
- Describe the special considerations concerning patient refusal of transport.
- Describe the special considerations concerning mass casualty incident documentation.
- Assume responsibility for self-assessment of all documentation.

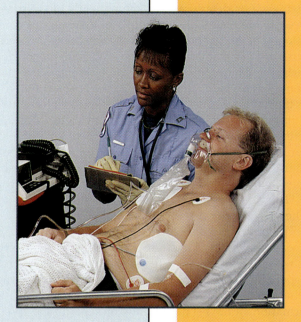

Affective Objectives
As an EMT-Intermediate you should be able to do the following:
- Advocate among peers the relevance and importance of properly completed documentation.
- Resolve the common negative attitudes toward the task of documentation.

Psychomotor Objectives
- None identified for this chapter.

INTRODUCTION

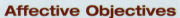 **Documentation** • The process of recording patient information.

Each prehospital care provider has an obligation and a responsibility to accurately document each emergency response. Proper **documentation** should describe the following:
- A record of the scene
- The patient's chief complaint
- The patient's condition
- The nature and extent of emergency care given
- Changes in the patient's condition

In addition, documentation should include patient information (such as the patient's name, address, age, and sex), as well as administrative information (such as the disposition of the call).

Reasons for Patient Care Documentation

The EMS run report facilitates the continuation of care from the prehospital setting to the hospital setting by supplying vital information to the emergency department staff.

It can point out improvement ("the patient became alert and oriented following the administration of 50% dextrose") or deterioration ("the patient's blood pressure dropped to 80/60 en route") in the patient's condition. The run report lists treatments administered, thus avoiding duplication of care in the emergency department. The report contains some information that would otherwise be unavailable to the hospital staff after the EMT–Intermediate (EMT–I) leaves, such as a description of the damage to an accident victim's car. A bent steering wheel or spider-webbed windshield can alert the hospital staff to look for injuries that might otherwise go unnoticed. As a link to subsequent care, documentation is an effective way for EMT–Is to represent themselves as professionals to other health care professionals.

The run report also serves as a legal record of each case. It may be used in court proceedings for a variety of reasons, including civil actions or criminal cases. Depending on the time that has passed since care was provided, the run report may be the sole source of information an EMT–I has to draw on regarding a given case. Trying to remember what happened several years previously could be challenging even for the best EMT–I.

Medical direction performs quality improvement audits to monitor a system's compliance with standing orders. Medical audits can be conducted through run review conferences or other educational forums. The EMS run report serves as an excellent source of information as to the care provided in the prehospital setting. EMT–Is practice, at least with regard to invasive procedures, under the auspices of a licensed physician. Documentation provides a record of these procedures, not only for the EMT–I, but also for the medical director and the EMS system as a whole. Proper documentation demonstrates that the EMT–I is adhering to appropriate protocols and that the care he or she is providing is in compliance with the law and meets the standard of care. It also provides a tally of the number of times the EMT–I performs various patient care procedures. When it is found that an EMT–I lacks sufficient skill repetition or is not able to perform the skills with sufficient success, additional skill practice can be provided in the laboratory or clinical setting.

System Need for EMS Documentation

The EMS run report is a key source for data collection. The data gleaned from run reports guide system improvements, training programs, revenue collection, and research. The billing and administrative data that are gathered can ensure the economic survival of an EMS agency. Operational statistics, such as the times calls were received, the distances traveled, and the times ambulances arrived on the scene, properly correlated with geographical and definitive care considerations, can help determine the most appropriate locations for stationing ambulances and other equipment. Properly written run reports can also be used as training tools by illustrating how to keep good records or how to handle unusual or uncommon cases. Run reports can also serve as an important source of data for research purposes.

Permanent Record

Once in the hospital, the run report usually becomes a permanent part of the patient's medical record. The length of time the medical record (including the run report) is kept by the hospital depends on statutes of limitations, accreditation, licensure, and other regulatory requirements. These requirements vary from state to state. Run reports concerning minors must be kept until the minor reaches legal age, plus any additional period of time as defined by statute or other requirements. Fear of lawsuits also influences the length of time a run report is kept. In some cases, lawsuits are filed years after the situation occurs.

EMT–Is may be called on to explain the content of a run report in a deposition or in a courtroom, even if the case does not involve them directly. Although many of today's lawsuits involve personal injury or product liability, the majority of cases against EMT–Is relate to improper care. In addition, the run report may be used as part of a criminal investigation. An EMT–I may have seen and recorded something that can reveal a person's innocence or guilt. In any circumstance, for all those involved, the best protection is a thorough and accurate run report.

TYPES OF RUN REPORTS

Present Types

There are many types of run reports in use today (Figure 14-1). The run report may be referred to as the prehospital care report, ambulance call report, EMS sheet, trip ticket, trip sheet, or any number of other names. The more traditional written form includes check boxes and sections for narrative. Some forms have an anatomical figure for labeling patient injuries or physical assessment findings. Scannable run reports, now used in many states, list treatments, assessment findings, past medical conditions, and so forth. A scannable run report is filled out by darkening circles or boxes (also called bubbles) to show which items apply to each case. Most scannable run reports also have a narrative section where the specifics of each case can be elaborated on.

A run report form usually consists of an original and two or three copies. At least one copy is left at the emergency department; the other copy and the original are used for EMS billing, quality assurance, or record-keeping purposes. Many systems use noncarbon reproduction (NCR) paper to keep expenses down and for its ease of use.

Although run reports may be different in design and length, the basic data are generally the same. The con-

> **HELPFUL HINT**
>
> For legal purposes, the original copy of the run report usually is kept by the EMS system. A copy is then provided to the hospital.

Illinois • Emergency Medical Services NARRATIVE

SERVICE NAME	SERVICE #	TODAY'S DATE
INCIDENT LOCATION	HOSPITAL DESTINATION	
PATIENT INFO: PATIENT LAST NAME / FIRST / M.I.	HOME PHONE # / AGE	DATE OF BIRTH
STREET ADDRESS		
CITY / STATE / ZIP CODE	LEGAL GUARDIAN	
ALLEGIES (MEDS)	○ NONE KNOWN	
CURRENT MEDICATIONS	○ NONE KNOWN	○ BROUGHT W/PT.
CHIEF COMPLAINT		
NARRATIVE		

NARRATIVE 1 OF ______

TIME	P	R	B/P	TEMP	BS	RHYTHM	TREATMENT	DOSE	ROUTE	02 SAT.	COMMENTS

LEFT	LUNG SOUNDS	RIGHT
T L	CLEAR	T L
T L	RHONCHI	T L
T L	RALES	T L
T L	WHEEZES	T L
T L	DIMINISHED	T L
T L	ABSENT	T L

SKIN TEMP (Initial / Last)	SKIN MOISTURE (Initial / Last)	SKIN COLOR (Initial / Last)	ABDOMEN (Initial / Last)
☐ NORMAL ☐	☐ NORMAL ☐	☐ NORMAL ☐	☐ NORMAL ☐
☐ COOL ☐	☐ MOIST ☐	☐ PALE ☐	☐ SOFT ☐
☐ COLD ☐	☐ DRY ☐	☐ CYANOTIC ☐	☐ RIGID ☐
☐ HOT ☐	☐ WET ☐	☐ FLUSHED ☐	☐ DISTENDED ☐
☐ WARM ☐		☐ JAUNDICED ☐	☐ TENDER ☐
		☐ MOTTLED ☐	
		☐ ASHENED ☐	

SIGNATURE OF PERSON RECEIVING PATIENT

X ______________________

514313

CREW SIGNATURES DRIVER COMPLETED REPORT

CREW MEMBER 1 ______________ D R

CREW MEMBER 2 ______________ D R

CREW MEMBER 3 ______________ D R

CREW MEMBER 4 ______________ D R

(Signatures should correspond with license numbers on back of data sheet.)

Service/Provider Copy

FIGURE 14-1 ▲ Many different types of run reports are used in EMS. (Courtesy EMS Data Systems, Inc., Phoenix; from Stoy W: *Mosby's EMT–Basic textbook,* St Louis, 1996, Mosby.)

Continued

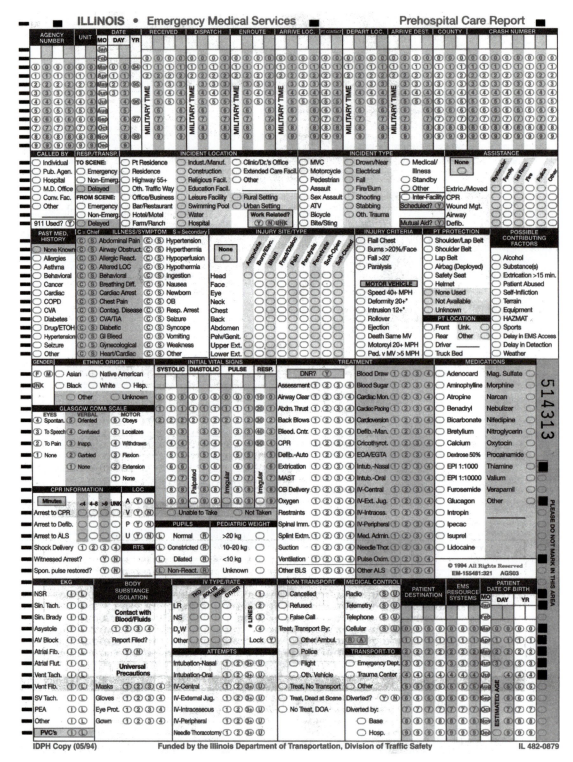

FIGURE 14-1, cont'd ▲ Many different types of run reports are used in EMS. (Courtesy EMS Data Systems, Inc., Phoenix; from Stoy W: *Mosby's EMT–Basic textbook,* St Louis, 1996, Mosby.)

tent of the run report includes both administrative and clinical data.

The Future

New technology has given us hand-held data entry and pen-based computers. These can be thought of as "elec-

tronic clipboards." Pen-based units automate much of the data entry by allowing the use of a touch screen to make selections from assessment and treatment lists. This expedites data entry. Some pen-based units allow wireless transfer of patient information to the hospital before the patient even arrives. Another benefit is that the transfer of the data from the field to administrative

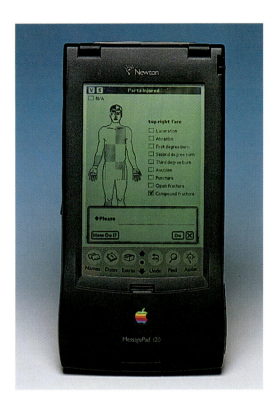

FIGURE 14-2 ▲ Computer-based reporting systems allow EMT–Is to transfer patient information to the receiving facility using wireless technology.

entities becomes significantly faster than when using paper-based systems. This allows the data to be analyzed and quality improvement activities performed much more quickly and efficiently. Although the technology is more advanced, the principles learned in this chapter can be easily applied to computer charting (Figure 14-2).

RULES FOR DOCUMENTING

Be Accurate

Document what actually occurred. Be precise and comprehensive. All check box sections of a document must show that they have been attended to. Blank boxes or lines render a report incomplete; they should be appropriately marked or contain an explanation as to why they are not marked. Sections that do not apply to a given patient or situation can be completed by writing "NA" across the entire box. Avoid simply drawing a line through a box; it may be misconstrued later as a stray mark.

Be Objective

When documenting any aspect of the emergency case, be objective and accurately describe what is seen. Be careful to avoid making assumptions about what has taken place.

Be Specific

Generalizations, such as "The patient was uncooperative," should be avoided. How was the patient uncooperative? Did the patient refuse care? Was he or she abusive toward you or your partner(s)? Describe the patient's behavior as specifically as possible; for example, "Patient refused to be carried, insisting on walking to the ambulance." Special attention should be given to calls involving domestic violence, suspected abuse, or other situations that must be reported to law enforcement agencies.

Write Legibly

An illegible run report breaks down the continuity of patient care; if physicians and nurses cannot glean important information from it, it is of no value. Write legibly, clearly, and concisely. Printed writing is often more readable than cursive writing. An important consideration is to avoid being placed in the embarrassing situation of being seated in a courtroom responding to questions from a plaintiff's attorney and being faced with documentation that is illegible. When marking check boxes, be clear and consistent from the top page of the document to all underlying pages.

Use A Ballpoint Pen

To make the record permanent, the run report should be filled out using a ball-point pen. This makes it difficult to tamper with or erase information on the run report and results in the second and third copies of the report being more legible.

> ### HELPFUL HINT
> - Felt-tip pens are impractical for use in the pre-hospital care setting. They do not press through NCR-type reports and tend to look sloppy, particularly if they get wet from rain or snow.

Use Correct Spelling

The first impression that hospital staff and other personnel have of EMT–Is is through their run reports. Be familiar with the meaning of common medical terms, along with their spelling. Misspelled words (especially medical words) reflect poorly on one's professionalism. If you do not know how to spell a word, find out, or use another word. It may be helpful to carry a small dictionary or stow one in the ambulance.

Acronym • A word that is formed by combining the first letter or letters of each word in a name or a phrase. Example: SOAP for *S*ubjective, *O*bjective, *A*ssessment, *P*lan.

Use Abbreviations and Acronyms With Care

Use of medical abbreviations and **acronyms** can increase the amount of information that can be included on the run report and can allow information to be written down more quickly. However, because abbreviations can have multiple meanings, only use those that are approved by your EMS system. Many EMS systems maintain a list of acceptable medical abbreviations and acronyms that can be used as part of the documentation (Table 14-1).

Avoid Soiling the Report With Blood, Body Fluids, or Other Liquids

In addition to looking bad, a soiled run report poses some health risks to the people who handle it. Take appropriate measures to prevent the run report from being contaminated with blood, body fluids, or other liquids. Avoid filling out the run report while still wearing gloves that were used to treat the patient. Also, do not place the run report close to where patient care is occurring.

TABLE 14-1

Common Abbreviations

NOTE: ABBREVIATIONS IN COMMON USE CAN VARY WIDELY FROM PLACE TO PLACE. EACH INSTITUTION'S LIST OF ACCEPTABLE ABBREVIATIONS IS THE BEST AUTHORITY FOR ITS RECORDS.

Abbr	Meaning	Abbr	Meaning
°C	degrees Centigrade	BMR	basal metabolic rate
°F	degrees Fahrenheit	BP	blood pressure
µg	microgram	BPH	benign prostatic hypertrophy
µm	micrometer	BRP	bathroom privileges
ʒ	dram	BSA	body surface area
@	at	BUN	blood urea nitrogen
aa	of each	c̄	with
ABG	arterial blood gas	c/o	complains of
ac	before meals	Ca	calcium, cancer, carcinoma
ad lib	freely as desired	CAD	coronary artery disease
ADL	activities of daily living	cap	capsule
Ag	silver, antigen	CAT	computed axial tomography
AIDS	acquired immunodeficiency syndrome	cath.	catheter, catheterize
ALS	amyotrophic lateral sclerosis	CBC	complete blood count
AM	morning	CBR	complete bed rest
a.m.a.	against medical advice	CC	chief complaint
AMI	acute myocardial infarction	cc	cubic centimeter
amp	ampule	CCU	coronary care unit, critical care unit
ARC	AIDS-related complex	CDC	Centers for Disease Control and Prevention
ARDS	adult respiratory distress syndrome	CFT	complement-fixation test
AS	aortic stenosis	cg	centigram
ASD	atrial septal defect	CHF	congestive heart failure
Ba	barium	CHO	carbohydrate
BE	barium enema	Cl	chlorine
bid	two times a day	cm	centimeter
BM, bm	bowel movement		

From Potter PA, Perry AG: *Fundamentals of nursing: concepts, process, and practice,* ed 4, St Louis, 1997, Mosby.

TABLE 14-1

Common Abbreviations—cont'd

NOTE: ABBREVIATIONS IN COMMON USE CAN VARY WIDELY FROM PLACE TO PLACE. EACH INSTITUTION'S LIST OF ACCEPTABLE ABBREVIATIONS IS THE BEST AUTHORITY FOR ITS RECORDS.

cm^3	cubic centimeter	grav I, II, III, etc	pregnancy one, two, three, etc.
CNS	central nervous system		
CO	carbon monoxide	gt, gtt	drop, drops
CO_2	carbon dioxide	GTT	glucose tolerance test
COPD	chronic obstructive pulmonary disease	GU	genitourinary
CPK	creatine phosphokinase	GYN,	
CPR	cardiopulmonary resuscitation	Gyn	gynecological
CSF	cerebrospinal fluid	H_2O	water
CT	computed tomography	h	hour
CVA	cerebrovascular accident, costovertebral angle	H^+	hydrogen ion
		h/o	history of
CVP	central venous pressure	H&P	history and physical examination
D&C	dilatation and curettage	HAV	hepatitis A virus
D5W	5% dextrose in water	Hb	hemoglobin
db, dB	decibels	HBAg	hepatitis B antigen
dc	discontinue	HBV	hepatitis B virus
DIC	disseminated intravascular coagulation	Hct, HCT	hematocrit
diff	differential blood count	Hg	mercury
dil	dilute	Hgb	hemoglobin
DJD	degenerative joint disease	HIV	human immunodeficiency (AIDS) virus
dl, dL	deciliter	hs	at bedtime
DM	diastolic murmur	HSV	herpes simplex virus
DNR	do not resuscitate	I&O	intake and output
DOE	dyspnea on exertion	IC	inspiratory capacity
dx, DX	diagnosis	ICP	intracranial pressure
EBV	Epstein-Barr virus	ICU	intensive care unit
ECF	extracellular fluid	IDDM	insulin-dependent diabetes mellitus
ECG	electrocardiogram	IE	immunoelectrophoresis
ECT	electroconvulsive therapy	Ig	immunoglobulin
EDC	estimated date of confinement	IgA, etc	immunoglobulin A, etc.
EDD	estimated date of delivery	IM	intramuscular
EEG	electroencephalogram	IOP	intraocular pressure
EKG	electrocardiogram	IPPB	intermittent positive pressure breathing
elix	elixir	IV	intravenous
EMG	electromyogram	IVP	intravenous push; intravenous pyelogram
ENG	electronystagmography	IVU	intravenous urogram
ER	emergency room	JRA	juvenile rheumatoid arthritis
ERG	electroretinogram	K	potassium
ESR	erythrocyte sedimentation rate	kg	kilogram
ESRD	end-stage renal disease	KUB	kidney, ureters, and bladder (radiograph)
EST	electroshock therapy	KVO	keep vein open
F℥	fluid ounce	L	liter
FANA	fluorescent antinuclear antibody test	L&A	light and accommodation
Fe	iron	LBBB	left bundle branch block
FEV	forced expiratory volume	LE	lupus erythematosus
FHR	fetal heart rate	LGV	lymphogranuloma venereum
FRC	functional residual capacity	LLL	left lower lobe
FUO	fever of unknown origin	LLQ	left lower quadrant
Fx, fx	fracture, fractional urine test	LMP	last menstraul period
g, gm, Gm	gram	LNMP	last normal menstrual period
		LP	lumbar puncture
Gc, GC	gonococcus	LUL	left upper lobe
GI	gastrointestinal	LUQ	left upper quadrant
gr	grain	LVH	left ventricular hypertrophy

Continued

TABLE 14-1

Common Abbreviations—cont'd

NOTE: **ABBREVIATIONS IN COMMON USE CAN VARY WIDELY FROM PLACE TO PLACE. EACH INSTITUTION'S LIST OF ACCEPTABLE ABBREVIATIONS IS THE BEST AUTHORITY FOR ITS RECORDS.**

m	meter	PEG	pneumoencephalography
m, min, ♏	minim	per	through, by way of
MAP	mean arterial pressure	PERRLA	pupils equal, round, and reactive to light and accommodation
mcg	microgram	PET	positron emission tomography
MCH	mean corpuscular hemoglobin	PG	prostaglandin
MCHC	mean corpusuclar hemoglobin concentration	pH	hydrogen ion concentration (acidity and alkalinity)
MCV	mean cell volume, mean corpuscular volume	PID	pelvic inflammatory disease
		PKU	phenylketonuria
mg	milligram	PM	postmortem
Mg	magnesium	PM	evening
MG	myasthenia gravis	PMS	premenstrual syndrome
MI	myocardial infarction	PND	paroxysmal nocturnal dyspnea, post-nasal drip
MICU	medical intensive care unit		
mL	milliliter	Po_2	partial pressure of oxygen
mm	millimeter	PO, po	orally
mm^3	cubic millimeter	PPD	purified protein derivative
mm Hg	millimeters of mercury	ppm	parts per million
MRI	magnetic resonance imaging	p.r.n.	when required, as often as necessary
MS	multiple sclerosis	PT	physical therapy; prothrombin time
MW	molecular weight	PTT	partial thromboplastin time
N	nitrogen	PUO	pyrexia of unkown origin
Na	sodium	PVC	premature ventricular contraction
NICU	neonatal intensive care unit	q	every
NIH	National Institutes of Health	q2h	every 2 hours
nm	nanometer	q3h	every 3 hours
NMR	nuclear magentic resonance	q4h	every 4 hours
NPO	nothing by mouth	qd	every day
NS	normal saline	qh	every hour
O_2	oxygen	qid	four times a day
OD	right eye; optical density; overdose	qn	every night
OL	left eye	qod	every other day
OOB	out of bed	qns	quantity not sufficient
ORIF	open reduction and internal fixation	R/O	rule out
OS	left eye	RA	rheumatoid arthritis
OT	occupational therapy	RBBB	right bundle branch block
OTC	over-the-counter	RDA	recommended daily (dietary) allowance
oz, ℥	ounce	RDS	respiratory distress syndrome
P&A	percussion and ausculation	Rh+	positive Rh factor
$Paco_2$	partial pressure of carbon dioxide (arterial blood)	Rh−	negative Rh factor
		RHD	rheumatic heart disease
Pao_2	partial pressure of oxygen (arterial blood)	RLL	right lower lobe
para I, II, etc	unipara, bipara, etc.	RLQ	right lower quadrant
		RML	right middle lobe
PAT	paroxysmal atrial tachycardia	ROM	range of motion
pc	after meals	ROS	review of systems
PCG	phonocardiogram	RS	Reiter's syndrome
Pco_2	partial pressure of carbon dioxide	RSV	Rous sarcoma virus
PCP	pulmonary capillary pressure, phencyclidine	RUL	right upper lobe
PCV	packed cell volume	RUQ	right upper quadrant
PCWP	pulmonary capillary wedge pressure	Rx	take; treatment
PD	interpupillary distance; postural drainage	s̄	without
PE	pulmonary embolism, physical examination	SB	sternal border
PEEP	positive end expiratory pressure	SC	subcutaneous

From Potter PA, Perry AG: *Fundamentals of nursing: concepts, process, and practice,* ed 4, St Louis, 1997, Mosby.

TABLE 14-1

Common Abbreviations—cont'd

NOTE: ABBREVIATIONS IN COMMON USE CAN VARY WIDELY FROM PLACE TO PLACE. EACH INSTITUTION'S LIST OF ACCEPTABLE ABBREVIATIONS IS THE BEST AUTHORITY FOR ITS RECORDS.

sib.	sibling	TIA	transient ischemic attack
SICU	surgical intensive care unit	TIBC	total iron-binding capacity
SIDS	sudden infant death syndrome	tid	three times a day
Sig	write on label	TKO	to keep open
SLE	systemic lupus erythematosus	TLC	total lung capacity; thin layer chromatography
sol	solution, dissolved		
sos	if necessary	TPN	total parenteral nutrition
sp. gr., SG, sg	specific gravity	TPR	temperature, pulse, and respirations
		tr, tinct	tincture
SQ, subq	subcutaneous	TST	triple sugar iron test
SR	sedimentation rate	UIBC	unsaturated iron-binding capacity
ss	half	URI	upper respiratory infection
SSS	sick sinus syndrome, specific soluble substance, short-stay surgery	UTI	urinary tract infection
		V&T	volume and tension
STAT	immediately	VC	vital capacity
STD	sexually transmitted disease	VD	venereal disease
STS	serologic test for syphilis	VDA	visual discriminatory acuity
susp	suspension	VDH	valvular disease of the heart
T_3	triiodothyronine	VDRL	Venereal Disease Research Laboratory (test for syphilis)
T_4	tetraiodothyronine		
T&A	tonsillectomy and adenoidectomy	VS	vital signs
TAB	typhoid and paratyphoid A and B	VSD	ventricular septal defect
TAH	total abdominal hysterectomy	V_T	tidal volume
TAT	tetanus antitoxin; thematic apperception test	W/V	weight/volume
		WBC	white blood cell, white blood count
TB, TBC	tuberculosis	WNL	within normal limits
TBG	thyroxin-binding globulin	WR	Wasserman reaction
TG	triglyceride		

Coffee, rain, and other liquids also can render a run report illegible. Again, take precautionary measures to prevent the report from getting wet. Many run report clipboards have a storage compartment that keeps completed forms dry and protected.

Promptly Record Information

Fill out the run report as soon as possible. The longer you wait before writing down the patient care information, the less likely you are to remember it, especially when responding to one call right after another. However, do not delay or compromise patient care in order to fill out the run report.

STREET WISE

Sometimes you can write down essential information, such as vital signs, on a piece of tape or other medium for later transcription.

❗ HELPFUL HINT

• When you have only a precious few minutes to get the patient to the ambulance, or when you must provide ongoing care (e.g., in situations such as shootings or cardiac arrest), wait to fill out the run report until after you arrive at the hospital.

Once you are at the hospital, you should complete the run report and leave copies with the emergency department staff.

Be Consistent

The run report must be consistent and accurate. If the patient's left arm is injured, take care to avoid citing the right arm as the location of injury elsewhere in the report.

Be Professional

Professional documentation is an obligation of the prehospital care provider. Remember that the run report can be subject to scrutiny by a variety of individuals, including hospital personnel, quality assurance personnel, supervisors, the court system, and the news media. Also, the patient or patient's family may request a copy of the run report. For these reasons, avoid making entries on the run report using jargon, street slang, bias, libel/slander, irrelevant opinions or impressions, or flippant or derogatory remarks, such as the patient is "faking it," or is "a drunk." These types of remarks can come back to haunt an EMT–I and his or her service. Likewise, complaints about being overworked, a lack of police protection, an unpleasant emergency department staff, and so forth, have no place on the run report. These are best documented on an incident or complaint form issued for use within the EMS system.

Check For Accuracy and Completeness

Once the report is done, take the necessary time to ensure that it is accurate and complete. Sometimes important facts are accidentally left out in the haste of providing patient care, transferring the patient over to the emergency department staff, and restocking the ambulance. Also, be sure to review the spelling of all words to ensure accuracy.

Practice the Skills

You can avoid pitfalls, enhance the delivery of patient care, reduce the risk of litigation, and promote your professional image by refining a few basic abilities such as grammar, spelling, and conciseness. It is often helpful to solicit feedback on the thoroughness and appearance of the run report from other members on the call before turning it in. Review of run reports is an important part of the quality improvement process.

SYSTEMS OF NARRATIVE WRITING

Information about the patient makes up a major portion of the EMS run report. This information may be acquired from the patient, family, bystanders, or the incident scene. It is made up of demographics, history, and physical examination data. To ensure thorough and consistent documentation, employ a system for gathering information. A standardized approach helps to prevent important data from being missed. Several formats are commonly used in the prehospital setting. Typically, these formats are based on either an assessment of the patient or the chronological progress of the call. No matter which format is used, the narrative documentation should start with the patient's age, sex, chief complaint, and how the patient was initially found.

The SOAP method is one way of documenting. It is based on patient assessment and includes the following components:

S—Subjective. This is what the patient experiences and tells you about his or her condition. Examples include "My chest hurts," I can't catch my breath," and I feel dizzy." Questions to answer include "How did it happen?" and "What was the patient doing when it started?" The SAMPLE history (symptoms, allergies, medications, pertinent past history, last meal, and events leading up to the injury or need for help) is included in this section.

O—Objective. This is a description of what you observed at the scene. It includes the mechanism of injury, results of the initial assessment, the focused and detailed examinations, and the vital signs (including an estimated weight). It may also include the results of such tests as the electrocardiogram (ECG) monitor, pulse oximetry, and blood glucose determination. Deformity or bleeding of an extremity, a blood pressure reading or pulse, and wheezing in a patient who is short of breath are also considered examples of objective findings.

A—Assessment. This is where you use the available information to sum up the patient's condition. The assessment may be a description of your examination findings, such as a fractured right humerus. The patient's symptoms may be an assessment, such as headache. Also, the assessment may be the most likely cause for a combination of symptoms and physical findings, such as "the patient is experiencing congestive heart failure."

P—Plan. This refers to the treatment provided or that which is refused by the patient. It includes medications, intravenous (IV) fluids, immobilization, reassessments, and any other interventions that are necessary. Also, this section includes the patient's status, response to treatment, and the transportation destination.

Head-to-Toe Method

Some EMS systems document patient assessment and management in a head-to-toe order. This approach documents the assessment the same way it was performed—head to toe. Start by noting the patient's age, sex, and level of consciousness, and how the patient was initially found. Then list the results of your initial assessment and focused history and examination. Describe your assessment findings of the head, chest, abdomen, pelvis, genitalia, lower extremities, upper extremities, and then the back. Conclude by describing the interventions and care delivered to the patient.

Body Systems Approach

Another format that can be used is the body systems approach. This narrative uses a comprehensive review of the primary body systems. It includes a detailed review of the skin, head, and endocrine, respiratory, cardiac, hematological, lymphatic, gastrointestinal, genitourinary, neurological, and psychiatric systems. Because it is time consuming, the body systems approach is better suited for nursing than for the prehospital setting.

Chronological Method

The chronological (start-to-finish) method is another way to document treatment. This documentation follows the care of the patient by identifying the steps taken in the order in which they were performed. It begins with the time of arrival on the scene. Each entry starts with a time notation followed by the pertinent information for that time period.

● ● ●

Although there are other formats that can be used in the prehospital setting, the bottom line is to use a system that helps you remember all the important information that is needed as part of every patient assessment and documentation. Follow the format applicable for your area.

INFORMATION INCLUDED IN THE RUN REPORT

This section lists the general information usually requested on a run report. Instruction on filling out the specific run report used by an EMS system will be provided by the individual service (Figure 14-3).

Dispatch Information

The first block of information on the run report is the information received from the dispatcher. This information includes the address, nature of the call, priority level, run number, and time of dispatch. This information usually is recorded while taking the call. In some EMS systems this information is recorded via mobile data terminals in the ambulance.

If the patient's condition is relatively stable, one EMT–I can do the patient assessment while the other fills out the run report. This way, important information is immediately captured. This also improves the legibility of the report and improves the EMS team's ability to provide care.

Care Being Provided Before Arrival

In some cases you may arrive at the scene to find care being provided by first responders or bystanders. In these cases you, as well as the first responders, must document the delivery of this care. Many first-responder agencies use a specific form to record assessment findings and treatments provided to patients before the arrival of EMTs. Two copies of this report should be given to you. Attach one of these copies to the run report, and give the other one to the emergency department staff. In some states this information is used to study the need for public education in cardiopulmonary resuscitation (CPR) or first aid.

✖ **Chief Complaint** • A brief statement describing the reason why the patient is seeking medical attention.

Chief Complaint

The **chief complaint** is the medical problem that prompted the patient, family member, friend, or bystander to call for EMS assistance. When the chief complaint comes directly from the patient, it is considered subjective information. When listing the patient's complaint, use the patient's own words, if possible, using quotation marks:

- Patient states, "My chest hurts."
- Patient states, "I can't catch my breath."
- Patient states, "I felt dizzy and fell to the floor."
- Patient states, "I feel sick to my stomach."
- Patient states, "My head is killing me and I can't bend my neck."

If the patient is unresponsive or in cardiac arrest, report the chief complaint as that. Obviously, this type of reporting is objective, because these conditions are directly observed.

Important Observations

Important observations that must be recorded might include child or elderly abuse or the presence of a suicide note, weapon, or mechanism of injury. Add quotation marks to any statement by patients or others that relate to possible criminal activity or admission of suicidal intent. If foul play is suspected, the surroundings must be examined more closely, because the scene can change before law enforcement personnel arrive. If a parent states, "My son fell off the swing in our backyard," your partner should check the backyard for a swing. If there is no swing, note this information. Also note the location where the injury occurred, such as on a roadway, sidewalk, and so forth. Some run reports also ask whether the patient was wearing or using safety equipment such as a helmet or seat belt. Whenever information is of a sensitive nature, note the source of that information.

When the patient refuses treatment or transport, the situation, including assessment findings (vital signs, physical examination, and so forth) and treatments provided, must be thoroughly documented. Clearly state the patient's reason for refusing treatment or transport. Record your explanation to the patient of the possible consequences of refusing treatment or transfer. Also

Use Blue/Black Ink - Press Firmly

SERVICE NAME COMMUNITY AMBULANCE	SERVICE # 02165	INCIDENT # 95-1379	TODAY'S DATE 03 16 96

INCIDENT LOCATION 123 MAIN STREET

PATIENT INFO

PATIENT LAST NAME SMITH	FIRST JANE	M.I. C.	PHONE 555-1212	AGE 68	DATE OF BIRTH 02 04 27	SEX F

STREET ADDRESS 123 MAIN STREET | SOCIAL SECURITY NUMBER 123-45-6789 | MEMBERSHIP ● Yes Ⓝ No

CITY ANYTOWN STATE PA ZIP CODE 15123 | INSURANCE CODE # | MILEAGE

PRIVATE PHYSICIAN DR. MARTINEZ | MEDICAID # | OUT 24652

○ BILL TO (COMPANY or NAME) PHONE | MEDICARE # | SCENE 24656

ADDRESS N/A STREET | GROUP INSURANCE # | DEST 24666

CITY STATE ZIP CODE | OTHER INSURANCE # | IN 24678

CHIEF COMPLAINT CHEST PAIN/DISCOMFORT

CURRENT MEDICATIONS ○ NONE KNOWN NTG, LANOXIN 0-125 MG. TENORNIM

ALLERGIES (MEDS) ● NONE KNOWN NKDA

PAST MEDICAL HISTORY ○ MI ○ CHF ○ COPD ●↑BP ○ DIABETES ○ CANCER ○ NONE KNOWN ● OTHER ANGINA

NARRATIVE 68 Y/O ♀ C/O CHEST PAIN/DISCOMFORT, IN MODERATE DISTRESS.
(HPI) PT. STATED THAT THE ONSET OF THE PAIN WAS WHILE WALKING. NO CHANGE IN PAIN ON PALPATION OR RESPIRATION. PT. DENIES RADIATION OF PAIN. ALSO DENIES SHORTNESS OF BREATH, NAUSEA OR VOMITING. PT. DESCRIBES THE PAIN AS CRUSHING IN NATURE. SEVERITY OF PAIN RATED AS A 6 ON A 1-10 SCALE. PT. STATED THAT THE PAIN BEGAN 1 HOUR PRIOR TO EMS NOTIFICATION. (PMH) HIGH BLOOD PRESSURE, ANGINA. (MEDS) NTG, LANOXIN 0.125 MG. & TENORNIM 10 MG. NKDA (PE) PT. CAOx3, ASSESSMENT OF CHEST UNREMARKABLE. LUNGS CLEAR & Ⓔ. ABDOMEN SOFT, NON-TENDER. SKIN PINK, WARM & DRY. GOOD PULSES, SENSATION & MOTOR FUNCTION ALL EXTREMITIES. ⊖ SACRAC OR PERIPHERAL EDEMA. VITAL SIGNS AS NOTED BELOW. (Rx) PT. WAS ALLOWED TO STAY IN A POSITION OF COMFORT. INITIAL ASSESSMENT COMPLETED. OXYGEN ADMINISTERED @ 15 LPM VIA NON-REBREATHER. FOCUSED HISTORY AND PHYSICAL EXAM COMPLETED. DR. JOHNSON @ COMMUNITY CONSULTED. ORDERS FOR ↑ SL NTG TABLET. PT. PLACED ON STRETCHER INTO AMBULANCE. ASSISTED WITH THE ADMINISTRATION OF NTG. PT. STATED THAT PAIN WAS RELIEVED. V/S REASSESSED. TRANSPORTED TO COMMUNITY HOSPITAL C̄ ON GOING ASSESSMENTS EN ROUTE.

● Narrative 1 of 1

TIME	P	R	B/P	RHYTHM	TREATMENT	PROVIDER ID #	RESPONSE/COMMENTS
1000					ASSESSMENT, O₂	067133	15 LPM VIA NON-REBREATHER
1005	88	18	128/76		FOCUSED Hx, P.E. VITALS	062247	
1008					STRETCHER	CREW	POSITION OF COMFORT
1010	88	16	128/76		VITALS / CONSULT	067133	ORDERS = ↑ SL NTG
1012					ASSISTED NTG	062247	PT. FELT RELIEF
1014	86	16	120/70		VITALS	062247	
1019	86	16	122/74		VITALS	062247	PT. PAIN FREE NOW

Signature of Person Receiving Patient _Bonnie Bolion_ Time

DR. JOHNSON 1234
Command Physician ID#

Crew Signatures:
A#1
A#2
A#3
A#4

Service Copy

FIGURE 14-3 ▲ A completed run report. (Courtesy EMS Data Systems, Inc., Phoenix; from Stoy W: *Mosby's EMT–Basic textbook*, St Louis, 1994, Mosby.)

note the number of times the patient was advised of the need to be transported, and list the names of the persons who witnessed the refusal.

✖ **History of Present Illness or Injury** • Events or complaints associated with the patient's complaint.

Present Medical History

Next, document the patient's **history of present illness or injury.** This history should be recorded in chronological order and should include the time of onset, frequency, location, quality, character of the problem, setting, and anything that aggravates or alleviates the problem. When recording the history of a patient with chest pain, you may write, "The patient states his chest pain started approximately 1 hour ago while he was watching his granddaughter roller skate. He reports it as a constant pain beneath his breastbone that radiates to his left arm. The patient describes it as an aching pain that is unrelieved with nitroglycerin, which he reports to have taken 10 minutes ago."

Pertinent positive and pertinent negative findings should also be recorded. A pertinent positive finding is the presence of a sign or symptom that helps substantiate or identify the patient's condition, or a response to treatment. A patient suspected of having a heart attack typically experiences chest pain and accompanying symptoms such as shortness of breath and nausea. The presence of these symptoms helps support the assessment that the patient may be having a heart attack. A pertinent negative finding is the absence of a sign or symptom that helps substantiate or identify a patient's condition, or a lack of response to treatment. A patient who is experiencing angina often responds to the administration of nitroglycerin with a cessation of chest pain. The failure of nitroglycerin to relieve chest pain should lead to a suspicion that the patient's chest pain is due to a more serious condition, such as acute myocardial infarction. Another consideration is that although pertinent negative findings may not warrant medical intervention, the fact that they are being sought shows evidence of the thoroughness of the examination and history taking of the event.

Record any statements made that may have an impact on subsequent patient care or resolution of the situation, including reports of the following:

- The mechanism of injury
- The patient's behavior
- Safety-related information, including disposition of weapons
- Information of interest to crime scene investigators
- Disposition of valuable personal property (e.g., watches, wallets)

✖ **Past Medical History** • Significant past medical illnesses or traumatic injury that the patient has experienced.

Past Medical History

After recording the patient's present history, document any significant **past medical history,** including surgeries, hospitalizations, illnesses, injuries, allergies, current medications the patient is taking, and the last meal the patient ingested. Also list the name of the patient's physician.

Physical Assessment Findings

Next, record the physical assessment findings. Begin by reporting how the patient was found on arrival (e.g., "Patient found sitting on edge of bed," "Patient ambulatory," or "Patient greeted us at his front door." This assessment includes the patient's vital signs, level of responsiveness, respiratory rate and character, pulse rate and character, blood pressure, skin color and temperature, capillary refill (if appropriate), and the findings of the secondary examination. Repeat vital signs provide important information regarding changes in the patient's condition over time and must be documented on the run report. The vital signs section usually includes space for recording multiple sets of vital signs and the time each was taken. This information is particularly important in situations in which the patient is seriously ill or injured or his or her condition is changing for the better or worse. Pertinent positive or negative findings, such as "Patient denies shortness of breath and nausea," also should be noted.

✖ **Narrative** • The portion of the run report that is written out.

Treatment Provided

Following documentation of the physical findings, record the treatment provided to the patient. Many treatments can be noted by checking a box, but others must be described in the **narrative** section of the run report. This documentation should include what procedure was performed, who performed it, and at what time. Delivered treatments should be described in appropriate detail. Instead of only stating "oxygen was administered," identify the liter flow rate, device used, and time initiated (e.g., "15 L of oxygen administered via nonrebreather mask, started at 2215").

Documentation of invasive or advanced treatments should note whether the treatment was performed with permission of on- or off-line medical direction.

The following are examples of proper narrative reports:

- IV of D_5W, 18-gauge needle to right antecubital fossa, microdrip administration set, run TKO, established at 1805 according to standing orders.
- Proventil, 0.25 mL by inhalation, administered at 0804 per medical direction (MD1).

Any advice or orders from medical direction should be noted, along with the results of implementing that advice or those orders. When documenting orders from on-line medical direction, list the identification number of the physician (or other medical professional) who authorized care to be given.

Treatments that are attempted without success and problems with delivering treatment should be noted on the run report. Include a brief description of the problem and your identification number or initials.

Response to Treatment • The patient's response or lack of response to the care that was rendered.

Response to Treatment

The patient's **response to treatment** should be noted, as well as any other changes, both positive and negative, in the patient's condition. These changes can reveal important information about the patient's condition.

The following are examples of a patient's response to treatment:

- Chest pain or shortness of breath that subsides with oxygen administration
- Severe leg pain that disappears after application of a traction splint
- Chest pain that subsides after the patient takes a nitroglycerin tablet
- A patient who goes from having a diminished level of responsiveness to being alert
- A patient who has trouble breathing when he or she is placed in a supine position

When completing the narrative portion of the run report, use a supplemental sheet if necessary. Do not sacrifice clarity for brevity.

Demographic Information • Information that includes the patient's name, address, age, phone number, and parent's name if the patient is a minor.

Demographic and Billing Information

Collect all patient **demographic information,** such as the patient's name, age, sex, date of birth, address, and phone number. In some systems you may also be required to obtain billing information, such as the patient's type of medical insurance. Some run reports even request the patient to sign his or her name as a means of expediting the billing process.

Use of Support Services

Record all support services or mutual aid services that were used. This includes helicopter or critical care transport, coroner, and rescue or extrication resources.

Anatomical Figure • A diagram of a human body, with anterior and posterior views. Part of some run reports, it is used to mark and label the patient's injuries or physical findings.

STREET WISE

When the patient's condition allows it, document pertinent patient information such as the patient's name, address, age, medical insurance information, and present and past medical histories before transporting the patient to the hospital. It often is difficult to hear the patient or complete the narrative portion of the report while the ambulance is moving.

Anatomical Figure

If applicable and included in the run report, circle or shade in the areas of the **anatomical figure** to represent the affected area(s) of the patient's body. Do not limit the use of this diagram to injuries, because certain medical conditions or physical assessment findings can be highlighted using this type of chart.

Run Times

In the administrative section of many EMS run reports, there is space to record the run times. Times that are recorded often include when the call occurred, dispatch, en route to the call, arrival at the scene, departure time from the scene, arrival at the hospital, transfer of care, and back in service (available for the next call). Some reports include a place to indicate when the patient is actually reached. This information helps show the actual time to treatment for each incident. These times are recorded using military times (Table 14-2).

Run Disposition

Note the disposition of the call, including whether the patient is gone on your arrival, refuses transportation, or is handed over to another ambulance crew. When applicable, also note to which hospital the patient is transported. Some EMS systems use numbers to denote the hospital identification. Any direct radio or cellular telephone communication with the hospital or your medical direction facility should be indicated on the run report as well.

Signatures

Last, all personnel responsible for the run usually sign the run report (or, at least, the names are clearly printed). This signature includes the first initial, last name, and professional credentials. Signatures must be legible. Some EMS systems, however, require only that EMT–Is record their identification number.

TABLE 14-2

Military Times

00 hours	=	12:00 AM
0100 hours	=	1:00 AM
0200 hours	=	2:00 AM
0300 hours	=	3:00 AM
0400 hours	=	4:00 AM
0500 hours	=	5:00 AM
0600 hours	=	6:00 AM
0700 hours	=	7:00 AM
0800 hours	=	8:00 AM
0900 hours	=	9:00 AM
1000 hours	=	10:00 AM
1100 hours	=	11:00 PM
1200 hours	=	12:00 PM
1300 hours	=	1:00 PM
1400 hours	=	2:00 PM
1500 hours	=	3:00 PM
1600 hours	=	4:00 PM
1700 hours	=	5:00 PM
1800 hours	=	6:00 PM
1900 hours	=	7:00 PM
2000 hours	=	8:00 PM
2100 hours	=	9:00 PM
2200 hours	=	10:00 PM
2300 hours	=	11:00 PM

WHEN A MISTAKE IS MADE

Fixing Mistakes

There is a right way and a wrong way to correct mistakes. Do not destroy the run report and start over again. Draw a single, horizontal line through the incorrect entry so that it is still legible (Figure 14-4). Indicate that the crossed-out entry is an error, and initial it. Then write the correct information beside it. You may want to document the reason for the correction and/or have it witnessed. Make every effort to ensure that your correction cannot be interpreted as tampering.

Documenting Late Entries

If a correction is made or an entry is added after a run report has been submitted, the time and date of the entry, as well as an explanation for its lateness, should be written next to it. Preferably make the correction using different-color ink. No attempt should be made to cover up the fact that it is a late entry.

An alternative way of revising a document is to put the information on a separate report form. Note the purpose of the revision and why the information did not appear on the original document, as well as the date and time of the revision. The original author of a document should make the revisions. When the need for revision is realized, it should be done as soon as possible.

If more information becomes available, a supplemental narrative can be written on a separate report form and attached to the original.

In any event, follow your local protocols for making corrections or revisions to the EMS run reports.

Documenting Deviations From Protocol

If the normal protocol or standard of care was not followed, document the reason why, and what steps were taken (if any) to correct the situation. Specify whether medical direction was notified of the problem. Also document any delays or problems responding, gaining access, or transporting the patient. Include an explanation of the problem (e.g., weather conditions, traffic congestion) and the length of the delay.

Alternatively, in some EMS systems, corrections are not made directly on the run report. Rather, corrections are documented on a supplemental form and attached to the run report.

Documenting Questionable Medical Direction

Occasionally EMT–Is may be directed by medical direction to administer a medication or dose that seems to be inappropriate or inconsistent with established protocols. In this event, record the facts of the incident and how it was handled.

Tampering With the Run Report

Tampering with the run report can cause serious trouble for an EMT–I. An incomplete, inaccurate, or illegible report may cause subsequent caregivers to provide inappropriate care to a patient. Changing or obliterating the run report can provide a plaintiff's attorney with information to use against the EMT–I, even though he or she may be completely innocent. Making erasures, scratching or crossing out an entry, tearing or cutting off a portion of a report, using correction fluid or ink markers, or squeezing an entry between the lines of a report may be interpreted as tampering, even if tampering was not the intent. In contrast, an attorney considering the merit of a potential lawsuit may be dissuaded from the case when the documentation is done correctly.

Falsifying Information

Falsifying information on the run report can have severe consequences. It can lead to suspension or revocation of one's certification or license, and it increases the risk of poor patient care. Paramedics or emergency department staff cannot provide accurate care if they are working with inaccurate information. Remember, your run report can be compared with the hospital chart.

NARRATIVE 68 y/o ♀ c/o CHEST PAIN/DISCOMFORT, IN MODERATE DISTRESS.
(HPI) PT. STATED THAT THE ONSET OF THE PAIN WAS WHILE WALKING. NO
CHANGE IN PAIN ON PALPATION OR RESPIRATION. PT. DENIES RADIATION
OF PAIN. ALSO DENIES SHORTNESS OF BREATH, NAUSEA OR VOMITING.
PT. DESCRIBES THE PAIN AS CRUSHING IN NATURE. SEVERITY OF PAIN
RATED AS A 6 ON A 1-10 SCALE. PT. STATED THAT THE PAIN BEGAN 1 HOUR
PRIOR TO EMS ~~ARRIVAL~~ (TB) NOTIFICATION. (PMH) HIGH BLOOD PRESSURE, ANGINA.
(MEDS) NTG, LANOXIN 0.125 mg. & TENORMIN 10 mg. NKDA (PE) PT. CAOX3 ASSESSMENT
OF CHEST UNREMARKABLE. LUNGS CLEAR & (=). ABDOMEN SOFT, NON-TENDER,
SKIN PINK, WARM & DRY. GOOD PULSES, SENSATION & MOTOR FUNCTION ALL
EXTREMITIES. (⊖) SACRAL OR PERIPHERAL EDEMA. VITAL SIGNS AS NOTED BELOW.
(RX) PT. WAS ALLOWED TO STAY IN A POSITION OF COMFORT. INITIAL ASSESSMENT
COMPLETED. OXYGEN ADMINISTERED @ 15 LPM VIA NON-REBREATHER. FOCUSED
HISTORY AND PHYSICAL EXAM COMPLETED. DR. JOHNSON @ COMMUNITY CONSULTED
ORDERS FOR ↑ SL NTG TABLET. PT. PLACED ON STRETCHER INTO AMBULANCE.
ASSISTED WITH THE ADMINISTRATION OF NTG. PT. STATED THAT PAIN WAS
RELIEVED. V/S REASSESSED. TRANSPORTED TO COMMUNITY HOSPITAL
c̄ ONGOING ASSESSMENTS EN ROUTE.

● Narrative 1 of 1

FIGURE 14-4 ▲ The proper way to correct a mistake on a run report. (Courtesy EMS Data Systems, Inc., Phoenix; from Stoy W: *Mosby's EMT–Basic textbook*, St Louis, 1994, Mosby.)

CONFIDENTIALITY

Maintaining patient confidentiality is one of the major responsibilities of the EMT–I—one that must be taken very seriously. Information recorded on the run report is considered confidential. For this reason, care is used to prevent unauthorized persons from having access to its contents. EMS systems have a responsibility to properly educate their membership (employees) on the importance of patient confidentiality. Some states have laws and regulations concerning the confidentiality of patient care records. Although the run report is a confidential document, multiple individuals routinely review it. Whether it is being used for continuity of care, reimbursement, legal issues, education, research, quality assurance, or other significant requirements, the run report is constantly being evaluated. As such, great care must be taken to protect the patient's right to confidentiality while allowing for necessary use of data contained on the form. During quality improvement and training activities, the patient's name should be crossed out or blackened.

Patient confidentiality, as well as patient refusal, is discussed further in Chapter 3.

DOCUMENTATION OF PATIENT REFUSAL

Competent adult patients have the right to refuse treatment. However, every effort must be made to persuade the patient to go to a hospital. It is absolutely essential to ensure that the patient is able to make a rational, informed decision. Patients under the influence of alcohol or other drugs or who are experiencing diminished mental capacity due to illness or injury should not be asked to sign a refusal. Document the process you have undergone to reach the conclusion that the patient refuses treatment or transport. This includes the following:

- The advice you give to the patient
- The advice given to the patient by medical direction by telephone or radio
- A complete narrative, including quotations or statements by others

If the patient absolutely refuses care or transport (and is able to make a rational, competent decision), document any assessment findings and emergency medical care given, and then have the patient sign a refusal form. Some EMS systems use a separate refusal form, whereas others include the refusal as part of the run report. Have a police officer or bystander sign the form as a witness. If the patient refuses to sign the refusal form, have a police officer or bystander sign the form, verifying that the patient refused to sign. If no other witnesses are available, it may be necessary to ask a family member to sign as a witness. When obtaining signatures from witnesses, record the correct spelling of each name, along with an address and phone number (if available), since it may be difficult to read the witness's signature.

DOCUMENTATION OF WHEN CARE IS NOT NEEDED

There are times when no care or transport is needed. These events must be documented thoroughly. This includes situations where the response is canceled en route. The canceling authority and time should be noted. If the response is canceled at the scene, note the canceling authority and any special circumstances (e.g., "fire officer on scene verified there are no injuries and cleared us to return to service—no patient contacts made").

DOCUMENTATION OF MULTIPLE-CASUALTY INCIDENTS

When treating more than one patient at a time, a run report must be completed for each patient. In the case of multiple-casualty incidents (MCIs), the documentation may need to be completed after the patients are delivered to the hospital. The local MCI plan typically provides instruction on how to temporarily record important medical information. The standard for completing the form in an MCI is not the same as for a typical call. Often, you must do the best you can with the limited information available.

SPECIAL SITUATION REPORTS

Special situations include suspected child abuse or abuse of the elderly, equipment failure, and/or complaints about the EMS providers' care or demeanor. EMT–Is may be obligated to report these or other situations to local authorities, and in some cases this requires a special report form. Other supplemental reports may include documentation of exposure to infectious disease, accident or injury reports, and hazardous materials reports.

Supplemental reports must be submitted in a timely manner and must be accurate and objective. When completing this type of report, keep a copy for your own records. The report and other copies should be submitted to the authority specified by local protocols.

IMPORTANCE OF ACCURATE DOCUMENTATION

Documentation is one of the less glamorous functions in EMS, but it is one of utmost importance for many reasons. EMS providers must conduct a self-assessment of all documentation to ensure legibility, accuracy, and completeness. This should be done immediately following completion of the EMS run report. Because of its importance, as an EMT–I, you must serve as an advocate for documentation that is properly completed. This means responding to negative attitudes regarding the task of documentation and encouraging professionalism among all those with whom you interact. All EMS providers can play a role in shaping the professional image of prehospital care providers by producing documentation that is thorough, accurate, and concise.

CASE HISTORY FOLLOW-UP ■ ■ ■

EMT–I Johnson becomes uneasy, then agitated, as he considers the documentation errors on the run report. He realizes that the errors in judgment could cost his employer thousands of dollars and possibly a great deal of negative publicity. They could also cost him his job and ruin his chances for promotion. After 2 years of experience as an EMT–I and some distance from the call, the errors are obvious to him.

First, when he recorded the patient's chief complaint as "SOB," EMT–I Johnson did not use an abbreviation approved by his service. Although *SOB* may mean "shortness of breath" to an EMT, it may mean something different—and demeaning—to a jury.

Second, he reported that the patient was "intoxicated on alcohol." Facing deposition, EMT–I Johnson is now aware that he had no way of knowing that the patient was intoxicated on alcohol because he had not seen her drinking any alcoholic beverages, nor did he have any confirming laboratory results.

Last, EMT–I Johnson reported that the patient was "combative" and that he had to restrain her with "hard restraints." Although restraining her was necessary, there was no documentation that she required only hand restraints, or that she had attempted to bite him and his partner, or that he had requested police assistance. Now, he realizes how hard it will be to justify to a jury restraining the patient with straps.

SUMMARY

Important points to remember from this chapter include the following:

- Learning to write organized, efficient run reports is an integral part of being an EMT–I. The EMT–I must accurately document all the events of each case. The run report should be a positive reflection on the excellence of the EMS system and the EMT–I. The run report provides for a continuum of care by communicating how the patient was found on the EMT–I's arrival, what care was provided, and how the patient's condition changed over time. Proper documentation also helps to protect the EMT–I against unfounded lawsuits and serves as an important data source for quality improvement activities.
- Although there are many different types of run reports in use today, they all include patient and ad-

ministrative information. The run report usually consists of an original and one or two copies. One copy is left with the patient at the hospital to be entered into his or her patient record, supplying the hospital staff with information they might not otherwise be able to access.

- The run report must be concise, accurate, and legible. When completing the report, the EMT–I should use a ballpoint pen and avoid using abbreviations unless they are approved by the EMS system.
- Key information includes the patient's demographic information (name, address, age, sex, phone number, etc.) and patient information (patient complaint, present history, past history, treatments delivered, etc.).

- When an error or omission occurs, the EMT–I must be sure to follow the appropriate procedure to correct the problem. False information must never be allowed to enter the patient record.
- The confidential nature of an EMS report must be respected. If a patient refuses care, the EMT–I documents this appropriately and gets signatures from both the patient and a witness. Patients experiencing diminished mental status must not be allowed to refuse care.
- The EMT–I must document information carefully and professionally. The run report becomes a part of patient's permanent medical record and may be viewed by many others both inside and outside the EMS system.

TRAUMA

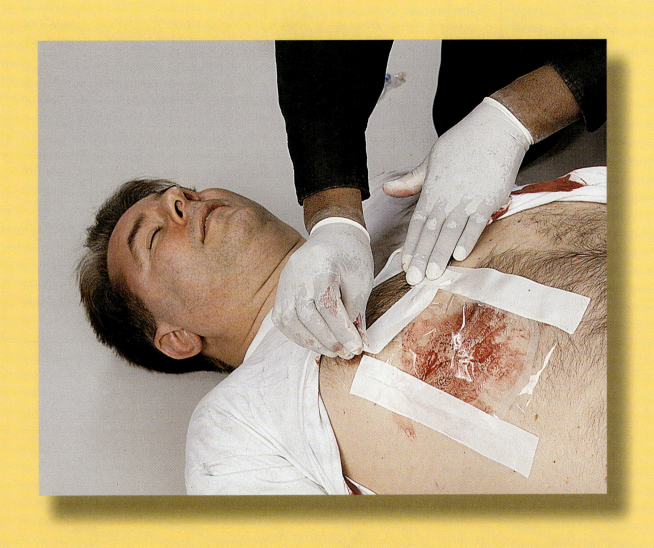

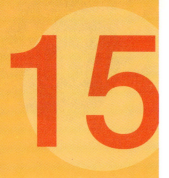

15

Trauma Systems and Mechanism of Injury

Key Terms

Blunt Trauma

Cavitation

Definitive Care

Kinematics

Penetrating Trauma

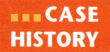

CASE HISTORY

It is 2:00 AM when EMT–Is Walker and Fox are awakened by the alarm. "Unit 53 . . . Respond to George's Corner Bar . . . Possible stabbing . . . Police are en route . . . Time out 02:03."

Within minutes, the EMT–Is are en route to the scene. EMT–I Walker's adrenaline is flowing.

EMT–I Walker knows the location of the bar well. In fact, he has been there a few times himself. It is not the nicest place, but it has always been a regular hangout for the "townies"—people like EMT–I Walker, who grew up in the area. As the EMT–Is approach the scene, they see lots of emergency lights and several police cars in the parking lot. Two men in handcuffs are being questioned by police officers.

The EMT–Is grab their gear and make their way through the crowd of people surrounding the victim. The victim is positioned on his right side and is guarding his stomach through a blood-stained shirt. EMT–I Walker and his partner place the victim supine to begin their assessment. As EMT–I Walker rolls the patient onto his back, he realizes that he knows him. He was a good friend from high school, and EMT–I Walker occasionally still plays ball on the same team as the victim. This call is the first time EMT–I Walker has taken care of someone he knows. The patient looks up at EMT–I Walker and says with a frightened voice, "Man, I'm glad it's you. I've been stabbed."

EMT–I Fox applies high-concentration oxygen by nonrebreather mask and gets a baseline set of vital signs while EMT–I Walker exposes his friend's abdomen. He sees a gaping 3-inch laceration just below the border of the patient's right rib cage. He finds a second, smaller wound just distal to the umbilicus. The abdominal wound is bleeding quite a bit, and EMT–I Walker knows the patient needs to get to the operating room. He prepares the pneumatic antishock garment (PASG) on the long board, positions his friend, and loads him in the ambulance for transport.

CHAPTER GOAL

Upon completion of this chapter, the EMT–Intermediate will be able to apply the principles of kinematics to enhance the patient assessment and predict the likelihood of injuries on the basis of the patient's mechanism of injury.

Cognitive Objectives

As an EMT–Intermediate you should be able to do the following:

- Describe the incidence and scope of traumatic injuries and deaths.

- List and describe the components of a comprehensive trauma system.

- Describe the role of and differences among levels of trauma centers.

- Describe the criteria and procedure for air medical transport.

- Describe the criteria for transport to a trauma center.

- Define energy and force as they relate to trauma.

- Describe the kinematics of blunt and penetrating injuries.

- Define laws of motion and energy, and understand the effect that increased speed has on injuries.

- Describe the following types of impact and the effect each has on an unrestrained victim: down and under, up and over, compression, and deceleration.

- Describe the pathophysiology of the head, spine, thorax, and abdomen that results from the above forces.

- List specific injuries and their causes as they relate to interior and exterior vehicle damage.

- Describe injury patterns associated with motorcycle and all-terrain vehicle crashes, as well as auto-pedestrian collisions.

- List the motion and energy considerations of mechanisms other than motor vehicle crashes.

- Define the role of kinematics as an additional tool for patient assessment.

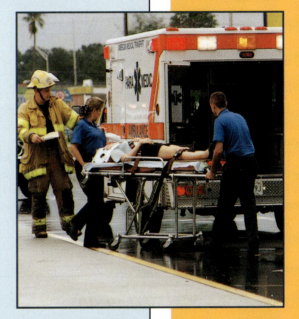

Affective Objectives

None identified for this chapter.

Psychomotor Objectives

None identified for this chapter.

INTRODUCTION

EMT–Intermediates (EMT–Is) who read the newspaper usually come across many stories related to injuries caused by trauma. Some type of traumatic event injured the man in the case history at the beginning of this chapter. How does this patient differ from someone who is lightheaded or who is having chest pain? The EMT–I must have an appreciation of trauma systems and be able to recognize mechanisms of injury to enhance patient assessment and emergency care.

EPIDEMIOLOGY OF TRAUMA

In 1998 there were approximately 92,000 accidental deaths in the United States. In that same year, trauma deaths were exceeded only by deaths from AIDS for persons 34 to 37 years of age and by deaths from cardiovascular disease and cancer among all other age-groups.

According to statistics, trauma[1,2]:

- Is the leading cause of death in people ages 1 through 44 years
- Is the fifth leading cause of death among all Americans
- Accounts for 60% of childhood deaths
- Accounts for 80% of teenage deaths
- Annually kills three times more Americans than died in Vietnam
- Temporarily disables 9 million people each year
- Permanently disables 350,000 people each year
- Has an economic effect of unintentional injuries in the United States that exceeds $480 billion each year

In the United States any given 10-minute period results in two deaths and about 370 disabling injuries from trauma. The cost of trauma amounts to more than 9 million dollars per year.

The top five causes of trauma deaths since 1970 are motor vehicle accidents, falls, poisoning by solids and liquids, fire and burns, and drowning (Figure 15-1). Deaths from unintentional injury increase yearly, which emphasizes the need for increased safety and health efforts (Box 15-1).

Phases of Trauma Care

There are three phases of trauma care: preincident, incident, and postincident.[1] EMT–Is have responsibilities in each phase, even though traditionally they have been trained primarily to function in the postincident phase.

In the preincident phase the focus is on prevention of intentional and unintentional trauma deaths. EMT–Is and other members of the health care team play a vital role in this phase. Public education (e.g., use of automobile occupant restraint systems and helmets, promotion of nonviolent conflict resolution, and appropriate use of the 9-1-1 system) and the promotion of legislation that supports injury prevention programs are activities that should be undertaken by all health care providers.

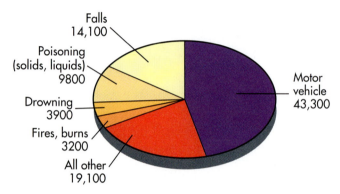

Falls
14,100

Poisoning
(solids, liquids)
9800

Drowning
3900

Fires, burns
3200

All other
19,100

Motor
vehicle
43,300

FIGURE 15-1 ▲ Deaths from unintentional injury by event, United States, 1996. (From National Safety Council: *Accident facts*, Chicago, 1997, The Council.)

BOX 15-1

PREVENTION OF TRAUMA DEATHS

Deaths from trauma occur in three periods: immediate, early, and late. Each period presents its own unique problems.[4]

IMMEDIATE

Immediate death occurs within seconds or minutes of the injury. Lacerations of the brain, brainstem, upper spinal cord, heart, aorta, or other large vessels usually cause these deaths. Few if any patients in this category can be saved. Effective injury prevention programs are the only way to reduce the number of these deaths.

EARLY

The second peak of death occurs within the first 2 to 3 hours after injury. The causes of these deaths usually are major head injury, hemopneumothorax, ruptured spleen, lacerated liver, pelvic fracture, or multiple injuries associated with significant blood loss. Most of these injuries are treatable with available techniques, but the time lapse between injury and definitive care is critical.

LATE

The third peak of death occurs days or weeks after the injury. These deaths most often result from sepsis, infection, or multiple-organ failure. Prehospital emergency care focused on early recognition and management of life-threatening injury can play an important role in preventing these late deaths from trauma.

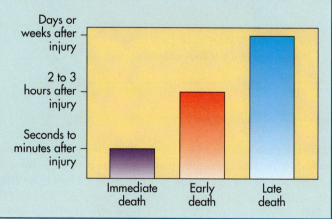

Days or
weeks after
injury

2 to 3
hours after
injury

Seconds to
minutes after
injury

Immediate
death

Early
death

Late
death

Baker C et al: Epidemiology of trauma deaths, *Am J Surg*, 40:144, 1980.

The actual traumatic event represents the incident phase. The role of EMT–Is should be to "practice what we preach"—using lap and diagonal seat belts when operating the ambulance, riding in the patient compartment, or driving in a personal vehicle and wearing a helmet when riding a bicycle. By exercising personal safety while on or off duty, the EMT–I can serve as a good role model for others.

The postincident phase is when the EMT–I traditionally uses the skills he or she has gained. Responsibilities in this phase include the following:
- Performing lifesaving procedures
- Properly preparing the patient for transport to an appropriate medical facility
- Promptly transporting the patient to the appropriate medical facility (Box 15-2)

TRAUMA SYSTEMS

✂ **Definitive Care** • In-hospital care that resolves the patient's illness or injury after a definitive diagnosis has been established.

There are eight components in a sophisticated trauma system[4]:
- Injury prevention
- Prehospital care, including treatment, transportation, and trauma triage
- Emergency department care
- Interfacility transportation as necessary
- **Definitive care**
- Trauma critical care
- Rehabilitation
- Data collection/trauma registry (Box 15-3)

Many of these components of a trauma system involve the EMT–I. Injury prevention, prehospital care, interfacility transport, data collection, and research are areas in which the EMT–I can positively influence the trauma patient's outcome.

Trauma Centers

In 1980 the U.S. Department of Health and Human Services (USDHHS) released the *Position Paper on Trauma Center Designation.* Since that time, many states have developed comprehensive trauma systems that include hospitals with a designated specialty in trauma.

The American College of Surgeons (ACS) has taken the lead in describing resources necessary to provide appropriate care to trauma patients. Since 1966 the ACS has published and updated a document now called *Resources for Optimal Care of the Injured Patient.* This document outlines the resources, personnel, equipment, and training necessary for an institution to provide quality trauma care.

Trauma centers are categorized on the basis of the resources and programs available at the facility (Tables 15-1 and 15-2). This categorization identifies those hospitals capable of handling trauma patients and enables EMS providers to rapidly transport patients to the most appropriate medical facilities.

In 1988 the American College of Emergency Physicians (ACEP) developed a position paper that described the components of a full trauma *system* (Table 15-3). This paper complemented the ACS document, which originally described only the hospital resources. Together, the two organizations have established the minimum criteria for a comprehensive trauma system. This system begins with access to emergency care via the prehospital phase and continues with the care provided in the emergency department, the operating room, the intensive care unit, and the general hospital floor, and finally through the rehabilitation component. For a patient to return to a full and productive life, all of these components must be present and work together in a coordinated fashion.

In addition to trauma centers, other specialized care facilities have been identified. These include pediatric trauma centers, burn centers, poison treatment centers, and burn centers.

BOX 15-2

THE GOLDEN HOUR

The first hour after severe injury is known as the *golden hour.* It is a critical period in which surgical intervention for the trauma patient can enhance survival and reduce complications. The EMT–I must recognize patients in this category and ensure that prehospital care activities do not unnecessarily delay patient transportation. These patients can be best served through rapid assessment, stabilization of life-threatening injuries, and rapid transportation to an appropriate medical facility for definitive care.

From Sanders MJ: *Mosby's paramedic textbook,* ed 2, St Louis, 2000, Mosby.

BOX 15-3

TRAUMA REGISTRIES

Trauma registries allow for the collection of injury data by individual hospitals or groups of hospitals on a local, regional, or state level. The American College of Surgeons (ACS) funded these registries (e.g., the *National Trauma Data Bank*) and software programs (e.g., *NATIONAL TRACS*) to provide for online data management and a national reciprocity of injury data for a variety of commercial registry programs. Trauma registries generate periodic standard reports that provide statistical data to allow facilities to compare trends and other important information regarding trauma care.

From Sanders MJ: *Mosby's paramedic textbook,* ed 2, St Louis, 2000, Mosby.

TABLE 15-1

Trauma Center Categories

LEVEL	DESCRIPTION	CAPABILITIES	WHERE
Level I	Regional resource center	Full spectrum of services from prevention programs to patient rehabilitation Serves as the leader in trauma care for a geographical area	Most are found in large university-based hospitals because of the requirements for patient care, education and teaching programs, and research
Level II	Provides initial definitive patient care	May not have all resources found in a Level I facility Some complex, critical patients may need to be transferred to a Level I facility Research is not an essential component	Usually a nonteaching or community hospital
Level III	Designed for communities that do not have immediate availability of a Level I or II institution	Provides evaluation, resuscitation, and operative intervention for stabilization When necessary, patients are transferred to a Level I or II trauma center for ongoing or more definitive care Should have preexisting relationships and transfer agreements in place with a Level I or II trauma center for rapid transfer when necessary	Usually a community hospital
Level IV	Created with rural and remote areas in mind	Provides initial stabilization and then transfer of the patient to a Level I, II, or III trauma center Should have preexisting relationships and transfer agreements in place with a Level I or II trauma center for rapid transfer when necessary	May not be a hospital but rather a clinic-type facility

Modified from National Association of Emergency Medical Technicians: *PHTLS: basic and advanced prehospital trauma life support,* ed 4, St Louis, 1999, Mosby.

Transport Considerations

The patient's needs and condition, as well as the advice of medical direction, determine the appropriate level of care and hospital destination. The EMT–I can then make decisions regarding whether the patient should be transported by ground or air ambulance.

Ground transportation should be used if the appropriate facility can be reached within a "reasonable time." This time frame is defined by national standards and local protocol. Factors that will affect this type of transport include the following:

- Geographical location
- Topographical area
- Population
- Weather
- Availability of resources
- Traffic conditions
- Time of day[3]

Ground transportation may also be used to move the patient from the location of the crash to a more accessible landing zone when air medical transport is used. Local protocols will determine appropriate landing sites.

Air medical services can provide rapid response time, high-quality medical care, and rapid transport to appropriate care facilities. Helicopters can also provide aerial surveillance, rescue for remote areas that cannot be reached by ground, and transportation of additional personnel and equipment to the emergency scene. EMT–Is should consult with medical direction and follow local protocols for use of air medical services.

Air transportation should be considered in the following situations:

- The time needed to transport a patient by ground to an appropriate facility poses a threat to the patient's survival and recovery.
- Weather, road, or traffic conditions would seriously delay the patient's access to definitive care.
- Critical care personnel and equipment not available from ground crews are needed to adequately care for the patient during transport.

TABLE 15-2

Essential (E) or Desirable (D) Characteristics of a Trauma Center

	LEVELS			
	I	**II**	**III**	**IV**
HOSPITAL ORGANIZATION				
Trauma service	E	E	E	—
Trauma service director	E	E	E	—
Trauma multidisciplinary committee	E	E	D	—
Hospital departments divisions/sections				
General surgery	E	E	E	D
Neurological surgery	E	E	D	—
Orthopedic surgery	E	E	D	—
Emergency services	E	E	E	D
Anesthesia	E	E	E	—
CLINICAL CAPABILITIES (SPECIALTY AVAILABILITY)				
In-house 24 hours a day				
General surgery	E	E	—	—
Neurological surgery	E	E	—	—
Emergency medicine	E	E	E	—
Anesthesiology	E	E	—	—
On call and promptly available				
Anesthesiology	—	—	E	D
Cardiac surgery	E	D	—	—
Cardiology	E	E	D	—
General surgery	—	—	E	D
Hand surgery	E	D	—	—
Infectious disease	E	D	—	—
Internal medicine	E	E	E	—
Microvascular surgery (replant/flaps)	E	D	—	—
Neurological surgery	—	—	D	—
Obstetric/gynecological surgery	E	E	D	—
Ophthalmic surgery	E	E	D	—
Oral/maxillofacial surgery	E	E	—	—
Orthopedic surgery	E	E	D	—

TABLE 15-3

Structure of a Trauma Care System

ENVIRONMENTS	COMPONENTS	PROVIDERS
Urban	Medical direction	System management
Rural	Prevention	Prehospital providers
	Communication	Acute care facilities
	Training	Rehabilitation/reconstructive services
	Triage	
	Prehospital care	
	Transportation	
	Hospital care	
	Public education	
	Rehabilitation	
	Medical evaluation	

From National Association of Emergency Medical Technicians: *PHTLS: basic and advanced prehospital trauma life support,* ed 4, St Louis, 1999, Mosby.

EMS Trauma System

Although the ACS has described the resources necessary for trauma centers, recent years have brought changes in the approach to trauma care. In the past, the main focus was on getting the critically injured trauma victim to a trauma center and on the preparation of the facility to be a trauma center. Recently, however, it has been recognized that the majority of trauma patients do not need the capabilities of a trauma center and that most trauma care can be provided at other acute care hospitals. Therefore all facilities should be part of the trauma system. Efforts in education and trauma care analysis should include all facilities, not just the trauma centers (Figure 15-2).

KINEMATICS OF TRAUMA

When dealing with trauma, there are several things the EMT–I must do before even touching a patient. First, he or she must look at the situation and get an idea as to what may have happened. The EMT–I must assess the kinematics of the trauma. **Kinematics** is the process of predicting injury patterns that may result from the forces and motions of energy.

Performing an overall assessment of the scene provides information as to what occurred when the patient was injured. In addition, safety can be determined for the patient and the rescuer(s). At the scene of a fall, for example, the following should be considered when assessing the kinematics of the situation:

- How many patients are involved?
- How far did the patient fall?
- On what type of surface did the patient land?
- Was the patient wearing any type of protective gear, such as a helmet, knee pads, or elbow pads?
- Was the patient secured by any type of rope, and did that rope injure him or her somehow in the fall?

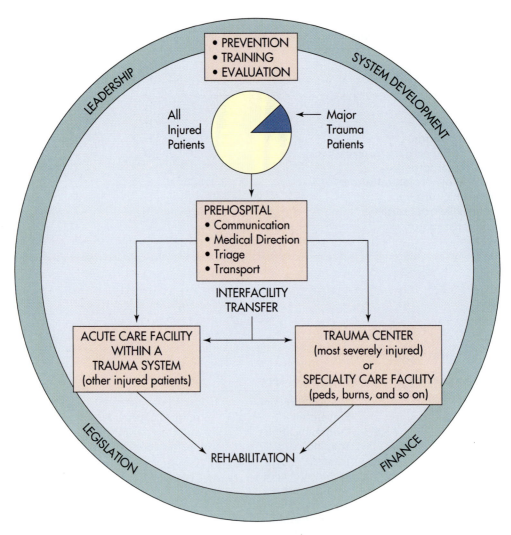

FIGURE 15-2 ▲ The integral nature of the EMS trauma system. (Modified from the Bureau of Health Services Resources, Division of Trauma and Emergency Medical Services: *Model trauma care system plan*, Rockville, Md, 1992, US Department of Health and Human Services.)

- What type of environment is present? Is the temperature cold or warm? Is it raining or sunny? Is it during the day or night?
- Are there any other things that may present a danger to the EMS personnel? Are there dangling ropes or wires, animals, hysterical bystanders, etc.?
- Did any material, such as rocks or stones, fall on top of the patient?
- Does the patient also have some underlying medical problem?

At the scene of a motor vehicle crash, the following should be considered when assessing the kinematics of the situation:

- How many vehicles are involved? What type of vehicles (cars, trucks, motorcycles) are involved? How fast were they traveling?
- What type of damage is present to the outside of the vehicles? Was it a head-on collision, or did the car flip over? Is there any damage to the inside of the vehicles, such as a sprung seat, cracked windshield, or deformed steering wheel?
- Are there any identifying marks at the scene, such as skid marks or broken glass? If skid marks are present, approximately how long are they?
- Are there any hazards in the area, such as gasoline or downed power lines?
- How many patients are involved? Are the patients still in the vehicles, or was anyone thrown from a vehicle or over the handlebars of a motorcycle? In what position was the patient found inside the vehicle?
- Are any patients entrapped, and is there easy access for patient extrication?
- Were the occupants in the vehicle(s) restrained? Did the occupants use shoulder belts or lap belts? Were air bags deployed? If any young children are involved, was some type of car seat used? Was the car seat properly restrained in the vehicle?

Energy

To better comprehend kinematics, a brief review of physics is necessary. *Newton's first law of motion* states that "a body at rest will remain at rest and a body in motion will remain in motion until acted upon by an equal and opposite force." For example, if a climber falls down a hill, he or she could remain in motion until the opposite force—the ground—is encountered. In the case of a motor vehicle crash, the vehicle is at rest until the engine starts. Once traveling down the road, it stays in motion until it hits another vehicle or slams into a stationary device, such as a telephone pole. Applying the brakes also stops the motion.

The second principle of physics is the *law of conservation of energy*. This law states that energy cannot be created or destroyed. It can, however, change its form. The forms of energy are mechanical, thermal, electrical, and chemical. For example, when a car crashes into a telephone pole, the energy is spread out over the frame of the car, the fenders, and other parts of the vehicle (mechanical). The more energy that is present, the greater the changes or damage will be to the structure of the car, as well as to the patient. If skid marks are noted, some of the energy of the car was transferred into the rubber, which burned onto the road from the tires (thermal). Electrical energy is displaced throughout the body during a lightning strike. If a corrosive hazardous material is spilled onto the skin, the chemical energy can destroy skin, muscle, and bones, depending on its strength and the duration of contact.

Newton's second law of motion involves force and the effects of acceleration or deceleration. Consider the following formulas:

Force (F) = Mass (M) × Acceleration (a), or F = M × a

Force (F) = Mass (M) × Deceleration (d), or F = M × d

Be aware that seat belts and air bags increase the distance over which the body stops its movement. This phenomenon can decrease the deceleration force considerably.

Kinetic energy also is involved; this refers to the object's weight and speed. When used to refer to people, the terms *weight* and *mass* are considered to be the same. Speed also is known as velocity. Therefore this relationship can be expressed by the formula:

Kinetic energy (KE) = $\frac{1}{2}$ Mass (M) × Velocity (V) squared,

or KE = $\frac{1}{2}$ M × V²

Speed, or velocity, is the determining factor in predicting the type of damage that occurs. If a patient weighing 120 pounds is traveling in a car at 30 miles per hour (mph), this results in 54,000 units of kinetic energy (known as *foot pounds*, calculated as pounds multiplied by miles per hour).

$$KE = \frac{1}{2} M \times V^2$$
$$= \frac{120}{2} \times 30^2$$
$$= 60 \times 900$$
$$= 54,000 \text{ units of energy}$$

If another person is also in the car and weighs 130 pounds, this increases the kinetic energy to 58,500 units.

$$KE = \frac{1}{2} M \times V^2$$
$$= \frac{130}{2} \times 30^2$$
$$= 65 \times 900$$
$$= 58,500 \text{ units of energy}$$

However, if the first patient is now traveling at 40 mph (only 10 mph faster), the kinetic energy increases significantly.

$$KE = \frac{1}{2} M \times V^2$$
$$= \frac{120}{2} \times 40^2$$
$$= 60 \times 1600$$
$$= 96,000 \text{ units of energy}$$

When the mass is increased from 120 to 130 pounds, the kinetic energy increases only from 54,000 to 58,500 units of energy. However, when the speed is increased by only 10 mph, the kinetic energy jumps from 54,000 to 96,000 units of energy. According to these calculations, an increase in speed is more deadly than an increase in mass.

In addition, since force equals mass multiplied by acceleration (Newton's second law of motion), the 120-pound driver is moving forward in the vehicle with about 7200 foot-pounds of force when he or she is stopped by the steering column. The energy of the body's motion causes tissue destruction as that energy is absorbed into the body cells when the body stops. This example illustrates the principle, but the actual total force also is determined by the true rate of deceleration (e.g., "g force") and several other factors.

TYPES OF TRAUMA

Trauma can be either blunt or penetrating. With blunt trauma, there may be no external signs of injury. Internal organs may be significantly damaged, whereas the skin remains intact. **Penetrating trauma** involves some type of invasive injury to the body in which an opening is created. At the time of impact, significant force may have been involved.

Blunt Trauma

Blunt trauma occurs from any type of impact resulting in two forces: compression and change of speed (shear). Direct compression, or pressure on a structure, is the most common type of force applied in blunt trauma.[2] The amount of injury depends on the length of time of compression, the force of compression, and the area compressed. For example, with blunt trauma to the chest, the heart is compressed between two rigid structures—the sternum and the spine (Figure 15-3). The myocardial muscle is injured as a result. Compression injuries can also include contusions and lacerations of solid organs and rupture of hollow (air-filled) organs.

During a change in speed, the body accelerates (increases) or decelerates (decreases), which may cause shearing or tearing injuries. An instance when the body

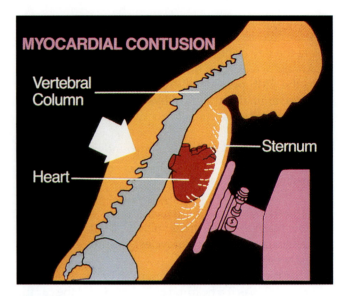

FIGURE 15-3 ▲   The heart or myocardium is injured from blunt trauma to the chest. (From National Association of Emergency Medical Technicians: *PHTLS: basic and advanced prehospital trauma life support*, ed 4, St Louis, 1999, Mosby.)

is going in a forward motion can be used as an example. When the head hits a stationary object, the brain slams against the front of the skull, which causes a bruise or laceration in the front and tearing of vessels in the back (Figure 15-4).

MOTOR VEHICLE COLLISIONS

The various injuries produced by blunt trauma are best illustrated through examination of motor vehicle collisions, although forces that cause blunt trauma can result from a variety of impacts. A motor vehicle collision involves three separate impacts as the energy is transferred: (1) the vehicle strikes an object, (2) the occupant collides with the inside of the car, and (3) the internal organs collide inside the body. The injuries that result from automobile accidents depend on the type of collision, the position of the occupant inside the vehicle, and the use or nonuse of active or passive restraint systems.

Motor vehicle collisions are classified by type of impact, including head-on, lateral, rear-end, rotational, and rollover. The forces of compression and change of speed produce predictable injury patterns in each type of collision.

Head-On (Frontal) Impact—Head-on collisions result when forward motion stops abruptly (e.g., when one automobile collides with another traveling in the opposite direction). The first collision occurs when the automobile hits the second vehicle, resulting in damage to the front of the car. As the vehicle abruptly stops, the occupant continues to move at the speed of the automobile before impact. The front seat

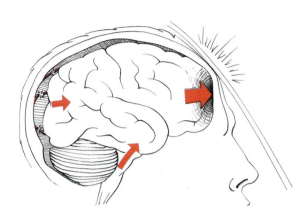

FIGURE 15-4 ▲ Even after the forward motion of the skull has stopped, the brain continues to move forward inside the skull, causing injury. (From Sanders MJ: *Mosby's paramedic textbook*, ed 2, St Louis, 2000, Mosby.)

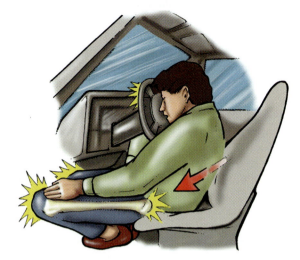

FIGURE 15-5 ▲ Down and under. (From American College of Emergency Physicians; Pons PT, Cason D, chief editors: *Paramedic field care: a complaint-based approach*, St Louis, 1997, Mosby for ACEP.)

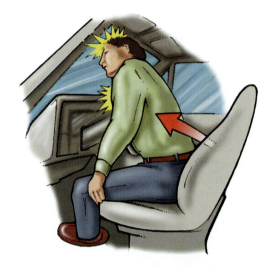

FIGURE 15-6 ▲ Up and over. (From American College of Emergency Physicians; Pons PT, Cason D, chief editors: *Paramedic field care: a complaint-based approach*, St Louis, 1997, Mosby for ACEP.)

occupant continues forward into the restraint system, steering column, or dashboard, resulting in the second collision. The occupant who is not restrained usually travels in one of two pathways in relationship to the dashboard: down and under or up and over. The precise course of this pathway determines how the organs collide inside the body and the extent of tissue damaged.

In the down-and-under pathway, the occupant travels downward into the vehicle seat and forward into the dashboard or steering column (Figure 15-5). The knees become the leading part of the body, striking the dashboard, with the upper legs absorbing most of the impact. Predictable injuries include knee dislocation, patellar fracture, femur fracture, fracture or posterior dislocation of the hip, fracture of the acetabulum, vascular injury, and hemorrhage. After the initial impact of the knees into the dashboard, the body rotates forward. As the chest wall hits the steering column or dashboard, the head and torso absorb energy as indicated in the description of the up-and-over pathway.

In the up-and-over pathway, as the body in forward motion strikes the steering wheel, the ribs and underlying structures absorb the momentum of the thorax (Figure 15-6). Predictable injuries from this transfer of energy include rib fracture, ruptured diaphragm, hemopneumothorax, pulmonary contusion, cardiac contusion, myocardial rupture, and vascular disruption (most notably, aortic rupture).

If the abdomen is the point of impact, compression injuries can occur to the hollow abdominal organs, solid organs, and lumbar vertebrae. The kidneys, liver,

and spleen are subject to vascular tears from supporting tissue, including the disruption of real vessels from their points of attachment to the inferior vena cava and descending aorta. Predictable injuries include liver laceration, spleen rupture, internal hemorrhage, and abdominal organ movement into the thorax (ruptured diaphragm).

If the occupant's head is the leading point of impact, the cervical vertebrae absorb the continued momentum of the body. Cervical flexion, axial loading, and/or hyperextension (further described in Chapter 19) can result in fracture or dislocation of the cervical vertebrae. In addition, severe angulation of the cervical vertebrae can damage the soft tissues of the neck and cause spinal cord injury and spinal instability, even without fracture. Other predictable injuries include trauma to the brain (e.g., concussion, contusion, shearing injury, edema) and intracranial vascular disruption, resulting in subdural or epidural hematoma.

Lateral or Side Impact—Lateral impact occurs when a vehicle is struck from the side. Injury patterns depend on whether the damaged automobile remains in place or moves away from the point of impact. The external shell of an automobile that remains in place after impact usually intrudes into the passenger compartment, directing force at the lateral aspect of the occupant's body (Figure 15-7). Predictable injuries result from compression to the torso, pelvis, and extremities. Examples of these injuries include fractured ribs, pulmonary contusion, ruptured liver or spleen (depending on the side involved), fractured clavicle, fractured pelvis, and head and neck injury (Figure 15-8). Some automobiles are equipped with side-impact air bags that can guard against injury in some lateral impacts.

If the damaged vehicle moves away from the point of impact, the occupant accelerates away from the point of impact, moving laterally with the car. The effects of inertia on the head, neck, and thorax produce lateral flexion and rotation of the cervical spine. This movement can result in neurological injury and tears or strains of the lateral ligaments and supporting structures of the neck. Injuries can also occur on the side of the passenger opposite the impact as the occupant is propelled toward the other side of the car. If other oc-cupants are in the automobile, secondary collisions with other passengers are likely.

Rear-End Impact—A vehicle struck from behind rapidly accelerates, causing the vehicle to move forward under the occupant. The greater the difference in the forward speed of the two vehicles, the greater the force and damaging energy of the initial impact. For example, if a vehicle traveling 50 mph strikes a stationary vehicle, the damaging energy is greater than when a vehicle traveling 50 mph strikes a vehicle traveling 30 mph. Thus in forward collisions the sum of both vehicles' speeds is the velocity that produces damage. In rear-end collisions the difference between the two speeds is the damaging velocity.

Predictable injuries in rear-end collisions include back and neck injuries and cervical strain or fracture caused by hyperextension. The cervical portion of the spine is particularly susceptible to secondary hyperextension, which is caused by the rapid forward acceleration of the vehicle and subsequent relative rearward forces on the occupant. For example, if the occupant has his or her headrest up, the head moves with the seat. If the headrest is down and not in a position to prevent hyperextension of the neck over the top of the seat, tearing of the neck's ligaments and supporting anterior structures often occurs (Figure 15-9). If the automobile undergoes a second collision by striking an object in front of it, injuries may occur in association with frontal impact.

If it can be proved that the victim's headrest was not properly positioned when the neck injury occurred, some courts consider reducing the liability of the party at fault in the collision on the grounds that the victim's negligence contributed to his or her injuries (contribu-

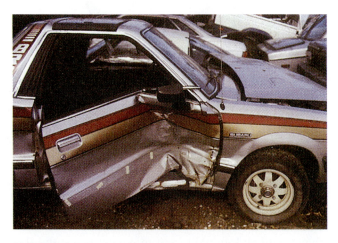

FIGURE 15-7 ▲ Intrusion of the side panels into the passenger compartment provides another source of basic injury. (From National Association of Emergency Medical Technicians: *PHTLS: basic and advanced prehospital trauma life support,* ed 4, St Louis, 1999, Mosby.)

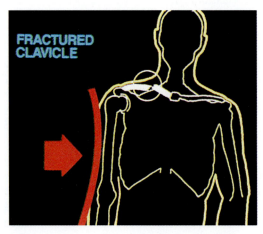

FIGURE 15-8 ▲ Compression of the shoulder against the clavicle produces midshaft fractures of this bone. (From National Association of Emergency Medical Technicians: *PHTLS: basic and advanced prehospital trauma life support,* ed 4, St Louis, 1999, Mosby.)

tory negligence). Similar measures have been considered in cases of failure to use occupant restraints.

Rotational Impact—Rotational impacts occur when an off-center portion of the automobile (usually the front quarter) strikes an immovable object or one that is moving more slowly or in the opposite direction. The part of the vehicle striking the object stops during impact. The remainder of the vehicle continues in forward motion until the energy is completely transformed. The occupant moves inside the vehicle with the forward motion and usually is struck by the side of the car as the vehicle rotates around the point of impact. A rotational impact results in injuries common to both head-on and lateral collisions.

Rollover Impact—In rollover crashes or collisions, the occupant tumbles inside the automobile and is injured wherever the body strikes the vehicle (Figure 15-10). The various impacts occur at many different angles, which can cause multisystem injuries. Predictable injuries sustained in roll-over collisions are difficult to categorize. These crashes can produce any of the injury patterns associated with other types of collisions.

RESTRAINTS

Public awareness programs in personal safety and various state laws regarding seat belt protection have increased automobile occupant use of personal restraints in recent years. According to the National Safety Council, among passenger vehicle occupants over 4 years of age,

seat belts saved an estimated 10,750 lives in 1997. An additional 9600 lives could have been saved if *all* passengers over 4 years of age had worn seat belts.[4]

A significant hazard to unrestrained occupants is ejection from the vehicle after impact. One of every 13 ejection victims suffers a spinal fracture, and ejected victims are killed six times more often than those who are not ejected.[1] The high mortality rate among ejected victims results in part from the occupant being subjected to a second impact as the body strikes the ground or another object outside the vehicle.

The four types of restraints available in the United States are lap belts, diagonal shoulder straps, air bags, and child safety seats, all of which significantly reduce injuries. If they are inappropriately worn, however, these protective devices also can produce injuries.

Lap Belts—The lap belt, used alone or in conjunction with a diagonal shoulder strap, is the most commonly used active restraint. When properly applied, the lap belt is directed at a 45-degree angle to the floor between the anterior-superior iliac spine and the femur (Figure 15-11). A lap belt worn tightly enough to remain in this position absorbs energy forces and protects the abdominal cavity by transferring energy to the strong, bony pelvis.

If the lap belt is worn incorrectly above the anterior-superior iliac spine, the forward motion of the body during impact is absorbed by vertebrae T12, L1, and L2 (Figure 15-12). As the thorax is propelled forward, the abdominal organs are compressed between the vertebral column and the lap belt, which can cause injury to the liver, spleen, duodenum, and pancreas. An indicator of these abdominal injuries is the presence of abrasions or a lap belt imprint over the abdomen.

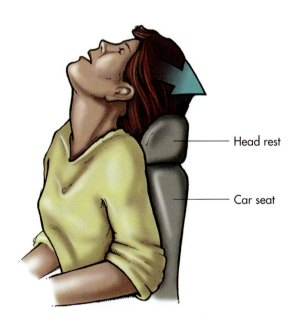

FIGURE 15-9 ▲ Hyperextension occurs from an improperly placed headrest. (From American College of Emergency Physicians; Pons PT, Cason D, chief editors: *Paramedic field care: a complaint-based approach,* St Louis, 1998, Mosby for ACEP.)

Head rest

Car seat

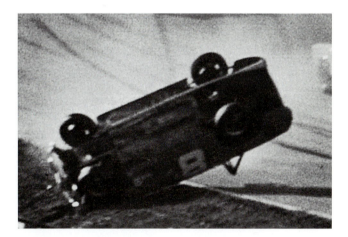

FIGURE 15-10 ▲ During a rollover, the unrestrained occupant can be wholly or partially ejected out of the car or can bounce around inside the car. This action produces multiple and somewhat unpredictable injuries, but they are usually severe. (From National Association of Emergency Medical Technicians: *PHTLS: basic and advanced prehospital trauma life support,* ed 4, St Louis, 1999, Mosby.)

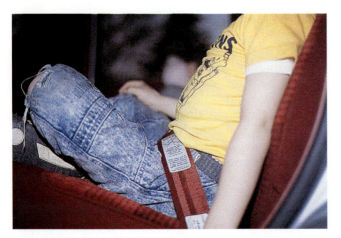

FIGURE 15-11 ▲ Correct position for lap belts on children. (From McSwain NE et al: *The basic EMT: comprehensive prehospital patient care,* ed 2, St Louis, 2001, Mosby.)

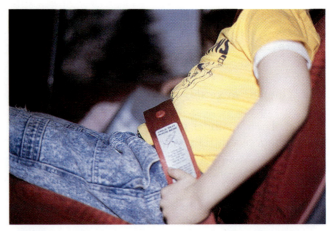

FIGURE 15-12 ▲ Incorrect position for lap belts on children. (From McSwain NE et al: *The basic EMT: comprehensive prehospital patient care,* ed 2, St Louis, 2001, Mosby.)

Significant injury can result even when the occupant uses a lap belt correctly. These injuries occur from angulation of the lumbar spine, pelvis, thorax, and head around the restraint system and from failure of the restraint system to sufficiently decrease the impact forces. In addition, the upper torso is not restrained, so head and neck injuries may be common. Injuries that can occur during high-speed impacts include sternal fractures, chest wall injuries, lumbar vertebral fractures, head injuries, and maxillofacial trauma.

Diagonal Shoulder Straps—Use of a diagonal shoulder strap helps absorb the forward motion of the thorax after impact. When the occupant wears the shoulder strap with the lap belt, the shoulder strap prevents the thorax, face, and head from striking the dashboard, windshield, or steering column. Clavicular fracture can result from the position of the shoulder strap. Organ collision inside the body with resultant internal organ injury, cervical fracture, and spinal cord injury can still occur during high-speed impacts, even when personal restraint systems are used.

Air Bags—Although some automobiles are equipped with side-impact air bags to protect against lateral impacts, the more common air bag is a frontal air bag that inflates from the center of the steering wheel or dashboard during frontal impact. These devices cushion the forward motion of the occupant when used with a lap and shoulder belt. Frontal air bags deflate rapidly and are effective only with an initial frontal collision. They are ineffective in lateral or roll-over impacts. These systems do not prevent movement in the down-and-under pathway. Thus the occupant's knees may still be the point of impact, resulting in leg, pelvis, and abdominal injuries.

An air bag can produce significant injury if it is deployed in close proximity (10 inches or closer) to the occupant. Deployment in these situations can produce spinal fractures, hand and eye injury, and facial and forearm abrasions (Figure 15-13). The following groups are at higher risk of injury from air bag deployment[5]:

- Infants and children under 12 years of age
- Adults less than 5 feet 2 inches tall
- Older adults
- Persons with special medical conditions

Children under 12 years of age, including infants in rear-facing safety seats, should not ride in the front seat of a vehicle with a passenger side air bag. Instead, they should ride in the rear seat.

Child Safety Seats—The leading cause of death in children under 4 years of age is injuries sustained in motor vehicle crashes. For each of these deaths, the U.S. Department of Health, Education, and Welfare estimates that thousands more suffer debilitating injury. The National Safety Council reports that an estimated 2894 lives have been saved by child restraints from 1975 through 1997, with 412 in 1997 alone.

All 50 states and the District of Columbia now require child safety seats for select age-groups of children. The seats are available in several shapes and sizes to accommodate the different stages of physical development, including infant carriers, booster seats, and toddler seats (Figure 15-14). Child safety seats use a combination of lap belts, shoulder belts, full-body harnesses, and harness-and-shield apparatus to protect the child during vehicle collision. Predictable injuries likely to occur even with the appropriate use of child safety seats include blunt abdominal trauma, change-of-speed injuries from deceleration forces, and neck and spinal injuries.

A significant amount of misuse of child safety seats (e.g., location, installation, and strapping) occurs. Public education in their correct use is an important prevention measure. Many ambulance services, fire departments, and other community agencies offer free car seat safety checks so that parents may have their child's seat inspected. The "inspectors" review proper use of the

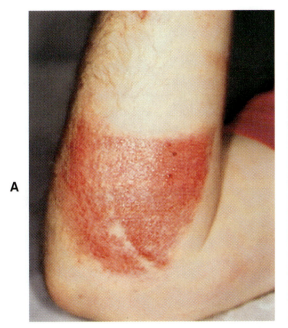

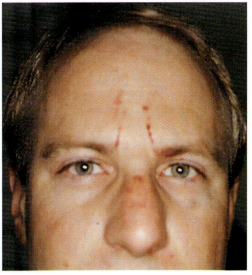

FIGURE 15-13 ▲ **A,** Abrasions of the forearm are secondary to rapid expansion of the air bag when the hands are tight against the steering column. **B,** Expansion of the air bag into eyeglasses produces abrasions. (From McSwain NE et al: *The basic EMT: comprehensive prehospital patient care,* ed 2, St Louis, 2001, Mosby.)

seat, where to position it in the vehicle, and how to properly secure it.

ORGAN COLLISION INJURIES

Organ motions and their injuries are a result of deceleration and compression forces. Recognition of these injuries requires a high degree of suspicion using the principles of kinematics.

Deceleration Injuries—When body organs are put into motion after an impact, they continue to move in opposition to the structures that attach them to the body. Therefore there is a risk of separation of body organs from their attachments. Injury to the vascular pedicle or mesenteric attachment can lead to brisk or exsanguinating hemorrhage. See later chapters for specific head, thoracic, and abdominal injuries.

Compression Injuries—Compressive forces can injure any portion of the body. See later chapters for specific injuries to the head, thorax, and abdomen.

OTHER MOTORIZED VEHICULAR COLLISIONS

Injuries from other motorized vehicular collisions include those involving motorcycles, all-terrain vehicles (ATVs), snowmobiles, motor boats, water bikes, jet skis, and farm machinery. This text discusses motorcycles and ATVs because of their common recreational use and popularity.

Small motorized vehicles are considered to be more dangerous than other motor vehicles because they

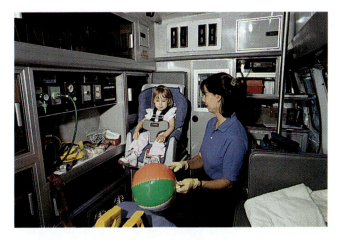

FIGURE 15-14 ▲ Child in child safety seat.

offer minimal protection to the rider from the transfer of energy associated with collisions. The injuries sustained in small motorized vehicle crashes usually are more severe than those received from automobile crashes. As with other types of motor vehicle collisions, predictable injuries depend on the type of collision that occurs.

Motorcycle Collision—According to the National Highway Traffic Safety Administration (NHTSA), about 55,000 motorcycle riders and passengers are injured each year, and more than 2000 die from their injuries. Common motorcycle collisions result from head-on impact, from angular impact, and from laying the motorcycle down.

Head-On Impact—A motorcycle's center of gravity is above the front axle, forward of the rider's seat. When the motorcycle strikes an object that stops its forward motion, the rest of the bike and the rider continue forward until acted on by an outside force (Figure 15-15). Typically, the motorcycle tips forward and the rider is propelled over the handlebars. Secondary impacts with the handlebars or other objects stop the forward motion of the rider.

Predictable injuries caused by these secondary impacts include head and neck trauma and compression injuries to the chest and abdomen. If the feet remain on the footrests during impact, the midshaft of the femur absorbs the rider's forward motion, which can result in bilateral fractures to the femur and lower leg (Figure 15-16). Severe perineal injuries can result if the rider's groin strikes the tank or handlebars of the motorcycle.

Angular Impact—When a motorcycle strikes an object at an angle, the rider often is caught between the cycle and the second object. Predictable injuries include crushing-type injuries to the patient's affected side, such as open fractures to the femur, tibia, and fibula, and fracture and dislocation of the malleolus.

Laying the Motorcycle Down—Professional racers and recreational riders often use the strategy of laying the motorcycle down before striking an object (Figure 15-17). This protective maneuver separates the rider from the motorcycle and the object by allowing the rider to slide away from the bike.

Predictable injuries include massive abrasions ("road rash") and fractures to the affected side as the rider slides on the ground or pavement. Although these injuries can be severe, they usually are less serious that those that occur from other types of impacts.

All-Terrain Vehicles—Injuries from crashes involving ATVs are different from those seen in motorcycle collisions. ATVs have a higher center of gravity than motorcycles (Figure 15-18). Those vehicles with three wheels have a large, flat front tire that makes them difficult to steer. A specific balance different than that required for riding motorcycles or bicycles is necessary to keep the "three-wheeler" from overturning.

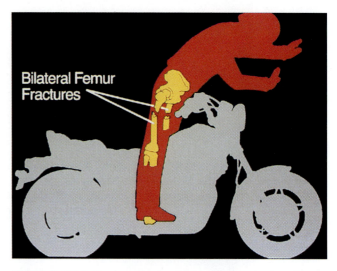

Bilateral Femur Fractures

FIGURE 15-16 ▲ The body travels forward and over the motorcycle, impacting the thighs and femurs into the handlebars. The driver can also be ejected. (From National Association of Emergency Medical Technicians: *PHTLS: basic and advanced prehospital trauma life support,* ed 4, St Louis, 1999, Mosby.)

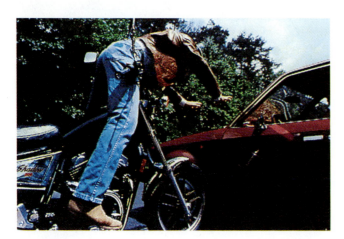

FIGURE 15-15 ▲ The position of a motorcycle driver is above the pivot point of the front wheel as the motorcycle impacts an object head-on. (From National Association of Emergency Medical Technicians: *PHTLS: basic and advanced prehospital trauma life support,* ed 4, St Louis, 1999, Mosby.)

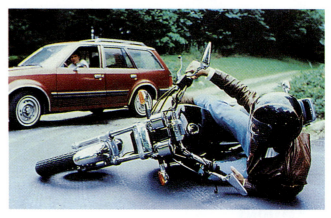

FIGURE 15-17 ▲ To prevent being trapped between two pieces of steel (motorcycle and automobile), the rider will frequently lay the motorcycle down to dissipate the injury. This often causes abrasions (road burns) as the rider's speed is slowed on the asphalt. (From National Association of Emergency Medical Technicians: *PHTLS: basic and advanced prehospital trauma life support,* ed 4, St Louis, 1999, Mosby.)

Many states now ban "three-wheelers" because of the injuries associated with these vehicles. "Four-wheelers" are more common because of the supposed increased stability with two front wheels as opposed to one.

The natural tendency of the rider to put a foot down to support the ATV when stopping can lead to the rear tire running over the rider's foot, catching the leg, and throwing the rider forward off the vehicle and onto his or her shoulder or crushing the rider. In addition, hidden wires can be a hazard as the rider goes through a presumed "empty" field and is caught across the neck or chest by the "invisible" wire.

Predictable injuries from ATV collisions include extremity injuries and fractures, and clavicular fractures. Serious head and neck injuries are also common. Other injuries can occur if the rider is thrown from the vehicle or the vehicle lands on top of the rider.

Personal Protective Equipment—Protective equipment for riders of small motorized vehicles include boots, leather clothing, eye protection, and helmets. Helmets are structured to absorb the energy of an impact, thereby reducing injuries to the face, skull, and brain. They are estimated to be 29% effective in preventing fatal injuries.[4] Injuries increase by more than 300% when helmets are not used.[1]

PEDESTRIAN INJURIES

In 1998, 145,000 people were injured in auto-pedestrian collisions in the United States. Of those injuries, 5900 were fatal.[4] All auto-pedestrian collisions can produce serious injuries and require a high degree of suspicion for multisystem trauma.

Three primary mechanisms of injury (multiple impacts) exist in auto-pedestrian collisions. The first impact occurs when the bumper of the vehicle strikes the body, the second occurs as the pedestrian strikes the hood of the vehicle, and the third occurs when the pedestrian strikes the ground or another object.

Predictable injuries depend on whether the pedestrian is an adult or a child. Variations in the height of the pedestrian in relation to the bumper and hood of the car affect the injury pattern. The velocity of the vehicle also is a major factor. However, even low speeds can result in serious trauma because of the mass of the vehicle and the transfer of energy. Another consideration in evaluating the auto-pedestrian incident is the possibility of the patient's suffering a second collision from another vehicle.

Adult Pedestrian—Most adult pedestrians threatened by an approaching vehicle attempt to protect themselves by turning away from the oncoming automobile (Figure 15-19). Therefore injuries often are a result of lateral or posterior impacts. During the initial impact, the adult usually is struck by the vehicle bumper in the lower legs, producing lower extremity fractures.

The second impact occurs as the pedestrian falls toward the hood of the vehicle. This impact can result in fractures to the femur, pelvis, thorax, and spine and produce intraabdominal or intrathoracic injuries. The head and spine also can be injured if the victim strikes the hood or windshield.

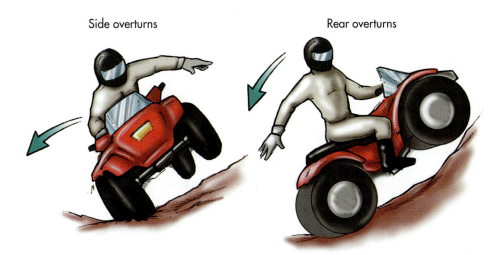

Side overturns   Rear overturns

FIGURE 15-18 ▲ All-terrain vehicles (ATVs) are prone to rollovers because of their high center of gravity and oversized wheels. (From American College of Emergency Physicians; Pons PT, Cason D, chief editors: *Paramedic field care: a complaint-based approach*, St Louis, 1997, Mosby for ACEP.)

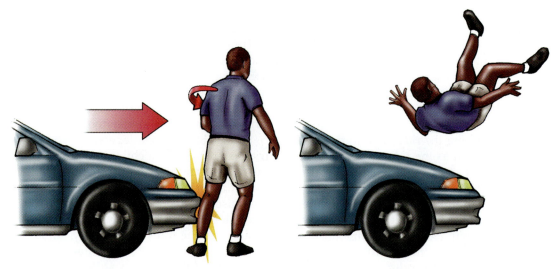

FIGURE 15-19 ▲ When an adult pedestrian is struck, he or she often turns, is struck on the side of the body, and is thrown onto the hood and/or windshield. (From American College of Emergency Physicians; Pons PT, Cason D, chief editors: *Paramedic field care: a complaint-based approach*, St Louis, 1997, Mosby for ACEP.)

The third impact occurs as the victim strikes the ground or is thrown against another object. This action can result in significant damage to the hip and shoulder of the affected side as the body makes contact with the surface on which it lands. Sudden deceleration and compression forces associated with this impact can cause fractures, internal hemorrhage, and head and spinal injuries.

Child Pedestrian—Unlike adults, who try to protect themselves from auto-pedestrian injury, children tend to face the oncoming vehicle. Therefore their injuries are often the result of a frontal impact. Because children are smaller than most adults, the initial impact of the automobile occurs higher on the body, usually above the knees or pelvis. Predictable injuries from the initial impact include fractures to the femur and pelvic girdle, as well as internal hemorrhage.

The second impact occurs as the front of the vehicle's hood continues forward, making contact with the victim's thorax. The victim immediately is thrown backward, forcing the head and neck to flex forward. Depending on the position of the child in relation to the automobile, the head and neck may contact the vehicle's hood. Predictable injuries include abdominal, pelvic, thoracic, and facial trauma, as well as head and neck injuries.

The third impact occurs as the child is thrown downward. Because of the child's smaller size and weight, he or she can fall under the vehicle and be dragged for some distance or fall to the side of the vehicle and be run over by the front or rear wheels. Predictable injuries consist of those previously described and may also include traumatic amputation.

OTHER CAUSES OF BLUNT TRAUMA

Blunt trauma can also be caused by vertical falls, sports injuries, and blast injuries.

Vertical Falls—In 1998, falls accounted for 16,000 deaths and were the second leading cause of accidental death in the United States.[4] More than half of all falls occur in the home, with four out of five involving a person 65 years of age or older.[4] In predicting injuries associated with falls, the EMT–I should evaluate the distance fallen, the body position of the patient on impact, and the type of surface on which the patient landed. Injuries associated with vertical falls are a result of deceleration and compression (Figure 15-20).

Although falls from some levels are rarely associated with fatal injury, falls from distances greater than three times the height of an individual (15 to 20 feet) are more likely to be associated with severe injuries. As a point of reference for these distances, the roof of a one-story house is about 15 feet from the ground, and the roof of a two-story house is about 30 feet from the ground.

Adults who have fallen more than 15 feet usually land on their feet. A predictable injury from this vertical fall is bilateral calcaneus fractures. As the energy is distributed from the initial impact, the head, torso, and pelvis push downward and force the body into flexion. When this pattern occurs, hip dislocation and compression fractures of the spinal column in the thoracic and lumbar areas are seen. About 10% of patients with calcaneal fracture have associated spinal fractures. If the patient leans forward or attempts to break the fall with outstretched hands, bilateral Colles' fractures to the wrists are likely.

If the distance fallen is less than 15 feet, most adults land in the position in which they fell. For example, an

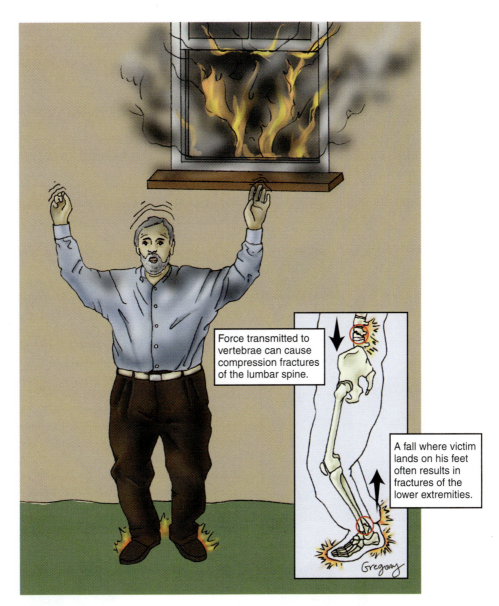

Force transmitted to vertebrae can cause compression fractures of the lumbar spine.

A fall where victim lands on his feet often results in fractures of the lower extremities.

FIGURE 15-20 ▲ Vertical falls produce deceleration and compression injuries.

adult who falls head first strikes the landing surface with the head, arms, or both. Predictable injuries depend on the body part that strikes the landing surface and the route of transfer of energy through the body. The EMT–I should suspect internal injuries if the trunk of the body is the initial impact area.

Because their heads are proportionally larger and heavier, children tend to fall head first, regardless of the distance fallen or body position during the fall. For this reason, children who experience a vertical fall usually have some type of head injury.

Remember that the ability of the landing surface to absorb energy influences the severity of an injury. For example, less damage is expected from a fall down steps onto a carpeted floor than from a fall onto a cement or tile floor.

Sports Injuries—People of all ages participate in sports. Common sports associated with frequent in-

juries include contact sports (e.g., football, basketball, hockey, and wrestling), high-velocity activity sports (e.g., downhill skiing, water skiing, bicycling, roller-blading, and skateboarding), racquet sports (e.g., tennis), and water sports (e.g., swimming and diving). Although sporting activities provide a variety of health benefits, they can also produce severe injury. Sports-related injuries account for 15% of all spinal cord injuries in the United States each year.[2]

The following forces cause sports-related injuries: acceleration, deceleration, compression, twisting, hyperextension, and hyperflexion. The EMT–I should think about the following principles of kinematics when trying to predict sports injuries:

● What energy forces were transferred to the patient?
● To what part of the patient's body was the energy transferred?

- What associated injuries should be considered as a result of the energy transfer?
- How sudden was the acceleration or deceleration?
- Was compression, twisting, hyperextension, or hyperflexion involved in the injury?

If the patient used protective equipment, the EMT–I should evaluate it to help determine the mechanism of injury. For example, the condition and structural stability of a helmet can provide clues as to the amount of energy transferred to the patient during the injury. Other examples include broken skis, broken hockey sticks, and structural deformities of bicycles.

Blast Injuries—Blast injury is damage to a patient exposed to a pressure field that is produced by an explosion of volatile substances. Explosions of this nature primarily have been a wartime concern. However, in recent years the number of blast injuries from homemade bombs used in social protests, terrorist activities, and general violent acts has increased. Other causes include the following:

- Exploding automobile batteries
- Industrial use of volatile substances
- Chemical reactions in undercover drug laboratories
- Explosions in mining
- Transportation incidents or accidents involving hazardous materials

Blasts release large amounts of energy in the form of pressure and heat. If this release of energy is confined in a casing (e.g., a bomb), the pressure ruptures the casing and ejects fragments of the housing at a high velocity. The remaining energy is transmitted to the surrounding environment and can severely injure bystanders. Blast injuries are classified as *primary, secondary, tertiary,* and *miscellaneous* (Figure 15-21).

Primary Blast Injuries—Primary blast injuries result from sudden changes in environmental pressure. These injuries usually occur in gas-containing organs and cause the most severe damage when poorly supported tissue is displaced beyond its elastic limit. The organs and tissues most vulnerable to primary blast injury are the ears, lungs,

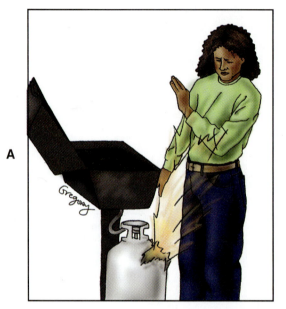

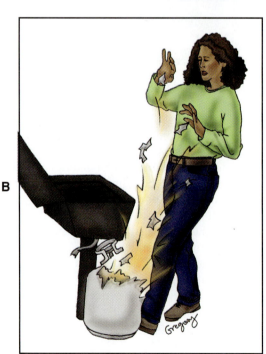

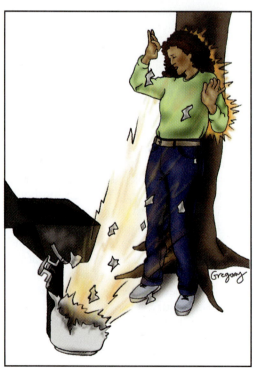

FIGURE 15-21 ▲ **A,** Primary blast injuries. **B,** Secondary blast injuries. **C,** Tertiary blast injuries.

central nervous system, and gastrointestinal tract. Predictable damage to these areas includes hearing loss, pulmonary hemorrhage, cerebral air embolism, abdominal hemorrhage, and bowel perforation. Thermal burns also can result from the release of energy in the form of heat (see Chapter 17 for more information on burns and emergency treatment). These injuries are likely to occur on unprotected areas that are close to the source of the explosion (e.g., the hands and face). In closed spaces, because of the blast reflection, victims farther from the explosion may be as severely injured as those close to the explosion.

Secondary Blast Injuries—Secondary blast injuries usually result when bystanders are struck by flying debris such as glass, metal, or falling mortar. In addition to the obvious injuries such as lacerations and fractures, flying debris can cause high-velocity, missile-type injuries if nails, screws, or casing fragments are part of the debris.

Tertiary Blast Injuries—Tertiary blast injuries occur when victims are propelled through space by an explosion and strike a stationary object. These injuries are similar to those sustained in vertical falls and ejections from automobiles or small motorized vehicles. In most cases the sudden deceleration from the impact causes more damage than the acceleration through space because the deceleration is more sudden. Injuries from these forces include damage to the abdominal viscera, central nervous system, and musculoskeletal system.

Miscellaneous Blast Injuries—Miscellaneous blast injuries result from radiation exposure and inhalation of dust and toxic gases. Predictable injuries include those to the eyes, lungs, and soft tissue.

Penetrating Trauma

With penetrating trauma, a permanent cavity is created when the skin is broken (e.g., an opening in the chest wall from a gunshot wound). This injury is usually more evident, because bleeding from the opening may be apparent.

Damage results from two types of forces: crushing and stretching. The character of the penetrating object, its speed of penetration, and the type of body tissue that it passes through or into determine which of the two mechanisms of injury predominates.

CAVITATION

Cavitation is an opening produced by a force that pushes body tissues laterally away from the tract of a projectile. The amount of cavitation produced by the transfer of energy is directly related to the density (number of particles) of tissue in a given body area and the ability of the body tissue to return to its original shape and position. For example, a person who receives a high-velocity blow to the abdomen experiences abdominal cavitation at the moment of impact (Figure 15-22, *A*). However, because of the lower density of the

abdominal musculature, the cavitation is temporary (lasting only a few milliseconds) even in the presence of severe intra-abdominal injury.

Permanent cavities are produced by penetrating injuries in which the transfer of energy exceeds the strength of the tissue (Figure 15-22, *B*). Tissues with high water density (e.g., liver, spleen, and muscle) or solid density (e.g., bone) are more prone to permanent cavitation. Certain injuries (stab wound to the abdomen) can produce cavitations as tissues are displaced in frontal and lateral directions.

ENERGY POTENTIAL

There are three energy levels to consider when discussing penetrating trauma: low energy, medium energy, and high energy.

Low Energy—Examples of weapons that have a low level of energy include those used by the attacker's hands, such as a knife, ax, needle, or ice pick (Figure 15-23). These weapons produce low-velocity injuries and can be determined by examining the path of the weapon into the body. The potential for more injury exists, however, if the attacker moves the weapon around once it has entered the body.

The more blunt the penetrating object, the more force that must be applied to cause penetration. The more force needed to cause penetration, the more tissue

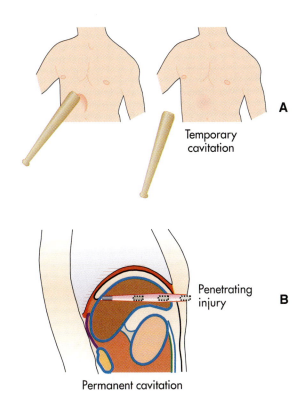

FIGURE 15-22 ▲ **A,** Temporary cavitation. **B,** Permanent cavitation. (From Sanders MJ: *Mosby's paramedic textbook,* ed 2, St Louis, 2000, Mosby.)

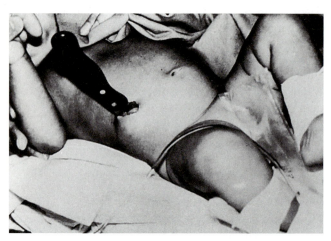

FIGURE 15-23 ▲ A stab wound is an example of a low-energy injury. (From Stoy W: *Mosby's EMT–Basic textbook,* St Louis, 1996, Mosby.)

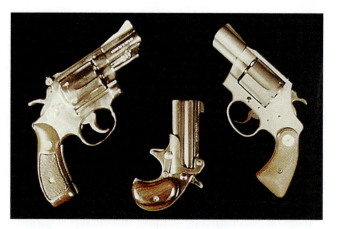

FIGURE 15-24 ▲ Medium-energy weapons are usually guns that have short barrels and contain cartridges with lesser power. High-energy weapons are assault rifles and hunting rifles. (From National Association of Emergency Medical Technicians: *Basic and advanced prehospital trauma life support,* ed 4, St Louis, 1999, Mosby.)

crushed. At the scene of a penetrating injury, the EMT–I should attempt to identify the type of wounding object and should consider the possibility of multiple wounds, embedded penetrating objects, extensive internal damage to organs of the thorax and abdomen, and penetration of multiple body cavities.

Stab wounds to the areas of the back and flank can cause penetrating hollow visceral injuries and injuries to retroperitoneal organs. Penetrating injuries of the thorax can involve the abdomen, just as abdominal injuries can involve the thorax.

Medium Energy—Handguns and some rifles are considered to have a medium level of energy (Figure 15-24). Whenever possible, the EMT–I should attempt to identify the type and caliber of the gun or rifle, as well as the approximate distance between the weapon and the patient (e.g., close range versus approximately 10 feet away). This information will help to estimate the amount of damage produced. In general, tissue will be damaged along the track of the bullet, as well as along the sides of the bullet's path (Figure 15-25).

High Energy—Hunting rifles, assault weapons, and any other type of weapon that discharges high-velocity missiles are considered to have a high level of energy (Figure 15-26). An increased amount of damage occurs to the sides of the path of the missile because of the increased energy.

ENTRANCE AND EXIT WOUNDS

With any type of penetrating injury, the EMT–I must determine the number of wounds present. Any entrance and exit wounds should be noted. Their presence is affected by several factors, including range, barrel length, caliber, powder, and weapon (Figure 15-27).

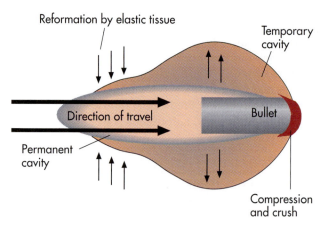

FIGURE 15-25 ▲ A bullet crushes tissues directly in its path. A cavity is created in the wake of the bullet. The crushed part is permanent. The temporary expansion can also produce injury. (From National Association of Emergency Medical Technicians: *Basic and advanced prehospital trauma life support,* ed 4, St Louis, 1999, Mosby.)

An entrance wound is usually round or oval and lies against the underlying tissue. It may be surrounded by an abrasion rim or collar. If the firearm is discharged at intermediate or close range, powder burns or tattooing may be present.

An exit wound, if present, is generally larger than an entrance wound because of the cavitational wave that occurs as the bullet passes through the tissues. As the bullet exits the body, the skin can "explode," resulting in ragged and torn tissue. This splitting and tearing often produce a starburst wound (Figure 15-28).

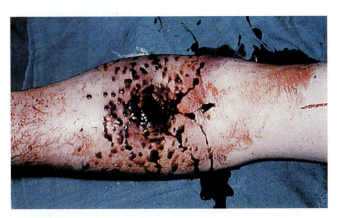

FIGURE 15-26 ▲ This entrance wound demonstrates a high-energy injury produced by a powerful shotgun. (From London PS: *A colour atlas of diagnosis after recent injury*, London, 1990, Mosby-Wolfe.)

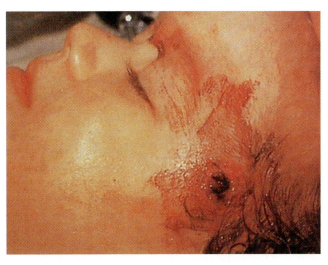

FIGURE 15-27 ▲ Wounds produced by handguns are examples of medium-energy injuries. (From London PS: *A colour atlas of diagnosis after recent injury*, London, 1990, Mosby-Wolfe.)

The EMT–I should treat all wounds, as well as describe and document their appearance, but refrain from commenting or speculating on which is the entry or exit wound. Identifying a wound as an entry or exit wound can result in the EMT–I's being served a subpoena to testify in court in an area that is beyond the scope of EMT–I practice.

GENERAL CONSIDERATIONS

Identification of ballistic injuries requires a thorough examination and a high degree of suspicion because penetrating trauma from high- and medium-velocity missiles is unpredictable. Whenever possible, precautions should be taken to preserve any evidence for any legal investigation (Box 15-4). However, lifesaving procedures always take precedence over forensic considerations.

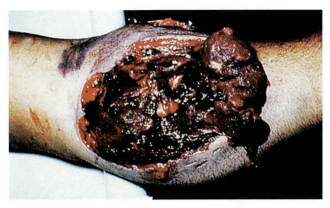

FIGURE 15-28 ▲ An exit wound caused by a powerful shotgun fired at close range. (From London PS: *A colour atlas of diagnosis after recent injury*, London, 1990, Mosby-Wolfe.)

IMPLICATIONS OF SOFT BODY ARMOR

Some EMS agencies have adopted the use of soft body armor (i.e., "bullet-proof" vests) as additional protection for emergency providers against blunt and penetrating trauma. Most agencies follow the U.S. Department of Justice guidelines to determine the type of body armor protection needed for the types of weapons most commonly found in their communities.

This equipment is effective against most handgun bullets and most knives. It provides protection by absorbing and distributing the impact of a ballistic missile or other penetrating object. However, it does not provide protection from high-velocity rifle bullets or thin or dual-edged weapons (e.g., ice picks). Like all other protective clothing, soft body armor is effective only when it is properly worn and when it is in good condition.

There are seven levels of body armor protection. Authorities generally recommend a type III or higher protection level for EMS providers.

When wearing body armor, the EMT–I should not develop a false sense of security from the device. *A general rule is never attempt a maneuver that would not normally be done without body armor.* In addition, be aware that body armor does not cover the entire body. Severe injury can still result from the forces of cavitation (in the absence of penetration) even when the vest is properly worn.

BOX 15-4

FORENSIC CONSIDERATIONS RELATED TO GUNSHOT WOUNDS

- Do not touch or move weapons or other environmental clues unless absolutely necessary for patient care procedures.
- Document the exact condition of the patient and wound appearance on arrival at the scene, including the environment of the patient and the body position in relation to objects and doorways.
- Disturb the scene as little as possible.
- If possible, cut or tear clothing along a seam to avoid altering tears made by a penetrating object.
- Avoid cutting through a bullet hole in the clothing.
- Do not shake clothing.
- Keep all clothing in a paper bag rather than a plastic bag that may alter evidence. Do not give these items to any of the victim's family members.
- Save any avulsed tissue for forensic pathology.
- If the bullet is retrieved, place it in a padded container to prevent any further damage.
- Secure all evidence until it is delivered to the authorities. Obtain a written receipt on delivery.

CASE HISTORY FOLLOW-UP ■ ■ ■

Before leaving the scene, EMT–I Fox talks with police officers to get a description of the knife and the assailant. She knows this information will be important in predicting the patient's internal injuries. The assailant was a man, and the knife had a 4-inch blade. The EMT–Is learned in EMT training that most men direct the knife upward when inflicting a stab wound. Based on the mechanism of injury, his knowledge of anatomy, and the length of the blade, EMT–I Walker suspects possible lacerations to his friend's liver, pancreas, lungs, bladder, and intestines.

Per protocol, en route, EMT–I Walker establishes two IV lines of lactated Ringer's solution, reassesses vital signs, and contacts medical direction. During the radio report, the patient tells EMT–I Walker that he feels faint and sick to his stomach. EMT–I Walker tells him to breathe slowly, but the patient starts to wretch and his intestines begin to eviscerate through the open wound in his abdomen. EMT–I Walker covers the protruding organs with wet, sterile dressings and secures the dressings in place. He prepares the suction and airway equipment and reassesses his friend's vital signs. The patient's blood pressure is dropping. He is now tachycardic and barely responsive. EMT–I Walker inflates the leg compartments of the PASG and elevates the foot of the backboard. He gives the trauma center an update and an estimated time of arrival of 5 minutes. They tell him they are waiting for their arrival and that the operating room staff is ready.

The EMT–Is deliver the injured patient to the emergency department. Before EMT–I Walker has had time to calm down from the call, his friend is on his way to surgery. On the way back to the base, the EMT–Is discuss the role of EMS in managing life-and-death situations, as well as routine interhospital transfers. They agree that both aspects are important in providing quality prehospital care. And yes, the EMT–Is both think the job is worth it.

SUMMARY

Important points to remember from this chapter include the following:

- Trauma is the leading cause of death among persons between 1 and 36 years of age and the fifth leading cause of death among all Americans.
- Trauma care is divided into three phases: preincident, incident, and postincident.
- Components of the trauma system include injury prevention, prehospital care, emergency department care, interfacility transportation if needed, definitive care, trauma critical care, rehabilitation, data collection, and trauma registry.
- Injuries are caused by a transfer of energy from some external source to the human body. The extent of injury is determined by the type of energy applied, how quickly it is applied, and to what part of the body it is applied.
- Blunt trauma is an injury produced by the wounding forces of compression and change of speed, which can disrupt tissues.
- The three restraining systems available in the United States are lap belts, diagonal shoulder straps, and air bags, all of which significantly reduce injuries. However, if they are inappropriately worn, these protective devices also can produce injuries.
- Organ motions and their injuries are a result of deceleration and compression forces. Recognition of these injuries requires a high degree of suspicion using the principles of kinematics.
- Small motorized vehicles, such as motorcycles, all-terrain vehicles (ATVs), snowmobiles, motor boats, water bikes, and farm machinery, are considered to be more dangerous than other motor vehicles because they offer minimal protection to the rider from the transfer of energy associated with collisions.

- All auto-pedestrian collisions can produce serious injuries and require a high degree of suspicion for multisystem trauma.
- Falls from greater than three times the height of an individual (15 to 20 feet) are associated with an increased incidence of severe injuries. In predicting injuries associated with falls, the EMT–I should evaluate the distance fallen, the body position of the patient on impact, and the type of landing surface struck.
- Blast injury is damage to a patient exposed to a pressure field that is produced by an explosion of volatile substances. Blasts release large amounts of energy in the form of pressure and heat.
- All penetrating objects, regardless of velocity, cause tissue disruption. The character of the penetrating object, its speed of penetration, and the type of body tissue it passes through or into determine whether crushing or stretching forces will cause injury.

REFERENCES

1. National Association of Emergency Medical Technicians: *PHTLS: basic and advanced prehospital trauma life support,* ed 4, St Louis, 1999, Mosby.
2. Sanders MJ: *Mosby's paramedic textbook,* ed 2, St Louis, 2000, Mosby.
3. US Department of Transportation, National Highway Traffic Safety Administration: *EMT–Intermediate national standard curriculum,* Washington, DC, 1998, The Department.
4. National Safety Council: *Injury facts,* Chicago, 1999, The Council.
5. American Heart Association: *Currents in emergency cardiac care,* vol 11, No. 3, Dallas, 2000, The Association.

16

Hemorrhage and Shock

Key Terms

...CASE HISTORY

EMT–Is Harris and Peters have been dispatched to a local residence for a medical emergency. En route, they are advised that a home-health nurse has requested transport of a patient to a nearby hospital. The patient is reported to be semiresponsive. No other information is available.

As the EMT–Is approach the neighborhood, they notice that all the homes look alike. The neighborhood is in an older, low-income area of town where most of the residents are elderly. The EMT–Is see the nurse waving them down at the front door. They pull into the driveway, gather their gear, and go into the house.

The nurse leads the EMT–Is to a back room where they find a frail, elderly woman lying on a bed. The room is dark and dingy. The nurse tells Harris and Peters that he was recently assigned this patient through social services. He knows little about the woman's medical history other than she is a cancer patient who had been treated at the city clinic for influenza last week. When he arrived 30 minutes ago, he found her in this condition. At that time, her vital signs were blood pressure 84/50, pulse 110, and respirations 24 and shallow. The patient's lung sounds revealed wheezing and fine crackles. She was hot to the touch with a fever of 101° F.

EMT–I Harris attempts to arouse the patient as EMT–I Peters inserts a nasal airway and applies high-concentration oxygen by nonrebreather mask. The woman groans and responds with purposeful movement. EMT–I Harris contacts medical direction and gives her patient report. The physician orders her to draw a "red top," perform a dextrose stick, and establish an intravenous (IV) line of lactated Ringer's solution. The woman's veins are difficult to see or palpate. EMT–I Harris attempts cannulation with a 16-gauge catheter in the patient's right forearm, but the vein blows and a hematoma quickly develops. A second attempt with an 18-gauge catheter in the left forearm is successful. The patient's serum glucose is normal. The EMT–Is prepare the pneumatic antishock garment, position the patient supine with her legs elevated 10 to 12 inches, package her, and move her to the ambulance. En route to the emergency department, EMT–I Harris sponges the patient's forehead with saline. Although she is not sure the woman can hear her, EMT–I Harris consoles her and tells her that she is in good hands.

CHAPTER GOAL

Upon completion of this chapter, the EMT–Intermediate will be able to use the assessment findings to formulate a field impression and implement the treatment plan for the patient with hemorrhage or shock.

Cognitive Objectives

As an EMT–Intermediate you should be able to do the following:

- Describe the epidemiology, including the morbidity, mortality, and prevention strategies for shock and hemorrhage.
- Discuss the anatomy and physiology of the cardiovascular system.
- Predict shock and hemorrhage based on mechanism of injury.
- Discuss the various types and degrees of hemorrhage and shock.
- Discuss the pathophysiology of hemorrhage and shock.
- Discuss the assessment findings associated with hemorrhage and shock.
- Identify the need for intervention and transport of the patient with hemorrhage or shock.
- Discuss the treatment plan for and management of hemorrhage and shock.
- Discuss the management of external hemorrhage.
- Differentiate between controlled and uncontrolled hemorrhage.
- Differentiate between the administration rate and amount of intravenous (IV) fluid in a patient with controlled versus uncontrolled hemorrhage.
- Relate internal hemorrhage to the pathophysiology of compensated and decompensated hemorrhagic shock.
- Relate internal hemorrhage to the assessment findings of compensated and decompensated hemorrhagic shock.
- Discuss the management of internal hemorrhage.
- Define shock based on aerobic and anaerobic metabolism.
- Describe the incidence, morbidity, and mortality of shock.
- Describe the body's physiologic response to changes in perfusion.
- Describe the effects of decreased perfusion at the capillary level.
- Discuss the cellular ischemic phase related to hemorrhagic shock.
- Discuss the capillary stagnation phase related to hemorrhagic shock.
- Discuss the capillary washout phase related to hemorrhagic shock.
- Discuss the assessment findings of hemorrhagic shock.
- Relate pulse pressure changes to perfusion status.
- Relate orthostatic vital sign changes to perfusion status.
- Define compensated and decompensated shock.
- Discuss the pathophysiological changes associated with compensated shock.
- Discuss the assessment findings associated with compensated shock.
- Identify the need for intervention and transport of the patient with compensated shock.
- Discuss the treatment plan and management of compensated shock.
- Discuss the pathophysiological changes associated with decompensated shock.
- Discuss the assessment findings associated with decompensated shock.

Continued

- Identify the need for intervention and transport of the patient with decompensated shock.
- Discuss the treatment plan and management of the patient with decompensated shock.
- Differentiate between compensated and decompensated shock.
- Relate external hemorrhage to the pathophysiology of compensated and decompensated hemorrhagic shock.
- Relate external hemorrhage to the assessment findings of compensated and decompensated hemorrhagic shock.
- Differentiate between the normotensive, hypotensive, and profoundly hypotensive patient.
- Differentiate between the administration of fluid in the normotensive, hypotensive, and profoundly hypotensive patient.
- Discuss the physiologic changes associated with the pneumatic anti-shock garment (PASG).
- Discuss the indications and contraindications for the application and inflation of the PASG.
- Apply epidemiology to develop prevention strategies for hemorrhage and shock.
- Integrate the pathophysiological principles to the assessment of a patient with hemorrhage or shock.
- Synthesize assessment findings and patient history information to form a field impression for the patient with hemorrhage or shock.

- Develop, execute, and evaluate a treatment plan based on the field impression for the hemorrhage or shock patient.

Psychomotor Objectives
As an EMT-Intermediate you should be able to do the following:

- Demonstrate the assessment of a patient with signs and symptoms of hemorrhagic shock.
- Demonstrate the management of a patient with signs and symptoms of hemorrhagic shock.
- Demonstrate the assessment of a patient with signs and symptoms of compensated hemorrhagic shock.
- Demonstrate the management of a patient with signs and symptoms of compensated hemorrhagic shock.
- Demonstrate the assessment of a patient with signs and symptoms of decompensated hemorrhagic shock.
- Demonstrate the management of a patient with signs and symptoms of decompensated hemorrhagic shock.
- Demonstrate the assessment of a patient with signs and symptoms of external hemorrhage.
- Demonstrate the management of a patient with signs and symptoms of external hemorrhage.
- Demonstrate the assessment of a patient with signs and symptoms of internal hemorrhage.
- Demonstrate the management of a patient with signs and symptoms of internal hemorrhage.

INTRODUCTION

Understanding and caring for the patient in shock is a challenge requiring keen assessment skills and the ability to make rapid, organized decisions. If treatment is performed inadequately or too late, the patient may die immediately from cardiac failure or may survive without brain function. The patient also may die in a few days to a few weeks, due to the failure of organs such as the lung, kidney, or liver.

This chapter addresses basics of oxygen intake and use and cardiovascular physiology, soft tissue injury, pathophysiology of hemorrhage and shock; and assessment and management of hemorrhage and shock.

Oxygen Intake and Use

Perfusion • The process by which oxygenated blood is delivered to the body tissues and wastes are removed from the tissues.

Diffusion • Movement of particles from an area of greater concentration to an area of lesser concentration.

All cells require oxygen to survive. The delivery of oxygenated blood to the tissues is known as **perfusion** (Figure 16-1). For oxygen to be delivered to the body's cells, four components must be in place. These factors are collectively known as the Fick principle (Figure 16-2).

1. *Inspiration of adequate oxygen in the atmospheric air.* This process requires adequate ventilation of the

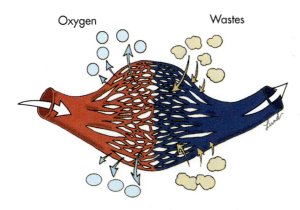

FIGURE 16-1 ▲ Perfusion is the delivery of oxygenated blood to the tissues. (Stacy Lund from Stoy W: *Mosby's EMT-Basic textbook,* St Louis, 1994, Mosby.)

lungs, a high concentration of inspired oxygen, and unobstructed flow through the air passageway.

2. *On-loading of oxygen to the red blood cells at the lungs.* This process requires minimal obstruction to the diffusion of oxygen across the alveolar/capillary membrane (i.e., no edema) and appropriate binding of oxygen to hemoglobin.

3. *Delivery of the red blood cells to the tissue cells.* This process requires normal hemoglobin levels, circulation of the oxygenated red blood cells to the tissues in need, adequate cardiac function, an adequate volume of blood flow, and proper routing of blood through the vasculature (blood vessels).

4. *Off-loading of oxygen from the red blood cells to the tissue cells.* This process requires close proximity of the tissue cells to the capillaries to allow for diffu-

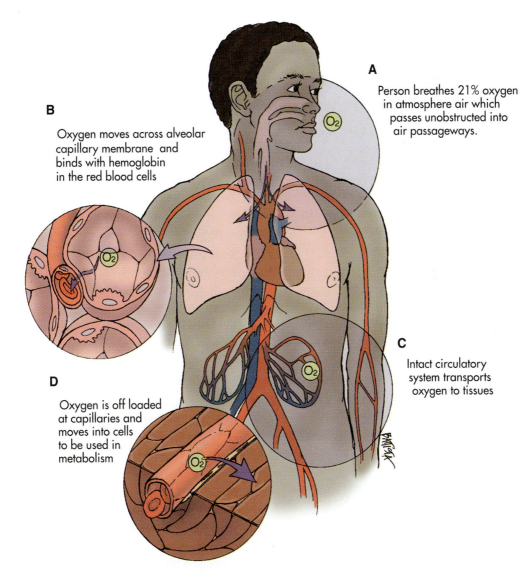

FIGURE 16-2 ▲ The four components of the Fick principle. **A,** Adequate ventilation of the lungs with a high concentration of oxygen. **B,** Oxygen binds with hemoglobin. **C,** Oxygen is transported via the circulatory system. **D,** Oxygen is off-loaded in the capillaries, and is used for metabolism.

sion of oxygen, and ideal conditions of pH and temperature.

The basic premise of the Fick principle is that the quantity of oxygen delivered to a body organ is equal to the amount of oxygen consumed by that organ plus the amount of oxygen carried away from the organ. For this process to function normally, there must be enough red blood cells available to deliver adequate amounts of oxygen to tissue cells.

Cellular Metabolism

The body is made up of billions and billions of cells. These cells require a continuous supply of oxygen and nutrients (e.g., the simple sugar glucose is the main energy source for the cells) to live. Depending on the workload and needs of the body, physiologic mechanisms ensure that appropriate nutrients and oxygen are available to allow the cells to carry out their life-sustaining functions.

Aerobic Metabolism • Metabolism that occurs with oxygen.

Cellular metabolism begins with food being broken down for energy in a series of reactions, called *cellular respiration.* The first part of this process can occur without oxygen; it is anaerobic. This step yields a very small amount of energy and produces a byproduct called *pyruvic acid.* In low-oxygen states, pyruvic acid is converted to lactic acid. Normally, lactic acid is produced in the muscles during periods of exertion and exercise. Although some small and primitive organisms, such as certain bacteria, can survive using anaerobic metabolism alone, humans cannot survive long with so little energy. A more complete use of food is necessary for survival. **Aerobic** (with oxygen) **metabolism** allows the human body to use food for energy more completely.

In aerobic metabolism the combination of oxygen and glucose fuels the individual cells and produces energy (Figure 16-3). Waste products such as carbon dioxide (CO_2) are produced as a by-product of this reaction and are moved away from the tissues into the blood. Wastes are excreted from the body by the lungs, kidneys, and liver. Oxygen also plays an important role in preventing the accumulation of lactic acid, a waste product that can cause muscle fatigue. The body can metabloize small amounts of lactic acid.

THE CARDIOVASCULAR SYSTEM

Under normal circumstances, the heart moves blood around inside a closed system of blood vessels (Figure 16-4). A closed system means that the blood is contained within the system with no opening to the outside. Oxygen is delivered to this system through the alveolar/capillary membrane of the lungs. It is then transported to the tissues. Absent or decreased delivery of

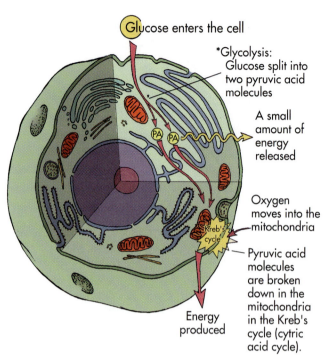

FIGURE 16-3 ▲ Aerobic metabolism occurs with oxygen and glucose to fuel the cell, and produce energy.

oxygen to the body's cells may occur if any of the components of the cardiovascular system are not functioning properly.

Stroke Volume

Stroke Volume • The amount of blood pumped into the cardiovascular system as a result of one heart contraction.

The amount of blood pumped into the cardiovascular system with each contraction of the heart is called the **stroke volume** (Figure 16-5). On average, the stroke volume amounts to 70 mL of blood with each contraction of the ventricles. The stroke volume is dependent on contractility, preload, and afterload.

Contractility

Contractility • The extent and velocity (quickness) of muscle fiber shortening.

The heart's function as a pump depends largely on its ability to contract. At the onset of contraction the ventricular walls begin squeezing the blood contained in the chamber. Pressure in the ventricle rises quickly and dramatically. When ventricular pressure exceeds pressure in the aorta and the pulmonary artery, the blood is ejected out of the ventricle. The rate at which the pressure rises in the ventricles is determined by how much and how fast the muscle fibers shorten. **Contractility** is the extent and velocity (quickness) of muscle fiber shortening.

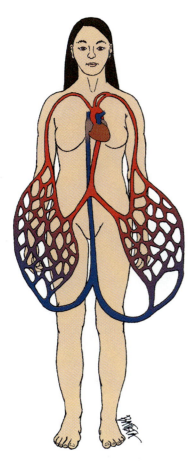

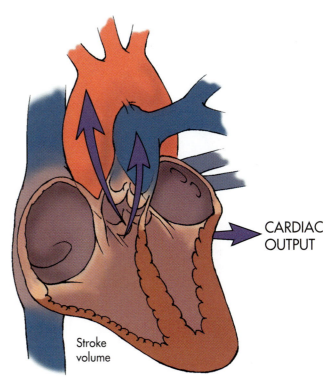

Stroke
volume

FIGURE 16-5 ▲ Stroke volume is the amount of blood output with each contraction of the heart.

CARDIAC
OUTPUT

FIGURE 16-4 ▲ Blood moves throughout the body in a closed system of blood vessels; the cardiovascular system. (Kimberly Battista from Stoy W: *Mosby's EMT-Basic textbook*, St Louis, 1994, Mosby.)

Myocardial contractility is influenced by oxygen supply and demand, degree of sympathetic stimulation, electrolyte balance, drug effects, and disease.

Calcium, an electrolyte, plays an important role in myocardial contraction. It triggers the action that causes muscle filaments to slide together, one on another. This action produces a shortening of the muscle fibers and subsequent myocardial contraction. Before the heart can contract, the myocardial cells must take in additional calcium ions through their cell membranes from the extracellular space.

Preload

✖ **Preload** • The passive stretching force exerted on the ventricular muscle at the end of diastole.

The heart muscle is stretched as the heart chambers fill with blood between contractions. This stretching of the muscle fibers before contraction increases the strength of the contraction (Figure 16-6). The volume of blood returning to the heart affects preload. More blood re-

turning increases preload, whereas less blood returning to the heart decreases preload. The more the myocardial muscles are stretched, the more forcefully they contract in systole. In certain pathologic processes there is an optimal point of stretch. If this point is exceeded, a decrease in the contractile state of the heart muscle results.

Afterload

✖ **Afterload** • The pressure the ventricular muscles must generate to overcome the higher pressure in the aorta.

Afterload (Figure 16-7) affects the stroke volume. The greater the afterload, the harder it is for the ventricles to eject blood into the arteries. To a large degree, afterload is dictated by the arterial blood pressure. Factors that increase afterload include obstruction of the aortic valve and circulatory fluid overload.

Blood Pressure

The **blood pressure** (Figure 16-8) is the force that blood exerts against the walls of the arteries as it passes through them. The blood pressure is equal to cardiac output times peripheral vascular resistance. Cardiac output is the amount of blood pumped by the heart each minute. It is a product of the heart rate times the stroke volume.

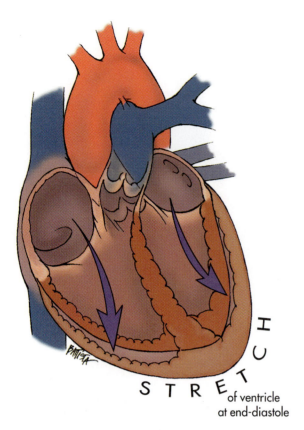

FIGURE 16-6 ▲ Preload is the heart's passive stretching force before it contracts.

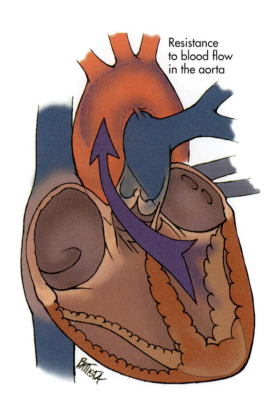

FIGURE 16-7 ▲ Afterload is the pressure necessary to overcome the pressure in the aorta.

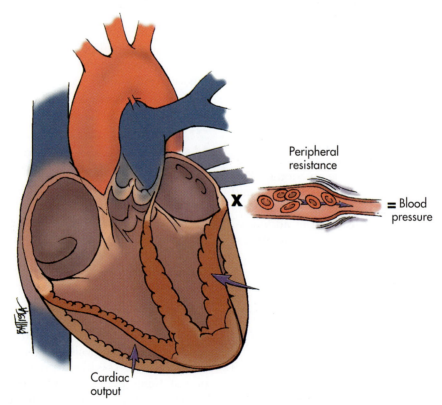

FIGURE 16-8 ▲ The elements of blood pressure: BP, cardiac output, peripheral resistance.

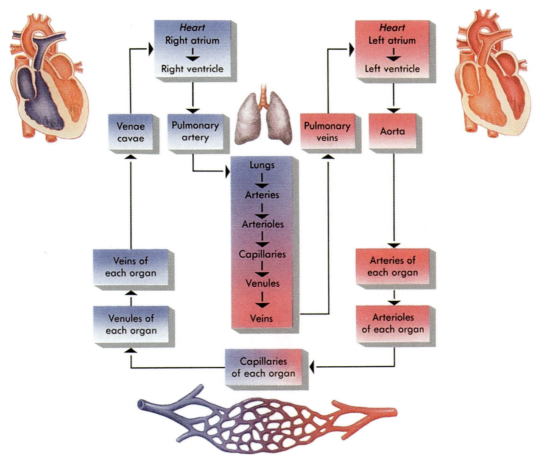

FIGURE 16-9 ▲ Blood flow through the cardiovascular system. (Rolin Graphics from Thibodeau GA, Patton KT: *The human body in health and disease,* St Louis, 1992, Mosby.)

Because the cardiovascular system is a closed system, increasing either cardiac output or peripheral vascular resistance increases blood pressure. Conversely, decreasing cardiac output or peripheral vascular resistance decreases blood pressure. Blood pressure also affects the perfusion of tissues. An abnormally low or high blood pressure can have an adverse effect on perfusion.

Blood Vessels

Collectively, the blood vessels are a continuous, closed, and pressurized pipeline moving blood throughout the body. Comprised of arteries, arterioles, capillaries, venules, and veins, the blood vessels make up the delivery system for the circulation (Figure 16-9).

The intravascular space is a closed system of blood vessels, sometimes referred to as the *container.* The blood vessels are elastic, and they change in size, adjusting the fluid volume of the container. The fluid volume of the container is directly related to the diameter of the blood vessels. Any dilation or constriction of the blood vessels will change the volume within the container. This change affects the amount

of blood returning to the heart and the amount of tissue oxygenation.

A number of regulatory mechanisms control blood flow to the tissues. First, microcirculation responds to local tissue needs. The blood vessels in the capillary network adjust their diameter to permit the microcirculation (Figure 16-10) to selectively supply undernourished tissue while temporarily bypassing tissues with no immediate need. The sympathetic nervous system also can directly stimulate the blood vessels to constrict or dilate, thereby redistributing blood to organs in need.

CLINICAL NOTES

A 70-kg adult man has a blood vasculature container size of about 5 liters. Though the size of any one person's container is relatively constant, the volume of the container is directly related to the diameter of the blood vessels (Figure 16-11).

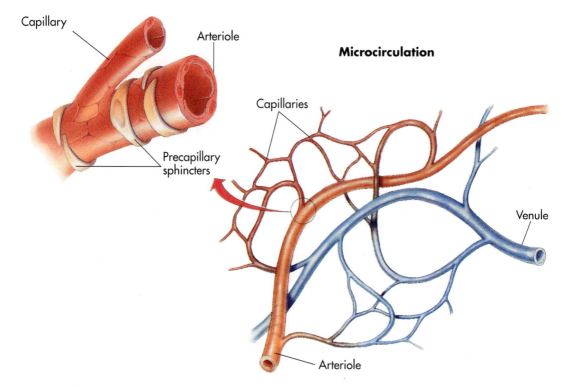

Microcirculation

FIGURE 16-10 ▲   The microcirculation system is composed of arterioles, capillaries, and venules. (Bill Ober; *inset,* Joan M. Beck from Thibodeau GA, Patton KT: *Anatomy and physiology,* ed 3, St Louis, 1996, Mosby.)

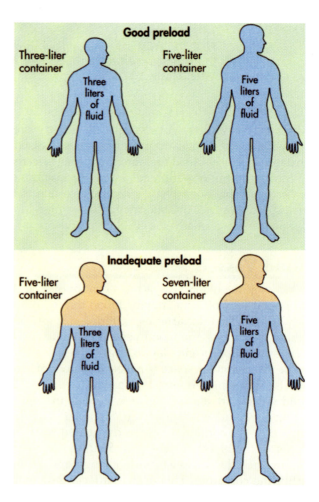

FIGURE 16-11 ▲   If the size of the human vascular container is greater than the amount of fluid, inadequate preload occurs, which leads to a decrease in cardiac output. (From Sanders M: *Mosby's paramedic textbook,* St Louis, 1994, Mosby.)

BLOOD

Blood has three functions: transportation, regulation, and protection. Blood delivers oxygen and nutrients to the cells and carries away waste products such as carbon dioxide. Buffers in the blood regulate the pH of the body. Finally, blood contains cells that protect the body against injury and disease. It is composed of cells, formed elements, and water.

Plasma ● The fluid or water portion of the blood.

The fluid, or water, portion of blood is called **plasma** and consists of approximately 55% of the total volume of blood. Plasma contains proteins, carbohydrates, amino acids, lipids, and mineral salts. The three major proteins of the plasma are albumin, globulin, and fibrinogen. Albumin is the most abundant plasma protein.

Erythrocytes ● Red blood cells.

Leukocytes ● White blood cells.

Hemoglobin ● A protein that binds oxygen to red blood cells.

The cells of the blood include **erythrocytes** (red blood cells) and **leukocytes** (white blood cells) (Figure 16-12). The erythrocytes are the most numerous of the blood's cells and have the ability to carry oxygen. **Hemoglobin,** a protein that contains iron, binds the oxygen to the red cells. This oxygen-hemoglobin complex makes it possible for the blood to efficiently transport large quantities of oxygen to the body cells. The combination of hemoglobin and oxygen gives blood its characteristic red color. The more oxygen there is, the brighter red the blood. Dark red blood has a decreased amount of oxygen.

Hematocrit ● The volume percentage of red blood cells in whole blood.

Hematocrit is a term used to identify the volume percentage of erythrocytes in whole blood (Figure 16-15). A hematocrit of 45 means that every 100 mL of whole blood has 45 mL of erythrocytes and 55 mL of plasma. The average hematocrit for a woman is 42 and 45 for a man. Leukocytes are outnumbered by erythrocytes 700 to 1 and tend to be colorless. The most important function of leukocytes is to destroy foreign organisms. They may accomplish this goal by producing antibodies or by directly attacking and killing bacterial invaders.

Platelets ● Formed elements suspended in plasma that are essential to blood clotting.

Platelets, which are not cells but formed elements, are suspended in the plasma. Platelets are essential for blood clotting. When blood comes into contact with something outside of the blood vessel, such as in an injury, platelets stick together and form a plug that seals the wound. Blood cells and platelets together comprise approximately 45% of total blood volume.

Blood is a viscous fluid, which is thicker and more adhesive than water. Because of this characteristic, it

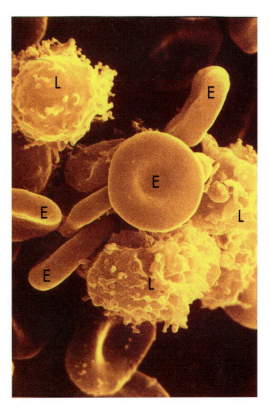

FIGURE 16-12 ▲ Erythrocytes *(E)* and leukocytes *(L).* (From NAEMT: *Prehospital trauma life support,* ed 3, St Louis, 1994, Mosby.)

flows more slowly than water. The viscosity (thickness) of the blood is determined by the ratio of plasma to cells and formed elements. The lesser the ratio of plasma to cells and formed elements, the greater the viscosity. Viscosity affects peripheral resistance—that is, the greater the viscosity, the greater the resistance. In shock, when there is a loss of plasma, peripheral resistance can be adversely increased.

The amount of blood in the body varies depending on the size of the individual. Blood accounts for approximately 8% of total body weight. In general, the average adult man who weighs 70 kg (154 lb) has approximately 5 L (5.2 quarts) of blood.

There must be enough blood to fill the container (the container is equal to the volume within the blood vessels of the cardiovascular system) and to carry oxygenated blood to the body's cells. Because the cardiovascular system is a closed system, the only way blood can escape is through a break in that system, such as in an injury. Even without blood being released from the system, the blood volume can fall due to an increase in the size of the system (increased diameter of the blood vessels).

SOFT-TISSUE TRAUMA

Soft-tissue trauma involves injury to the skin and surrounding structures. Injury can occur to the outer layer

Percentage by
body weight

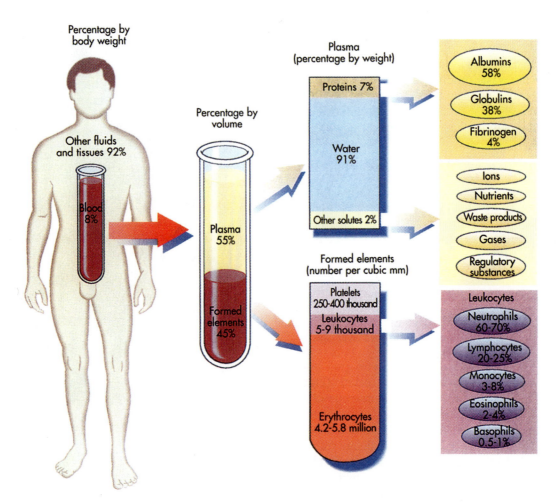

FIGURE 16-13 ▲ Composition of whole blood. (From Thibodeau GA, Patton KT: *Anatomy & physiology,* ed 3, St Louis, 1996, Mosby.)

(epidermis) or the inner layer (dermis). Nerves, blood vessels, subcutaneous tissue, muscles, ligaments, and so forth can be affected depending on the mechanism of injury.

It is important for the EMT–I to focus his or her skills on identifying and treating life-threatening injuries. Blood loss is the most serious complication of soft-tissue injury and can represent a direct threat to life. Adequate steps should be taken to control bleeding to combat the onset of hypovolemic shock and its associated hypoxemia. Without the presence of major bleeding, most soft-tissue injuries do not require immediate treatment. The EMT–I should not become distracted and waste precious time treating a soft-tissue injury if the patient has any multisystem trauma.

Closed Wounds

�֎ **Contusion** • Bruising below the dermis caused by blunt trauma.

✖ **Hematoma** • Swelling caused by leaking blood vessels below the dermis, caused by blunt trauma.

CONTUSIONS AND HEMATOMAS

Contusions and hematomas are caused by blunt trauma. With these injuries the blood vessels are torn beneath the dermis. Bruising or a contusion may result. The blood also may leak into deeper tissues and lead to swelling or a hematoma. A hematoma also may cause pain. Treatment includes applying cold to the area to encourage vasoconstriction, compressing the area to decrease bleeding, elevating the injured part whenever possible, and immobilizing when applicable to prevent motion.

CRUSH INJURIES

Crush injuries are caused by a crushing force applied to the body. They usually involve the extremities, torso, or pelvis (Figure 16-16). Crush injuries can result in blood vessel injury and internal organ rupture. Symptoms include pain, paresis, or weakness (late finding), paresthesia, pallor, and pulselessness in the extremity (late finding). Treatment for a patient who has a crush injury includes airway and breathing mangement, high-concentration oxygen, fluid replacement as needed (en

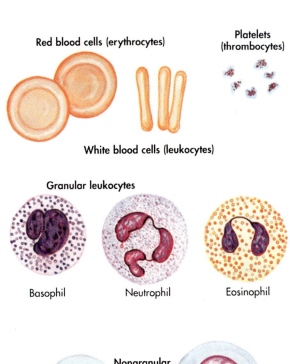

Red blood cells (erythrocytes)

Platelets (thrombocytes)

White blood cells (leukocytes)

Granular leukocytes

Basophil   Neutrophil   Eosinophil

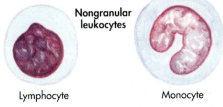

Nongranular leukocytes

Lymphocyte   Monocyte

FIGURE 16-14 ▲ **The formed elements of blood.** (From Thibodeau GA, Patton KT: *Anatomy & physiology,* ed 3, St Louis, 1996, Mosby.)

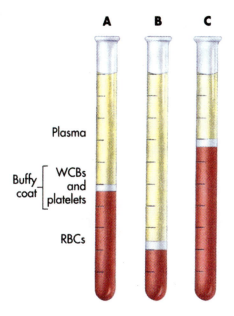

FIGURE 16-15 ▲ **Hematocrit tube showing normal percent of red blood cells.** (From Thibodeau GA, Patton KT: *Anatomy & physiology,* ed 3, St Louis, 1996, Mosby.)

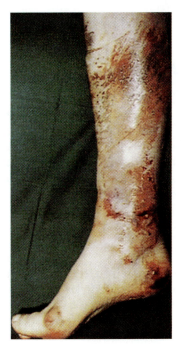

FIGURE 16-16 ▲ **The appearance of a crush injury to the leg.**

route unless the patient is entrapped), immobilization, and rapid transport to a trauma center.

COMPARTMENT SYNDROME

Compartment syndrome is considered a surgical emergency. It is caused by blunt trauma or compressive forces to areas with a minimal ability to stretch. It develops as bleeding and swelling, increased pressue in a closed area, which comprises circulation and leads to ischemia of the tissues. Ischemia causes tissue, muscle, and nerve damage. Signs and symptoms include extreme pain, swelling, tenderness, weakness of involved muscle groups, pain on passive stretching, and signs of ischemia at the site. Treatment is the same as for a crush injury; definitive care is necessary to restore circulation and correct metabolic abnormalities.

CRUSH SYNDROME

Crush syndrome is a life-threatening condition caused by prolonged compression or immobilization (beyond

4 to 6 hours). This condition is rare and the exact mechanism is unknown. Signs and symptoms appear after the patient is released from the crushing mechanism or immobilzation. Shock and possible metabolic acidosis occur due to release of toxins and end products of anaerobic metabolism. Treatment includes airway and ventilatory support, high-concentration oxygen, maintenance of body temperature, rehydration, some pharmacologic agents or arterial tourniquets (controversial), and

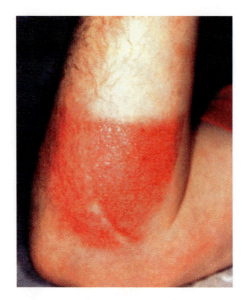

FIGURE 16-17 ▲ An abrasion of the forearm. (From McSwain NE et al: *The basic EMT: comprehensive prehospital care,* St Louis, 1997, Mosby.)

surgical amputation (by a physician) if extrication is not possible.

Open Wounds

ABRASIANS

An abrasian occurs when the outermost layer of skin is rubbed away by friction from a hard object or surface. Signs and symptoms include pain and minimal bleeding. Abrasions may involve loss of body fluids and/or blood depending on the size, depth, and location of the injury. Treatment includes cleaning the surface and removing any contaminants (Figure 16-17).

LACERATIONS

A laceration is caused by a tear, split, or incision into the skin. Blunt or penetrating forces can cause it. Signs and symptoms include pain and bleeding. The amount of bleeding may be minimal or major depending on the site and mechanism. Treatment is directed at controlling hemorrhage and monitoring for signs and symptoms of hemorrhagic shock (Figure 16-18, *A-C*).

PUNCTURES

Puncture wounds are caused by contact with sharp, pointed objects. Because of their nature, they may involve underlying tissues, and internal bleeding may be severe. Signs and symptoms include pain and bleeding (the amount will depend on the mechanism). Treatment for punture wounds includes controlling hemorrhage and monitoring for signs and symptoms of hemorrhagic shock. If an object is impaled, the EMT–I SHOULD NOT REMOVE IT. He or she should control

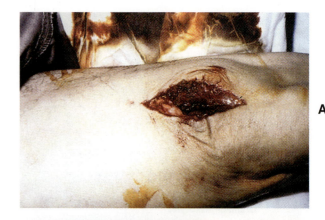

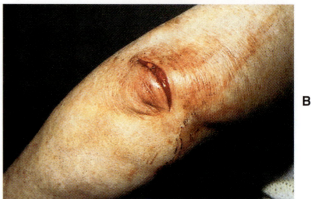

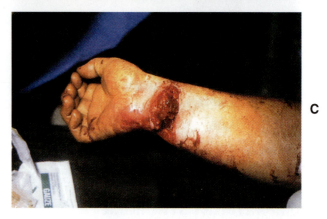

FIGURE 16-18 ▲ Lacerations. **A,** Deep lacerations to the thigh caused by a circular saw. **B,** Laceration of the elbow caused by a fall on the street. **C,** Laceration to the wrist. (From Henry MC, Stapleton ER: *EMT–prehospital care,* ed 2, Philadelphia, 1997, Saunders.)

bleeding and stabilize the object. The object should only be removed if there is interference with airway management, ventilation, or chest compressions if needed (Figure 16-19).

AVULSION

An avulsion is the loss of full thickness of skin and usually is not repaired. Most commonly this injury involves fingertips, ear lobes, and nose tips. Signs and symptoms include pain and bleeding. If the tissue is still attached,

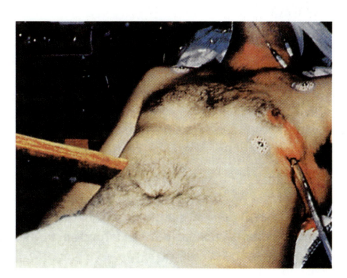

FIGURE 16-19 ▲ Punctures. Piece of wood impaled in the right chest, piercing the diaphragm and lacerating the spleen, stomach, and liver. (From London PS: *A colour atlas of diagnosis after recent injury,* Ipswich, England, 1990, Wolfe Medical Publications.)

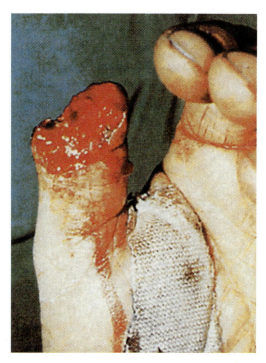

FIGURE 16-20 ▲ Amputation of thumb. (From London PS: *A colour atlas of diagnosis after recent injury,* Ipswich, England, 1990, Wolfe Medical Publications.)

the EMT–I should cleanse the area, return the skin to its normal position as much as possible, control bleeding, and apply a bulky dressing. If the tissue is separated, it should be treated as an amputation.

AMPUTATION

An amputation involves partial or complete loss of a limb due to some type of mechanical force. Major bleeding is the most serious side effect and can be fatal. Signs and symptoms include pain, bleeding, and associated injuries dependent on the mechanism. The EMT–I should control bleeding and save the amputated part (Figure 16-20).

Care of an amputated body part begins with retrieving the part and placing it in a sterile dressing. The dressing may be dry or moistened with lactated Ringer's solution or normal saline depending on local protocol. Next, the part and dressing should be placed inside a plastic bag. The plastic bag is then placed on ice. The amputated part should be transported to the hospital with the patient whenever possible. However, transport of a critically injured patient should not be delayed to look for the amputated part. Someone else at the scene can look for the part, retrieve it, and meet the EMT–Is at the hospital. If fire or police personnel are left at the scene, they should be provided with the proper equipment and directions for saving the amputated part.

HEMORRHAGE

Hemorrhage (bleeding) occurs when there is a break in the body's vascular system. Hemorrhage may be external, from obvious cuts, punctures, or other wounds, or it can occur internally, in which case no obvious signs of hemorrhage will be evident. Internal bleeding, even when not apparent, may still be critical, leading to shock or death.

External Bleeding

External bleeding occurs when there is soft tissue injury. Each year in the United States it results in around 10 million emergency department visits. Most soft tissue trauma is accompanied by mild bleeding and is not life threatening. However, it can carry significant risks of patient morbidity and disfigurement. The effects an injury has on a patient depends on the anatomical source of the hemorrhage (arterial, venous, capillary), degree of vascular disruption, and amount of blood loss that the patient can tolerate.

Bleeding is classified in the following ways (Figure 16-21):

- *Arterial*—Blood is bright red and, if the artery is exposed, the blood may escape in spurts synchronized with the pulse. This type of bleeding is the least frequent but the most serious.
- *Venous*—Blood is dark red and flows slowly and steadily. This is the type of bleeding associated with deeper cuts.

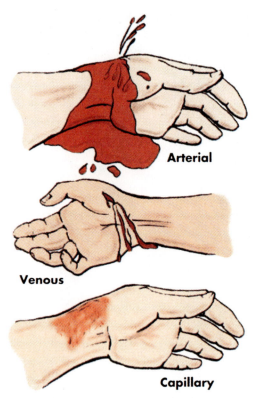

FIGURE 16-21 ▲ Arterial, venous, and capillary bleeding. (From Stoy WA: *Mosby's EMT—basic textbook*, St Louis, 1996, Mosby.)

- *Capillary*—Blood is medium red and oozes slowly. This type of bleeding is associated with minor scrapes and cuts.

External bleeding from an ordinary cut or puncture usually can be controlled with direct pressure. Whenever tissue is cut, the body releases chemicals that interact with blood components to promote clotting (coagulation) while constricting or narrowing the blood vessels. Internal bleeding often is not readily apparent, although in some cases there may be coughing or vomiting of blood or bleeding from the rectum, urethra, or vagina, depending on the location and nature of the injury. Other warning signs are those of hypovolemic shock (described later in this chapter).

An adult can lose 500 mL of blood without any harm, but the loss of 300 mL might cause death in an infant. Most bleeding can be controlled by direct pressure, but if it becomes uncontrolled, then it may be necessary to apply pressure to the pressure points. Hemorrhage can be related to trauma but may also have nontrauma origins such as a bleeding ulcer or aneurysm.

Stages of Hemorrhage

STAGE 1
- Up to 15% intravascular loss
- Compensated by constriction of vascular bed
- Blood pressure maintained
- Normal pulse pressure, respiratory rate, and renal output

- Skin pallor
- Low to normal central venous pressure
- Anxiety

STAGE 2
- Up to 15% to 25% intravascular loss
- Cardiac output cannot be maintained by arteriolar constriction
- Reflex tachycardia
- Increased respiratory rate
- Blood pressure maintained
- Catecholamines increase peripheral resistance
- Increased diastolic pressure
- Narrow pulse pressure
- Diaphoresis from sympathetic stimulation
- Renal output almost normal
- Anxiety and confusion

STAGE 3
- Up to 25% to 35% intravascular loss
- Classic signs of hypovolemic shock:
  - Marked tachycardia
  - Marked tachypnea
  - Decreased systolic pressure
  - 5 to 15 mL/hr urine output
  - Alteration in mental status
  - Diaphoresis with cool, pale skin

STAGE 4
- Loss of greater than 35%
- Extreme tachycardia
- Pronounced tachypnea
- Significantly decreased systolic blood pressure
- Confusion, lethargy, and unconsciousness
- Skin is diaphoretic, cool, and extremely pale

Assessment

The amount of visible blood loss is not a good way to judge the severity of an injury. Serious injuries do not always bleed heavily, and some relatively minor injuries such as scalp wounds bleed profusely. The blood of people who take blood-thinning medication or who have a bleeding disorder such as hemophilia may not clot easily. Although puncture wounds usually do not bleed much, they carry a high risk of infection. Procedures should be taken to prevent tetanus or other infection.

PHYSIOLOGICAL RESPONSE TO HEMORRHAGE

The body's first response to bleeding is to stop it by chemical means (hemostasis). This vascular reaction involves: local vasoconstriction, formation of a platelet plug, coagulation, and the growth of fibrous tissue into the blood clot that permanently closes and seals the injured vessel. If hemorrhage is severe, these mechanisms may fail, resulting in shock (hypoperfusion).

Management

To manage an injury that is bleeding and progressively causing shock, the EMT–I should do the following:

1. Employ body substance isolation precautions.
2. Apply direct pressure to the wound with a gloved hand. Direct pressure will stop most bleeding (Figure 16-22, *A*).
3. If the bleeding is uncontrolled elevate the wound (if it is on an extremity) (Figure 16-22, *B*).
4. Apply additional dressings if the wound continues to bleed (Figure 16-22, *C*).
5. If the bleeding continues apply a pressure dressing and bandage the wound (Figure 16-22, *D*).
6. Locate and apply pressure to the appropriate arterial pressure point if the wound continues to bleed (Figure 16-22, *E*). These are found on the main artery above the wound (Figure 16-22, *F*).

When bleeding has been controlled, remove pressure to the point and reapply direct pressure to the wound.

If the injury mechanism or signs indicate the victim is in compensatory shock:

7. Properly position the patient (supine with his or her legs elevated).
8. Apply a high concentration oxygen.
9. Take steps to prevent heat loss (cover the patient as appropriate).
10. Initiate immediate transport of the patient.
11. Reassess the patient's vital signs.

Occasionally, in major limb injuries such as partial amputations and shark attack, severe bleeding cannot be controlled by direct pressure. Only then, it may be necessary to resort to the application of a constrictive bandage (tourniquet) above the elbow or knee. Splinting of an extremity, packing of large gaping wounds with sterile dressing and/or the application and inflation of the pneumatic anti-shock garment (PASG) can also be used to help control uncontrolled arterial bleeding.

Internal Bleeding

Internal bleeding can result from blunt or penetrating trauma, and acute or chronic medical illnesses. Internal bleeding that can cause hemodynamic instability usually occurs in one of four body cavities—the chest, abdomen, pelvis, or retroperitoneum. Intracranial hemorrhage can also cause grave hemodynamic instability. Internal hemorrhage is associated with higher mobility and mortality than external hemorrhage.

ASSESSMENT

A patient suspected of internal bleeding may have signs and symptoms of:

- Coughing up red, frothy blood
- Vomiting blood the color of coffee grounds or bright red. The blood may be mixed with food.
- Passing of feces with a black, tarry appearance. This is referred to as melena.
- Passing of red blood through the rectum. This is referred to as hematochezia.
- Passing urine which has a red appearance
- Dizziness or syncope on sitting or standing
- Orthostatic hypotension
- Pain
- Tenderness
- Rigidity of abdominal muscles
- Faintness or dizziness
- Restlessness
- Nausea
- Thirst
- Weak, rapid pulse
- Cold, clammy skin
- Rapid, gasping breathing
- Sweating

MANAGEMENT

The treatment of internal hemorrhage centers on the delivery of definitive care such as surgical intervention to stop the bleeding. This emphasizes the need to rapidly transport the patient who is experiencing internal hemorrhage to an appropriate medical facility. A patient who is hemorrhaging internally must be kept warm and treated for shock. Management of shock will be discussed later in this chapter.

SHOCK

Shock • The body's response to poor perfusion.

Loss of blood or body water can lead to decreased tissue perfusion. When tissue perfusion falls below a level necessary to sustain life, **shock** occurs. Shock is sometimes referred to as hypoperfusion (hypo means deficient or low) or hypoperfusion syndrome. Shock cannot be defined simply in terms of blood pressure, pulse rate, and respiration, or by superficial symptoms, such as cool and clammy skin. These indicators are some of the signs and symptoms of shock, but they do not tell what is happening on the cellular level and can also be caused by other conditions.

Baroreceptors • Sensory nerve endings that sense changes in blood pressure as a result of vasodilation or vasoconstriction.

When the oxygen concentration of the blood circulating in the body decreases, the body compensates by sending blood to the top priority organs—the heart, brain, and lungs. The body does this by shunting (moving) blood away from less essential systems, such as the liver, intestines, muscle, bone, and skin. Compensatory adjustments begin with the **baroreceptors** (Figure 16-23) detecting a drop in arterial blood pressure.

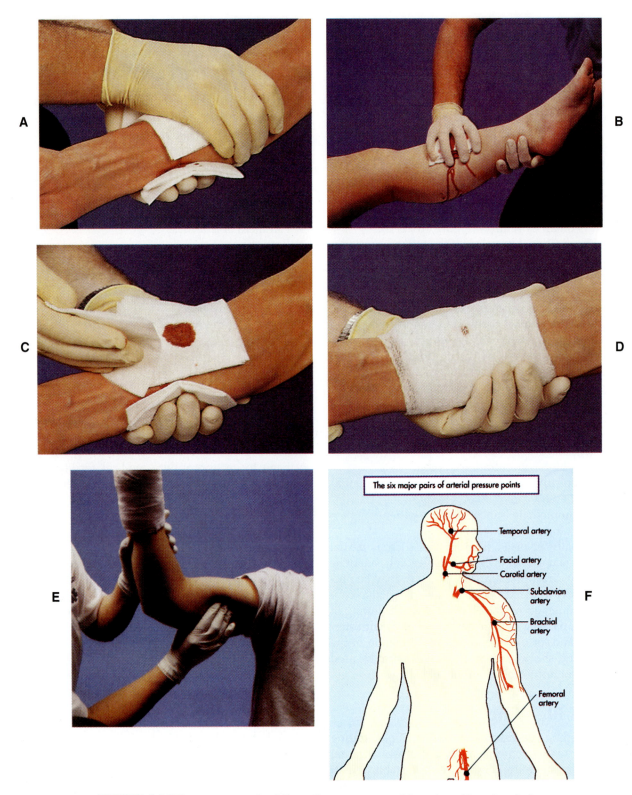

FIGURE 16-22 ▲ **A,** Apply diffuse direct pressure with a gloved hand and absorbent dressing. **B,** Attempt to control bleeding by direct pressure. Check the entire extremity for other injuries; if there are signs or symptoms of skeletal injuries, do not elevate the extremity until it is splinted. **C,** If blood soaks through the dressing place additional dressings on top. **D,** Continue to apply manual pressure until you apply a dressing that will keep pressure on the injury. **E,** Pressure point control. **F,** Arterial pressure points. (**A** to **D,** From Stoy WA: *Mosby's EMT—basic textbook,* St Louis, 1996, Mosby; **E,** From Sanders MJ: *Mosby's paramedic textbook,* ed 2, 2001, Mosby; **F,** from doCarmo P: *Basic EMT skills and equipment,* St Louis, 1988, Mosby.)

The baroreceptors (sensory nerve endings) are found in the carotid sinus, aortic arch, atrial walls of the heart, and vena cava. Baroreceptors reflexes help sustain blood pressure by two negative feedback mechanisms: first they lower the blood pressure in response to increased arterial pressure, second they increase blood pressure in response to decreased arterial pressure.

Normal blood pressure partially stretches the arterial walls so that baroreceptors produce a constant, low-level stimulation. When the blood pressure increases, impulses from the baroreceptors inhibit the vasoconstrictor center of the medulla and excite the vagal center. This leads to vasodilation in the peripheral circulatory system and a decrease in the heart rate and force of contraction. The combined effect is a decrease in arterial pressure.

A fall in arterial pressure decreases the stretch of the arterial wall and leads to a decrease in baroreceptor stimulation. This produces several important cardiovascular responses. First, fewer inhibitory impulses are transmitted via the vagus, Hering's, and glossopharyngeal nerves to the vasomotor center. This leads to an increase in vasomotor activity. A regulatory center in the brain then activates the sympathetic nervous system.

Stimulation of the sympathetic nervous system causes a release of norepinephrine from sympathetic nerve endings and epinephrine (also called adrenalin) from the adrenal glands (Figure 16-24). These hormones stimulate the beta 1 receptors causing the heart to beat faster (increased dromotropy and chronotropy) and more forcefully (increased inotropy). They also stimulate the beta 2 receptors leading to bronchodilation and gut smooth muscle dilation and stimulate the alpha 1 receptors leading to the constriction of the smooth muscles in the peripheral arterioles and venules. (Figure 16-25). This constriction increases the blood pressure (by increasing peripheral vascular resistance) and decreases the container size shunting blood from the peripheral vasculature to the internal organs. The result is

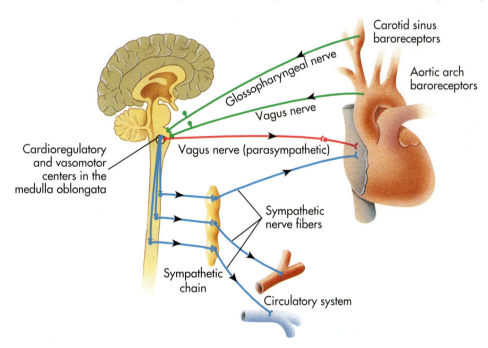

FIGURE 16-23 ▲ **Baroreceptors detect changes in blood pressure and send messages to a regulatory center in the brain. The central nervous system is then activated, which tells the heart to beat faster or slower. (Christine Oleksyk from Seeley R:** *Anatomy and physiology,* **ed 3, St Louis, 1995, Mosby.)**

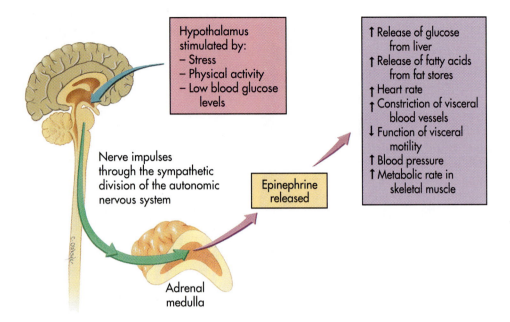

Hypothalamus stimulated by:
– Stress
– Physical activity
– Low blood glucose levels

Nerve impulses through the sympathetic division of the autonomic nervous system

Epinephrine released

↑ Release of glucose from liver
↑ Release of fatty acids from fat stores
↑ Heart rate
↑ Constriction of visceral blood vessels
↓ Function of visceral motility
↑ Blood pressure
↑ Metabolic rate in skeletal muscle

Adrenal medulla

FIGURE 16-24 ▲ Sympathetic nervous system stimulation causes norepinephrine to be released into the body. (Modified from Seeley R: *Anatomy and physiology,* ed 3, St Louis, 1995, Mosby.)

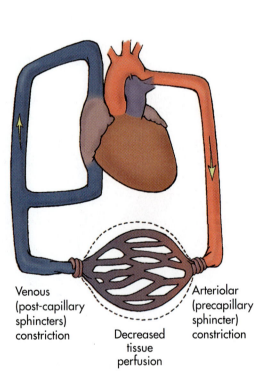

Venous (post-capillary sphincters) constriction

Decreased tissue perfusion

Arteriolar (precapillary sphincter) constriction

FIGURE 16-25 ▲ The release of norepinephrine causes the peripheral arterioles and venules to constrict, decreasing tissue perfusion.

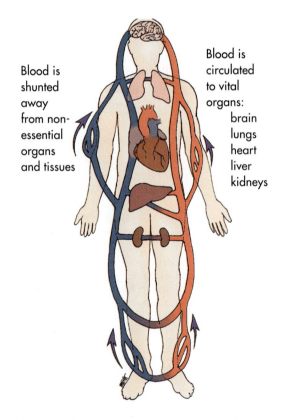

Blood is shunted away from non-essential organs and tissues

Blood is circulated to vital organs:
brain
lungs
heart
liver
kidneys

FIGURE 16-26 ▲ Peripheral vasoconstriction causes blood pressure to increase, and blood is shunted to the internal, more essential organs such as the heart, the lungs, and the brain.

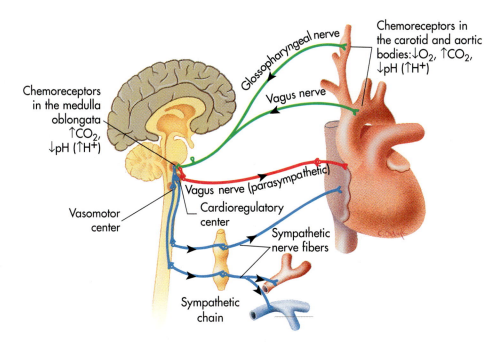

FIGURE 16-27 ▲ During the compensatory stage of shock, chemoreceptors attempt to maintain the body's acid-base balance by stimulating and increasing the rate and depth of respirations, increasing oxygen and decreasing carbon dioxide. (Christine Oleksyk from Seeley R: *Anatomy and physiology*, ed 3, St Louis, 1995, Mosby.)

improved circulation to the vital organs and decreased circulation to the rest of the body (Figure 16-26).

During this time changes in the concentration of oxygen, carbon dioxide, and pH also activate the sympathetic nervous system. A group of specialized receptors, the chemoreceptors (Figure 16-27), detect these changes in the blood. Like the baroreceptors, the chemoreceptors are located in the walls of the atria of the heart, vena cava, aortic arch, and carotid sinus. Increases in carbon dioxide and/or decreases in oxygen typically initiate a sympathetic response that increases the rate and depth of respirations. The increased respiratory volume brings in more oxygen and removes more carbon dioxide. Initially this compensatory hyperventilation helps to maintain the acid-base balance in early shock by creating a respiratory alkalosis that acts to offset the metabolic acidosis, resulting in a shift of the pH back toward normal.

CAPILLARY AND CELLULAR CHANGES—THE BODY'S RESPONSE TO SHOCK

✂ **Anaerobic Metabolism** • Metabolism without oxygen.

Ischemia

With vasoconstriction there is minimal blood flow to the capillaries resulting in stagnation. This leads to tissue is-

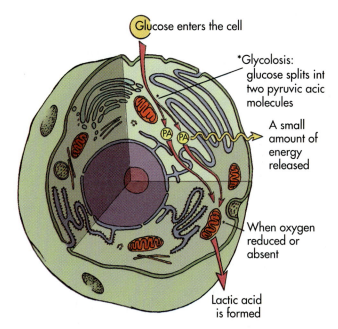

FIGURE 16-28 ▲ Anaerobic metabolism occurs without oxygen, and produces lactic acid.

chemia and the cells shift from aerobic to **anaerobic metabolism** (Figure 16-28). In prolonged anaerobic metabolism, there is an excess of lactic acid, which the body is unable to handle. This excess causes an increase in hydrogen ions in the blood. As a result, the pH in the blood decreases, and metabolic acidosis occurs. Unresolved acidosis eventually results in cellular death.

As shock progresses, even the cells of the vital organs suffer from the lack of perfusion. For instance, following severe hemorrhage, cardiac output decreases and the myocardium itself is deprives of blood. As coronary artery perfusion declines the heart becomes ischemis causing it to weaken. This further decreases cardiac output.

Precapillary Sphincter Relaxation

Arteries that are deprived of their blood supply cannot remain constricted (Figure 16-29). The precapillary sphincters start relaxing in response to lactic acid, vasomotor failure, and increased carbon dioxide. However, the postcapillary sphincters remain constricted causing the capillaries to become engorged with fluid. As the arteries dilate, venous return decreases, which in turn decreases cardiac output.

As anaerobic metabolism continues it produces more lactic acid. The red blood cells begin to clump together, or aggregate, forming columns of coagulated cells (microemboli) called rouleaux. Also, during this time the lining of the capillary loses its ability to retain large molecular structures within its walls, permitting protein-containing fluid to leak into the interstitial spaces. This is known as the *leaky capillary syndrome.* Additionally, plasma is pushed into the interstitial spaces by hydrostatic pressure. This increases the distance from the capillaries to the cells thus decreasing oxygen transport and further aggravating tissue hypoxia.

> **CLINICAL NOTES**
>
> An oxygen deficiency does not have to be extreme to cause the body to be less efficient; i.e., anaerobic metabolism does not produce as much energy as aerobic metabolism.

Washout

The building acidosis from the accumulating lactic acid and carbon dioxide acts as a potent vasodilator leading to relaxation of the postcapillary sphincters. This allows the accumulated hydrogen, carbon dioxide, potassium (released by the cells to help maintain a neutral environment due to the building acidosis), and columns of coagulated erythrocytes to *washout* into the venous circulation. Metabolic acidosis worsens and cardiac output drops further.

STAGES OF SHOCK

The development of shock occurs in three principal stages, which merge with one another. At each stage,

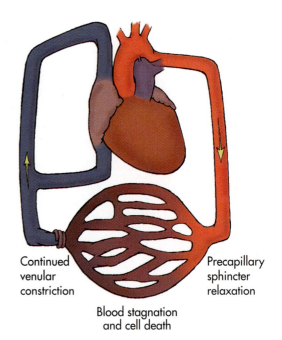

FIGURE 16-29 ▲ As shock progresses, arteries deprived of their blood supply dilate, decreasing venous return. Decreased cardiac output is the result.

Labels in figure: Continued venular constriction — Precapillary sphincter relaxation — Blood stagnation and cell death

certain signs and symptoms are present that may alert the EMT–I to the presence of shock.

Compensated (Nonprogressive) Shock

The earliest phase of shock is called the *compensated (nonprogressive) stage.* During this stage, the body recognizes the catastrophic event that is occurring and triggers corrective action in an attempt to return cardiac output and arterial blood pressure to normal.

> **CLINICAL NOTES**
>
> Following a small bleed, the heart rate increases, the blood vessels constrict, and the kidneys decrease urinary output to conserve water. These responses help preserve blood volume and maintain blood pressure, cardiac output, and blood flow to the tissues. In an otherwise healthy individual, acute blood loss of as much as 10% of the total blood volume can be handled by compensatory mechanisms.

Signs and symptoms are minimal in this stage of shock and if certain parts of the cardiovascular system compensate, no serious damage will result. It is important that the EMT–I learn to recognize the subtle clues that the body gives off, indicating the development of shock. They are as follows:

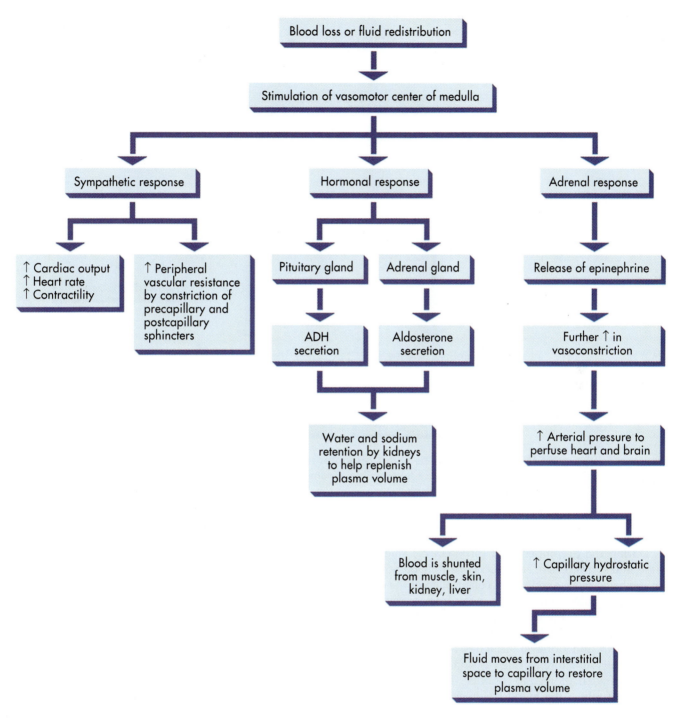

FIGURE 16-30 ▲ The body's response to compensatory shock. (From Sanders M: *Mosby's paramedic textbook,* St Louis, 1994, Mosby.)

- Altered mental status, usually restlessness
- Increased pulse rate
- Increased respiratory rate
- Pale, cool skin

If the initiating cause (i.e., the hemorrhage) does not worsen, a full recovery typically follows. Figure 16-30 shows the body's various reactions to shock during the compensatory stage.

Decompensated (Progressive) Shock

If blood volume drops more than 15% to 25%, the shock becomes steadily worse because compensatory mechanisms are no longer able to maintain perfusion. As the cardiovascular system progressively deteriorates, cardiac output falls dramatically. This condition can lead to further reductions in blood pressure and cardiac function.

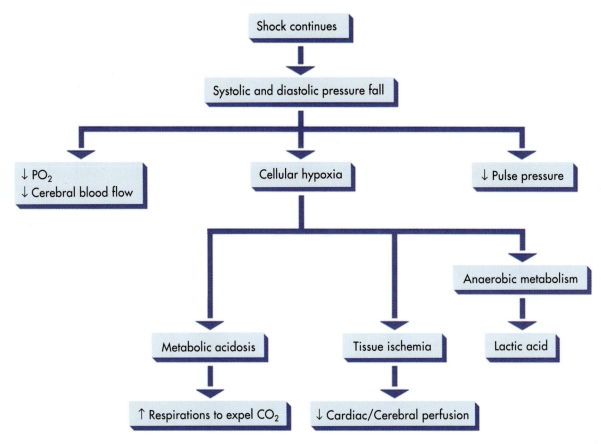

FIGURE 16-31 ▲ The body's responses to uncompensated (or progressive) shock. This stage of shock is reversible. (From Sanders M: *Mosby's Paramedic textbook*, St Louis, 1994, Mosby.)

During the decompensated (progressive) stage, the signs and symptoms of shock become more obvious. As epinephrine release continues, constriction of the arterioles and venules shunts blood away from certain nonvital organs (e.g., the skin, muscles, and gastrointestinal tract) and directs it toward the vital organs (i.e., the heart, brain, and kidneys). Although helping to keep the vital organs functioning, this vasoconstriction has a disastrous effect if allowed to continue. The cells in the tissues from which the blood has been diverted become hypoxic, leading to anaerobic metabolism. This condition causes the production of harmful acids, eventually bringing about metabolic acidosis.

Immediate medical intervention is required to reverse the changes during the decompensated stage of shock. (Figure 16-31). Treatment at this stage will sometimes result in recovery. If this intervention fails, shock progresses to the third stage.

The signs and symptoms of progressive shock include the following:

- Additional increases in pulse and respirations
- Cool, clammy skin
- Decreased capillary refill
- Thirst (the body's call for increased volume)

- Narrowing of the pulse pressure. The pulse pressure is the difference between systolic and diastolic blood pressure. It reflects the tone of the arterial system and is more sensitive to changes in perfusion than the systolic or diastolic pressure. The normal value is 40 mm Hg. Narrowing of the pulse pressure indicates an impairment of circulation.
- Sweating
- Increased anxiety and confusion
- Nausea and vomiting (caused by shunting of blood from the abdominal organs)

Eventually patients in the decompensated (progressive) stage of shock will develop hypotension. Hypotension is a late sign of shock. By the time hypotension develops, the body's compensatory mechanisms have failed. Failure to quickly halt the progress of hypotension will lead to irreversible shock.

HELPFUL HINT

Decreased blood pressure is a late sign of shock. Children often lose 30% of their blood supply before experiencing a drop in blood pressure.

Irreversible Shock

In the third stage of shock, a rapid deterioration of the cardiovascular system occurs that cannot be helped by compensatory mechanisms or medical intervention. As the shock cycle continues, the heart deteriorates to the point that it can no longer effectively pump blood and life-threatening reductions in cardiac output, blood pressure, and tissue perfusion occur. The body shunts blood away from the liver, kidneys, and lungs to keep the heart and brain perfused. These organs begin to falter, eventually becoming ineffective. Their malfunction accelerates the overall decline of the body. The cells begin to die and so do the organs (Figure 16-32).

If the shock syndrome progresses to the point at which the cells in the vital organs begin to die because of inadequate perfusion, the shock syndrome is said to be irreversible. Even if the cause of the shock syndrome was then treated and reversed, the damage to the vital organs could not be repaired, and the patient would eventually die. The "golden hour" theory holds that after 1 hour, the chances of developing irreversible shock increase dramatically. Some signs and symptoms of impending irreversible shock include the following:

● Marked decrease in level of responsiveness (Glasgow coma scale 7 or below)
● Decreased respiratory rate and effort
● Profound hypotension and inability to palpate a pulse, even in a responsive patient
● Decrease in the pulse rate from too fast to too slow

Except in the case of hemorrhagic shock, it may be several days before progression to irreversible shock becomes apparent in the form of adult respiratory distress syndrome, renal failure, liver failure, and sepsis. Rapid assessment and immediate transportation are essential to preserve any chance of patient survival.

Shock develops in three successive stages: compensated, decompensated, and irreversible. The keys to the successful recognition and care of the patient in shock include:

1. Have a high level of suspicion. THINK SHOCK!
2. Anticipate the potential for shock from the scene survey.

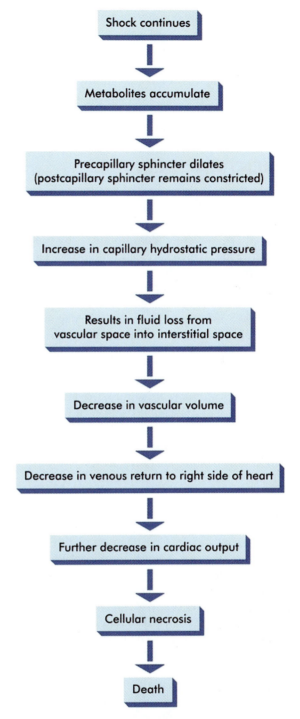

FIGURE 16-32 ▲ The body's responses to irreversible shock. (From Sanders M: *Mosby's paramedic textbook*, St Louis, 1994, Mosby.)

3. Remember the subtle signs and symptoms of shock that are present in the compensatory stage.
4. The "golden hour" begins at the time of the incident. The guiding philosophy is to get the right person (a patient in shock) to the right place (the appropriate hospital) at the right time (less than 1 hour).

5. Do not rely on any one sign or symptom to judge the degree of shock.
6. Hypotension is a late sign of shock. Other abnormalities indicating poor blood flow (tachycardia, abnormal mental status, or cold/clammy skin) precede hypotension. The EMT–I should be able to recognize shock without having to rely on the presence of low blood pressure.

PATIENTS AT RISK

There are several classes of patients for whom the development of the three stages of shock may be particularly devastating. The trauma patient with multiple injuries may be severely compromised by decreased tissue perfusion, which can lead to hypoxic damage to organs already injured by the trauma. Elderly patients also are particularly susceptible to the effects of low tissue blood flow. These patients may have previously compromised tissue perfusion secondary to atherosclerotic vascular disease, and even small decreases in perfusion may make the blood flow inadequate to meet their metabolic needs.

Shock poses the greatest danger to pregnant women. During shock, the body sees the fetus as just another piece of peripheral tissue to which the blood flow should be decreased to maintain perfusion of the mother's vital organs. This may be fatal to the fetus if the blood flow is not quickly restored.

TYPES OF SHOCK

Although shock may have a number of different origins, it is usually caused by one or more of three primary mechanisms: (1) fluid loss, (2) significant vasodilation, (3) pump failure.

Knowing the types of shock allows the EMT–I to anticipate these differences. The EMT–I should know the five major types of shock but should remember that one type may overlap another. The most important point is that all types of shock occur due to an underlying lack of tissue perfusion.

Hypovolemic Shock

✖ **Hypovolemic Shock** • A form of shock caused by the loss of blood or fluid volume from the body.

Hypovolemic shock (Figure 16-33) is caused by the loss of blood or fluid volume from the body. This state commonly occurs after internal or external hemorrhage due to trauma or medical conditions such as gastrointestinal bleeding or a ruptured aortic aneurysm. Hypovolemic shock also results from other conditions associated with fluid volume loss without bleeding, such as burns and severe dehydration. Burns cause the loss of plasma through the damaged skin. Dehydration can occur following severe vomit-

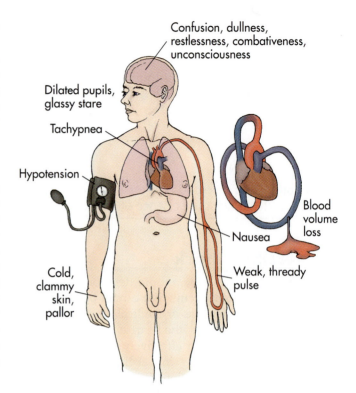

FIGURE 16-33 ▲ The body experiencing hypovolemic shock, resulting from a large blood or fluid loss in the body.

ing, diarrhea, profuse sweating, diabetic ketoacidosis, or inadequate fluid intake.

Hypovolemic shock is the most common type of shock seen in the prehospital setting. It should be suspected in any injured or ill patient whose clinical circumstances suggest the possibility of volume loss (e.g., an accident, fall, severe nausea, and vomiting).

✖ **Orthostatic Hypotension** • A decrease in blood pressure resulting from a patient being moved to a standing or sitting position from a sitting or supine position.

Cardiogenic Shock

✖ **Cardiogenic Shock** • A form of shock caused by profound failure of the heart.

Cardiogenic shock (Figure 16-34) is caused by profound failure of the heart, primarily the left ventricle. When more than 40% of the left ventricle is nonfunctional, the heart loses its ability to efficiently pump blood into the circulatory system. Hence, blood will not be adequately circulated (perfused) to the body. In cardiogenic shock there is good peripheral vascular resistance and adequate blood volume but the heart is not pumping properly.

Cardiogenic shock can be caused by several factors, including severe myocardial infarction, and severe heart failure.

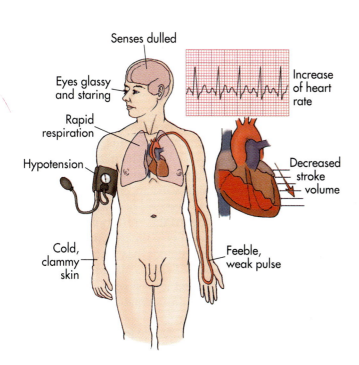

FIGURE 16-34 ▲ The body experiencing cardiogenic shock, resulting from profound heart failure.

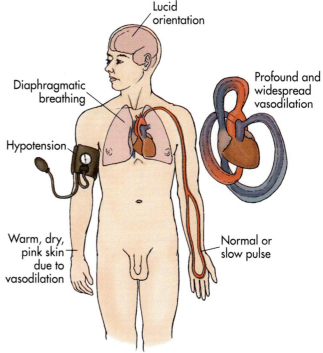

FIGURE 16-35 ▲ Neurogenic shock is caused by the nervous system's inability to control the diameter of blood vessels in the body.

CLINICAL NOTES

A diagnostic test for early hypovolemia by assessing for orthostatic vital sign changes is known as the tilt test.

The procedure for dealing with orthostatic hypotension is as follows:
1. Place the patient in a supine position and assess vital signs.
2. Sit the patient up and reassess vital signs after 2 minutes of sitting.

An abnormal, or positive, tilt test result is present if the pulse rate increases by 20 beats per minute and/or the systolic blood pressure drops by greater than 10 to 20 mm Hg. The test also is considered positive if the patient complains of dizziness, feels very weak, or faints with the change of position. Positive findings may indicate **orthostatic hypotension**. The presence of orthostatic changes implies a volume loss of at least 500 mL. Do not perform the tilt test on patients with suspected spinal injury.

In a myocardial infarction, for example, there may be damage to the wall of the heart. The heart is not able to contract as forcefully as it once did, and cardiac output decreases, leading to shock. Many diseases, if allowed to go untreated, may eventually do enough damage to the heart to cause cardiogenic shock.

Cardiogenic shock can also be caused by a lack of filling or obstruction of blood flow out of the heart. Cardiac tamponade, tension pneumothorax, or other such conditions put excessive pressure on the heart, impairing its ability to contract or push blood through the major arteries. Bradycardia, significant tachycardia, and severe irregularities in the heart rhythm can also reduce cardiac output to the point that it produces shock.

In addition to the general signs and symptoms of shock, patients in cardiogenic shock may experience severe respiratory distress due to a backup of fluid from the left side of the heart into the lungs. They also may have chest pain if there has been an associated myocardial infarction or blunt trauma to the heart.

Neurogenic Shock

Neurogenic Shock • A form of shock in which the nervous system is no longer able to control the diameter of the blood vessels.

Neurogenic shock, also called distributive, vasogenic, and spinal shock is seen with spinal cord injury, drug overdose, sepsis, and anaphylaxis (Figure 16-35). With neurogenic shock the nervous system is no longer able to control the diameter of the blood vessels. Without this control, the blood vessels dilate, increasing the volume of the cardiovascular system. There is no longer enough blood to fill the entire system, and blood will pool in the blood vessels in certain areas of the body. Venous return to the heart decreases, and shock results.

�֍ **Priapism** • Sustained erection.

Neurogenic shock due to a spinal or severe brain injury is referred to as spinal shock. Damage to the brain or spine prevents nerve impulses from the brain's regulatory center from reaching the vital organs. A disruption in the sympathetic nervous system prevents secretion of epinephrine, resulting in profound vasodilation and shock. Although no actual blood loss occurs, vasodilation leads to relative hypovolemia. Blood volume is present but not in the necessary places. With spinal shock there is flaccid paralysis distal to the injury site and loss of autonomic function that results in (in addition to hypotension and vasodilation) loss of bladder and bowel control, **priapism,** and loss of thermoregulation. Spinal shock does not always involve a permanent primary injury.

Spinal shock is a rare occurrence. Shock presentation in trauma is usually due to hidden volume loss such as that produced by chest, abdominal, or other violent injury.

The signs and symptoms of neurogenic shock differ somewhat from those of hypovolemic shock. Due to decreased epinephrine secretion, the patient may not exhibit tachycardia (in some cases a relative bradycardia will be seen), sweating, or a pale skin color. The vasodilation may cause the skin to appear pink or flushed, warm and dry. Altered mental status and hypotension may be the only signs of neurogenic shock. Treatment of neurogenic shock is focused primarily on volume replacement.

CLINICAL NOTES

Psychogenic shock is simple fainting. The blood vessels dilate, allowing blood pooling. If blood flow falls to the point at which perfusion is momentarily interrupted, the victim will feel faint or pass out. Psychogenic shock usually corrects itself when the victim falls to the ground, restoring circulation to the brain. If the victim is responsive, remaining in the supine position for a few minutes usually returns perfusion to normal.

Anaphylactic Shock

✖ **Anaphylactic Shock** • A form of shock caused by exposure to a substance to which the patient is extremely allergic.

✖ **Antigen** • A protein found on the membrane of red blood cells that triggers the formation of an antibody.

✖ **Antibody** • A protein developed in the body in response to an antigen.

✖ **Histamine** • A compound released in the body during an allergic reaction.

In anaphylactic shock the body reacts to a substance to which the patient is extremely allergic (Figure 16-36). Anaphylactic shock is a severe response to a foreign substance (antigen) entering the body. Antigens may enter the body through numerous channels:

- *Skin contact*—Poison ivy, poison oak, skin creams
- *Injections*—Medications given by injection (e.g., penicillin), insect bites, and stings
- *Inhalation*—Molds, pollen, perfumes
- *Ingestion*—Chocolate, shellfish, peanuts, oral penicillin

When an antigen to which the patient is sensitive enters the body, it is attacked by an antibody. Antibodies function to destroy foreign substances. In the event of anaphylaxis, the antibody does not destroy the antigen. Instead, the reaction between the antigen and the antibody triggers a series of events in the patient's body that leads to shock. After the antibody has reacted with the antigen, there is a release of chemicals from a specialized type of leukocyte called a mast cell. The most important substance released from mast cells during anaphylactic shock is histamine.

The release of histamine causes the following responses:
- Sudden, severe bronchoconstriction, which can cause airway compromise
- Intense vasodilation (resulting in distributive shock)
- Leaking of fluid from vessels due to a change in permeability

Responses can range from mild to extreme, sometimes causing death.

The signs and symptoms of anaphylactic shock (Figure 16-37) differ somewhat from other forms of shock and may develop rapidly or gradually. Anaphylactic shock presents a special problem because profound airway compromise can develop quickly. Signs and symptoms of anaphylactic shock include the following:
- A sense of uneasiness or agitation; this is often the first symptom noticed by the patient
- Swelling of the soft tissues such as the hands, tongue, and pharynx; patients may feel as if their tongue is swelling and their throat is closing up
- Skin flushing and hives
- Tachycardia
- Coughing, sneezing, or wheezing due to spasms of the upper and lower airway
- Tingling, burning, and itching of the skin
- Abdominal pain
- Profound hypotension (late sign)
- Decreased level of responsiveness

Septic Shock

✖ **Septic Shock** • A form of shock caused by an infection resulting in a massive vasodilation of the circulatory system.

Septic shock (Figure 16-38) is caused by an overwhelming infection (usually bacterial) that leads to massive vasodilation (distributive shock). The blood

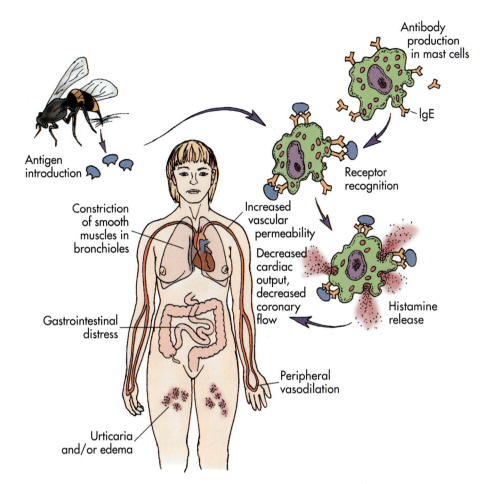

Antibody
production
in mast cells

IgE

Receptor
recognition

Antigen
introduction

Constriction
of smooth
muscles in
bronchioles

Increased
vascular
permeability

Decreased
cardiac
output,
decreased
coronary
flow

Histamine
release

Gastrointestinal
distress

Peripheral
vasodilation

Urticaria
and/or edema

FIGURE 16-36 ▲   The effects of histamine release in the body.

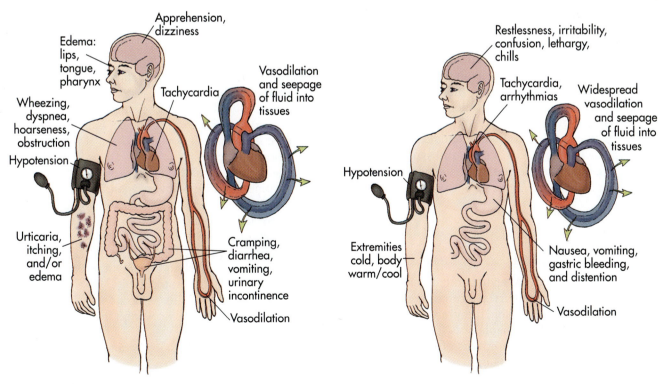

Apprehension,
dizziness

Edema:
lips,
tongue,
pharynx

Tachycardia

Vasodilation
and seepage
of fluid into
tissues

Wheezing,
dyspnea,
hoarseness,
obstruction

Hypotension

Urticaria,
itching,
and/or
edema

Cramping,
diarrhea,
vomiting,
urinary
incontinence

Vasodilation

FIGURE 16-37 ▲   The body experiencing anaphylactic shock.

Restlessness, irritability,
confusion, lethargy,
chills

Tachycardia,
arrhythmias

Widespread
vasodilation
and seepage
of fluid into
tissues

Hypotension

Extremities
cold, body
warm/cool

Nausea, vomiting,
gastric bleeding,
and distention

Vasodilation

FIGURE 16-38 ▲   The body experiencing septic
shock.

vessels dilate due to toxins being released into the bloodstream. As in neurogenic shock, the amount of blood available for effective circulation is decreased because it is pooled or trapped in the dilated veins. In addition, blood plasma is lost through blood vessel walls, causing an additional loss in blood volume. Therefore, poor tissue perfusion results.

Until recently, septic shock was rarely seen in the prehospital environment. With expanded long-term care facilities and increased use of emergency medical services (EMS) by the elderly, EMS personnel are beginning to see septic shock more often.

The patient in septic shock may have a fever. The trunk of the body is often warm, but the extremities are cold due to shunting of blood from the skin of the arms and legs. As septic shock progresses, the entire body becomes cool; this is an ominous sign.

DIFFERENTIAL SHOCK ASSESSMENT FINDINGS

Shock should be assumed to be hypovolemic until proven otherwise. Cardiogenic shock can be differentiated from hypovolemic shock by the presence of one or more of the following:

- Chief complaint (chest pain, dyspnea, tachycardia)
- Heart rate (bradycardia or excessive tachycardia)
- Signs of congestive heart failure (jugular vein distention, rales)
- Dysrhythmia

Distributive shock can be differentiated from hypovolemic shock by the presence of one or more of the following:

- Mechanism that suggests vasodilation, e.g., spinal cord injury, drug overdose, sepsis, or anaphylaxis
- Warm, flushed skin, especially in dependent areas
- Lack of tachycardia response (not reliable though, since many hypovolemic patients never bceome tachycardic)

Obstructive shock can be differentiated from hypovolemic shock by presence of signs and symptoms suggestive of cardiac tamponade or tension pneumothorax.

ASSESSMENT AND MANAGEMENT OF THE PATIENT IN SHOCK

The EMT–I must always keep in mind that shock can result from any illness or injury and can present itself in a variety of ways. Hypotension, tachycardia, hyperventilation, pallor (pale skin), diaphoresis (sweating), thirst, and weakness are classic indicators of shock. These indicators, however, are only signs and symptoms. The condition of shock may exist long before any of these indicators appear.

The body's compensatory efforts to maintain an adequate blood pressure and to perfuse the vital organs can mask the signs and symptoms of shock. Shock can be hidden by compensatory mechanisms such as generalized vasoconstriction and/or an increase in heart rate. These compensatory mechanisms work to maintain an adequate blood pressure and to perfuse the vital organs. Rapid assessment and immediate transportation are essential for the survival of the patient. Although measuring blood pressure is the most frequent monitoring device for patient care, it is not the most important factor in the management of shock. Evaluation of the patient in shock is directed at assessing oxygenation and perfusion of the various body organs. Goals of prehospital care include the following:

1. Ensuring a patent airway
2. Providing adequate oxygenation and ventilation
3. Restoring perfusion
4. Repair the cause or stop the cause.

The EMT–I's initial approach to the patient often can yield a great deal of information. Before reaching the patient's side, his or her mental status, respiratory effort, and skin color can be observed. In situations in which the patient is obviously in shock, the EMT–I must be aggressive with assessment and management. This chapter addresses only the assessment and management of patients experiencing shock related to volume depletion. Assessment and management of other forms of shock are covered in other chapters in this book.

HELPFUL HINT

- Some tips for caring for a patient in shock include the following:
  - Conducting the initial assessment (primary survey) and detecting shock early; finding the mechanism of injury may lead the EMT–I to suspect shock
  - Securing and maintaining a patent airway
  - Administering high-flow oxygen; if available, the EMT–I should use a pulse oximeter and adjust the oxygen concentration to raise saturation above 90%
  - Controlling external bleeding
  - Applying and inflating pneumatic antishock garment per local protocols
  - Administering IV fluids per local protocols
  - Preserving warmth by covering the patient with a blanket
  - Monitoring the vital signs frequently, at least every 5 minutes
  - Promptly transporting the patient

Level of Responsiveness

The level of responsiveness should be assessed throughout the initial survey. In fact, the level of responsiveness is probably a better indicator of decreased tissue perfusion throughout the body than most other signs. Because of the high energy requirements of the brain, any reduction in cerebral blood flow may be manifested by any of the following:

- Restlessness
- Agitation
- Disorientation
- Confusion
- An inability to respond to questions or commands appropriately
- Belligerent or combative behavior
- Unresponsiveness

Any significant alteration in the level of responsiveness must be viewed as an indication of critical hypoperfusion or hypoxia. Additionally, with an increased secretion of norepinephrine and epinephrine, the patient often becomes anxious or apprehensive. Mind-altering substances also may be involved in trauma-related shock. When alcohol or drugs interfere with the patient's normal thought processes it is extremely difficult to get an accurate picture of the patient's mental status. The EMT–I must keep in mind, however, that just because a patient has been drinking or taking drugs does not mean that a serious underlying injury does not exist. Whenever the likelihood of serious trauma exists, it is probably best to assume that any altered mental status is due to decreased cerebral perfusion.

Airway
ASSESSMENT

The EMT–I begins the assessment by looking for and assuring a patent airway. The airway must be opened and maintained to ensure adequate air movement. This is done using appropriate cervical spine stabilization for any patient who is likely to have suffered a spinal injury. Sounds that point to the presence of upper airway obstruction include snoring (obstruction by the tongue); gurgling (obstruction by liquids such as blood or vomitus); and stridor (obstruction due to foreign body or swelling).

MANAGEMENT

An airway adjunct should be inserted to prevent the tongue from obstructing the airway in any patient with decreased responsiveness and no gag reflex. The EMT–I might use an oropharyngeal airway, nasopharyngeal airway, multilumen airway, or endotracheal tube. When dealing with the patient in shock who is unresponsive, particularly those who are bleeding into the pharynx, endotracheal intubation is the preferred airway technique, because the trachea can be sealed to prevent aspiration of blood.

Blood or fluids should be cleared with appropriate suctioning techniques, taking care not to stimulate the gag reflex or create inadvertent hypoxia. Larger foreign objects such as teeth should be removed using the finger sweep technique. In the presence of ongoing fluid accumulation in the pharynx it may be necessary to place the patient on his or her side. Although this positioning is effective because fluids will seek the lowest point and drain out, it is cumbersome to maintain cervical spine support and assist ventilations while the patient is in this position.

Breathing and Oxygenation
ASSESSMENT

Once an open airway is assured, the adequacy of air exchange should be checked. The rate and depth of ventilation may be increased to reduce the carbon dioxide content of the blood and to compensate for metabolic acidosis. This condition is referred to as *compensatory hyperventilation.* Although compensatory hyperventilation tends to occur in early shock, the unresponsive shock patient will often hypoventilate. Hypoventilation occurs when the respiratory center of the brain becomes depressed due to hypoperfusion. When evaluating the ventilatory status, the EMT–I should check both the rate and depth of respirations, watching for patients who exhibit rapid, shallow breathing. This type of breathing is just as ineffective as slow or irregular respirations. Rapid, shallow breathing results in reduced air volume because not enough air is being exchanged.

MANAGEMENT

Any indication of hypoventilation should prompt the EMT–I to assist the patient's breathing with a bag-valve-mask or other ventilatory device. Other conditions that produce respiratory compromise must be managed with the appropriate means as local protocols allow. This might include relieving an obstructed airway, covering an open chest wound with an occlusive dressing (with three sides taped down), stabilizing an unstable chest wall, or performing needle decompression of tension pneumothorax to improve breathing and cardiac output.

Once the airway and breathing have been ensured, the patient should receive 100% oxygen. A nonrebreather mask with an airflow of 10 to 15 L/min should be applied. The EMT–I must be sure to pay attention to the amount of oxygen that remains in the reservoir of the device at the end of each inspiration. Patients experiencing compensatory hyperventilation can deplete the reservoir, in which case, a simple face mask should be employed to prevent suffocation. If the patient becomes nauseous or is frightened by the mask, a nasal cannula with a liter flow of 6 to 8 L/min can be employed.

When there is a need to assist ventilation, such as during hypoventilation or when an endotracheal tube has been placed, 100% oxygen should be delivered via a bag-valve-mask or automatic ventilator device. A pulse oximeter will assist the EMT–I in determining the oxygen content of the patient's blood. After patency of the airway and ventilatory effectiveness have been ensured, attention should be turned to evaluating circulation.

Circulation

ASSESSMENT

The EMT–I should begin by examining the patient for obvious external bleeding. Usually direct pressure is sufficient to contain blood loss. In cases in which hemorrhage cannot be controlled by direct pressure, other measures must be employed, including using a pressure point over a major artery or, as a last resort, the use of a tourniquet. Application of the pneumatic antishock garment may be helpful in controlling intraabdominal (e.g., aorta, liver, spleen, retroperitoneal, pelvic) and lower extremity hemorrhage.

Once major bleeding is controlled, the rate and character of the pulse should be assessed. Compensatory mechanisms can maintain a normal pulse rate even in the presence of a 10% to 15% volume deficit. A fast, weak, or thready pulse suggests decreased circulatory volume. The location of a palpable pulse also will give a rough estimate of the systolic blood pressure. In the case of profound shock in which severe vasoconstriction is present, the EMT–I may not be able to feel a pulse.

The color, appearance, and temperature of the skin also provide useful information about circulatory effectiveness. In early shock, the skin may appear normal. Then, as compensatory mechanisms such as vasoconstriction take effect and blood is routed to the central circulation, the skin becomes pale (decreased perfusion); cyanotic; mottled (combination of pale and cyanotic skin; a late sign of shock); cool to the touch; and diaphoretic (sweaty). Often, the appearance of the skin suggests shock even before there are any noticeable changes in the blood pressure.

Another procedure used to assess the circulation (in children less than 6 years of age) is capillary refill. Capillary refill testing is performed by applying pressure to the nail bed of one of the patient's fingers. This pressure should cause a blanching, or whitening, of the nail bed. When the pressure is released, the nail bed should return to its normal pink color in less than 2 seconds. The EMT–I can approximate this time period by saying "capillary refill." If the normal pink color does not return to the nail bed or the capillary refill is slow, it can be assumed that there is decreased perfusion to this area.

Because the nail bed is the most distal part of the circulation, poor capillary refill is an early indicator of decreased perfusion to the whole body. However, use of the capillary refill test has limited value in the prehospital setting due to poor lighting conditions and other environmental factors. Low skin temperature also may slow capillary refill time. Therefore as with other signs, delayed capillary refill is just one of the possible signs of shock.

MANAGEMENT

Decreased circulation is treated with elevation of the patient's legs, placement of intravenous lifelines, and applying and if necessary inflating the pneumatic antishock garment. Also, the EMT–I must be able to recognize the need for expeditious transport of patients experiencing suspected cardiac tamponade to a definitive care facility where pericardiocentesis can be performed. Last, positive cardiac inotropes and rate-altering medications may be called for in certain conditions.

POSITIONING

The preferred position for the patient in shock is supine with his or her legs elevated 10 to 12 inches. This position promotes increased venous return to the heart and increased cerebral perfusion. In some situations, elevation of the legs alone is enough to raise the blood pressure. However, in cases in which the patient is experiencing respiratory compromise (e.g., acute pulmonary edema secondary to cardiogenic shock), an upright, sitting position should be used to ease respirations. If it is necessary to place a patient experiencing respiratory compromise in a supine position, steps must be taken to assure appropriate air exchange. This might include using a bag-valve-mask device to assist the patient's breathing.

Fluid Replacement

IV lines are used to counter blood loss by introducing fluid into the intravascular space. These fluids act to restore the circulatory volume until the body is able to manufacture more blood. A patient in hypovolemic shock may require at least two IV lines using large bore catheters (14 to 16 gauge).

Three of the most commonly used solutions in prehospital care are lactated Ringer's solution, 0.9% sodium chloride (normal saline), and 5% dextrose in water (D_5W). Lactated Ringer's solution is an isotonic electrolyte solution containing sodium chloride, potassium chloride, calcium chloride, and sodium lactate in water. The lactate of this solution, when metabolized by the liver, is broken down to bicarbonate, a buffer.

Normal saline is an electrolyte solution containing sodium chloride in water, which is isotonic with the extracellular fluid. Both lactated Ringer's solution and normal saline are used to replace fluid volume in patients experiencing shock, because their administration causes an immediate expansion of the circulatory volume. The other solution, 5% dextrose in water, is a hypotonic glucose solution, used to keep a vein open and to supply calories necessary for cell metabolism.

Fluid resuscitation for the shock patient should be guided by medical direction and established protocol. Generally, fluid replacement initiated in the prehospital setting should continue until indicators of adequate tissue perfusion are present, such as, improved blood pressure, improved skin color, a capillary refill less than 2 seconds in nonhypothermic or normothermic pediatric patients, and normal pulse oximetry readings.

CLINICAL NOTES

The EMT–I must keep in mind that overhydration of trauma patients can occur. It is particularly important in patients with closed head injury or pulmonary or cardiac contusion to avoid "fluid overload."

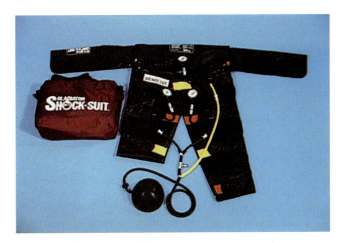

FIGURE 16-39 ▲ The PASG can be effective in managing shock patients. (Jobst Institute, Inc.; Toledo, Ohio from Sanders M: *Mosby's paramedic textbook*, St Louis, 1994, Mosby.)

Blood Preparations

Blood for transfusion can be processed into packed erythrocytes, plasma, and other products such as platelets, or used as whole blood. Erythrocytes can be stored for approximately 35 days before deterioration, depending on the type of preservative used. Blood is administered to restore circulating red cell volume due to an acute loss of blood from trauma or internal hemorrhage. Plasma, the fluid portion of the blood, is transfused in patients who suffer massive burns or in trauma in which large volumes of red blood cell replacement is required. Packed erythrocytes used for transfusion are erythrocytes that have been separated from the plasma. Packed erythrocyte transfusion improves the oxygen-carrying capacity of the blood in various types of anemia.

Erythrocytes have no substitutes. Therefore once the oxygen-carrying capacity is diminished by a massive loss of erythrocytes, only the infusion of additional erythrocytes replenishes the oxygen supply to the body.

For the proper procedures for starting an IV and using necessary equipment and sites for peripheral venous cannulation.

Pneumatic Anti-Shock Garment

✖ **Pneumatic Anti-Shock Garment (PASG)** • An inflatable garment sometimes used on patients with severely low blood pressure or unstable pelvic fractures.

The **pneumatic anti-shock garment (PASG)** (Figure 16-39) is a garment consisting of three air-containing rubber bladders covered with cloth. Two of the compartments wrap around the patient's legs, and one wraps around the stomach. A manual air pump is at-

tached to the bladders of the PASG by hoses. Velcro closures hold the sections in place when the PASG is applied to the patient. Initially, only the leg compartments are inflated. If the patient needs additional assistance, the abdominal compartment is then inflated. Studies suggest that the pneumatic anti-shock garment is not indicated in the prehospital setting with the possible exception of pelvic fracture with hemodynamic instability or when prolonged transport is anticipated.

Originally, the PASG was thought to increase blood pressure by compressing the vessels of the legs and abdomen, thus squeezing 500 to 1000 mL of blood to the trunk and upper extremities. More recent studies suggest that this "autotransfusion effect" is minimal—less than 250 mL. The PASG probably works by increasing resistance in the blood vessels it encloses, leading to an increase in the blood pressure. It is likely that the mechanism by which hypotension is reversed differs depending on the clinical situation. It is possible that several mechanisms may operate together.

The PASG also helps control bleeding. When the garment is inflated, pressure is exerted on the blood vessels. The same internally transmitted pressure that increases the resistance also serves to decrease blood flow in a bleeding vessel. The PASG increases intraabdominal pressure and may be able to tamponade or slow intraabdominal bleeding.

Indications

The most common indication for the use of the PASG is hypovolemic shock, whether caused by bleeding, trauma, sepsis, a ruptured aneurysm, or ectopic pregnancy. The garment may be of help in hypotension secondary to decreased cardiac output.

Another use is stabilization of fractures of the femur, lower leg, and pelvis. A final very helpful role is the PASG's prophylactic placement in air and ground ambulance transfers of potentially unstable patients. If the patient's condition deteriorates, the garment only needs to be inflated.

The criteria for the PASG includes a systolic blood pressure below 90 mm Hg when obvious signs and symptoms of shock are present.

In some EMS systems, the PASG is used based solely on the mechanism of injury and patient presentation rather than blood pressure measurement. Other EMS systems require physician direction for inflation. The EMT–I should check with his or her EMS system for guidelines concerning PASG use and inflation.

Contraindications

Pulmonary edema is an absolute contraindication to the use of the PASG. Increased venous return (preload) and/or an increase in afterload (arterial resistance) is detrimental to the failing heart. It is also contraindicated in ruptured diaphragm and cardiogenic shock. The inflation of the abdominal compartment is contraindicated in pregnancy, respiratory distress of any nature, evisceration, and when there is an impaled object in the abdomen.

Complications

A major complication in the use of the PASG involves chest injuries. Studies have shown that PASG use in the presence of open or closed chest injuries can cause further complications by increasing bleeding into the intrathoracic cavity, thus leading to a tension hemopneumothorax (both blood and air in the chest cavity). It also can cause undue pressure on an injured heart, whether it be a cardiac contusion or pericardial tamponade (blood surrounding the heart). A patient who has a flail segment and is having difficulty breathing will have increased difficulty because the garment is putting added pressure on the diaphragm.

Some other complications may include vomiting, urination, and defecation. If vomiting occurs, the EMT–I must remember to protect the patient's airway.

TECHNIQUES FOR APPLYING AND REMOVING THE PNEUMATIC ANTI-SHOCK GARMENT

Three methods for positioning the PASG under the patient are as follows:

1. Spread the garment on top of the long spine board prior to placing the patient on the board. Use this method when anticipating the need for the PASG (Figure 16-40, *A*).

2. Slide the garment under the patient.
3. Loosely wrap the garment around your arms and slide it on in a pants-type fashion. Do not use this method when spinal injury is suspected.

When positioning the garment ensure that you have done the following:

1. Apply it with the inside portion facing toward the patient and the pump connections on the outside. The inside midline is marked to help prevent confusion. Placing the garment on inside-out will not benefit the patient.
2. Position the garment so that the top is just below the rib cage. If placed too high, it will interfere with respirations.
3. Wrap the three sections around the patient. Secure the device by attaching the Velcro pieces together. If they are too tight or too loose they will be less effective.
4. Connect the foot pump to the pump connections on the leg and abdominal sections. Keep the stopcocks closed until ready to inflate.

When you are ready to inflate the PASG, perform the following:

1. Open both leg compartment stopcocks and ensure that the abdominal compartment is closed (Figure 16-40, *B*). Some local protocols call for inflation of all three chambers at the same time, some call for inflation of one at a time.
2. Quickly compress the foot pump until (Figure 16-40, *C*): (a) the vents on the stopcocks begin to leak or (b) you hear tearing sounds ("crackling") from the Velcro.
3. Close the leg compartment stopcocks and reassess the patient (Figure 16-40, *D*).
4. If the systolic blood pressure has not reached 100 to 110 mm Hg systolic or severe shocklike symptoms still exist, inflate the abdominal compartment.

HELPFUL HINT

- Indications and contraindications for PASG use can vary among EMS systems. The EMT–I should check with his or her instructor, EMS physician, or EMS system concerning local guidelines. Local protocols take precedence over all else. Although the PASG helps control bleeding under the garment, areas near the femoral artery may require additional manual direct pressure to control bleeding.

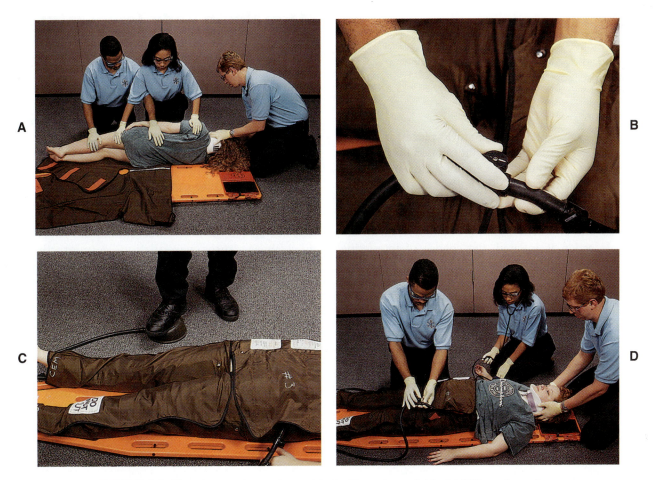

FIGURE 16-40 ▲ Applying the PASG. **A,** Place the unfolded PASG on the spine board and logroll the patient onto the spine board. **B,** Check all valves to ensure the leg compartments are open and the abdominal compartment is closed. **C,** Inflate the garment. **D,** Close all valves and reassess the patient. (Vincent Knaus from Stoy W: *Mosby's EMT-Basic textbook,* St Louis, 1996, Mosby.)

5. Continue inflating the abdominal compartment as you did the leg section.
6. Reassess the patient's vital signs.

TECHNIQUES FOR REMOVING THE PNEUMATIC ANTI-SHOCK GARMENT

Rapid removal of the PASG may cause irreversible shock in some patients. The PASG is rarely deflated in the field. If, however, severe respiratory compromise or pulmonary edema develops, the emergency department physician may order deflation before the patient reaches the hospital.

● HELPFUL HINT

● Deflation of the PASG in the prehospital setting is done only by direct physician order.

The procedures for PASG deflation are as follows:
1. Ensure that the emergency department physician has ordered PASG deflation.
2. Disconnect the stopcock from the abdominal section tubing of the foot pump. Slowly open the stopcock and allow a small amount of air to escape. Reassess vital signs every 5 minutes.
3. If the blood pressure has dropped by more than 5 mm Hg systolic or the patient's condition has deteriorated, discontinue deflation. After additional intervention (IV fluids) reassess the patient.
4. Continue to slowly deflate the abdominal section. Reassess vital signs every 5 minutes. If the patient's condition quickly deteriorates, the abdominal section may be reinflated.
5. If the patient's condition permits, slowly deflate each leg segment. The deflated garment may be left in place until further stabilization occurs.

The PASG may have to remain in place for several hours. The garments are often left inflated until the patient is in the operating room. Endotracheal intubation, blood gases, radiograph, and Foley catheter (urinary collection bag) placement may be accomplished with the PASG applied and inflated.

Pay close attention to respiratory status. When the abdominal section is inflated, the chance of interfering with respiratory effort increases significantly. Some EMS systems have chosen not to use the abdominal section on pediatric patients unless it is absolutely necessary. Prehospital use of the PASG is currently being debated. Some EMS systems have eliminated or restricted the use of PASG. The information presented in this chapter is meant to explain the actual use of the PASG. The EMT–I should check with his or her instructor, EMS physician, or EMS system on local policies regarding PASG's use.

Maintaining Body Temperature

When treating the patient in shock the body temperature must be maintained as close to normal as possible. Attention must be paid to factors that affect the body temperature, including environmental/weather conditions, temperature of the oxygen and intravenous fluids, and the location where the patient is found, to name a few. Patients lying on the ground, particularly during inclement weather, may experience hypothermia.

Body temperature can be maintained by protecting the patient from the elements and by removing any wet clothing. Additionally, cover the patient to avoid heat loss but be careful not to overbundle the patient. Too much heat causes vasodilation, counteracting the body's vasoconstrictive compensatory efforts.

Focused History and Physical Examination

After completing the initial assessment and initiating necessary treatment modalities, a focused history and physical examination and detailed assessment should be performed. The thoroughness of the focused history and physical examination and detailed assessment depends on the severity of the patient's condition. Obvious life-threatening problems that cannot be corrected in the prehospital care setting warrant rapid transportation of the patient to an appropriate definitive care facility. Ideally, when assessing the seriously injured patient, the EMT–I should expose and inspect the head, neck, chest, and abdomen.

Throughout the focused history and physical examination and detailed assessment and while providing treatment and transporting the patient to the hospital, the EMT–I must continually reassess the patient's level of responsiveness, temperature and moistness of the skin, blood pressure, pulse rate, and respiratory rate. The potential for cardiac dysrhythmias exists in shock, and appropriate defibrillation devices should be nearby.

Additional information can be obtained in the detailed assessment by asking the patient appropriate questions to find out how he or she feels. Is the patient thirsty, weak, nauseous, dizzy, etc.? Does the patient have a history of significant medical conditions or take any medications? These answers will give the EMT–I additional information from which he or she can base the treatment modalities.

Transport Considerations

The EMT–I must recognize the indications for rapid transport of the patient experiencing shock to an appropriate medical facility by ground or air ambulance. Guidelines established by local protocol and medical direction in determining the appropriate prehospital level of care for patients and in identifying the appropriate medical facility for patient transport should be followed. Last, the receiving hospital should be provided advance notification of the incoming patient so appropriate provisions can be made to treat the patient.

PREVENTION

The best ways to avoid significant trauma are education and prevention before the event occurs. The EMT–I can play an active role in community education (e.g., use of seat belts), enforcement (e.g., helmet laws) and environment and engineering (e.g., installing "walk signals" at a busy intersection). These and other prevention strategies can help reduce the occurrence of significant injury.

En route to the emergency department (ED), EMT–I Harris reassesses the patient's vital signs and contacts medical direction. Aside from a slight increase in blood pressure, the patient's condition is unchanged. The EMT–Is deliver the patient to the ED and begin to replenish their supplies. As they are cleaning and restocking the ambulance, they are dispatched to a motor vehicle accident at an intersection near the hospital. This call was the second of what was to be a very busy shift.

Later that evening the EMT–Is stop by the ED to check on a few patients that they had transported that day. They are particularly curious about the elderly woman with the fever. The nurse in charge tells the EMT–Is that the woman was diagnosed with pneumonia and septicemia. According to the nurse, the patient developed shaking chills and began to hyperventilate shortly after arrival in the ED. She was later intubated and placed on a ventilator to manage her respiratory failure. Her blood cultures confirmed bacteremia infection for which she was receiving IV antibiotics. The EMT–Is know that pneumonia is a major cause of death in the elderly and that anti-cancer drugs can markedly reduce normal defense mechanisms to combat illnesses like influenza, but they have never really seen a patient like this before.

The nurse said that the patient was moved to the intensive care unit where she wasn't doing very well. Despite fluid resuscitation and vasopressors, she is still hypotensive. Her condition remains guarded.

SUMMARY

Important points to remember from this chapter include the following:

- Shock develops in three successive stages: compensatory, decompensated, and irreversible.
- The first stage occurs when the body fails to compensate for the insult. Signs and symptoms of shock are more apparent at this stage. Survival often depends on prompt recognition in the field, rapid care, and prompt transport to the hospital.
- As shock progresses, the oxygen supply to the cells decreases and the cells resort to anaerobic metabolism. This form of metabolism is far less effective than the normal state of aerobic metabolism.

Anaerobic metabolism produces several abnormal acids, the best known of which is lactic acid. Accumulation of acids changes the pH of the body, resulting in a condition known as acidosis. Untreated shock progresses to the irreversible stage, when the tissues die.

- Evaluation of the trauma patient for shock is begun in the initial assessment, during which the most obvious signs of decreased tissue perfusion may be present. It is continued during the focused and detailed survey, when more subtle clues may be found. The patient is then continually assessed for signs of developing shock until he or she is placed in the hands of the receiving medical personnel.

- Treatment for shock includes adequate ventilation and oxygen and further prevention of the shock process. Rapid transport to the medical facility is imperative.

- Low blood pressure (below 90 mm Hg) is a late sign of shock and therefore is not the sole indicator that shock is present. Evaluation begins with the scene survey, mechanism of injury, and history. If any of these factors indicate that shock is or could be present, the EMT–I should already be taking measures to counter the effects of shock.

- Long-term survival of the body as a whole is dependent on the delivery of adequate amounts of oxygen and glucose to the individual cells by the blood.

- Shock is a condition in which there is inadequate perfusion to the tissues and cells of the body. This creates a lack of tissue oxygenation, leading to anaerobic metabolism.

- Decreased blood flow, which is common in shock syndromes, may occur secondary to hemorrhage, pump failure, or inappropriate systemic vascular resistance. Because of decreased perfusion, the body's tissues become damaged. Even the cardiovascular system deteriorates, worsening the severity of the shock state.

- The body tries to compensate for this damage by utilizing several mechanisms. These mechanisms will only work until the body can no longer maintain perfusion to the vital organs: the heart, lungs, and brain.

- Anaerobic metabolism produces several abnormal acids, the best known of which is lactic acid.

- Accumulation of acids changes the pH of the body, resulting in a condition known as acidosis. Untreated shock progresses to the irreversible stage, when the tissues die.

17

Burns

Key Terms

Alternating Current (AC)

Carboxyhemoglobin (COHb)

Contracture

Direct Current (DC)

Emergent Phase

Entrance Wound

Eschar

Escharotomy

Exit Wound

Fluid Shift Phase

Fourth-Degree Burn

Full-Thickness Burn

Hemoglobinuria

Hemolysis

Inhalation Injury

Myoglobin

Myoglobinuria

Partial-Thickness Burn

Rhabdomyolysis

Rule of Nines

Rule of Palms

Superficial Burn

Tetany

Zone of Coagulation

Zone of Stasis

Zone of Hyperemia

...CASE HISTORY

EMT–Is Baker and Knoll are called to the scene of a house fire. En route, they listen to the radio traffic describing the scene and discuss what equipment they will need. Firefighters are already bringing victims outside, and a triage area has been established.

On arrival at the house, police officers direct the ambulance to a safe area for parking. EMT–I Baker places an oxygen tank, the portable suction unit, the adult airway/intubation bag, a long backboard, cervical collars, head immobilizer, and straps on the stretcher. She also grabs the jump kit. They leave the vehicle and wheel the stretcher to the triage area. Two firefighters bring over a 16-year-old male who is coughing and gasping for air. The triage officer assigns this patient to EMT–Is Baker and Knoll.

EMT–I Baker begins to assess the boy while EMT–I Knoll holds manual, in-line cervical spine stabilization. Initial examination reveals superficial burns to the face and neck, as well as singed eyebrows and facial hair. The young man is complaining of pain on his face and difficulty "catching his breath." Breath sounds reveal scattered wheezes throughout all lung fields.

LEARNING OBJECTIVES

CHAPTER GOAL
Upon completion of this chapter, the EMT-Intermediate will be able to utilize the assessment findings to formulate a field impression and implement the management plan for the patient with a burn injury.

Cognitive Objectives
As an EMT-Intermediate you should be able to do the following:
- Describe the incidence, patterns, and sources of burn injury.
- Describe the pathophysiology of local and systemic responses to burn injury.
- Identify the types of burns according to the depth, extent, and severity of the burn based on established standards.
- Discuss the pathophysiology of burn shock as a basis for key signs and symptoms.
- Describe the physical examination of a patient with burns.
- Describe the out-of-hospital management of a patient with burn injury.

- Discuss pathophysiology as a basis for key signs, symptoms, and management of the patient with an inhalation injury.
- Outline the general assessment and management of the patient who has a chemical injury.
- Describe specific complications and management techniques for selected chemical injuries.
- Describe the physiological effects of electrical injury as they related to each body system based on an understanding of key principles of electricity.
- Outline assessment and management of the patient with electrical injury.
- Describe the distinguishing features of radiation injury and considerations in the prehospital management of these patients.

Affective Objectives
As an EMT–Intermediate you should be able to do the following:
- Value the changes of a patient's self-image associated with a burn injury.
- Value the impact of managing a patient with a burn injury.
- Advocate empathy for a patient with a burn injury.
- Characterize morbidity and mortality based on the pathophysiology and assessment findings of a patient with a burn injury.
- Value and defend the sense of urgency in burn injuries.
- Serve as a model for universal precautions and body substance isolation.

Psychomotor Objectives
As an EMT–Intermediate you should be able to do the following:
- Take body substance isolation (BSI) procedures during assessment and management of patients with a burn injury.
- Perform assessment of a patient with a burn injury.
- Perform management of a thermal burn injury, including airway and ventilation, circulation, pharmacologic, nonpharmacologic, transport considerations, psychological support/communication strategies, and other management described by local protocol.
- Perform management of an inhalation burn injury, including airway, ventilation, and circulation.

INTRODUCTION

Burn injuries are a form of trauma that can be very distracting to the EMT–Intermediate (EMT–I) because of the look and smell of the burn. In addition, these injuries have high mortality rates and can result in lengthy rehabilitation, cosmetic disfigurement, psychosocial problems, and permanent physical disabilities for the patient. The EMT–I should focus on the treatment of life-threatening injuries if they are present even though the burn may consume his or her attention. The burn should be treated only when the EMT–I is sure there is no threat to the patient's airway, breathing, circulation, or neurological status.

INCIDENCE OF BURN INJURY

Each year, more than 2 million Americans seek medical attention for burns. Of these, 70,000 are hospitalized and as many as 10,000 die as a result of thermal injury or burn-related infection.[1]

Fires rank fifth among unintentional injuries following motor vehicle–related crashes, poisonings, falls, and drownings.[2] Deaths from residential fires are most commonly caused by careless use of cigarettes. Heating equipment malfunction ranks second, and electrical equipment malfunction is the third most common cause of residential fires. Approximately 2% of those fatalities are caused by children playing with ignition sources such as matches or cigarette lighters. The consumption of alcohol has been shown to be the strongest independent risk factor for death after the fire begins.[2]

Morbidity and mortality rates from burn injury depend on gender, age, and socioeconomic status. For example, two thirds of all fire fatalities are men; the death rate from thermal injury is highest among children and older adults; and three fourths of all fire deaths occur in the home, with the highest incidence in lower-income households.

PATHOPHYSIOLOGY OF BURN INJURY

Direct contact with either a flame or hot liquid such as water or grease will cause thermal burns. Exposure and length of contact with the substance or flame determine the extent of the burn injury. Factors that influence the body's ability to resist burn injury include the following:
- Water content of the skin tissue
- Thickness and pigmentation of the skin
- Presence or absence of insulating substances such as skin oils or hair
- Peripheral circulation of the skin that affects dissipation of the heat

Local Response

When the burn occurs, cells are immediately destroyed or have their metabolic functions disrupted so that cellular death results. This injury is distributed around the area of direct contact. Some of these cells are destroyed instantly, some of them are irreversibly injured, and others may survive if rapid and appropriate intervention is provided in the out-of-hospital and in-hospital settings.

Major burns have three distinct zones of injury that usually appear in a "bull's-eye" pattern (Figure 17-1). The central area of the burn wound that has sustained the most intense contact with the thermal source is called the **zone of coagulation.** Necrosis of the cells has occurred, and the tissue is no longer viable. The **zone of stasis** surrounds the critically injured area and consists of potentially viable tissue despite the serious thermal injury. In this area, cells are ischemic because of clotting

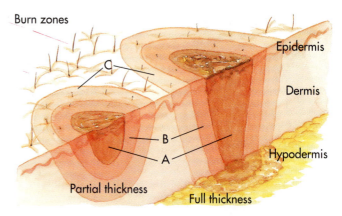

FIGURE 17-1 ▲ Three zones of intensity: *A*, zone of hyperemia (peripheral); *B*, zone of stasis (intermediate); and *C*, zone of coagulation (central). (From Sanders MJ: *Mosby's paramedic textbook,* ed 2, St Louis, 2000, Mosby.)

and vasoconstriction. These cells die within 24 to 48 hours after injury if no supportive measures are taken. The **zone of hyperemia** is at the periphery of the zone of stasis and has increased blood flow as a result of the normal inflammatory response. The tissues in this area recover in 7 to 10 days if infection or profound shock does not develop.

The wound caused by the burn usually swells rapidly, causing an increase in capillary permeability and a fluid shift from the intravascular space into the injured tissue. Sodium moves into the injured cells, causing an increase in osmotic pressure. This increase causes an inflow of vascular fluid into the wound, which results in oozing of fluid from the wound and eventually hypovolemia.

The temperature of the burn source and the age of the patient are major determinants in burn severity. In young children, for example, exposure to water temperatures above 130° F will cause a full-thickness burn in less than 5 seconds. This same exposure by older children and adults will take 15 seconds to cause the same severity of burn.

Systemic Response

While the burn is causing injury at the site of contact, other organ systems become involved as a general response to stress caused by the burn. A large thermal injury can cause hypovolemic shock with a decrease in venous return due to oozing of intravascular fluid at the site of the injury, decreased cardiac output, and increased vascular resistance except in the hyperemic zone. This hypovolemic state, when combined with the breakdown of red blood cells or **hemolysis, rhabdomyolysis** (breakdown of striated or skeletal muscle), and subsequent **hemoglobinuria** (hemoglobin in the urine) and **myoglobinuria** (myoglobin in the urine) seen with major burns and electrical injury, can lead to renal fail-

SYSTEMIC RESPONSES TO MAJOR BURN INJURY

PULMONARY RESPONSE
Hyperventilation to meet increased metabolic needs

GASTROINTESTINAL RESPONSE
Decrease in splanchnic perfusion that may lead to mucosal hemorrhage and transient adynamic ileus
Vomiting and aspiration
Stress ulcers

MUSCULOSKELETAL RESPONSE
Decreased range of motion from immobility and edema
Possible osteoporosis and demineralization (late)

NEUROENDOCRINE RESPONSE
Increased amounts of circulating epinephrine and norephinephrine, as well as transient elevation of aldosterone levels.

METABOLIC RESPONSE
Elevated metabolic rate, particularly with infection or surgical stress

IMMUNE RESPONSE
Altered immunity, resulting in increased susceptibility to infection
Depressed inflammatory response

EMOTIONAL RESPONSE
Physical pain
Isolation from loved ones and familiar surroundings
Fear of disfigurement, deformities, and disability
Altered self-image
Depression

ure. **Myoglobin** is the molecular complex responsible for the red color of muscle and its ability to store oxygen. See Box 17-1 for other systemic responses that occur with major burn injury.

CLASSIFICATION OF BURNS

Burns are classified according to the depth of the burn. Various terminology exists to identify the classes of burns.

Superficial

A **superficial burn** involves only the epidermis (Figure 17-2, *A*). These burns typically occur secondary to prolonged exposure to low-intensity heat or a short-duration flash exposure to a heat source. The skin is usually reddened, and the patient complains of pain. The dead epidermal cells usually peel away or slough off from the healthy tissue beneath the wound in 2 to 3 days without any scarring. The other term commonly used for this type of injury is a *first-degree burn*. An example of a superficial burn is sunburn.

Partial Thickness

A **partial-thickness burn** involves the epidermis and dermis but no underlying tissue. This burn also may be called a *second-degree burn.* There is intense pain; and the skin may appear white or red, moist, and mottled. Blisters usually are present.

These burns are usually divided into two groups: superficial partial thickness and deep partial thickness. The superficial group is characterized by blisters and is commonly caused by skin contact with hot (but not boiling) water or other hot liquids, explosions producing flashburns, hot grease, and flame (Figure 17-2, *B*). The injury extends through the epidermis to the dermis, but the basal layers of the skin are not destroyed. Edematous fluid infiltrates the dermal-epidermal junction, creating the blisters characteristic of this depth of wound. Intact blisters provide a seal that protects the wound from infection and excessive fluid loss. It is for this reason that the blisters should not be broken in the out-of-hospital setting. The injured area usually is red, wet, painful, and may blanch when the tissue around the injury is compressed. As long as infection does not occur, the skin regenerates within a few days to a week and heals without scarring.

A deep partial-thickness burn involves the basal layer of the dermis (Figure 17-2, *C*). Edema still forms at the epidermal-dermal junction so that blisters again should not be broken. Sensation in and around the wound may be diminished because of the destruction of basal-layer nerve endings. The injury may appear red and wet or white and dry, depending on the degree of vascular injury. Wound infection with subsequent sepsis and fluid loss are major complications of these injuries. If uncomplicated, deep partial-thickness burns usually heal within three to four weeks. Skin grafting may be necessary to promote timely healing and minimize thick scar tissue formation, which may severely restrict joint movements and cause persistent pain and disfigurement.

Full Thickness

A **full-thickness burn** extends through all of the dermal layers. This burn is also called a *third-degree burn.* Subcutaneous tissue, muscle, bone, and/or organs also may be involved (Figure 17-2, *D*). There is no pain associated with this burn because nerves have been burnt away. However, there may be extreme pain in some areas due to partial-thickness burns surrounding the full-thickness burns. The skin may look very dry and leathery or appear

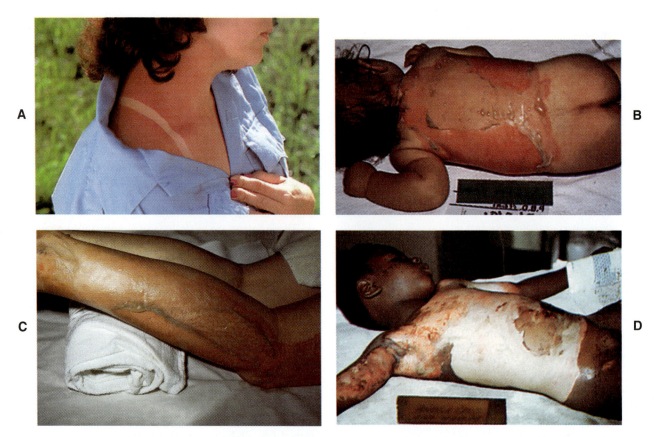

FIGURE 17-2 ▲ Classification of burns. **A,** A superficial burn involves only the epidermis. **B,** A partial-thickness burn involves the epidermis and dermis. No damage occurs to the underlying skin tissues. **C,** Deep partial-thickness burn. **D,** A full-thickness burn involves all layers of the dermis, and may involve bones, muscle, or underlying organs. (**A,** From Stoy W: *Mosby's EMT-Basic textbook,* St Louis, 1996, Mosby; **B** and **D,** Courtesy of St Johns Mercy Medical Center, St Louis from Stoy W: *Mosby's EMT-Basic textbook,* St Louis, 1996, Mosby.; **C,** Courtesy of St John's Mercy Medical Center, St Louis.)

white, dark brown, or charred. **Eschar,** a tough, nonelastic coagulated collagen of the dermis, is present in these injuries. Large plasma volume loss, infection, and sepsis frequently occur after these types of burns. Natural wound healing may produce a **contracture** (permanent condition of a joint characterized by flexion and fixation) deformity, and severe scarring (Figure 17-3). Therefore, surgical intervention with skin grafting is necessary to close full-thickness wounds, minimize complications, and allow restoration of maximal function.

Some burn classifications also include a **fourth-degree burn** to describe a full-thickness injury that penetrates the subcutaneous tissue, muscle, fascia, periosteum, or bone. These burns usually result from incineration-type exposure and electrical burns in which heat is sufficient to destroy tissues below the skin.

Extent and Severity

When assessing a burn, it is important to consider the severity. This information is needed to make a decision on the patient's final destination (local emergency department, burn center, and so on). The EMT–I should use a method for determining the extent of burn injury approved by medical direction.

Elements that are used to categorize the severity of a burn include the following:
- The depth or degree of the burn
- The percentage of body surface affected
- Locations on the body that affect function such as the face and upper airway, hands, feet, and genitalia
- Preexisting medical conditions

Patients who are under 5 or older than 55 years of age should be evaluated immediately at a burn or trauma center if they have serious burns. Medical direction should be consulted to make this referral.

RULE OF NINES

The **rule of nines** commonly is used in the out-of-hospital setting. This measurement divides the total body surface area into segments that are multiples of

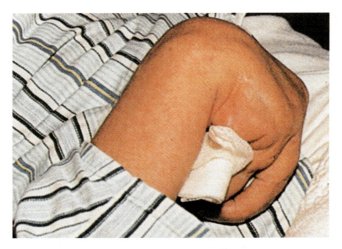

FIGURE 17-3 ▲ This joint is in a permanent state of flexion and fixation known as a contracture.

9%. It provides a rough estimate of burn injury size and is most accurate for adults and children older than 10 years of age (Figure 17-4).

RULE OF PALMS

If the burn is irregularly shaped or has a scattered distribution throughout the body, the rule of nines is difficult to apply. In these situations, burn size can be estimated by visualizing the patient's palm as an indicator of percentage (**rule of palms**). The surface of the patient's palm equals about 1% of the total body surface area.

AMERICAN BURN ASSOCIATION CATEGORIZATION

Using criteria established by the American Burn Association, burn injuries are categorized as major, moderate, and minor. Box 17-2 shows the three categories and their characteristics.

PATHOPHYSIOLOGY OF BURN SHOCK

With large body surface area burns, shock occurs from local and systemic responses to thermal trauma. These responses lead to edema and accumulation of vascular fluid in the tissues in the area of the injury. Locally there is a brief initial decrease in blood flow to the area known as the **emergent phase.** This response is followed by a marked increase in arteriolar vasodilation. The **fluid shift phase** occurs when the concurrent release of vasoactive substances from the burned tissue cause increased capillary permeability, producing intravascular fluid loss and wound edema. The fluid loss into the injured tissues and the marked increase in evaporative fluid loss secondary to the break in the epithelial barrier contribute to produce hypovolemia.

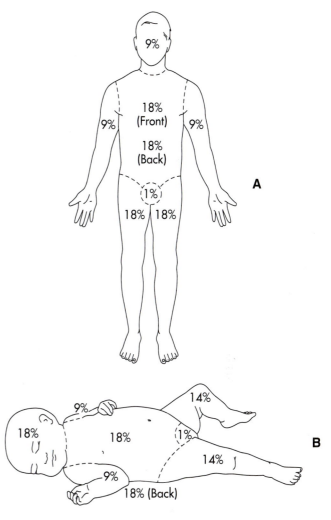

FIGURE 17-4 ▲ The rule of nines. **A,** Adult. **B,** Infant. (From Rosen P, Barkin R: *Emergency medicine: concepts and clinical practice,* ed 4, St Louis, 1998, Mosby.)

STREET WISE

Hypovolemia secondary to burn trauma is usually not seen in the prehospital setting because burn edema develops over the first several hours after the burn. A patient with burns and hypovolemia should be evaluated at the scene for other injuries that may be responsible for the loss of volume.

Within minutes of a major burn injury, all capillaries in the circulatory system (not just those in the area of the burn) lose their capillary seal. This increase in capillary permeability prevents the creation of an osmotic gradient between the intravascular and extravascular spaces, allowing colloid solutions to quickly equilibrate across the capillary barrier and into the interstitium.

BOX 17-2

AMERICAN BURN ASSOCIATION CATEGORIZATION

MAJOR BURN
Twenty-five percent of body surface or greater
Functionally significant involvement of hands, face, feet, or perineum
Electrical or inhalation injury
Concomitant injury
Severe, preexisting medical problems

MODERATE BURN
Fifteen percent to 25% of body surface area
No complications or involvement of hands, face, feet, or perineum
No electrical injury, inhalation injury, concomitant injury, or severe preexisting medical problem

MINOR BURN
Fifteen percent or less of body surface area
No involvement of face, hands, feet, or perineum
No electrical burns, inhalation injury, severe preexisting medical problems, or complications

Therapy for burn shock is aimed at supporting the patient through the period of hypovolemic shock. Crystalloid solution (e.g., lactated Ringer's solution) is usually considered the fluid of choice in initial resuscitation.

! HELPFUL HINT

- Fluid resuscitation in burns in controversial. Medical control may recommend that fluid resuscitation not be initiated in the prehospital setting if transport to a hospital can be made within 30 minutes.[1] Whatever the decision, transport should not be delayed to initiate intravenous (IV) therapy.

ASSESSMENT

During assessment, the dramatic appearance of the burns, the patient's intense pain, and the characteristic odor of burned flesh may easily distract the EMT–I from life-threatening problems. Concentrate on locating life-threatening circumstances *before* turning attention to the burn. Confidently assess and direct efforts toward the patient as a whole. Remember that personal and scene safety is the number one priority!

Initial Assessment

Evaluate the patient's airway, particularly for the patient with an actual or potential inhalation injury. Upper

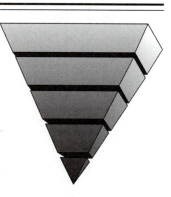

- Burns around nose or mouth
- Soot in mouth or nose: singed nasal hairs
- Intraoral burns: burned tongue
- Intraoral swelling (no stridor)
- Hoarseness of voice
- Visible pharyngeal edema
- **Inspiratory stridor**

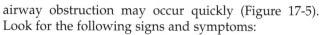

FIGURE 17-5 ▲ Probability of upper airway obstruction. (From Sanders MJ: *Mosby's paramedic textbook,* ed 2, St. Louis, 2000, Mosby.)

airway obstruction may occur quickly (Figure 17-5). Look for the following signs and symptoms:
- Stridor (an ominous sign that indicates the patient's upper airway is at least 80% narrowed)
- Facial burns
- Soot in the mouth or nose
- Singed facial or nasal hair
- Edema of the lips and oral cavity
- Coughing/wheezing
- Inability to swallow secretions in the pharynx
- Hoarse voice
- Circumferential neck burns

Evaluate breathing for rate, depth, and the presence of wheezes, crackles, or rhonchi. Evaluate the circulatory status by assessing the presence, rate, character, and rhythm of pulses; capillary refill; skin color and temperature; pulse oximetry, which may be inaccurate in the presence of carbon monoxide; and obvious arterial bleeding.

Determine the patient's neurological status by using the AVPU scale (alert, responds to verbal stimuli, responds to painful stimuli, unresponsive) or a similar method. Evaluate any deviations for an underlying cause. These include hypoxia, decreased cerebral perfusion from hyovolemia, and cerebral injury resulting from head trauma.

After the initial assessment, obtain an accurate history from the patient or bystanders. Ask the following:
- What is the patient's chief complaint (e.g., pain, dyspnea)?
- What were the circumstances of the injury?
- Did it occur in an enclosed space?
- Were explosive forces involved?
- Were hazardous chemicals involved?
- Was there electricity involved in the burn?
- Is there related trauma?
- What was the source of the burning agent?
  - Flame
  - Metal
  - Liquid

- Chemical
- Electrical
- Does the patient have any significant medical history?
- What medications does the patient take (including any recent ingestions of illegal drugs or alcohol)?
- Did the patient lose consciousness at any time? If so, suspect inhalation injury.
- What is the status of the patient's tetanus immunization?
- Does the patient smoke?

Physical Examination

Obtain a complete set of vital signs, including a blood pressure in an unburned extremity if possible. If all extremities are burned, place sterile gauze under the blood pressure cuff and try to auscultate a blood pressure. Use an electrocardiogram (ECG) monitor for patients with severe burns or those with preexisting medical or cardiac illnesses. Modify lead placement if necessary so as not to place electrodes over burned areas.

MANAGEMENT

The first step in management of the patient with burns is to treat any life-threatening injuries. Specific burn management should occur *after* airway, breathing, circulation, and neurological problems have been treated.

Goals for managing severe burns include the following:
- Stopping the burning process
- Preventing further tissue injury
- Maintaining the airway
- Administering oxygen and providing ventilatory support
- Providing fluid resuscitation (as per local protocol)
- Providing rapid transport to an appropriate medical facility
- Providing pain management as appropriate
- Using clean technique to minimize the patient's exposure to infectious agents
- Providing psychological and emotional support

Stopping the Burning Process

The first step in managing any burn is to stop the burning process. This step must be accomplished with the safety of the emergency crew in mind because it often occurs in close proximity to the source that caused the burn. For minor burns, the burning process can be terminated by cooling the local area with cold water. Ice, snow, or ointment should not be applied to the burn because these agents may increase the depth and severity of thermal injury. In addition, ointments may impair or delay assessment of the injury when the patient arrives in the emergency department.

In the case of severe burns, the patient should be rapidly and safely moved from the burning source to an

area of safety if possible. A person whose clothing is in flames or who is smoldering should be placed on the floor or ground and rolled in a blanket to smother the flames and/or doused with large quantities of the cleanest available water. Use cold water whenever possible to rapidly decrease the skin temperature. However, be aware that cold water may contribute to hypothermia. Avoid contaminated water sources such as a lake or river. Remove the burnt, hot clothes and any jewelry such as rings and necklaces that may become constrictive once swelling occurs.

Airway, Oxygen, and Ventilation

High-concentration humidified oxygen should be administered to any patient with severe burns, and ventilation should be assisted as needed. If inhalation injury is suspected, the patient should be closely observed for signs of impending airway obstruction. Life-threatening laryngeal edema may be progressive and may make tracheal intubation difficult if not impossible. The decision to intubate these patients should not be delayed. Every attempt should be made to intubate the patient's lungs with a normal (not smaller) sized endotracheal tube. These patients are often difficult to ventilate even with an appropriately-sized tube.

Circulation

The need for fluid resuscitation is based on the severity of the injury, the patient's vital signs, and transport time to the hospital. Some authorities believe that prompt intervention of IV therapy in the patient with critical burns is essential to prevent long-term complications such as burn shock and renal failure. Consult with medical direction and follow local protocols regarding fluid replacement.

If IV therapy is to be performed, initiate a large-bore catheter in a peripheral vein in an unburned extremity, preferably the arm. If an unburned site is not available, insert the catheter through burned tissue, although the risk of subsequent infection is greater. Secure the catheter with a dressing as tape may not adhere to the injured area as it begins to leak fluid.

Pain Management

Consider pain medication as an early intervention. Patients with large burns may require IV morphine or meperidine (Demerol) as per local protocols and medical direction.

General Wound Care

Wound care for partial-thickness and full-thickness burns consists of first removing the burning process by cutting away clothes or removing the chemical in the case of a chemical burn. If blisters are present, the EMT–I should not break them open. Cover the burned area with a clean, dry dressing. Some controversy exists regarding the use of wet versus dry dressings. It generally is recommended that wet dressings be used on up to 10% of the body surface area burned. The EMT–I should check with medical direction for specific treatment guidelines.

Other Procedures

If transport is delayed or a lengthy interfacility transport is anticipated, other patient care procedures may be required. These include the placement of a nasogastric tube to prevent gastric distention or vomiting, as well as the placement of an indwelling urinary catheter to measure urine output and to maintain patency of the urethra in patients with burns to the genitalia.

Special Considerations

Burns to the face and extremities, as well as circumferential burns, require special consideration. Burns of the face swell rapidly and may be associated with airway compromise. As long as spinal trauma is not present, elevate the head of the stretcher at least 30 degrees to minimize edema. Avoid using a pillow if the patient's ears are burned so as not to cause additional injury to the area.

If burns involve the extremities or large areas of the body, remove all rings, watches, and other jewelry as soon as possible to prevent vascular compromise with increased wound edema. Inventory any personal belongings (including the jewelry), place it in a labeled bag, and document to whom the bag is given. Reassess peripheral pulses frequently, and elevate the burned limb above the patient's heart if possible.

Circumferential burns of an extremity may produce a tourniquet-like effect that may quickly compromise circulation and cause irreversible damage to the limb. Circumferential burns of the chest can severely restrict movement of the thorax and may significantly impair chest wall compliance. If this occurs, the depth of respirations is reduced, tidal volume is decreased, and the patient's lungs may become difficult to ventilate, even by mechanical means. Definitive treatment for circumferential burns includes an **escharotomy.** This procedure involves incisions made through deep burns to reduce compartment pressure and allow adequate blood volume to flow to and from the affected limb or thorax. This procedure is most commonly performed by paramedics, flight nurses, and physicians depending on local protocols.

Burn Center Referral Criteria

According to the Committee on Trauma of the American College of Surgeons and the American Burn Association, burn injuries usually requiring referral to a burn center include 11 guidelines (Box 17-3). Medical direction usually will determine by protocol how this standard is applied and used by an emergency medical services (EMS) agency.

SPECIFIC TYPES OF BURN INJURY

Inhalation Burn Injury

Smoke inhalation injury is present in about 20% to 35% of all patients admitted to burn centers.[3] In addition, more than 50% of the 12,000 fire deaths each year are directly related to smoke inhalation or **inhalation injury.** Prehospital considerations in caring for patients with inhalation injury include recognition of the dangers inherent in the fire environment, pathophysiology of inhalation injury, and early detection and treatment of impending airway or respiratory problems.

Smoke inhalation most commonly occurs in a closed environment such as a building, an automobile, or an airplane and is caused by the accumulation of toxic byproducts of combustion. Inhalation injury also can occur in an open space; therefore all burn victims should be evaluated for this injury. Dangers that contribute to inhalation injury in a fire environment are as follows:

- Heat
- Consumption of oxygen by the fire
- Production of carbon monoxide
- Production of other toxic gases

GUIDELINES FOR REFERRAL TO A BURN CENTER

Partial- and full-thickness burns that in combination cover more than 10% of the body surface area in patients under 10 or over 50 years of age

Partial- and full-thickness burns that in combination cover more than 20% of the body surface area of patients in other age groups

Partial- and full-thickness burns that involve the face, hands, feet, genitalia, or perineum or those that involve skin overlying major joints

Full-thickness burns over more than 5% body surface area in any age group

Significant electrical burns, including lightning injury

Significant chemical burns

Inhalation injury

Burn injury in patients with pre-existing illnesses that could complicate management, prolong recovery, or affect mortality

Burns in any patient in whom concomitant trauma poses an increased risk of morbidity or mortality and who may be initially treated in a trauma center until stable before transfer to a burn center

Burns in children seen in hospitals without qualified personnel or equipment for their care (they should be transferred to a burn center with these capabilities)

Burn injuries in patients who require special social and emotional or long-term rehabilitative support, including cases involving suspected child abuse and neglect

CLINICAL NOTES

Inhalation injury may also occur in the absence of significant thermal injury from exposure to toxic gases (e.g., carbon monoxide).

PATHOPHYSIOLOGY

Smoke inhalation and inhalation injury compose a broad group of consequences secondary to combustion. These consequences may be classified as carbon monoxide poisoning, *supraglottic* (inhalation injury above the glottis), and *infraglottic* (inhalation injury below the glottis).

Carbon Monoxide Poisoning—Carbon monoxide is a colorless, odorless, tasteless gas produced by incomplete combustion of carbon-containing fuels. Carbon monoxide does not physically harm lung tissue, but it causes a reversible displacement of oxygen on the hemoglobin molecule, forming **carboxyhemoglobin (COHb)**. The result is low circulating volumes of oxygen despite normal partial pressures. In addition, the presence of COHb requires that tissues be very hypoxic before oxygen is released from the hemoglobin to fuel the cells.

Carbon monoxide has about 250 times the affinity for hemoglobin that oxygen has. Therefore small concentrations of carbon monoxide in inspired air can result in severe physiological impairments including tissue hypoxia, inadequate cellular oxygenation, inadequate cellular and organ function, and eventually death. The physical effects of carbon monoxide poisoning are related to the level of COHb in the blood (Table 17-1).

CLINICAL NOTES

Tachypnea and cyanosis usually are not present in patients with carbon monoxide poisoning because arterial oxygen tension is normal. Patients with high COHb levels may have a skin appearance that is bright red, but more commonly, the patient has normal or pale skin and lip coloration.

Treatment includes the following:
● Ensure a patent airway
● Provide adequate ventilation
● Administer high-concentration oxygen

STREET WISE

The half-life of carbon monoxide at room air is about 4 hours. This time frame can be reduced to 30 to 40 minutes if 100% oxygen and adequate ventilation are provided.

Supraglottic Inhalation Injury (Above the Glottis)—The structure and function of the airway above the glottis make it particularly susceptible to injury if exposed to high temperatures. The upper airway is very vascular and has a large surface area, which allows it to normalize temperatures of inspired air. Because of this design, the upper airway sustains the impact of injury when environmental air is superheated.

Thermal injury to the airway can result in immediate edema of the pharynx and larynx, which can rapidly progress to complete airway obstruction (Figure 17-6). Signs and symptoms include the following:
● Facial burns
● Singed nasal or facial hairs
● Carbonaceous sputum
● Edema of the face, oropharyngeal cavity, or both
● Signs of hypoxemia
● Hoarse voice
● Stridor

TABLE 17-1

Physical Effects of Carbon Monoxide Poisoning

CARBON MONOXIDE LEVEL	SIGNS AND SYMPTOMS
Less than 10%	Not usually significant
	Commonly found in smokers, traffic police, truck drivers, and others who are chronically exposed to carbon monoxide
20%	Headache
	Nausea and vomiting
	Loss of manual dexterity
30%	Lethargy and confusion
	Electrocardiogram abnormalities
Between 40% and 60%	Coma may develop
More than 60%	Often fatal

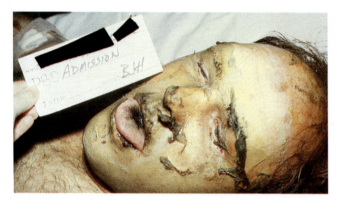

FIGURE 17-6 ▲ Inhalation injury. (From Sanders MJ: *Mosby's paramedic textbook,* ed 2, St Louis, 2000, Mosby.)

- Brassy cough
- Grunting respirations

Prompt recognition and protection of the airway are critical in these patients. If impending airway obstruction is suspected, early nasotracheal or orotracheal intubation may be warranted because progressive edema can make emergency intubation extremely hazardous if not impossible.

Infraglottic Inhalation Injury (Below the Glottis)—The two primary mechanisms of direct injury to the lung parenchyma are heat and toxic material inhalation. Thermal injury to the lower airway is rare. Causes include inhalation of superheated steam, which has 4000 times the heat-carrying capacity of dry air; aspiration of scalding liquids; and explosions, which occur as the patient is breathing high concentrations of oxygen under pressure.

Most fire-related lower airway injuries result from the inhalation of toxic chemicals such as the gaseous by-products of burning materials. Signs and symptoms of lower-airway injury may be immediate but more frequently are delayed, beginning several hours after the exposure.

These include the following:
- Wheezes
- Crackles or rhonchi
- Productive cough
- Signs of hypoxemia
- Spasm of bronchi and bronchioles

Prehospital care should be directed at ensuring a patent airway and providing high-concentration oxygen and ventilatory support. Specific airway and ventilatory management, which may include nasal or oral tracheal intubation and pharmacological therapy with bronchodilators, should be coordinated with on-line/direct medical control.

Chemical Burn Injury

Caustic chemicals are often present in the home and workplace, and unintentional exposure is common. Three types of caustic agents frequently are associated with burn injuries are alkalis, acids, and organic compounds (Table 17-2). The severity of chemical injury is related to the chemical agent, concentration and volume of the chemical, and duration of contact (Figure 17-7).

ASSESSMENT

Exposure factors often can be assessed during the patient history. When dealing with a chemical exposure, the EMT–Intermediate should ascertain the following:
- Type of chemical substance—if container is available and can be safely transported, take it to the medical facility
- Concentration of chemical substance
- Volume of chemical substance
- Mechanism of injury (local immersion of a body part, injection, or splash)
- Time of contamination
- First aid administered before EMS arrival
- Appearance (chemical burns vary in color)
- Pain

TABLE 17-2

Types of Caustic Agents Associated With Burn Injuries

TYPE OF CAUSTIC AGENT	EXAMPLES
Alkalis (strong bases with a high pH)	Hydroxides and carbonates of sodium, potassium, ammonium, lithium, barium, and calcium Found in the following: • Oven cleaners • Household drain cleaners • Fertilizers • Heavy industrial cleaners • Structural bonds of cement and concrete
Acids	Found in many household cleaners such as rust removers, bathroom cleaners, and swimming pool acidifiers
Organic compounds (chemicals that contain carbon; may be absorbed by the skin causing serious side effects)	Those that can produce caustic injury to human tissue are phenols, creosote, and petroleum products such as gasoline NOTE: Most organic compounds such as wood and coal are harmless chemicals.

MANAGEMENT

As with all burn injuries, the safety of the rescuers must be the first consideration in managing the victim of chemical injury. Law enforcement, fire service, and special rescue personnel may be needed to secure the scene before entry.

The EMT–I must consider the use of protective gear before approaching the scene. Depending on the scene and chemical agent(s) involved, personal protection may include gloves, eye shields, protective garments, and appropriate breathing apparatus.

The treatment of chemical burns varies little from that of thermal burns during the initial assessment. Treatment is directed at stopping the burning process and can be best accomplished by doing the following:

1. Remove all clothing, including shoes, which can trap concentrated chemicals.
2. Brush off powdered chemicals.
3. Irrigate the affected area with copious amounts of water:
   • In otherwise stable patients, irrigation takes priority over transportation unless irrigation can be continued en route to the emergency department.
   • If a large body surface area is involved, a shower should be used for irrigation, if readily available.

Although the primary treatment for most chemical burns is copious irrigation with water, several specific chemical injuries warrant further treatment. These include petroleum, hydrofluoric acid, phenols, ammonia, and alkali metals (Table 17-3).

Chemical Burn Injury to the Eyes—Chemical burns to the eyes (e.g., from mace, pepper spray, or other irritants) may cause damage ranging from chemical conjunctivitis (superficial inflammation) to severe burns. Patients with these conditions have local pain,

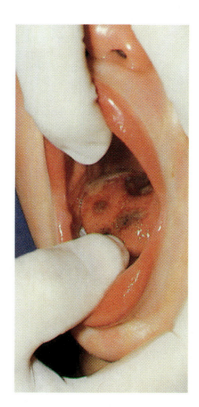

FIGURE 17-7 ▲ Intraoral chemical burns sustained by a boy who has ingested bleach. (From Beattie TF, Hendry GM, Duguid KP: *Pediatric emergencies*, London, 1997, Mosby-Wolfe.)

visual disturbance, lacrimation (tearing), edema, and redness of surrounding tissues.

Management guidelines include flushing the eyes with water by using a mild flow from a hose, IV tubing, or water from a container. The affected eye should be irrigated from the medial to the lateral aspect to avoid

TABLE 17-3

Chemicals, Injuries, and Treatment

TYPE OF CHEMICAL	DESCRIPTION	SIGNS AND SYMPTOMS	TREATMENT
Petroleum	Prolonged gasoline and diesel fuel contact in absence of flame	Initially appears as only superficial or partial-thickness burn when in fact it may be full-thickness The following systemic effects may result from absorption: • Central nervous system (CNS) depression • Organ failure • Death • Lead toxicity if gasoline contained tetraethyl lead	Conduct copious irrigation with water.
Hydrofluoric acid	One of the most corrosive materials known Used in industry for cleaning fabrics and metals, glass etching, and manufacture of silicone chips for electronic equipment Fluoride ion inhibits several chemical reactions essential to cell survival; continues to penetrate and kill cells when it is neutralized by binding to calcium or magnesium	Has the potential to produce very-deep, painful, and severe injuries If large body surface area is involved or there has been exposure to high concentrations of the acid, severe hypocalcemia and even death may occur. NOTE: Even the most minor-appearing wounds that involve hydrofluoric acid should be evaluated at an appropriate medical facility.	Irrigate exposed area with copious amounts of water before transport. On arrival at the emergency department, treatment may include subcutaneous administration of a 10% calcium gluconate solution directly into the burn site.
Phenol (carbolic acid)	Aromatic hydrocarbon derived from coal tar Widely used in industry as a disinfectant in cleaning agents and in the manufacture of plastics, dyes, fertilizers, and explosives	Local tissue coagulation with skin contact; may be painless because of agent's anesthetic properties Minor exposures may cause CNS depression and dysrhythmias Systemic toxicity if agent absorbed	Conduct copious irrigation with large volumes of water. After irrigation, medical direction may recommend swabbing wound with a suitable solvent such as glycerol, vegetable oil, or soap and water to bind phenol and prevent systemic absorption. Patients with significant exposures (10 to 15% total body surface area) may require systemic support and should be carefully observed for signs of respiratory failure.

TABLE 17-3

Chemicals, Injuries, and Treatment—cont'd

TYPE OF CHEMICAL	DESCRIPTION	SIGNS AND SYMPTOMS	TREATMENT
Ammonia	Noxious, irritating gas Strong alkali that is very soluble in water Extremely hazardous solution if introduced into the eye; may result in necrosis and blindness	If eyes affected, there will be swelling or spasm of the eyelids. Respiratory injury from ammonia vapors depends on concentration and duration of exposure. Short-term, high-concentration exposure results in upper airway edema. Long-term, low-concentration exposure results in damage to lower respiratory tract.	Irrigate eye injuries with water or a balanced salt solution. Supply high-concentration oxygen and ventilatory support as needed for respiratory exposure. Rapid transport to an appropriate medical facility
Alkali metals	Sodium and potassium are highly reactive metals that can ignite spontaneously	Local tissue damage	Water is generally contraindicated when these metals are imbedded in the skin because they react with water and produce large amounts of heat. Physically remove the metal or cover it with oil to minimize the thermal injury

flushing the chemical into the unaffected eye. Irrigation should continue during transport. In addition, contact lenses, if present, should be removed.

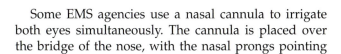

CLINICAL NOTES

When retracting the lids to irrigate the eyes, the EMT–Intermediate should be careful to apply pressure only to the bony structures surrounding the eye and avoid pressure on the globe.

Some EMS agencies use a nasal cannula to irrigate both eyes simultaneously. The cannula is placed over the bridge of the nose, with the nasal prongs pointing

STUDENT ALERT

A chemical burn to the eye can be frightening for the patient who fears loss of sight from the injury. The EMT–I should attempt to calm the patient and explain the importance of thorough eye irrigation, which may be uncomfortable. This explanation may help to improve the patient's cooperation.

down toward the eyes. The cannula is attached to an IV administration set using either normal saline or lactated Ringer's solution and run continually into both eyes (Figure 17-8).

USE OF ANTIDOTES OR NEUTRALIZING AGENTS

According to the American Burn Association, no agent has been found to be superior to water for treating most chemical burns.[3] Therefore the use of antidotes or neutralizing agents should be avoided in initial prehospital management of most burn injuries. Many neutralizing agents produce heat and may increase injury when applied to the wound.

In special circumstances such as when an industrial complex is located within the EMS agency's response area and they are known to use a chemical agent with a specific antidote, medical direction may elect to have the EMS stock the neutralizer. In this situation, the EMT–I should receive special training on the indications, contraindications, use, and side effects of these agents.

Electrical Burn Injuries

Electrical injuries account for 4% to 6.5% of admissions to burn centers and are responsible for about 500 deaths

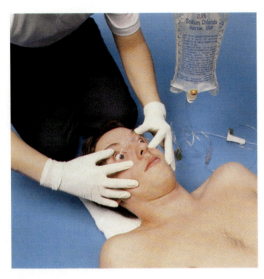

FIGURE 17-8   ▲   Use of nasal cannula for eye irrigation. (From Sanders MJ: *Mosby's paramedic textbook*, ed 2, St Louis, 2000, Mosby.)

each year.[4] An understanding of the principles of current and the path of destruction it may produce in the body is essential for good patient care and personal safety at the scene of an electrocution.

TYPES OF ELECTRICAL INJURY

Three basic types of injury may occur as a result of contact with electric current. These are outlined in Table 17-4.

> **CLINICAL NOTES**
>
> The entrance site of an electrical injury can "hide" and may be difficult to find, especially in a patient with an altered level of consciousness. Look for the wound in the "not-so-common" places such as between the fingers and toes and in the patient's hairline.

EFFECTS OF ELECTRICAL INJURY

Electrical injuries often are unpredictable and vary according to the parameters described previously. However, certain physiological effects should be anticipated by the EMS crew.

The skin is almost always the first point of contact with electrical current. Direct contact and passage of current through tissue may produce extensive areas of coagulation necrosis. The entrance site or **entrance wound** is often a characteristic "bull's-eye" wound and may appear dry, leathery, charred, or depressed. The **exit wound** may be ulcerated and may have an "exploded" appearance where areas of tissue are missing.

Oral burns are frequently seen in children under 2 years of age. These wounds are typically caused by chewing or sucking on a low-tension electrical cord. Oral burns may be associated with injury to the tongue, palate, and face.

Hypertension and tachycardia associated with a large release of catecholamines is a common finding in electrical injury. Electrical current also may cause significant dysrhythmias (including ventricular fibrillation and asystole) and damage to the myocardium as it passes through the body. If the patient has suffered cardiac arrest and early rescue and resuscitation can be initiated by the EMT–I, success rates are high.

Nerve tissue is an excellent conductor of electrical current and may therefore be commonly affected in electrical injuries. Central nervous system (CNS) damage may result in seizures or coma with or without focal neurological findings. Peripheral nerve injury may lead to motor or sensory deficits, which may be permanent. If the current passes through the brain stem, respiratory arrest or depression, cerebral edema, or hemorrhage may rapidly lead to death.

Ventilation may be impaired when electrical burns produce CNS injury or chest wall dysfunction. If the respiratory center is disrupted, hypoventilation can lead to immediate patient death. Contact with any **alternating current (AC)** sources has also been documented to produce respiratory arrest and death from **tetany** (violent muscle spasm) of the muscles of respiration.

Electrical injury can cause extensive necrosis of blood vessels. These injuries, although they may not be evident on EMS arrival, can cause immediate or delayed internal hemorrhage or arterial or venous thrombosis and embolism with subsequent complications.

Damage within the extremities after an electrical burn is similar to crush injury in that severe muscle necrosis releases myoglobin, and hemolysis releases hemoglobin, which can precipitate in the renal tubules causing acute renal failure. Some patients may require amputation of the affected extremity as a result of decreased circulation and compartment syndrome. Severe muscle spasms can produce bony fractures and dislocations, even of major joints. In addition, a patient may fall after the electrical shock and sustain significant skeletal trauma, including damage to the cervical spine.

Numerous other internal structures may be damaged secondary to electrical injury including the abdominal organs and urinary bladder. Submucosal hemorrhage may occur in the bowel, and various forms of ulceration are possible. Each patient requires a thorough physical assessment and a high degree of suspicion for associated trauma.

ASSESSMENT AND MANAGEMENT

Patient assessment should begin by ensuring that no hazards exist for the rescuers or bystanders. If the patient is still in contact with the electrical source, the electric company, fire department, or other specially trained personnel should be summoned before ap-

TABLE 17-4

Types of Electrical Injury

TYPE OF ELECTRICAL INJURY	DESCRIPTION	SIGNS AND SYMPTOMS
Direct contact burns	Occur when electric current directly penetrates resistance of skin and underlying tissues	Greatest tissue damage occurs directly under and adjacent to contact points; may include fat, fascia, muscle, and bone
	Hand and wrist are common entrance sites (Figure 17-9, *A*) Foot is common exit site (Figure 17-9, *B*)	Tissue destruction may be massive at entrance and exit sites
	Although skin may initially resist current flow, continued contact with source lessens resistance and permits increased current flow	Area affected between the wounds that poses greatest threat to patient's life
Arc injuries	Occur when person is close enough to high-voltage source	As described above
	Current between two contact points near skin overcomes resistance in air, passing current flow through air to bystander Temperatures may be as high as 2000° C to 4000° C (3632° F to 7232° F) Arc may jump as far as 10 feet.	
Flash burns	Occur when heat of electric current ignites a nearby combustible source Clothes may ignite or cause fire in surrounding environment No electrical current passes through body	Common injury sites include face and eyes Local tissue injury can occur

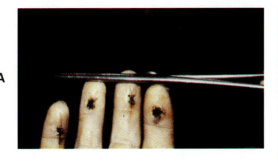
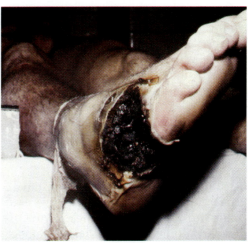

FIGURE 17-9 ▲ Direct contact burn. **A,** Entry wound (hand). **B,** Exit wound (foot). (From Sanders MJ: *Mosby's paramedic textbook,* ed 2, St Louis, 2000, Mosby.)

proaching the patient. Once the scene is safe, patient intervention may begin.

Initial assessment should proceed as for all other trauma patients with particular care taken to immobilize the cervical spine. If the patient is not breathing, assisted ventilation should begin immediately. Intu-

bation should be performed as soon as possible because apnea may persist for lengthy periods. A patient who is breathing should have a patent airway maintained and respirations supported with supplemental high-concentration oxygen. If the patient is in cardiac arrest, resuscitation efforts should be implemented ac-

cording to protocol. If possible, obtain the following history:
- Chief complaint (e.g., injury, disorientation, chest pain, and so on)
- Source, voltage, and amperage of the electrical injury
- Duration of contact
- Level of consciousness before and after the injury
- Past significant medical history

> **HELPFUL HINT**
>
> The source, voltage, and type of current (AC versus DC) are essential information for the attending physician to estimate internal damage from external wounds. However, DO NOT delay transport trying to gather this information.

During the physical examination, search for entrance and exit wounds or any associated trauma caused by tetany or a fall. Remember that there may have been multiple pathways of current and therefore multiple wounds. Remove all clothing and jewelry, and examine the areas between the patient's fingers and toes for sites of entry or exit. Assess distal pulses, motor function, and sensation of all extremities to monitor possible development of compartment syndrome. Cover entrance and exit wounds with sterile dressings, and appropriately manage any other associated trauma.

Frequent reassessment is necessary because of the progressive nature of electrical injury and the fact that the internal damage may be much more significant than external wounds. Implement ECG monitoring at the scene and continue during transport due to the potential for dysrhythmias.

Early fluid resuscitation is critical in managing patients with severe electrical injury to prevent hypovolemia and subsequent renal failure. If possible, establish two large-bore IV lines in an extremity without entry or exit wounds. Use lactated Ringer's solution or normal saline without glucose, and determine the flow rate based on the patient's clinical status.

Lightning Injury

Lightning strikes the earth about 7.4 million times each year and accounts for about 90 deaths each year.[3] It comprises **direct current (DC)** of up to 200,000 amps at a potentional of 100 million or more volts, with temperatures that vary between 16,000° F and 60,000° F (8871° C and 33,315° C). Lightning injuries can occur from a direct strike or by a side flash (splash) between a victim and a nearby object that has been struck by lightning. About 30% of those struck by lightning die. Lightning strikes are most common in Florida, Texas, and North Carolina.

Lightning strikes produce tissue injuries that differ from other types of electrical injury because the path-

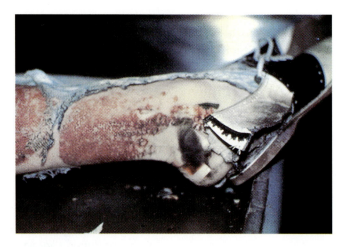

FIGURE 17-10 ▲ Lightning injury. (Courtesy of Michael Graham, MD.)

way of tissue damage often is *over* rather than *through* the skin (Figure 17-10). Because the duration of lightning is short (1/100 to 1/1000 second), skin burns are less severe than those seen with other high-voltage current. Full-thickness burns are rare.

Common lightning burns are linear, feathery, and pinpont in appearance. In addition, depending on the severity of the strike, the patient may experience cardiac and respiratory arrest, which are the most common causes of death in lightning injuries. The injuries are classified as minor, moderate, or severe (Table 17-5).

> **CLINICAL NOTES**
>
> Depending on the severity of the strike, cardiac and respiratory arrest are the most common causes of death in lightning strikes.

ASSESSMENT AND MANAGEMENT

Scene safety is the first priority. If the electrical storm is still in progress, all patient care activities should take place in a safe, sheltered area. To prevent injury from subsequent lightning strikes, the EMS crew should stay away from objects that project from the ground, including trees, fences, and high buildings, and should avoid areas of open water. If rescue attempts in an open area are necessary, the EMS crew should stay low on the ground.

Prehospital management is the same as for other severe electrical injuries. Initial patient care is directed at the following:
- Airway and ventilatory support
- Basic and advanced life support
- Patient immobilization
- Fluid resuscitation to prevent hypovolemia and renal failure

TABLE 17-5

Lightning Injuries

CLASSIFICATION OF LIGHTNING INJURY	SIGNS AND SYMPTOMS
Minor	May see no change in level of consciousness
	May also see confusion and amnesia
	Vital signs stable
	Burns or other signs of injury are rare
Moderate	Combative or comatose
	May have associated injuries from impact of lightning strike
	Superficial and partial-thickness burns are common
	Tympanic membrane rupture common
	May have serious internal organ damage; should be carefully observed for signs and symptoms of cardiorespiratory dysfunction
Severe	Immediate brain damage
	Seizures
	Respiratory paralysis
	Cardiac arrest

- Pharmacological therapy per protocol to manage seizures if present, promote excretion of myoglobin, and treat dysrhythmias
- Wound care
- Rapid transport to an appropriate medical facility

CLINICAL NOTES

Cardiopulmonary resuscitation should be initiated immediately for patients who appear "dead" because resuscitation is possible after lightning injury.

Radiation Exposure

The most common radiation accidents involve sealed radioactive sources used in industrial radiography and nondestructive testing. Victims of these types of accidents rarely require emergency care. However, EMS personnel may be summoned to building fires and

STREET WISE

Safety issues regarding radiation have been excellent overall throughout the world. However, hazards associated with radiation became well known as a result of the disastrous accident at the Chernobyl Nuclear Power Station in the Soviet Union in 1986 and the serious potential for disaster that occurred at Three Mile Island in Pennsylvania in 1979.

transportation crashes potentially involving radioactive materials, so an understanding of the hazards of radiation exposure is important.

HARMFUL EFFECTS FROM RADIATION EXPOSURE

STREET WISE

Radiation is a hazardous material. The EMS crew should not enter the scene until the scene has been made safe by the proper authorities.

Radioactive particles generally are classified into three types: alpha, beta, and gamma. These types are outlined in Table 17-6.

Nonionizing radiation includes radio waves and microwaves and usually is not considered dangerous. Ionizing radiation is produced by nuclear weapons, reactors, radioactive material, and x-ray machines. Although it is rare, the exposure to ionizing radiation poses a threat to victims and rescue personnel.

STUDENT ALERT

An object or a person who has been exposed to radiation is not "radioactive." It is only the *presence* of radioactive residue that poses a threat to rescuers.

TABLE 17-6

Types of Radioactive Particles

CLASSIFICATION OF RADIOACTIVE PARTICLE	DESCRIPTION
Alpha	Large; travel only a few millimeters
	Have minimal penetrating ability
	May be stopped by paper, clothing, or skin
	Considered least dangerous external radiation source
	May damage internal organs and interfere with body's chemical functions if inhaled, ingested, or absorbed
	Internal exposure to alpha radiation is considered the most dangerous form of internal radiation exposure
	Protection requires full protective clothing, including a positive-pressure SCBA
Beta	1/7000 the size of alpha particles
	Have considerably more energy and penetrating power
	Can penetrate subcutaneous tissue
	Usually enter the body through damaged skin, ingestion, or inhalation
	Protection requires full, protective clothing, including a positive-pressure SCBA
Gamma	Most dangerous forms of penetrating radiation
	Protective clothing does not stop gamma rays; require lead shields for protection
	Have 10,000 times the penetrating power of beta particles
	Possess internal and external hazards
	May produce localized skin burns and extensive internal damage

Sanders MJ: *Mosby's EMT—Paramedic,* ed 2, St Louis, 2000, Mosby.

EMERGENCY RESPONSE TO RADIATION ACCIDENTS

If the EMS crew has been advised that radioactive materials are present at an emergency scene, they should approach the site with caution and not enter the scene until it has been secured by proper authorities. Rescue personnel, emergency vehicles, and the command post should be positioned 200 to 300 feet upwind of the site. Emergency workers should not eat, drink, or smoke at the accident site or in any rescue vehicle. Contact the appropriate local authorities (e.g., state radiological health office, local specialists, and so on), and notify medical control. Wear protective clothing suitable for other hazardous material releases and have dose meters available for all rescue personnel. Use self-contained breathing apparatus (SCBAs) if fire, smoke, or gas are present.

Basic radiation protection for both the rescuer and patient are recommended by the Federal Emergency Management Agency (FEMA). These guidelines are outlined in Table 17-7.

EMERGENCY CARE FOR VICTIMS OF RADIATION ACCIDENTS

Patients who have been irradiated are not radioactive. However, when external contamination occurs and radioactive material remains on the patient's clothing and skin or in open wounds, the rescuer should consult with medical direction and follow agency protocol. The effects of radiation may be immediate, as with burns, or delayed.

With the exception of dealing with contaminants and containing their spread, there are no emergency care procedures specific to radiation injury. Ensure an adequate airway and breathing rate. All external bleeding should be controlled, the spine immobilized, open wounds covered, and fractures stabilized in routine fashion. The EMS crew should move the patient away from the radiation source as soon as possible. Lifesaving care should not be delayed for patient transfer or decontamination procedures. IV fluid replacement should be initiated if indicated, using strict aseptic technique. If an IV line is not needed for specific therapy, avoid its use to prevent introducing contaminants into the patient's body.

RADIATION DECONTAMINATION PROCEDURES

Radiation emergencies involving patients may be defined as either *clean,* meaning that the patient was exposed but not contaminated, or *dirty,* meaning that the patient was contaminated. Only properly trained personnel (e.g., haz mat teams and qualified county, state, or federal health department personnel) should attempt to decontaminate radiation victims at the scene. A patient who is to be transported to a hospital for decontamination should be isolated from the environment, and all patient effects should be transported with the patient.

TABLE 17-7

Radiation Protection Recommended by the Federal Emergency Management Agency (FEMA)

FACTOR	DESCRIPTION
Time	Less time spent in radiation field is less radiation exposure
	Use rotating team approach if adequate personnel available to keep individual radiation exposure to a minimum
Distance	The farther a person is from the source of radiation, the lower is the radiation dose
	Moving several feet away from a radioactive source greatly reduces the level of exposure
Shielding	The denser the material, the greater its ability to stop passage of radiation
	Lead shields provide best protection from exposure
	Vehicles, mounds of dirt, and pieces of heavy equipment placed between radiation source and rescuer/victim also diminish exposure levels
	Protective clothing and SCBAs may provide adequate protection from all alpha and some beta radiation
	Protective clothing does not prevent penetration of gamma rays
	If adequate shielding not available, use time and distance factors to reduce radiation exposure
Quantity	Limiting amount of radioactive material in a specific area lessens radiation exposure
	Examples include the following:
	• Removing contaminated clothing
	• Bagging all contaminated items
	• Moving containers of radioactive material from area

PRIMARY INJURY PREVENTION

The EMT–I has a unique opportunity to prevent burns and decrease the risks for burn injuries. In many instances, the EMT–I will see the patient's home and observe various behaviors and socioeconomic factors. Look for things like smoke detectors, improperly stored flammable materials, and children's access to lighters. Use that time to tactfully educate the patient and his or her family regarding safe practices in the home.

Participate in programs that aim to decrease the likelihood of injury. Go to local schools or churches in the area, and present an injury prevention educational session. Many prepackaged materials are available from organizations such as the American Trauma Society and the National SAFEKIDS Coalition.

CASE HISTORY FOLLOW-UP ■■■

The initial examination reveals a potential airway injury that needs immediate treatment. The mechanism of injury was a blast to the face so the young man probably inhaled hot air and potentially noxious gases.

EMT–I Knoll continues to hold manual cervical stabilization while EMT–I Baker gets a nonrebreather oxygen mask and the oxygen tank. After filling up the reservoir bag, EMT–I Baker places the face mask on the patient.

EMT–I Baker sees the triage officer, tells her that this patient needs immediate transport, and provides a brief report. The triage officer notifies the nearby trauma center that a patient with a probable inhalation injury will be en route.

EMT–I Baker quickly applies a rigid cervical collar while a police officer brings over the long backboard.

The EMT–Is rapidly immobilize the young man to the long backboard and prepare for transport. Once the patient is moved onto the stretcher, the head of the backboard is elevated slightly to optimize ventilatory effort.

Once inside the ambulance, EMT–I Knoll puts the patient on cool, humidified oxygen to minimize tracheal swelling. The patient is secured, and transport is started. This EMS team was on the scene for eight minutes.

During transport, EMT–I Baker again evaluates the patient's respiratory status. The humidified oxygen has eased the patient's dyspnea. EMT–I Baker assesses vital signs and examines the rest of the boy's body. No other injuries are found.

SUMMARY

- Each year more than 2 million Americans seek medical attention for burns. Morbidity and mortality rates from burn injury depend on the patient's gender, age, and socioeconomic status.
- A burn injury is caused by an interaction between thermal, chemical, electrical, or radiation energy and biological matter.
- Tissue damage depends on the degree of heat and duration of exposure to the thermal source. As local events occur at the injury site, other organ systems become involved in a general response to the stress caused by the burn.
- Burns are classified in terms of depth as superficial, partial thickness, and full thickness. The rule of nines provides a rough estimate of burn injury size (extent) and is most accurate for adults and for children older than 10 years of age. Severity of burn injury and burn center referral guidelines are based on standards that take into account the depth, extent, and severity of the burn wound; the source of injury; patient age; presence of concurrent medical or surgical problems; and the body region that is burned.
- Shock after thermal injury results from edema and accumulation of vascular fluid in the tissues in the area of injury and systemic hypovolemia if the burn is large.
- Emergency care for a patient with burns begins with the initial assessment to recognize and treat life-threatening injuries.

- Goals for out-of-hospital management of the patient with severe burns include preventing further injury, maintaining the airway, administering oxygen and ventilatory support, providing fluid resuscitation, providing rapid transport to an appropriate medical facility, using clean technique to minimize the patient's exposure to infectious agents, managing pain, and providing psychological and emotional support.

REFERENCES

1. National Institute of General Medical Sciences, National Institutes of Health: *Trauma, burn, shock, and injury facts and figures,* Bethesda, Md, 1999, The Institute.
2. Centers for Disease Control and Prevention, National Center for Injury Prevention and Control: *Fire and burn injuries fact sheet,* Atlanta, 1993, The Centers.
3. Sanders, M: *Mosby's paramedic textbook,* ed 2, St Louis, 2000, Mosby.
4. National Safety Council: *Injury Facts,* Itasca, Ill., 1999, The Council.

18

Thoracic Trauma

Key Terms

Flail chest

Hemothorax

Hemopericardium

Hemopneumothorax

Pneumothorax

Tension pneumothorax

Traumatic asphyxia

■■■ **CASE HISTORY** EMT-Is Bailey and Hanson are called to the scene of a pedestrian struck by a car. Having just completed a Prehospital Trauma Life Support provider course 2 weeks ago, they began to talk about the mechanism of injury en route to the scene. The information received by the dispatcher was limited so they do not know if the patient was an adult or a child.

Evaluating the scene will reveal important information. Does anyone know how fast the car was driving? Where was the person when he or she was struck? How far was the patient thrown? Upon what did he or she land: gravel, concrete, or grass? Was the person riding a bicycle or enjoying some other recreation in which there was any protective gear such as a helmet, knee pads, and so on? Is there a chance that a medical event may have caused a lapse in judgment? For example, did this person walk into the street in a stupor because of hypoglycemia? Was this someone with a seizure disorder who was postictal? Was the person under the influence of drugs or alcohol and not thinking clearly?

Knowing if the patient is an adult or child is also crucial. A child has less body fat, connective tissue is more elastic, and the organs are much closer together. In addition, the child's skeleton is not completely calcified and has many active growth centers. Once struck, the child usually bounces up over the car and then lands on the ground, usually on the head due to its large size. Injuries occur during the initial impact, during the impact on the automobile, and during the impact with the ground when the child lands.

Children, as opposed to adults, usually sustain head and chest injuries from the initial impact because of their size. Adults usually have hip and leg injuries because they are taller and the automobile hits them lower on their body. Children also tend to face the car because they may not realize the danger involved. If an adult sees the impending situation, he or she will turn away from the vehicle and try to get out of the way, again resulting in a different mechanism of injury.

At the scene, they find a crowd of people on the side of the road hovering over a 14-year-old girl. EMT-I Bailey immediately stabilizes the cervical spine while EMT-I Hanson examines the girl. She is sleepy and crying softly. Airway is patent, respirations are regular at 28, and the radial pulse is weak at 122. No bleeding is noted.

The police officer tells the EMT-Is that the girl walked right into the street without looking. The car was going about 25 miles per hour, and she landed about 10 feet away in the neighbor's grassy front yard. Skid marks are seen on the road and are being measured by another police officer.

At this point, the mother comes on the scene and tells you that her daughter has a seizure disorder. Sometimes she wanders around incoherently after she has had a seizure.

Further examination is benign. The EMT-Is apply a nonrebreather face mask at 15 liters per minute oxygen and a rigid cervical collar. The girl weakly tries to take off the mask. EMT-I Bailey reassures her and lets her mother sit by her on the grass to hold her hand. The child is log-rolled onto a long backboard. Padding is placed in all open areas, and the straps are secured. She is moved to a stretcher and placed in the back of the ambulance.

EMT-I Hanson asks the mother if she wants to ride along in the back of the ambulance. The EMT-Is recognize the value of family-centered care and encourage participation of the mother. A policy was developed by their service a few months ago that outlines how parents can accompany their injured or ill children. EMT-I Hanson assists the mother with her seat belt.

Vitals show respirations of 20, a barely palpable radial pulse of 126, and a blood pressure of 80/50. She continues to be sleepy but can be aroused when her mother calls out her name. Reassessment reveals a firm abdomen now that had been soft at the scene. Vitals are monitored every five minutes during transport. She now tolerates the nonrebreather face mask. Electrocardiogram shows a sinus tachycardia without dysrhythmias.

The medical control physician is contacted and diverts the EMT-Is to the nearby trauma center based on the mechanism of injury and reassessment. EMT-I Hanson gives report to the physician at the receiving hospital.

LEARNING OBJECTIVES ✓

CHAPTER GOAL

Upon completion of this chapter, the EMT–Intermediate will be able to integrate pathophysiological principles and the assessment findings to formulate a field impression and implement a treatment plan for the patient with thoracic trauma.

Cognitive Objectives

As an EMT–Intermediate you should be able to do the following:

- Describe the incidence, morbidity, and mortality of thoracic injuries in the trauma patient.
- Predict thoracic injuries based on mechanism of injury.
- Discuss the types of thoracic injuries.
- Discuss the pathophysiology of thoracic injuries.
- Discuss the assessment findings associated with thoracic injuries.
- Discuss the management of thoracic injuries.
- Identify the need for rapid intervention and transport of the patient with thoracic injuries.
- Describe mechanism of injury, signs and symptoms, and management of the following:
  - Clavicular fracture
  - Rib fracture
  - Sternal fracture
  - Closed or simple pneumothorax
  - Open pneumothorax
  - Tension pneumothorax
  - Hemothorax
  - Pulmonary contusion

INTRODUCTION

Chest injuries account for about 16,000 deaths per year in the United States and are directly responsible for more than 20% of all traumatic deaths, regardless of the mechanism of injury.[1] They are the second leading cause of trauma deaths and can be caused by blunt or penetrating mechanisms such as motor vehicle crashes, falls from heights, blast injuries, blows to the chest, chest compression, gunshot wounds, and stab wounds.

PATHOPHYSIOLOGY

The most commonly fractured bone is the clavicle, yet an isolated clavicular fracture is not usually a significant injury (Figure 18-1). It is common in children who fall on an outstretched arm or shoulder and in athletes involved in contact sports. It can, however, be an indicator of potential underlying trauma such as vascular or pulmonary injuries. Other thoracic injuries are outlined below.

Thoracic Injuries That Interfere With Ventilation

It is vital for the EMT–Intermediate (EMT–I) to initially recognize injuries that interfere with ventilation before the patient suffers any lack of oxygen to the tissues. Several examples of these injuries are described below.

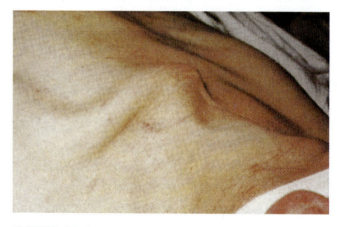

FIGURE 18-1 ▲ Fracture of the left clavicle seen from above the left shoulder. (From London PS: *A colour atlas of diagnosis after recent injury,* Ipswich, England, 1990, Wolfe Medical Publications.)

RIB FRACTURE

A rib can be broken depending on the amount of force exerted on the thoracic cavity and most commonly occurs on the lateral aspect of ribs three through eight. It is those areas that are least protected by musculature. They are more likely in adults than children because children have more cartilage than bone in the chest.

A simple fracture usually is not a threat to life. It becomes more serious when underlying tissue, blood vessels, and/or organs are damaged from the force of the injury or the broken end of a bone. The patient's age and the number and location of the fractures also influence morbidity and mortality.

STERNAL FRACTURE

Even though sternal fractures are not common, when they do occur they are serious. The mortality rate is between 25% and 45%.[1] They are usually caused by a direct blow to the chest as in a massive crush injury, line-drive baseball to the middle of the chest, or when the chest strikes the steering wheel of a motor vehicle during a head-on crash. They are usually painful and can be associated with an unstable chest wall, myocardial injury, or cardiac tamponade.

FLAIL CHEST

A **flail chest** occurs when two or more ribs are broken in two or more places. At least one section of the chest wall will move in a direction opposite that of the remainder of the chest, which is called *paradoxical motion*. It hinders the patient's breathing and produces hypoxia and hypercarbia (Figure 18-2). More importantly, there may be a serious injury (pulmonary contusion) to the lung under the area of the broken ribs, which further leads to decreased oxygenation.

PULMONARY CONTUSION

A pulmonary contusion usually occurs as a result of blunt trauma and is seen frequently under a flail chest. Rapid deceleration forces such as those occurring in motor vehicle crashes cause the lung to contact the chest wall. Bleeding occurs in the interstitial and alveolar areas of the lung. It also can be caused by penetrating

trauma in the area around the initial injury. Over 50 percent of patients with blunt chest trauma have pulmonary contusion.[2]

Because the contused area of the lung is not able to function properly after an injury, profound hypoxemia may develop. The degree of respiratory complication is directly related to the size of the contused area.

STUDENT ALERT _____

Pulmonary contusion can result from flail chest and can lead to profound hypoxemia.

CLOSED OR SIMPLE PNEUMOTHORAX

When air is present in the pleural space, a closed or simple **pneumothorax** exists. Air enters the pleural space through an opening in the lung. The lung begins to collapse as the pressure in the pleural space increases (Figure 18-3). This injury occurs in 10% to 30% of patients with blunt chest trauma.[2] It may become life-threatening if it develops into a tension pneumothorax, occupies more than 40% of the hemothorax, or occurs in a patient with shock or preexisting pulmonary or cardiovascular disease.[3]

A common cause of pneumothorax is a fractured rib that penetrates the underlying lung. This injury may also occur in the absence of rib fractures from excessive pressure on the chest wall against a closed glottis (known as the *paper-bag effect*).

A rupture or tear of the lung parenchyma and visceral pleura with no demonstrable cause may also result in a spontaneous pneumothorax. Many times a bleb or cystic lesion on the lobe of a lung ruptures, allowing air to enter the pleural space from within the

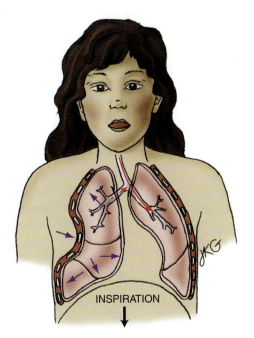
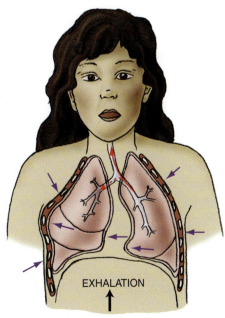

INSPIRATION

EXHALATION

FIGURE 18-2 ▲ Flail chest.

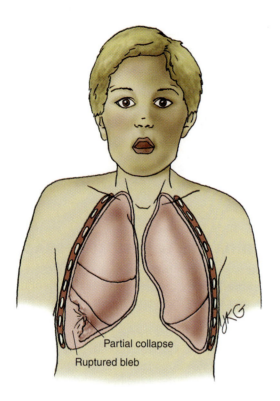

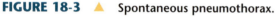

FIGURE 18-3 ▲ Spontaneous pneumothorax.

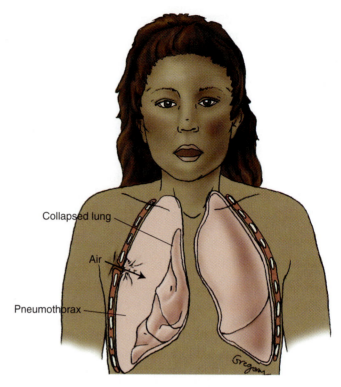

FIGURE 18-4 ▲ Open pneumothorax.

lung. This condition usually occurs in apparently healthy persons between the ages of 20 and 40 years.[3] Commonly, these persons are men who are tall and thin and have long, narrow chests. Other examples include people with acquired immunodeficiency syndrome (AIDS) who have pneumonia and drug abusers who deeply inhale free-base cocaine, marijuana, or inhalants such as glue or solvents.

OPEN PNEUMOTHORAX (SUCKING CHEST WOUND)

This open injury to the chest is caused by penetrating trauma. It creates an opening between the intrathoracic cavity and the outside of the body. The wound allows air to freely enter and exit the pleural cavity (Figure 18-4). The severity of the injury is directly proportional to the size of the wound and may result in severe ventilatory dysfunction, hypoxemia, and death unless it is rapidly recognized and corrected.

Depending on the mechanism of injury, some wounds may seal independently (such as a small stab wound). Others such as those caused by a shotgun blast will create an opening. Air enters through the wound, producing a "sucking" sound.

TENSION PNEUMOTHORAX

When air enters the pleural space but does not exit, pressure builds inside the chest. This condition is a **tension**

pneumothorax and is considered to be life threatening (Figure 18-5). Because of the tension created, the lung on the side of the injury collapses, the mediastinum shifts away from the injury, and the heart becomes compressed, resulting in a decrease of blood flow back to the heart. Breathing becomes increasingly labored, and the blood pressure drops as cardiac output decreases.

STREET WISE

Tension pneumothorax is a true emergency that results in profound hypoventilation and death if it is not immediately recognized and managed.

ESOPHAGEAL AND TRACHEAL/ BRONCHIAL INJURIES

When blunt or penetrating trauma occurs, any part of the esophagus, trachea, or bronchial tree can be injured. Rupture of these structures may produce a hemothorax, pneumothorax, and/or subcutaneous emphysema.

Penetrating trauma usually causes esophageal injuries yet they can also occur from spontaneous perforation caused by cancer and anatomic irregularities such as diverticulae or gastric reflux.[1] Violent emesis may result from the last two causes.

Injuries to the trachea or bronchial tree occur in less than three percent of victims of blunt or penetrating

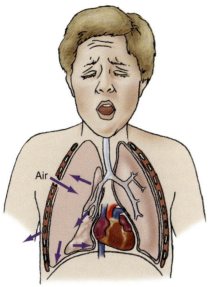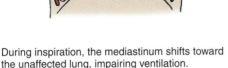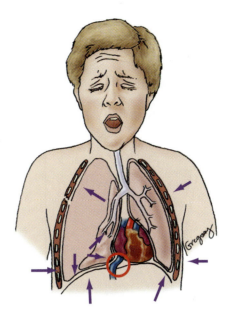

During inspiration, the mediastinum shifts toward the unaffected lung, impairing ventilation.

On expiration, the mediastinum shift distorts the vena cava and reduces venous return.

FIGURE 18-5 ▲ Tension pneumothorax.

chest trauma. However, they carry a mortality rate greater than 30%.[4] Most injuries occur within 3 cm of the carina, but they can be seen anywhere along the tracheobronchial tree.

DIAPHRAGMATIC RUPTURE

The diaphragm is a sheet of voluntary muscle that separates the abdominal cavity from the thoracic cavity. When rapid compression of the abdomen results in a sharp increase in intraabdominal pressure such as blunt trauma to the trunk, the pressure differences may cause abdominal contents to rupture through the thin diaphragmatic wall and enter the chest cavity (Figure 18-6). This rupture is detected more on the left side than on the right. Ruptures on either side, however, may allow intraabdominal organs to enter the thoracic cavity, where they may cause compression of the lung with a reduction in ventilation, a decrease in

venous return, a decrease in cardiac output, and shock. Multiple injuries are often present in patients with diaphragmatic rupture because of the mechanical forces involved.

TRAUMATIC ASPHYXIA

Traumatic asphyxia describes a severe crushing injury to the chest and abdomen (Figure 18-7). It usually results from an increase in intrathoracic pressure that forces blood from the right side of the heart into the veins of the upper thorax, neck, and face. Although the forces involved in this phenomenon may produce lethal injury, traumatic asphyxia is not life threatening. However, brain hemorrhages, seizures, coma, and death have been documented as occasional sequelae.[3]

Thoracic Injuries That Interfere With Circulation

HEMOTHORAX

A **hemothorax** occurs when blood collects within the pleural space (Figure 18-8). Causes include bleeding from the lung or from blood vessels within the chest. The most critical symptoms are the loss of blood and associated hypotension. Remember that each side of the thorax can hold 30% to 40% (2 to 3 L) of the patient's blood volume.[2] For example, a severed intercostal artery can easily bleed 50 mL per minute.

STREET WISE

Diaphragmatic ruptures may allow intraabdominal organs to enter the thoracic cavity, where they may cause compression of the lung with a reduction of ventilation, a decrease in venous return, a decrease in cardiac output, and shock.

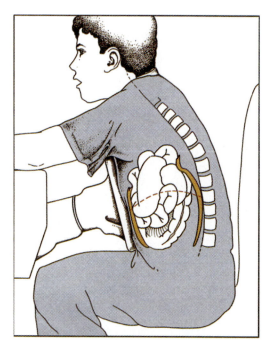

FIGURE 18-6 ▲ Diaphragmatic rupture. A rapid compression of the abdomen may increase intraabdominal pressure, causing the abdominal contents to rupture through the thin diaphragmatic wall and enter the chest cavity. (From Moylan EE: *Principles of trauma surgery*, ed 2, New York, 1992, Gower Medical Publishing.)

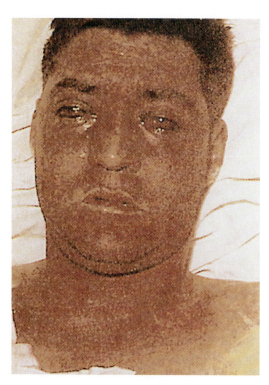

FIGURE 18-7 ▲ Discoloration of traumatic asphyxia, which results from forcible compression of the chest. (From London PS: *A colour atlas of diagnosis after recent injury*, Ipswich, England, 1990, Wolfe Medical Publications.)

A hemothorax that is associated with great vessel or cardiac injury carries a high mortality rate. Approximately 50% of these patients will die immediately. Another 25% will live for 5 to 10 minutes while another 25% may live longer than 30 minutes.[3]

HEMOPNEUMOTHORAX

A **hemopneumothorax** is present when air and blood accumulate in the pleural cavity. It most often occurs with penetrating trauma.

MYOCARDIAL CONTUSION

Whenever blunt trauma occurs to the chest, the heart is at risk for injury. It can be compressed between the sternum and the spinal column, as seen when the patient strikes the steering wheel in a frontal motor vehicle crash. Injuries can involve a disturbance to the cardiac electrical system, bruising of the cardiac wall, or a complete rupture of the myocardium. This injury occurs in 16% to 76% of all patients who experience blunt trauma to the chest and must be suspected with any mechanism suggesting blunt trauma to the chest.[3]

The extent of injury may vary from a localized bruise to a full-thickness injury to the wall of the heart with hemorrhage and edema. A **hemopericardium** (blood in the pericardium) may occur from a lacerated epicardium or endocardium, resulting in cardiac rupture or a traumatic myocardial infarction. The fibrinous reaction at the contusion site may lead to delayed rupture or a ventricular aneurysm.

PERICARDIAL TAMPONADE

The pericardium is a membranous inelastic sac that encloses the heart. There is a potential space, the pericardial space, between the heart and the pericardium. This space can fill with blood, yet not expand with an increase in volume. As the space fills, the heart is compressed and cannot adequately expand to receive blood from the body. Cardiac output is decreased, leading to hypotension. This situation occurs despite the fact that the patient may have an adequate circulating blood volume (normovolemia) (Figure 18-9).

MYOCARDIAL RUPTURE

When the blood-filled chambers of the ventricles are compressed with sufficient force to rupture the chamber wall, septum, or valve, myocardial rupture occurs. This injury is nearly always immediately fatal, yet death may

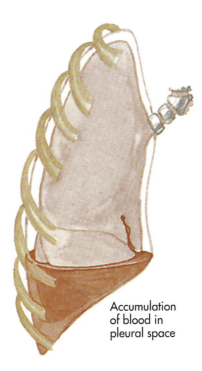

Accumulation
of blood in
pleural space

FIGURE 18-8 ▲ Hemothorax. (From Sanders MJ: *Mosby's paramedic textbook,* ed 2, St Louis, 2000, Mosby.)

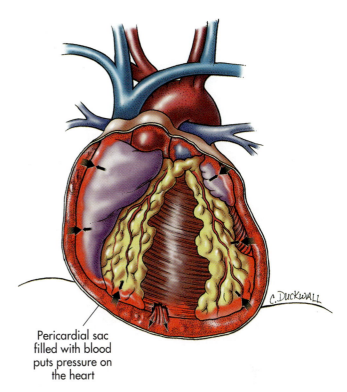

C. DUCKWALL

Pericardial sac
filled with blood
puts pressure on
the heart

FIGURE 18-9 ▲ Pericardial tamponade results from a collection of blood in the pericardial sac which leads to compression of the heart muscle and ineffective pumping. (From Pons P: *Paramedic field care,* ed 1, St Louis, 1997, Mosby.)

be delayed for two to three weeks after blunt trauma.[1] Motor vehicle crashes are responsible for most cases. Other possible mechanisms include the following:

- Deceleration or shearing forces that disrupt the inferior and superior vena cava
- Upward displacement of blood (causing an increase in intracardiac pressure) after abdominal trauma
- Direct compression of the heart between the sternum and vertebrae
- Laceration from a rib or sternal fracture
- Complications of myocardial contusion

> **STREET WISE** ✳
>
> *Myocardial rupture* refers to an acute traumatic perforation of the ventricles or atria. It is nearly always immediately fatal, but death may be delayed for several weeks after blunt trauma.

AORTIC RUPTURE

The aorta can be ruptured or torn in incidents involving high energy. Shear forces will tear the heart and aortic arch away from the descending aorta, which is fixed to the thoracic vertebrae (Figure 18-10). Most of these patients bleed to death within the first hour after the injury.

> **STREET WISE** ✳
>
> Aortic rupture is a severe injury with an 80% to 90% mortality in the first hour. The EMT-I should consider aortic rupture in any trauma patient who has unexplained shock after rapid deceleration injury.

ASSESSMENT

The index of suspicion for thoracic injury should be based on the mechanism of injury and on outward signs such as ecchymosis or marks of collision. Consider the following indicators for establishing the index of suspicion for thoracic injury:

- Mechanism of injury or damage to the passenger compartment of a motor vehicle (e.g., bent steering wheel)
- Outward signs of trauma
- Presence of dyspnea or cyanosis
- Level of shock greater than explained by other injuries

Expose the chest and look for contusions, abrasion, penetration, impaled object(s), and/or obvious bleeding. Palpating the chest can reveal defects or elicit pain

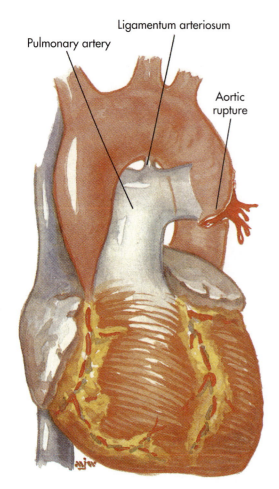

Pulmonary artery

Ligamentum arteriosum

Aortic rupture

FIGURE 18-10 ▲ Aortic rupture. (From Sanders MJ: *Mosby's paramedic textbook*, ed 2, St Louis, 2000, Mosby.)

in the area palpated. Voluntary or involuntary guarding and/or tenderness may be indicative of rib fractures or underlying injury. Be aware that alcohol or drugs may mask the signs and symptoms of thoracic injury.

Physical Examination

Auscultation of breath sounds will reveal potential injury to one or both lungs. See Table 18-1 for a review of signs and symptoms related to specific thoracic injuries.

MANAGEMENT

Management of airway and respiratory complications is a priority in the patient with thoracic trauma. Specific strategies are outlined below.

Airway, Oxygen, and Ventilation

High-concentration oxygen should be administered to any patient with possible thoracic injuries, and ventila-

tion should be assisted as needed. Consider endotracheal intubation as necessary.

Intubation may also be indicated if the chest injury is associated with shock, other severe injuries, head injury, and pulmonary disease. Many patients with significant chest injury develop respiratory failure and require long-term ventilatory support and ongoing hospitalization. Some protocols may use positive end-expiratory pressure (PEEP) to keep alveoli open at the end of exhalation. Be aware that PEEP may produce adverse circulatory effects including decreased venous return, decreased cardiac output, and pulmonary barotraumas. This procedure requires special equipment and training, as well as authorization from medical control.

POSITIVE END-EXPIRATORY PRESSURE

Positive end-expiratory pressure (PEEP) maintains a degree of positive pressure at the end of exhalation to keep alveoli open and to push fluid from the alveoli back into the interstitium or capillaries. Ventilatory support with PEEP can be done in the prehospital setting through intubation and the use of a Boehringer valve, a cylinder in which a metal ball is suspended (Figure 18-11). This valve is connected to the expiratory port of a bag-valve device and creates PEEP by forcing the patient to exhale against the weight of the metal ball. It is available in 5-, 10-, and 15-cm water pressures.

Circulation

Monitoring of the electrocardiogram (ECG) is routine for patients who have experienced an injury to the chest that could ultimately affect the patient's cardiac status. Premature ventricular contractions resulting from myocardial contusions should be treated as per local protocols. Any intervention that increases myocardial oxygen demand should be avoided.

The need for fluid resuscitation is based on the severity of the injury, the patient's vital signs, and transport time to the hospital. If hypovolemic shock is present, consider direct transport to a trauma center and initiation of intravenous (IV) lines of lactated Ringers solution en route. Consult with medical direction and follow local protocols regarding fluid replacement.

STREET WISE

Patients with multisystem trauma require rapid transport to an appropriate facility for definitive care. Rapid transport means that no more than 10 minutes (or less whenever possible) should be spent in the field with these patients.

TABLE 18-1

Signs and Symptoms of Thoracic Injuries

INJURY	SIGNS AND SYMPTOMS
Clavicular fracture	Pain Point tenderness Evident deformity Injury to subclavian vein or artery or lung from bony fragment penetration, producing a hematoma or venous thrombosis (rare)
Rib fracture	Pain when moving Decreased chest expansion due to discomfort Local tenderness Occasionally movement or crepitus may be palpated
Sternal fracture	Chest pain (may be severe) Tenderness over sternum Abnormal motion or crepitation over sternum
Flail chest	Dyspnea Pain with movement (may be severe) Local tenderness Bony crepitus on palpation Paradoxical motion (late sign) Patient may try to splint the area with his or her arm to avoid moving much air in and out of the lungs NOTE: This injury may not be detected in the prehospital setting because of the muscle spasm that accompanies the injury. Within 2 hours after the injury, the muscle spasm subsides and the injured segment of the chest wall may begin to move in a paradoxical motion.
Pulmonary contusion	Dyspnea, tachypnea, and/or tachycardia Cyanosis Cough Hemoptysis Decreased breath sounds on side of injury
Closed or simple Pneumothorax	Chest pain Dyspnea and tachypnea Decreased or absent breath sounds on the affected side
Open pneumothorax (sucking chest wound)	Dyspnea Pain at the site of injury May be a sucking or bubbling sound as air moves in and out of the pleural space through the open chest wound (hence the term, *sucking chest wound*)
Tension pneumothorax	*EARLY SIGNS* Decreased or absent breath sounds on the injured side Dyspnea and/or tachypnea despite any treatment *PROGRESSIVE SIGNS* Increasing tachypnea and dyspnea Tympany (low-pitched sound heard on percussion; may be difficult to hear in the prehospital setting) Tachycardia *LATE SIGNS* Tracheal deviation away from the injured side Jugular vein distention (absent if patient is hypovolemic) Signs of acute hypoxia, tympany, and narrowing pulse pressure
Esophageal or tracheal/ bronchial injuries	Severe dyspnea Hemoptysis (coughing up bright red blood)
Diaphragmatic rupture	Abdominal pain Dyspnea Decreased breath sounds Presence of bowel sounds in the affected hemithorax (due to abdominal contents displaced into the chest)

Continued

TABLE 18-1

Signs and Symptoms of Thoracic Injuries—cont'd

INJURY	SIGNS AND SYMPTOMS
Traumatic asphyxia	Reddish purple discoloration of the face and neck (skin below the area remains pink)
	Jugular vein distention
	Swelling or hemorrhage of the conjunctiva
Hemothorax	Signs and symptoms related primarily to the loss of blood (e.g., confusion, anxiety, and other signs of hypovolemic shock)
	Dyspnea and tachypnea
	Cyanosis (often not evident in hemorrhagic shock)
	Diminished or decreased breath sounds on the side of the injury (causing dullness on percussion)
Hemopneumothorax	Same as pneumothorax and hemothorax
Myocardial contusion	Possible to have no signs or symptoms
	Chest pain
	Tachycardia
	Palpitations with dysrhythmias on the cardiac monitor
Pericardial tamponade	Dyspnea
	Signs and symptoms of shock
	Tachycardia
	Cyanosis of the head, neck, and upper extremities
	As the pressure inside the pericardium increases, blood pressure drops and jugular venous distention may appear.
	Pulsus parodoxus (systolic blood pressure that drops more than 10 to 15 mm Hg during inspiration compared with expiration; difficult to measure in prehospital setting)
	Beck's triad (seen in only 30% of cases)[1]
	Jugular vein distention due to elevated central venous pressure (single best way to distinguish pericardial tamponade from hemorrhagic shock)
	Muffled heart sounds
	Hypotension
Myocardial rupture	Chest pain
	Signs and symptoms of shock, congestive heart failure, and/or cardiac tamponade
Aortic rupture	Chest pain
	Signs and symptoms of shock
	Upper extremity hypertension with absent or decreased amplitude of femoral pulses
	Generalized hypertension secondary to increased sympathetic discharge

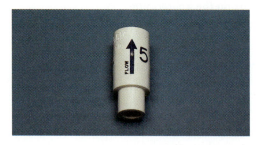

FIGURE 18-11 ▲ Boehringer valve. (Courtesy of Boehringer Laboratories; Norristown, Pa.)

Other Treatment

For rib fractures, splint the chest using a sling and swathe around the patient's arm on the affected side. The EMT–I should make sure the patient can continue to take a deep breath and maintain an adequate tidal volume. The chest should not be restricted with tape or any other type of band.

Specific treatment for a flail chest is controversial. One method is to splint the flail segment in the inward position with simple hand pressure or bulky dressings or towels taped to the chest wall. Sandbags are NEVER used. This treatment may increase the efficiency of ventilation but reduce the vital capacity of the affected lung. Another recommendation is intubation and positive pressure ventilation, which provides internal splinting. This strategy is usually reserved for those patients in respiratory distress from a flail chest.

STUDENT ALERT

Remember an occlusive dressing is used to treat an open pneumothorax.

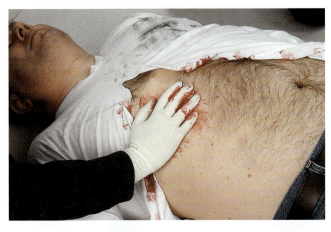

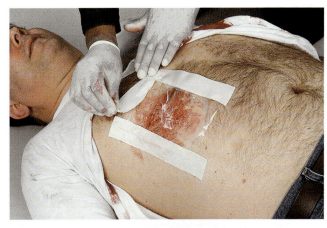

FIGURE 18-12 ▲ **A,** Cover open area with gloved hand. For an open pneumothorax, the EMT-I should immediately cover the open area with a gloved hand. **B,** Cover open area with occlusive dressing. Once materials are available, cover the open area with an occlusive dressing and tape three sides of the dressing.

For an open pneumothorax, the EMT–I should immediately cover the open area with a gloved hand (Figure 18-12, *A*). Once materials are available, cover the open area with an occlusive dressing; and tape three sides of the dressing (Figure 18-12, *B*). This method creates a one-way valve, allowing the escape of air through the fourth, untaped side. It does not allow air back into the wound. Any impaled objects should be left in place and stabilized for transport unless they directly interfere with cardiopulmonary resuscitation. Always consult medical control if there is any question as to whether to remove an impaled object.

> **STREET WISE**
>
> Options for an occlusive dressing may include Vaseline gauze covered with its own package, aluminum foil, or plastic wrap. Follow local protocols.

To relieve the tension pneumothorax, the EMT–I should perform a needle thoracentesis. This skill should be performed under the auspices of proper medical direction and occur *only* after a thorough and proper assessment. To perform this technique, the EMT–I should do the following:

1. Assemble and prepare the necessary equipment (Figure 18-13, *A*):
   - Needle (10- to 14-gauge)
   - Roll of 1/2-inch adhesive tape
   - Several alcohol or Betadine (povidone-iodine) swabs
   - One-way valve or equivalent
   - Syringe (10 mL)
2. Locate the second or third intercostal space on the midclavicular line. Cleanse this area with an alcohol or Betadine (povidone-iodine) swab (Figure 18-13, *B*).

3. Insert the needle and gently slide it over the rib (Figure 18-13, *C*). In this manner, interference with the blood vessels and nerves that run along the underside of the rib will not occur. A rush of air may be felt or heard.
4. Remove the needle from the catheter while being careful not to kink the catheter.
5. Attach the one-way valve to the catheter, and secure the entire device to the anterior chest (Figure 18-13, *D*).
6. Auscultate breath sounds.
7. If the tension is not relieved with initial decompression, insertion of a second or third needle may be indicated.

Remember that an open pneumothorax that has been sealed with an occlusive dressing may result in a tension pneumothorax. In that instance, the increase in pleural pressure can be relieved by briefly removing the dressing. Once it is lifted, there should be an audible release of air from the thoracic cavity. If that release does not occur or the patient's condition remains unchanged, gently spread the chest wound open with a gloved hand, allowing the trapped air to escape. After the pressure has been released, seal the wound again.

Specific diagnosis for aortic rupture only can be made by an aortogram or specialized radiograph done at the hospital, and surgical repair is the only definitive

> **STREET WISE**
>
> Unresponsive patients should be transported in a supine position immobilized on a long backboard. After control of airway, breathing, and circulation, one or two large-bore (14- to 16-gauge) IV lines using normal saline or lactated Ringer's solution and macroadministration sets may be started en route.

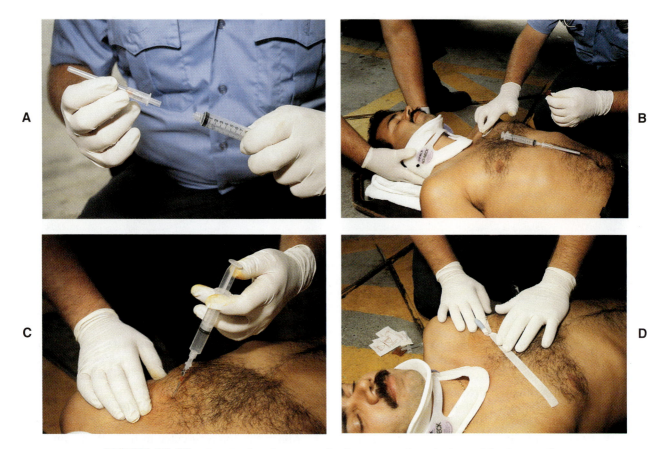

FIGURE 18-13 ▲ Performing a needle decompression. **A,** Assemble the needle. **B,** Carefully cleanse the area over the second or third intercostal spaces. **C,** Insert the needle, and slide it over the rib. **D,** Attach a one-way valve to the catheter, and secure it in place. (From National Association of Emergency Medical Technicians: *Prehospital trauma life support,* ed 4, St Louis, 1999, Mosby.)

care that will prevent most deaths. If the patient has unexplained shock and the mechanism indicates blunt trauma to the chest, aortic rupture should be suspected. The EMT–I should rapidly transport this patient to definitive care at a trauma center.

Once airway, breathing, and circulation have been addressed, connect the patient to the cardiac monitor. Evaluation of the ECG may show premature ventricular contractions from a myocardial contusion.

For thoracic injury, it is important to document the mechanism of injury, especially if no signs and symptoms are demonstrated. A broken steering wheel or bruising of the chest should be reported to medical direction and personnel at the receiving facility.

PREVENTION

Prevention of thoracic trauma is also another important role for the EMT–I. Assess the pattern of injuries in the community and develop injury prevention projects aimed at reducing those types of injuries. Become involved in violence prevention efforts to decrease the incidence of penetrating trauma to the chest (e.g.,

"knife and gun clubs"). Advocating the use of proper restraints when riding in motor vehicles may help to reduce the incidence of blunt chest trauma from motor vehicle crashes.

CASE HISTORY FOLLOW-UP ■ ■ ■

On arrival, the girl's carotid pulse is 140, and a radial pulse cannot be palpated. She is barely arousable with respirations of 12, and her blood pressure is 74/44. She is quickly moved into the trauma room where the staff in the Emergency Department takes over her care. EMT–I Hanson provides an updated report while EMT–I Bailey restocks the ambulance.

Once back at the station, the EMT–Is receive a call from the trauma center. This girl had a closed head injury and a lacerated liver. She had surgery to repair the liver laceration and was transferred to the trauma Intensive care unit. They are monitoring her neurological status and vital signs. The EMT–Is were encouraged to stop in and see her if they brought in another patient.

SUMMARY

- Thoracic trauma is caused by blunt or penetrating injuries due to motor vehicle crashes, falls from heights, blast injuries, blows to the chest, chest compression, gunshot wounds, and stab wounds.
- A simple or closed pneumothorax may become life threatening if it develops into a tension pneumothorax, occupies more than 40% of the hemithorax, or if it occurs in a patient with shock or preexisting pulmonary or cardiovascular disease. Tension pneumothorax is a true emergency that results in profound hypoventilation and death if it is not immediately recognized and managed.
- An open pneumothorax may result in severe ventilatory dysfunction, hypoxemia, and death unless it is rapidly recognized and corrected.
- Hemothorax may result in massive blood loss, leading to hypovolemia and hypoxemia.
- Pulmonary contusion results when trauma to the lung causes alveolar and capillary damage. Severe hypoxemia may develop and is directly related to the size of the contused area.
- Traumatic asphyxia occurs when forces cause an increase in intrathoracic pressure. When it occurs alone, it is often not lethal. However, brain hemorrhages, seizures, coma, and death have been reported following this type of injury.
- The extent of injury from myocardial contusion may vary from a localized bruise to a full-thickness injury to the wall of the heart, resulting in cardiac rupture, ventricular aneurysm, or a traumatic myocardial infarction. Pericardial tamponade occurs if 150 to 200 mL of blood enters the pericardial space, resulting in a decrease in stroke volume and cardiac output.
- Myocardial rupture refers to an acute traumatic perforation of the ventricles or atria. It is nearly always immediately fatal, but death may be delayed for several weeks after blunt trauma.
- Aortic rupture is a severe injury with an 80- to 90-percent mortality in the first hour. The EMT-I should consider aortic rupture in any trauma patient who has unexplained shock after rapid deceleration injury.

- Esophageal injuries are most frequently caused by penetrating trauma. Tracheobronchial injuries are rare yet carry a mortality rate greater than 30%.
- Diaphragmatic ruptures may allow intraabdominal organs to enter the thoracic cavity, where they may cause compression of the lung with a reduction of ventilation, a decrease in venous return, a decrease in cardiac output, and shock.
- Care for patients with thoracic trauma begins with careful airway management, with close attention given to protecting the cervical spine. The next step is to provide ventilatory support and administer high-concentration oxygen.
- Bleeding is controlled by broad manual pressure, and open wounds are dressed. Impaled objects should be left in place.
- Unresponsive patients should be transported in a supine position immobilized on a long backboard. One or two large-bore (14- to 16-gauge) IV lines using normal saline or lactated Ringer's solution and macroadministration sets may be started en route.
- Patients with multisystem trauma require rapid transport to an appropriate facility. Rapid transport means that no more than 10 minutes (or less whenever possible) should be spent in the field with these patients. By performing a skilled assessment, the EMT–I can identify trauma situations and their proper management.
- Prevention of thoracic trauma is another important role for the EMT–I.

REFERENCES

1. Rosen P, Barkin R: *Emergency medicine: concepts and clinical practice,* ed 4, St Louis, 1998, Mosby.
2. US Department of Transportation National Highway Traffic Safety Administration: *EMT-intermediate national standard curriculum,* Washington, DC, 1998, The Department.
3. Sanders M: *Mosby's paramedic textbook,* ed 2, St Louis, 2000, Mosby.
4. National Association of Emergency Medical Technicians. *PHTLS: basic and advanced prehospital trauma life support,* ed 4, St Louis, 1999, Mosby.

19

Head and Spinal Trauma

Key Terms

Antegrade Amnesia

Battle's sign

Cheyne-Stokes Respirations

Cushing Reflex or Triad

Decerebrate Posturing

Decorticate Posturing

Hemiplegia

Intracranial Pressure (ICP)

LeFort Fracture

Paraplegia

Quadriplegia

Raccoon Eyes

Retrograde Amnesia

Spinal Shock

...CASE HISTORY

Two EMT-Is volunteer with an ambulance service in a rural community. They are called to a farm where kids often race on all-terrain vehicles. On arrival, a 14-year-old boy is lying beside a hard dirt path. He was riding a very old three-wheeler, was caught by a wire line along the front of the neck, and was thrown off the vehicle. He has been unconscious since the event and was not wearing a helmet. The scene is safe, and several of his friends are available to help.

The boy is supine on the ground. EMT-I Mills holds cervical stabilization while EMT-I Taylor starts the assessment. The boy's face is cyanotic, and he is breathing about four times per minute. There is a red line across his anterior neck, yet no other signs of trauma are present. There is no bleeding.

EMT-I Taylor assembles the bag-valve-mask device and connects it to 15 liters of oxygen. After inserting an oral airway and ventilating with the bag-valve-mask device, there is only a slight improvement in the boy's skin color. EMT-I Mills holds the boy's head between her knees (to maintain stabilization) and takes over ventilation. EMT-I Taylor listens to his breath sounds and notices diminished sounds throughout all fields despite aggressive ventilation. EMT-I Taylor connects him to the cardiac monitor and sees a sinus rhythm at about 82 beats per minute.

EMT–I Taylor prepares the intubation equipment. After EMT–I Mills hyperventilates the patient, EMT–I Taylor attempts intubation. It is difficult to visualize the cords but finally they are in view and the tube is inserted. EMT–I Mills ventilates the endotracheal tube, but no breath sounds are audible. While adjusting the tube, the boy's heart rate decreases. EMT–I Mills again attempts ventilation, knowing that EMT–I Taylor saw that tube go through the cords. The heart rate continues to drop, and subcutaneous emphysema appears in the upper chest. At that point, EMT–I Taylor makes the decision to extubate him and continues ventilations via the bag-valve-mask device.

EMT–I Taylor updates the medical control physician and requests air transport to the trauma center. EMT–I Taylor applies a rigid cervical collar and rapidly immobilizes the boy on a long backboard with the help of the boy's friends while EMT–I Mills continues bag-valve-mask ventilation. The patient is transported to the helipad at the local community hospital while bag-valve-mask ventilation continues. Report is given to the air medical staff, and the boy is flown to the trauma center.

LEARNING OBJECTIVES ✓

CHAPTER GOAL

Upon completion of this chapter, the EMT-Intermediate will be able to utilize the assessment findings to formulate a field impression and implement the management plan for the patient with a head or neck injury.

Cognitive Objectives

As an EMT-Intermediate you should be able to do the following:

- Describe the mechanisms of injury, assessment, and management of the following:
  - Maxillofacial injuries
  - Ear, eye, and dental injuries
  - Anterior neck injuries
  - Scalp or cranial nerve injuries
  - Skull fractures
- Identify the types of traumatic brain injury based upon an understanding of pathophysiology and assessment findings.
- Describe the out-of-hospital care of the patient with a traumatic brain injury.
- Calculate a Glasgow coma scale and pediatric trauma score when given appropriate patient information.
- List four mechanisms of spinal injury.
- List three types of devices used to assist with spinal immobilization.
- Identify four instances in which rapid extrication techniques may be necessary.
- Identify one difference between open and closed bone injuries.
- List three signs or symptoms of a bone or joint injury.
- Identify three complications of musculoskeletal trauma.
- List three complications of splinting.

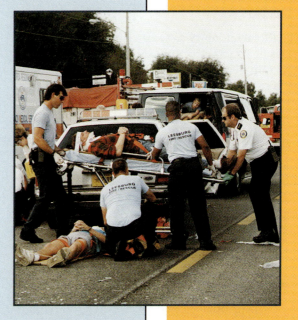

Affective Objectives

As an EMT-Intermediate you should be able to do the following:

- Advocate the use of a thorough assessment to determine a differential impression and treatment plan for head and neck trauma.
- Advocate the use of a thorough scene survey to determine the forces involved in head and neck trauma.
- Value the implications of failing to properly suspect head and neck trauma.
- Value the implications of failing to initiate timely interventions to patients with head and neck trauma.

Psychomotor Objectives

As an EMT-Intermediate you should be able to do the following:

- Demonstrate a clinical assessment for a patient with suspected head and/or neck trauma.
- Demonstrate the following techniques of management for head and neck injuries:
  - Oxygenation and ventilation
  - Cervical spine stabilization and immobilization
  - Helmet removal

INTRODUCTION

Head injuries affect nearly 4 million people each year in the United States, and about 50,000 patients with severe head trauma die each year before reaching the emergency department.[1] The categories of head trauma discussed in this chapter include maxillofacial trauma; ear, eye, and dental trauma; anterior neck trauma; and trauma to the skull and brain. See Chapter 4 for a review of head, neck, spine and nervous system anatomy and physiology.

Head, face, neck, and spinal injuries are closely related. Trauma to one area is likely to involve injury to several areas. A force to the face also can injure the head, neck, and/or spine. In addition, these injuries may be difficult to treat because the patient may be unresponsive and/or unable to provide a past medical history or details surrounding the incident. The EMT–Intermediate (EMT–I) should assume that any patient who receives an injury to the upper torso also has an injury to any of these areas until proven otherwise.

MAXILLOFACIAL INJURY

Maxillofacial injury may be classified as soft tissue injuries and facial fractures. Major causes of this type of injury, in descending order of frequency, are motor vehicle crashes, home accidents, athletic injuries, animal bites, intentional violent acts, and industrial injuries.

Soft Tissue Injuries

The face receives its blood supply from the branches of the internal and external carotid arteries. Because of this rich blood supply, soft tissue injuries to the face often appear to be quite serious (Figure 19-1). With the exception of a compromised upper airway and the potential

CLINICAL NOTES

Soft tissue injuries to the nose and mouth are common with facial injuries. Ensure that these patients have a clear and open airway.

for significant bleeding, damage to the tissues of the maxillofacial area is seldom life threatening.

PATHOPHYSIOLOGY

A closed soft-tissue injury to the scalp occurs after a fall or following direct trauma such as an assault or motor vehicle crash. Closed injuries to the head should provoke a high index of suspicion that the brain or neck also may be injured. The EMT–I should assume a patient with a closed scalp injury has a cervical spine and brain injury until proven otherwise.

Open soft tissue injuries to the scalp occur similarly to closed injuries. A knife, gunshot wound, or a sharp or blunt object can cause this type of injury. For individuals with long hair, the scalp can be avulsed if the hair is caught in and pulled by a mechanical device. The EMT–I should look for items as described previously for closed soft-tissue injuries.

ASSESSMENT

Depending on the mechanism of injury, facial trauma may range from minor cuts and abrasions to more serious injuries involving extensive soft tissue lacerations and avulsions. If possible, the EMT–Intermediate should obtain a thorough history from the patient, including mechanism of injury; events leading up to the injury; time of injury; associated medical problems; and allergies, medications, and last oral intake.

MANAGEMENT

Management of soft tissue injuries includes the following:
- Use spinal precautions/stabilization.
- Assess the airway for obstruction caused by blood, vomitus, bone fragments, broken teeth, dentures, and damage to the anterior neck.

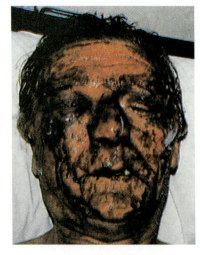 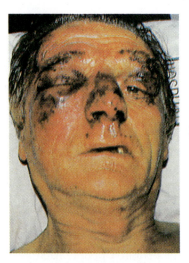

FIGURE 19-1 ▲ **A,** Appearance of a patient after being attacked. **B,** Appearance of same man after cleansing. (From London PS: *A colour atlas of diagnosis after recent injury,* London, 1990, Wolfe Medical Publications.)

- Use suction as necessary.
- Secure and maintain the airway through oral or nasal adjuncts or tracheal intubation.
- Ensure adequate ventilation and oxygenation.
- Control bleeding through direct pressure and pressure bandages. A bulky, bloody dressing should not be removed to examine the wound because clots adhered to the dressing may be helping to control the bleeding. The dressing should be left in place and reinforced as necessary.
- Examine the wound when possible, but do not probe it with fingers.
- Apply pressure over a broad area with gauze pads in the palm of a gloved hand (Figure 19-2). Do not use fingers to stop the bleeding as this action may drive bony fragments into the brain if there is any fracture.
- If the scalp is avulsed, the skin flap should be replaced to its normal position. Wrap the avulsed tissue in dry or moistened sterile gauze, depending on local protocol, and transport it with the patient to the hospital.

💡 HELPFUL HINT

- The EMT–I should not delay transport while searching for an avulsed part. Someone from the scene should continue to search for the part and bring it to the hospital if found.

Facial Fractures

PATHOPHYSIOLOGY

Although facial bones can withstand tremendous forces from energy impact, facial fractures are common after blunt trauma. The anatomical structure of the facial bones allows a "stepwise" fracture to absorb the impact of blunt trauma. These injuries may be classified anatomically as fractures to the mandible, midface, zygoma, orbit, and nose.

Fractures of the Mandible—The mandible is the single facial bone in the lower third of the face. Because of its prominence, fractures to this bone rank second in frequency after nasal fractures. Signs and symptoms include malocclusion (patients may complain that their teeth do not "feel right" when their mouths are closed), numbness in the chin, and inability to open the mouth. The patient also may have difficulty swallowing and excessive salivation.

Fractures of the Midface—The middle third of the face includes the maxilla, zygoma (cheekbone), floor of the orbit, and nose. Fractures to this region result from direct or transmitted force (e.g., blunt trauma to the mandible transmitted to produce fractures to the maxilla). They often are associated with central nervous system injury and spinal trauma.

A **LeFort fracture** is a fracture pattern that can be produced in the midface region (Figure 19-3). The LeFort I fracture involves the maxilla up to the level of the nasal fossa. The LeFort II involves the nasal bones and medial orbits and generally is shaped like a pyramid. The LeFort III (i.e., "floating face") entails craniofacial dislocation involving all of the bones of the face.

Fractures of the Zygoma—The zygoma (cheekbone) articulates with the frontal, maxillary, and temporal bones. It is seldom fractured because of its study construction. When fractures do occur, they usually result from physical assaults and motor vehicle crashes. Zygomatic fractures are often associated with orbital fractures and manifest similar clinical signs (Figure 19-4).

Fractures of the Orbit—The orbital contents are protected by a bony ring that resembles a pyramid, with the apex pointed toward the back of the head. The bones of the walls, floor, and roof of the orbit are quite thin and are easily fractured by direct blows and transmitted forces. In addition, many orbital fractures are associated with other facial injuries, such as LeFort II and III fractures. Injuries to the orbital contents is common and should be suspected with any facial fracture.

A blowout fracture to the orbit can occur when an object of greater diameter than that of the bony orbital rim strikes the globe of the eye and surrounding soft tissue (Figure 19-5). This impact pushes the globe into the orbit, compressing the orbital contents. The sudden increase in intraocular pressure is transmitted to the orbital floor, the weakest part of the orbital structure.

Fractures of the Nose—Of all the facial bones, the nasal bones have the least structural strength and are fractured the most often. Fractures to the orbit also may be present. In children, minimal displacement of nasal bones can result in growth changes and ultimate deformity.

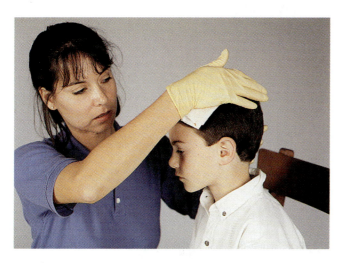

FIGURE 19-2 ▲   Use an open-palmed hand when using pressure to control bleeding of the scalp.

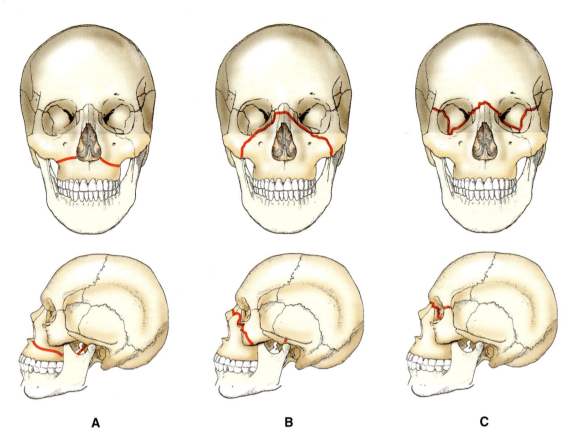

FIGURE 19-3 ▲ **A,** Lefort I facial fractures (lateral and frontal views). **B,** LeFort II fractures (lateral and frontal views). **C,** LeFort III fractures (lateral and frontal views). (From Sheehy S: *Emergency nursing,* ed 3, St Louis, 1992, Mosby.)

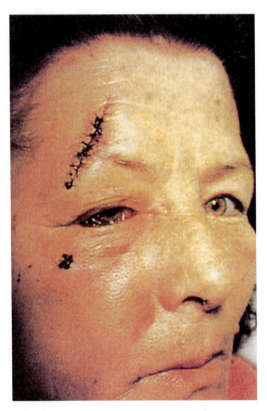

FIGURE 19-4 ▲ Fracture of the zygomatic bone. (From London PS: *A colour atlas of diagnosis after recent injury,* London, 1990, Wolfe Medical Publications.)

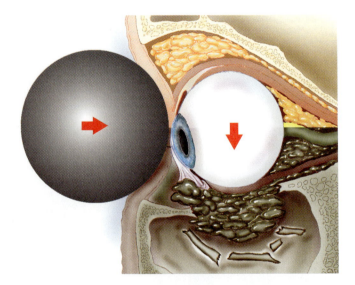

FIGURE 19-5 ▲ Artist's impression of a blowout fracture caused by the impact of a ball. (From Ragge N: *Immediate eye care,* London, 1990, Wolfe Medical Publications.)

ASSESSMENT

Signs and symptoms of facial fractures include the following:

- Pain
- Swelling
- Ecchymosis
- Lacerations and bleeding
- Numbness
- Dental malocclusion
- Limitation of mandibular excursion
- Visual disturbances
- Limited ocular movements
- Asymmetry of cheekbone prominences
- Discontinuity of the orbital rim
- Crepitus

Signs and symptoms of midface fractures include midfacial edema, unstable maxilla, lengthening of the face ("donkey face"), epistaxis, numb upper teeth, nasal flattening, and cerebrospinal fluid (CSF) rhinorrhea (CSF leakage caused by ethmoid cribriform plate fracture). These patients, especially those with LeFort II and III fractures, are at risk of having a seriously compromised airway and of having nasograstric or even nasotracheal tubes placed intracranially. Therefore nasal airways, nasogastric tubes, and nasotracheal intubation are contraindicated in patients who have fractures of the basal skull or facial bones.

Signs and symptoms of zygomatic fractures include flatness of a usually rounded cheek area, numbness of the cheek, nose, and upper lip (particularly if an orbital fracture is involved); and epistaxis. Altered vision may also be present.

Signs and symptoms of a blowout fracture of the orbit include periorbital edema, subconjunctival ecchymosis, double vision, recessed globe, epistaxis, and anesthesia in the region of the anterior cheek. Double vision and impaired extraocular movements may also be present.

Injuries to the nose may depress the nose or displace it to one side. In some instances, nasal fractures may result only in epistaxis and swelling without apparent skeletal deformity.

MANAGEMENT

When confronted with a patient with facial fractures, airway and ventilation remain the ultimate priority. Management should include the following:

1. Assume that the spine has been injured and use spinal precautions. Facial fractures are associated with a high percentage of concomitant cervical spine fractures.
2. Assess the airway for obstruction caused by blood, vomitus, bone fragments, broken teeth, dentures, and damage to the anterior neck.
3. Suction the airway as needed.
4. Secure and maintain the airway through oral adjuncts, nasal adjuncts (in the absence of suspected midface or basal skull fracture), tracheal intubation, or cricothyroidotomy as indicated.
5. Ensure adequate ventilation and oxygenation.
6. Control bleeding through direct pressure and pressure bandages.
7. Control epistaxis, which may be severe, by external direct pressure (compression of the anterior nares).

CLINICAL NOTES

To prevent blood from draining down the throat, mild epistaxis is best controlled in the conscious patient by instructing the patient to sit upright or to lean forward (if spinal precautions are not indicated) while compressing the nares. An unconscious patient should be positioned on the side (if not contraindicated by injury) or tilt the backboard to the side if spinal immobilization has been done. If bleeding is severe, the patient should be evaluated for hemorrhagic shock.

EYE, EAR, AND DENTAL TRAUMA

The ears, eyes, or teeth may be injured separately or in association with other forms of head trauma. Injury to these regions may be minor or may result in permanent sensory function loss and disfigurement. Regardless of the severity, these injuries should only be treated after life-threatening situations have been addressed.

Ear Trauma

Trauma to the ear may include lacerations and contusions, thermal injuries, chemical injuries, and traumatic perforations. Barotitis may occur when an individual is exposed to changes in barometric pressure great enough to produce inflammation and injury to the middle ear such as flying at high altitudes or scuba diving.

PATHOPHYSIOLOGY

Lacerations and contusions usually result from blunt trauma and are particularly common in victims of domestic violence (Figure 19-6). These injuries may produce a great deal of bleeding.

Thermal injuries may occur from prolonged exposure to extreme cold or in exposure of lesser duration to extreme heat. Contact with hot liquids or electrical currents also can lead to thermal injury (see Chapter

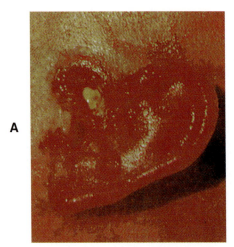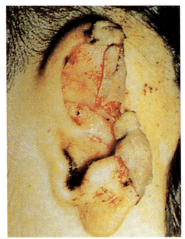

FIGURE 19-6 ▲ **A,** Partially detached pinna. **B,** Loss of rim. (From London PS: *A colour atlas of diagnosis after recent injury,* London, 1990, Wolfe Medical Publications.)

17). Chemical injuries occur with strong acids or alkali produce burns when they come in contact with the skin. Chapter 17 reviews these types of injuries as well.

Traumatic perforations to the tympanic membrane can be caused by penetrating objects such as a cotton-tipped applicator or from great pressure differentials resulting from blast injuries (explosions) or barotraumas (scuba diving). Serious complications include facial nerve palsy frequently accompanied by temporal bone fractures, hearing loss, and vertigo.

Barotitis occurs when an individual is exposed to changes in barometric pressure great enough to produce inflammation and injury to the middle ear. Gas pressure in the air-filled spaces of the middle ear is normally in equilibrium with the environment. During ascent, this gas expands; and it contracts during descent.

ASSESSMENT

The following signs and symptoms are present with ear trauma:

- Bleeding and tissue swelling occur with lacerations and avulsions.
- Thermal and chemical injuries produce burns to the tissue, depending on the mechanism of injury and length of contact.
- Traumatic perforations cause ear pain. Depending on the mechanism of injury, there may be temporary loss of hearing or a high-pitched ringing in the ear.
- When trapped gas cannot reach equilibrium with the outside pressure (barotitis), pain and the sensation of a blocked ear may develop.

MANAGEMENT

Management of ear trauma depends on the specific injury. Direct pressure should be applied to lacerations and contusions to control bleeding. Ice or cold com-

presses may help to decrease soft tissue swelling. If any portion of the outer ear has been avulsed, retrieve that tissue whenever possible. Wrap the avulsed tissue in moist gauze, seal it in a plastic bag, place it on ice, and transport it with the patient for possible surgical repair.

☀ STUDENT ALERT

Do not delay transport looking for an avulsed body part if the patient has any life-threatening injuries.

Prehospital treatment of thermal injuries is usually limited to soft tissue dressing to prevent contamination. Transport the patient for further medical evaluation.

Chemical injuries to the ear require copious irrigation. After irrigation, bathe the ear and ear canal with saline or sterile water. Allow the irrigation liquid to remain in the ear canal for 2 to 3 minutes. Repeat this procedure three to four times, dry the ear, and then cover it to prevent contamination. Transport the patient for further medical evaluation.

If a traumatic perforation has occurred, cover the ear to prevent further contamination. If the patient was swimming or used a foreign object to cause the perforation, antibiotics are often prescribed at the hospital.

For barotitis, efforts to equalize the pressure in the middle ear include asking the patient to bear down as if he or she was having a bowel movement (Valsalva maneuver), yawn, swallow, or move the lower jaw. These methods may cause the Eustachian tube to open, equalizing pressure in the middle ear cavity.

Eye Trauma

More than 2000 eye and orbital injuries are estimated to occur each day in the United States.[2] These injuries may result in a range of temporary blurred vision to complete blindness.

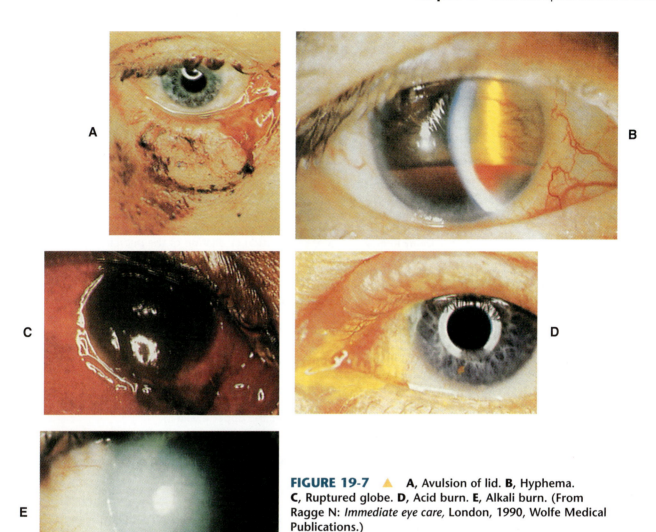

FIGURE 19-7 ▲   **A**, Avulsion of lid. **B**, Hyphema. **C**, Ruptured globe. **D**, Acid burn. **E**, Alkali burn. (From Ragge N: *Immediate eye care*, London, 1990, Wolfe Medical Publications.)

PATHOPHYSIOLOGY

Common causes of eye and orbital injuries are blunt and penetrating trauma from motor vehicle crashes, sport and recreational activities, violent altercations, chemical exposure from household and industrial accidents, and foreign bodies. Animal bites and scratches may also be common mechanisms of injury (Figure 19-7).

Blunt injury may be associated with other serious injuries such as an orbital fracture, vitreous hemorrhage, and dislocation of the lens. Conversely, penetrating injury may be associated with embedded foreign bodies, lid avulsions, and lacerations to the lids, sclera, or cornea. These injuries can damage retinal structures and cause a loss of vitreous humor and subsequent blindness.

Corneal injuries may be associated with loss of corneal epithelial tissue, globe perforation, and scarring and deformation of eyelids and conjunctiva. These injuries represent true emergencies.

Corneal abrasion occurs when the outer layers of the cornea are rubbed away. The injury often results from a foreign body scratching the cornea, and it is also common in those who wear contact lenses.

ASSESSMENT

Acute eye injuries may be difficult to identify because a patient with normal vision may still have a serious underlying injury. The following symptoms require a high index of suspicion:

- Obvious trauma with eye injury
- Visual loss or blurred vision that does not improve with blinking, indicating possible damage to the globe, ocular contents, or optic nerve

☀STUDENT ALERT

Evaluation of the patient's vision will be a rough estimation while in the prehospital setting. It will be evaluated again in the emergency department under controlled circumstances.

TABLE 19-1

Assessment of the Eye

ASSESSMENT	ITEMS TO INCLUDE
Assess history	Exact mechanism of injury
	Previous ocular, medical, and drug history
	Any cataracts, glaucoma, or presence of hepatitis or human immunodeficiency virus
	Use of eye medications
	Use of corrective glasses or contact lenses
	Presence of ocular prostheses (e.g., glass eye from previous injury)
Assess pupil reaction	Unequal pupils
	Any interruption in the circumference of the pupil
	Delay in or absence of constriction or dilation of the pupil in response to light
Look for extraocular movements	Ask the patient to track movement of an object (e.g., finger, pen, or penlight) up, down, to the right, and to the left
	Document any times in which the patient cannot follow the object or blurred vision
Contusion injury suspected	Traumatic dilatation or constriction of the pupil
	Pain
	Photophobia (abnormal light sensitivity)
	Blurred vision
	Tears of the iris (tear-shaped pupil)
Corneal abrasion suspected	Pain
	Foreign body sensation under the upper eyelid
	Photophobia
	Decrease in visual acuity
Foreign body	Foreign body sensation, especially when opening and closing the eyelids
	Profuse tearing
Traumatic hyphema suspected	Traumatic dilation or, less commonly, constriction of the pupil
	Decrease in visual acuity
	Blood in the anterior chamber (may be visible with penlight)
Globe or scleral rupture suspected	Decrease in visual acuity to hand movements or light perception
	Lowered intraocular pressure (soft eye)
	Pupil irregularity
	Hyphema (bleeding into anterior chamber)

• Loss of a portion of the visual field, indicating possible detachment of the retina, hemorrhage into the eye, or optic nerve injury

Other items related to the assessment of the eye are outlined in Table 19-1.

MANAGEMENT

All patients with ocular trauma should be evaluated by a physician even though many of them are not urgent. If a serious injury requiring specialized care (i.e., an ophthalmologist) is suspected, notify medical direction as soon as possible. The specialist will be available on arrival of the patient, or the patient may be diverted to another hospital with those capabilities.

Treatment for eye injuries is specific to the injury. See Table 19-2 for management of individual injuries.

If management of an eye injury is complicated by the presence of contact lenses (e.g., chemical burns to the eyes), medical direction may recommend that the lenses be removed. If the patient is unable to do so, the EMT–I may be instructed to do so (Box 19-1).

Dental Trauma

Each tooth consists of two sections: the crown, which projects above the gingival (portion of the oral mucosa surrounding the tooth), and the root, which fits into the bony socket (alveolus) of the maxilla or mandible. The hard tissues of the teeth are made up of three layers: the enamel, the dentin (ivory) and the cementum.

CLINICAL NOTES

Some services may carry a topical ophthalmic anesthetic such as *tetracaine* (Pontocaine). Consult with medical direction to see if this medication may be used to decrease the patient's discomfort.

TABLE 19-2

Management of Eye Injuries

INJURY	MANAGEMENT
Foreign body	Inspect the inner surface of the upper and lower lids and the conjunctiva. Attempt to remove the foreign body by gentle, copious irrigation with clear fluid (e.g., tap water, normal saline, or sterile water).
Corneal abrasion	Gently irrigate affected eye with clear fluid. Apply a double patch to both eyes to prevent movement of both eyes and resulting discomfort (Figure 19-8).
Blunt trauma	Control bleeding with gentle, direct pressure. Protect affected eye with a metal shield or cardboard cup. Immobilizae spine if traumatic hyphema or globe/scleral rupture; then elevate head of long backboard about 40 degrees to decrease intraocular pressure; instruct patient to avoid any activity that might increase intraocular pressure (e.g., straining or coughing). Rapid transport for physician evaluation.
Penetrating injury	Control bleeding with gentle, direct pressure. Protect the globe from dehydration or contamination from foreign bodies by covering the orbital area with plastic or dame, sterile dressings and an eye shield. Stabilize and cover any protruding intraocular foreign bodies with a cardboard cup secured with tape; cover the unaffected eye to prevent consensual movement. DO NOT ATTEMPT TO REMOVE THE OBJECT. If necessary, *carefully* shorten the penetrating object to facilitate transport after consult with medical direction. Oxygen and IV fluids may also be indicated.
Chemical injury	Continuously irrigate both eyes with a neutral fluid for 20 minutes before patient transport *only if* effective irrigation can be done. Continue irrigation while en route to the hospital.

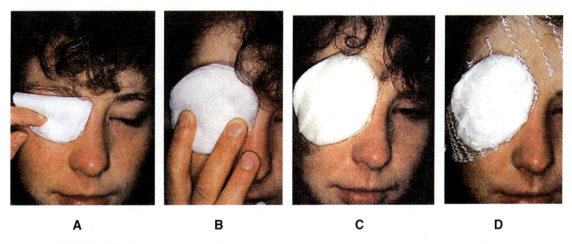

A   B   C   D

FIGURE 19-8 ▲ **A,** A folded pad is placed over the closed eye. **B,** A second unfolded pad is placed over the top of the first pad. **C,** Tape is applied along the length of the pad. **D,** The pads are secured firmly in place. (From Ragge N: *Immediate eye care,* London, 1990, Wolfe Medical Publications.)

The soft tisssues of the teeth include the pulp and the periodontal membrane (Figure 19-9).

PATHOPHYSIOLOGY

The teeth and associated alveolar process may be injured alone or in combination with fractures of the jaw or facial bones. The two most common types of dental trauma involve fractures and avulsions of the anterior teeth. Lacerations and avulsions to the tongue and surrounding mucous membranes also routinely occur with dental trauma.

Tooth avulsions are common, and many teeth can be saved with proper emergency treatment.[3] Permanent teeth that have been avulsed have a good survival rate if reimplanted and stabilized within one hour.

REMOVAL OF CONTACT LENSES

REMOVAL OF HARD AND RIGID GAS-PERMEABLE LENSES

With gloved hands, separate the eyelids so that the margins of the lids are beyond the top and bottom edges of the lens.

Gently pass the eyelids down and forward to the edges of the lens.

Move the eyelids toward each other, forcing the lens to slide out between them.

Store the lens in a container with water or saline and label the container with the patient's name. If a contact lens container is not available, store each lens in a separate container and label as left or right.

If lens removal is difficult, the lens should be gently moved downward from the cornea to the conjunctiva overlying the sclera until arrival in the emergency department.

NOTE: Special suction cups are also available for the removal of hard and rigid contact lenses. This device should be moistened with saline or sterile water before contacting the lens.

REMOVAL OF SOFT LENSES

With gloved hands, pull down the lower eyelid.

Gently slide the soft lens down onto the conjunctiva.

Using a pinching motion, compress the lens between the thumb and index finger.

Remove the lens from the eye.

Store the lens in a container (marked right or left) with water or saline and label the container with the patient's name.

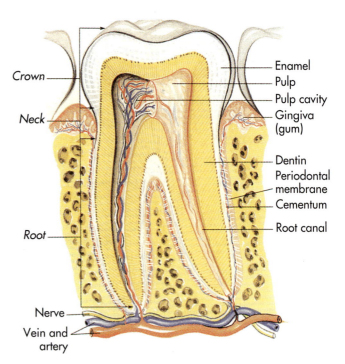

FIGURE 19-9 ▲ Longitudinal section of a tooth. (From Thibodeau GA, Patton KT: *Structure and function of the body,* ed 9, St Louis, 1992, Mosby.)

ASSESSMENT

Look in the mouth for any evidence of bleeding or missing teeth. Look for loose teeth or pieces of a fractured tooth in the mouth or posterior pharynx that may interfere with a patent airway and breathing. Lacerations and avulsions are often painful, may bleed profusely, and may also compromise the patient's airway.

MANAGEMENT

Remove any teeth or fragments to reduce the risk of aspiration and obstruction of the airway. Suction the airway if blood is in the posterior oropharynx.

If an avulsed tooth has been extraoral for less than 15 minutes, medical direction may recommend reimplanting the tooth into the original socket. The EMT–I should be careful not to reimplant the tooth backwards and be alert for possible aspiration. If reimplantation is not possible, the EMT–I should follow the guidelines established by the American Dental Association and the American Association of Endodontists (Box 19-2).

Anterior Neck Trauma

Anterior neck injuries are caused by blunt and penetrating trauma (see Figure 19-8). These injuries may result in damage to the skeletal structures, vascular structures, nerves, muscles, and glands of the neck. In addition, cervical spine injury must be assumed until ruled out by clinical examination and cervical x-rays.

PATHOPHYSIOLOGY

Injuries to the base of the neck (from the sternal notch to the top of the clavicles or cricoid cartilage) carry the highest mortality rate. It is in this area where there is a risk of injury to major vascular and thoracic structures (subclavian vessels, jugular veins, lungs, esophagus, trachea, cervical spine, and cervical nerve roots).

Injuries between the clavicles or cricoid cartilage and the angle of the mandible may affect the carotid artery, jugular vein, trachea, larynx, esophagus, and cervical spine. These injuries are more common but have a lower mortality rate.

The last part of the neck is above the angle of the mandible. Structures in this area include the distal carotid artery, salivary glands, and pharynx.

Blood vessels are the most commonly injured structures in the neck and may be caused by blunt or penetrating trauma. Vessels at risk of injury include the carotid, vertebral, subclavian, innominate, internal mammary arteries, and the jugular and subclavian veins.

GUIDELINES FOR CARE OF THE AVULSED TOOTH

Never place an avulsed tooth in anything that can dry or crush the outside of the tooth.

Do not handle the tooth roughly. Do not rinse it off or rub, scrape, or disinfect the outside of the tooth in any way. Any adherent membrane or fibrous tissue should be left in place to avoid stripping off the periodontal membrane and ligament, which are critical to the survival of a reimplanted tooth.

Place the tooth in a nurturing, break-resistant storage device with a tightly fitted top and soft inner walls.

Store the tooth in a pH-balanced, isotonic, glucose-, calcium-, and magnesium-enriched cell-preserving fluid (e.g., Hank's solution). Use refrigerated fresh whole milk as the best alternative storage medium (powdered milk is not suitable). For very short periods of one hour or less, use sterile saline. Do not use tap water because it damages the periodontal ligament.

Advise medical direction of avulsed teeth so that appropriate services will be available when the patient arrives in the emergency department.

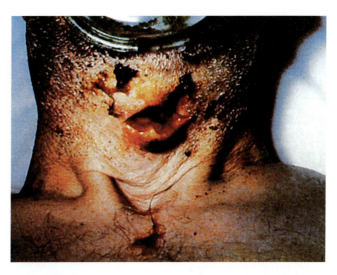

FIGURE 19-10 ▲ A self-inflicted stab wound that had entered the pharynx. (From London PS: *A colour atlas of diagnosis after recent injury,* London, 1990, Wolfe Medical Publications.)

Laceration of these major vessels can result in rapid exsanguination if bleeding is not controlled.

Injury secondary to blunt or penetrating trauma to the anterior neck may cause fracture or dislocation of the laryngeal and tracheal cartilages, hemorrhage, or swelling of the air passages. These may all significantly compromise the airway and cause respiratory distress. Other injuries associated with laryngeal and tracheal trauma include the following:

1. Fracture of the hyoid bone resulting in laceration and distortion of the epiglottis
2. Separation of the hyoid and thyroid cartilages resulting in epiglottis dislocation, aspiration, and subcutaneous emphysema
3. Fractures of the thyroid cartilage resulting in epiglottis and vocal cord avulsion, arytenoids dislocation, and aspiration of blood and bone fragments
4. Dislocation or fracture of the cricothyroid resulting in long-term laryngeal stenosis, laryngeal nerve paralysis, and laryngotracheal avulsion
5. Fracture to the trachea resulting in tracheal avulsion, complete airway obstruction, and subcutaneous emphysema

Common mechanisms of anterior neck injury include the following:
- Motor vehicle crashes
- Neck striking dashboard or steering column
- Hyperextension and hyperflexion injuries
- Sport and recreational activities
- Contact sports (boxing, karate, basketball, football, hockey)
- All-terrain vehicles (ATVs) and other small motor vehicles ("clothesline" injuries to the neck from running into wires, ropes, and fences)
- Water sports (jet skiing and water skiing)
- Snow skiing
- Horseback riding
- Industrial accidents
- "Strangulation" injuries from clothing, jewelry, or personal equipment getting caught in machinery
- Violent altercations
- Stab wounds (knives, screwdrivers, and ice picks) (Figure 19-10)
- Missile injury from firearms
- Blows to the neck
- Hangings

ASSESSMENT

Soft tissue injuries often produce hematomas and associated edema, or direct laryngeal or tracheal injury. These injuries can result in airway compromise.

Penetrating trauma may produce lacerations and puncture wounds with resultant vascular, laryngeal-tracheal, or esophageal injury. Signs and symptoms of significant penetrating neck trauma include the following:
- Shock
- Active bleeding
- Tenderness to palpation
- Mobility and crepitus
- Large or expanding hematoma
- Pulse deficit
- Neurological deficit (e.g., stroke, brachial plexus injury, or spinal cord injury)

- Dyspnea
- Hoarseness
- Stridor
- Subcutaneous emphysema
- Hemoptysis
- Dysphagia
- Hematemesis

Esophageal injuries should be suspected in patients with trauma to the neck or chest. This problem is difficult to assess in the field and may be overlooked as the EMT–I focuses on more obvious life-threatening injuries. Signs and symptoms include subcutaneous emphysema, neck hematoma, and oropharyngeal or nasogastric blood (indicating esophageal perforation).

CLINICAL NOTES

Esophageal perforation is associated with a high mortality rate from mediastinitis, caused by the release of gastric contents into the thoracic cavity. If not contraindicated by mechanism of injury, place the patient with a suspected esophageal tear in a semi-Fowler's position to prevent reflux of gastric contents.

MANAGEMENT

Stabilize the head and neck, and provide high-concentration oxygen via a nonrebreather face mask. The administration of cool, humidified oxygen may help to minimize edema of the airway.

Clear blood and vomitus from the airway with suction. Turn the patient to the side (using spinal precautions) if the patient continues to vomit or have heavy bleeding from the mouth.

If the airway is compromised (i.e., presence of dyspnea, inspiratory stridor, cyanosis, or changes in voice quality), consider oral or nasal intubation with spinal precautions. Intubation will stabilize the damaged areas of the neck, protect the airway, and provide a means for ventilatory support. A slightly smaller endotracheal tube may be needed to ensure passage through the airway, especially if there is edema of the larynx or trachea from the injury.

Hemorrhage control by direct pressure may be indicated to stop the bleeding. Consider fluid replacement using large-bore catheters and isotonic crystalloids if signs of shock are present. Fluids may need to be started en route if rapid transport is indicated.

When bleeding is present from a vascular injury, apply direct, constant pressure. Only apply pressure to the affected side so that blood flow to the brain is not blocked. If traumatized vessels can be visualized, consult medical direction for further suggestions for stopping the hemorrhage. DO NOT use hemostats in the prehospital setting because of the risk of damage to critical vascular structures and permanent nerve injury.

If a venous injury is suspected, keep the patient supine or in a slight Trendelenburg position to prevent air embolism. If this lethal complication is suspected, tilt the long backboard so that the patient is on his or her left side. Keep the head lower than the feet to try to trap the air embolus in the right ventricle.

Regardless of the injury, treatment priorities are as follows:

- Secure the airway (using spinal precautions)
- Provide adequate ventilatory support
- Control hemorrhage
- Treat for shock
- Provide rapid transport to an appropriate medical facility for definitive surgical care

---

STREET WISE

Assume that the patient has a cervical spine injury any time blunt or penetrating injuries occur to the neck. Maintain cervical stabilization during treatment, and fully immobilize the patient for transport.

HEAD TRAUMA

The anatomical components of the skull are the scalp, followed by the cranial vault, under which are the dural membrane, the arachnoid membrane, the pia, and the brain (Figure 19-11). Injuries to the skull may be classified as soft tissue injuries to the scalp and skull fractures.

Soft Tissue Injuries to the Scalp

The most common scalp injury is an irregular linear laceration. Like the face, the scalp is very vascular.

PATHOPHYSIOLOGY

Profuse bleeding and subsequent hypovolemia may result from scalp lacerations, particularly in infants and children. Other, less frequent scalp injuries include wounds, avulsions, and hematomas.

ASSESSMENT

Assume that the patient has a spinal injury when any head trauma is present. Utilize spinal precautions when completing the assessment.

Visually survey the head looking for any bleeding or the origin of the bleeding. Remember that even small wounds to the scalp can bleed profusely (Figure 19-12).

MANAGEMENT

Use direct pressure or pressure dressings to decrease blood loss. Use caution not to press too hard in case of

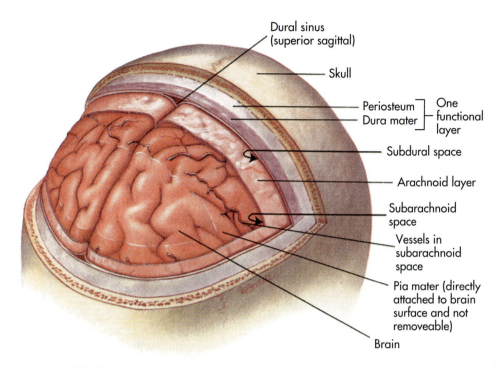

FIGURE 19-11 ▲ The skull, protective membranes, and the brain.

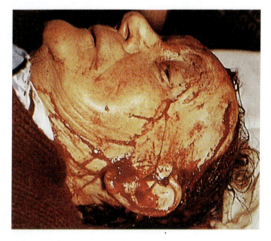

FIGURE 19-12 ▲ Scalp lacerations can produce severe bleeding. (From London PS: *A colour atlas of diagnosis after recent injury,* London, Wolfe Medical Publications.)

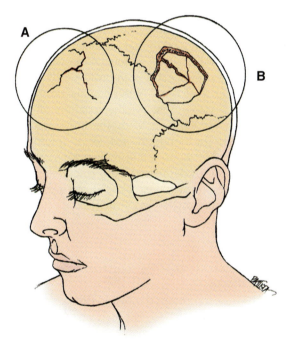

FIGURE 19-13 ▲ **A,** A nondepressed skull fracture. **B,** A depressed skull fracture. (From National Association of Emergency Medical Technicians: *Prehospital trauma life support,* ed 4, St Louis, 1999, Mosby.)

underlying skull fracture and possible brain trauma. It is best to use an open-palmed hand so that increased pressure does not push skull fragments into the brain (see Figure 19-2). Prevent contamination of open wounds by covering them, and consider fluid replacement as necessary.

Skull Fractures

A skull fracture is a break in the continuity of any of the bones of the skull. Generally, skull fractures cannot be def-initely diagnosed without a radiograph. Uncomplicated skull fractures are often of minor significance. However, damage to underlying brain tissue or vascular structures of the meninges can be life threatening.

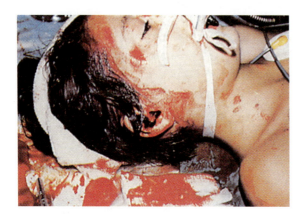

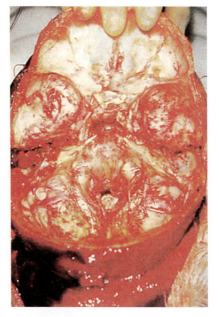

FIGURE 19-14 ▲ Severe fracture of the base of the skull. (From London PS: *A colour atlas of diagnosis after recent injury,* London, 1990, Wolfe Medical Publications.)

PATHOPHYSIOLOGY

Skull fractures are classified as open or closed. An open skull fracture involves skin that has been disrupted, exposing the central nervous system. A closed skull fracture means the skin has not been broken.

Skull fractures also are described as depressed or nondepressed, depending on the location of fracture fragments in comparison with the uninjured bones (Figure 19-13). In nondepressed skull fractures, the pieces of fractured bone retain their normal alignment within the skull. In depressed skull fractures, the bony fragments have been forced inward toward the brain and may press on underlying structures.

ASSESSMENT

The EMT–I should suspect a skull fracture if the patient has the following:
- A history of trauma to the head with or without unresponsiveness
- An altered level of responsiveness
- Pupils sluggish to react or dilated
- Obvious penetrating or impalement injury
- Deformity of the skull (Figure 19-14)
- Blood or cerebrospinal fluid draining from the nose or ears
- Raccoon eyes (may be a late sign)
- Battle's sign (may be a late sign)

Blood and Cerebrospinal Fluid Drainage—Normally, the brain and spinal cord are contained within a closed system consisting of the meninges and cerebrospinal fluid (CSF). If the meninges are disrupted,

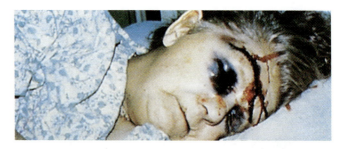

FIGURE 19-15 ▲ "Raccoon eyes" may be seen with a basilar skull fracture.

CSF may leak and drain into the nostrils or ear canal. CSF is normally clear and watery in appearance. Because bleeding can occur from a bone fracture, blood may mix with the CSF. Thus, drainage may appear watery or bloody. The EMT–I should consider any type of clear or bloody drainage from the nostrils or ears following head trauma an indication of a possible skull fracture.

Raccoon Eyes—Raccoon eyes are a black and blue discoloration that results from the collection of blood in the tissue around the eye sockets. Raccoon eyes suggest the presence of a basilar skull fracture and may not occur until 12 hours or more after the injury (Figure 19-15).

Battle's sign—Battle's sign is a discoloration of the skin at the mastoid region behind the ear. This sign is caused by an accumulation of blood after a basilar skull fracture and may not occur until 12 hours or more after the injury (Figure 19-16).

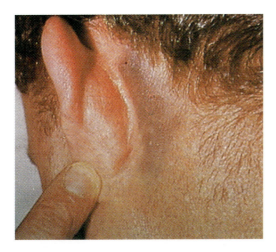

FIGURE 19-16 ▲ "Battle's sign" may be present after a basilar skull fracture. (From London PS: *A colour atlas of diagnosis after recent injury,* London, 1990, Wolfe Medical Publications.)

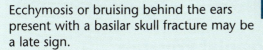

CLINICAL NOTES

Ecchymosis or bruising behind the ears present with a basilar skull fracture may be a late sign.

MANAGEMENT

Patients suspected of having skull fractures and possible trauma to the central nervous system, including the brain and spinal cord, should be monitored closely during transport so that any changes in their level of responsiveness can be rapidly identified. In addition, any related injuries such as facial and intracranial trauma, compromised airway, and spinal injuries should be anticipated by the EMT–I.

Brain Injuries

A *brain injury* is defined by the National Head Injury Foundation as "a traumatic insult to the brain capable of producing physical, intellectual, emotional, social, and vocational change."[3] Categories include mild and moderate diffuse injury, diffuse axonal injury, and focal injury.

PATHOPHYSIOLOGY

Types of brain injuries include concussion, contusion, open injuries, hematoma, and hemorrhage.[2] It is far more important for the EMT–I to recognize the *presence* of a brain injury than it is that he or she determine its *precise nature.*

Bleeding within and around the brain can compress brain tissue, impair neurological function, and lead to death. It is difficult to distinguish the different types of intracranial bleeding in the field.

ASSESSMENT

The patient's level of responsiveness is extremely important in the evaluation of any brain injury. A change in the level of responsiveness is the most significant sign to follow when monitoring the patient with a brain injury. Patients who develop a sudden loss of responsiveness or decrease in their level of responsiveness should be transported immediately.

Signs and symptoms of brain injury can range from the brief loss of responsiveness seen with a concussion (usually 5 minutes or less) to the longer period of unresponsiveness (from 5 minutes to 1 hour) seen with a contusion.

The patient with an altered level of responsiveness may be disoriented or confused or have garbled speech. The Glasgow Coma Scale (GCS) (Table 19-3) helps evaluate and describe the patient's level of responsiveness.

Other specific signs and symptoms may include the following:
- Headache
- Unequal, dilated, or nonreactive pupils; occasional eye deviation to one side
- Loss of consciousness followed by periods of drowsiness, restlessness, and confusion
- Presence of alcohol on the patient's breath or other evidence of drug intoxication (This finding is important because the presence of drugs and/or alcohol complicates the assessment and masks serious injuries. If the mechanism of injury suggests a brain injury, the EMT–I should initially attribute abnormal behavior to the injury and not to drugs or alcohol.)
- **Retrograde amnesia** (no recall of events before the injury)
- **Antegrade amnesia** (no recall of events immediately after recovery of consciousness)
- Vomiting
- Blood or clear fluid (or a mixture) coming from the nose or ears, indicating a CSF leak
- Raccoon eyes or Battle's sign, suggesting a co-existing fracture
- Combativeness
- Transient visual disturbances (e.g., light flashes and wavy lines)
- Defects in equilibrium and coordination
- Exposed brain tissue or fractured bone fragments if an open injury has occurred
- Abnormal body posturing (The patient may be in this position during the assessment, or this posturing may follow the application of painful stimuli.)
- **Decorticate posturing** (position of a patient in which the upper extremities are flexed at the elbows and wrists; legs also may be flexed [Figure 19-17, *A*])
- **Decerebrate posturing** (position in which the arms are extended and internally rotated and the legs are

TABLE 19-3

Glasgow Coma Scale (GCS)

EYE OPENING		MOTOR RESPONSE	
Spontaneous	4	Obeys command	6
To voice	3	Localizes pain	5
To pain	2	Withdrawn (pain)	4
None	1	Flexion (pain)	3
		Extension (pain)	2
		None	1
VERBAL RESPONSE		**TOTAL GCS POINTS**	
Oriented	5	14-15 = 5	
Confused	4	11-13 = 4	
Inappropriate words	3	8-10 = 3	
Incomprehensible	2	5-7 = 2	
None	1	3-4 = 1	

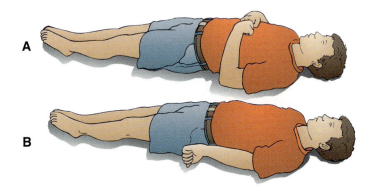

FIGURE 19-17 ▲ **A,** Abnormal flexion (decorticate posturing). **B,** Abnormal extension (decerebrate posturing). (From Sheehy S: *Emergency nursing,* ed 3, St Louis, 1992, Mosby.)

extended with the feet in forced plantar flexion; later sign of increasing ICP [Figure 19-17, *B*])
- The presence of either decorticate or decerebrate posturing suggests the presence of severe neurologic damage, and these patients should be transported quickly.

Patients with brain injury may have paralysis of any or all limbs. If the right side of the brain is injured, the patient's left side will be affected and vice versa. The injury may result in muscle weakness or paralysis of one or both sides of the body. Paralysis on one side of the body is called **hemiplegia.** Paralysis of the lower extremities is called **paraplegia.** Paralysis of all four extremities is **quadriplegia.**

The EMT–I must not allow a patient to attempt to move if a cervical spine injury is suspected. Movement without spinal immobilization may further aggravate the injury or cause an unstable fracture to sever the spinal cord. Once the spine has been immobilized appropriately, the EMT–I may proceed to check hand-grips, foot motion, and sensation.

Intracranial Pressure

Continuous assessment of patients with potential or known brain injuries is important in order to detect signs of deterioration. The pressure within the intracranial compartment, the **intracranial pressure (ICP),** may increase. This increase can lead to further brain injury and death due to compression of vital brain structures. Several findings should suggest that the ICP is rising (Box 19-3):
- A deterioration in the level of responsiveness (the most important sign to follow)
- Progressive neurologic deficits, especially paralysis
- Vomiting, especially if projectile in nature
- Unequal pupils, especially if one pupil is normal size and the other is markedly dilated
- A repetitive pattern of slow, shallow breathing to rapid, deep ventilations back to slow, shallow breaths followed by a period of apnea, known as **Cheyne-Stokes respirations,** an early sign of increased ICP
- Progressive increases in the blood pressure, especially the systolic reading, an increase in the respiratory rate, and a decreasing pulse rate (known as **Cushing reflex or triad,** a late sign of increased ICP)

LEVELS OF INCREASING INTRACRANIAL PRESSURE

CEREBRAL CORTEX AND UPPER BRAINSTEM
Blood pressure rises, pulse rate slows
Pupils remain reactive
Cheyne-Stokes respirations may be present
Patient will initially try to localize and remove painful stimuli (eventually withdraws and flexion occurs).

MIDDLE BRAINSTEM
Wide pulse pressure and bradycardia
Pupils become nonreactive or sluggish
Central neurogenic hyperventilation develops
Abnormal posturing (extension)
Few patients function normally with injury at this level.

LOWER PORTION OF BRAINSTEM/MEDULLA
Pupil "blown" (fixed and dilated) on same side of injury
Respirations become ataxic
Patient will be flaccid
Irregular pulse rate
QRS, ST-, and T-wave changes will be present
Blood pressure will fluctuate
These patients generally do not survive.

MANAGEMENT

The goal of treatment for a brain injury is to maintain cerebral oxygenation and perfusion while protecting the cervical spine. An oropharyngeal airway or endotracheal tube may be inserted if the patient is unresponsive and has no gag reflex. Insertion of a nasopharyngeal airway and nasotracheal intubation are both contraindicated if a basilar skull fracture is suspected. The American College of Surgeons Committee on Trauma recommends intubation for any patient with a GCS score of 8 or less.[2]

Arterial carbon dioxide causes blood vessels to dilate, which takes up more intracranial space. Decreasing the carbon dioxide will cause the vessels to constrict and take less space, thus decreasing the ICP. Patients with signs and symptoms of increasing intracranial pressure should be ventilated with high-concentration oxygen at a rate *not to exceed 30 breaths/minute*. Routine hyperventilation is no longer widely recommended.

CLINICAL NOTES
Some current research raises questions about the use of hyperventilation in the management of acute head injury. Check your local protocols for direction.

As previously mentioned, the face and scalp are highly vascular and can produce a great deal of bleeding. Obvious bleeding should be controlled. Suction equipment should be readily available to manage vomiting. An intravenous (IV) line of normal saline or Ringer's lactate also should be established at a keep vein open rate whenever possible. The rate can be adjusted if signs of hypovolemic shock are present.

If fluid or blood is coming from the nose or ears, the EMT–I should loosely cover the nostrils and/or ears with a clean dressing. The EMT–I should allow slight leaking to occur because this will prevent a complete tamponade of the fluid. If the fluid is not permitted to drain, the ICP may increase, thus increasing the amount of damage to the brain.

The care for all sources of bleeding in the brain is the same: support the patient's oxygenation as well as ventilatory and circulatory functions while maintaining spinal precautions. Get the patient to definitive care, which can only be provided at the trauma center. It is important to document the patient's current level of responsiveness, any previous loss of responsiveness, ongoing neurological status, and memory deficits at the scene and en route to the hospital.

Serial vital sign determinations and frequent reassessments help detect signs of ICP as they occur. Any changes that suggest a progressive rise in ICP should be immediately reported to medical direction and/or the receiving hospital. In addition, this type of patient should be transported immediately.

Patients with head injuries should be immobilized based on the mechanism of injury. Forces significant enough to cause a brain injury also will traumatize the spinal cord. Cervical spine immobilization and use of a long backboard are appropriate. Whenever possible, the long backboard should be raised so that the head is elevated. This positioning may help decrease ICP.

PRIMARY INJURY PREVENTION

The EMT–I has a unique opportunity to prevent head injuries. Participate in bicycle safety and brain injury reduction efforts. Be a good role model and wear a helmet when riding a bike or roller blading. Use safety equipment that protects the head, eyes, and face when taking part in sports activities.

SPINAL TRAUMA

Spinal injuries are physical trauma to the spinal cord, vertebral column, or surrounding connective tissues. Injury to any of these structures can affect the passage of nerve impulses to and from the spinal cord. Injury to any section of the spinal cord can affect the communication between the brain and the rest of the body. The cord itself may be damaged directly, or injury can result from swelling around the cord or improper movement of the spine. If the cord is severed, it cannot be repaired because the central nervous system does not regenerate.

Anyone sustaining a head injury causing a loss of responsiveness, significant blunt trauma to the torso, significant injury above the clavicles, or a major fall must be considered also to have a spinal injury. A patient with spinal injury may be neurologically intact or may have deficits of movement and/or sensation. When nerve damage occurs, it may be partial or complete. With proper care, however, substantial recovery may be possible.

Although spinal injury can occur at any time, it is most common in patients between 16 and 35 years of age. It is during this age range when people are involved in the most violent types of activity. This trauma can leave the patient with devastating effects if not properly managed in the prehospital setting. EMT–Is must work to preserve as much function as possible for the patient.

Stable Versus Unstable Spinal Injuries

Nerve damage may or may not occur immediately following spinal injury. If deficits are present, the EMT–I's responsibility is to prevent further damage from taking place. If an injury exists but no nerve damage is present, the EMT–I must prevent such damage from occurring. It is impossible to determine in the field if any injury is stable or not, so the EMT–I must always care for the patient with any suspected spinal injury as though the injury was unstable.

Types of Spinal Injuries

Injury can occur to any part of the spinal column. Although isolated injuries can occur, most often, trauma affects several different structures, such as vertebrae, ligaments, intervertebral disks, and the spinal cord.

Any portion of the spinal cord may be injured by direct or indirect trauma. Often the damage occurs from indirect trauma when a segment of vertebra presses against the cord (Figure 19-18). In addition, the spinal cord can be contused or compressed when nearby injured tissues swell and constrict the cord. Injury also can be due to direct trauma, such as damage that occurs from a gunshot wound.

In all forms of spinal injury, the bottom line is whether the spinal cord is affected. If cord injury has occurred, the EMT–I must take steps to prevent additional damage. If the cord is not injured, the patient should be treated so that the risk of spinal cord damage is minimized. Because it usually is difficult to know if true spinal cord damage has occurred, the EMT–I should use every precaution for all suspected spinal injuries.

Mechanisms of Spinal Injury

Major causes of spine injury in adults include car crashes, shallow-water diving accidents, motorcycle crashes, and all other injuries and falls. In children, most injuries occur from falls from heights, falls from a tricycle or bicycle, and being struck by a motor vehicle. Remember that injury can occur to the cervical spine any time a significant force meets the head. This area of the spine is flexible and may not withstand the force of the impact. The cervical spine is, therefore, compressed directly, hyperextended, or hyperflexed. The forces that lead to spinal injury are flexion, rotation, extension, and compression. Many times, these forces occur in combination.

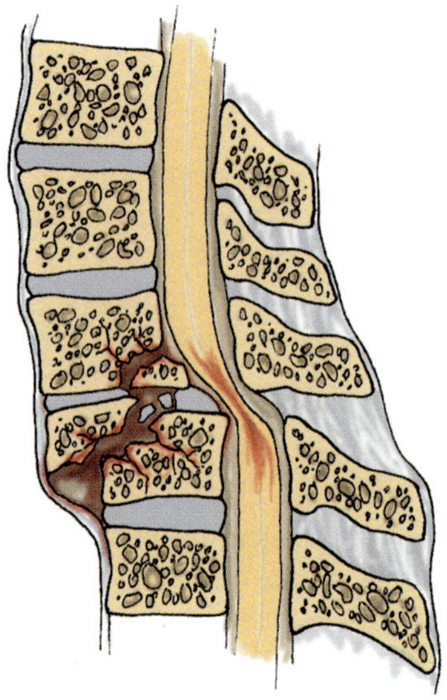

FIGURE 19-18 ▲ An example of a spinal injury caused by a vertebra pressing against the spinal cord.

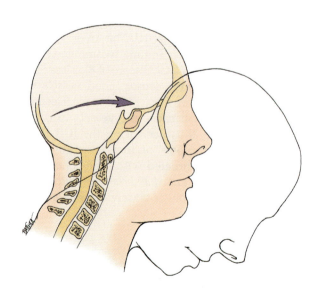

FIGURE 19-19 ▲ Flexion injuries to the spinal column occur when the spinal structures are flexed forward violently.

FLEXION

Flexion injuries occur when the spinal structures are flexed violently forward such as when hitting one's head while diving. As a result, the supporting ligaments of the posterior spine are abnormally stretched, leading to tears or avulsions of the spinous processes of the vertebrae.

Mechanical pressure of one vertebra on another leads to "wedge" fractures of the body of the vertebra (Figure 19-19). In the lumbar spine region, flexion forces, often after a fall, cause V-shaped compression fractures (Figure 19-20).

ROTATION

Rotation injuries of the cervical spine seldom occur as isolated events. Rather, a combination of flexion and rotation of the spine causes dislocation of the intervertebral joints. A pure rotational force applied to the lumbar spine can result in an unstable fracture of the lumbar vertebrae.

EXTENSION

Tears of the ligaments and vertebral instability occur with hyperextension of the head (Figure 19-21). Additionally, the skull may be forced down on the posterior aspects of the upper vertebrae, leading to fracture and patient death.

A combination of flexion and extension is responsible for many spinal injuries after motor vehicle crashes. One example is the classic "whiplash" injury. In this injury pattern, the head is "whipped" forward in a flexion motion and then back in an extension motion or vice versa. The spine, spinal cord, and adjacent structures are exposed to both types of forces.

VERTICAL COMPRESSION

Vertical compression injuries occur when a force is directed along the axis of the spine. The intervertebral disk is compressed into the body of the vertebra, leading to spinal cord damage. This type of injury occurs following a fall, especially when landing on the feet or if the head is hit by a heavy object (Figure 19-22).

Lateral bending also can contribute to spinal injuries when the patient is hit from the side. Examples include a side-impact motor vehicle crash or someone hit from the side while riding a bicycle or other riding toy. The chest and thoracic spine move sideways while the head stays in place until pulled along by the cervical attachments. Dislocations and bony fractures may occur.

Lastly, the spine may be pulled apart, causing the spinal cord to be stretched and torn. For example, this mechanism can occur to the cervical spine after a hanging, hence the term hangman's fracture. The force of the object around the neck and the weight of the body contribute to the injury.

Assessment of the Patient With Spinal Injuries
PATIENT HISTORY

Assessment of the patient with spinal injuries must include a thorough review of the mechanism of injury. If there is any possibility that the patient may have a spinal injury, the spine must be immobilized. As the EMT–I moves the patient to complete the assessment, in-line spinal immobilization must be maintained. The following clues are indicative of possible spinal trauma:
- Mechanism of injury regardless of the absence of any other signs and symptoms

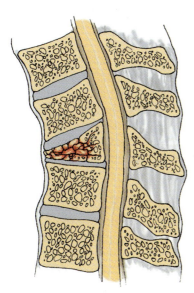

FIGURE 19-20 ▲ Flexion forces can cause V-shaped compression fractures in the lumbar spine region.

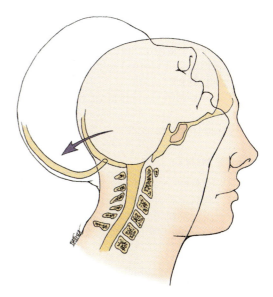

FIGURE 19-21 ▲ Hyperextension injuries to the spinal column can occur when the spinal structures are forced back violently.

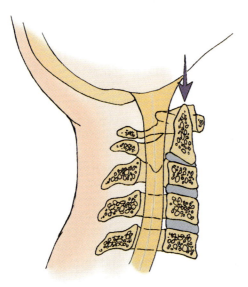

FIGURE 19-22 ▲ A vertical compression injury occurs when force is exerted along the axis of the spine, compressing the vertebral disk into the body of the vertebra.

- Motor vehicle and motorcycle crashes
- Diving accidents
- Wounds of the face, head, neck, or shoulders
- Falls greater than 15 feet (for an adult)

> **HELPFUL HINT**
> - The EMT–I should always assume that patients with severe injuries to the head or face also have injury to the spine.

- Pain, especially pain on movement
- Point tenderness
- Deformity
- Guarding of the spine area
- Paralysis, paresis, numbness, or tingling in the legs or arms at any time after injury
- Presence of gunshot wound to head, trunk, or back
- Unexplained shock
- Priapism (continuing erection of the penis) in male patients
- Loss of urine (incontinence)

> **HELPFUL HINT**
> - The ability to walk after an accident does not exclude the existence of significant spinal trauma. Some patients with serious spinal injury initially are able to walk without difficulty.

If there is any doubt whether spinal cord injury exists, the patient should be immobilized. If the mechanism of injury is such that a spinal cord injury may have occurred, the patient should be immobilized. If other people were seriously injured or killed in the same

> **HELPFUL HINT**
> - Although spinal injuries may cause unexplained shock, the EMT–I should always assume that shock is caused by bleeding (hypovolemia) until proven otherwise.

crash, the EMT–I should immobilize the patient's spine. Immobilizing the patient does no harm and could preserve neurologic function or prevent further injury if spinal trauma is present.

Complications of Spinal Injury

Patients with spinal injury may develop several complications. If the cervical spinal cord is damaged, the patient may have difficulty breathing or be in respiratory arrest. The EMT–I should prepare to provide respiratory support to patients with possible spinal injuries.

Injury to the spinal cord may lead to partial or complete paralysis. Some patients may have a "pins and needles" feeling in their extremities. Others may experience weakness in the arms and/or legs without specific paralysis. If the patient is responsive and any of these signs or symptoms are present, strong emotional support is recommended. The patient may be scared or upset at the possibility of present or future paralysis and the associated disability.

Spinal shock is a form of neurogenic shock that results from complete transection of the spinal cord. There is complete loss of sensation and voluntary movement below the injury. The patient in spinal shock is hypotensive because of the loss of vascular control caused by the injury. As a rule, the patient will not have an elevated pulse rate. The patient's skin will be pink, warm, and dry and possibly even flushed due to vasodilation below the level of the injury. Hypotension from spinal shock is difficult to treat.

The most common cause of shock and hypotension after trauma is hemorrhage. The EMT–I should assume that a trauma patient who is in shock has significant bleeding. The EMT–I should not attribute shock to spinal shock even if the patient appears to be paralyzed. These patients usually have life-threatening injuries and need immediate transport.

Emergency Care

As with all other emergencies, the EMT–I should perform initial and ongoing assessments as previously described. Life-threatening conditions such as airway obstruction, respiratory arrest, cardiac arrest, or severe bleeding take precedence over spinal injuries. If spinal injury is suspected, movement of the spine should be limited whenever possible while treating critical injuries.

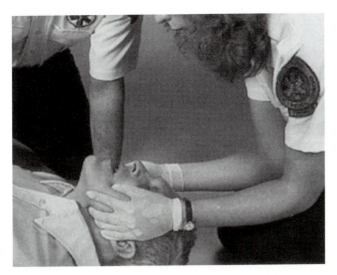

FIGURE 19-23 ▲ **Use a trauma jaw-thrust maneuver to open the airway on a patient with a suspected cervical spine injury.** (From the National Association of Emergency Medical Technicians: *Prehospital trauma life support*, ed 4, St Louis, 1999, Mosby.)

Patients with known or suspected spinal injuries present challenges for airway management. The EMT–I should not move or hyperextend the head of a patient with a possible spinal injury. To open the airway a jaw-thrust maneuver should be performed (Figure 19-23).

The EMT–I should administer high-concentration oxygen and assist breathing as necessary. Suction may be necessary. Accompanying injuries should be treated and spinal immobilization maintained throughout treatment. One to two large-bore IV lines of normal saline or Ringer's lactate solution should be inserted once transport has been initiated.

Many people activate the EMS system for lower back pain even in the absence of trauma. Many conditions can cause back pain, and some of these, such as an abdominal aneurysm, can be life-threatening. If there is doubt about the severity of a patient's condition, the EMT–I should immobilize the spine.

Spinal Immobilization

Anyone with the potential for spinal injury must be completely immobilized using the *joint above/joint below* theory. The joint above is the head, whereas the joint below is the pelvis. Essentially, the full body should be immobilized to prevent movement of the spine.

Spinal immobilization is a method of splinting the spine to prevent movement and additional injury to the vertebral column and spinal cord. The process has two steps: immobilization of the neck and immobilization of the body.

Neck Immobilization

Immobilization of the cervical vertebrae is performed in two steps: manual stabilization and application of a rigid cervical spine immobilization device. The EMT–I should perform manual, in-line stabilization immediately when cervical spine injury is suspected. Manual stabilization aids with the following:

- Helps establish and maintain the patient's airway.
- Places the head and neck into neutral alignment, which is the splinting position for the spine.
- Minimizes the risk of additional damage to the cervical spine.

MANUAL STABILIZATION

The EMT–I should get into position at the top of the patient's head (if the patient is lying down) or behind the patient (if the patient is seated). The EMT–I should place his or her hands at the corner of the patient's jaw on both sides. The EMT–I should grasp the corner of the jaw and provide stabilization of the neck by wrapping his or her hands around the posterior portion of the neck. The patient's head should be placed in the neutral position to align the spine. If the patient complains of pain, if the head is not easily moved into position, if muscle spasm occurs, or if the airway becomes compromised, the EMT–I should not attempt this positioning. A second EMT–I should apply a rigid cervical spine immobilization device. Constant manual in-line stabilization should be maintained until the patient is properly secured to a backboard with the body and head immobilized.

Cervical Spine Immobilization Devices

While maintaining manual stabilization, the EMT–I should quickly inspect and palpate the neck area. A rigid cervical spine immobilization device should be applied, which reduces movement of the cervical spine and helps maintain neutral alignment of the head and neck. However, the device does not immobilize on its own, and movement of the head can still occur.

Soft cervical spine immobilization devices provide little, if any, stabilization of the injured spine. They are not strong enough to support the head nor do they prevent movement of the neck. The EMT–I should not use these soft devices.

STREET WISE

Some EMT–Is prefer to apply a rigid cervical spine immobilization device on the patient who is leaning forward before any movement. Others prefer to manually stabilize the neck and apply the device once the patient is moved upright. As long as the end goal is the same, the EMT–I should use whatever technique is most comfortable for him or her as the rescuer.

There are many varieties of rigid cervical spine immobilization devices available for prehospital use. EMT–Is should consult their instructor and the manufacturer's written directions for the use of any particular device.

To apply a one-piece cervical spine immobilization device, the EMT–I must do the following:

1. Continue to provide manual stabilization during application of the device.
2. Properly measure the patient to determine the appropriate-sized device. Remove the patient's earrings, if present, and move the hair out of the way as much as possible. Place your fingers flat against the patient's neck under the corner of the mandible (jaw) to determine the height to the shoulder. Size the device to the same measurement as the patient's neck. The sizing depends on the type and the design of the type used.

3. Place the back portion of the device behind the patient's head (Figure 19-24, A). Slide the front portion upward along the sternum until the device is around the neck.
4. Secure the device in place. Sometimes it is necessary to firmly mold the device around the neck while securing the Velcro to ensure a proper fit (Figure 19-24, B).
5. Make sure the device is snug and the head is in neutral alignment.

To apply a two-piece cervical spine immobilization device, the EMT–I must do the following:

1. Continue to provide manual stabilization during application of the device.
2. Properly measure the patient to determine the appropriate-sized device. Remove the patient's earrings, if present, and move the hair out of the way as much as possible.
3. Place the anterior section under the patient's jaw and secure the Velcro around the back of the neck (Figure 19-25, A).
4. Position the posterior piece behind the patient's neck, and connect it to the anterior piece using the Velcro straps (Figure 19-25, B).
5. Make sure the device is snug and the head is in neutral alignment.

A rigid cervical spine immobilization device alone for spinal immobilization should never be used. It should always be combined with an appropriate body immobilization device, such as a long backboard, and some type of head immobilization to prevent lateral movement. The head immobilization device is used in conjunction with the rigid cervical spine immobilization device to immobilize the patient's head to the long backboard. Sandbags should not be used to help immobilize the head because the weight of the sandbags can cause lateral pressure and movement of the patient's head if the board is tilted.

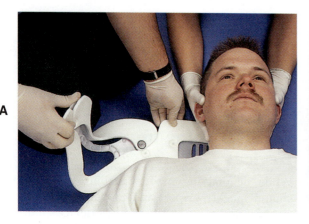
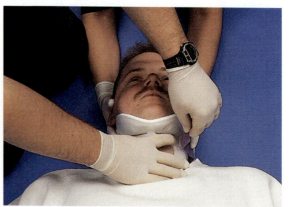

FIGURE 19-24 ▲ Applying a one-piece cervical spine immobilization device. **A,** Carefully slide the back portion of the collar behind the patient's neck. **B,** Secure the collar with the Velcro straps to make a snug fit.

Body Immobilization

After manual neck stabilization and application of a rigid cervical spine immobilization device, the rest of the body and the spine should be immobilized. The patient's position will determine which immobilization device is best. Although techniques vary from device to device, some general guidelines apply, and the EMT–I should conduct the following:

- Keep the patient's airway open.
- Maintain access to the patient to perform suctioning, oxygenation, ventilation, cardiopulmonary resuscitation, and bleeding control.
- Secure the patient firmly to any device used while keeping the spine in neutral alignment.
- Secure the head immobilization device to minimize lateral movement.
- Ensure that the patient will remain immobilized during transportation.
- Make the patient comfortable enough to cooperate as best as possible.

The techniques used to immobilize the spine depend on whether the patient is supine or seated. Outlined in the following sections are several methods to be used based on how the patient is found.

THE SEATED PATIENT

Some patients with a suspected spine injury may be in a seated position. Examples include patients who have sustained injury from motor vehicle crashes or falls and those patients who have moved after their injury.

During the scene assessment, the EMT–I should note if the patient is entrapped. If in doubt, he or she should call for assistance early. Patients found in the seated position must be immobilized in a short (half) spine board, vest-type, or similar device before being transferred to a full-body immobilization device as long as their overall condition is stable. Doing so will maintain neutral alignment and prevent movement of the patient's head and neck.

When employing a half spine board or vest-type device, several important rules must be followed. First, as soon as the EMT–I is at the patient's side, he or she immediately should provide manual stabilization. The head should be stabilized in a neutral, in-line position unless pain is encountered when moving the head to the neutral position. If the patient has too much pain, the head can be stabilized with towels or blankets in the position where movement is stopped. The EMT–I should apply a rigid cervical spine immobilization device if the head is in a neutral position. The EMT–I must avoid releasing manual stabilization before it is maintained with the immobilization device. The patient's head should be secured to the immobilization device *only* after the device has been secured to the torso. The apparatus used to secure the head must not obstruct the airway. During use of the device, the EMT–I should continually maintain neutral alignment. He or she should tightly secure the device while allowing for sufficient chest expansion. The EMT–I should avoid moving the patient excessively while applying the device, and should not pull on it to move the patient.

For demonstration purposes, the Kendrick extrication device (KED) is reviewed. Several vest-type models are available, so the EMT–I should review the equipment he or she has available to understand the general

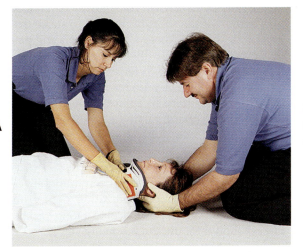 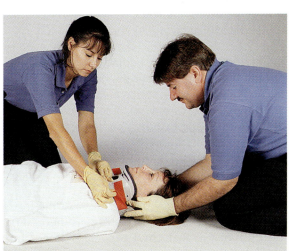

FIGURE 19-25 ▲ Applying a two-piece cervical spine immobilization device. **A,** Place the anterior section under the patient's jaw and secure the Velcro around the back of the neck. **B,** Position the posterior piece behind the patient's neck, and connect it to the anterior piece using the Velcro straps.

design and application sequence. To apply a vest-type device, the EMT–I should use the following procedure:

1. After ensuring scene safety, move to the patient and begin the initial assessment. Whenever possible, assume a position in front of the patient to minimize the patient's natural response to turn the head toward the EMT–I's voice. Throughout assessment and management of the patient, be sure to employ body substance isolation procedures.
2. Move behind the patient. Place one hand on each side of the head, fingers spread wide, with the thumbs on the occipital area.
3. Place/maintain the patient's head in a neutral, in-line position. If the patient complains of extreme pain or if resistance is felt, do not move the head. Pad around it in that position.
4. Open the airway, if necessary, using the trauma jaw-thrust. Do not tilt the patient's head. Continue maintaining the head in a neutral position to ensure an open airway while preventing hyperextension. (If a partner or another EMT has completed steps 2 through 4, assess the manual immobilization of the patient's head.)
5. If the patient is stable, assess motor, sensory, and distal circulation in all four of the patient's extremities.
6. Select a rigid cervical spine immobilization device of the appropriate size and apply it, without moving the patient. Remember to quickly inspect and palpate the neck before applying the device (Figure 19-26, A to C).
7. Carefully move the patient forward and position the immobilization device behind him or her (Figure 19-26, D and E).
8. Bring the patient to the device. Stabilize the head while a partner slowly moves the patient backward (Figure 19-26, F).
9. Secure the immobilization device to the patient's torso so that it cannot move up or down, left or right. When using the KED, be sure that it is snug against the axillae (armpits) (Figure 19-26, G).
10. Secure the device using the color-coded belts (Figure 19-26, H). When pulling the straps tight, hold the buckles to prevent the device from rotating. Typically, the chest straps are applied first and then the groin straps. As the torso straps are tightened, be careful not to jerk or move the patient unnecessarily. Secure the leg straps so that the legs are not pulled upward (Figure 19-26, I). In some EMS systems, use of the leg straps is optional. Check with medical direction to be sure.
11. Reevaluate the position and tightness of the torso straps (torso fixation), adjusting as necessary. Check to ensure that chest expansion is not impaired by the tightness of the torso straps. On smaller patients, the chest section may interfere with respirations. In these cases, fold the chest section back to avoid interfering with breathing.
12. Evaluate and pad behind the patient's head as necessary (Figure 19-26, J).
13. Secure the patient's head to the device being sure to maintain a neutral, in-line position (Figure 19-26, K). Wrap the headpiece around the patient. Pad any gaps between the patient and the device to ensure neutral alignment.
14. Secure the patient's head to the device using cravats, adhesive tape, or commercially prepared straps.
15. Reassess the patient before moving him or her to the long backboard; be certain that the patient is securely fastened to the device. Reassess motor, sensory, and distal circulation in all four extremities (Figure 19-26, L).
16. Move the patient to a long backboard.
17. Reassess motor, sensory, and distal circulation in all four extremities.

To apply the short (half) backboard, the EMT–I should use the following steps:

1. Complete steps 1 through 6 as described for the KED. Then, with the rigid cervical spine immobilization device already in place, continue to keep the patient in neutral alignment.
2. Slide the short backboard into position (Figure 19-27, A). Ensure that the top of the board is even with the top of the patient's head.
3. Secure the patient's body to the board with 9-ft or larger straps (Figure 19-27, B). Several techniques are acceptable.
4. Pad behind the head to ensure neutral alignment.
5. Secure the patient's head to the board with cravats or strong 2-inch or wider adhesive tape (Figure 19-27, C).
6. Secure the wrists, knees, and ankles.
7. Reassess the patient before moving him or her to the long backboard; also be certain that the patient is securely fastened to the short backboard.
8. Transfer the patient to a long backboard. Be sure to lift the patient when transferring. Do not allow the bottom of the short backboard to strike the surface of the long backboard, because this will place additional pressure on the patient's head and neck. It may be necessary to loosen the leg straps to lower the patient's legs onto the long backboard.
9. If it is necessary to adjust the head portion of the short backboard, maintain manual stabilization.

TRANSFERRING TO A BACKBOARD

To transfer a patient who has been immobilized with a rigid cervical spine immobilization device and short backboard (or vest-type device) to a long backboard, the EMT–I should follow the following steps:

1. Make sure the short device is secure.
2. Move the ambulance cot with a long backboard on it next to the patient (in a motor vehicle crash, use the door opening of the vehicle).

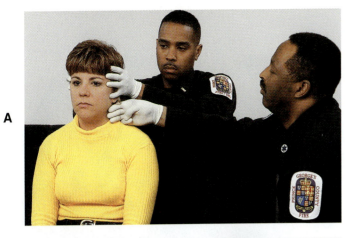

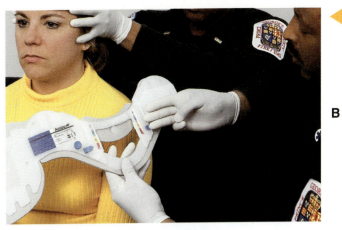

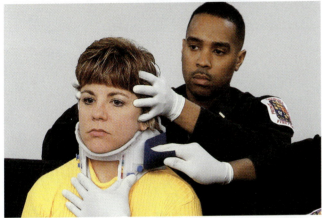

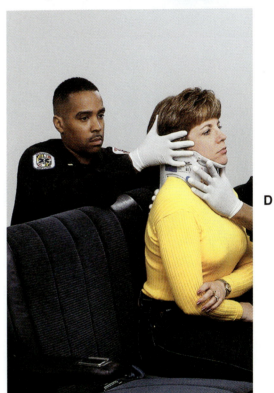

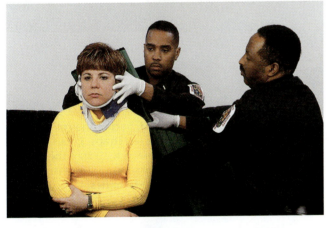

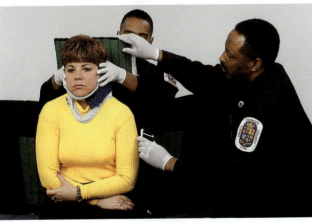

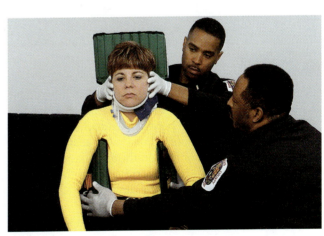

FIGURE 19-26 ▲ Applying the vest-type device. **A,** Measure the patient's neck.
B, Measure the cervical collar. **C,** Apply the cervical collar. **D,** Move the patient forward. **E,** Slide the device behind the patient. **F,** Bring the patient to the device.
G, Position the device snugly against the patient's armpit while positioning the groin straps.

Continued

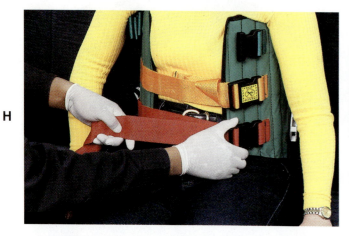

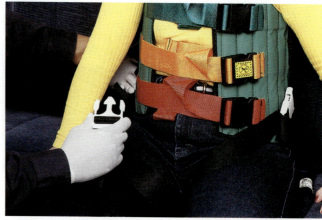

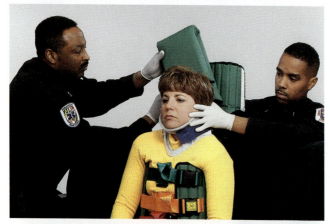

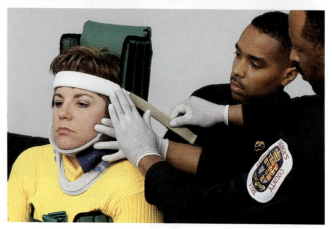

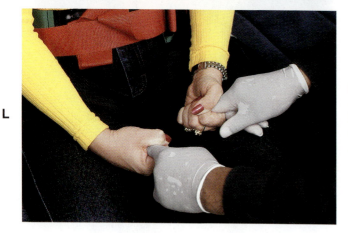

FIGURE 19-26, cont'd ▲ **H,** Secure the color coded chest straps. **I,** Secure the leg straps. **J,** Pad behind the patient's head as necessary. **K,** Secure the patient's head to the device. **L,** Reassess motor, sensory, and distal circulation in all four extremities.

3. Position the long backboard as close to the patient as possible. Place the end of the long backboard next to or under the patient's buttocks so that one end is securely supported on the car seat, chair, and so on, and the other end on the ambulance cot. The backboard should be perpendicular to the cot.

4. Rotate the patient (with the device in place) and elevate his or her legs (Figure 19-28, *A*).

5. Lower the patient to a supine position on the long backboard.

6. Lower the patient's legs onto backboard (in some patients it may be necessary to loosen the groin straps).

7. Slide the patient up until properly positioned on the long backboard. Avoid using the short backboard or vest-type device as a handle to move the patient. Keep the upper and lower body in line as much as possible.

8. Position the patient onto the long backboard (Figure 19-28, *B*). If the patient is taller than the long backboard, let the feet extend beyond the device.

9. Secure the patient to the long backboard.

10. Position the long backboard onto the ambulance cot.

11. Securely fasten the device to the backboard.

12. Immobilize the patient's legs to the long backboard.

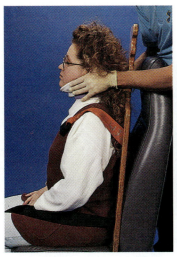 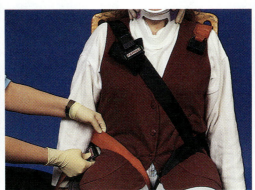 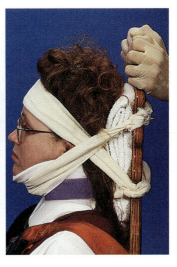

A   B   C

FIGURE 19-27 ▲ Applying a short backboard cervical spine immobilization device. **A,** Slide the short backboard into place, with the top of the board even with the patient's head. **B,** Secure the patient's torso to the board. **C,** Secure the patient's head to the board.

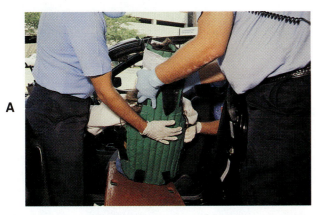 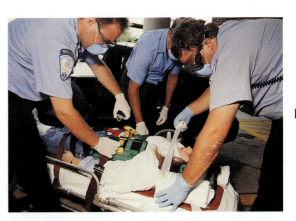

A   B

FIGURE 19-28 ▲ Transferring an immobilized patient to a backboard. **A,** Rotate the patient in place and elevate the legs. **B,** Position the patient onto a long backboard and secure in place. (From National Association of Emergency Medical Technicians: *Prehospital trauma life support,* ed 4, St Louis, 1999, Mosby.)

13. Secure the long backboard and the patient to the cot.
14. If the ambulance cot is not available, the long backboard can be held by others while the patient is lifted out of the seat and placed on the long backboard.

HELPFUL HINT

● If the patient is prone, stabilize the head while logrolling the patient into a supine position.

THE SUPINE PATIENT

Many patients who are likely to have spinal injury are found lying down. Ideally, four people should be used to immobilize the spine of patients who are found in

this position, but two to three people can accomplish the task. To perform this maneuver, the EMT–Is should follow these steps:

1. After ensuring scene safety, move to the patient and begin the initial assessment.
2. Employ body substance isolation procedures throughout assessment and management of the patient.
3. Approach the patient from the top of his or her head to limit the patient's motion before beginning cervical stabilization.
4. Place one hand along each side of the patient's head.
5. Carefully move the patient's head into a neutral in-line position (Figure 19-29, *A*). If the patient com-

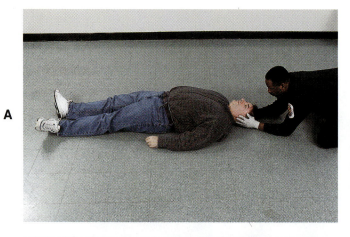

A

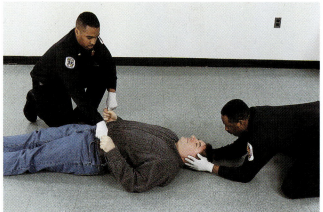

B

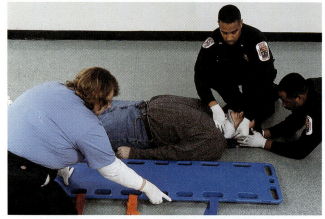

C

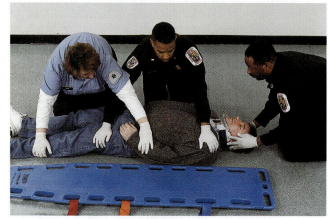

D

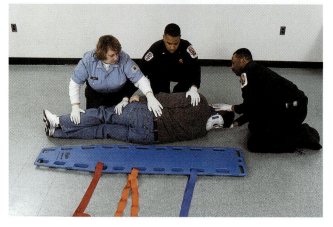

E

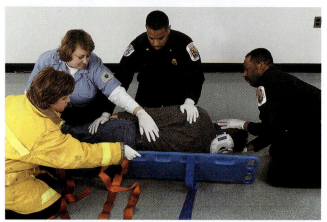

F

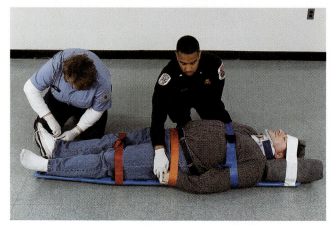

G

FIGURE 19-29 ▲ Immobolizing the supine patient onto a long backboard. **A,** Carefully move the patient's head into in-line position. **B,** Evaluate motor, sensory, and distal circulation in all of the patient's extremities. **C,** Position the long backboard alongside the patient. **D,** Assume correct position next to the patient. **E,** Slowly roll the patient to the side. **F,** Slide the backboard close to the patient. **G,** Reassess motor, sensory, and distal circulation in all four extremities.

plains of extreme pain or resistance is felt, do not move the head. Continue to maintain the airway and manual stabilization of the head.

6. Open the airway, if necessary, using the trauma jaw thrust. Do not tilt the patient's head.

7. If the patient is stable, evaluate motor, sensory, and distal circulation in all four of the patient's extremities (Figure 19-29, *B*).

8. Select an appropriately-sized rigid cervical spine immobilization device and apply it without moving the patient. Use the largest device that does not cause hyperextension.

9. Position a long backboard alongside the patient (Figure 19-29, *C*).

10. Kneel next to the patient's midthorax.

11. The second partner should kneel next to the patient's knees. Each EMT–I should kneel within 1 inch of the patient, which allows the patient to be rolled and reduces excessive movement.

12. Straighten the patient's arms so that they are in a "palm-in" position next to the torso, and direct the second EMT–I to bring the legs together into neutral alignment. Do not raise the patient's arm to assist with the log roll, because this action causes movement of the cervical and thoracic vertebrae.

13. Grasp the far side of the patient at his or her shoulder and wrist.

14. Direct the second EMT–I to grasp the patient's hip with his or her left hand just distal to the wrist and tightly grasp both pant cuffs at the ankles with his or her right hand (Figure 19-29, *D*). (If the patient is wearing shorts or a skirt or no pants are available, a cravat tied around both ankles can be used instead.)

15. Usually the EMT–I at the head decides when the patient is logrolled. The other EMT–Is should follow the directions of the person at the patient's head.

16. With the patient's arms locked firmly at his or her sides, slowly roll the patient to the side (toward the EMT–Is) only until there is enough room to insert the long backboard (Figure 19-29, *E*). Elevate the ankles as necessary to maintain lateral alignment. This must be done without compromising the integrity of the spine.

17. Slide the backboard close to the patient, and instruct the other EMT–Is as to when the patient will be rolled back down (Figure 19-29, *F*).

18. On command, roll patient back onto the board. This must be done without compromising the integrity of the spine.

19. Keeping the patient in neutral alignment, adjust the patient's position so that he or she is centered on the board and proper space exists between the top of the board and the patient's head.

20. Ensure alignment by padding gaps or voids between the long backboard and the patient's body.

Carefully place padding under the head as necessary to assist with neutral alignment.

21. Immobilize the patient's torso to the long backboard so that it cannot move up or down or laterally. Place one strap over the nipple line and one strap over the iliac crests or use an X-strap technique.

22. Secure the patient's legs to the long backboard with one strap just above the knees and one strap midway between the ankles and knees.

23. If moving the patient over rough terrain or on steps, secure his or her feet to the board.

24. Place the patient's arms palm-in along his or her sides and secure them to long backboard.

25. Immobilize the patient's head to the device in a neutral, in-line position by placing pads or rolled blankets on each side of patient's head and fastening a strap tightly over the pads and patient's lower forehead. Place a second strap over the pads and rigid cervical spine immobilization device, and secure it to the long backboard.

26. Reassess motor, sensory, and distal circulation (Figure 19-29, *G*).

27. If the immobilized patient vomits, turn the entire board onto its side and suction as needed.

Patients found in a prone position require employment of a special technique to maintain the airway and provide in-line support as the patient is being logrolled (Figure 19-30, *A* to *C*). The EMT–I stabilizing the head places one hand over the other, twisted about the patient's head. This puts the hands in the correct position after the roll. The prone patient is rolled into a supine position while carefully immobilizing the head, neck, and body. In extreme emergencies, when only two EMT–Is are available, the second EMT–I must control the entire body.

RAPID EXTRICATION TECHNIQUES

There are times when a patient with a spine injury must be rapidly removed from a vehicle without the benefit of full immobilization. These techniques only are used when the patient's life is clearly at risk. Rapid extrication techniques are used in two instances: an unsafe scene or patients with life-threatening injuries.

During the scene assessment, the following conditions are examples that justify rapid extrication:

- Presence or threat of fire
- Rising water
- Danger of explosion
- Danger of structure collapse

Patients with life-threatening injuries also may require rapid removal. Some examples include the following:

- Patients in cardiac or respiratory arrest
- Patients whose airways cannot be maintained while in a sitting position
- Patients in whom bleeding cannot be controlled

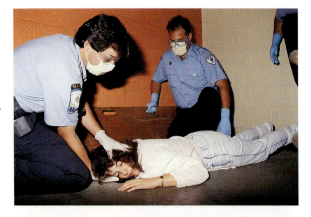

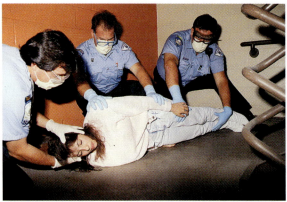

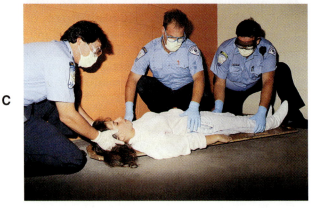

FIGURE 19-30 ▲ Providing in-line stabilization for a patient found in the prone position. **A,** The EMT–I at the patient's head places his or her hands on the patient's head so that they will be in proper position after the logroll is complete. **B,** Roll the patient while carefully immobilizing head, neck, body, and spine. **C,** Roll the patient down onto a long backboard, and continue neutral alignment. (From National Association of Emergency Medical Technicians: *Prehospital trauma life support,* ed 4, St Louis, 1999, Mosby.)

STREET WISE

The decision to employ rapid extrication techniques is not easy to make. The best guideline is, "Must this be done to save a life?"

• Patients who exhibit signs and symptoms of severe shock
• Patients whose mechanism of injury indicates the potential for rapid decompensation

Rapid extrication requires a combination of three EMT–Is. A bystander can substitute for one EMT–I if necessary. Procedure is as follows:

1. The first EMT–I stabilizes the patient's head.
2. The second EMT–I ensures that necessary equipment is gathered.
3. The third EMT–I applies a rigid cervical spine immobilization device (Figure 19-31, *A*).
4. The second EMT–I places the long backboard on the stretcher and positions the stretcher at the door of the vehicle.
5. The first EMT–I directs the other EMT–Is to begin turning the patient toward the long backboard (Figure 19-31, *B* and *C*). The EMT–Is must maintain neutral alignment and avoid sudden or jerking movements.

6. The third EMT–I takes control of the head, while the first and second EMT–Is slide the patient onto the long backboard (Figure 19-31, *D*).
7. Move the patient to a safe area where additional care is provided.

MOTORCYCLE, FOOTBALL, AND OTHER HELMETS

For the EMT–I to properly manage the airway and cervical spine, access to the head is essential. If additional equipment (e.g., shoulder pads or other protective equipment) is in place, the EMT–I must be careful to keep the head in neutral alignment (Figure 19-32, *A* to *C*).

The EMT–I should remove helmets unless the following is true:

• The patient is obviously dead.
• The helmet is entangled into the patient's head.
• An impaled object penetrates the helmet and head.

Many experts disagree over whether protective helmets should be removed in the field. The EMT–I should review the types of protective equipment that are worn for various sports in addition to a helmet and work with medical direction and the athletic trainers in the area before an emergency occurs to establish the best policy and procedure for helmet removal.

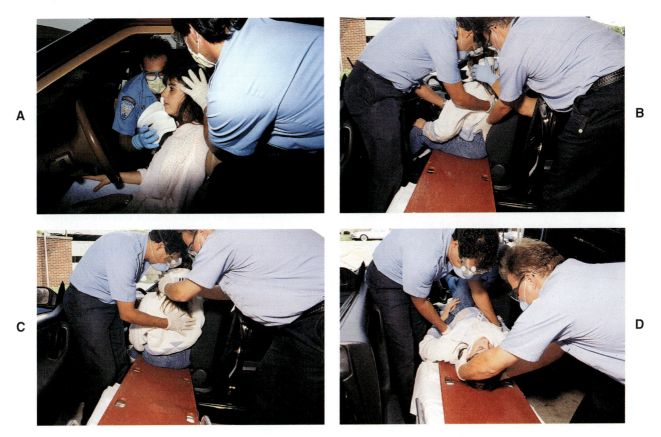

FIGURE 19-31 ▲ Steps involved in rapid patient extrication. **A,** Apply a rigid cervical collar. **B,** Begin rotating the patient toward the long backboard. **C,** Continue to rotate the patient onto the long backboard, maintaining neutral alignment. **D,** Slide the patient onto the long backboard. (From National Association of Emergency Medical Technicians: *Prehospital trauma life support,* ed 4, St Louis, 1999, Mosby.)

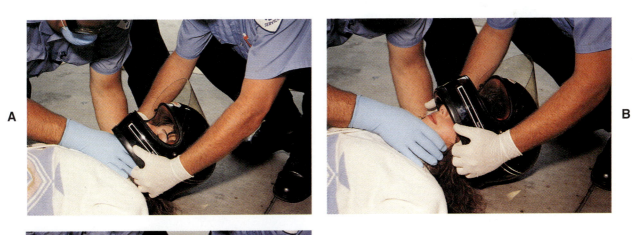

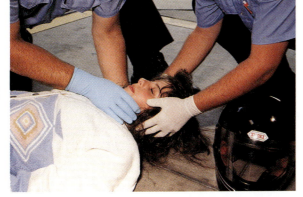

FIGURE 19-32 ▲ Removing a motorcycle helmet from a suspected spinal trauma patient. **A,** Perform manual immobilization of the head and neck. **B,** The EMT–I above the patient's head pulls the sides of the helmet apart, while pulling the helmet off of the patient. **C,** The other EMT–I maintains immobilization of the patient's cervical spine. (From National Association of Emergency Medical Technicians: *Prehospital trauma life support,* ed 4, St Louis, 1999, Mosby.)

At the hospital, it is determined that the boy's trachea was transected when he struck the wire line. The trauma surgeon does a tracheostomy and inserts an endotracheal tube into the distal end of the transected trachea. The boy is then taken to the operating room where his trachea is repaired. After one week or so in the hospital, he is discharged with no neurological deficits.

Quick thinking to stop intubation efforts, use basic life support, and transport him rapidly by air contributed to this positive outcome. In this case, it was appropriate to concentrate all efforts on management of airway and ventilation.

SUMMARY

- Spinal injuries are trauma to the spinal cord, vertebral column, or surrounding tissues. The spinal cord itself may or may not be damaged.
- Stable spinal injuries have a low likelihood of further nerve damage. Unstable spine injuries are high risk.
- Improper patient movement or handling can lead to further neurologic damage. It is impossible to distinguish stable from unstable spinal injuries in the field. Consequently, all patients with suspected spinal trauma are handled as though there is an unstable injury.
- Major causes of maxillofacial trauma are motor vehicle crashes, home accidents, athletic injuries, animal bites, intentional violent acts, and industrial injuries.

- With the exception of compromised airway and the potential for significant bleeding, damage to the tissues of the maxillofacial area is seldom life threatening. Blunt trauma injuries may be classified as fractures to the mandible, midface, zygoma, orbit, and nose.
- Injury to the ears, eyes, or teeth may be minor or may result in permanent sensory functional loss and disfigurement. Trauma to the ear may include lacerations and contusions, thermal injuries, chemical injuries, traumatic perforation, and barotitis.
- Injuries to the skull may include soft tissue injuries to the scalp and skull fractures.
- Out-of-hospital management of the patient with head injuries is determined by a number of factors including the mechanism and severity of injury, the patient's level of consciousness, and associated injuries that affect the priorities of care.

REFERENCES

1. National Association of Emergency Medical Technicians: *PHTLS: basic and advanced prehospital trauma life support,* ed 4, St Louis, 1999, Mosby.
2. Sanders, M: *Mosby's paramedic textbook,* ed 2, St Louis, 2000, Mosby.
3. US Department of Transportation National Highway Traffic Safety Administration: *EMT–Intermediate national standard curriculum,* Washington, DC, 1998, The Department.

20

Abdominal Trauma

Key Terms

Evisceration

Hematuria

Hemoperitoneum

Kerr's Sign

Peristalsis

Peritonitis

Retroperitoneal Space

Supine Hypotension Syndrome

...CASE HISTORY

A call comes in for a boy beat up at a local repair garage in town. Upon arrival at the scene, EMT–Is Casciola and George find a 17-year-old patient lying on his side on the sidewalk in front of the garage. He tells the EMT–Is that he was struck in the abdomen with a large wrench during a fight. Upon assessment, he is awake and appropriate; has a respiratory rate of 20; a weak, thready pulse at a rate of 126; a blood pressure of 90/78; and cool, pale, diaphoretic skin. Auscultation of the chest reveals clear bilateral lung sounds. Bruising and rigidity of the upper right abdominal quadrant is evident. No other injuries are found.

Upon further questioning, the boy states that he was "roughed up pretty good" during the fight. EMT–I Casciola immediately stabilizes the cervical spine while EMT–I George places a rigid cervical collar around the boy's neck. After getting the long backboard, EMT–I George quickly examines the back and finds no injuries. He then places the backboard behind the patient's back, and he logrolls the patient onto the board with the help of two bystanders.

EMT–I George applies a nonrebreather face mask with a reservoir on the patient, and turns up the flow to 15 liters/minute. Suspecting a possible internal injury, EMT–I Casciola suggests transporting the boy to the trauma center and starting the IV line en route.

The boy is quickly immobilized, placed on the cot, and moved to the ambulance. Another set of vitals reveals a respiratory rate of 22, a weak pulse of 132, and a blood pressure of 86/72. Pulse oximeter shows a pulse rate of 130 with a saturation of 98%. The neurological status is unchanged. Skin remains pale, cool, and diaphoretic.

EMT–I Casciola remains in the back compartment with the patient and contacts the medical control physician en route. She provides an update and gives an estimated time of arrival. She also inserts a large bore IV catheter into the patient's left antecubital vein and begins infusing lactated Ringers solution. Vital signs are monitored and remain unchanged.

LEARNING OBJECTIVES ✓

CHAPTER GOAL

Upon completion of this chapter, the EMT-Intermediate will be able to integrate pathophysiological principles and the assessment findings to formulate a field impression and implement a treatment plan for the patient with abdominal trauma.

INTRODUCTION

The abdomen is a region of the body where it is most difficult to correctly identify traumatic injuries that require surgical repair. When unrecognized, abdominal injury is one of the major causes of death in the trauma patient. It is also the second leading cause of preventable trauma deaths.[1] The EMT–Intermediate (EMT–I) must have a high degree of suspicion based on the mechanism of injury because death usually results from continuing hemorrhage and/or delay of surgical repair.

PATHOPHYSIOLOGY/MECHANISM OF INJURY

Injuries to this area of the body are caused by blunt or penetrating mechanisms (see Chapter 14). Penetrating trauma is usually obvious, and blunt trauma can be particularly challenging to the EMT–I. It is important to assess the mechanism of injury and suspect abdominal trauma when there is unexplained shock.

Loss of blood into the abdominal cavity, regardless of its source, will contribute to or be the primary cause of the development of shock. The release of acids, enzymes, or bacteria from the gastrointestinal tract into the peritoneal cavity will result in additional organ damage and **peritonitis** (inflammation of the peritoneum).

Blunt Trauma

Blunt abdominal trauma is usually the result of compression or shear injuries. During compression mechanisms, organs of the abdomen are crushed between solid objects. Shear incidents create rupture of the solid organs or rupture of blood vessels in the cavity because of the tearing forces exerted against their stabilizing ligaments and vessels.

The degree of injury caused by blunt forces is related to the quantity and duration of force applied, as well as the type of abdominal structure injured (i.e., fluid filled, gas filled, solid, or hollow). The aorta, liver, and spleen bleed easily, so blood loss can occur at a rapid rate. Pelvic fractures may be associated with bladder or urethral injuries and are usually associated with a loss of large volumes of blood. See Chapter 4 for a review of the abdominal cavity and organs.

The automobile is the major cause of blunt abdominal trauma. Automobile-to-automobile and automobile-pedestrian accidents have been cited as causes in 50% to 75% of cases, blows to the abdomen in about 15% of cases, and falls in 6% to 9% of cases. Other causes include injuries from the use of personal restraints, assaults, and blast injuries[2] (Figure 20-1).

Penetrating Trauma

Penetrating trauma is more visible that blunt trauma and can be caused by stab wounds, gunshot wounds, or impaled objects. Multiple organ damage can occur although it is less likely with a stab wound than with a gunshot wound. The trajectory of a missile such as a bullet or the path of a knife blade can frequently be visualized and can help identify possible injured organs. As a rule, injuries from penetrating trauma do not have as high a mortality rate as those that result from blunt trauma.[3]

Penetrating injury to the thorax may also cause abdominal injury. In addition, penetrating wounds of the flanks and buttocks may involve organs in the abdominal cavity. These penetrating injuries may cause bleeding from a major vessel or solid organ and perforation of a segment of the intestine—the most frequently injured organ in penetrating trauma.[2]

SPECIFIC ABDOMINAL INJURIES

Abdominal injury may be classified as solid organ, hollow organ, retroperitoneal organ, pelvic organ, or vascular injury (Figure 20-2). Specific patterns are discussed in this chapter.

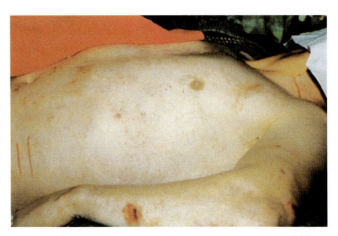

FIGURE 20-1 ▲ Marks of impact sustained by the front-seat passenger in a car crash. The victim suffered rupture of the diaphragm and spleen. (From Sanders MJ: *Mosby's paramedic textbook,* ed 2, St Louis, 2000, Mosby.)

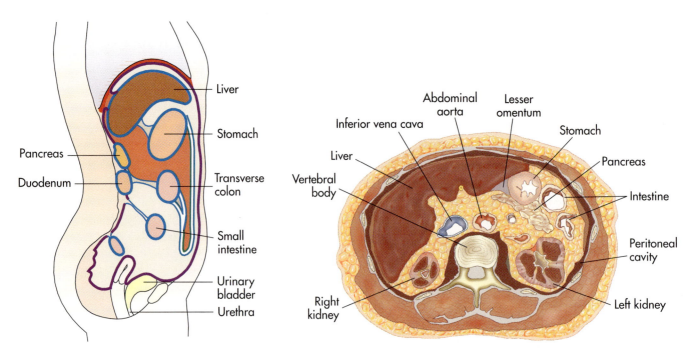

FIGURE 20-2 ▲ Hollow, solid, retroperitoneal, and pelvic organs. (From Sanders MJ: *Mosby's paramedic textbook,* ed 2, St Louis, 2000, Mosby.)

Solid Organ Injury

Injury to solid organs usually results in rapid and significant blood loss. The two solid organs commonly injured are the liver and spleen. Both of these are primary sources of exsanguinations. Injury to the liver should be suspected in any patient with a steering wheel injury, lap belt injury, or history of epigastric trauma. After injury, blood and bile escape into the peritoneal cavity, producing signs and symptoms of shock and peritoneal irritation.

Injury to the spleen is commonly associated with other intraabdominal injuries. It should be suspected in motor vehicle crashes and in falls or sport injuries in which there was an impact to the lower left chest, flank, or upper left abdomen. Although about 40% of patients with splenic injuries have no symptoms, the patient may complain of pain in the left shoulder (**Kehr's sign**), thought to be caused by referred pain secondary to irritation of the adjacent diaphragm from splenic hematoma or **hemoperitoneum** (blood in the peritoneum).

Hollow Organ Injury

Injuries to the hollow abdominal organs may result in sepsis, wound infection, and abscess formation, particularly if trauma to the intestine remains undiagnosed for an extended period. In contrast to solid organ injury, in which hemorrhage is the major cause of symptoms, injury to the hollow organs results in symptoms from spillage of their contents, resulting in peritonitis (Box 20-1).

The stomach is usually protected during blunt mechanisms because of its location in the abdomen. Gastric transection or laceration can, however, occur with penetrating trauma. Leakage of acidic gastric contents will quickly cause signs of peritonitis. The stomach is damaged in about 1% of blunt abdominal trauma and in about 19% of cases of penetrating trauma.[4]

The colon is injured in about 6% of cases of blunt trauma and 16% of cases of penetrating trauma. The small intestine sustains injury in about 7% of blunt trauma cases and 25% of penetrating trauma.[4] The large and small bowel may be injured by compression forces in high-speed motor vehicle crashes and in deceleration injuries associated with wearing personal restraints. Because of the amount of force required to injure the colon and small intestine, other injuries are usually present. Peritoneal contamination with bacteria is a common problem.

Retroperitoneal Organ Injury

The **retroperitoneal space** (potential space behind the "true" abdominal cavity) can sustain injury from blunt or penetrating trauma to the anterior abdomen, posterior abdomen (particularly the flank area), or thoracic spine. Hemorrhage within the retroperitoneal space may be massive and usually results from pelvic and/or lumbar fractures.

Retroperitoneal structures are damaged in about 9% of cases of blunt abdominal injuries and in about 11% of cases of penetrating trauma.[4] Injuries to the kidneys involve contusion fractures and lacerations, resulting in hemorrhage, urine extravasation, or both. Ureters are usually injured from penetrating abdominal or flank wounds. Pancreas injuries are rare, yet they can be caused by compressive or penetrating forces to the upper left quadrant, as in steering wheel and bicycle handlebar impalement.

When great force from blunt trauma or penetrating injury occurs, the duodenum may be crushed or lacerated. Injury to this organ usually is associated with concurrent pancreatic trauma, which can only be confirmed during surgery.

Pelvic Organ Injury

Injury to pelvic organs usually results from motor vehicle crashes that produce pelvic fractures. Other, less frequent causes of pelvic organ injury are penetrating trauma, straddle-type injuries from falls, pedestrian accidents, and some sexual acts. Because the pelvis provides support and protection for multiple organ systems, there is great potential for associated injury. The most common associated injuries are those to the urinary bladder and urethra.

Pelvic fractures often are associated with severe retroperitoneal hemorrhage. In addition, they carry a mortality rate that ranges from 6.4% to 19%.[4]

Injury to the bladder is more likely if the bladder is distended at the time of injury. With rupture, the in-

---

BOX 20-1

PERITONEAL IRRITATION

Peritonitis usually is acute and quite painful and may be delayed for hours or days after a hollow-organ injury. It results from the spillage of enzymes, acids, and bacteria into the abdominal cavity that produces a chemical irritation to the peritoneum, the membrane that lines the wall of the abdomen and covers the abdominal organs. (Blood is not a chemical irritant to the abdomen.) The pain of peritonitis usually is localized (via somatic nerve fibers) but also may be diffuse. Signs and symptoms of peritonitis include the following:
1. Pain
2. Tenderness on percussion or palpation
3. Guarding, rigidity
4. Fever (if untreated)
5. Distention (a late finding)

NOTE: The adult abdomen can accommodate 1.5 L of fluid with no abdominal distention.

tegrity of the peritoneum may be broken, and urine may leak into the peritoneal cavity. Gross **hematuria** (blood in the urine) may be present, or the patient may complain that he or she is unable to void.

Urethral disruption occurs more often in men and is usually secondary to blunt trauma associated with pelvic fracture. Placement of an indwelling urinary catheter is contraindicated in these patients.

Vascular Structure Injury

Intraabdominal arterial and venous injuries may be life threatening because of their potential for massive hemorrhage. These injuries usually occur from penetrating trauma but may also occur from compression or deceleration forces applied to the abdomen. As in solid organ injury, vascular injury usually presents as hypovolemia and occasionally is associated with a palpable abdominal mass.

The major vessels most frequently injured are the aorta; the inferior vena cava; and the renal, mesenteric, and iliac arteries and veins. Vascular structure injury carries a high mortality rate if it is not surgically repaired soon after the traumatic event.

ASSESSMENT

The index of suspicion for injury should be based on the mechanism of injury and on outward signs such as ecchymosis or marks of collision. Consider the following indicators for establishing the index of suspicion for abdominal injury:

- Mechanism of injury or damage to the passenger compartment of a motor vehicle (e.g., bent steering wheel)
- Outward signs of trauma
- Shock with unexplained cause
- Level of shock greater than explained by other injuries
- Presence of abdominal rigidity, guarding, or distention (a rare finding)

Expose the abdomen and look for distention, contusions, abrasion, penetration, evisceration, impaled object(s), and/or obvious bleeding. Palpating the abdomen can reveal abdominal wall defects or elicit pain in the area palpated. Voluntary or involuntary guarding, rigidity, and/or rebound tenderness may be indicative of bruising, inflammation, or hemorrhage. Avoid deep palpation of an obviously injured abdomen so that existing hemorrhage or other injuries are not worsened.

Auscultation of bowel sounds will not change the out-of-hospital management of this patient and is not considered a valuable assessment tool in the field. Do not waste time trying to determine their presence or absence.

Assess pelvic instability by gently applying pressure to the pelvic girdle. Any instability is associated with pelvic fractures that are usually accompanied by significant hemorrhage. DO NOT rock the pelvis as this action may cause further injury or an increase in bleeding.

Intraabdominal bleeding should be suspected when the following signs and symptoms are present:
- External bruising
- Pain
- Abdominal tenderness
- Abdominal rigidity or distention

Remember that many patients with substantial intraabdominal hemorrhage do not demonstrate these signs and symptoms. The most reliable indicator of intraabdominal bleeding is the presence of shock from an unexplained source.

Response to physical examination of the abdomen in the conscious patient may or may not be reliable. Pelvic or rib fractures produce pain not necessarily association with intraabdominal injury, whereas alcohol, drugs, or spinal fracture may mask such symptoms. Fresh blood in the abdomen is not an irritant to the peritoneum and in most cases will not cause any signs of peritonitis. The adult abdominal cavity can hold up to 1.5 L of fluid before showing any signs of distention.

Evisceration

An **evisceration** is the protrusion of an internal organ or peritoneal contents through a wound or surgical incision, particularly in the abdominal wall. The presence of an evisceration from abdominal trauma usually is associated with major intraperitoneal injury.

TRAUMA IN PREGNANCY

Pregnancy causes anatomical and physiological changes to the body's system, and these changes affect

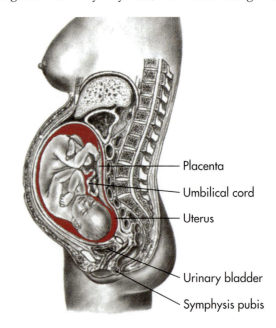

Placenta

Umbilical cord

Uterus

Urinary bladder

Symphysis pubis

FIGURE 20-3 ▲ In a pregnant patient, as the uterus and fetus enlarge above the symphysis pubis, the fetus becomes more susceptible to both blunt and penetrating trauma. (From Wong DL, Perry SE: *Maternal child care nursing,* St Louis, 1998, Mosby.)

the potential patterns of injuries. Two or more patients are involved, and the EMT–I must be alert to what occurs during pregnancy. The protruding uterus, high blood flow, and its contents are more susceptible to injury including rupture, penetration, abruption of the placenta, and premature rupture of membranes. The abdominal organs remain essentially unchanged with the exception of the uterus (Figure 20-3).

When assessing the pregnant patient, keep in mind the changes to the respiratory, cardiovascular, and gastrointestinal systems. Table 20-1 reviews these changes.

Management

Stabilize the patient and prepare for rapid transport to an appropriate medical facility that can provide surgical intervention. This patient needs definitive care that cannot be provided in the out-of-hospital setting.

Airway, Oxygen, and Ventilation

Maintain a patent airway, and administer high-concentration oxygen. Consider bag-valve-mask ventilation or endotracheal intubation if necessary to control the airway and maximize oxygenation.

Circulation

Control obvious bleeding or hemorrhage with direct pressure. Depending on local protocols, consider using the pneumatic anti-shock garment (PASG). Fluid replacement should be started en route to the hospital. Do not waste precious time at the scene trying to start an intravenous (IV) line.

OTHER PROCEDURES

If spinal injury is suspected, immobilize the patient on a long backboard. Again, do not waste time or delay transport due to this procedure.

Rapidly package the patient and begin transport as quickly as possible. Choose the receiving hospital based on its ability to provide rapid surgical management.

During transport, perform a comprehensive physical examination and ongoing assessment to include a focused history, vital sign assessment and reassess-

---

TABLE 20-1

Changes During Pregnancy[1]

SYSTEM	CHANGES	GENERAL CONSIDERATIONS
Respiratory	Rate not altered by pregnancy During the third trimester, diaphragm is elevated; may cause mild dyspnea, especially when the patient is supine	During third trimester, dyspnea may be caused by the position of the mother Maintain spinal precautions and consider elevation of the head of the long backboard once immobilization is complete
Cardiovascular	Heart rate (HR) increases throughout pregnancy HR rises 15 to 20 beats per minute above normal by the third trimester Blood pressure drops 5 to 15 mm Hg during the second trimester but is usually normal at term **Supine hypotension syndrome** occurs when mother is on her back; large uterus compresses the inferior vena cava, restricting blood return to the heart Cardiac output increases by 1 to 1.5 L/min after the tenth week of pregnancy; 48% increase in blood volume by term	Interpretation of tachycardia may be more difficult Slight hypotension in the second trimester may be normal Hypotension in the later stages of pregnancy may be caused by the mother lying on her back; usually relieved by placing the mother on her left side (left lateral decubitus position) Because of increased cardiac output, 30% to 35% of blood volume can be lost before signs and symptoms of hypovolemia become apparent
Gastrointestinal	**Peristalsis** (propulsive, muscular movements of the intestines) slow so food may remain in stomach many hours after eating	Vomiting and subsequent aspiration may occur

From National Association of Emergency Medical Technicians: *PHTLS: basic and advanced prehospital trauma life support,* ed 4, St Louis, 1999, Mosby.

ment. Inspect and palpate the abdomen, and estimate any increase in the abdominal girth. Listening to bowel sounds may be difficult in a moving vehicle and will not change the care given in the out-of-hospital setting.

Impaled Objects

Do not move or remove an impaled object as severe bleeding and further abdominal trauma may be caused. In addition, the distal end of the object may actually be controlling internal bleeding. Generally, the object needs to be identified by radiographic evaluation at the hospital where blood replacement and a surgical team are available.

Support the impaled object and immobilize it manually or mechanically to prevent further movement. Apply direct pressure around the object if bleeding occurs.

Do not palpate the abdomen, since this action may cause additional tearing or intrusion by the distal end of the object. The PASG is also contraindicated in a patient with an impaled object.

Do not attempt to replace the eviscerated contents into the peritoneal cavity as this action would increase the risk of infection and complicate surgical evaluation of the injury. Instead, leave the viscera on the abdomen or protruding as found. Cover them with a moist, sterile gauze or trauma dressing to prevent further contamination and drying. Use regular normal saline IV fluid, and remoisten the dressings periodically to prevent them from drying out.

Trauma in Pregnancy

In this instance, priority should be given to treating the mother. Signs and symptoms of shock may be present, and the patient should be transported as quickly as possible in an effort to save the mother and the fetus. High-concentration oxygen should be applied immediately. Some systems will authorize inflation of the legs of the PASG with proper medical direction.

Once the pregnant patient has been immobilized to the long backboard, the board should be tilted to the left approximately 10 to 15 degrees. This positioning will take pressure off the inferior vena cava and assist with blood return to the heart (Figure 20-4).

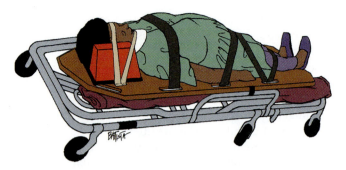

FIGURE 20-4 ▲ Once a pregnant patient is fully immobilized, tilt the backboard approximately 10 to 15 degrees to the left. (Kimberly Battista from Stoy W: *Mosby's EMT-Basic textbook,* St Louis, 1996, Mosby.)

PRIMARY INJURY PREVENTION

Like most other types of trauma, many abdominal injuries can be prevented. The EMT–I should participate in community efforts that promote safety such as those that emphasize the need for using personal restraints when in motor vehicles. Working with law enforcement officials to promote gun safety is another opportunity to prevent injuries.

CASE HISTORY FOLLOW-UP ■ ■ ■

At the trauma center, EMT–I Casciola gives report to the trauma team. They thank her for getting the boy to the hospital so quickly.

As the EMT–Is are restocking the ambulance, the boy's father arrives. They understand the importance of family-centered care and spend a few minutes giving the father a brief report about what was done at the scene.

The next day EMT–Is Casciola and George are delivering another patient to the trauma center and find out what happened to this boy. He had a Grade II liver laceration that was repaired in the operating room and is resting in the Trauma Intensive Care Unit in stable condition. They were told the boy would have bled to death if he had not been so efficiently managed at the scene. The EMT–Is pat each other on the back for a job well done.

SUMMARY

- Blunt trauma to abdominal organs usually results from compression or shearing forces.
- Penetrating injury may result from stab wounds, gunshot wounds, or impaled objects.
- The two solid organs most commonly injured are the liver and spleen. Both are primary sources of exsanguinations. Injuries to the hollow abdominal organs may result in sepsis, wound infection, and abscess formation.
- Injury to the kidneys, ureters, pancreas, and duodenum (retroperitoneal organs) may cause massive hemorrhage.
- Injury to the pelvic organs (bladder and urethra) usually results from motor vehicle crashes that produce pelvic fractures.
- Abdominal vascular structure injuries may be life threatening because of their potential for massive hemorrhage.
- The most significant indicator of severe abdominal trauma is the presence of unexplained shock.
- Emergency care of patients with abdominal trauma involves stabilizing the patient and rapid transport to an appropriate medical facility for surgical intervention.

REFERENCES

1. National Association of Emergency Medical Technicians: *PHTLS: basic and advanced prehospital trauma life support*, ed 4, St Louis, 1999, Mosby.
2. Sanders MJ: *Mosby's paramedic textbook*, ed 2, St Louis, 2000, Mosby.
3. US Department of Transportation National Highway Traffic Safety Administration: *EMT–Intermediate national standard curriculum*, Washington, DC, 1998, The Department.
4. Rosen P, et al: *Emergency medicine: concepts and clinical practice*, ed 4, St Louis, 1998, Mosby.

21

Extremity Trauma

Key Terms

Closed Injury
or Fracture

Compartment
Syndrome

Dislocations

Formable Splint

Fractures

Open Injury or Fracture

Position of Function

Rigid Splint

Traction Splint

...CASE HISTORY

EMT–Is Criss and Miller are called to the scene of a park for a man injured. When they arrive on the scene, several young men are sitting in the middle of a baseball field. One of the bystanders explains that everyone was playing a game of softball at the company picnic. The man who was pitching was hit with a line drive to his left thigh. The man's wife is holding a bag of ice over his thigh.

EMT–I Criss assesses the patient while EMT–I Miller speaks with the patient's wife. On initial examination, a large deformity is noted in the left thigh area. The skin is red and cold, presumably from the ice pack. After removing his shoe, EMT–I Criss notices that he does not have a left pedal pulse. Nail beds are pale on his left foot, capillary refill is delayed, and the man can barely feel his toes. The left popliteal pulse is weakly palpable.

LEARNING OBJECTIVES

CHAPTER GOAL

Upon completion of this chapter, the EMT-Intermediate will be able to integrate pathophysiological principles and the assessment findings to formulate a field impression and implement a treatment plan for the patient with extremity trauma.

Cognitive Objectives

As an EMT-Intermediate you should be able to do the following:

- Identify one difference between open and closed bone injuries.
- List three signs or symptoms of a bone or joint injury and internal/external bleeding.
- Describe the treatment of closed fractures, open fractures, internal and external arterial bleeding, circulation compromise, pelvic fractures, and compartment syndrome.
- Identify three complications of extremity trauma.
- List one example of a rigid splint, a formable splint, and a traction splint.
- Describe the process of immobilizing a suspected upper extremity fracture, lower extremity fracture, and pelvic fracture.
- List three complications of splinting.

Affective Objectives

As an EMT-Intermediate you should be able to do the following:

- Advocate the use of thorough assessment to determine a differential impression and treatment plan for extremity trauma.

- Advocate the use of a thorough scene survey to determine the forces involved in extremity trauma.
- Value the implications of spending too much time on extremity injuries when head, thoracic, or abdominal injuries may be present.

Psychomotor Objectives
As an EMT–Intermediate you should be able to do the following:
- Demonstrate a clinical assessment for a patient with suspected extremity trauma.
- Demonstrate the following techniques for extremity immobilization:
  - Application of a rigid splint.
  - Application of a formable splint.
  - Application of a traction splint.

INTRODUCTION

Extremity trauma involves injury to muscles and bones and can occur by a variety of mechanisms. Violence, sports, and other recreational activities, as well as daily routines, can cause damage to muscles, bones, and the related tissues.

The EMT–Intermediate (EMT–I) will often see patients with these types of injuries. They are seldom life threatening unless circumstances such as uncontrolled bleeding are present. A fractured femur is one such injury that may produce severe internal bleeding. Fractures may be "limb threatening" if significant nerve damage is present or circulation is compromised to the injured extremity.

PATHOPHYSIOLOGY

Extremity or musculoskeletal trauma can be a single injury or can occur with other injuries.

Fractures and Dislocations

Fractures occur when there is any break in the continuity of bone or cartilage.

There are two types of bone injuries or fractures. An **open injury or fracture** occurs when there is a break in the bone and a disruption of the skin. The skin may be perforated by the ends of the broken bone. The skin may also be cut by a crushing mechanism or a laceration at the time of the injury (Figure 21-1).

A **closed injury or fracture** is present when there is a break in the bone but no disruption of the skin. There may be swelling of the skin or a deformity in an extremity (Figure 21-2).

A **dislocation** occurs when there is a separation of two bones at the joint (Figure 21-3). The dislocation may cause an area of instability that may produce a large amount of pain. It may be difficult to distinguish between a fracture and a dislocation.

The following complications can occur from extremity trauma:
- Excessive bleeding due to tissue damage caused by bone ends
- Restriction of blood flow as a result of bone ends compressing blood vessels
- Damage to muscles, nerves, or blood vessels caused by broken bones
- Conversion of a closed fracture to an open fracture
- Increased pain associated with movement of bone ends
- Paralysis of extremities due to damage to the spine
- Compartment syndrome

Arterial hemorrhage is the most serious complication and can be difficult to confirm when it occurs internally only. Internal or external hemorrhage can be life-threatening events. The following two types of closed fractures can cause major hemorrhage:
- *Closed femur fracture*—Blood loss of approximately 500 mL per fracture may accumulate in the thigh with a potential total loss of up to 2000 mL. The femur is the

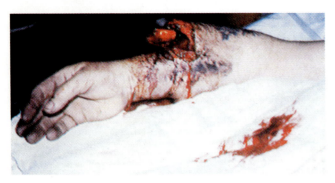

FIGURE 21-1 ▲ Open fracture. (National Association of Emergency Medical Technicians: *PHTLS: basic and advanced prehospital trauma life support,* ed 4, St Louis, 1999, Mosby.)

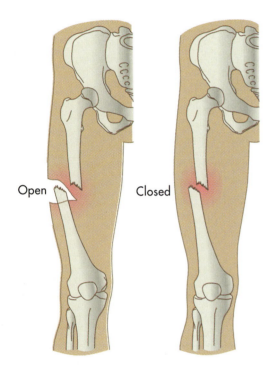

Open Closed

FIGURE 21-2 ▲ Open versus closed fracture. (National Association of Emergency Medical Technicians: *PHTLS: basic and advanced prehospital trauma life support,* ed 4, St Louis, 1999, Mosby.)

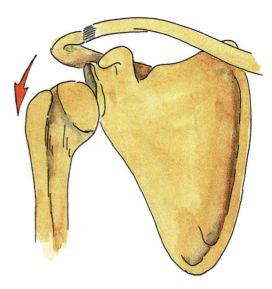

FIGURE 21-3 ▲ A dislocation is a separation of two bones at the joint. (National Association of Emergency Medical Technicians: *PHTLS: basic and advanced prehospital trauma life support,* ed 4, St Louis, 1999, Mosby.)

Compartment syndrome is ischemia and compromised circulation that occur from a vascular injury. The structures in an enclosed space, such as the forearm, are deprived of oxygen due to the compression that occurs from bleeding into that space. The hematoma or any other space-occupying mass reduces the amount of space that can be used by other structures. The pressure causes the cells to become anoxic, swell, and exert more pressure on surrounding structures. When a blood vessel is involved, the vessels collapse, blood flow is decreased, more cells are deprived of oxygen, and the cycle continues. The peripheral nerves are usually the first to feel the effects of this ischemic cycle. If not recognized and treated, the limb will be compromised and lead to a limb-threatening situation. In addition, distal tissue will be affected by the ischemia.

ASSESSMENT

Signs and symptoms of a bone or joint injury include the following:

- Deformity or abnormal position of an extremity
- Pain and tenderness
- Grating
- Swelling
- Bruising or discoloration
- Guarding
- Exposed bone ends
- Joint locked into position

When bleeding has occurred, it is critical to estimate the blood loss. All clothes should be removed from that extremity so that an adequate assessment can be con-

largest bone in the body, and fractures of the femur can result in life-threatening bleeding. In addition, the muscles in the thigh are strong and may cause the fractured bone ends to override, which creates a "third space" into which bleeding can occur leading to hemorrhage. The bleeding and pain from the overriding bones can contribute to hypovolemic shock.

- *Pelvic fracture*—Large blood loss can occur due to the large blood supply in the pelvis and possible disruption of vascular plexes that are located adjacent to the pelvis.

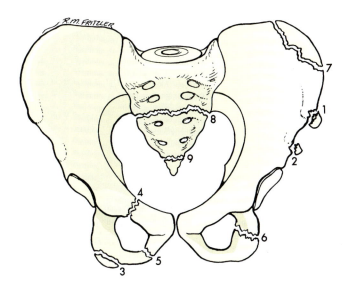

FIGURE 21-4 ▲ **Fractures of individual pelvic bones.** *(1)* Avulsion of anterosuperior iliac spine, *(2)* avulsion of anterioinferior iliac spine, *(3)* avulsion of ischial tuberosity, *(4)* fracture of superior pubic ramus, *(5)* fracture of inferior pubic ramus, *(6)* fracture of ischial ramus, *(7)* fracture of iliac wing, *(8)* transverse fracture of sacrum, *(9)* fracture of coccyx. (National Association of Emergency Medical Technicians: *PHTLS: basic and advanced prehospital trauma life support,* ed 4, St Louis, 1999, Mosby.)

ducted. Factors that can complicate this estimation include the following:

1. External bleeding
   • The patient may have been moved from the original site of the incident so that the EMT–I cannot see the amount of blood previously lost.
   • The patient may be wearing dark clothing or waterproof material that will conceal the actual blood loss.
   • The blood loss may have been washed away by rain or other water at the scene or concealed in the surface upon which the patient is lying.
2. Internal bleeding
   • Bleeding inside an extremity is difficult to assess.
   • Any continued swelling of an extremity should be considered as an increasing hematoma due to hemorrhage from arterial bleeding until proven otherwise.

A great deal of blood can hemorrhage into the large pelvic cavity space without many external signs of a problem (Figure 21-4). This bleeding is a major complication of pelvic fractures. Often times, the first symptom is the onset of shock.

When assessing for a pelvic fracture, *do not rock the pelvis!* This type of motion may aggravate existing fractures, cause additional fractures if the pelvis is already unsteady, and, most importantly, may cause additional bleeding due to rupture of blood vessels or disruption of an existing hematoma. Apply gentle pressure inward

from both sides of the pelvis. If there are any fractures, pain will most likely be elicited.

Signs and symptoms of compartment syndrome include the following:
• Pain greater than expected from the original injury
• Pain increases when the involved muscles are stretched
• Decreased sensation distal to the injury
• Tense swelling of the injured area
• Paresthesias of the web space between the thumb and first finger or first and second toes
• Weakness or paralysis of involved muscles (late sign)
• No distal pulse (late sign)

When a patient presents with any of the previous chief complaints, a thorough examination should still be completed. However, the EMT–I should rule out any life-threatening or limb-threatening injuries first.

TREATMENT

The goals of treating patients with extremity trauma are as follows:
• Control bleeding
• Treat for shock if indicated
• Prevent further injury
• Minimize permanent damage
• Reduce pain

After protecting against any body substances, the EMT–I should focus initial treatment on controlling bleeding and treating life-threatening injuries. If no life-threatening injuries are present, any limb-threatening injuries should be treated next. The injured limb should be returned to its anatomic position to restore sensory function unless severe pain or further damage results. Oxygen administration and intravenous (IV) fluid therapy may be indicated, depending on the severity of the patient's condition.

External arterial hemorrhages should be controlled by the following:
• Direct pressure (apply additional dressings if bleeding continues through the original dressing; do not remove the original dressing.)
• Elevation (for patients who are immobilized, raise the long back board)
• Pressure points

For internal hemorrhage, direct pressure to the outside of the body over the injured area is thought to help decrease the bleeding. An air splint can be used on the upper extremities. The pneumatic anti-shock garment (PASG) can be used on lower extremities or suspected pelvic fractures and should only be inflated to control the hemorrhage. Inflation of either an air splint or the PASG does not usually lead to compartment syndrome until after four to six hours.

If no immediate threats are found, the extremity should be splinted and prepared for transport. Application of cold items such as ice or cold packs may provide some assistance in reducing swelling and providing pain relief. Remember to reevaluate motor, sensory, and circulation in the extremity after splinting to assess for changes in distal neurovascular function.

PELVIC FRACTURES

When the pelvic fracture is unstable, it may be difficult to move the patient to the ambulance. Using a scoop stretcher with padding to stabilize the pelvis may be helpful if internal hemorrhage is not suspected. The PASG can also be used for initial stabilization even without internal hemorrhage.

COMPARTMENT SYNDROME

Compartment syndrome should be managed in the field as a fracture. If limb-threatening signs and symptoms are present, rapid transport should be initiated. Document the following:

* Position in which the extremity was initially found (if known)
* Neurovascular status upon arrival (pulses, movement, sensation including level of pain, and skin color)
* Neurovascular changes during treatment and transport

CIRCULATION COMPROMISE

Consider the extremity to be in jeopardy if the circulation is impaired or absent. Repositioning may initially restore the distal pulse and does not significantly delay transport. Use caution not to fully extend or fully flex the extremity.

If two attempts are made at repositioning without a return in the distal pulse, quickly immobilize the extremity and begin transport. At that point, the limb-threatening condition warrants rapid transport. Communicate the situation to personnel at the receiving hospital.

SPLINTING

Splinting can be a very useful tool in controlling the injury until further evaluation is possible at a healthcare facility. It is important to prevent motion of any bony fragments, the bone ends, or abnormally positioned joints that may be present. Various options available for splinting a fracture or suspected fracture are listed in Table 21-1.

Open and Closed Fractures

Once bleeding from an open wound has been controlled, apply a sterile pressure dressing to continue to control the bleeding. Immobilize the extremity as discussed below.

With an open fracture, a traction splint may cause the bone ends to retract back into the skin. Communicate this fact to the physicians and nurses at the receiving hospital and include it in any written documentation.

Rigid or air splints can be used for open and closed fractures. Once the air splint is inflated, it should not be

---

TABLE 21-1

Types of Splints and Splinting Material

TYPE	DEFINITION	EXAMPLES
Rigid splint (Figure 21-5)	Requires positioning of body part to fit the splint's shape Cannot be changed in shape	Board splints Wood (includes long back board [LBB]) Plastic Metal Inflatable "air splints"
Formable splints (Figure 21-6)	Accommodates the shape of the injured extremity Can be molded into various shapes and combinations	Vacuum splints Pillows Blankets Cardboard splints Wire ladder splints Foam-covered moldable metal splints
Traction splints (Figures 21-7)	Designed to maintain mechanical in-line traction to help realign fractures Most commonly used to stabilize femur fractures	Hare-traction splint Sager splint

From National Association of Emergency Medical Technicians: *PHTLS: Basic and advanced prehospital trauma life support,* ed 4, St Louis, 1999, Mosby.

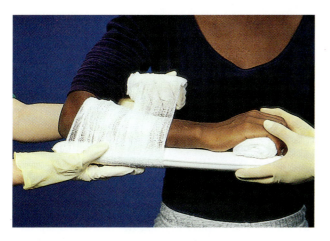

FIGURE 21-5 ▲ Rigid splint. (National Association of Emergency Medical Technicians: *PHTLS: basic and advanced prehospital trauma life support,* ed 4, St Louis, 1999, Mosby.)

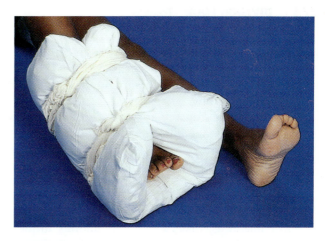

FIGURE 21-6 ▲ Formable splint. (National Association of Emergency Medical Technicians: *PHTLS: basic and advanced prehospital trauma life support,* ed 4, St Louis, 1999, Mosby.)

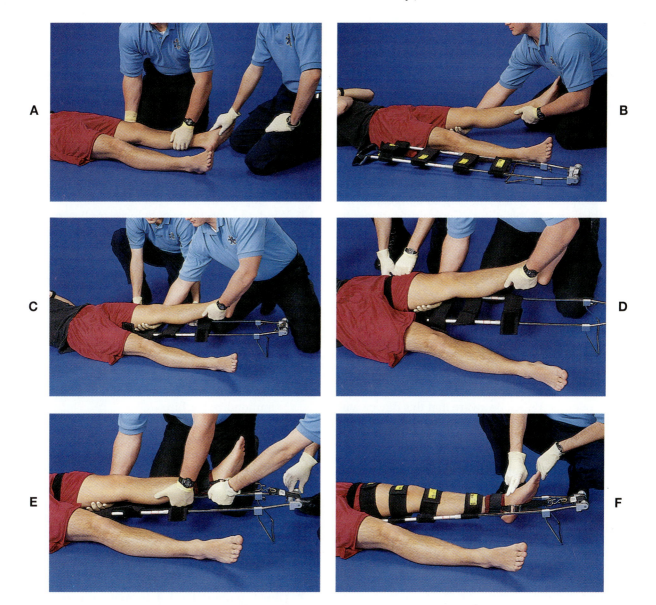

FIGURE 21-7 ▲ Applying a traction splint. **A,** Provide manual stabilization to the injured leg. **B,** Applying manual traction to the injured leg may relieve some of the patient's pain. **C,** Slide the splint under the patient's leg. **D,** Apply ischial strap around the patient. **E,** Attach the distal securing device, and wind the ankle hitch for manual traction. **F,** Secure the support straps, and release manual traction. Reassess motor, sensory, and distal circulation. (**A** to **D,** Vincent Knaus from Stoy W: *Mosby's EMT–Basic textbook,* St Louis, 1996, Mosby.)

deflated for reassessment of the wound by the EMT–I. Rigid splints, therefore, may be easier to use. To limit movement of the injured extremity on the rigid splint, use adequate padding.

Reassess the neurovascular status of the injured extremity after any immobilization procedures. If a pulse is no longer present when it was originally detected, rapid transport is indicated.

Dislocations and Joint Injuries

In most instances, dislocations and injuries to joints should be splinted in the position in which they are found. If distal circulation is compromised, move the joint slightly to attempt to return the blood flow. Warn the patient before moving the extremity, since a great deal of pain may occur with any manipulation of the injured or dislocated joint.

Use whatever splint is available to splint the injury. Improvise if necessary. A formable splint may be appropriate for this situation. Reassess the extremity's neurovascular status after splinting, and communicate the information to personnel at the receiving facility.

FEMUR INJURIES

Using traction for a femur fracture, whether it is manual or with the assistance of a mechanical device, will decrease the patient's pain and help to tamponade internal "third-space" bleeding. Contraindications to traction splinting include the following:

- Fractured pelvis
- Hip injury with gross displacement
- Any significant injury to the knee
- Avulsion or amputation of the ankle and foot

The PASG can be also be used for femur fractures. Apply manual traction before inflating the leg of the injured extremity. Inflate that leg first to full pressure. The remainder of the garment can be inflated per usual procedures and indications. If mechanical traction is still necessary and there is adequate time, the splint can be placed over the PASG. Be aware that this device will create a space between the patient's extremity and the garment leading to the possible formation of an internal capsule with trapped blood, soft tissue damage, and potential collapse of circulation. Reassess the foot frequently to determine ongoing neurovascular status.

Traction Splinting

Two traction splints are most commonly used. The Hare traction splint and Sager splint are detailed in the following section.

HARE TRACTION SPLINT

To apply a Hare traction splint, the EMT–I should do the following:

1. Employ body substance isolation (BSI) precautions. If the patient is wearing pants, cut the trouser leg to expose the injury site and remove the shoe and sock.
2. Direct another EMT–I to manually stabilize the injured leg so that no motion occurs at the site of pain and/or swelling (Figure 21-7, A).
3. Assess motor, sensory, and distal circulation in the injured extremity.
4. Direct the other EMT–I to pull on the distal leg to apply manual traction (Figure 21-7, B). This action may provide some pain relief.
5. Measure the splint against the uninjured leg (typically, the pad is at the ischial tuberosity and the end of the splint extends approximately 8 to 12 inches beyond the foot) and lock it in place.
6. Move the splint into position at the injured leg.
7. Open and adjust the four Velcro support straps (midthigh, above the knee, below the knee, and above the ankle).
8. While the other EMT–I lifts the injured leg, apply the splint by sliding it under the patient's injured limb so that the ischial pad is seated well against the ischial tuberosity (Figure 21-7, C). Gently lower the leg.
9. Apply the proximal ischial strap (Figure 21-7, D).
10. Apply the ankle hitch.
11. With the other EMT–I maintaining gentle manual traction on the patient's injured extremity, connect the S hook of the ratchet mechanism of the splint to the loops of the ankle hitch.
12. Wind the mechanism, which applies mechanical traction (Figure 21-7, E). Without releasing manual traction, continue until the patient's pain is relieved.
13. Secure the splint support straps around the leg and release manual traction once mechanical traction is adequate (Figure 21-7, F).
14. Reevaluate proximal/distal securing devices.
15. Reassess vital signs as well as motor, sensory, and distal circulation.
16. Secure the patient to a long backboard as follows:
    - Logroll the patient onto the board.
    - Secure the patient's torso to a long backboard to immobilize the hip.
    - Secure the splint to the long backboard to prevent movement of the splint.
17. Pay careful attention to the injured leg in the ambulance, because it may extend past the end of the stretcher.

SAGER TRACTION SPLINT

To apply a Sager splint, the EMT–I should do the following:

1. Employ BSI precautions, cut the trouser leg to expose the injury site, and remove the shoe and sock.
2. Direct another EMT–I to manually stabilize the injured leg so that no motion occurs at the fracture site.
3. Assess motor, sensory, and distal circulation in the injured extremity.

4. Place splint medially between the legs.
5. Seat the perineal cushion against the groin and ischial tuberosity.
6. Apply the thigh strap snugly around the thigh of the injured leg.
7. Extend the inner shaft of the splint until the pulley wheel or crossbars are even with the patient's heel.
8. Apply the ankle harness(es) firmly around the ankle(s) above the medial and lateral malleoli.
9. Pull the control tabs on the ankle harness to shorten the ankle sling, pulling it up against the sole of the foot.
10. Pull out the inner shaft of the splint.
11. Extend the splint shaft to achieve the desired traction while observing the amount registered on the traction scale.
12. Check the thigh strap. Retighten to keep a snug fit.
13. Open and secure the three Velcro support straps (midthigh, below the knee, and above the ankle) around both legs.
14. Strap ankles and feet together.
15. Reevaluate proximal/distal securing devices.
16. Reassess motor, sensory, and distal circulation.
17. Secure the patient to a long backboard.

When immobilizing a patient with a suspected femur injury, the EMT–I must first remember that traction must be kept in place at all times once it has been applied. Avoid rotating or extending the foot. The ischial strap or thigh strap must be applied before instituting mechanical traction. The EMT–I should avoid applying supporting straps over the knee or injury site or applying the supporting straps too tightly. He or she also should avoid pulling too hard on the leg when applying mechanical traction. Motor, sensory, and distal circulation should be reassessed after splinting.

Long Bone Fractures

To immobilize various injuries and dislocations of the long bones, the EMT–I should do the following:

LOWER EXTREMITY IMMOBILIZATION

1. Employ BSI precautions, cut the trouser leg to expose the injury site, and remove the shoe and sock.
2. Direct another EMT–I to apply manual stabilization to the injured lower extremity (Figure 21-8, A).
3. Assess motor, sensory, and distal circulation in the injured extremity.
4. Measure the splint(s) to the end of the leg (Figure 21-8, B).
5. Place one padded board splint medially and one laterally (Figure 21-8, C).
6. Pad the voids.
7. Immobilize the joint above and below the injury (Figure 21-8, D).
8. Immobilize the foot in the position of function.

9. Secure the entire injured extremity by placing the patient onto a long backboard.
10. Reassess motor, sensory, and distal circulation in the injured extremity.

The EMT–I should handle the injured extremity carefully and not allow gross movement. Immobilize adjacent joints. Check motor, sensory, and distal circulation before and after splinting. Do not apply the splint too tightly or too loosely.

UPPER EXTREMITY IMMOBILIZATION

To immobilize the upper extremities, the EMT–I should do the following:

1. Employ BSI precautions.
2. Direct another EMT–I to apply manual stabilization to the injured upper extremity (Figure 21-9, A).
3. Assess motor, sensory, and distal circulation in the injured extremity.
4. Move the patient's hand into the position in which one most comfortably holds a baseball. This position is called a **position of function.** To attain this position, dorsiflex the wrist approximately 20 degrees to 30 degrees with all fingers flexed slightly. Place a soft roller bandage into the palm of the patient's hand for immobilization (Figure 21-9, B).
5. Measure the splint and immobilize the joint below the fracture by applying the splint to the palmar side of the hand and wrist. Secure it with a soft roller bandage throughout the length of the splint, making sure areas above and below the fracture are immobilized.
6. Secure the entire injured extremity by applying a sling and swathe (Figure 21-9, C). A pillow may be placed between the arm and chest for patient comfort.
7. Reassess motor, sensory, and distal circulation in the injured extremity.

The EMT–I should handle the injured extremity carefully and not allow gross movement. Immobilize joints above and below the injury. Check motor, sensory, and distal circulation of the injured extremity before and after splinting. Do not apply the splint too tightly or too loosely.

IMMOBILIZATION OF A SHOULDER INJURY

To immobilize a shoulder injury, the EMT–I should do the following:

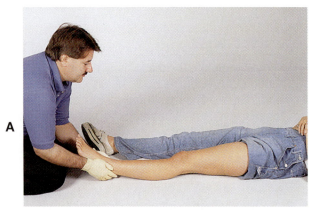
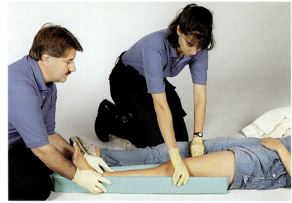
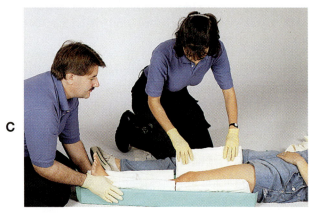
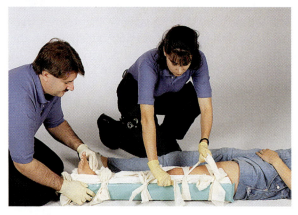

FIGURE 21-8 ▲ Immobilizing a lower extremity. **A,** Apply manual stabilization to the injured lower extremity. **B,** Measure for the appropriate size splint. **C,** Place one splint medially and one laterally for complete stabilization and place padding between any voids. **D,** Immobilize the joint above and below the injury.

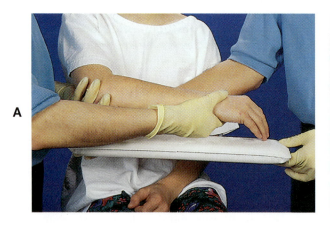
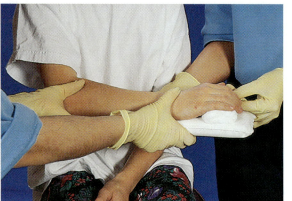
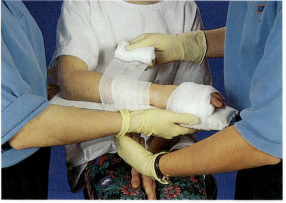

FIGURE 21-9 ▲ Immobilizing an upper extremity. **A,** While performing manual stabilization of the extremity, measure the splint. **B,** Pad any voids to limit movement of the extremity. **C,** Secure the extremity to the board using gauze or cravats. (Vincent Knaus from Stoy W: *Mosby's EMT–Basic textbook,* St Louis, 1996, Mosby.)

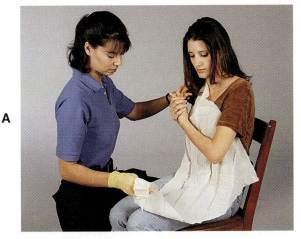
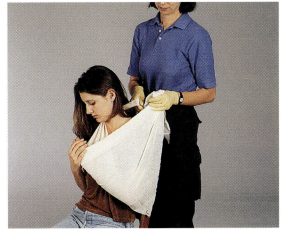
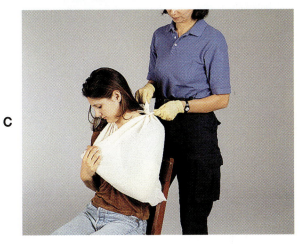
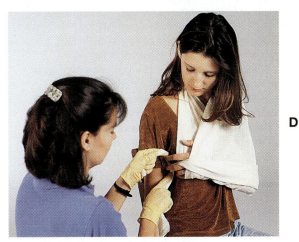

FIGURE 21-10 ▲ Immobilizing a shoulder injury. **A,** Position the sling over the patient's chest. One point should be behind the elbow, one point over the shoulder, and the third point lying across the patient's lap. **B,** Bring the bottom point over the patient's arm over the injured shoulder. **C,** Tie the two ends of the sling together. **D,** Secure the arm in place using a swathe.

1. Employ BSI precautions.
2. Direct another EMT–I to apply manual stabilization to the injured shoulder. If this is not possible, have the patient apply stabilization with the other hand.
3. Assess motor, sensory, and distal circulation of the arm on the same side as the injured shoulder.
4. Select proper splinting materials. A sling, swathe, and pillow are effective for immobilizing an injury in which the patient presents with the upper arm positioned at his or her side while supporting the lower arm at a 90-degree angle across the chest with the uninjured arm.
5. Immobilize site of injury:
   - Position the sling over the top of the patient's chest with one point of the triangle extending behind the elbow on the injured side, one point over the shoulder, and one point lying across the patient's lap (Figure 21-10, *A*).
   - Bring the bottom point of the triangle up over the patient's arm, taking the end up over the top of the patient's injured shoulder (Figure 21-10, *B*).

- Draw up on the ends of the sling so that the patient's hand is approximately 4 inches above the elbow.
- Tie the two ends of the sling together, making sure that the knot does not press against the back of the patient's neck (Figure 21-10, *C*).
- Take hold of the point of material at the patient's elbow and fold it forward, pinning it to the front of the sling. If a pin is not available, twist the excess material and tie a knot in the point.
6. Place a pillow between the patient's arm and chest to make it more comfortable for the patient.
7. Secure the arm in place by tying a swathe around the chest and injured arm over the sling (Figure 21-10, *D*).
8. Reassess motor, sensory, and distal circulation in the immobilized arm.

Immobilize bones above and below the injured joint. Support the joint so that it does not bear distal weight. Assess motor, sensory, and distal circulation before and after splinting. Do not place the swathe over the patient's arm on the uninjured side. Pad the area where the knot is tied (against the back of the patient's neck) with bulky dressings if undue pressure is being applied. Leave the patient's fingertips exposed to detect any color or skin temperature changes that indicate a lack of circulation.

It is important to be careful when splinting an extremity. If the splint is too tight, complications can occur, including compression of nerves, tissues, and blood vessels. Distal circulation can be compromised, or the bone or joint injury can become worse because of improper treatment. Surrounding tissue, nerves, blood vessels, or muscles can be damaged from excessive movement.

If the patient complains of numbness or tingling of the extremity or if the feet or fingers become cool and/or mottled, the splint should be loosened. The EMT–I should reapply the splint and reassess the extremity.

CASE HISTORY FOLLOW-UP ▪▪▪

EMT–I Miller finds out from the patient's wife that the patient is 55 years old and had several beers today at the picnic. He takes some type of antihypertensive for his high blood pressure. No other pertinent past medical history was discovered.

Vital signs are as follows: pulse of 122, respirations of 26, and a blood pressure of 110/68. The patient complains of significant pain in his left leg and feels slightly dizzy. He is unable to wiggle the toes on his left foot.

EMT–I Miller places the patient on 10 liters (L) of oxygen via a nonrebreather face mask while EMT–I Criss prepares the PASG. EMT–I Miller holds traction on the left leg as EMT–I Criss applies the PASG and inflates the left leg compartment.

Once in the ambulance, EMT–I Criss places the patient on the cardiac monitor. The electrocardiogram reveals a sinus tachycardia without any ectopics.

The patient is transported to the emergency department without incident. Repeat vital signs are stable, and there is no worsening of the neurovascular status to his left foot. EMT–I Criss gives report to personnel at the hospital and documents all findings on the trip sheet, which is left at the hospital.

SUMMARY

- Extremity trauma alone is not a life-threatening injury. If the patient has sustained other multisystem injuries, those injuries take priority.
- Attention should focus on first treating life-threatening or limb-threatening injuries including internal and external bleeding.
- Do not be distracted by the appearance of an open fracture when the patient may have other critical injuries.
- Once the EMT–I knows the patient is stable and has an isolated extremity injury, treatment should focus on supporting the extremity and keeping the patient comfortable.
- In the field, all deformities and painful extremities should be treated as fractures until the patient receives a definitive diagnosis at the hospital.

MEDICAL

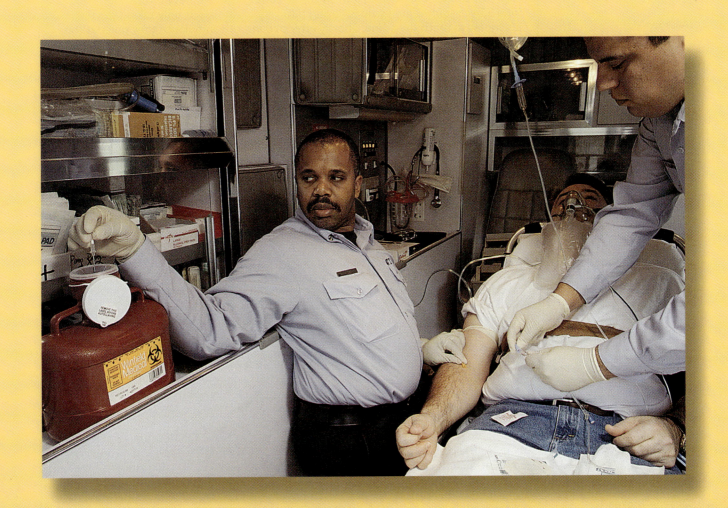

Respiratory Emergencies

...CASE HISTORY

It is a humid Sunday morning and EMT–Is Morgan and Lithe have finished the daily beginning-of-the-shift inspection of their ambulance. The two have been assigned together at the same station for the past 5 years and have developed a good working relationship. Just as they are pouring a fresh cup of coffee, a call comes in from a local church for a 35-year-old woman who is having difficulty breathing. It only takes the crew 3 minutes to reach the scene. Shortly after parking the ambulance they pull out the cot and quickly load their jump kit, oxygen unit, drug box and electrocardiogram (ECG) monitor onto it.

As they enter the church they are directed to the front where their patient is sitting on a pew between two elderly women who are dressed in nurse uniforms. They tell EMT–I Morgan that the patient, Mrs. Claypool, is having "trouble catching her breath." Morgan asks, "Have you ever had this problem before?" She responds by nodding her head. While he is pulling out the oxygen unit and attaching a nonrebreather mask, he asks several key questions to determine the patient's present and past histories. At the same time, EMT–I Lithe takes her blood pressure and applies the pulse oximeter clip to her finger.

The patient is in obvious distress, gasping for air, and is only able to speak incomplete sentences as she attempts to respond to Morgan's questions. She has a blood pressure of 164/100; a regular pulse at a rate of 140 beats per minute; and cool, pale, diaphoretic skin. She is breathing at a rate of 26 breaths per minute, and the pulse oximeter reading is 86%. She has inspiratory wheezes and diminished breath sounds in all her lung fields.

Morgan begins administering 15 liters (L) of oxygen to the patient via nonrebreather mask while Lithe sets up a macrodrip administration set with a 1000-milliliter (mL) bag of normal saline and clears the line of air. Morgan applies a tourniquet above the patient's elbow, cleans the site with povidone-iodine and wipes it with an alcohol wipe. Lithe hands him an 18-gauge catheter-over-needle and he easily cannulates a vein on the dorsal aspect of the patient's hand. Morgan disposes of the needle in a "sharps" container in the jump kit.

"Mrs. Claypool, does it feel like the oxygen is helping?" asks EMT–I Lithe. The patient nods her head to indicate that it is. Morgan has been able to determine the patient has a history of respiratory problems that recur a couple times a year. She uses a pocket inhaler but ran out of medication over the weekend.

"Let's go ahead and set up a nebulizer," Morgan says to Lithe. Lithe is already pouring the medication into the base of the nebulizer mask, and Morgan contacts medical command. After giving a brief report, he is given permission to administer the medication. As the oxygen tubing is attached to the regulator and the flow meter is turned up, the medication mist starts flowing from the mask. Lithe applies the nebulizer mask to the patient's face. "Mrs. Claypool, we need you to take some deep breaths," she tells the patient.

LEARNING OBJECTIVES ✓

CHAPTER GOAL

Upon completion of this chapter, the EMT–Intermediate will be able to use assessment findings to formulate a field impression and carry out a treatment plan for the patient with respiratory emergencies.

Cognitive Objectives

As an EMT–Intermediate you should be able to do the following:

- Identify and describe the function of the structures in the upper and lower airway.
- Discuss the physiology of ventilation and respiration.
- Identify common pathological events that affect the pulmonary system.
- Discuss abnormal assessment findings associated with pulmonary diseases and conditions.
- Compare various airway and ventilation techniques used in the management of pulmonary diseases.
- Review the pharmacological preparations that EMT–Is use for management of respiratory diseases and conditions.
- Review equipment used during the physical examination of patients with respiratory complaints.
- Identify the assessment findings and management for the following respiratory diseases and conditions: (1) bronchial asthma; (2) chronic obstructive pulmonary disease (chronic bronchitis, emphysema); (3) pneumonia; (4) pulmonary edema; (5) spontaneous pneumothorax; (6) hyperventilation syndrome.

Affective Objectives

As an EMT–Intermediate you should be able to do the following:

- Recognize and value the assessment and treatment of patients with respiratory diseases.
- Indicate appreciation for the critical nature of accurate field impressions of patients with respiratory diseases and conditions.

Psychomotor Objectives

As an EMT–Intermediate you should be able to do the following:

- Demonstrate and record pertinent assessment findings associated with pulmonary diseases and conditions.
- Review proper use of airway and ventilation devices.
- Conduct a simulated history and patient assessment, record the findings, and report appropriate management of patients with pulmonary diseases and conditions.

Continued on p. 582

Key Terms—cont'd

Pleuritic Chest Pain	Pulmonary Thromboembolism	Status Asthmaticus	Thromboembolism
Pneumonia	Respiration	Stridor	Thrombophlebitis
Pulmonary Embolus	Spontaneous Pneumothorax	Tachypnea	Tripod Position
Pulmonary Edema		Tension Pneumothorax	Ventilation

INTRODUCTION

Respiratory emergencies are extremely common. They are divided into two categories: acute and chronic. Both chronic and acute respiratory problems can present as life-threatening situations (Figure 22-1). Patients with chronic respiratory problems such as chronic obstructive pulmonary disease (COPD) (see pp. 594-598) usually present with an acute worsening of their chronic condition. In this sense, nearly all persons with respiratory problems who come to the attention of the EMT–Intermediate (EMT–I) will have an acute condition. Many persons, however, are completely healthy before developing the problem. In these situations, it is truly a new and acute respiratory emergency.

ANATOMY AND PHYSIOLOGY

The respiratory system is responsible for filtering, warming, humidifying, and exchanging more than 10,000 liters (L) of air per day in an adult. It is divided into two parts: the upper respiratory system (mouth, nasal cavity, oral cavity, larynx, and vocal cords) and the lower respiratory system (trachea, bronchi, bronchioles, and alveoli) (Figure 22-2). For a detailed review of airway anatomy see Chapter 8.

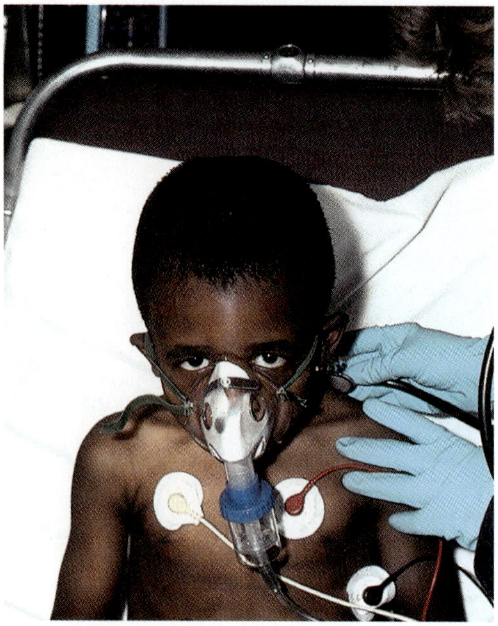

FIGURE 22-1 ▲ Both chronic and acute conditions can lead to life-threatening respiratory distress. (From Sanders MJ: *Mosby's paramedic textbook*, ed 2, St. Louis, 2000, Mosby.)

NOTE: Breathing, or **respiration,** involves inspiring oxygen-containing air and exhaling carbon dioxide. **Ventilation** refers specifically to exchange of carbon dioxide, whereas **oxygenation** refers only to the exchange of oxygen. Both cross the thin capillary membrane at the capillary-alveolar junction; this process is known as **diffusion** (Figure 22-3). In this text, respiration and ventilation will be used interchangeably.

Oxygen diffuses from the alveolar air into capillary blood where it is distributed via the bloodstream for use in cellular metabolism. Carbon dioxide diffuses from the capillary blood into the alveoli and is excreted from the body via the respiratory system. **Perfusion** is the process where oxygenated blood is pumped to the tissues and waste products are returned to the lungs for expulsion (Figure 22-4).

GENERAL RESPIRATORY SYSTEM PATHOPHYSIOLOGY, ASSESSMENT, AND MANAGEMENT

Pathophysiology

A variety of problems can affect the respiratory system's ability to achieve gas exchange. A general understanding of these problems enables the EMT–I quickly and effectively to pinpoint probable causes and perform necessary interventions.

Overall, respiratory abnormalities can affect ventilation, diffusion, or perfusion. Many conditions involve more than one process.

Those primarily affecting ventilation (exchange of oxygen and carbon dioxide) include the following:

- Upper airway obstruction (e.g., trauma, epiglottitis, foreign body obstruction, tonsillitis)
- Lower airway obstruction (e.g., trauma, obstructive lung disease, mucus accumulation, smooth muscle spasm [bronchospasm], airway edema)
- Impairment of chest wall movement (e.g., trauma, hemothorax, pneumothorax, empyema [pus in the pleural space], pleural inflammation, neuromuscu-

lar diseases such as multiple sclerosis or muscular dystrophy)

- Problems in neurological control, involving either the central nervous system (CNS) (e.g., CNS-depressant drugs, stroke, other medical condition, or trauma) or the peripheral nervous system (phrenic or spinal nerve dysfunction due to trauma or neuromuscular diseases)

Diffusion-related (movement of gases across membranes) conditions include the following:

- Inadequate oxygen concentration in the ambient air
- Alveolar pathology (e.g., asbestosis, blebs from COPD, inhalation injuries)
- Interstitial space pathology either due to elevations of hydrostatic pressure (water pressure) in the pulmonary circulation (e.g., pulmonary edema, pulmonary hypertension) or secondary to abnormal permeability of the pulmonary vessels (e.g., adult respiratory distress syndrome [ARDS], environmental lung diseases, near-drowning, hypoxia, inhalation injuries)

Perfusion-related (pumping of blood from the heart to the tissues) factors may also impair gas exchange. These include the following:

- Inadequate blood volume or hemoglobin levels (e.g., hypovolemia, anemia)
- Impaired circulatory blood flow (e.g., pulmonary embolus, cardiac tamponade)
- Chest wall pathology (trauma)

Assessment Findings

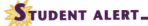

STUDENT ALERT_____

Scene size-up always comes first!

Pulmonary complaints may be associated with a variety of toxin exposures including carbon monoxide, products of combustion, or oxygen-deficient environments (e.g., silos, enclosed storage spaces). Assuring a

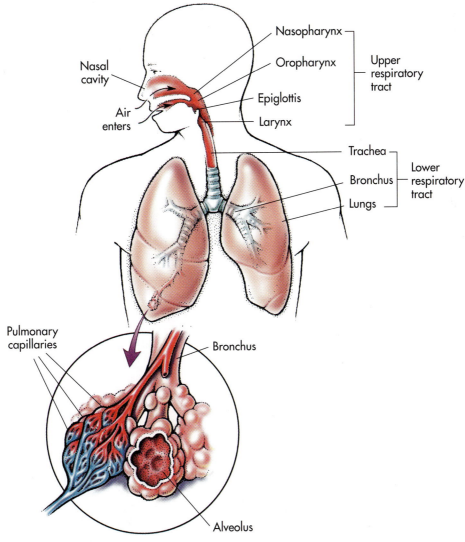

FIGURE 22-2 ▲ The respiratory system. (From Duckwall Productions.)

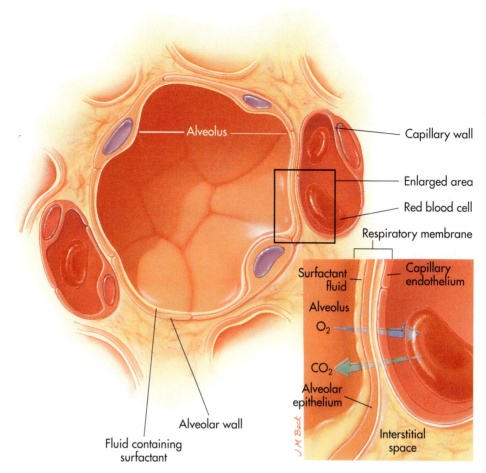

FIGURE 22-3 ▲ The gas exchange structures of the lungs. Insert, a magnified view of the respiratory membrane. (Joan M. Beck from Thibodeau GA, Patton KT: *Anatomy and physiology,* ed 3, St Louis, 1996, Mosby.)

FIGURE 22-4 ▲ Exchange of gases in lung and tissue capillaries. The diagram shows oxygen diffusing out of alveolar air into blood and associating with hemoglobin in lung capillaries to form oxyhemoglobin. In tissue capillaries oxyhemoglobin dissociates, releasing oxygen, which diffuses from the red blood cells and then crosses the capillary wall to reach the tissue cells. At the same time, carbon dioxide diffuses in the opposite direction (into red blood cells) and associates with hemoglobin to form carbaminohemoglobin. As shown in the inset, some carbon dioxide combines with water to form carbonic acid, which dissociates to form hydrogen and bicarbonate ions. Back in the lung capillaries, carbon dioxide diffuses out of blood into alveolar air. (From Thibodeau, GA: *Structure and function of the body,* ed 9, St Louis, 1992, Mosby.)

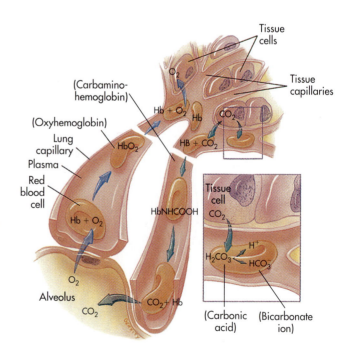

safe environment for all emergency medical services (EMS) personnel before initiating patient contact is crucial. If necessary, use individuals with specialized training and equipment to remove the patient from a hazardous environment.

A major focus of the *initial assessment* is recognition of life-threatening conditions. Many pulmonary diseases present a very real risk for patient death. Recognition of immediately life-threatening conditions and prompt initiation of resuscitation takes priority over detailed assessment. Always consider early administration of oxygen therapy, if indicated.

The following are signs of potential life-threatening respiratory distress in adults (listed from most ominous to least severe) (Figure 22-5):

- Alterations in mental status
- Severe **cyanosis**
- Absent breath sounds
- Audible stridor
- 1 to 2 word dyspnea
- Tachycardia of greater than 130 beats per minute
- Pallor and diaphoresis
- The presence of retractions or the use of accessory muscles of respiration

The *focused history and physical examination* is aimed at the patient's specific respiratory complaints. The *chief complaint* may include dyspnea, chest pain, cough (productive, non-productive, bloody [hemoptysis]); wheezing; or signs of infection (e.g., fever, chills). Especially relevant areas to explore in the patient's history are as follows:

- Has the patient had experiences with similar or identical symptoms? If the current problem represents an exacerbation of a chronic condition, the patient's subjective description of the acuity may be helpful. Ask the patient, "What happened the last time you had an attack this bad?"

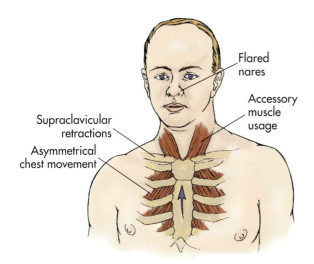

FIGURE 22-5 ▲ **Signs of respiratory distress: nasal flaring, asymmetric chest movements, and the use of accessory muscles to breathe.**

▶ NOTE: Some asthmatics lose their ability to sense dyspnea and present for help only when they are critically ill. In these patients, their assessment of acuity may be incorrect.

- Does the patient have a known pulmonary diagnosis? If you are not familiar with the specific entity, try to learn if it is primarily related to ventilation, diffusion, perfusion, or a combination.
- Has the patient ever required intubation? History of previous intubation is an accurate indicator of severe pulmonary disease, and suggests that intubation may be required again.
- What medications does the patient take? Be certain to ask not only how the medications were prescribed (i.e., what is supposed to be taken by the patient) but how and when the patient actually takes them. Also determine if the patient has any medication allergies.
- Common pulmonary medications and their trade names are summarized in Table 22-1. Persons who are on oral corticosteroids typically have severe, chronic disease. Inhaled steroid use is now common in both asthma and COPD, even in patients with mild disease (see below).
- Determine details of the present episode.
- Determine any possible toxic exposures, especially cigarette smoke or toxic gases.

During the physical examination, pay special attention to the following:

1. *General impression*—Form a general impression of the patient's condition based on your assessment of the following (Figure 22-6):
   - *Position*—The patient's position often indicates the degree of respiratory difficulty. Dyspneic persons often sit, leaning forward on their hands, with the feet dangling. This is known as the **tripod position** and suggests moderately severe respiratory distress is present (Figure 22-7).
   - *Mentation*—Confusion suggests hypoxemia or hypercarbia (carbon dioxide retention) until proven otherwise; both fear and hypoxemia can cause restlessness and irritability. Severe lethargy or coma is a sign of severe hypoxia or hypercarbia.
   - *Ability to speak*—A good indicator of breathing difficulty is a patient's ability to speak freely, without having to stop and breathe. Persons with the ability to speak one or two words have **dyspnea** (i.e., visibly short of breath after speaking only one or two words) have severe respiratory distress. Rapid, rambling speech often indicates anxiety and fear, though many other conditions may be responsible (e.g., **pulmonary embolus,** drug intoxication).
   - *Respiratory effort*—Patients who look as if they are working to breathe usually are! Often, the presence of retractions or the use of accessory muscles of respiration suggests obstruction to expiratory airflow. Any condition resulting in dyspnea, however, may lead to these findings.

TABLE 22-1

DYSPNEA-RELATED PATIENT MEDICATIONS

CLASSIFICATION	SPECIFIC DRUG	INDICATION	THERAPEUTIC ACTION	SIDE EFFECTS AND PRECAUTIONS
BRONCHODILATORS				
Oral	Aminophylline Theodur Somophylline Elixophylline Brethine	Asthma	Dilates the bronchi	Cardiac dysrhythmias Tachydysrhythmias Nervousness N/V
Inhalants	Proventil Ventolin Alupent Albuterol			
ANTICOAGULANTS	Coumadin Heparin Persantine	Pulmonary embolism DVT Thrombo-phlebitis AMI	Increased clotting time	Hemorrhage
ANTIINFLAMMATORY				
Steroid	Medrol Prednisone	Arthritis Asthma Allergies Inflammation	Reduces inflammation from severe disease	Masks symptoms of other diseases Mood swings Weight gain
ANTIHYPERTENSIVE				
Diuretics	Lasix (furosemide) Esidrex (hydro-chlorothiazide) Hydrodiuril Diuril Oretic Aldactone	HTN CHF	Increases urinary output Decreases circulating volume	Dehydration Electrolyte imbalances Hypotension Hypokalemia
CARDIOTONICS	Digitalis (digoxin)	CHF	Increases force of contraction	Bradycardia
	Lanoxin	A-fib/A-flutter/PSVT	Slows conduction through the AV node; decreases heart rate	Digitalis toxicity

AMI, Acute myocardial infarction; *AV,* atrioventricular; *CHF,* congestive heart failure; *COPD,* chronic obstructive pulmonary disease; *DVT,* deep vein thrombosis; *HTN,* head, throat, and nose; *N/V,* nausea/vomiting; *PSVT,* paroxysmal supra-ventricular tachycardia. (From American College of Emergency Physicians; Pons PT, Cason D, chief editors: *Paramedic field care: a complaint-based approach,* St Louis, 1997, Mosby.)

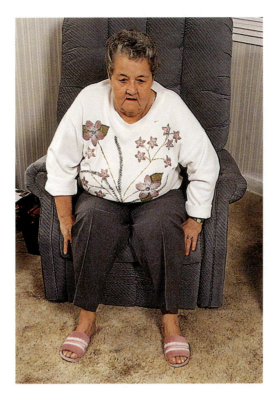

FIGURE 22-6 ▲ A patient whose breathing is audibly abnormal or silent may be experiencing an acute COPD episode. (Vincent Knaus from Stoy W: *Mosby's EMT–Basic textbook,* St Louis, 1996, Mosby.)

FIGURE 22-7 ▲ The tripod position suggests moderately-severe respiratory distress.

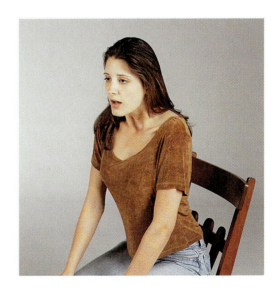

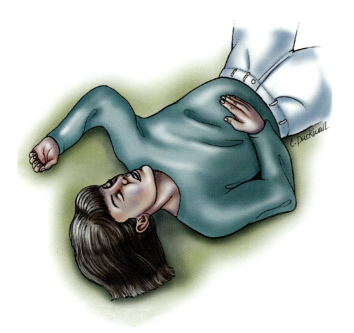

FIGURE 22-8 ▲ Cyanosis is a late sign of respiratory difficulty. (Courtesy of Duckwall Productions.)

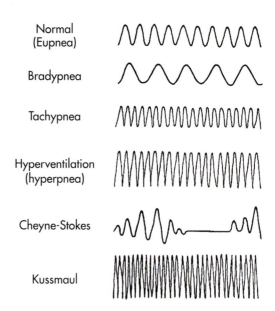

Normal (Eupnea)

Bradypnea

Tachypnea

Hyperventilation (hyperpnea)

Cheyne-Stokes

Kussmaul

FIGURE 22-9 ▲ Common breathing patterns. (From Sanders M: *Mosby's paramedic textbook*, St Louis, 1994, Mosby.)

- *Skin color and appearance*—Diaphoresis is a nonspecific finding but typically indicates that the patient is in more distress than someone who is not diaphoretic. Cyanosis, either peripherally or centrally, is always worrisome (Figure 22-8).

2. *Vital signs*—Obtain baseline vital signs; use these in combination with other findings, as follows, to evaluate the severity of the patient's condition:
   - *Pulse*—Tachycardia is a sign of hypoxemia and fear. It may also occur because of sympathomimetic medication use, such as inhaled bronchodilators. In the face of a respiratory problem, bradycardia is an ominous sign of severe hypoxemia and suggests imminent cardiac arrest, especially in pediatric patients.
   - *Blood pressure*—Hypertension may be associated with fear, anxiety, dyspnea, use of sympathomimetic medications, or a combination of factors.
   - *Respiratory rate*—Isolated measurement of a patient's respiratory rate is an inaccurate measurement of respiratory status unless it is very slow (less than 8 to 10 breaths per minute in an adult). More helpful are changes in the measured respiratory rate. Trends are essential in evaluating any patient. A slowing respiratory rate in the face of an unimproved condition suggests patient exhaustion and impending respiratory failure.
   - *Respiratory patterns*—Various terms are used to describe breathing patterns in the medical literature. Distinguishing them clinically is not always possible. See Box 22-1 for helpful descriptives (Figure 22-9).

BOX 22-1

RESPIRATORY PATTERNS

Eupnea—Normal breathing rate
Tachypnea—Rapid breathing rate
Bradypnea—Slower than normal breathing rate
Cheyne-Stokes breathing—Abnormal pattern of breathing, characterized by alternating period of apnea and deep, rapid breathing. Although once thought to indicate only neurological disease, congestive heart failure is the most common cause in elderly patients. It may also occur in healthy persons during hyperventilation and high altitude exposure.
Central neurogenic hyperventilation—A pattern of breathing marked by rapid and regular respirations at a rate of about 25 per minute. Increasing regularity, rather than rate, is an important diagnostic sign of increasing depth of coma.
Kussmaul respirations—Abnormally deep, very rapid sighing respirations often due to the presence of metabolic acidosis (e.g., diabetic ketoacidosis).
Ataxic (Biot's) breathing—Type of breathing characterized by a series of several short inspirations followed by long, irregular periods of apnea. This breathing pattern usually indicates increased intracranial pressure.
Apneustic breathing—Pattern of respirations characterized by a prolonged inspiratory phase followed by expiration apnea. The respiratory rate averages 1.5 cycles per minute.
Apnea—Absence of breathing

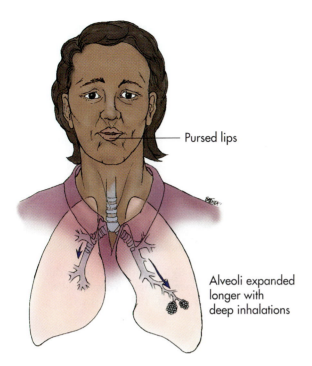

Pursed lips

Alveoli expanded
longer with
deep inhalations

FIGURE 22-10 ▲ Pursed lips may indicate that a patient is having trouble breathing.

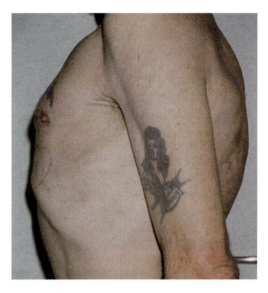

FIGURE 22-11 ▲ A barrel-shaped chest is a sign that a patient is experiencing COPD. (Vincent Knaus from Stoy W: Mosby's EMT–Basic textbook, St Louis, 1996, Mosby.)

3. *Head and neck*—observe for the presence of pursed lip breathing (Figure 22-10) often present in asthma and COPD. Also look for retractions of the neck muscles and jugular venous distention (JVD). JVD may accompany right-sided heart failure, which may be caused by pulmonary disease. The presence of sputum may suggest a potential cause for the patient's problem:
   • Increasing amounts suggest infection.
   • Thick green or brown sputum suggests infection, possibly pneumonia.
   • Yellow or pale gray sputum may be caused by allergy or inflammation.
   • Pink, frothy sputum is usually associated with cardiac disease, often acute pulmonary edema.

▶ NOTE: Do not completely rely on the presence or type of sputum in forming a field impression. The above suggestions are merely guidelines. A diagnosis is based on far more than just sputum color and quantity.

4. *Chest*—Observe the chest for the following:
   • Symmetry
   • Signs of trauma
   • **Barrel chest** *deformity*—Suggests the presence of long-standing COPD (Figure 22-11)
   • Retractions

   • Auscultate the lungs and determine if the breath sounds are:
      • Normal
      • Abnormal (e.g., **stridor,** [abnormal high-pitched sound suggestive of upper airway obstruction], wheezes, crackles)
5. *Extremities*—Evaluation of the extremities may reveal peripheral cyanosis or carpopedal spasm (Figure 22-12). **Carpopedal spasm** is associated with decreased carbon dioxide levels (hypocapnia) resulting from periods of rapid, deep respirations—whatever the cause. It is not just a sign of "anxiety-hyperventilation" (see below).
6. *Diagnostic testing*—Field diagnostic tests help confirm your clinical impression of disease severity. An EMT–I should *not* allow a test to convince him or her that a sick-appearing patient is fine. Keeping this caveat in mind, potentially helpful field diagnostic tests include the following:
   • *Pulse oximetry*—This is used to evaluate or confirm the adequacy of oxygen saturation. It may be inaccurate in the presence of conditions that abnormally bind hemoglobin (e.g., carbon monoxide poisoning, methemoglobinemia).
   • *Peak flow*—Peak flow meters are easy to use and provide a baseline assessment to follow therapy. Isolated readings on their own are potentially misleading; follow trends instead.

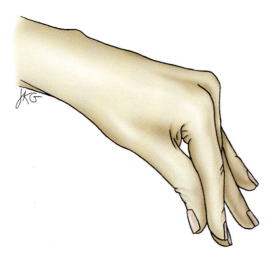

FIGURE 22-12 ▲ Carpopedal spasm.

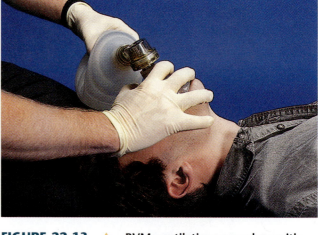

FIGURE 22-13 ▲ BVM ventilation procedure with one rescuer. (From Vincent Knaus from Stoy W: *Mosby's EMT–Basic textbook,* St Louis, 1996, Mosby.)

- *Capnometry*—Capnometry provides ongoing assessment of endotracheal tube position; the end-tidal carbon dioxide drops almost immediately when the tube is displaced from the trachea. Quantitative monitoring meters may be more accurate than qualitative colorimetric devices but are also far more expensive. As long as you monitor trends, the device used is not as important as the thought processes of the EMT–I interpreting the results.

Management

Management of respiratory emergencies first requires careful attention to details. Provide airway, ventilatory, and circulatory support, as required, by a combination of the following devices and techniques (see Chapter 8) (Figures 22-13 to 22-15):
- Manual airway opening maneuvers
- Oropharyngeal airway
- Nasopharyngeal airway
- Nasal cannula
- Simple oxygen mask
- Nonrebreather mask
- Multilumen airway
- Bag-valve-mask device
- Suctioning
- Endotracheal tube
- Oxygen-powered manually triggered ventilators
- Automatic transport ventilator

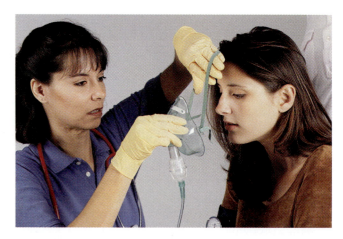

FIGURE 22-14 ▲ Treating a patient with an inhaled beta-2 agonist medication.

Provide necessary circulatory and respiratory support via both nonpharmacological and pharmacological interventions:
- Place the patient in a position of comfort, usually sitting.
- Use medications as indicated (e.g., albuterol, epinephrine)

Monitor patients appropriately and transport them to the appropriate facility, using the appropriate mode (e.g., emergency, nonemergent). Remember that a cardinal part of treating persons with respiratory problems is providing psychological support; fear and anxiety are usually present.

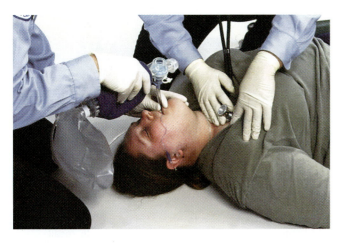

FIGURE 22-15 ▲ Placement of an endotracheal tube.

OBSTRUCTIVE AIRWAY DISEASE

Obstructive airway disease is a generic term for a spectrum of diseases that affect many individuals worldwide. The most common diseases include asthma and COPD. COPD is sometimes subdivided into emphysema and chronic bronchitis, although many patients have clinical features of both.

Epidemiology and Causes of Obstructive Airway Disease

Obstructive airway disease is a significant health problem in the United States and consumes a large portion of medical expenses each year. Asthma affects 4% to 5% of the U.S. population, and the death rate from severe attacks continues to rise. Experts estimate that nearly 20% of adult males have evidence of chronic bronchitis.

The most common cause of COPD is cigarette smoking. Genetic predisposition and exposure to environmental toxins contribute to many asthma attacks.

Factors that may exacerbate underlying conditions include the following:

• *Stress*—Stress is a significant exacerbating factor, particularly in adults.
• *Infection*—Upper respiratory infection is a common precipitant of acute exacerbation of both asthma and COPD.
• *Exercise*—Although exercise may exacerbate any respiratory condition, exercise-induced wheezing and asthma is especially common.

External stimuli, as indicated in the following, may also play a significant contributory role:

• *Tobacco smoke*—Smoking increases the chances of developing COPD and heart disease. In addition, exposure of others to second-hand smoke affects them similarly. Children with asthma who are surrounded by parental cigarette smoke have an increased frequency of asthmatic attacks.
• **Allergens**—Various substances (e.g., foods, animal dander, dusts, molds, pollens) in the personal environment may precipitate or worsen obstructive lung disease. One purported reason for the increased incidence of asthma in inner city children is exposure to cockroaches.
• *Drugs*—Allergic reactions to any medication may lead to wheezing. Certain drugs (e.g., beta blockers) affect the ability of the sympathetic nervous system to cause bronchodilation and may provoke or worsen obstructive disease.
• *Occupational hazards*—Many occupational exposures have been shown to cause or worsen obstructive lung disease. One of the most significant to health care providers is latex allergy. Many health care workers have developed a latex allergy because of widespread use of latex-containing products, especially gloves. Patients may also be latex sensitive; failure to have equipment that is latex-free may place an EMS system in a serious medicolegal situation.

Pathophysiology Review

The underlying pathophysiology of all forms of obstructive lung disease is decreased expiratory airflow and air trapping primarily due to obstruction in the small bronchioles. Obstruction is usually a result of several factors including the following:

• *Smooth muscle spasm*—Various irritants cause bronchiolar wall smooth muscle to contract, resulting in bronchospasm, obstruction, and wheezing. These muscles contain **beta receptors** that respond to sympathetic stimulation, resulting in bronchodilation. Bronchoconstrictors have the opposite effect (e.g., beta blockers).
• *Mucus*—**Goblet cells** line the respiratory tract and normally produce a layer of mucus that is continuously swept out of the lungs by **cilia,** moving hairs (Figure 22-16). Anything that disrupts the movement of cilia leads to accumulation of excess mucus in the airways. Abnormal ciliary movement occurs in obstructive lung disease and in many other conditions, such as cystic fibrosis. Sometimes, the disruption is temporary but damage sometimes (e.g., chronic bronchitis, cystic fibrosis) is permanent.

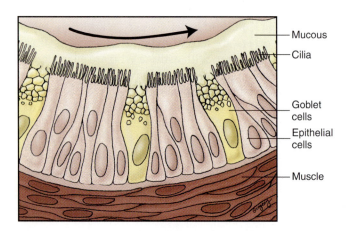

FIGURE 22-16 ▲ Layer of mucus that is continuously swept out of the lungs by cilia, moving hairs.

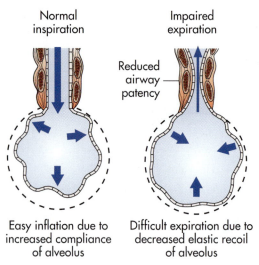

FIGURE 22-17 ▲ Mechanisms of air trapping in COPD: Mucus plugs and narrowed airways cause air trapping and hyperinflation on expiration. During inspiration, the airways enlarge, allowing gas to flow past the obstruction. This mechanism of air trapping occurs in asthma and chronic bronchitis. Mechanism of air trapping in emphysema: Damaged or destroyed alveolar walls no longer support and hold open the airways, and alveoli lose their property of elastic recoil. Both of these factors contribute to collapse during expiration. (From Wilson SF: *Respiratory disorders,* St Louis, 1990, Mosby.)

- *Inflammation*—Obstructive lung disease occurs in the face of both acute and chronic inflammation. This finding has completely changed our approach to the treatment of asthma in recent years. Data also suggest that chronic inflammation underlies COPD. Acutely, infection leads to inflammation that may exacerbate any form of obstructive lung disease.

Despite the mechanism, obstruction may be reversible or irreversible. Typically, asthmatics improve between attacks, although some never achieve normal pulmonary function. However, at least part of the damage in COPD is irreversible, leading to continuous air trapping, as detailed in the following:

- Bronchioles dilate naturally on inspiration as they fill with air.
- Dilation enables air to enter the alveoli even if the lumen (opening) of the bronchiole is narrowed due to obstruction.
- Bronchioles naturally constrict on expiration.
- Air becomes trapped distal to the site of obstruction during exhalation (Figure 22-17).

▶ NOTE: The sections directly following cover disease-specific aspects *excluding* patient assessment and management. Making a definitive field diagnosis of asthma versus COPD (chronic bronchitis or emphysema) is often difficult. Consequently, the authors have chosen to discuss patient assessment and management in one unified section below, rather than separately for each entity.

ASTHMA

Acute **asthma** is a recurring condition of completely or partially reversible acute airflow obstruction in the lower airway. About 8.9 million people in the United States suffer from asthma, with thousands dying each year. It is the most common chronic disease of childhood.

Pathophysiology—Asthma is a chronic disease that involves the lower airway, beyond the level of the trachea and mainstem bronchi. It occurs when the bronchial airways narrow, making breathing difficult. It is not contagious and cannot be cured, but it can be controlled. Acute episodes of worsening, usually called an *attack,* are the most likely reason these persons will seek emergency medical assistance.

People with asthma have hypersensitive bronchial airways that are easily irritated. When the airways become irritated, a series of events occurs (Figure 22-18):

- **Bronchospasm**—Tiny muscle layers surrounding the bronchioles go into spasm and narrow the lumen of the airways. Bronchospasm is similar to pinching a drinking straw; it limits the movement of air. The result is wheezing as air is forced through the narrowed airways. Shortness of breath follows because not enough air reaches the alveoli.

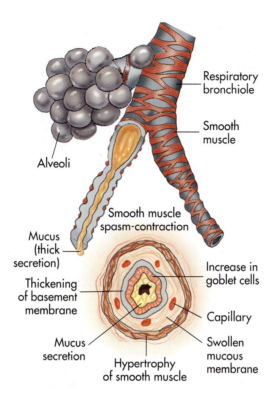

FIGURE 22-18 ▲ With bronchial asthma, the bronchiole is obstructed on expiration, particularly by muscle spasm, edema of the mucosa, and thick secretions. (From Wilson SF: *Respiratory disorders*, St Louis, 1990, Mosby.)

• *Increased mucous production*—Because of the irritation, the bronchial airways produce an abnormal amount of mucus. This secreted mucus is particularly thick, making it difficult to remove with coughing. Since mucus is no longer being removed through normal processes, it clogs the smaller bronchioles, further decreasing airway diameter. This makes breathing even more difficult.
• *Swelling and edema*—Fluid collects in the lining of the irritated airways, causing them to swell, which further blocks the flow of air.
• *Inflammatory cell proliferation*—White blood cells accumulate in the airway. These cells secrete substances that worsen the muscle spasm and increase mucus production.

The patient develops shortness of breath, wheezing, and cough. With proper care, many of these changes are reversible. A severe asthma patient may have ongoing inflammation in the lungs, despite appearing clinically normal. The patient may depend on daily medication to prevent attacks.

Epidemiology—It is not known exactly why some people have asthma and others do not. However, heredity plays a role. If one member of a family has asthma, hay fever, or an allergic skin condition called *eczema*, another family member is more likely to develop asthma than someone who has no such family history.

Asthma can begin at any age, but it is most common in children and young adults. Approximately one third of the people who have asthma develop the condition before 5 years of age. About one third of the children who have asthma outgrow it before they reach adulthood. Conversely, adult asthma is usually persistent. One fourth of all asthma cases begin after age 50.

Classification of asthma—The two kinds of asthma are as follows (Figure 22-19):
• **Extrinsic asthma**—Some specific outside substance such as pollen causes the bronchioles to narrow. The onset of extrinsic asthma is more common in childhood.
• **Intrinsic asthma**—No specific substance can be identified as causing the air tubes to narrow. Intrinsic asthma more commonly has an adult onset.

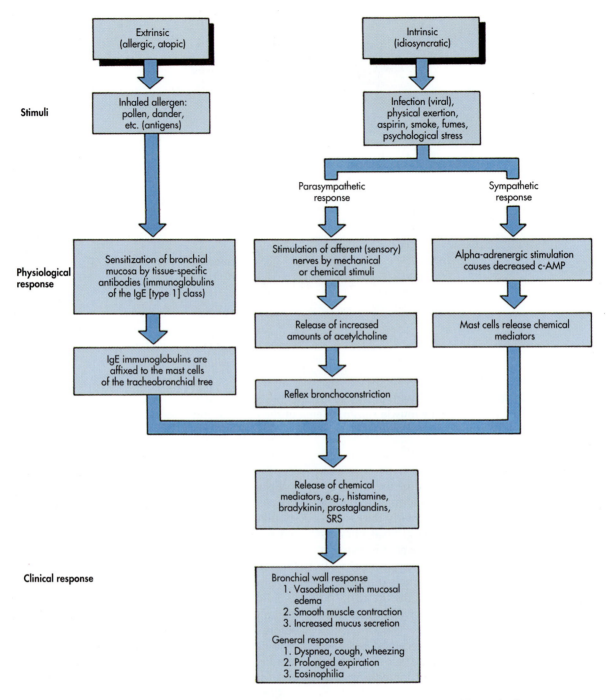

FIGURE 22-19 ▲   Proposed pathogenesis of extrinsic and intrinsic bronchial asthma. (From Wilson SF: *Respiratory disorders,* St Louis, 1990, Mosby.)

Causes of asthma—The cause of an asthma attack is not always easy to identify. In people with asthma, a wide range of substances ranging from chemicals, odors, and smoke to physical activity can irritate the bronchial airways. These items are called *triggers* because they cause bronchospasm, mucus production, and swelling—an asthma attack. Seven groups of common asthma triggers are as follows (Figure 22-20):

• Respiratory infections—Respiratory infections are the most common asthma triggers. They include: colds,

the flu, sinus infections, etc. These illnesses trigger asthma attacks because they temporarily inflame and damage the lining of the air tubes causing bronchospasm, increased mucus production, and swelling. Asthma attacks that occur with a respiratory infection are usually worse than those that occur at other times.

• *Allergens*—Allergens are substances that can trigger an allergic reaction that irritates the bronchial airways. Children are more likely to have allergies that trigger attacks than are adults who develop asthma

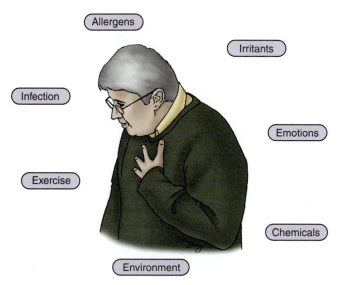

FIGURE 22-20 ▲ Seven groups of common asthma triggers.

which are often used to preserve fruits and vegetables and are found on food and salad bars.

- Changes in environmental conditions—cold, wind, humidity.

A few people experience asthmatic crises only once or twice a year. However, most people with asthma have some discomfort on a regular basis. Most experience at least some increased discomfort in the fall and spring when pollen levels are highest. Occasionally, hormonal variations during pregnancy or menstruation may make asthma either better or worse.

Status asthmaticus is a severe, prolonged asthma attack that does not respond to standard medications. Its onset may be sudden or insidious and is frequently precipitated by a viral respiratory infection. Status asthmaticus requires immediate transport as the patient is in imminent danger of respiratory failure. Prehospital treatment is the same as for acute asthma; however, rapid transport is more important. Patients should be closely monitored and the EMT–I should anticipate the need for intubation and aggressive ventilatory support.

CHRONIC OBSTRUCTIVE PULMONARY DISEASE

Chronic **obstructive pulmonary disease (COPD),** is a progressive and irreversible disease of the airway marked by decreased inspiratory and expiratory capacity of the lungs. COPD may result from **chronic bronchitis** (excess mucus production) or **emphysema** (lung tissue damage with loss of elastic recoil of the lungs). COPD patients usually suffer from a combination of chronic bronchitis and emphysema (Figure 22-21).

Patients with COPD function at a certain baseline level until an event occurs which causes decompensation. This is known as an acute COPD episode (exacerbation) and is usually when EMS is called for help.

Pathophysiology—Chronic bronchitis results from overgrowth of the airway mucus glands and excess secretion of mucus that blocks the airway. These patients have a productive cough for at least three months per year for two or more consecutive years (Figure 22-22).

Emphysema results from destruction of the walls of the alveoli (Figure 22-23). Normally, exhalation is a passive process resulting from elastic recoil of the lungs after they have expanded, similarly to air coming out of a balloon after it has been blown up. The loss of normal alveolar structure leads to a decrease in elastic recoil, which creates resistance to expiratory airflow. Air is trapped within the lungs, resulting in poor air exchange.

Most patients with COPD have a combination of the features of both chronic bronchitis and emphysema. They have marked resistance within their airways to air movement. The work required to breathe is considerable.

After a time, the right side of the heart may develop failure due to the effort required to move blood through

later in life. The most common allergens are pollen, dust, animal dander, lint, insecticides, food, mold and drugs (e.g., aspirin, penicillin, local anesthetics, antiinflammatory drugs such as ibuprofen).

- *Drugs*—Street drugs such as cocaine may cause acute asthmatic attacks in sensitive individuals. Contrary to popular belief, food allergies are very rare. Nuts and seafood are the most common causes of food allergies that trigger asthma attacks.
- *Irritants*—Irritant triggers are substances that can irritate everyone's bronchi but in persons who have asthma, they can trigger an attack. Examples include odors, cigarette smoke, air pollution, and fumes. Work place irritants are particularly common among people who work in factories where heavy dust or fumes are present.
- *Exercise*—Exercise, or fast breathing, especially during cold weather, irritates the bronchial airways. They become more sensitive and produce more mucus, which can lead to an asthma attack. Another common trigger among children is exercise. It is natural for children to run and exercise outdoors, especially in the spring and fall when pollen fills the air.
- *Emotions*—Any strong, subjective feeling or reaction may cause an asthma attack. Although there has been less research conducted in this area than on other asthma triggers, examples of emotions that might trigger an attack include crying, yelling, or even laughing. Stress from personal or work related worry is a particularly powerful trigger.
- *Chemicals*—Many people have severe asthma reactions to specific chemicals. Common examples include red and yellow dye (not only in food but also in colored pills); sulfur dioxide in red wine; aspirin (and other antiinflammatory drugs); and sulfites,

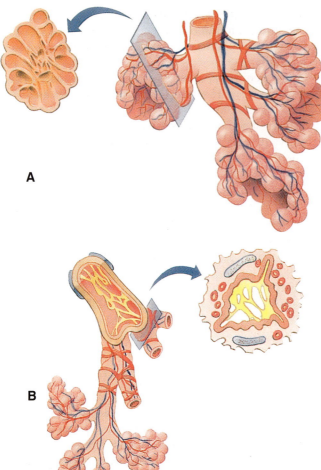

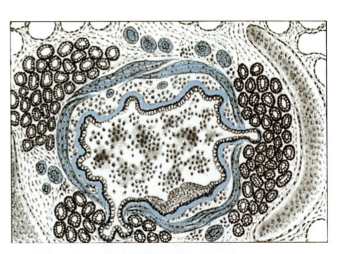

FIGURE 22-22 ▲ Chronic bronchitis. Bronchi are filled with excess mucus. (From Wilson SF: *Respiratory disorders,* St Louis, 1990, Mosby.)

FIGURE 22-21 ▲ **A,** Chronic bronchitis. Air tubes narrow as a result of swollen tissues and excessive mucus production. **B,** Emphysema. Walls of alveoli are torn and cannot be repaired. Alveoli fuse into large air spaces. (From Thibodeau GA: *Anatomy and physiology,* ed 4, St Louis, 1999, Mosby.)

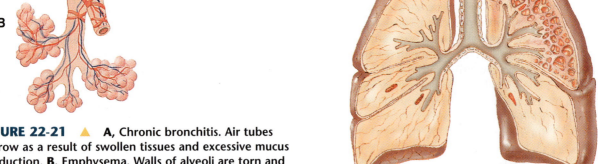

FIGURE 22-23 ▲ Cystic changes of labor emphysema resulting from destruction of alveoli. (From Wilson SF: *Respiratory disorders,* St Louis, 1990, Mosby.)

diseased lungs. This condition is known as chronic **cor pulmonale** and indicates severe COPD.

Causes—The major cause of COPD is cigarette smoking. Industrial inhalants such as asbestos and coal dust, air pollution, and tuberculosis also contribute to the condition.

Assessment Findings

Many asthmatics keep medications at home to care for attacks. Usually, they try these remedies before calling EMS. Victims will often report a recent upper respiratory infection, often with a cough. Their symptoms often come on relatively quickly, as compared with persons with COPD. The patient with an acute COPD episode will complain of shortness of breath with symptoms gradually increasing over a period of days.

CLINICAL NOTES

Some patients with COPD call their disease "asthma." This use of terms is a misnomer, since patients with COPD never have totally normal airway function.

Patients may report the following:
- New cough or a change in their previous pattern of cough and sputum production
- Stopped medications (without the doctor's advice) because they were "feeling better"
- Use of home oxygen
- Use of a home **nebulizer** to give themselves breathing treatments, which may have failed to improve the situation

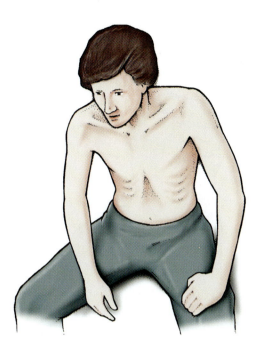

FIGURE 22-24 ▲ **A patient who is using accessory muscles to breathe is experiencing respiratory distress. (Courtesy of Duckwall Productions.)**

Given that many patients die of asthma and COPD, careful assessment and intervention in the field are essential. Often the patient is found sitting upright, leaning forward with hand on knees (tripod position), using accessory muscles to breathe, and in obvious respiratory distress. Breathing is loud and audible wheezing often present, even without a stethoscope. In the later stages, patients airways may become so severely constricted that wheezing is minimal—the airways are "too tight to wheeze."

▶ NOTE: A quiet-sounding chest in a patient who is obviously short of breath is an ominous sign.

Other common signs and symptoms of obstructive lung disease include the following:
- *Shortness of breath*—Patients may speak in short sentences because they are unable to get enough air to talk in longer phrases.
- *Coughing*—They may or may not be productive of sputum.
- Cyanosis
- *Anxiety, agitation, anxiousness*—Patients often feel as though they are suffocating.
- Diaphoresis and pallor
- *Cigarette stains on the fingertips, especially in patients with COPD*—This suggests that the patient has been a heavy smoker for many years.
- Tachycardia
- Hypertension
- Tachypnea

- Hyperinflated or "barrel-shaped" chest
- *Use of accessory breathing muscles*—Normally, most of the breathing effort is done by the diaphragm. A person in respiratory distress may use the supraclavicular and intercostal muscles of the rib cage. Use of accessory muscles causes the inward movement of these muscles during inspiration. This is a sign of straining severely to breathe (Figure 22-24).
- *Audible abnormal breath sounds*—Wheezing is the most common. A silent chest indicates that the patient is too tight to wheeze, a serious sign.
- Decreased oxygen saturation on pulse oximetry

If the patient also has cor pulmonale, the following additional features are likely to be seen:
- Marked neck vein distention (although this finding may occur from COPD or asthma alone)
- Abdominal bloating (from fluid in the abdominal cavity)
- Leg edema

▶ Use the pulse oximeter to document hypoxemia and monitor the patient's response to therapy. Use a peak flow meter to establish the patient's baseline airflow, and to follow the therapeutic response.

▶ *All that wheezes is not asthma!* Wheezes may also be present with other diseases that cause dyspnea, such as COPD, heart failure, pulmonary embolism, pneumothorax, toxic inhalation, foreign body aspiration, and other pathological states. Always consider the possibility of a foreign body in the airway, especially in young children with wheezing and no history of asthma. A complete history and thorough patient examination are necessary for appropriate emergency care decisions (Figure 22-25).

Certain signs show that a patient is in very serious condition. Manage these individuals as "priority" patients. These include the following (Figure 22-26):
- Altered level of consciousness such as sluggishness, exhaustion, agitation, and confusion—This indicates that insufficient oxygen is getting to the brain, and a build-up of carbon dioxide in the blood. The victim may be agitated or drowsy.
- *"Silent chest"*—An absence of breath sounds when auscultating the chest of the asthma patient means that there is severe narrowing of the bronchial passageways. These patients are said to be "too tight to wheeze." It indicates air flow through the respiratory passageways is severely limited. The partial or complete absence of lung sounds is also a sign of danger in COPD patients.
- Marked diaphoresis
- Cyanosis
- If patients state they are "too tired to breathe anymore."

All that wheezes is not asthma!

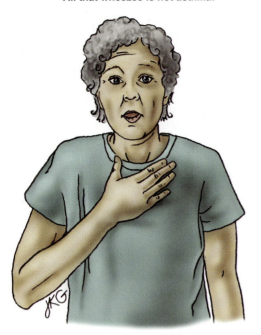

Consider...

- COPD
- CHF
- Pulmonary embolism
- Toxic inhalation
- Foreign body aspiration

FIGURE 22-25 ▲ **Not all wheezing is asthma.**

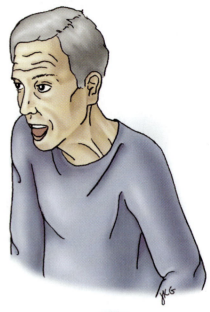

- Altered LOC
- Silent chest
- Marked diaphoresis
- Cyanosis
- "Too tired to breathe"

FIGURE 22-26 ▲ **Priority patients.**

Management of Obstructive Lung Disease (COPD or Asthma)

Initial patient management in the out-of-hospital setting should include the following:

1. Perform endotracheal intubation and ventilate using high-concentration oxygen if the following is present:
   - Unable to maintain an airway
   - Ventilatory assistance is needed
   - Severe respiratory distress
   - Significant cyanosis is present
   - Significant hypotension (blood pressure less than 70 mm Hg systolic)

2. If the patient is likely experiencing respiratory distress but breathing adequately, provide a high concentration of humidified supplemental oxygen:
   - The patient should receive 10 to 15 L using a nonrebreather mask (85% to 100%) if he or she can tolerate the mask.
   - A nasal cannula delivering a 44% concentration of oxygen (flow rate of 6 L/ min.) may be used if the patient is afraid of or agitated by the oxygen mask. Assist ventilation if necessary.
   - The patient should be placed in a position of comfort. This is typically sitting upright, if he or she is having trouble breathing.
   - The patient should be calmed and reassured.

HELPFUL HINT

- Never withhold high-concentration oxygen from ill or injured patients based on the unlikely possibility that they may be carbon dioxide retainers.

3. Provide timely transport with treatment en route.

4. Monitor vital signs, including pulse oximetry, frequently.

5. Monitor the electrocardiogram (ECG) for cardiac rhythm disturbances.

6. Treat the bronchospasm as follows (Figure 22-27):
   - Administer an aerosolized bronchodilator such as **albuterol** (Proventil), isoetharine (Bronkosol), or metaproterenol (Alupent) *and/or*
   - Administer **epinephrine** (Adrenalin) at a dose of 0.1 to 0.5 milliliters (mL) of a 1:1000 solution subcutaneously *and/or* Terbutaline (Brethine) at 0.25 mL subcutaneously.

▶ NOTE: Inhaled beta-2 agonists (e.g., albuterol) are the first agent of choice in patients with an exacerbation of obstructive lung disease. Other modalities are mentioned for completeness sake (alternatives are good). Epinephrine or terbutaline in an older patient or a person with cardiac disease may be harmful. Always follow local protocols.

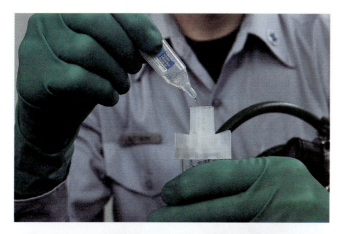

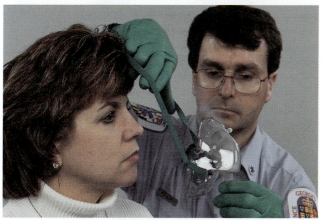

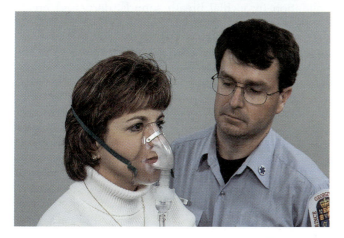

FIGURE 22-27 ▲ **Administration of medication via a hand-held nebulizer.**

Unfortunately, there is still some disagreement among EMS systems about giving oxygen to patients with COPD. The basis for this argument is the fact that there are two separate respiratory drives:

■ *The* **carbon dioxide drive**—When a person holds his or her breath, carbon dioxide accumulates in the blood. After a period, the level of carbon dioxide gets high enough to stimulate breathing centers in the brain. The reflex response is to take a breath. The accumulation of carbon dioxide in our blood is the major stimulus that normally causes us to breathe.

■ *The* **hypoxic drive**—A secondary mechanism that stimulates breathing is a lack of oxygen in the blood. If the level of oxygen in the blood goes very low, brain breathing centers are stimulated, leading to the reflex response of breathing.

A small number of patients with COPD do not effectively excrete carbon dioxide from their lungs. Carbon dioxide is always elevated in their bloodstream. These patients are called *carbon dioxide retainers.* These patients have lost their carbon dioxide drive to breathe. The only thing that stimulates breathing is the low level of oxygen in their blood (the hypoxic drive).

If a high level of oxygen is given to a carbon dioxide retainer, hypoxia, the only remaining stimulus for breathing, will be eliminated. The patient could develop hypoventilation and eventually respiratory arrest. Based on this logic, some EMS protocols limit the use of oxygen to low concentration. Others recommend the field use of Venturi masks to give precise oxygen concentrations.

Only a few COPD patients are at risk for developing respiratory arrest from too high an oxygen concentration. Unfortunately, determining in the field who these patients are is impossible. As a rule, the EMT–I should give the patient the amount of oxygen considered necessary for his or her condition. High-concentration oxygen should not be withheld when required only because the patient *might* be a carbon dioxide retainer and stop breathing. In reality, this is quite unusual.

7. Place an intravenous (IV) lifeline of normal saline or Ringer's lactate or 5% dextrose in water according to local protocols. Sometimes, IV hydration helps patients bring up secretions, although experts are not as emphatic on this point as they once were.

8. Identify priority patients and make an appropriate transport/backup decision.

9. Provide ongoing psychological encouragement and support.

● **HELPFUL HINT**

• Oxygen without humidification may not be as beneficial, but it is better than none at all.

PNEUMONIA

Pneumonia is an acute inflammatory condition of the lungs, usually caused by either bacterial or viral infection. It is the fifth leading cause of death in the United States.

Epidemiology

Pneumonia is not a single disease but a *group* of infections due to many different agents. Several risk factors, including the following, make some individuals more likely to get the disease:

- *Cigarette smoking*—Cigarette smoke directly inhibits the normal movement of mucus via bronchial cilia out of the lung. As a result, the lung is unable to clear pathogens (e.g., bacteria, viruses) as effectively. Allowed to remain, these infectious agents multiply, resulting in pneumonia.
- *Alcoholism*—Drinkers are especially likely to get aspiration pneumonia (inhaling their vomit) during passing-out spells. Even without aspiration, chronic alcoholics have an increased risk of acquiring infections because of weakened immune systems due to ethanol.
- *Cold exposure*—Although it is a myth that mild cold exposure causes pneumonia, prolonged acute or chronic hypothermia exerts a severe toll on the body's immune system. Pneumonia is especially common in elderly patients who are chronically hypothermic, often under less than ideal living conditions.
- *Extremes of age*—Both the very young and the elderly are more susceptible to pneumonia than other groups of people.
- *Abnormal immune systems*—Diseases such as acquired immunodeficiency syndrome (AIDS) predispose victims to severe infections, including pneumonia. Other potential high-risk patients include those on chronic steroid therapy (especially oral), cancer chemotherapy, or antirejection drugs following a transplant.

Pathophysiology

Pneumonia is primarily a disorder of ventilation due to infection of the lung parenchyma. It is most commonly bacterial, although viruses and fungi may also cause pneumonia. Causative agents vary somewhat, depending on whether the infection is community acquired or hospital acquired. Community-acquired pneumonia is often caused by *Diplococci* or *Mycoplasma pneumoniae* organisms. These do not tend to be as severe infections as hospital-acquired ones, which are more commonly due to gram-negative bacteria such as *Pseudomonas* (Figure 22-28).

Sometimes infection causes alveolar collapse **(atelectasis),** which prevents the body from adequately "clearing the invaders" from the system. Localized inflammation or infection may become systemic, leading to overwhelming infection (sepsis) and potentially fatal septic shock.

Assessment Findings

The "typical" picture of bacterial pneumonia is heralded by acute onset of fever and chills. Cough productive of purulent (rust-colored or green) sputum soon fol-

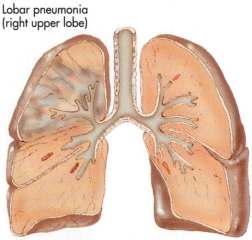

Lobar pneumonia
(right upper lobe)

Pneumococcal pneumonia

FIGURE 22-28 ▲ **Pneumonia is an inflammatory process of the respiratory bronchioles and alveoli that is caused by infection. (From Wilson SF: *Respiratory disorders*, St Louis, 1990, Mosby.)**

lows. Depending on the location of the infection, the patient may have **pleuritic chest pain,** or pain that worsens with deep breathing or moving due to inflammation near the external lung surface. Physical findings vary widely, although crackles and signs of pulmonary consolidation (bronchial breath sounds, decreased breath sounds) are often present (see Chapter 10).

"Atypical" symptoms are more common in viral pneumonia and in the very young or very old. These include the following:

- Nonproductive cough
- Headache
- Myalgias (muscle aches)
- Fatigue
- Sore throat
- Nausea, vomiting, diarrhea
- Fever and chills (continuous, versus a dramatic onset as in "typical" pneumonia)

Management

Consider any patient with possible pneumonia to be contagious and act accordingly (Figure 22-28). Once assuring the safety of the EMS team, provide airway and ventilatory support. Often, high-concentration oxygen is sufficient. At times, either assisted ventilation or intubation may be required.

Provide circulatory support via the administration of IV fluids, according to local protocols. Often, these patients are dehydrated due to fever and fluids are of great benefit. They may also help thin and mobilize pulmonary mucus. Septic shock is commonly caused by pneumonia, so valuate the patient carefully and treat for shock as necessary (see Chapter 16). If the patient has a high fever and is very uncomfortable, consider the combination of cool cloth sponging and fanning to reduce the temperature.

At times, inhaled beta-2 agonists (e.g., albuterol) may be helpful, especially if the patient has accompanying obstructive lung disease (follow local protocols). Generally, antibiotics are not given by EMTs of any level in the field. Similarly, the use of aspirin and acetaminophen for pain and fever by the EMT–I is not part of the United States Department of Transportation (DOT) EMT–I curriculum.

Monitor patients appropriately and transport them to the appropriate facility, using the appropriate mode (e.g., emergency, nonemergent). Remember that a cardinal part of treating persons with respiratory problems is providing psychological support; fear and anxiety are usually present.

PULMONARY EDEMA

Epidemiology

Pulmonary edema refers to filling of the lungs with fluid in the interstitial spaces, the alveoli, or both. It is not a disease in itself but rather a pathophysiological condition resulting from many possible causes.

Anatomy and Physiology

Mechanistically, pulmonary edema is classified as either **high-pressure** or **high-permeability pulmonary edema.** The origin of this differentiation is based on a law described early last century by the physiologist Starling. He noted that two factors determine the flow into or out of a fluid-filled biological tube, such as a pulmonary capillary:

- The permeability of the tube's walls
- The hydrostatic pressure ("water pressure") of the fluid inside (Figure 22-29)

Thus the classification of pulmonary edema is based on whether the pressure is elevated (high pressure) or whether the permeability is abnormal (high permeability). Although the physiology is fascinating, it is often difficult to distinguish clinically (especially in the field) one form from the other.

▶ NOTE: The osmotic pressure (protein pressure or oncotic pressure) also helps determine the net fluid flow into or out of a capillary. The authors have deleted this component to avoid unnecessary confusion since osmotic pressure is not usually clinically-relevant to the EMT-I in the field.

With due regard to the often incorrect use of the terms *cardiogenic* and *noncardiogenic* pulmonary edema (see NOTE above), this text follows the classification system used in the DOT EMT–I curriculum: high-pressure (cardiogenic) and high-permeability (noncardiogenic) pulmonary edema.

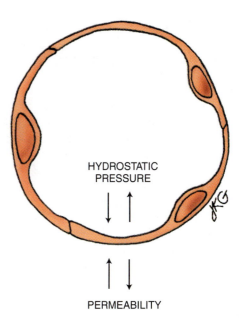

FIGURE 22-29 ▲ The hydrostatic pressure ("water pressure") of the fluid inside.

High-pressure, or cardiogenic, pulmonary edema most commonly results from acute myocardial ischemia. This may be due to acute myocardial infarction (AMI) or just as commonly severe ischemia, without infarction. Distinguishing the difference in the field is nearly impossible. Heart valve disease, chronic hypertension, or myocarditis (viral infection of the heart muscle) may also result in **cardiogenic pulmonary edema,** although far less commonly than ischemia due to coronary artery disease.

▶ The most common causes of high-pressure pulmonary edema are cardiac, though other diseases (scorpion bites, brain injury, diving accidents) may also raise the hydrostatic pressure in the lungs. Consequently, many people often, albeit incorrectly, refer to high-pressure pulmonary edema as *cardiogenic.* Similarly, the term **noncardiogenic pulmonary edema** is often used for high-permeability edema when, in reality, noncardiac factors can *also* raise the hydrostatic pressure, as noted earlier.

Many processes alter lung capillary permeability, leading to high-permeability (noncardiogenic) pulmonary edema. These include the following:

- Acute hypoxemia (for any reason)
- Near-drowning
- Cardiac arrest
- Shock
- High altitude exposure
- Inhalation of pulmonary irritants (e.g., chlorine gas)
- **Adult respiratory distress syndrome (ARDS)**

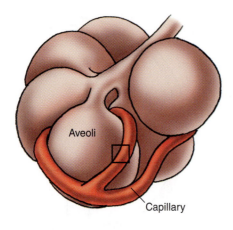

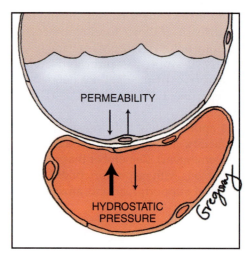

FIGURE 22-30 ▲ In high pressure (cardiogenic) pulmonary edema.

Sometimes, health care providers incorrectly classify *all* noncardiogenic pulmonary edema as ARDS. ARDS is a highly specific diagnosis consisting of high-permeability pulmonary edema, due to any of a number of causes, *and* the inability to adequately oxygenate the patient despite 100% FiO$_2$. Administering 100% oxygen often requires a ventilator in a hospital setting, and arterial blood gas measurements are needed to confirm the diagnosis. The proper classification of acute pulmonary edema is based purely on mechanism—that is, high pressure or high permeability.

Pathophysiology

The underlying pathophysiology and anatomical changes vary between the two types of pulmonary edema. Despite different mechanisms, both result in impairment of gas diffusion, particularly oxygen. In high-pressure (cardiogenic) pulmonary edema (Figure 22-30) the following may occur:

- Ischemia leads to acute failure of the left ventricle.
- Inability of the ventricle to pump blood adequately results in an increase in ventricular pressure.
- Increased ventricular pressure is back-transmitted to the left atrium and then the pulmonary vessels, causing an increase in the pulmonary venous pressure.
- Elevated pulmonary venous pressure results in increased pulmonary capillary hydrostatic pressure.

- The engorged vessels leak fluid into the interstitial space due to the elevated hydrostatic pressure (Starling's mechanism).
- As cough and lymphatic drainage fail to drain the excess fluid, it accumulates in the interstitial space.
- Fluid accumulation causes expansion of the interstitial space that impairs diffusion of gases.
- If the amount of interstitial fluid is significant, alveoli are ruptured by the pressure and fill with fluid.

During high-permeability (noncardiogenic) pulmonary edema, the alveolar-capillary membrane is disrupted by any of the following causes:
- Severe hypotension
- Severe hypoxemia (postdrowning, post–cardiac arrest, severe seizure, prolonged hypoventilation)
- High altitude
- Environmental toxins (e.g., chlorine gas inhalation)
- Septic shock

Because of membrane disruption, fluid leaks into the interstitial space (Figure 22-31).

Widening of the interstitial space by fluid impairs diffusion. Although possible, alveolar filling in high-permeability (noncardiogenic) pulmonary edema is less frequent than in high-pressure (cardiogenic) pulmonary edema.

Assessment Findings

The most common presentation of pulmonary edema, whatever the cause, is an acute onset of shortness of breath. In high-permeability cases, symptoms may develop over a longer period, but an acute onset is still common. For further details on acute cardiogenic pulmonary edema, refer to Chapter 23 (Figure 22-32).

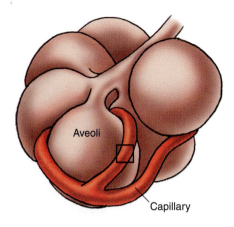

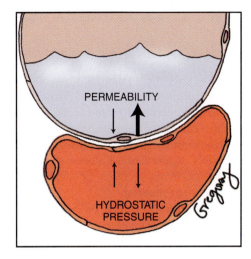

FIGURE 22-31 ▲ Because of membrane disruption, fluid leaks into the interstitial space.

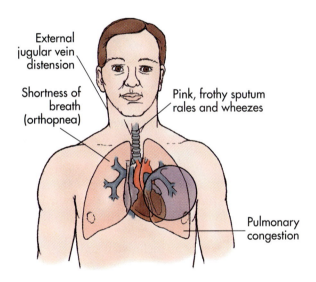

FIGURE 22-32 ▲ **Left-sided congestive heart failure results in a buildup of fluids in the lungs.**

Evaluate the patients history concerning the following factors associated with pulmonary edema:
- Cardiac history
- Chest pain
- Hypoxic episode
- Shock (hypovolemic, septic, neurogenic)
- Chest trauma
- Recent acute inhalation of toxic gases or particles
- Recent ascent to high altitude without acclimatizing

Typically, patients will complain of dyspnea. It may worsen when lying down (orthopnea). Fatigue and reduced exercise capacity are common.

Auscultation of the chest reveals "wet"-sounding lungs, often with diffuse crackles and wheezes. Especially in acute cardiogenic pulmonary edema, noisy lung sounds are often evident without use of a stethoscope. Diagnostic testing may show decreased pulse oximetry values and cardiac dysrhythmias. Signs of myocardial ischemia or stress may also be present on a 12-lead ECG.

Management

Airway and circulatory support form the core treatment approach to *any* patient, regardless of the problem. High-flow oxygen is preferable, but persons in acute pulmonary edema often refuse a mask. The reason is that they are already markedly short of breath; putting a mask over their face may make them feel like they are suffocating. This worsens patient anxiety and causes the release of epinephrine from the patient's adrenal gland. Epinephrine causes the heart to work harder, worsening myocardial function. Therefore unless the patient can be easily to convinced to wear the mask, a nasal cannula should be used initially. However, if a patient's condition is deteriorating, assisted ventilation and intubation as required must be performed.

An IV should be started according to local protocol; the American Heart Association recommends normal saline as the fluid of choice, although the IV flow rate should be kept low. Alternatively, an intermittent device can be placed to avoid the need to provide a continuous infusion of IV fluids but yet allow the administration of medications if indicated (see Chapter 6). The patient should be in an upright position with the legs dangling. Continued reassurance and encouragement will go a long way to benefit the patient.

In case of a suspected environmental toxin, the patient should be removed from the hazard as soon as possible *without* risking your own safety. If high-altitude pulmonary edema is suspected, rapid descent is recommended; this may involve use of aeromedical evacuation in some cases.

PHARMACOLOGICAL MANAGEMENT

The DOT EMT–I curriculum adds the use of nitroglycerin, furosemide, and morphine sulphate for the treatment of high-pressure (cardiogenic) pulmonary edema. These are also discussed in Chapter 23. General information, and commonly administered doses of each drug are listed in the following sections. Specific local protocols should always be followed.

Nitroglycerin—Nitroglycerin dilates both the veins and the arteries. Vasodilation decreases the amount of blood returned to the heart (preload), thus decreasing the amount it must pump out with each stroke. Arterial dilation decreases the workload against which the heart must pump (afterload). Generally, if the patient's systolic blood pressure is greater than 100 mm Hg, then sublingual (one [1] $\frac{1}{150}$-grain tablet) or spray nitroglycerin (one [1] spray) is a first-line drug in cardiogenic pulmonary edema. The dose may be repeated every 5 minutes, up to a limit of three doses, as needed.

Furosemide (Lasix)—Furosemide has several effects in acute pulmonary edema. It vasodilates, causing a decrease in the cardiac preload. In addition, furosemide increases lymphatic flow from the lungs back into the circulatory system, helping drain the lungs of fluid. Finally, the **diuretic** effect causes the kidneys to eliminate the excess fluid from the body. Furosemide is usually given intravenously (initial dose: 20 to 40 milligrams (mg) slow IV push; may be repeated in 10 to 20 minutes as needed) in acute pulmonary edema.

Morphine sulfate (MS)—A narcotic analgesic (painkiller) that also has significant effects on the CNS, causing dilation of both veins and arteries. As with nitroglycerin, both cardiac preload and afterload are reduced, allowing the heart to work more efficiently. MS also allays patient anxiety. It is usually given intravenously (2 mg IV every 5 minutes as needed) in acute pulmonary edema.

PULMONARY THROMBOEMBOLISM

Epidemiology

Pulmonary embolism is the blockage of a pulmonary artery by foreign matter. Usually, the obstruction is due to a piece of a blood clot that has broken away from a pelvic or deep leg vein. The term **thromboembolism**

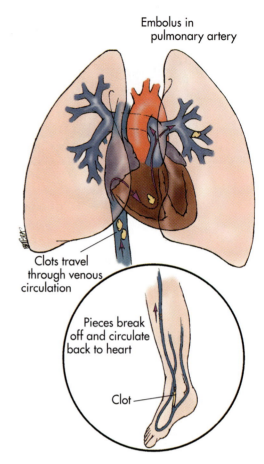

FIGURE 22-33 ▲ Pulmonary embolism is the blockage of a pulmonary artery by foreign matter.

refers to a combination of two processes: the formation of a venous thrombus (clot), followed by a fragment breaking off into the venous circulation (embolus) (Figure 22-33).

Other foreign matter include include fat, amniotic fluid, air, or tumor tissue. Pulmonary emboli are responsible for nearly 50,000 deaths annually in the United States and account for 5% of sudden death cases. Despite these frightening numbers, less than 10% of pulmonary emboli result in death.

> ❗ **HELPFUL HINT**
>
> Pulmonary embolism is common, potentially lethal, and highly underdiagnosed. It is the third most common cause of death in the United States. There are about 650,000 cases annually. Of these, 10% die within 1 hour of the event. Among survivors, the diagnosis is missed in two of three cases.

Risks for pulmonary embolism include the following (Figure 22-34):

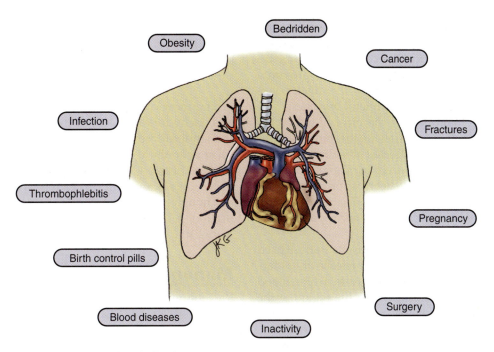

FIGURE 22-34 ▲ Risks for pulmonary embolism.

- *Sedentary lifestyle (prolonged inactivity or being bedridden)*—Pulmonary embolism is common in hospitalized patients and in those who have completed long auto or airplane trips.
- Obesity
- Infection
- *Cancer*—Certain tumors (e.g., kidney, lung) produce substances that make the blood more coagulable ("thicker") and increase the risk of embolism.
- **Thrombophlebitis,** an inflammation of the veins.
- Oral contraceptives (birth control pills).
- *Fracture of a long bone (femur, humerus)*—The source of emboli is fat released from the bone marrow.
- *Pregnancy*—Amniotic fluid embolism may occur during delivery. It is often fatal.
- *Recent surgery*—Patients may remain in the same position on the operating table for several hours, leading to blood clot formation in the veins of the pelvis and legs.
- *Blood diseases*—Rare blood disorders can make a patient's blood more likely to clot.

Pathophysiology

Pulmonary embolism (PE) results in a perfusion disorder—that is, the blood supply to some lung is blocked. The result is that the area is oxygenated but not perfused. Most PEs arise from deep veins in the pelvis and thighs.

Typical development of a PE follows this progression (Figure 22-35):
- Blood flow is altered in the peripheral vein, due to injury to the vein wall, decreased movement of the patient, or other factors that increase the coagulability of the blood.

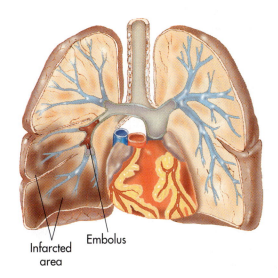

Infarcted area — Embolus

FIGURE 22-35 ▲ Pulmonary embolism is the blockage of a pulmonary artery by foreign matter, such as a thrombus, that usually arises from a peripheral vein, fat, air, or tumor tissue. The blockage obstructs blood supply to the lung tissue. (From Wilson SF: Respiratory disorders, St Louis, 1990, Mosby.)

- Altered blood flow leads to platelet aggregation and activation of the body's coagulation system.
- A thrombosis or clot forms in the deep vein.
- For unknown reasons, pieces of the clot dislodge into the venous circulation and return to the heart as emboli.
- Emboli pass from the right atria through the tricuspid valve to the right ventricle. From there, they transverse the pulmonic valve and lodge in the pulmonary arterial circulation.

- As the clot passes through progressively smaller and smaller branches of the pulmonary circulation, it becomes lodged and a blockage occurs.
- Larger emboli occlude larger, more proximal branches of the pulmonary artery, while smaller ones travel to the smaller, more peripheral branches.
- The lung tissue supplied by the blocked artery becomes ischemic. If circulation to the lung is sufficiently compromised, the affected area dies (infarcts).
- If large pulmonary emboli occlude major branches of the pulmonary arteries, the heart is forced to pump blood against very high pressures. The result is often acute right-sided heart failure (acute cor pulmonale), syncope, shock, or cardiac arrest.
- Occlusion of the artery not only results in decreased blood supply, but also leads to the release of vasoactive substances (e.g., histamine) from white blood cells. This causes bronchospasm in the region of the clot and may be responsible for localized wheezing sometimes heard during the physical examination.

Other materials may obstruct the pulmonary circulation including air, fat, foreign objects (e.g., venous catheters), and amniotic fluid. The process within the lungs is similar, regardless of whether the embolism consists of blood clot, fat, tissue, air, or other foreign matter.

Assessment Findings

Patients with massive pulmonary emboli often experience cardiac arrest or a syncopal spell as the first symptom of the illness. Altered mentation, severe cyanosis, or profound hypotension also suggests the presence of a life-threatening embolus in a proximal location.

Patients with smaller emboli may have the following signs and symptoms:

- Sudden, unexplained onset of chest pain increases in intensity with a deep breath (pleuritic chest pain). The pain may be localized to the area of the chest overlying the involved lung tissue.
- *Respiratory distress and shortness of breath*—The patient's respiratory rate is usually increased, and he or she may hyperventilate.
- Wheezing or coughing up of blood **(hemoptysis)**
- Anxiety
- Hypotension
- Shock

> **HELPFUL HINT**
> - The signs and symptoms of pulmonary embolism are often similar to myocardial infarction or spontaneous pneumothorax.

> **HELPFUL HINT**
> - Pleuritic chest pain is sharp discomfort felt when taking a deep breath.

The most common physical findings are tachypnea and tachycardia. Breath sounds are usually normal, though localized wheezing is heard occasionally. After several hours, a grating sound (pleural friction rub) may be heard. Clinical evidence of deep vein thrombophlebitis is found in less than 50% of patients.

Though pulse oximetry often reveals low oxygen saturation, a normal value does *not* exclude pulmonary embolism.

Management

Prevention plays a strong role in the management of pulmonary emboli. Early ambulation of surgical patients and identification and treatment of predisposing medical disorders, as follows, is also helpful:

- Maintain the patient's airway, ventilate with high-concentration oxygen, and assist breathing if necessary.
- Start an IV lifeline; watch for shock and provide care as necessary.
- Place the patient on a cardiac monitor.
- Transport the patient in a position of comfort using the appropriate mode to the appropriate facility.
- Support the patient psychologically as best as possible.

SPONTANEOUS PNEUMOTHORAX

Spontaneous pneumothorax is a sudden accumulation of air in the pleural space. This condition is due to the rupture of a weak area on the lung surface. As the air enters the pleural space, the lung on the involved side collapses (Figure 22-36). Tension pneumothorax can also develop.

Epidemiology

Spontaneous pneumothorax is a common cause of sudden-onset shortness of breath and chest pain in a young individual. It is more common in men than in women. The incidence is 18 per 100,000 persons.

The most frequent cause of spontaneous pneumothorax is rupture of a congenital defect **(bleb)** on the surface of the lung. A congenital bleb is an air-filled sac that has been present since birth. Young, tall, thin male smokers are most likely to develop pneumothorax from rupture of a congenital bleb.

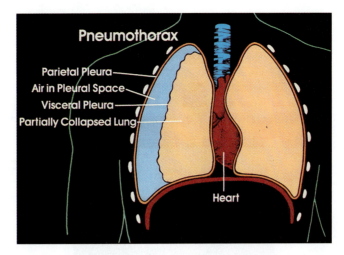

FIGURE 22-36 ▲ A spontaneous pneumothorax is caused by a sudden accumulation of air in the pleural space of the lungs. (From National Association of Emergency Medical Technicians: *Prehospital trauma life support,* St Louis, 1994, Mosby.)

Other less common causes of spontaneous pneumothorax include the following:

- *Menstruation*—Spontaneous pneumothorax associated with menstruation is usually right-sided and occurs in women aged 20-30 years. It is thought to be secondary to the presence of endometrial tissue in the lung or pleura that ruptures after swelling during the menstrual cycle.
- Lung disease involving connective tissues of the lung
- *COPD*—Spontaneous pneumothorax associated with COPD is usually secondary to rupture of defects that have formed from the destruction of normal lung tissue that results from COPD **(bullae).**

Assessment Findings

Patients with spontaneous pneumothorax complain of the sudden onset of sharp chest pain accompanied by shortness of breath. The pain is often localized to the side of the lung involved. Decreased breath sounds are present on the involved side and the patient's respiratory rate is increased. The patient may be coughing and be anxious or agitated.

Often, the patient has only a simple spontaneous pneumothorax. An EMT–I should always, however, be on the watch for development of tension pneumothorax.

The signs and symptoms of **tension pneumothorax** are as follows:

- Increasing respiratory distress
- Weak pulse

- Cyanosis
- Hypotension
- Decreased breath sounds on the same side
- Distended neck veins
- Tracheal deviation away from the side of the pneumothorax. *This is a late sign.*
- *Subcutaneous emphysema*—Crepitus may be felt in the skin of the chest wall overlying the collapsed lung.

Management

Provide the following emergency care for a patient with suspected spontaneous pneumothorax:

- Maintain the patient's airway; give high concentrations of oxygen and assist breathing as necessary.
- Start an IV lifeline.
- Place the patient on a cardiac monitor.
- Transport the patient in the most comfortable position. Some EMS physicians feel that lying with the affected side down is more comfortable for the patient.
- If evidence of tension pneumothorax develops and emergency service personnel are authorized to do so, immediately perform needle decompression as described in Chapter 18 (trauma).

HYPERVENTILATION SYNDROME

Hyperventilation is a respiratory rate greater than that required for normal body function. It is the result of an increased frequency of breathing, an increased

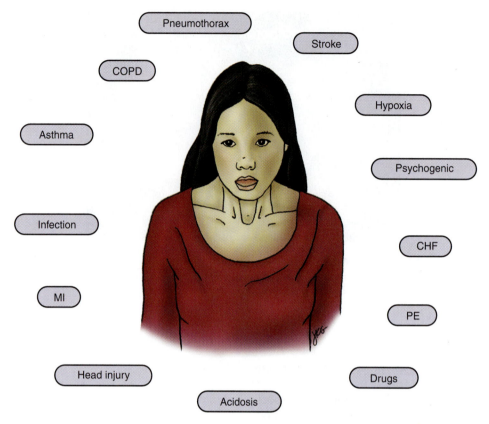

FIGURE 22-37 ▲ Many disease states can result in hyperventilation.

volume of air moved, or both. Hyperventilation causes an excessive intake of oxygen and the excessive elimination of carbon dioxide. Many disease states cause hyperventilation. **Anxiety-hyperventilation syndrome** results in tachypnea without physiologic demand for increased oxygen, leading to respiratory alkalosis.

Pathophysiology

Excessive excretion (blowing off) of carbon dioxide results in low blood levels (hypocapnia), which disturbs the normal blood acid-base balance by increasing the pH. These pH changes can interfere with the normal function of other body systems.

Many disease states can result in hyperventilation. These include the following (Figure 22-37):
- Asthma attack
- COPD
- Myocardial infarction
- Pulmonary embolism
- Spontaneous pneumothorax
- Congestive heart failure
- *Increased metabolism*—Exercise, fever, hyperthyroidism, infection

- *Central nervous system lesions*—Stroke, encephalitis, head injury, meningitis
- Hypoxia
- *Accumulation of metabolic acids in the body*—Kidney failure, diabetic ketoacidosis, alcohol poisoning (methanol, ethanol)
- *Drugs*—Cocaine, amphetamines, aspirin, epinephrine
- *Psychogenic factors*—Acute anxiety or pain

> **! HELPFUL HINT**
> - Many diseases cause patients to hyperventilate. Do not assume that the hyperventilating patient simply has anxiety.

Assessment Findings

Signs and symptoms of hyperventilation include the following:
- *Chest pain*—The pain is usually in the center of the chest and is often described as sharp. The discomfort of hyperventilation may appear similar to myocardial ischemia.
- *Dizziness, faintness*—Although loss of unconsciousness is possible, this is rare.

- Numbness and tingling of the face, fingers, and toes
- Tightness or a lump in the throat
- Spasm of the fingers and toes (carpopedal spasm)
- Altered mental status
- Abnormal lung sounds
- *Tachycardia*—This is a common sign; the patient may complain of palpitations.

Management

The major risk in caring for a patient with hyperventilation is to assume that anxiety is the basis of the symptoms. Many serious and life-threatening medical illnesses can cause hyperventilation. The patient can appear identical to someone with only a simple anxiety attack. A conservative approach demands the assumption that the patient is seriously ill until the case is proven otherwise.

A discarded method of caring for hyperventilation is to have patients breathe into a paper bag. The theory was that having patients breathe their own carbon dioxide increases the level of that gas in the bloodstream, allowing the normal respiratory control mechanisms to bring breathing down to a normal rate and depth. Plugging the portals of an oxygen mask was also used in the past for the same purpose.

> ▶ Rebreathing is no longer an acceptable practice. Many patients who appear to have simple hyperventilation actually have serious illness. Having the patient breathe into a paper bag causes a marked decrease in the available oxygen. Dangerous hypoxia can result.

Use the following guide to care for patients with hyperventilation:
- Assume that there is an underlying medical cause of the hyperventilation.
- Give oxygen, generally 3 to 4 L/min nasal cannula. Follow pulse oximetry.
- If isolated anxiety hyperventilation is suspected, ask the patient to control his or her breathing. Suggest that the patient breathes only when instructed to by EMS personnel or have him or her count to five between breaths. Do not force patients if they have obvious respiratory difficulty.
- Do not have the patient breathe in a paper bag.
- Do not plug the portals of an oxygen mask in an attempt to have a patient recreate carbon dioxide.

- If patients have chest pain, place them on a cardiac monitor and start an IV lifeline.
- Transport to the hospital according to local protocols; provide ongoing psychological support.

> **HELPFUL HINT**
> - Do not use a paper bag or a blocked-off oxygen mask to care for hyperventilation. Give the patient the benefit of the doubt and administer oxygen.

CASE HISTORY FOLLOW-UP ▪▪▪

Mrs. Claypool responds favorably to the treatment. So far, she has received oxygen at 15 L/min via nonrebreather mask, an IV of normal saline delivered at a TKO rate, and an albuterol breathing treatment. Reassessment by EMT–I Morgan reveals the patient has a respiratory rate of 18; a pulse rate of 120; a blood pressure of 128/84; and warm, dry skin. Auscultation of her chest reveals that there is still bilateral wheezing, but she is moving air much better. The ECG monitor reveals sinus tachycardia with occasional PVCs and the pulse oximetry shows a SaO2 of 92%.

As they carry Mrs. Claypool out of the church on the cot, the music and singing start up again. On the way to the hospital Mrs. Claypool, who is breathing a lot easier, tells EMT–I Morgan. "That minister sure gets me worked up, I haven't been singing like that for years." Morgan replies, "I don't know if I would go to his sermon without your pocket inhaler. He seems like he is really good at getting people worked up." "Well, you come again next Sunday and I will show you how its done," Mrs. Claypool tells Morgan. With a slight laugh Morgan responds, "I might just be there."

SUMMARY

- The respiratory system is responsible for filtering, warming, humidifying, and exchanging more than 10,000 L of air per day in an adult. It is divided into the upper and lower respiratory parts.
- Both chronic and acute respiratory problems can present as life-threatening situations.
- Abnormalities of ventilation, diffusion, perfusion, or a combination can lead to respiratory problems.
- Because pulmonary complaints may be associated with many toxin exposures, assure a safe environment for all EMS personnel before initiating patient contact.
- The major focus of the *initial assessment* is recognition of life-threatening conditions.

- The *focused history and physical examination* is aimed at the patient's specific respiratory complaints. Previous respiratory history and use of medications are particularly important to determine.
- Specific conditions may be difficult to diagnose in the field. Remember that maintenance of airway, breathing, and circulation always form the basis of excellent patient care.

  Common respiratory problems include the following:
- *Obstructive airway disease*—The underlying common denominator in all obstructive conditions is decreased expiratory airflow due to obstruction of the bronchioles and air trapping. Although many things can precipitate obstructive lung disease, the most common are cigarette smoke and allergen exposure. Treatment centers around airway management and treatment of bronchospasm, often with inhaled beta-2 agonist drugs (e.g., albuterol).
- *Pneumonia*—A group of diseases resulting in acute inflammation of the lungs, pneumonia is usually caused by either bacterial or viral infection. Airway maintenance and IV hydration form the basis of emergency care.
- *Pulmonary edema*—A filling of the lungs with fluid in the interstitial spaces, the alveoli, or both, pulmonary edema is not a disease in itself, but rather a pathophysiological condition. It is classified as either high pressure or high permeability. The result in both types of pulmonary edema is a diffusion defect—that is, lung tissue is distended by fluid, impairing gas exchange (primarily oxygen). General treatment involves maintenance of the airway, breathing, and circulation. Specific pharmacological treatment by the EMT–I for cardiogenic pulmonary edema encompasses nitroglycerin, furosemide, and morphine sulphate.
- *Pulmonary thromboembolism*—Pulmonary embolism is the blockage of a pulmonary artery by foreign matter. Usually, pulmonary emboli are due to a piece of a blood clot that has broken away from a pelvic or deep leg vein (thromboembolism). The most common underlying causes are patient inactivity (sedentary lifestyle or being bedridden). Signs and symptoms vary from sudden death to cough with pleuritic chest pain. Prehospital treatment consists of careful attention to the airway, breathing, and circulation and appropriate transport to the appropriate facility.

• *Spontaneous pneumothorax*—A sudden accumulation of air in the pleural space. This condition is due to the rupture of a weak area ("bleb") on the lung surface. As the air enters the pleural space, the lung on the involved side collapses. Spontaneous pneumothorax is most common in young, tall, and thin male smokers. Symptoms are sudden onset of shortness of breath and pleuritic chest pain. Physical examination reveals decreased breath sounds on the involved side and an increased respiratory rate. Prehospital treatment consists of careful attention to the airway, breathing, and circulation and appropriate transport to the appropriate facility. If a tension pneumothorax develops, and EMS personnel are authorized to do so, needle decompression should be immediately performed.

• *Hyperventilation syndrome*—Hyperventilation is a respiratory rate greater than that required for normal body function. It is the result of an increased frequency of breathing, an increased volume of air moved, or both. Anxiety-hyperventilation syndrome results in tachypnea without physiological demand for increased oxygen, leading to respiratory alkalosis. Many serious and life-threatening medical illnesses can cause hyperventilation. Give the patient the benefit of the doubt and administer oxygen. Having the patient breathe into a paper bag causes a marked decrease in the available oxygen. Dangerous hypoxia can result.

23 Cardiovascular Emergencies

CASE HISTORY

At 2:21 PM EMT–Is Adams and Graham are dispatched to 832-A Margaret Street for a "patient with chest pain." The EMT–Is had taken care of Mr. Molino, age 73 years, several times previously. Three months ago he had a acute myocardial infarction (MI), and he has had several episodes of congestive heart failure (CHF) since that time.

The EMT–Is arrive at the patient's house 9 minutes later and find him sitting in his living room chair. "Hi, Mr. Molino, remember us? We're the crew that came here before for you," EMT–I Adams says.

The patient looks up at the EMT–Is and nods his head with recognition, but holds his fist over his chest and says, "I can't catch my breath."

"How long have you had the pain this time?" EMT–I Adams asks.

"About a half hour. I took two nitro pills. They aren't working," he responds.

EMT–I Adams gives the patient oxygen and attaches the electrocardiographic (ECG) leads while EMT–I Graham takes the patient's blood pressure. EMT–I Adams prepares to start an intravenous (IV) line of normal saline while his partner takes the patient's vital signs.

LEARNING OBJECTIVES

CHAPTER GOAL

Upon completion of this chapter, the EMT-Intermediate will be able to use assessment findings to formulate a field impression, as well as implement and evaluate a management plan for the patient experiencing a cardiac emergency.

Cognitive Objectives

As an EMT-Intermediate you should be able to do the following:

- Describe the incidence, morbidity, and mortality of cardiovascular disease.
- Discuss prevention strategies that may reduce morbidity and mortality of cardiovascular disease.
- Identify the risk factors most predisposing to coronary artery disease.
- Identify and describe the components of the focused history as it relates to the patient with cardiovascular compromise.
- Explain and defend the purpose for electrocardiographic (ECG) monitoring.
- Describe how ECG waveforms are produced.

- Correlate the electrophysiological and hemodynamic events occurring throughout the entire cardiac cycle with the various ECG waveforms, segments, and intervals.
- Identify how heart rates may be determined from ECG recordings.
- List the limitations to the ECG.
- Describe a systematic approach to the analysis and interpretation of cardiac dysrhythmias.
- Explain how to confirm ventricular fibrillation and asystole using the three-lead ECG.
- Define the term *defibrillation.*
- List the clinical indications for defibrillation.
- Identify the specific mechanical, pharmacological, and electrical therapeutic interventions for patients with dysrhythmias causing compromise.
- List the clinical indications for an implanted defibrillation device.
- Define the terms *angina pectoris* and *myocardial infarction (MI).*
- List other clinical conditions that may mimic signs and symptoms of angina pectoris and MI.
- List the mechanisms by which MI may be produced by traumatic and nontraumatic events.
- List and describe the assessment parameters to be evaluated in a patient with chest pain.
- Identify what is meant by the OPQRST of chest pain assessment.
- List and describe the initial assessment parameters to be evaluated in a patient with chest pain that may be myocardial in origin.
- Identify the anticipated clinical presentation of a patient with chest pain that may be angina pectoris or MI.
- On the basis of the pathophysiology and clinical evaluation of the patient with chest pain, list the anticipated clinical problems according to their life-threatening potential.
- Describe the pharmacological agents available to the EMT–I for use in the management of dysrhythmias and cardiovascular emergencies.
- Describe the "window of opportunity" as it pertains to reperfusion of myocardial injury or infarction.
- Develop, execute, and evaluate a treatment plan based on the field impression for the patient with chest pain that may be indicative of angina or MI.
- Define the terms *congestive heart failure (CHF)* and *pulmonary edema.*
- Define the cardiac and noncardiac causes and terminology associated with CHF and pulmonary edema.
- Describe the early and late signs and symptoms of CHF.
- Explain the clinical significance of paroxysmal nocturnal dyspnea.
- List and describe the pharmacological agents available to the EMT–I for use in the management of a patient with cardiac compromise.
- Define the term *hypertensive emergency.*
- Describe the clinical features of the patient in a hypertensive emergency.
- List the interventions prescribed for the patient with a hypertensive emergency.
- Define the term *cardiogenic shock.*
- Identify the clinical criteria for cardiogenic shock.
- Define the term *cardiac arrest.*
- Describe the incidence, morbidity, and mortality of cardiac arrest.

Continued on p. 614

LEARNING OBJECTIVES—cont'd

- Define the term *resuscitation*.
- Identify local protocols dictating circumstances and situations where resuscitation efforts would not be initiated.
- Identify local protocols dictating circumstances and situations where resuscitation efforts would be discontinued.
- Identify the critical actions necessary in caring for the patient in cardiac arrest.
- Synthesize the patient history and assessment findings to form a field impression of the patient with chest pain and cardiac dysrhythmias that may be indicative of a cardiac emergency.

Affective Objectives

As an EMT-Intermediate you should be able to do the following:

- Value the sense of urgency for initial assessment and intervention as it contributes to the treatment plan for the patient experiencing a cardiac emergency.
- Defend patient situations where ECG rhythm analysis is indicated.
- Value and defend the sense of urgency necessary to protect the "window of opportunity" for reperfusion in the patient with chest pain and dysrhythmias that may be indicative of angina or MI.
- Value and defend the urgency in rapid determination and rapid intervention of patients in cardiac arrest.

Psychomotor Objectives

As an EMT-Intermediate you should be able to do the following:

- Demonstrate how to set and adjust the ECG monitor settings to varying patient situations.
- Demonstrate a working knowledge of various ECG lead systems.
- Demonstrate how to record an ECG.
- Perform, document, and communicate a cardiovascular assessment.
- Set up and apply a transcutaneous pacing system.
- Given the model of a patient with signs and symptoms of heart failure, position the patient to afford comfort and relief.
- Demonstrate satisfactory performance of psychomotor skills of basic and advanced life support techniques according to the current American Heart Association Standards and Guidelines, including cardiopulmonary resuscitation, defibrillation, and transcutaneous pacing
- Complete a communication patch with medical direction and law enforcement for termination of resuscitation efforts.
- Demonstrate how to evaluate major peripheral arterial pulses.

Key Terms—cont'd

Nitroglycerin	Complexes (PVCs)	Circulation (ROSC)	Tricuspid Valve
Norepinephrine	Procainamide	Sinus Arrhythmia	U Wave
Normal Sinus Rhythm (NSR)	Progressive Angina	Sinus/Sinoatrial (SA) Node	Unstable Angina
Orthopnea	Pulmonary Circulation	ST Segment	Vagal Maneuvers
P Wave	Pulmonary (Semilunar) Valve	Stable Angina	Vasopressin
Paroxysmal Nocturnal Dyspnea (PND)	Pulseless Electrical Activity (PEA)	Starling's Law of the Heart	Veins
Pericardium	Purkinje's Fibers	Stroke Volume	Ventricles
Polarized	QRS Complex	Survival	Ventricular Conduction Disturbances
PR Segment	Relative Refractory Period	Systemic Circulation	
Preexcitation Syndromes	Repolarization	Systole	Ventricular Fibrillation (VF)
Preinfarction Angina	Resuscitation	Tachycardia	Ventricular Tachycardia (VT)
Preload	Retractions	Threshold	Verapamil
Premature Ventricular	Return of Spontaneous	Torsade de Pointes	
		Transcutaneous Pacing (TCP)	

INTRODUCTION

Cardiovascular disease is a common cause of medical problems. Patients may present with symptoms ranging from chest pain to sudden collapse. The EMT–Intermediate (EMT–I) should be familiar with the most important causes of cardiovascular emergencies: angina, heart attack (acute myocardial infarction), congestive heart failure, pulmonary edema, cardiogenic shock, dysrhythmias, hypertensive emergency, and cardiac arrest. In the absence of any obvious trauma, the EMT–I should assume that a patient with chest pain has myocardial ischemia until proven otherwise. A cardinal point is to always treat the patient, *not* the monitor. Even if the cardiac monitor displays a dysrhythmia, the astute EMT–I should always evaluate the clinical status of the patient *before* reaching any conclusions or administering treatment.

EPIDEMIOLOGY

Since 1900 cardiovascular disease (CVD) has been the number 1 killer in the United States every year but 1918. More than 2600 Americans die each day of CVD—an average of one death every 33 seconds. According to current estimates, 59,700,000 Americans have one or more types of CVD. These include high blood pressure, coronary heart disease, acute myocardial infarction (AMI), angina pectoris, stroke, rheumatic heart disease, congenital cardiovascular defects, and congestive heart failure (CHF). One in five men and women together has some form of CVD. Major CVD before age 60 occurs in 1 in 3 men; the odds for women are 1 in 10.

Ischemic heart disease (IHD) includes coronary heart disease **(coronary artery disease)**, AMI, angina pectoris, and CHF (due to coronary artery disease) (Box 23-1). Between 1963 and 1995 there was a 50% decrease in the death rate from IHD in the United States. The basis for this trend likely reflects a combination of the following:
- Better prevention efforts, including dietary changes, decreased cigarette smoking, control of hypertension (high blood pressure)
- Improved methods of treatment (e.g., thrombolytic therapy [early reperfusion] for AMI—see later discussion)
- Improved public education with earlier recognition of symptoms
- Prevention of recurrences in patients with previous cardiac ischemic events

Despite improvements in the outcome, IHD remains a major public health challenge. About every 29 seconds an American will suffer a coronary event. This year, an estimated 1,100,000 Americans will have a new or recurrent coronary attack (defined as MI or fatal IHD). About 650,000 of these will be first attacks, and 450,000 will be recurrent attacks. More than 40% of the people who experience a heart attack in a given year will die of it. About 225,000 people a year die of IHD without being hospitalized. Many of these are sudden deaths caused by cardiac arrest, usually resulting from ventricular fibrillation.[1]

Risk Factors

Numerous risk factors that predispose a person to IHD have been identified. These include the following (Box 23-2):
- *Age*—Age is a dominant influence. Although not clinically evident until middle age or later, atherosclerosis ("hardening of the arteries"; in the heart, coronary artery disease) is a slowly progressive condition that begins in childhood. Death rates rise with each decade of life. Between age 40 and age 60 there is a fivefold increase in the rate of AMI (heart attack).
- *Family history*—There is a well-established familial predisposition to IHD. It may relate to familial tendencies toward other risk factors, such as hypertension or diabetes or may be completely independent.
- *Hypertension*—**Hypertension** is a major risk factor, especially after age 45. Men ages 45 to 62 whose blood pressure exceeds 170/95 mm Hg have more than a fivefold greater risk of IHD.
- *Lipids*—**Hypercholesterolemia** (elevated serum cholesterol levels) is a far greater risk than hypertriglyceridemia (elevated triglycerides). The main component of the total serum cholesterol associated with increased risk is low-density lipoprotein (LDL) cholesterol ("bad cholesterol"). High-density lipoprotein

---

BOX 23-1

ISCHEMIC HEART DISEASE

Ischemic heart disease includes the following:
- Coronary heart disease (coronary artery disease)
- Acute myocardial infarction
- Angina
- Congestive heart failure
- Acute pulmonary edema

BOX 23-2

MAJOR RISK FACTORS FOR ISCHEMIC HEART DISEASE

- Age
- Family history
- Hypertension
- Sex
- Hypercholesterolemia
- Smoking
- Diabetes mellitus

(HDL) cholesterol ("good cholesterol") levels, on the other hand, are inversely associated with risk—higher HDL levels are protective. LDL levels reflect cholesterol that is deposited into the walls of the blood vessels, leading to atherosclerosis. HDL levels represent cholesterol that is *removed* from the walls of the vessels, thus *lessening* the degree of atherosclerosis.

In adults, total cholesterol levels of 240 mg/dL or higher are considered high. Levels from 200 to 239 mg/dL are considered borderline high. The risk of AMI in both men and women is highest at lower HDL cholesterol levels and higher total cholesterol levels. However, those with lower levels of HDL cholesterol (37 mg/dL or lower in men and 47 mg/dL or lower in women) are at a high risk regardless of their total cholesterol level. Conversely, those with high levels of total cholesterol have lower risks of AMI when accompanied by higher levels of HDL cholesterol (53 mg/dL or greater in men and 67 mg/dL or greater in women). This suggests the importance of screening for both total and HDL cholesterol levels in adults.[1]

- *Sex*—Men are far more prone to IHD than are women. IHD is uncommon in premenopausal women unless they have diabetes, severe hypertension, or some form of hyperlipidemia (elevated cholesterol, triglycerides, or both). Following menopause the gap narrows, and the risks are similar after ages 60 to 70. Postmenopausal hormone replacement therapy offers women some protection, however.
- *Smoking*—This is a well-established risk. Smoking one or more packs of cigarettes per day for several years increases a person's risk of death from IHD up to 200%. About one in five deaths from CVD is attributable to smoking. About 37,000 to 40,000 nonsmokers die each year of IHD as a result of exposure to environmental tobacco smoke. Cessation of smoking decreases the increased risk by 50% within 1 to 5 years after stopping.
- *Diabetes mellitus*—Diabetes accelerates atherosclerosis and is associated with a marked increased in the risk of IHD. The incidence of AMI in persons with diabetes is twice as high as in nondiabetic persons.

Other factors have been associated with an increased risk of IHD, but to a lesser degree. These include the following:
- Diet
- Obesity
- Oral contraceptive use
- Sedentary living
- Personality type
- Psychosocial tension

The risk factor of obesity is related to sedentary living. Thirty-three percent of overweight men and 41% of overweight women are not physically active during their leisure time. The relative risk of coronary heart disease associated with lack of physical activity ranges from 1.5 to 2.4, an increase in risk comparable to that observed for high blood cholesterol, high blood pressure, or cigarette smoking. According to the American Heart Association, as many as 250,000 deaths per year in the United States (about 12% of total deaths) are attributed to a lack of regular physical activity.

ANATOMY AND PHYSIOLOGY REVIEW

Heart

The *heart* is a muscular, cone-shaped organ, and its function is to pump blood throughout the body. It is located behind the sternum (breastbone) and is about the size of a closed fist. Roughly two thirds of the heart lies in the left side of the chest cavity. Functionally, the heart is divided into right and left sides, which are separated by a thick wall called the *interventricular septum*. The heart muscle is referred to as the **myocardium.** The inner lining cells of the heart form the *endocardium*.

Surrounding the heart is a thick set of two membranes, the **pericardium.** Together, these membranes form the pericardial sac around the heart. The inner portion of the pericardial membrane is the *visceral pericardium*, which lies close to the outside of the heart, or **epicardium.** The outside pericardial membrane is the *parietal pericardium*. Normally, the pericardial sac contains only a small amount of clear *serous* ("like serum") lubricating fluid, which allows the heart to contract and expand smoothly within the chest cavity.

The normal human heart consists of two upper chambers (the **atria**) and two lower chambers (the **ventricles**). The atria receive blood returned to the heart from other parts of the body, and the ventricles pump blood out of the heart. The atria and ventricles are separated by valves that prevent backward flow of blood. Other valves are located between the ventricles and the arteries into which they pump blood.

Deoxygenated blood returns to the *right atrium* via the *superior* and *inferior vena cava*, the largest veins in the body. It passes through the **tricuspid valve** into the *right ventricle*, situated inferiorly. Blood then flows from the right ventricle through the **pulmonary (semilunar) valve** into the *main pulmonary artery*. This vessel branches, taking blood to both the left and right lungs. Blood is oxygenated in the lungs and returned to the *left atrium* via the pulmonary veins. Blood then transverses the **mitral (bicuspid) valve** into the *left ventricle*. It is then pumped through the **aortic (semilunar) valve** into the aorta (Figure 23-1).

CARDIAC CYCLE

The **cardiac cycle** is the repetitive pumping process of blood that begins with the onset of cardiac muscle contraction and ends with the beginning of the next contraction. Myocardial contraction leads to pressure changes within cardiac chambers, causing blood movement. Blood moves from areas of high pressure to areas of low pressure.

Contraction of the atria and ventricles, with concomitant pumping of blood vessels, is known as **systole.** The *systolic blood pressure* is the pressure within the arteries during this time. **Diastole** is the relaxation phase. It is during this time that the heart receives most of its blood supply from the coronary arteries. Thus *diastolic blood pressure* not only reflects the pressure in the heart during the relaxation phase but is an indication of myocardial perfusion (see Figure 23-1).

CARDIAC OUTPUT

The amount of blood pumped through the circulatory system in 1 minute is referred to as the **cardiac output.** It is expressed in liters per minute. The cardiac output equals the heart rate multiplied by the **stroke volume,** or amount of blood (volume) pumped with each heartbeat:

Cardiac output = Stroke volume × Heart rate

Factors that influence the heart rate, the stroke volume, or both, will affect cardiac output and thus tissue oxygen delivery (perfusion).

To a point, increased venous return to the heart stretches the ventricles, leading to increased cardiac contractility. This relationship was first described by the British physiologist Dr. E.H. Starling and has become known as **Starling's law of the heart.** Starling noted that if a muscle is stretched a little bit before it is stimulated to contract, it contracts harder. So if the heart is stretched, the muscle contracts harder. This is a *normal defense mechanism.* The amount of blood returning to the right atrium varies somewhat from minute to minute, yet the normal heart continues to pump out the same *percentage* of blood returned. This is called the **ejection fraction.** If more blood returns to the heart, rather than having it back up into the veins, the stretched heart pumps harder. The result is that more blood is pumped with each contraction, yet the ejection fraction remains unchanged (the amount of blood pumped out increases, but so does the amount returned). It is this relationship that maintains normal cardiac output when a person changes positions, coughs, breathes, or moves.

Vascular System and Circulation

Arteries are blood vessels that carry blood away from the heart to the body. **Veins** transport blood from the body back to the heart. Arteries decrease in size as they move away from the heart, branching into many small

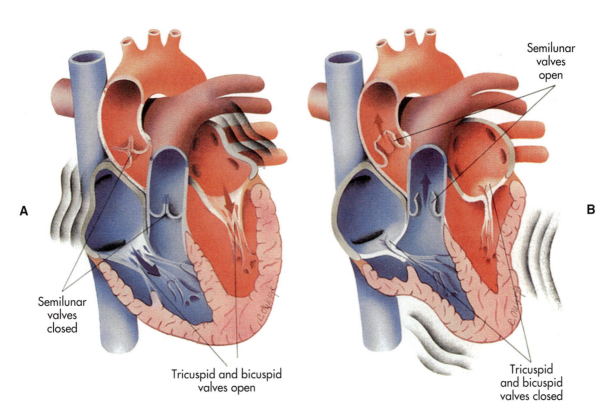

FIGURE 23-1 ▲ Heart action. **A,** During diastole the heart fills with blood. **B,** During systole the heart contracts. (From Thibodeau GA: *Structure and function of the human body,* ed 11, St Louis, 2000, Mosby.)

arterioles. Arterioles then divide many times until they form **capillaries.** Capillaries are microscopic thin-walled vessels through which oxygen, carbon dioxide, and other nutrients and waste products are exchanged.

To return deoxygenated ("used") blood to the heart, groups of capillaries gradually enlarge to form *venules.* Venules then merge together, forming larger and larger veins. Eventually, the veins merge together into the immense *superior vena cava* and *inferior vena cava,* which empty into the *right atrium.*

The total resistance within the arteriolar bed determines the **afterload,** or workload against which the heart must pump. The capacitance within the venules gives rise to the **preload,** or venous return to the heart. Essentially, the preload is the amount of blood that the heart must pump out. It is determined by the patient's intravascular volume status, gravity (patient position), and a number of nervous system–related factors.

Deoxygenated blood returned to the right atrium from the superior and inferior vena cava passes through the tricuspid valve into the right ventricle. From here, it is pumped through the pulmonary valve into the pulmonary artery. This is the beginning of the **pulmonary circulation,** which is designed to transport deoxygenated blood through the lungs, oxygenate it, and return it back to the left side of the heart so that the left ventricle may pump it out to the body via the **systemic circulation.**

The main pulmonary artery branches to each lung. In the lungs the blood is oxygenated and waste products are removed. Freshly oxygenated blood is returned to the left atrium via the pulmonary veins. Blood then flows into the left ventricle, which pumps the oxygenated blood through the aorta and then to the entire body. The aorta consists of three distinct portions: ascending, thoracic, and abdominal.

CORONARY CIRCULATION

The heart receives most of its blood supply directly from the **coronary circulation.** The first branches of the aorta, immediately as it leaves the heart, are the *right* and *left main coronary arteries.* These then branch into several smaller divisions, each of which supplies a particular portion of the myocardium. The major branches of the main coronary arteries are as follows (see Figure 4-42):

- *Right main coronary artery*—Consists of the nodal artery (supplies the sinoatrial node), the descending right artery (supplies the anterior right ventricle), and the posterior descending artery (supplies the posterior heart wall).
- *Left main coronary artery*—Consists of the left anterior descending artery (supplies the anterior wall of the left ventricle), the diagonal artery (usually supplies the lateral left ventricular wall), and the circumflex

artery (usually supplies the superior left ventricle).

The blood supply to the atrioventricular node is variable. In about 60% of persons, it arises from the right side. Deoxygenated venous blood from the heart drains into five different coronary veins that empty into the right atrium via the coronary sinus.

CARDIAC CONDUCTION PATHWAY

Contraction of myocardial tissue is initiated within the heart itself in a group of electrical tissues called the **sinus** or **sinoatrial (SA) node.** The electrical impulse then goes through the cardiac conduction system, which is a complex grouping of specialized tissues that form a network of connections, much like an electrical circuit, throughout the heart. This network carries the electrical nerve impulse that causes the heart muscle to contract.

The initial electrical impulse begins high in the right atrium, in the SA node. It travels through the atria via *intraatrial pathways* to the **atrioventricular (AV) node.** The stimulus then passes into the **bundle of His,** where the conduction system divides into two portions: the *right bundle branch* and the *left bundle branch.* The left bundle branch divides further into the *left anterior fascicle* and the *left posterior fascicle.* These fibers spread out to their respective sides of the heart. Finally, very small **Purkinje's fibers** take the current from the bundle branches to the individual myocardial cells. Normal depolarization of the myocardium progresses from atria to ventricles in an orderly fashion (see Figure 4-45).

INHERENT RATES AND BACKUP PACEMAKERS

Although the SA node is the primary pacemaker site, other cardiac cells can act as a "fail-safe" mechanism for initiating electrical impulses. The "backup" (intrinsic) pacemakers are arranged in cascade fashion—the farther from the SA node, the slower the intrinsic firing rate. In order, the location of cells with pacemaker capabilities and rates of spontaneous discharge are as follows (Figure 23-2):

1. SA node (60 to 100 beats per minute)
2. AV junctional tissue (40 to 60 beats per minute)
3. Ventricles, including the bundle branches and Purkinje's fibers (20 to 40 beats per minute)

ELECTROPHYSIOLOGY

Myocardial cells possess four unique characteristics:

- **Automaticity**—The ability to self-generate electrical activity (action potential) without the need for extraneous nerve stimulation.
- **Excitability**—The ability to respond to an appropriate electrical stimulus.

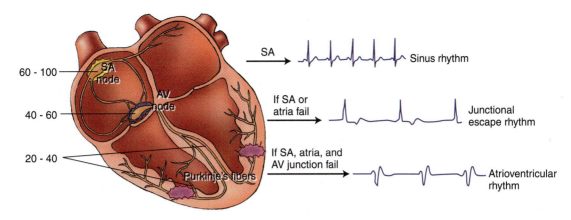

FIGURE 23-2 ▲ Inherent pacemaker rates of the heart.

- **Conductivity**—The ability to transmit an appropriate electrical stimulus from cell to cell throughout the myocardium.
- **Contractility**—The ability of the myocardial cell to contract when stimulated by an appropriate electrical stimulus.

The interior of the heart cell (myocyte) is negatively charged (−90mV) during the resting (*nondepolarized*) phase. This is referred to as the *resting membrane potential (RMP)*. When depolarization begins, sodium, calcium, and potassium ions move from their "resting" locations in and out of the cell. The net result is that the interior of the myocyte becomes more positively charged. When a certain level, or **threshold,** is reached, depolarization of the entire cell occurs. After a period of time, each cell returns back to the resting state (repolarizes), again as a result of the movement of sodium, calcium, and potassium, waiting for the next stimulus (Figure 23-3).

The term for the electrical process of depolarization and repolarization is **action potential** (Figures 23-4 and 23-5). As one cell is depolarized, it chemically passes the signal to the next one, causing similar changes to occur, and the "wave of depolarization" (followed by repolarization) progresses through the heart.

During the repolarization phase, the heart is less amenable to receiving new electrical stimuli. During early repolarization, there is a time when *no* stimulus, no matter how strong, will depolarize the myocyte. This is the **absolute refractory period.** A sufficiently strong stimulus, however, *will* depolarize the myocardium during the **relative refractory period.**

REGULATION OF HEART FUNCTION

Control of the heart rate (**chronotropic state**), rate of electrical conduction (**dromotropic state**) Box 23-3, and strength of contraction (**inotropic state**) comes partially from the brain (via the autonomic nervous system), from hormones of the endocrine system, and

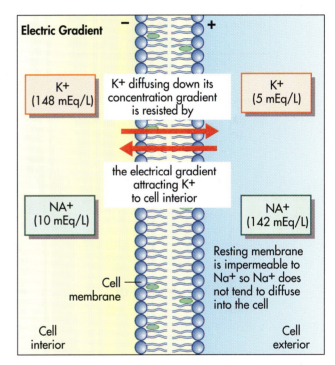

FIGURE 23-3 ▲ At equilibrium (resting conditions), the tendency for potassium ions to diffuse out of the cell is opposed by the potential difference (electrical gradient) across the cell membrane. Because the resting membrane is not permeable to sodium ions, sodium ions do not tend to diffuse into the cell. (Rusty Jones from Sanders MJ: *Mosby's paramedic textbook,* ed 2, St Louis, 2000, Mosby.)

from the heart tissue. Receptors in the blood vessels, kidneys, brain, and heart constantly monitor body homeostasis. **Baroreceptors** respond to changes in pressure, usually within the heart or the main arteries. **Chemoreceptors** sense changes in the chemical composition of the blood. If abnormalities are sensed, nerve signals are transmitted to appropriate target organs, leading to release of hormones or neurotransmit-

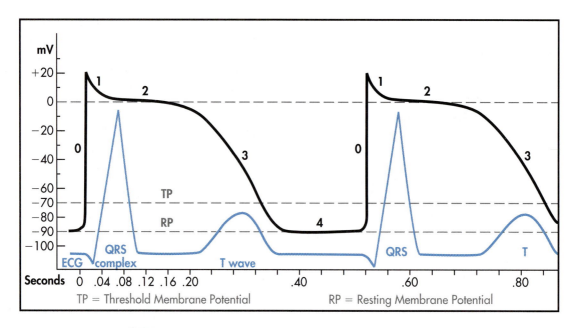

FIGURE 23-4 ▲ Cardiac action potential of myocardial cells.

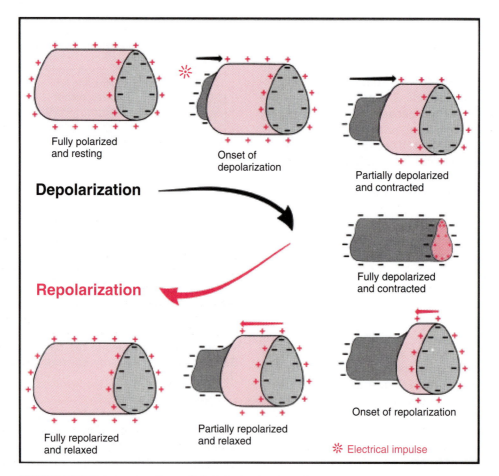

FIGURE 23-5 ▲ Cardiac cell depolarization/repolarization. (From Huszar R: *Basic dysrhythmias,* ed 2, St Louis, 1994, Mosby.)

ters to rectify the situation. Once conditions normalize, the receptors stop firing and the signals cease.

Often, stimulation of receptors leads to activation of either the parasympathetic or the sympathetic branches of the autonomic nervous system. These affect both the heart rate and the strength of heart muscle contraction (**contractility**). Parasympathetic stimulation slows the heart rate, primarily by affecting the AV node. Sympathetic stimulation has several potential effects, depending on which nerve receptor is stimulated:

- **Alpha effects**—Stimulation of alpha receptors leads to vasoconstriction.
- **Beta effects**—Stimulation of beta receptors leads to increased heart rate, cardiac conduction, and contractility (increased inotropic, dromotropic, and chronotropic states).

Epinephrine and **norepinephrine** are naturally occurring hormones that may also be given as cardiac drugs. Epinephrine has a greater stimulatory effect on beta receptors, whereas norepinephrine has predominant alpha stimulatory actions.

For example, if a patient is bleeding, baroreceptors sense abnormally low blood volume. Although several different body responses occur at once, a major one is the release of epinephrine and norepinephrine from the adrenal glands. These cause sympathetic (adrenergic) stimulation, resulting in an increased heart rate, as well as increased contractility. On the other hand, simple fainting often results because of parasympathetic stimulation leading to a slow heart rate (**bradycardia**).

INITIAL CARDIOVASCULAR ASSESSMENT

During the initial assessment, after ensuring your own safety, pay particular attention to the patient's level of consciousness and the ABCs (airway, breathing, and circulation):

- *Level of consciousness*—As a rule, persons who are alert and responsive are in better condition than those who are either dizzy or unresponsive. However, the fact that a person is "A&O × 3"does not necessarily mean that "all is well." Most patients with potentially life-threatening problems (e.g., AMI) have a normal level of consciousness.
- *Airway*—As always, rapidly assess the patient's airway, ensuring that it is patent. Note and clear debris

and blood, if present. The presence of pink-tinged, frothy sputum may suggest acute pulmonary edema.

- *Breathing*—If breathing is absent, immediately begin appropriate resuscitative measures. If breathing is present, rapidly determine the rate and depth, as well as the adequacy. Note the patient's respiratory effort—is he or she breathing calmly or working hard to breathe? Note the presence of extraneous breath sounds, either audible to the "naked" ear or with the stethoscope. For example, wheezing that is easy to hear even without a stethoscope is likely to be more severe than if a stethoscope is required.
- *Circulation*—Assessment of the circulation involves three phases (pulse, skin, and blood pressure). First, check the pulse. If absent, immediately begin cardiopulmonary resuscitation (CPR) and apply electrocardiographic (ECG) monitoring (automated external defibrillator or standard defibrillator-monitor, according to local protocols). If the pulse is present, note the rate and quality. Ensure that pulses are equal and symmetrical (carotids, brachials, radials, femorals, pedals). If required by local protocols, auscultate the heart to obtain an apical pulse rate.

Evaluate the skin in terms of color, temperature, moisture, turgor, mobility, and the presence of edema. Finally, determine the patient's blood pressure.

FOCUSED HISTORY

Obtain a focused history using the SAMPLE acronym:
 S—Signs and symptoms
 A—Allergies
 M—Medications
 P—Pertinent past medical history
 L—Last oral intake, fluid or solid
 E—Events leading to the present situation

The most common symptom of cardiac problems is chest pain. Cardiac chest pain typically is described as a squeezing, dull pressure often radiating (moving) down the arms or to the jaw. The acronym OPQRST should be used to ask questions concerning chest pain:

O—Onset; what was the patient doing when the pain started? Was the patient sitting, sleeping, or exercising? Was there a period of emotional distress (such as a fight or the receipt of bad news)? Has the patient ever had pain like this before?

P—Provocation; what makes the pain better or worse? What effect does breathing or movement have on the pain? Is the pain exertional, nonexertional, or a combination of the two?

Q—Quality; what does the pain feel like? Is it dull, aching, sharp, pressing, or constricting? Is the patient able to describe the pain using a common metaphor, such as pressure "like an elephant is standing on my chest" or like a "hot knife is going through me"?

R—Radiation/relief; does the pain go anywhere? Does it radiate to the neck, jaw, teeth, back, arms, or legs?

Does anything make the pain better (e.g., nitroglycerin, rest)?

S—Severity; how bad is the pain? On a scale of 0 to 10 (0 = no pain, 10 = the worst pain possible), how does the patient rate the discomfort?

T—Time; how long has the pain been present? Has it been continuous, or does it come and go? What is the pain like now, compared with when it started?

Atypical Cardiac Pain

Pain is not always felt in the chest. Quite commonly, persons with angina or AMI have discomfort in the epigastrium (pit of the stomach), jaw, arm, or shoulder. They may actually complain of indigestion as the first symptom of a heart attack. Any person with pain in the anterior portion of the body from the umbilicus (navel) to the jaw should be assumed to have cardiac problems until proven otherwise (Box 23-4). Diabetic and elderly patients often present with atypical cardiac pain.

Other signs and symptoms may accompany cardiac chest pain or by themselves may indicate possible cardiac disease:

- *Sweating (diaphoresis)*—The sudden onset of profuse sweating without preceding heavy activity can indicate a cardiac problem.
- *Breathing difficulty (dyspnea)*—An underlying heart or respiratory condition should be suspected in any person with shortness of breath. Important factors to determine include whether the dyspnea is continuous or intermittent, exertional or not. Is it worse or only present with lying down **(orthopnea)?** Has the patient been awakened at night with severe shortness of breath **(paroxysmal nocturnal dyspnea [PND])?** Either of these findings suggests that the patient has CHF, although he or she may also have other cardiovascular problems. Finally, determine whether or not the patient has had a cough. If so, was it dry or productive? If productive, what was produced? Were the secretions frothy or bloody?

- *Anxiety and irritability*—Patients who are uncomfortable for any reason, and especially those who are hypoxic, will feel anxious. By itself, the presence of anxiety or irritability does not necessarily indicate a cardiac condition, but it often is found in combination with other signs and symptoms noted in this section.
- *Feeling of impending doom*—Pay close attention to any patient who feels like he or she is about to die, because it is quite common for persons to have this sensation before cardiac arrest.
- *Nausea and vomiting*—Although these conditions are unlikely to be the sole manifestation of a cardiac problem, nausea quite commonly accompanies MI. Vomiting is less frequent.
- *Abnormal pulse rate*—If the pulse is irregular, either too fast or too slow, the presence of a potential cardiac condition should always be suspected. However, numerous other problems (such as pain, bleeding, and neurological problems) also can result in an abnormal pulse. Most patients complain of "feeling their heartbeat" or palpitations, rather than of an "abnormal pulse rate."
- *Abnormal blood pressure*—Many persons have high or low blood pressure for many different reasons. These findings by themselves do not necessarily indicate cardiac disease. However, in combination with other cardiac signs and symptoms, abnormally high or low blood pressure should suggest the possibility of a cardiac problem. As with other abnormal vital signs, patients rarely complain of the abnormality itself, but of the associated symptoms (fatigue, headache, syncope, activity limitations).

Past Medical History

Determine whether the patient or close family members (mother, father, brothers, sisters) have a history of the following:

- Coronary artery disease (angina, previous AMI, CHF, pulmonary edema)
- Previous cardiac surgery
- Elevated cholesterol levels
- Congenital heart disease
- Hypertension
- Valvular or inflammatory heart disease (e.g., myocarditis)
- Aneurysm
- Lung disease
- Kidney disease
- Diabetes
- Vascular disease (e.g., atherosclerosis of the leg arteries)

Medications

As in any patient, determine past and current medications, whether prescribed, borrowed, over the counter, or recreational, and any allergies. Attempt to discover if the patient takes the medications as prescribed (compliance).

BOX 23-4

FINDINGS SUGGESTIVE OF MYOCARDIAL ISCHEMIA

- Chest pain (or pain in the anterior body from the umbilicus to the jaw, inclusive)
- Diaphoresis
- Dyspnea
- Anxiety and irritability
- Nausea and vomiting
- Feeling of impending doom
- Abnormal heart rate or rhythm
- Abnormal blood pressure

DETAILED PHYSICAL EXAMINATION

Inspection

NECK VEINS AND TRACHEA

The trachea should be midline. Normally, the neck veins are barely visible. Their level of distention is called the **jugular venous pressure.** If they appear to be bulging outward, they are considered distended. Neck vein distention may be seen in conditions such as CHF and cardiac tamponade (Figure 23-6). Venous pulsations are rarely palpable—if a pulse is felt, it is most likely the carotid artery. In addition, venous pulsations are eliminated by light pressure on the vein just above the sternal end of the clavicle; arterial (carotid) pulsations are not eliminated by this pressure. Finally, the level of venous pulsations changes with position, dropping as the patient becomes more upright. Carotid pulsations are not changed by position.

THORAX

If not already done, expose the chest and observe for symmetrical breathing. Observe the rate, rhythm, depth, and effort of breathing; always check for cyanosis. Along with the rate, assess the depth and quality of respirations. Inspect the chest for the following:

- *Deformities or asymmetry*—Check for "barrel chest deformity" (increased anterior-posterior diameter), traumatic flail chest, open wounds, and other evidence of trauma.
- *Impairment of respiratory movement*—Listen to the patient's breathing. Are abnormal signs present (e.g., wheezing, stridor) even without the aid of a stethoscope?
- *Abnormal* **retractions**—Inward movements of the skin between the rib interspaces during inspiration. They may also be seen in the area above the clavicles, the *supraclavicular fossa.* Although sometimes seen in normal thin persons, the presence of retractions, especially if the patient is short of breath, indicates increased work of breathing. Normally, diaphragmatic contraction is sufficient for adequate ventilation and oxygenation. Retractions represent contraction of the accessory muscles of respiration, such as the intercostal muscles, to help in inspiration.

EPIGASTRIUM

Note pulsations and distention. In thin individuals it is sometimes possible to see the abdominal segment of the aorta as it pulsates. Otherwise, pulsations are not normally visible in the epigastrium. If pulsations are present, suspect either a markedly enlarged heart or an aortic aneurysm.

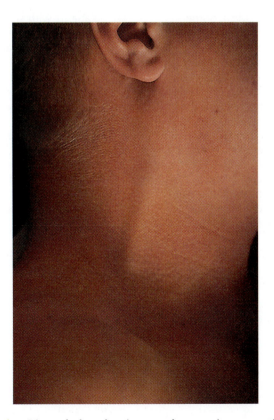

FIGURE 23-6 ▲ **Distended neck veins may be seen in congestive heart failure.**

AORTIC ANEURYSM

An aneurysm is an abnormal dilation of any portion of an artery. The types of aneurysm likely to be encountered in the field setting are a dissecting thoracic aortic aneurysm and a leaking abdominal aortic aneurysm.

DISSECTING THORACIC AORTIC ANEURYSM

Dissecting thoracic aortic aneurysms are most commonly due to hypertension, although the weakness can be congenital (present at birth). They are more common in men than in women. Patients typically have a history of poorly controlled hypertension.

An aneurysm develops as blood enters a tear in the intimal lining of the vessel, causing a separation of weakened elastic and fibromuscular elements in the medial layer. The blood causes cystlike dilation of the media, resulting in a false passage for blood. Essentially, the walls of the aorta tear apart, much like layers of an onion, as the dissection proceeds. The most severe complications occur when the dissection involves various arteries that arise from the aorta. Blood is unable to flow properly into these arteries, resulting in impaired blood supply to the tissues that they supply. Life-threatening conditions such as pericardial tamponade, AMI, and stroke may occur.

When dissection occurs, the patient suffers excruciating pain, usually starting in the anterior chest and moving downward and toward the back. A key symptom many patients complain of when describing the onset of their pain is a "tearing" sensation (especially between the shoulder blades). Some patients do not feel anterior chest pain; their symptoms are limited to severe pain between the shoulder blades. The pain may exactly mimic that of AMI.

The physical examination findings vary greatly, depending on the severity and location of the dissection. If peripheral arteries are compromised, there often will be asymmetry of pulses between the right and left sides of the body. Check carotid, radial, and femoral pulses, as well as color, temperature, and neurological signs, on *both* sides in patients with suspected dissection. If the carotids are involved, the patient may have neurological symptoms, similar to those of stroke. If the femoral arteries are affected, the femoral pulse will be decreased or absent on one side and the leg, foot, or toes may be white or cyanotic and are often cooler than the other side.

RUPTURED OR LEAKING ABDOMINAL AORTIC ANEURYSM

An abdominal aortic aneurysm is a saclike widening in the abdominal portion of the aorta, usually caused by a combination of atherosclerosis and hypertension. Most of these aneurysms are totally asymptomatic and are discovered on routine physical examination. Aneurysms that leak or rupture can lead to catastrophic circumstances. Patients have a 35% mortality rate if emergency surgery is required to attempt to repair the rupture. Abdominal aortic aneurysms are present in 2% to 4% of the adult population, the majority occurring in elderly men.

Unless the aneurysm is leaking or has actually ruptured, the patient is likely to be asymptomatic. Symptoms include back and/or abdominal pain, nausea, vomiting, and signs of shock (the patient appears quite ill and is very diaphoretic). With rupture, the symptoms come on quickly. The onset of severe abdominal pain is rapid, often radiating to the back and scrotum. Nausea and vomiting are common. A pulsating abdominal mass may be present. If the aorta has already ruptured, the most common finding is a markedly distended, tender abdomen and shock. Femoral pulses may be decreased. Occasionally, blood will dissect through the abdominal cavity into the groin, resulting in massive swelling of the scrotum with bluish discoloration, the so-called blue scrotum sign.

Patients with suspected aortic aneurysm are "priority" patients. They require gentle but rapid transport to a medical facility. While en route to the hospital, provide the following care:

- Secure and maintain a patent airway.
- Administer high-concentration oxygen.
- Initiate one to two large-bore intravenous (IV) lines of normal saline. As long as the patient's blood pressure is greater than 90 mm Hg systolic, keep the fluid rate TKO ("to keep open"). *Do not* increase the IV rate without medical direction.
- Monitor the cardiac rhythm.
- Monitor the vital signs, pulse oximetry, and peripheral pulses frequently, at least every 5 minutes.

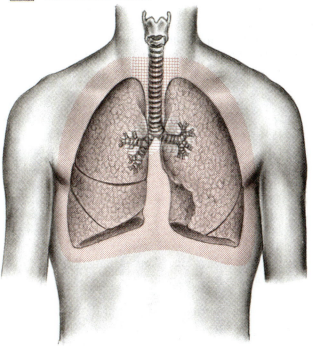

Percuss each side, alternately, from top to bottom.

FIGURE 23-7 ▲ Six sites on posterior chest for auscultating lung sounds.

KEY:

☐ Bronchovesicular over main bronchi

☐ Vesicular over lesser bronchi, bronchioles, and lobes

☐ Bronchial over trachea

Auscultation

Auscultation of the chest for *normal lung sounds* (also called *breath sounds*) is vital for assessment of airflow through the airways. It involves listening to the sounds generated by breathing, checking for symmetry, and then determining whether additional abnormal sounds (*adventitious lung sounds*) are present. The chest should be auscultated in at least six different areas (Figure 23-7). Ascertain that breath sounds are equal on each side. If cervical spine injury is not suspected, perform both anterior and posterior auscultation.

The easiest way to understand the normal lung sounds is to practice with a partner. Four normal patterns are heard, depending on the area auscultated (Figure 23-8):

- *Vesicular*—A normal sound of rustling or swishing heard with the stethoscope over the lung periphery; these are usually higher pitched during inspiration and fade rapidly during expiration.
- *Bronchial*—Normal if heard over the anterior sternum; otherwise, an abnormal sound heard with a stethoscope over the lungs, indicating *consolidation* (filled with fluid) or compression of normal lung. Expiration and inspiration produce loud, high-pitched sounds with a short silent period between the inspiratory and expiratory sounds. Expiration lasts longer.
- *Bronchovesicular*—Intermediate sounds between tracheal sounds and vesicular sounds. These may be normal in the first and second interspaces anteriorly and between the scapulae but otherwise suggest fluid in the lungs.

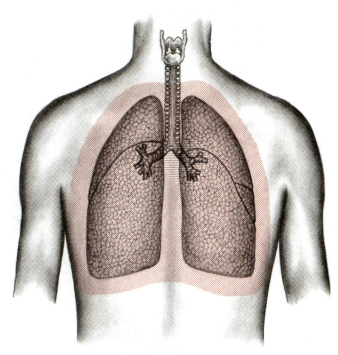

FIGURE 23-8 ▲ Lung sounds heard. (From Thompson J: *Clinical nursing,* St Louis, 1986, Mosby.)

- *Tracheal*—A normal breath sound heard during auscultation over the trachea. Inspiration and expiration are equally loud, the expiratory sound being heard during the greater part of expiration, whereas the inspiratory sound stops abruptly at the height of inspiration, with a pause before the sound of expiration is heard.

Adventitious lung sounds are additional sounds heard during auscultation of the chest and are usually *abnormal.* There has been much debate over the use of terms, and experts continue to disagree. The most practical way to classify added sounds is by their duration throughout the respiratory cycle:

- *Discontinuous sounds*—These are sounds that are, by definition, not present for the entire respiratory cycle (full inspiration to full exhalation). These intermittent sounds may follow a pattern, such as being present only during inspiration, or may occur in a random fashion. If the patient's condition is serious enough, some usually discontinuous sounds may become continuous (e.g., crackles in severe CHF).

The general term for discontinuous sounds is *crackles.* Some use the term *rales* to indicate a similar sound, but "crackles" is a far more descriptive and understandable term. Crackles are crackling or bubbling sounds that represent fluid in the alveoli and are present in heart failure or pneumonia. Some further differentiate crackles into *fine crackles* (quieter, higher pitched) and *coarse crackles* (louder, higher pitched). One way to get an idea of the sound of crackles is to rub two pieces of hair together between the thumb and index finger close to the ear.

- *Continuous sounds*—Again, there is some overlap between continuous and noncontinuous sounds. Wheezes and rhonchi tend to be more continuous than crackles. *Wheezes* are squeaking, high-pitched sounds that may occur on inspiration, expiration, or both. They represent spasms in the airways and are present in asthma, chronic obstructive pulmonary disease (COPD), and heart failure. *Rhonchi* are coarser and sound like "gurgling." They are often present over the larger airways only and may be present on both inspiration and expiration. Rhonchi indicate mucus or other material in the larynx, trachea, or bronchi; they are often present in upper respiratory infections, such as bronchitis.

As in the rest of the body, symmetry is important. Lung sounds should be relatively similar on both sides of each part of the chest. *Diminished* or *absent lung sounds* suggest pleural effusion (fluid), consolidation (fluid in the lungs for any reason), a collapsed lung, or a surgically removed lung.

Palpation

Palpate the chest. Begin with the clavicles, and then palpate the rib cage. Note pain, tenderness, possible fractures, or subcutaneous emphysema. Then palpate the epigastrium, paying particular attention to abnormal distention or pulsations.

ELECTROCARDIOGRAPHIC MONITORING

STREET WISE

Because guidelines for the treatment of cardiac emergencies have changed and it is unclear if this will affect the current curriculum and/or educational programs for EMT–Is (also, various communities use the EMT–I differently, depending on local need), this textbook includes most of the medications that are recommended for the advanced-level treatment of cardiac emergencies. This is not intended to require you to learn and/or administer all of these treatments. Ask your instructor which medications you are responsible for learning. Then follow your local protocols when determining which medications you may deliver.

Components of the Normal Adult Electrocardiogram

The **electrocardiogram (ECG)** is a record of the electrical activity within the heart. Electrodes placed on the patient's skin detect the activity. These impulses, which appear as a series of waves, or "blips," are then transferred to the ECG machine and displayed via a screen (oscilloscope) or printed onto moving graph paper.

The printed paper shows heavy vertical lines and smaller vertical lines. These lines divide the tracing into big and small "boxes," respectively (Figure 23-9). The distance between the lines, or boxes, represents time. The time between two large lines is 0.2 second. Four smaller lines divide the large 0.2-second box into five smaller 0.04-second boxes. These standardized distances can be used to determine the length of any portion of an ECG complex.

The machine records positive electrical impulses as upward deflections and negative impulses as downward deflections. A flat, or *isoelectric,* line is produced if no electrical impulse is present. This series of waves and complexes is commonly known as the P wave, QRS complex, and T wave and represents the normal cardiac conduction pattern (Figure 23-10).

As the electrical impulse passes through the heart cells, it causes chemical changes within the cell **(depolarization),** causing it to become more positively charged. As the cell depolarizes, muscle fibers are stimulated to contract. Following depolarization and contraction, the chemical balance within the cell returns to

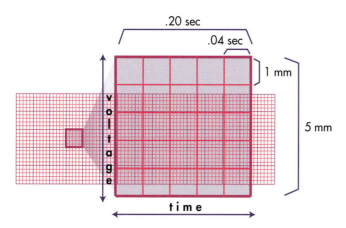

FIGURE 23-9 ▲ ECG paper is a grid composed of standardized line distances and markings.

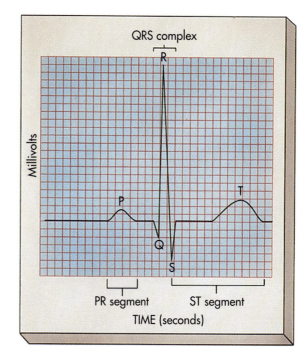

FIGURE 23-10 ▲ An ECG is composed of P waves, QRS complexes, and T waves.

the way it was before depolarization, or to the resting state (baseline, repolarization). The cardiac muscle relaxes during repolarization.

The **P wave** occurs first and represents movement of the electrical impulse (depolarization) through the atria, resulting in atrial contraction. It is normally upright and round in appearance. Following this wave is a flat line, or electrical pause, called the **PR segment,** which represents the time delay that occurs as the impulse passes through the AV node.

Next is a larger wave, the **QRS complex,** which represents movement of the electrical impulse (depolarization) through the ventricles. This wave corresponds to ventricular contraction, or systole. The Q wave is the first downward deflection, the R wave is the first upward deflection after the P wave, and the S wave is the first negative deflection after the R wave. Another pause then occurs, known as the **ST segment.** During this period, repolarization of the ventricles is beginning. The T wave follows, representing completion of repolarization. Sometimes a small wave is seen following the T wave but before the next P wave. This is known as a **U wave.** Generally, it is not present. Atrial repolarization occurs during the QRS complex and is not visible on the regular ECG (Figure 23-11).

The normal ECG, representing a normal cardiac rhythm (normal sinus rhythm; Figure 23-12), consists of the following:

- Upright and round P waves occurring at regular intervals with a rate of 60 to 100 beats per minute
- A PR segment of normal duration (0.12 to 0.20 second) followed by a QRS complex of normal upright contour, duration (less than 0.12 second), and configuration
- A flat ST segment followed by a T wave of normal contour and configuration

The QT interval is the distance from the onset of the QRS complex until the end of the T wave. It measures the time of ventricular depolarization and repolarization and may be altered by numerous factors (e.g., drugs [tricyclics], electrolyte abnormalities, arsenic poisoning).

Electrocardiographic Leads and Principles

ECG machines monitor voltage changes between electrodes that are placed in different places on the body. Each pair of electrodes is called a **lead.** Each lead consists of two surface electrodes of opposite electrical polarity (negative and positive, or positive and reference [ground]). Settings on the ECG machine allow any electrode to be made either positive or negative, depending on the required lead. Although the 12-lead ECG is becoming increasingly more popular in the out-of-hospital setting, a three- or four-lead system is sufficient in many cases.

Multilead ECGs are like a televised sporting event. Although there is just one game taking place on the field, modern-day television uses multiple cameras to view the "action" from many different angles. Each view looks different, even though the actual action is still the same. The same is true for the 12-lead (or 3- or 4-lead) ECG. The "game" here is the electrical depolarization of the heart that normally follows a predictable pathway from atria to ventricles. All the multilead ECG does is place multiple "cameras" (called leads) to view the *same* electrical activity of the heart from *different* vantage points.

▶ NOTE: Despite the potential value of an ECG, a normal test does not mean a normal patient. There are limitations to any test, including the ECG.

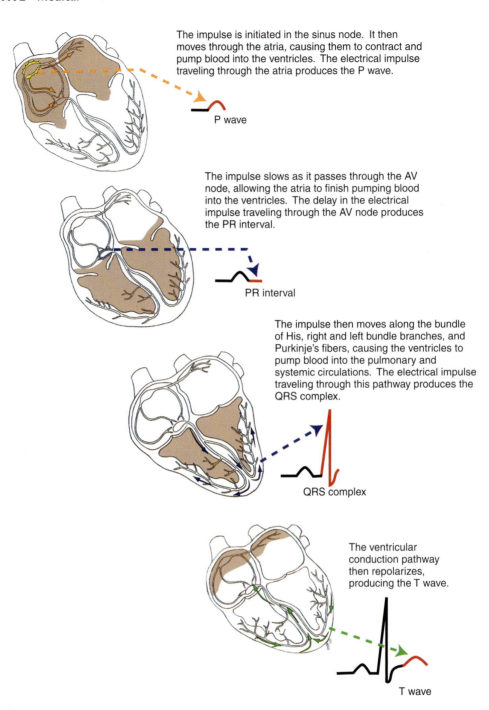

The impulse is initiated in the sinus node. It then moves through the atria, causing them to contract and pump blood into the ventricles. The electrical impulse traveling through the atria produces the P wave.

P wave

The impulse slows as it passes through the AV node, allowing the atria to finish pumping blood into the ventricles. The delay in the electrical impulse traveling through the AV node produces the PR interval.

PR interval

The impulse then moves along the bundle of His, right and left bundle branches, and Purkinje's fibers, causing the ventricles to pump blood into the pulmonary and systemic circulations. The electrical impulse traveling through this pathway produces the QRS complex.

QRS complex

The ventricular conduction pathway then repolarizes, producing the T wave.

T wave

FIGURE 23-11 ▲ Conduction of an electrical impulse through the heart.

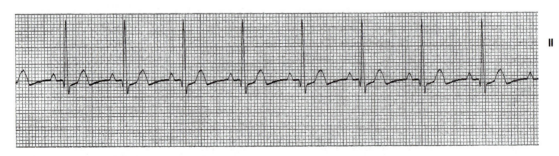

II

FIGURE 23-12 ▲ Normal sinus rhythm. (From Sanders MJ: *Mosby's paramedic textbook*, ed 2, St Louis, 2000, Mosby.)

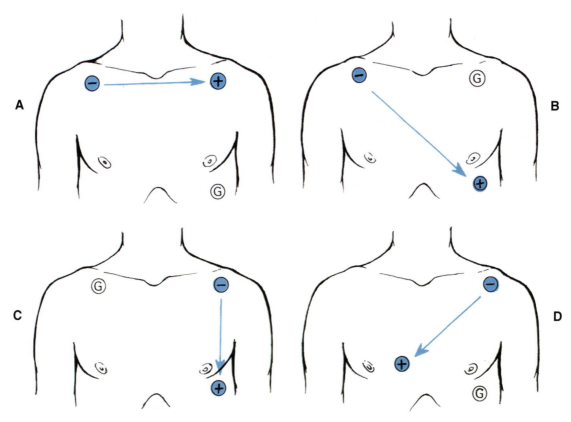

FIGURE 23-13 ▲ **A,** Lead I placement. **B,** Lead II placement. **C,** Lead III placement. **D,** Lead MCL₁ placement.

Application of Electrocardiographic Leads

In a typical prehospital situation, the ECG tracing is monitored in one of four leads. Three electrodes are placed on the patient: positive, negative, and ground. Depending on the lead position, either lead I, lead II, lead III, or lead MCL₁ may be monitored (Figure 23-13).

Routinely, lead II most commonly is used for continuous patient monitoring in the prehospital setting. This single lead shows the rate and regularity of the heartbeat—it does *not* give information about the pumping capability of the heart or the presence/location of AMI. Some jurisdictions also use MCL, follow your local protocol.

The following guidelines should be followed to obtain the best possible tracing:

* Avoid large muscle masses and large quantities of hair.
* Cleanse the area first with alcohol.
* Use the inner surfaces of the arms and legs whenever possible.
* Shave excess body hair if necessary.
* Attach the electrodes to the prepared site.
* Attach the ECG machine cables to the electrodes; follow the markings at the end of each cable.
* Turn the ECG machine on to obtain a baseline tracing.

Electrocardiogram Analysis

There are two commonly used methods to analyze ECG tracings. One method is to observe the rhythm directly on the monitor screen or oscilloscope. In this manner the basic rhythm usually can be identified, but it may be difficult to ascertain details such as PR-segment measurement or QRS-complex duration. The other method is to print out a rhythm strip on paper. In this way the specific ECG components can be measured and plotted.

EMT–Is must be able to recognize a host of cardiac dysrhythmias. Some present no problem to the patient, whereas others are life threatening. Each ECG rhythm should be approached in a logical and systematic manner using the steps listed below every time an ECG rhythm is interpreted. If a dysrhythmia is present, this finding should be compared with the assessment of the patient. This will determine the significance of the dysrhythmia and assist in any decision regarding patient treatment.

STEP 1: EVALUATE THE RATE

Several methods are available to calculate the heart rate. The following are most practical for use in the prehospital setting:

* Method 1: Identify a 6-second interval on the ECG paper by identifying two 3-second marks at the top of the ECG paper. Count the number of QRS com-

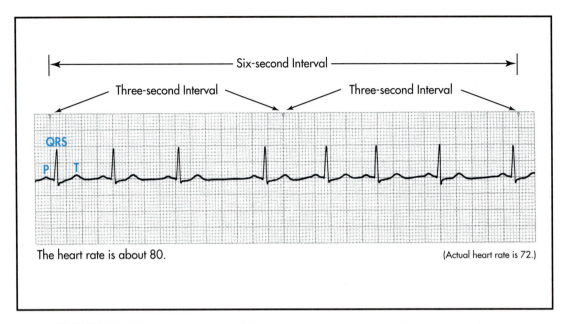

FIGURE 23-14 ▲ The patient's heart rate can be estimated by counting the number of QRS complexes in a 3- or 6-second period and then multiplying by 20 or 10, respectively.

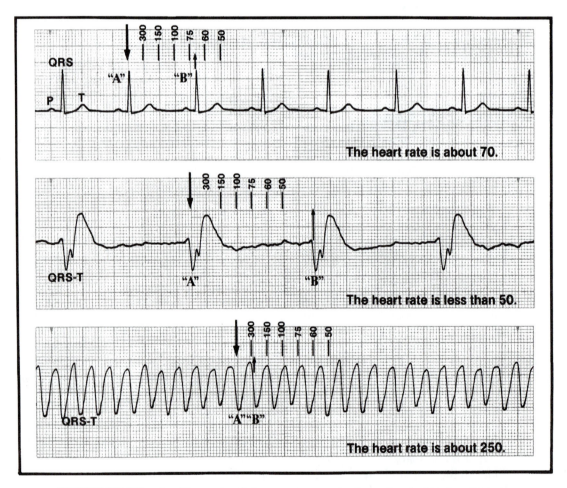

FIGURE 23-15 ▲ The patient's heart rate can also be estimated by locating an R wave on a dark line and assigning the proceeding dark lines 300, 150, 100, 75, 60, and 50 until a second R wave is located.

plexes, and multiply by 10. This number will be the estimated heart rate per minute (Figure 23-14).
- Method 2: Locate an R wave on the dark line of a large box on the ECG paper. Give numbers to the next six dark lines to the right in the following order: 300, 150, 100, 75, 60, and 50. The line (and corresponding number) closest to the next R wave is an approximation of the heart rate per minute (Figure 23-15). NOTE: This method is accurate only if the rhythm is regular.

STEP 2: EVALUATE THE P WAVES

First and foremost, are P waves present? Are they regular, and is one present before every QRS complex? Are they upright or inverted as compared with the QRS complex? Do they all look the same? A normal, rounded P wave indicates that the impulse has originated in the SA node and denotes a "sinus" rhythm. The P waves should appear mostly upright in any of the leads used in out-of-hospital cardiac monitoring. Normally, a QRS complex should follow each P wave (separated, of course, by the PR interval). This relationship should be consistent (Figure 23-16).

STEP 3: EVALUATE THE PR INTERVAL

Measure the PR interval. Is it within the range of 0.12 and 0.20 second? Is the interval constant? A prolonged PR interval is abnormal and suggests delay of AV conduction, possibly as a result of cardiac ischemia. Note any prolongation of the PR interval, whether constant or progressive (Figure 23-17).

STEP 4: EVALUATE THE QRS COMPLEX

Are all complexes alike? Measure the QRS complex. Is it less than 0.12 second in duration? NOTE: The rhythm is considered "normal" sinus only when these standards are met. If the QRS complexes are widened, whether identical or not, there is an abnormality present (Figure 23-18).

STEP 5: EVALUATE THE RHYTHM

Measure the R-R interval (ventricular rate), and determine if it is regular. Is there an occasional irregular beat, or is there a pattern of irregular beats (in other words, a cycle that seems to repeat itself over and over

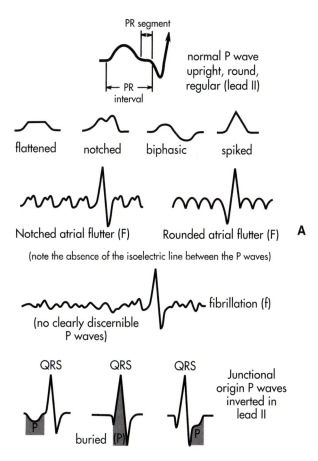

FIGURE 23-16 ▲ **A,** Abnormal P waves. (**A,** From American College of Emergency Physicians; Pons PT, Cason D, chief editors: *Paramedic field care: a complaint-based approach,* St Louis, 1997, Mosby for ACEP.) *Continued*

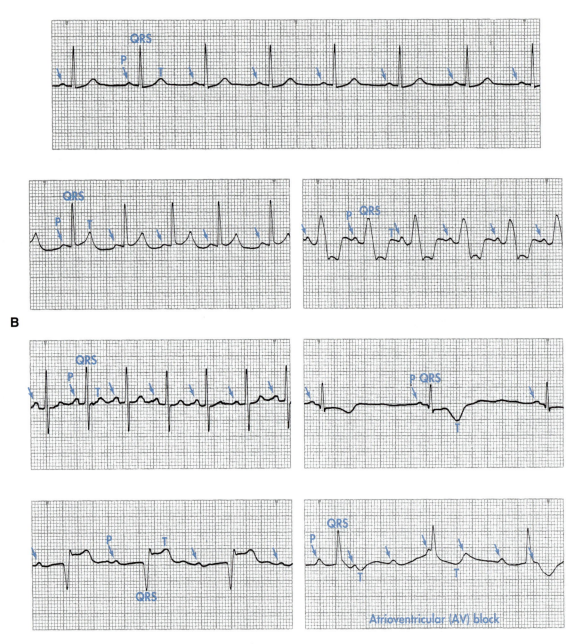

FIGURE 23-16, cont'd ▲ **B,** Normal P waves. (**B,** From Huszar R: *Basic dysrhythmias,* ed 2, St Louis, 1994, Mosby.)

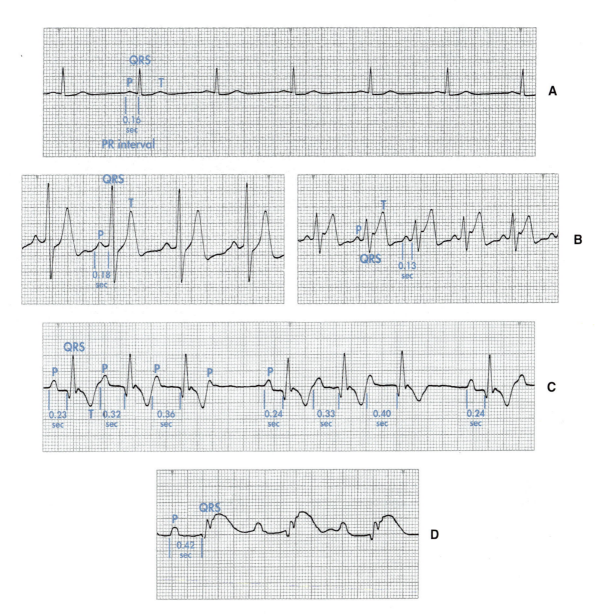

FIGURE 23-17   ▲   **A** and **B**, Normal PR intervals. **C** and **D**, Abnormal PR intervals. (From Huszar R: *Basic dysrhythmias,* ed 2, St Louis, 1994, Mosby.)

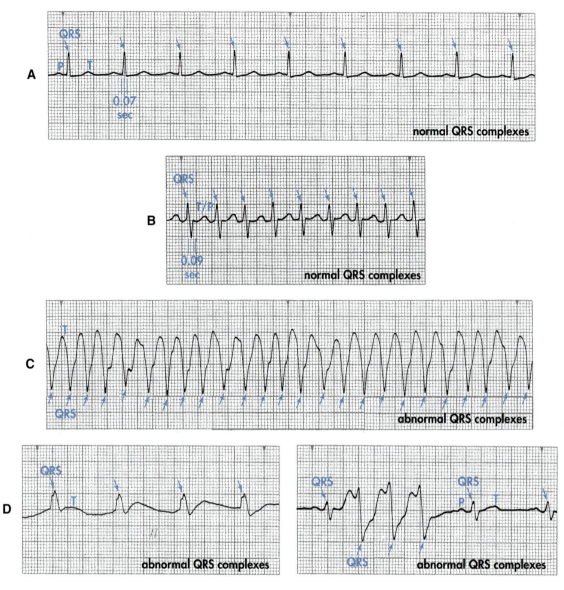

FIGURE 23-18 ▲ **A** and **B**, Normal QRS complexes. **C** to **E**, Abnormal QRS complexes. (From Huszar R: *Basic dysrhythmias,* ed 2, St Louis, 1994, Mosby.)

again)? Is it "irregularly irregular," in which case there is no relationship between the R-R intervals? Also measure the P-P interval (atrial rate). Determine if it is regular and constant. Slight irregularities in rhythm that vary with a person's breathing are common (**sinus dysrhythmia**). As a rule, however, the R-R interval should not vary by more than one small box every few (three to five) beats. A rhythm that is more irregular than this is abnormal until proven otherwise (Figure 23-19).

STEP 6: EVALUATE THE ST SEGMENT

Normally, ST segments should be *isoelectric* (on the same baseline level) with the PR segment (the line from the end of the P wave to the beginning of the QRS complex). If the ST segment is either too high (ST-segment

elevation) or too low (ST-segment depression), cardiac ischemia or AMI may be present (Figure 23-20).

STEP 7: EVALUATE THE QT INTERVAL

Although helpful in determining a predisposition to dysrhythmias, the normal QT interval varies with the heart rate. Rather than memorizing formulas and performing calculations in the field, a general rule helps much of the time. The normal QT interval is usually less than one half of the R-R interval. Use this as a rough guide only.

STEP 8: EVALUATE THE T WAVES

In the commonly used field leads, T waves should be upright. If they are biphasic (part upward, part down-

The distances between the
R waves are determined:

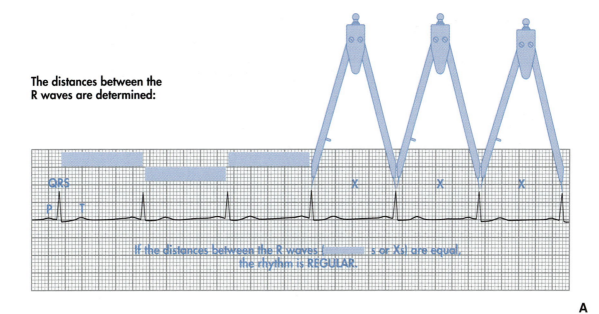

QRS

P   T

If the distances between the R waves (s or Xs) are equal,
the rhythm is REGULAR.

A

1. by estimating the
   R-R intervals,

2. by measuring the R-R intervals
   with ECG calipers,* or

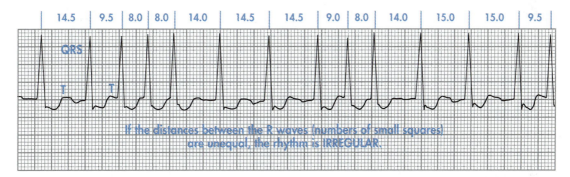

| 14.5 | 9.5 | 8.0 | 8.0 | 14.0 | 14.5 | 14.5 | 9.0 | 8.0 | 14.0 | 15.0 | 15.0 | 9.5 |

QRS

T   T

If the distances between the R waves (numbers of small squares)
are unequal, the rhythm is IRREGULAR.

3. by counting the small squares
   between the R waves.

* If calipers are not available, mark off the
  distance between two R waves on a piece of
  paper and compare this distance with the other
  R-R intervals.

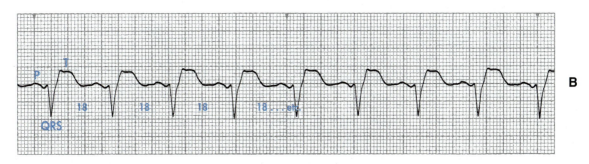

P   T

18   18   18   18 . . . etc.

QRS

B

FIGURE 23-19 ▲ **A,** Determining the rhythm. **B,** Regular rhythm. (From
Huszar R: *Basic dysrhythmias,* ed 2, St Louis, 1994, Mosby.)   *Continued*

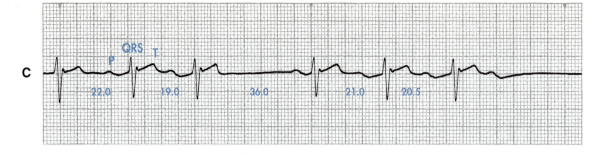

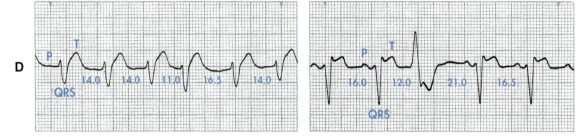

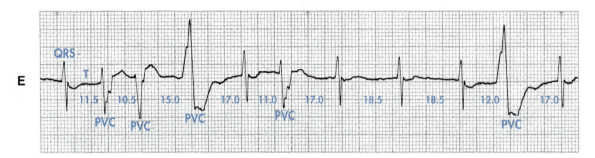

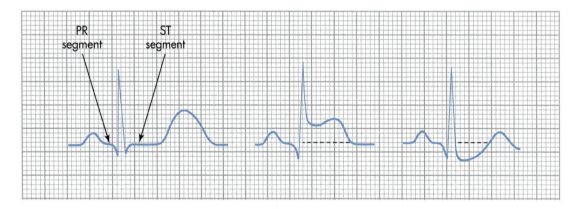

FIGURE 23-19, cont'd ▲ **C**, Regularly irregular rhythm. **D**, Occasionally irregular rhythm. **E**, Irregularly irregular rhythm. (From Huszar R: *Basic dysrhythmias,* ed 2, St Louis, 1994, Mosby.)

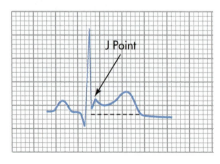

FIGURE 23-20 ▲ ST-segment deviations. **A**, Use of the PR segment as a baseline. **B**, The ST segment is elevated with respect to the PR-segment baseline. **C**, The ST segment is depressed with respect to the PR-segment baseline. **D**, J point (ST-segment elevation). (From Grauer K: *Practical guide to ECG interpretation,* St Louis, 1992, Mosby.)

ward) or inverted, suspect cardiac ischemia. Note that numerous factors may influence the T-wave configuration. The most acutely dangerous, however, is myocardial ischemia.

STEP 9: LOOK FOR U WAVES

Although U waves may be normal variants, they more likely signify either an electrolyte (e.g., potassium) abnormality or cardiac ischemia.

• • •

Sometimes other markings are present on the ECG tracing that are not related to the heart's electrical activity. These are known as artifacts and can be caused by patient movement, shivering, muscle tremors, or 60-cycle current interference (Figure 23-21). In addition, the electrodes may be loose or improperly placed, the machine may not be functioning properly, or electrical interference may be present. Before finalizing the ECG interpretation, reassess the patient and inspect the ECG machine. This step is especially important before treating potentially lethal dysrhythmias.

Dysrhythmias

Summarized here, along with their causes, ECG findings, clinical features (when applicable), and treatment (if necessary), are the common dysrhythmias.

Cardiac **dysrhythmias** are irregularities in the heart rhythm. Dysrhythmias can result from a number of physiological, pharmacological, and disease processes, including the following:

- Myocardial ischemia or necrosis
- Autonomic nervous system imbalance
- Distention of heart chambers
- Acid-base abnormalities
- Hypoxemia
- Electrolyte imbalance
- Drug effects or toxicity
- Electrical injury
- Hypothermia
- Central nervous system injury

Some cardiac rhythm disturbances are normal, even in patients who have healthy hearts. An example is sinus bradycardia seen with athletes or tachycardia that results from stress or anxiety. Despite the cause or type of dysrhythmia, management is focused on the patient and the underlying cause, not merely the dysrhythmia.

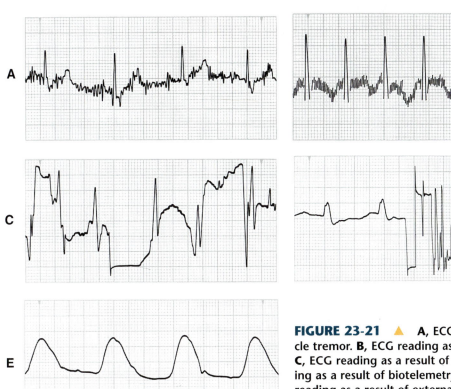

FIGURE 23-21 ▲ **A,** ECG reading as a result of a muscle tremor. **B,** ECG reading as a result of AC interference. **C,** ECG reading as a result of loose electrodes. **D,** ECG reading as a result of biotelemetry-related interference. **E,** ECG reading as a result of external chest compressions.

TABLE 23-1

Dysrhythmias Originating in the Sinus Node

TYPES OF DYSRHYTHMIAS ORIGINATING IN THE SINUS NODE	COMMON FEATURES
Normal sinus rhythm	Upright, round P waves (one preceding each QRS complex)
Sinus bradycardia	
Sinus tachycardia	Normal QRS complexes
Sinus arrhythmia, or dysrhythmia	PR intervals are within normal duration of 0.12-0.20 sec and
Sinus arrest	constant

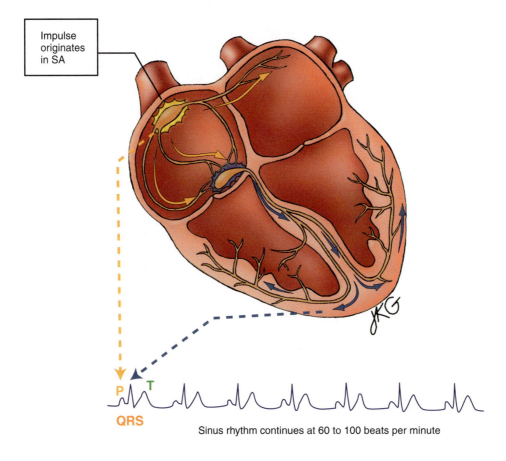

Impulse originates in SA

Sinus rhythm continues at 60 to 100 beats per minute

Sinus bradycardia continues at less than 60 beats per minute

Sinus tachycardia continues faster that 100 beats per minute

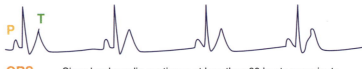

FIGURE 23-22 ▲ Sinus rhythms.

TABLE 23-2

Sinus Bradycardia

CAUSES	ECG FINDINGS*	SIGNIFICANCE
Intrinsic sinus node disease	Rhythm is regular	Persons who are aerobically
Increased parasympathetic vagal tone	**Rate is less than 60 beats per minute**	conditioned often have slower than usual heart rates (40-50 beats per minute)
Hypothermia	P waves are rounded and upright; each is followed by a QRS complex	In some patients the decreased rate associated with sinus
Hypoxia		bradycardia may compromise
Drug effects (e.g., digitalis, beta blockers, calcium channel blockers)	PR intervals are within normal duration of 0.12-0.20 sec and constant	cardiac output, resulting in hypotension, angina pectoris, and central nervous system
Acute myocardial infarction (MI)	QRS complexes are usually less than 0.12 sec, provided no conduction block occurs in the bundle branches	symptoms (lightheadedness, vertigo, syncope)
May also serve as one of the body's protective mechanisms by reducing myocardial oxygen consumption in the setting of MI (provided the patient is well perfused)		If a patient is symptomatic (e.g., short of breath, chest pain, dizziness), the presence of sinus bradycardia should be considered abnormal and potentially significant

MANAGEMENT

Patients experiencing symptomatic bradycardia (chest pain, hypotension, etc.) should receive high-concentration oxygen, an IV infusion of normal saline administered at a TKO rate, and prompt treatment.
Administer atropine (a drug used to speed the heart rate) at a dose of 0.5-1.0 mg IV push. In unresolved bradycardia the atropine dose may be repeated every 3-5 min to a maximum dose of 0.03 to 0.04 mg/kg (average of 3.0 mg) (Figure 23-23).
The use of transcutaneous pacing is another alternative—always follow local protocols.

* Bold type indicates key characteristic(s) identifying dysrhythmia.

Each dysrhythmia carries with it certain characteristics. Learning which characteristics are associated with each dysrhythmia makes interpreting the ECG rhythm easier. Instead of trying to remember what each rhythm looks like (the ECG examples included in this or other textbooks are only samples; the patient's ECG will not look exactly like them), all effort should go into memorizing the characteristics associated with the various dysrhythmias. These characteristics can then be matched up with what is seen on the ECG monitor or printout.

Rhythms originating from the SA node are called sinus rhythms. The key characteristics for these rhythms are listed in Table 23-1.

Normal sinus rhythm (NSR) (Figure 23-22) is the name given to what is considered the normal electrical activity of the heart. It is a regular rhythm with a heart rate of 60 to 100 beats per minute (in an adult). Each P wave is followed by a normal QRS complex, which is then followed by a normal T wave. The PR intervals are within the normal range of 0.12 to 0.20 second in duration and are constant (each PR interval is the same).

Sinus bradycardia has all the characteristics of NSR, but the heart rate is less than 60 beats per minute. It looks like a slow NSR. It results from a slowing of the pacemaker rate of the SA node (Table 23-2).

Sinus tachycardia is an ECG rhythm having the same characteristics as NSR but with a rate greater than 100.

It looks like a fast NSR and results from an increase in the rate of sinus node discharge (Table 23-3, p. 641).

Sinus dysrhythmia (Figure 23-24, p. 642), has all the characteristics of sinus rhythm (normal P waves, QRS complexes, and T waves) except there is a patterned irregularity to the rhythm. Some describe the rhythm as "slowing, then speeding up, then slowing again." This cycle continually repeats itself (Table 23-4, p. 642).

> **PALPITATIONS AND SYNCOPE**
> Palpitation is a sensation of pounding or racing of the heart. Syncope is a transient state of unresponsiveness due to inadequate perfusion of the brain from which the patient has recovered. These symptoms may occur together or individually.
> Palpitations and syncope result from cardiac dysrhythmias, other types of heart disease, nervous system disorders, anxiety, and thyroid disease. The conditions can also be caused by a variety of drugs, such as caffeine, cocaine, or amphetamines. The most common form of syncope is the simple fainting spell. Once the patient assumes the recumbent position, he or she rapidly regains responsiveness. The possibility of acute cocaine intoxication should be considered in a young patient with tachycardia,

Continued

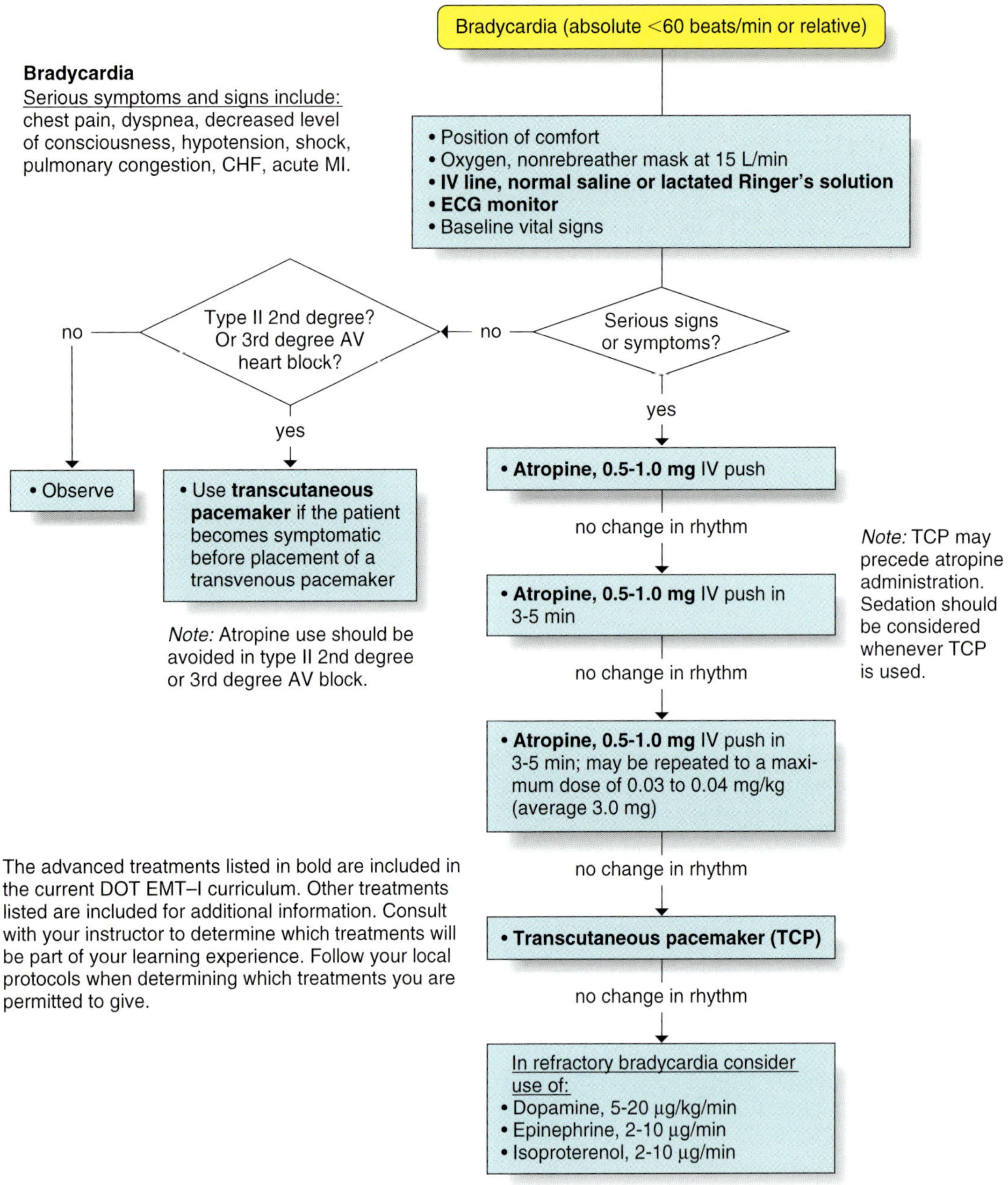

Bradycardia (absolute <60 beats/min or relative)

Bradycardia

Serious symptoms and signs include: chest pain, dyspnea, decreased level of consciousness, hypotension, shock, pulmonary congestion, CHF, acute MI.

- Position of comfort
- Oxygen, nonrebreather mask at 15 L/min
- **IV line, normal saline or lactated Ringer's solution**
- **ECG monitor**
- Baseline vital signs

Type II 2nd degree? Or 3rd degree AV heart block? ← no ← **Serious signs or symptoms?**

no →
- Observe

yes →
- Use **transcutaneous pacemaker** if the patient becomes symptomatic before placement of a transvenous pacemaker

Note: Atropine use should be avoided in type II 2nd degree or 3rd degree AV block.

yes →
- **Atropine, 0.5-1.0 mg** IV push

no change in rhythm

- **Atropine, 0.5-1.0 mg** IV push in 3-5 min

no change in rhythm

- **Atropine, 0.5-1.0 mg** IV push in 3-5 min; may be repeated to a maximum dose of 0.03 to 0.04 mg/kg (average 3.0 mg)

no change in rhythm

- **Transcutaneous pacemaker (TCP)**

no change in rhythm

In refractory bradycardia consider use of:
- Dopamine, 5-20 µg/kg/min
- Epinephrine, 2-10 µg/min
- Isoproterenol, 2-10 µg/min

Note: TCP may precede atropine administration. Sedation should be considered whenever TCP is used.

The advanced treatments listed in bold are included in the current DOT EMT–I curriculum. Other treatments listed are included for additional information. Consult with your instructor to determine which treatments will be part of your learning experience. Follow your local protocols when determining which treatments you are permitted to give.

FIGURE 23-23 ▲ Bradycardia algorithm.

PALPITATIONS AND SYNCOPE—cont'd
palpitations, diaphoresis, and chest pain. Cocaine can also cause acute MI.

Some people, particularly the elderly, experience fainting while straining on the toilet. This event is called vasovagal syncope. It results when increased abdominal pressure stimulates the vagus nerve, which travels near the stomach. Increasing the abdominal pressure while the breath is held is called the Valsalva maneuver.

To assess the patient who may have suffered a loss of responsiveness or feels dizzy, consider the following questions:

- How long was the patient unresponsive? Patients who have had a simple fainting spell recover almost immediately after "hitting the ground."

- In what position was the patient when the syncopal episode occurred? Patients who have syncope while in the supine or recumbent position may have a cardiac dysrhythmia.
- Does the patient feel lightheaded when going from lying down to sitting or from sitting to standing? If so, the patient may have orthostatic hypotension.
- Is the patient pregnant? Women in the second and third trimesters of pregnancy may have syncope if they lie flat, allowing the uterus to compress the inferior vena cava. This compression decreases venous return to the heart, and syncope may result. This is called the supine hypotension syndrome of pregnancy.
- Did the patient appear to have a seizure?

TABLE 23-3

Sinus Tachycardia

CAUSES	ECG FINDINGS*	SIGNIFICANCE
Following exercise or with pain, fear, excitement, anxiety, ingestion of caffeine or alcohol, smoking, or fever, persons often develop a slight sinus tachycardia (110-120 beats per minute) Rates more than 120 beats per minute in an adult may indicate some type of underlying illness, such as hypovolemia, hyperthyroidism, anemia, respiratory distress, or congestive heart failure Administration of atropine or any vagolytic or sympathomimetic drug such as epinephrine (Adrenalin) or isoproterenol (Isuprel) Intrinsic sinus node disease	Rhythm is regular **Rate is greater than 100 beats per minute** P waves are rounded and upright; each is followed by a QRS complex PR intervals are within normal duration of 0.12-0.20 sec and constant QRS complexes are usually less than 0.12 sec, provided no conduction block occurs in the bundle branches	Increases myocardial oxygen consumption, which can aggravate ischemia and infarction Can predispose the patient to more serious rhythm disturbances

MANAGEMENT

Treatment of patients experiencing sinus tachycardia is directed at correcting the underlying cause. When the underlying cause is removed, the tachycardia usually resolves gradually and on its own.

* Bold type indicates key characteristic(s) identifying dysrhythmia.

PALPITATIONS AND SYNCOPE—cont'd

Following even a simple fainting spell, the blood supply to the brain is transiently decreased. This decrease may result in one or two jerking movements. These movements are not actually a true seizure; however, a nonmedically trained person observing the event may report that the patient "fainted and had a seizure."

- Are the patient's vital signs normal? The vital signs may be normal, especially if the patient has recovered. The pulse may be normal, rapid, slow, or irregular.

Although a patient has recovered from a syncopal episode, he or she should be transported to the hospital for evaluation.

The care for a patient with palpitations or syncope includes the following:
- Administer high-concentration oxygen. Assist ventilations or intubate as necessary, according to local protocols.
- Monitor the cardiac rhythm. Cardiac dysrhythmias are a common cause of syncope.
- Start an IV line of normal saline at a TKO rate.
- Monitor the patient's vital signs and pulse oximetry.
- Transport the patient to the hospital for evaluation.

Sinus arrest occurs when the SA node stops firing transiently. It results from a marked depression in SA node automaticity. Failure of the sinus node causes short periods of cardiac standstill until lower-level pacemakers discharge (escape beats) or the sinus node resumes its normal function. The usual result of sinus arrest is a brief pause in all electrical activity that is not usually clinically significant (Figure 23-25, p. 643). The ECG rhythm looks like normal sinus except there is a pause in the rhythm or an absence of the P, QRS, and T waveforms until a pacemaker site reinitiates the rhythm (Table 23-5, p. 643).

DYSRHYTHMIAS ORIGINATING IN THE ATRIA

Dysrhythmias may originate in the atrial tissue or in the internodal pathways. They are called atrial rhythms. The most common causes include ischemia, hypoxia, and atrial stretching (dilation), usually due to either CHF, mitral valve disease, or increased pulmonary artery pressures. Features common to all dysrhythmias in this group are summarized in Table 23-6 on p. 644.

Tables 23-7 to 23-11 summarize key features for dysrhythmias originating in the atria.

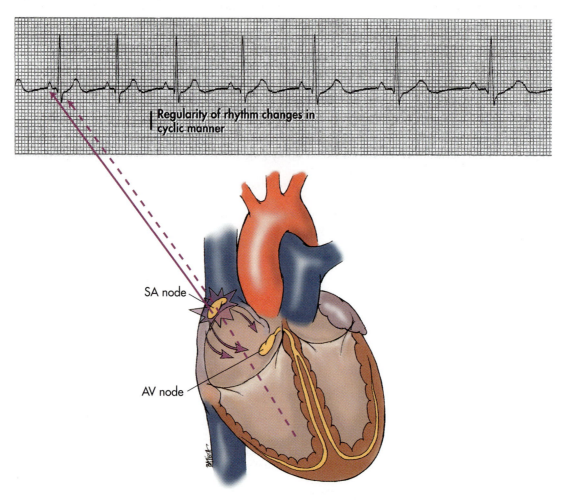

FIGURE 23-24 ▲ Sinus dysrhythmia. (Modified ECG strip from Sanders MJ: *Mosby's paramedic textbook,* ed 2, St Louis, 2000, Mosby.)

TABLE 23-4

Sinus Dysrhythmia

CAUSES	ECG FINDINGS*	SIGNIFICANCE
The beat-to-beat variation corresponds with the respiratory cycle and changes in intrathoracic pressure; heart rate increases during inspiration and decreases during expiration Can also occur in patients with heart disease or acute myocardial infarction and in those receiving certain drugs such as digitalis and morphine	**Rhythm is irregular (patterned)** Rate is between 60 and 100 beats per minute P waves are rounded and upright; each is followed by a QRS complex PR intervals are within normal duration of 0.12-0.20 sec and constant QRS complexes are usually less than 0.12 sec, provided no conduction block occurs in the bundle branches	Common in children, young adults, and older adults and may be associated with palpitations, dizziness, and syncope Usually is of no clinical significance

MANAGEMENT

Usually no treatment is required.

* Bold type indicates key characteristic(s) identifying dysrhythmia.

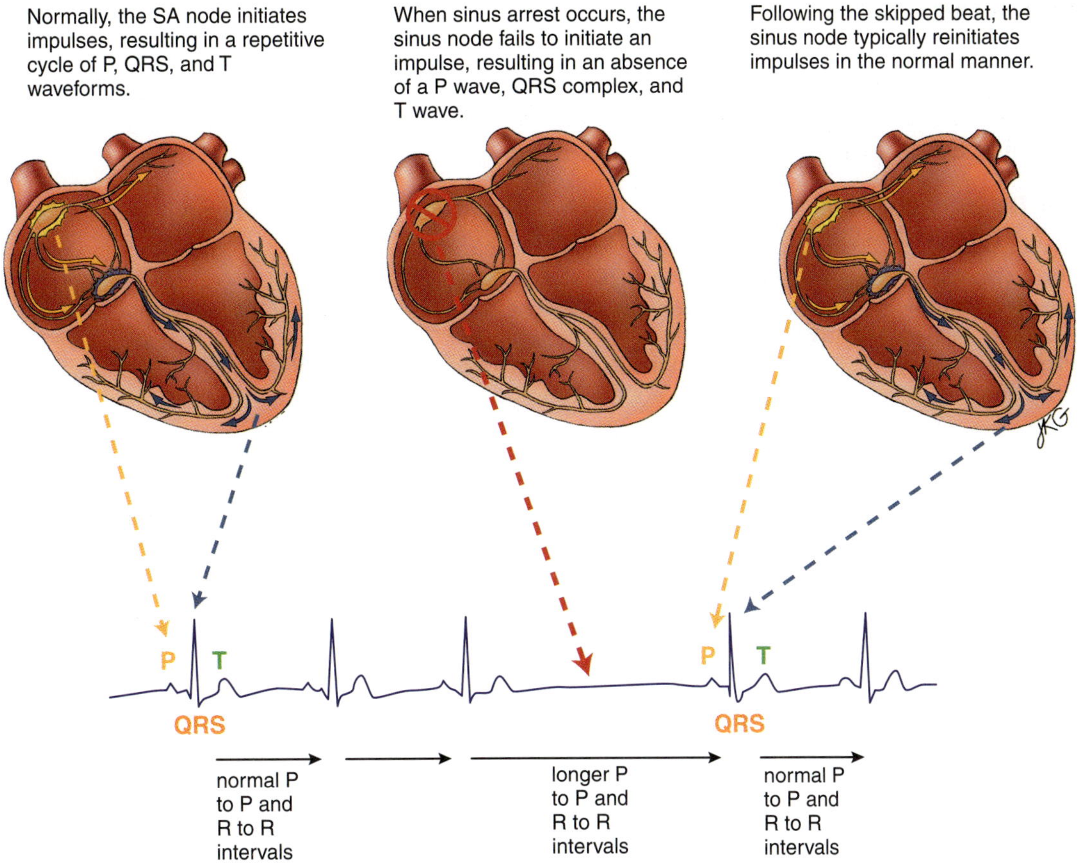

Normally, the SA node initiates impulses, resulting in a repetitive cycle of P, QRS, and T waveforms.

When sinus arrest occurs, the sinus node fails to initiate an impulse, resulting in an absence of a P wave, QRS complex, and T wave.

Following the skipped beat, the sinus node typically reinitiates impulses in the normal manner.

P T QRS
normal P to P and R to R intervals

longer P to P and R to R intervals

P T QRS
normal P to P and R to R intervals

Sinus arrest appears as regular sinus rhythm that is interrupted by a pause or absence of an impulse. The sinus node then reinitiates sinus rhythm, or an escape pacemaker takes over.

FIGURE 23-25 ▲ Sinus arrest.

TABLE 23-5

Sinus Arrest

CAUSES	ECG FINDINGS*	SIGNIFICANCE
An increase in parasympathetic tone on the SA node	**Rhythm is irregular because of the pause in the rhythm**	Rhythm typically resumes its normal appearance after this transient pause in the rhythm unless an escape pacemaker resumes the rhythm
Hypoxia or ischemia	Rate may be normal or is less than 60 beats per minute (depending on the frequency of recurrence)	
Excessive administration of digitalis or propranolol (Inderal) hyperkalemia	P waves are rounded and upright; each is followed by a QRS complex	Depending on the frequency and duration of sinus arrest, the rate may be normal to slow
Damage to the SA node (acute myocardial infarction, degenerative fibrotic disease)	PR intervals are within normal duration of 0.12-0.20 sec and constant	Rhythm is irregular when sinus arrest is present
	QRS complexes are usually less than 0.12 sec, provided no conduction block occurs in the bundle branches	Frequent or prolonged episodes of sinus arrest may compromise cardiac output by decreasing the heart rate and abolishing the atrial contribution to ventricular filling
		There is danger that sinus node activity will completely cease and an escape pacemaker may not take over pacing (resulting in asystole)

MANAGEMENT

If the patient is asymptomatic, close observation is all that is required.

Patients who are symptomatic (chest pain, hypotension, etc.) should receive high-concentration oxygen, an IV infusion of normal saline administered at a TKO rate, and prompt treatment.

In symptomatic patients with marked bradycardia, management may include the administration of atropine or transcutaneous pacing.

* Bold type indicates key characteristic(s) identifying dysrhythmia.

TABLE 23-6

Dysrhythmias Originating in the Atria

TYPES OF DYSRHYTHMIAS ORIGINATING IN THE ATRIA	COMMON FEATURES
Wandering pacemaker	Normal QRS complexes
Premature atrial complex (PAC)	P waves (if present) that differ in appearance from normal sinus P waves
Supraventricular tachycardia (SVT)	
Atrial flutter	Abnormal, shortened, or prolonged PR intervals
Atrial fibrillation	

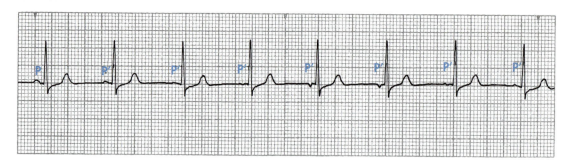

FIGURE 23-26 ▲ Wandering atrial pacemaker. (From Huszar R: *Basic dysrhythmias,* ed 2, St Louis, 1994, Mosby.)

TABLE 23-7

Wandering Atrial Pacemaker

CAUSES	ECG FINDINGS*	SIGNIFICANCE
Generally, caused by the inhibitory vagal effect of respiration on the SA node and AV junction	**Rhythm is slightly irregular**	May be nonpathological in the very young, the older adult, and well-conditioned athletes
	Rate is usually normal: 60-100 beats per minute	
Associated underlying heart disease	**Change in P wave morphology from beat to beat is the most distinguishing feature**	Not usually significant
Digitalis administration	P waves may be upright, inverted, rounded, notched, biphasic, or buried in the QRS complex	
	PR interval often varies	
	QRS complexes are usually less than 0.12 sec, provided no conduction block occurs in the bundle branches	

MANAGEMENT

Usually no treatment is required.
Atropine may help if the heart rate slows excessively.

* Bold type indicates key characteristic(s) identifying dysrhythmia.

Wandering atrial pacemaker (Figure 23-26) is a rhythm in which the pacemaker site switches from beat to beat. The transient shift of pacemaker sites is from the sinus node to other latent pacemaker sites in the atria. The shift is usually back and forth along the SA node, atria, and AV junction (Table 23-7).

Premature atrial complexes (PACs) (Figure 23-27) are ectopic beats. They can originate from a single ectopic pacemaker site or from multiple sites in the atria. They can be brought about by enhanced automaticity or a reentry mechanism. On the ECG, PACs appear as early beats, causing the R-R interval to be shorter between the preceding beat and the early beat (as compared with the underlying rhythm) (Table 23-8).

Supraventricular tachycardias (SVTs) (Figure 23-28, p. 646) arise either in the atria or in the AV junction as a

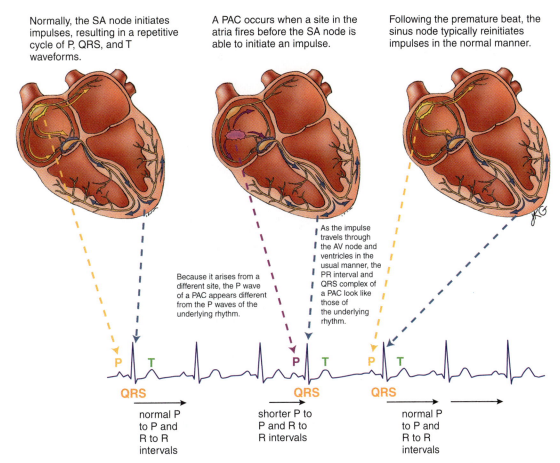

Normally, the SA node initiates impulses, resulting in a repetitive cycle of P, QRS, and T waveforms.

A PAC occurs when a site in the atria fires before the SA node is able to initiate an impulse.

Following the premature beat, the sinus node typically reinitiates impulses in the normal manner.

Because it arises from a different site, the P wave of a PAC appears different from the P waves of the underlying rhythm.

As the impulse travels through the AV node and ventricles in the usual manner, the PR interval and QRS complex of a PAC look like those of the underlying rhythm.

normal P to P and R to R intervals

shorter P to P and R to R intervals

normal P to P and R to R intervals

With a premature atrial complex the regularity of the underlying rhythm is interrupted by an impulse that occurs earlier than normal. This causes a shortening of the P to P and R to R intervals.

FIGURE 23-27 ▲ Premature atrial complex.

TABLE 23-8

Premature Atrial Complexes

CAUSES	ECG FINDINGS*	SIGNIFICANCE
Increased catecholamines and sympathetic tone Use of caffeine, tobacco, or alcohol Use of sympathomimetic drugs: epinephrine (Adrenalin), isoproterenol (Isuprel), norepinephrine (Levophed) Electrolyte imbalance Hypoxia Digitalis toxicity Cardiovascular disease In some cases, no apparent cause	**Early beat causes the underlying rhythm to be irregular** P wave, often with different morphology (appearance) than normal, occurs early QRS accompanying the premature beat is usually less than 0.12 sec PR interval accompanying the premature beat is within normal limits of 0.12-0.20 sec Premature atrial complexes (PACs) are usually not followed by a compensatory pause	Isolated PACs in patients with healthy hearts are not significant Frequent PACs may predispose the patient to serious atrial dysrhythmias PACs with aberrant ventricular conduction may cause a wide QRS complex and be confused with premature ventricular complexes (PVCs) Asymptomatic patients usually require observation only

MANAGEMENT

Usually no treatment is required.
If nonconducted PACs are frequent and the patient becomes symptomatic from bradycardia (rare), transcutaneous pacing or atropine may be indicated (see text).

* Bold type indicates key characteristic(s) identifying dysrhythmia.

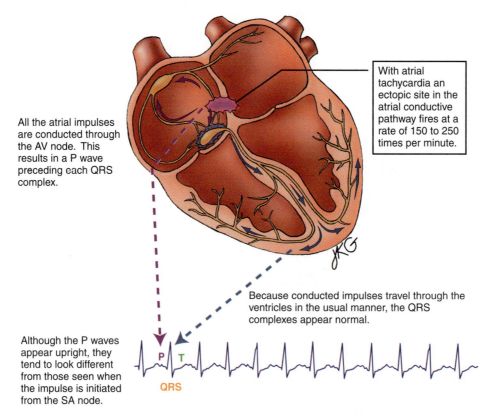

All the atrial impulses are conducted through the AV node. This results in a P wave preceding each QRS complex.

With atrial tachycardia an ectopic site in the atrial conductive pathway fires at a rate of 150 to 250 times per minute.

Because conducted impulses travel through the ventricles in the usual manner, the QRS complexes appear normal.

Although the P waves appear upright, they tend to look different from those seen when the impulse is initiated from the SA node.

P T
QRS

FIGURE 23-28 ▲ Atrial tachycardia.

CLINICAL NOTES

A variation of wandering atrial pacemaker is multifocal atrial tachycardia (MAT). It looks like wandering atrial pacemaker, but rates are frequently in the range of 120 to 150 beats per minute. It is always considered pathological. MAT is most often found in patients with severe COPD and may respond to management of this underlying disorder. MAT is often misdiagnosed as atrial fibrillation with rapid ventricular response. Rules for interpretation in lead II monitoring include the following:

- QRS complexes are usually less than 0.12 second, provided no conduction block occurs in the bundle branches.
- P waves change in morphology (appearance) from beat to beat. In lead II the P waves may be upright, rounded, notched, inverted, biphasic, or buried in the QRS complex.
- MAT may be precipitated by acute exacerbation of emphysema, CHF, or acute mitral valve regurgitation. Management is aimed at the underlying cause.

result of rapid depolarization that overrides the SA node. This group of tachycardias can include paroxysmal supraventricular tachycardia (PSVT), nonparoxysmal atrial tachycardia, multifocal atrial tachycardia, junctional tachycardia, atrial flutter, and atrial fibrillation. Distinguishing among these tachycardias is often difficult, since the ventricular rate is so fast it is hard to tell if there are P waves or PR intervals (Figure 23-29).

PSVT is a supraventricular tachycardia that begins abruptly. It may originate in the atria (paroxysmal atrial tachycardia [PAT]) or AV junction (paroxysmal junctional tachycardia [PJT]). It is characterized by repeated episodes (paroxysms) of atrial tachycardia, which often have a sudden onset (lasting minutes to hours) and an abrupt termination. It looks like an extremely fast rate with narrow QRS complexes (Table 23-9, p. 648).

STUDENT ALERT

In some cases of supraventricular tachycardia, the QRS complexes appear wide, making the assessment of supraventricular tachycardia difficult, since it looks like ventricular tachycardia. This is called wide-complex tachycardia of unknown origin. The mechanisms of this appearance are described under Disturbances of Ventricular Conduction.

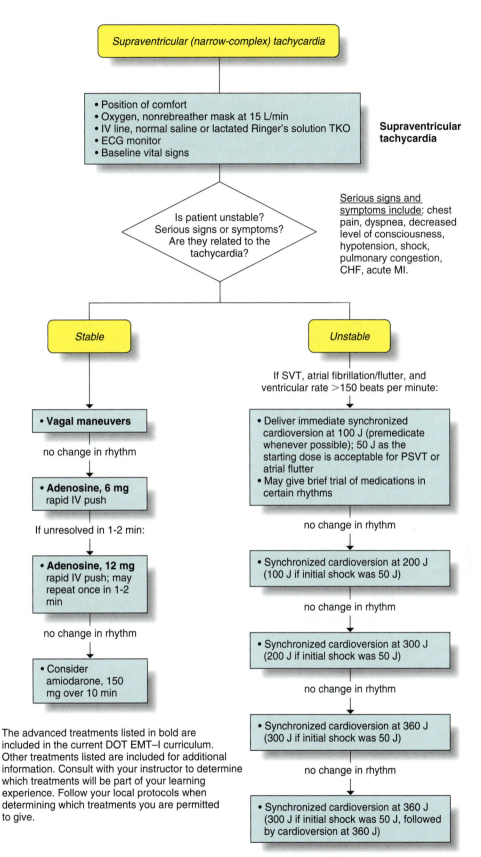

FIGURE 23-29 ▲ Supraventricular tachycardia algorithm.

TABLE 23-9

Supraventricular Tachycardias

CAUSES	ECG FINDINGS*	SIGNIFICANCE
Stress Overexertion Tobacco use Caffeine consumption Paroxysmal supraventricular tachycardia (PSVT) is also common in patients who have Wolff-Parkinson-White syndrome Rare in patients with acute myocardial infarction	Rhythm is regular (except if there is an onset and termination, as seen with PSVT) **Atrial and ventricular rate is 150-250 beats per minute** There is one P wave preceding each QRS complex; the P wave is typically buried in the T wave of the preceding beat; if present, the P waves may be flattened or notched Because the P waves tend to be buried, the PR intervals are typically indeterminable; if visible, the PR interval is often shortened but may be normal or rarely prolonged **QRS complexes are narrow (less than 0.12 sec)**, provided no ventricular conduction disturbance is present With multifocal atrial tachycardia (MAT) there are at least three distinct atrial foci associated with supraventricular tachycardia	Can occur at any age and is not commonly associated with underlying heart disease Palpitations, nervousness, and anxiety frequently accompany PVST Short bursts are well tolerated in otherwise normal people With sustained rapid ventricular rates, ventricular filling may not be complete during diastole Can significantly compromise cardiac output in patients with underlying heart disease (vertigo, lightheadedness, syncope, angina pectoris, hypotension, congestive heart failure) Increases cardiac oxygen requirements, which may increase myocardial ischemia and the frequency and severity of the patient's chest pain It is difficult to differentiate the exact origin most of the time; thus the term *PSVT* One variant, MAT, has unique features and prognostic implications

MANAGEMENT

Synchronized cardioversion starting at 50 J is indicated if the ventricular rate is greater than 150 beats per minute and the patient is symptomatic. If this fails to convert the rhythm, the energy level may be increased to 100, 200, 300, and finally 360 J.

Patients who are symptomatic (chest pain, hypotension, etc.) should receive high-concentration oxygen, an IV infusion of normal saline administered at a TKO rate, and prompt treatment.

If the heart rate is less than 150 beats per minute, or if the patient is tolerating the dysrhythmia, vagal maneuvers and drug therapy may be attempted before synchronized cardioversion. Adenosine, at a dose of 6 mg, is delivered by rapid IV push (in 1-3 sec). If, after 1-2 min, cardioversion does not occur, administer 12 mg by rapid IV push (in 1-3 sec). The higher dose may be repeated once if necessary. Attach a second syringe to a stopcock or through the port with the adenosine, and immediately deliver a 20-mL flush of normal saline after administering the drug.

EMT–Is in some EMS systems may be permitted to deliver verapamil or diltiazem in patients with persistent tachycardia.

Lidocaine, amiodarone, or electrical therapy (cardioversion) can be considered in *wide*–QRS complex tachycardia.

MAT usually represents either severe underlying heart or lung disease; the primary therapy is treatment of the underlying condition.

* Bold type indicates key characteristic(s) identifying dysrhythmia.

Atrial flutter (Figure 23-30) is a rapid atrial depolarization (250 to 350 beats per minute) with a typical "sawtooth" flutter wave or "picket fence" pattern visible (Table 23-10).

Atrial fibrillation (Figure 23-31, p. 650) occurs when multiple areas fire simultaneously within the atria, completely suppressing normal SA node output. Numerous impulses bombard the AV node and are conducted to the ventricles only in an irregular and sporadic fashion (Table 23-11, p. 651).

DYSRHYTHMIAS ORIGINATING IN THE ATRIOVENTICULAR JUNCTION

Rhythms that start in the AV node or AV junctional area are considered junctional rhythms. These typically occur when the SA node and atria are unable to generate sufficient electrical impulses to depolarize. The most common causes are hypoxia, ischemia, MI, and drug toxicity (e.g., digitalis preparations). In these cases the next lower pacemaker (the AV junction) takes over.

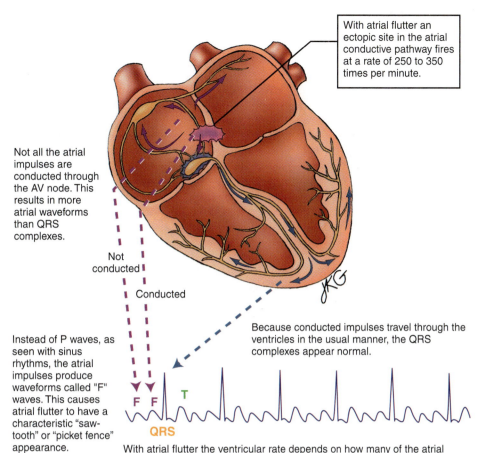

With atrial flutter an ectopic site in the atrial conductive pathway fires at a rate of 250 to 350 times per minute.

Not all the atrial impulses are conducted through the AV node. This results in more atrial waveforms than QRS complexes.

Not conducted

Conducted

Instead of P waves, as seen with sinus rhythms, the atrial impulses produce waveforms called "F" waves. This causes atrial flutter to have a characteristic "sawtooth" or "picket fence" appearance.

Because conducted impulses travel through the ventricles in the usual manner, the QRS complexes appear normal.

With atrial flutter the ventricular rate depends on how many of the atrial impulses are conducted through the AV node. The ventricular rate may be normal, slow, or fast.

FIGURE 23-30 ▲ Atrial flutter.

TABLE 23-10

Atrial Flutter

CAUSES	ECG FINDINGS*	SIGNIFICANCE
Occasionally occurs in patients with healthy hearts Commonly associated with other conditions: Cardiomyopathy Cardiac hypertrophy Digitalis toxicity (rare) Hypoxia Congestive heart failure Pericarditis and myocarditis	**Atrial rhythm is regular** Depending on conduction ratio, ventricular rhythm may be regular or irregular **Atrial rate is 250-350 beats per minute** Ventricular rate depends on ventricular response; may be normal, slow, or fast **Normal P waves are absent; "sawtooth" flutter waves are present** 1:1 AV conduction is rare; AV conduction is usually 2:1, 3:1, or 4:1 Conduction ratios may be constant or variable PR interval is usually constant QRS complexes are usually normal (less than 0.12 sec, unless ventricular conduction disturbance [aberrancy] is present)	Often well tolerated 2:1 conduction may result in loss of "atrial kick" and signs of decreased cardiac output Signs and symptoms of decreased cardiac output from a rapid ventricular response may occur

MANAGEMENT

Vagal maneuvers may make flutter waves more visible by transiently increasing the degree of the block.

Patients who are symptomatic (chest pain, hypotension, etc.) should receive high-concentration oxygen, an IV infusion of normal saline administered at a TKO rate, and prompt treatment.

Drugs that may be used for rates of 120-140 beats per minute with relative stability include propranolol, diltiazem, verapamil, and digoxin.

Rates greater than 150 beats per minute and/or hemodynamic instability require immediate cardioversion. The initial attempt at cardioversion for atrial flutter should consist of a synchronized shock of 50 J. If necessary, the energy may be increased to 100, 200, 300, and 360 J.

* Bold type indicates key characteristic(s) identifying dysrhythmia.

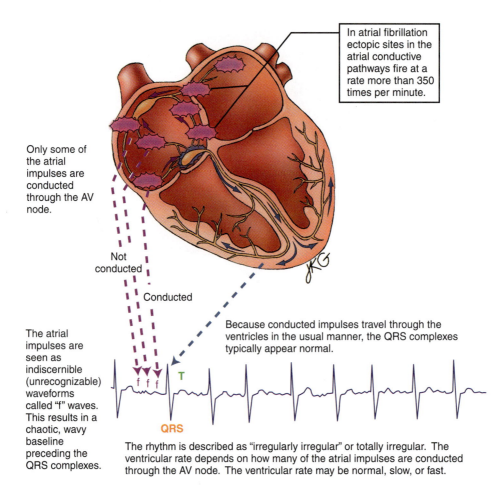

In atrial fibrillation ectopic sites in the atrial conductive pathways fire at a rate more than 350 times per minute.

Only some of the atrial impulses are conducted through the AV node.

Not conducted

Conducted

The atrial impulses are seen as indiscernible (unrecognizable) waveforms called "f" waves. This results in a chaotic, wavy baseline preceding the QRS complexes.

Because conducted impulses travel through the ventricles in the usual manner, the QRS complexes typically appear normal.

f f f   T

QRS

The rhythm is described as "irregularly irregular" or totally irregular. The ventricular rate depends on how many of the atrial impulses are conducted through the AV node. The ventricular rate may be normal, slow, or fast.

FIGURE 23-31 ▲ **Atrial fibrillation.**

In junctional rhythms, electrical impulses travel in a normal pathway from the AV junction through the bundle of His and bundle branches to Purkinje's fibers, ending in the ventricular muscle. Because conduction through the ventricles proceeds normally, the QRS complex is usually within normal limits of 0.04 to 0.12 second. The impulse that depolarizes the atria travels in a backward or retrograde direction, resulting in inverted P waves in lead II with a short PR interval, absent P waves (as they are buried by the QRS complex), or retrograde P waves.

These rhythms are generally not lethal; always, however, the entire picture must be considered. Features common to all dysrhythmias in this group are summarized in Table 23-12 on p. 651 (Figure 23-32, p. 652).

Tables 23-13 to 23-16 summarize cardinal features for dysrhythmias originating in the AV junction.

Premature junctional complex (PJC) (Figure 23-33) is a single premature electrical impulse originating in the AV junction. It occurs before the next expected sinus impulse. PJCs are thought to result from enhanced automaticity or a reentry mechanism. On the ECG, PJCs appear as "early beats." This causes the R-R interval to be shorter between the preceding beat and the early beat (as compared with the underlying rhythm) (Table 23-13, p. 652).

Junctional escape complexes or *rhythms* is an isolated complex (escape complex) or series of impulses (escape rhythm) that occur when the rate of the primary pacemaker (SA node) falls below that of the AV junctional area (Table 23-14, p. 653).

Accelerated junctional rhythm is faster than the usual junctional rate of 40 to 60 beats per minute because of increased excitability (automaticity, irritability) of the AV junction (Table 23-15, p. 654).

Junctional tachycardia is faster than the usual junctional rate because of increased excitability (automaticity, irritability) of the AV junction. Because this rhythm is faster than 100 beats per minute, it is referred to as tachycardia (Table 23-16, p. 654).

DYSRHYTHMIAS ORIGINATING IN THE VENTRICLES

Most ventricular dysrhythmias are potentially life threatening. These typically result when the atria, AV junction, or both, are unable to initiate an electrical impulse or in the face of enhanced excitability of the ventricular myocardium. In the latter case, myocardial ischemia is the most common cause. Features common to all dysrhythmias in this group are summarized in Table 23-17, p. 655.

Text continued on p. 655

TABLE 23-11

Atrial Fibrillation

CAUSES	ECG FINDINGS*	SIGNIFICANCE

Often associated with other conditions:
  Rheumatic heart disease
  Congestive heart failure (atrial dilation)
  Atherosclerotic heart disease
Less commonly, atrial fibrillation may occur with:
  Cardiomyopathy
  Acute myocarditis and pericarditis
  Chest trauma
Rarely caused by digitalis toxicity, but a very slow, regular ventricular response with atrial fibrillation should raise suspicion of digitalis toxicity
Paroxysmal atrial fibrillation, which occurs in young adults after heavy alcohol ingestion (the "holiday heart" syndrome) or because of acute stress, is a self-limited phenomenon, usually resolving without management
	Rhythm is totally (grossly) irregular; also referred to as irregularly irregular
	Atrial rate is too rapid to be counted (350-700 beats per minute)
	Ventricular rate depends on AV conduction; may be normal, slow, or fast
	There are no discernible P waves; the baseline is chaotic, since the atrial activity is represented by "fibrillatory" waves, or "f" waves
	No PR intervals are present
	QRS complexes are usually normal (less than 0.12 sec, provided no conduction block occurs in the bundle branches)
	An irregularly irregular supraventricular rhythm is atrial fibrillation until proven otherwise
		"Atrial kick" is lost, decreasing cardiac output by up to 25%
		Patients experiencing atrial fibrillation may develop intraatrial emboli, since the atria are not contracting and blood stagnates in the atrial chambers; this predisposes the patient to systemic emboli—particularly stroke
		Rapid ventricular response may lead to angina, acute myocardial infarction, congestive heart failure, or cardiogenic shock
		Moderate ventricular response is often well tolerated.

MANAGEMENT

If the rate of ventricular response is normal (often seen in patients taking digitalis), the dysrhythmia is usually well tolerated and requires no immediate intervention.

Patients who are symptomatic (chest pain, hypotension, etc.) should receive high-concentration oxygen, an IV infusion of normal saline administered at a TKO rate, and prompt treatment.

If the patient is stable with a ventricular response of 120-150 beats per minute, consider drug treatment as for atrial flutter.

For rates over 150 beats per minute and/or hemodynamic instability, consider immediate cardioversion (initially start at 100 J).

* Bold type indicates key characteristic(s) identifying dysrhythmia.

TABLE 23-12

Dysrhythmias Originating in the Atrioventricular Junction

TYPES OF DYSRHYTHMIAS ORIGINATING IN THE ATRIOVENTRICULAR JUNCTION	COMMON FEATURES
Premature junctional complex (PJC) Junctional escape complexes or rhythms Accelerated junctional rhythm Junctional tachycardia	QRS duration usually normal Retrograde (inverted) P waves common PR interval usually greater than 0.12 sec

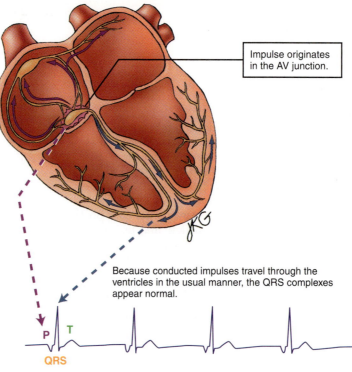

Impulse originates in the AV junction.

The atria are stimulated via retrograde conduction.

Because there is one pacemaker site, these rhythms are regular.

The P waves are often inverted (although they may be upright). They may precede, be buried in, or follow the QRS complex.

The PR interval, if present, is less than 0.12 sec in duration.

Because conducted impulses travel through the ventricles in the usual manner, the QRS complexes appear normal.

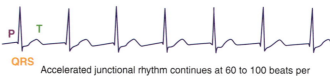

Junctional escape continues at 40 to 60 beats per minute.

Accelerated junctional rhythm continues at 60 to 100 beats per minute.

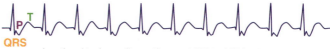

Junctional tachycardia continues at 100 to 180 beats per minute.

FIGURE 23-32 ▲ Junctional rhythms.

TABLE 23-13

Premature Junctional Complexes

CAUSES	ECG FINDINGS*	SIGNIFICANCE
Digitalis toxicity Other cardiac medications (quinidine, procainamide) Increased vagal tone on the SA node Sympathomimetic drugs (cocaine, methamphetamine) Hypoxia Congestive heart failure Damage to the AV junction	**Rhythm is irregular (underlying rhythm is disrupted by presence of early beats)** Rate is dependent on the rate of the underlying rhythm P waves typically are present with the underlying rhythm but not with the premature beats; if present, the P waves are usually inverted PR intervals are typically present with the underlying rhythm; if present with the premature beats, they will be less than 0.12 sec QRS complexes of premature beats are narrow (less than 0.12 sec) and look the same as QRS complexes of the underlying rhythm T waves of the premature beats are of the same direction as the R waves Premature junctional complexes (PJCs) are not usually followed by a compensatory pause	Isolated PJC is of little clinical significance Frequent (more than 4-6 beats per minute) PJCs portend more serious dysrhythmias

MANAGEMENT

No specific management is required.

* Bold type indicates key characteristic(s) identifying dysrhythmia.

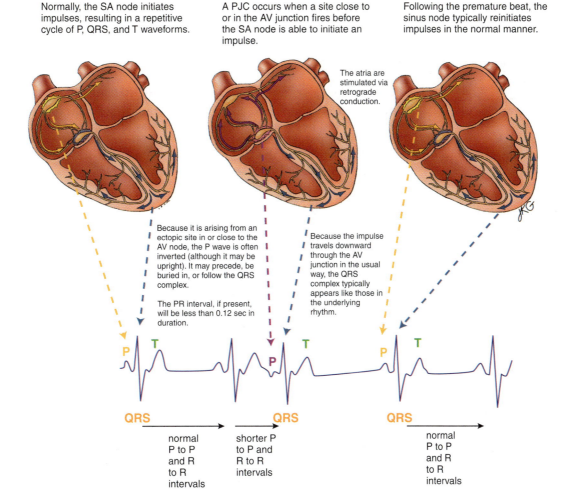

Normally, the SA node initiates impulses, resulting in a repetitive cycle of P, QRS, and T waveforms.

A PJC occurs when a site close to or in the AV junction fires before the SA node is able to initiate an impulse.

Following the premature beat, the sinus node typically reinitiates impulses in the normal manner.

The atria are stimulated via retrograde conduction.

Because it is arising from an ectopic site in or close to the AV node, the P wave is often inverted (although it may be upright). It may precede, be buried in, or follow the QRS complex.

The PR interval, if present, will be less than 0.12 sec in duration.

Because the impulse travels downward through the AV junction in the usual way, the QRS complex typically appears like those in the underlying rhythm.

P   T   QRS   normal P to P and R to R intervals

P   T   QRS   shorter P to P and R to R intervals

P   T   QRS   normal P to P and R to R intervals

With a premature junctional complex the regularity of the underlying rhythm is interrupted by an impulse that occurs earlier than normal. This causes a shortening of the P to P and R to R intervals.

FIGURE 23-33 ▲ Premature junctional complex.

TABLE 23-14

Junctional Escape Complexes or Rhythms

CAUSES	ECG FINDINGS*	SIGNIFICANCE
Usually due to digitalis toxicity	Rhythm is regular if it is an escape rhythm but irregular if it is an isolated escape complex	Escape complex or rhythm is a safety mechanism to prevent cardiac standstill
Increased vagal tone on the SA node	**Rate is between 40 and 60 beats per minute**	Occurs when the SA node fails to transmit a normal impulse to the AV junction within 1.0-1.5 sec
Pathological slowing of the SA discharge	**P waves may precede, be lost in (absent), or follow the QRS complex; when present, the P wave will be inverted**	Rates of greater than 50 beats per minute are usually well tolerated
Complete AV block	**PR interval, if present, will be less than 0.12 sec**	Junctional rhythms can cause decreased cardiac output because of their slow rate
Following open heart surgery	QRS complexes are within normal limits (less than 0.12 sec)	Junctional rhythms may lead to symptoms (lightheadedness, hypotension, syncope)
No specific management is required.		

MANAGEMENT

Stable patients require no immediate intervention.
Patients who are symptomatic (chest pain, hypotension, etc.) should receive high-concentration oxygen, an IV infusion of normal saline administered at a TKO rate, and prompt treatment.
If the patient is symptomatic (or if ventricular irritability is present), atropine administration is indicated.
In severe cases and in patients unresponsive to atropine, external transcutaneous pacing may be necessary.

* Bold type indicates key characteristic(s) identifying dysrhythmia.

TABLE 23-15

Accelerated Junctional Rhythm

CAUSES	ECG FINDINGS*	SIGNIFICANCE
Excessive catecholamine administration Damage to the AV junction Inferior-wall myocardial infarction Rheumatic fever Often the result of digitalis toxicity, especially if any type of block is also present Following open heart surgery	Rhythm is regular **Rate is 60-100 beats per minute** **P waves may precede, be lost in (absent), or follow the QRS complex; when present, the P wave will be inverted** **PR interval, if present, will be less than 0.12 sec** QRS complexes are within normal limits (less than 0.12 sec)	Usually well tolerated May predispose patient with myocardial ischemia to more serious dysrhythmias

MANAGEMENT
Generally, no specific immediate intervention is required.

* Bold type indicates key characteristic(s) identifying dysrhythmia.

TABLE 23-16

Junctional Tachycardia

CAUSES	ECG FINDINGS*	SIGNIFICANCE
Commonly the result of digitalis toxicity Other causes: Excessive catecholamine administration Anxiety Hypoxia Damage to the AV junction Acute myocardial infarction Following open heart surgery	Rhythm is regular (except if there is an onset and termination, as seen with paroxysmal supraventricular tachycardia [PSVT]) **Rate is 100-180 beats per minute** **P waves may precede, be lost in (absent), or follow the QRS complex; when present, the P wave will be inverted** **PR interval, if present, will be less than 0.12 sec** QRS complexes are within normal limits (less than 0.12 sec)	Can occur at any age with no patient history of underlying heart disease Palpitations, nervousness, and anxiety frequently accompany it Short bursts are well tolerated in otherwise normal people With sustained rapid ventricular rates, ventricular filling may not be complete during diastole Can significantly compromise cardiac output in patients with underlying heart disease (vertigo, lightheadedness, syncope, angina pectoris, hypotension, congestive heart failure) Increases cardiac oxygen requirements, which may increase myocardial ischemia and the frequency and severity of the patient's chest pain

MANAGEMENT
Treatment depends on the severity of the patient's signs and symptoms.
Patients who are symptomatic (chest pain, hypotension, etc.) should receive high-concentration oxygen, an IV infusion of normal saline administered at a TKO rate, and prompt treatment.
Synchronized cardioversion starting at 50 J is indicated if the ventricular rate is greater than 150 beats per minute and the patient is symptomatic. If this fails to convert the rhythm, the energy level may be increased to 100, 200, 300, and finally 360 J.

* Bold type indicates key characteristic(s) identifying dysrhythmia.

TABLE 23-17

Dysrhythmias Originating in the Ventricles

TYPES OF DYSRHYTHMIAS ORIGINATING IN THE VENTRICLES	COMMON FEATURES
Premature ventricular complex (PVC)	QRS complexes wide, bizarre in appearance, and greater than
Ventricular escape complexes or rhythm	0.12 sec in duration
Ventricular tachycardia	P waves not visible (hidden in the QRS complex)
Ventricular fibrillation	
Asystole	
Artificial pacemaker rhythm	

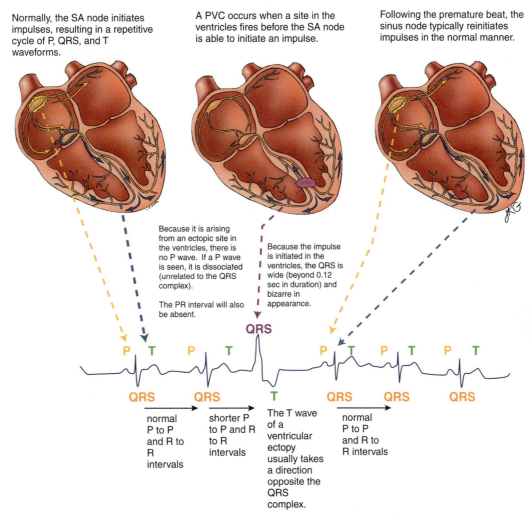

Normally, the SA node initiates impulses, resulting in a repetitive cycle of P, QRS, and T waveforms.

A PVC occurs when a site in the ventricles fires before the SA node is able to initiate an impulse.

Following the premature beat, the sinus node typically reinitiates impulses in the normal manner.

Because it is arising from an ectopic site in the ventricles, there is no P wave. If a P wave is seen, it is dissociated (unrelated to the QRS complex).

The PR interval will also be absent.

Because the impulse is initiated in the ventricles, the QRS is wide (beyond 0.12 sec in duration) and bizarre in appearance.

normal P to P and R to R intervals

shorter P to P and R to R intervals

The T wave of a ventricular ectopy usually takes a direction opposite the QRS complex.

normal P to P and R to R intervals

With a premature ventricular complex the regularity of the underlying rhythm is interrupted by an impulse that occurs earlier than normal. This causes a shortening of the P to P and R to R intervals.

FIGURE 23-34 ▲ Premature ventricular complex.

Tables 23-18 to 23-23 summarize cardinal features for dysrhythmias originating in the ventricles.

Premature ventricular complexes (PVCs) (Figure 23-34) are extra beats originating from the ventricle, which interrupt the normal rhythm. Sometimes, PVCs all originate from one place in the ventricle. These beats look the same and are referred to as uniform (unifocal)

PVCs. Other times, PVCs arise in several areas of the ventricles. These beats tend to appear different from each other and are called multiformed (multifocal) PVCs (Figure 23-35 and Table 23-18).

PVCs may occur singly or more frequently. PVCs that are interspersed between normal beats are named depending on their frequency. *Bigeminal PVCs* are said

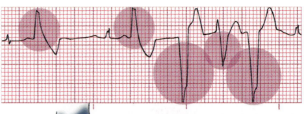

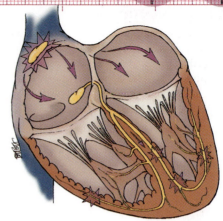

FIGURE 23-35 ▲ Multiformed premature ventricular complexes appear differently because they arise from several areas of the ventricle.

TABLE 23-18

Premature Ventricular Complexes

CAUSES	ECG FINDINGS*	SIGNIFICANCE
Pathological premature ventricular complexes (PVCs) are usually a result of one or more of the following: Myocardial ischemia Hypoxia Acid-base and electrolyte imbalance Hypokalemia Congestive heart failure Increased catecholamine and sympathetic tone (as in emotional stress) Ingestion of stimulants (alcohol, caffeine, tobacco) Drug toxicity Sympathomimetic drugs (cocaine; stimulants such as phencyclidine, epinephrine, isoproterenol)	**Rhythm is irregular, since underlying rhythm is disrupted by presence of the early beat(s)** Rate is dependent on the rate of the underlying rhythm P waves are typically present with the underlying rhythm but not with the premature beats PR intervals are typically present with the underlying rhythm but not with the premature beats **On the monitor, a wide (greater than 0.12 sec), usually bizarre-looking QRS complex** is seen, which is *not* preceded by a P wave; appears earlier in the cycle than the normal set of complexes would be expected to occur QRS complexes of the PVCs differ from QRS complexes of the underlying rhythm **T waves of the premature beats take an opposite direction to the R waves** **Following each PVC is a pause, called a compensatory pause**	Occur in healthy individuals without apparent cause and are usually of no significance Require special attention in persons with acute myocardial ischemia (angina, acute myocardial infarction) Isolated PVCs that occur in patients without underlying cardiovascular disease are usually of no significance Patients frequently experience the sensation of "skipped beats" PVCs that occur with myocardial ischemia may indicate the presence of enhanced automaticity, a reentry mechanism, or both, and may trigger lethal ventricular dysrhythmias PVCs do not permit complete ventricular filling and may produce a diminished or nonpalpable pulse (nonperfusing PVC) If the PVCs are frequent enough and occur early enough in the cardiac cycle, cardiac output is compromised Warning signs of the potential development of serious ventricular dysrhythmias in patients with myocardial ischemia: Frequent PVCs Presence of multifocal PVCs Early PVCs (R-on-T) Patterns of grouped PVCs

MANAGEMENT

Asymptomatic patients seldom require management.

In patients with myocardial ischemia, treatment of frequent PVCs includes administration of high-concentration oxygen, placement of an IV line, and prompt transport.

Some protocols may call for the EMT–I to administer lidocaine or other antidysrhythmics (e.g., amiodarone) by IV push and continue maintenance infusion. Follow local protocols or consult with medical direction.

* Bold type indicates key characteristic(s) identifying dysrhythmia.

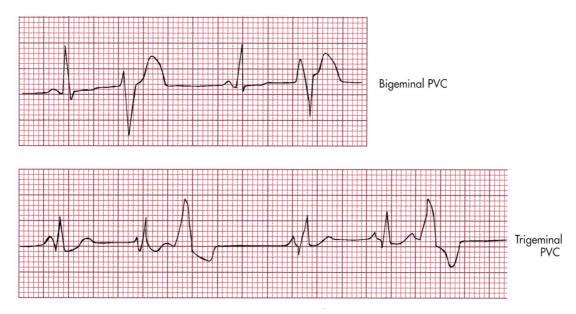

FIGURE 23-36 ▲ Premature ventricular complexes (PVCs) present after every other beat are bigeminal PVCs. If every third beat is a PVC, the result is trigeminal PVC, or ventricular trigeminy.

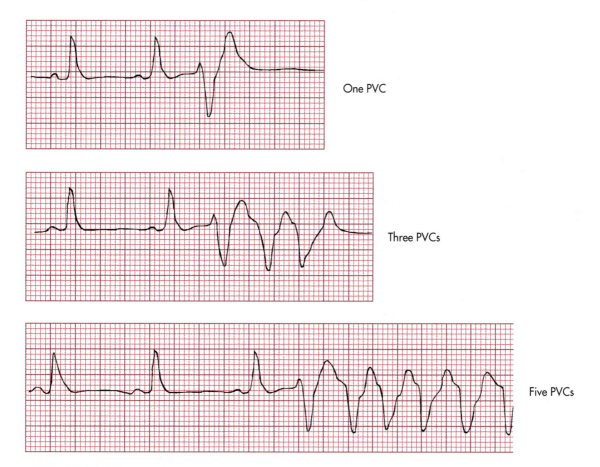

FIGURE 23-37 ▲ Premature ventricular complexes (PVCs) can appear singularly or many times. Three or more PVCs in a row are called ventricular tachycardia.

to be present when every other beat is a PVC, regardless of whether the PVC is unifocal or multifocal. If every third beat is a PVC, the condition is called *trigeminal PVCs* or ventricular trigeminy. Similarly, a PVC every fourth beat is *ventricular quadrigeminy.* Regular PVCs at greater intervals than every fourth beat have

no special name and are simply referred to as frequent PVCs (Figure 23-36).

PVCs may occur one after the other. Two PVCs in a row are a couplet, or pair. Three or more PVCs in a row constitute an abnormal rhythm known as ventricular tachycardia (Figure 23-37).

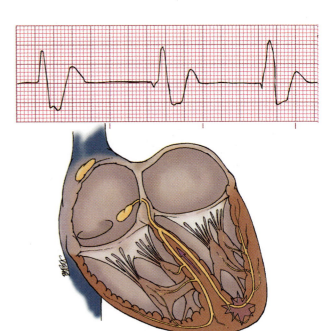

FIGURE 23-38 ▲ Idioventricular rhythm.

TABLE 23-19

Ventricular Escape Complexes or Idioventricular Rhythm

CAUSES	ECG FINDINGS*	SIGNIFICANCE
Occurs when the rate of impulse formation of the dominant pacemaker (usually the SA node) and the escape pacemaker in the AV junction falls below that of the escape pacemaker in the ventricles or when the stimuli of the dominant and escape pacemakers fail to reach the ventricles Frequently seen as the first organized rhythm after defibrillation	Rhythm is usually regular (becomes irregular as the heart dies) **Rate is usually 20-40 beats per minute; may be slower** **QRS complexes are wide (greater than 0.12 sec) and bizarre; the T wave typically takes the opposite direction of the R wave** P waves may be present or absent; if present, there is no predictable relationship between P waves and QRS complexes (AV dissociation) PR interval, if present, is variable and irregular	Escape complex or rhythm is a safety mechanism to prevent cardiac standstill Generally symptomatic (hypotension, decreased cardiac output) Decreased perfusion of the brain and other vital organs results in syncope and shock Patient assessment is essential because the escape rhythm may be perfusing or nonperfusing (pulseless electrical activity [PEA])

MANAGEMENT

Patients who are symptomatic (chest pain, hypotension, etc.) should receive high-concentration oxygen, an IV infusion of normal saline administered at a TKO rate, and prompt treatment.
If patient is perfusing, give atropine and consider transcutaneous pacing.
Lidocaine and amiodarone are *contraindicated* and may be lethal (by suppressing any remaining cardiac activity).
If there is no perfusion, treat as PEA.

* Bold type indicates key characteristic(s) identifying dysrhythmia.

Frequent PVCs, especially if bigeminal, trigeminal, or couplets or runs of ventricular tachycardia, may forecast the development of ventricular fibrillation. PVCs occurring on or near the previous T wave *(R-on-T PVCs)* are also a harbinger of worse ventricular dysrhythmias (e.g., ventricular fibrillation).

Ventricular escape complexes or *rhythm* (Figure 23-38) is an isolated complex (escape complex) or series of impulses (escape rhythm) that occur when stimuli from higher pacemakers (SA node, AV junction) fail to reach the ventricles or their rate falls to less than that of the ventricles (Table 23-19).

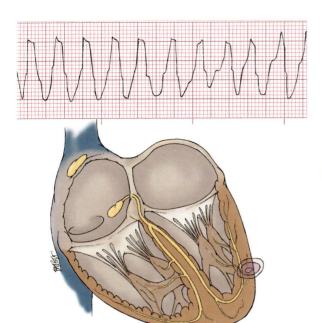

FIGURE 23-39 ▲ Ventricular tachycardia.

Sometimes a rhythm having all the characteristics of idioventricular rhythm will have a rate between 40 and 100 beats per minute. This is referred to as accelerated idioventricular rhythm.

Ventricular tachycardia (VT) (Figure 23-39) is three or more PVCs in a row. It may come in bursts of 6 to 10 complexes or may persist (sustained VT) (Table 23-20, p. 660).

A unique variant of polymorphic VT, **torsade de pointes,** literally meaning "twisting about the pointes" is seen frequently. It is characterized by QRS complexes that alternate (usually gradually) between upright deflections and downward deflections (Figure 23-40, p. 660). Unless the patient is in cardiac arrest, torsade de pointes often responds to infusion of magnesium sulfate. Standard antidysrhythmic drugs (e.g., procainamide) can *worsen* the condition, leading to cardiac arrest. Of course, if the patient is in cardiac arrest, the treatment of choice is prompt defibrillation.

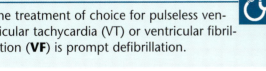

CLINICAL NOTES

The treatment of choice for pulseless ventricular tachycardia (VT) or ventricular fibrillation (**VF**) is prompt defibrillation.

Ventricular fibrillation (VF) (Figure 23-42, p. 662) is erratic firing of multiple sites in the ventricle. On the cardiac monitor, VF appears as a wavy line, undulating without logic (Table 23-21, p. 665).

Ventricular fibrillation, asystole, and pulseless electrical activity result in cardiac arrest and require prompt treatment. The universal algorithm is the starting point for managing patients suspected to be experiencing cardiac arrest (Figure 23-43, p. 663).

Asystole is the absence of any cardiac activity (Figure 23-45, p. 665). Asystole appears as a flat (or nearly flat) line on the monitor screen (Table 23-22, p. 667).

The presence of asystole in two leads should always be verified before treatment is initiated. Many nonmedical conditions, such as misplacement of a lead or a loose wire, can mimic asystole (or VF) on the monitor screen. Before concluding that a patient is actually in asystole, assess for mechanical causes of this appearance on the monitor. The following checks should be done if a patient is in cardiac arrest and appears to be in asystole:
- Make sure all the leads are attached in the proper places to both the machine and the patient.
- Make sure the correct lead (e.g., I, II, III) is selected on the monitor.
- Check the rhythm in more than one lead.
- Make sure that the monitor batteries are functioning appropriately.

Pulseless electrical activity (**PEA**) (Figure 23-47, p. 667) is a condition in which there is a rhythm noted on the monitor that *should* result in adequate perfusion, but the patient is pulseless and apneic. In other words, there is electrical activity in the heart that is *not* generating effective cardiac contraction. The primary characteristic associated with this condition is the presence of an electrical rhythm without a corresponding pulse (Table 23-23, p. 669).

TABLE 23-20

Ventricular Tachycardia

CAUSES	ECG FINDINGS*	SIGNIFICANCE

Usually occurs in the presence of myocardial ischemia or significant cardiac disease
 	
Other causes:
  Acid-base and electrolyte imbalance
  Hypokalemia
  Hypoxia
  Exercise
  Congestive heart failure
  Increased catecholamine and sympathetic tone (as in emotional stress)
  Ingestion of stimulants (alcohol, caffeine, tobacco)
  Drug toxicity (digitalis, tricyclic antidepressants)
  Sympathomimetic drugs (cocaine, methamphetamine)
  Prolonged QT interval (may be caused by drugs or metabolic problems or may be congenital)
  Ventricular aneurysm
  Rheumatic heart disease
	Rhythm is typically regular
	Ventricular rate is between 150-250 beats per minute; if the rate is between 100 and 150 beats per minute, it is referred to as slow ventricular tachycardia (VT); if the rate is greater than 250, it is referred to as ventricular flutter
	Typically, P waves are not discernible (if seen, they are dissociated)
	Rhythm consists of frequent wide (greater than 0.12 sec) and bizarre QRS complexes
	Rate is 150-220 beats per minute
	T waves may or may not be present and typically are of the opposite direction of the R waves
	VT may be *monomorphic* (the appearance of each QRS complex is similar) or *polymorphic* (the appearance varies considerably from complex to complex); either is potentially life threatening
		Clinically, VT is *always* significant; even if the rhythm results in a pulse, it should be considered potentially *unstable* (i.e., patients are very likely to develop worse rhythms and cardiac arrest)
		Usually indicates significant underlying cardiovascular disease
		Rapid rate and concurrent loss of "atrial kick" associated with VT result in compromised cardiac output and decreased coronary artery and cerebral perfusion
		Severity of symptoms varies with the rate of the VT and the presence or absence of underlying myocardial dysfunction
		VT may be perfusing or nonperfusing
		May initiate or degenerate into ventricular fibrillation (VF)

MANAGEMENT

Treatment of a patient experiencing VT includes maintaining a patent airway, administering high-concentration oxygen, placing an IV line, and prompt transport.

A patient who has a decreased level of consciousness, chest pain, shortness of breath, low blood pressure, shock, pulmonary congestion, heart failure, or acute myocardial infarction should be considered clinically unstable.

Initially these patients are managed with immediate cardioversion, followed by antidysrhythmics. The initial energy level for VT (with a pulse) is 100 J, followed by 200, 300, and 360 J. Polymorphic VT cannot be reliably synchronized and should be managed like VF, with an initial unsynchronized shock of 200 J (Figure 23-41).

Some protocols may allow the EMT–I to administer lidocaine (at a dose of 1.0-1.5 mg/kg IV push) or other drugs (e.g., amiodarone at a dose of 150 mg over 10 minutes).

Patients with pulseless VT should be treated as though they are in VF.

* Bold type indicates key characteristic(s) identifying dysrhythmia.

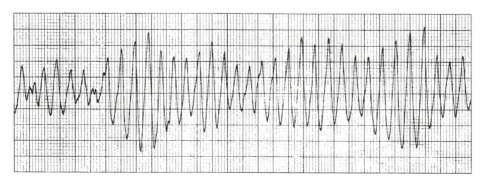

FIGURE 23-40 ▲ Torsades de pointes. (From Aehlert B: *ACLS quick review study guide,* St Louis, 1994, Mosby.)

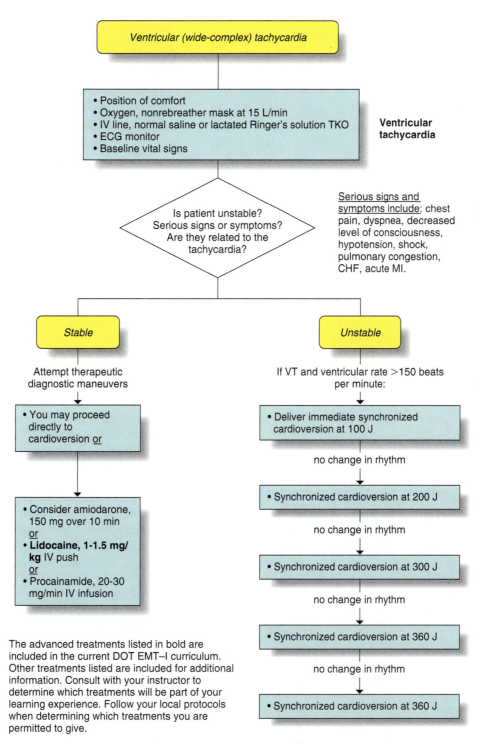

Ventricular (wide-complex) tachycardia

• Position of comfort
• Oxygen, nonrebreather mask at 15 L/min
• IV line, normal saline or lactated Ringer's solution TKO
• ECG monitor
• Baseline vital signs

Ventricular tachycardia

Is patient unstable?
Serious signs or symptoms?
Are they related to the tachycardia?

Serious signs and symptoms include: chest pain, dyspnea, decreased level of consciousness, hypotension, shock, pulmonary congestion, CHF, acute MI.

Stable

Attempt therapeutic diagnostic maneuvers

• You may proceed directly to cardioversion or

• Consider amiodarone, 150 mg over 10 min or
• **Lidocaine, 1-1.5 mg/ kg** IV push or
• Procainamide, 20-30 mg/min IV infusion

Unstable

If VT and ventricular rate >150 beats per minute:

• Deliver immediate synchronized cardioversion at 100 J

no change in rhythm

• Synchronized cardioversion at 200 J

no change in rhythm

• Synchronized cardioversion at 300 J

no change in rhythm

• Synchronized cardioversion at 360 J

no change in rhythm

• Synchronized cardioversion at 360 J

The advanced treatments listed in bold are included in the current DOT EMT–I curriculum. Other treatments listed are included for additional information. Consult with your instructor to determine which treatments will be part of your learning experience. Follow your local protocols when determining which treatments you are permitted to give.

FIGURE 23-41 ▲ Ventricular tachycardia algorithm.

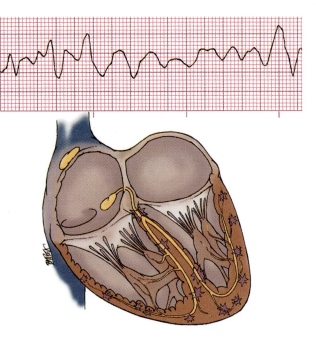

FIGURE 23-42 ▲ Ventricular fibrillation is an erratic firing of multiple sites in the ventricles.

DYSRHYTHMIAS THAT ARE DISORDERS OF CONDUCTION

Heart Blocks—*Heart blocks* are partial delays or complete interruptions in the cardiac conduction pathway. The most common causes are ischemia, myocardial necrosis, degenerative disease of the conduction system, and drugs (especially digitalis preparations). Abnormal conduction pathways exist in the preexcitation syndromes. Features common to all dysrhythmias in this group are summarized in Table 23-24 on p. 669.

Tables 23-25 to 23-28 summarize cardinal features for AV blocks (heart blocks).

First-degree AV block (Figure 23-49, p. 670) is not a true block, but rather a delay of conduction at the level of the AV node. It results in fixed prolongation of the PR interval (Table 23-25, p. 669).

❗ HELPFUL HINT

> • Some describe the pathophysiology of second-degree AV block, Mobitz type I, as a weakened AV junction that grows more and more tired with each heartbeat (thus producing a progressively longer PR interval following each P wave). Finally, the AV junction is too tired to carry the impulse and a QRS complex is dropped (only a P wave appears). The lack of conduction through the AV junction allows it to rest; thus the next PR interval is shorter. Then as each subsequent impulse is generated and transmitted through the AV junction, there is a progressively longer PR interval until, again, a QRS is dropped. This cycle can repeat itself over and over again.

Second-degree AV block, Mobitz type 1 (or Wenckebach) (Figure 23-50, p. 671), is an intermittent block at the level of the AV node. The PR interval (representing AV conduction time) increases until a QRS complex is dropped. By then, AV conduction recovers and the sequence repeats itself (Table 23-26, p. 672).

Second-degree AV block, Mobitz type II (Figure 23-51, p. 672), is an intermittent block at the level of the AV node when atrial impulses are not conducted to the ventricles. It differs from Mobitz type I in that the PR interval is *constant* before a beat being "dropped" (Table 23-27, p. 673).

Third-degree heart block (Figure 23-52, p. 673) is a complete electrical block at or below the AV node. The SA node serves as the pacemaker for the atria while an ectopic focus paces the ventricles. P waves and QRS complexes occur rhythmically, but the rhythms are unrelated to each other *(AV dissociation)* (Table 23-28, p. 674).

A helpful approach to differentiating the heart blocks is summarized in Figure 23-53 on p. 674.

Artificial pacemaker rhythm is shown in Figure 23-54 and summarized in Table 23-29 both on p. 675.

Disturbances of Ventricular Conduction—**Ventricular conduction disturbances** involve delays in electrical conduction through either the bundle branches (right or left) or the fascicles (anterior or posterior). Developing an ability to understand these interesting disturbances requires a detailed knowledge of cardiac vectors, a subject beyond the intended scope of this text (a number of excellent texts are available on the subject). Here, the principles of the ventricular conduction system and its abnormalities, as recognized on a field three- to four-lead ECG, are summarized.

The bundle of His divides to form the left and right bundle branches. The right bundle branch continues toward the apex, spreading throughout the right ventricle. The left bundle branch subdivides into the anterior and posterior fascicles and spreads throughout the left ventricle. Normally, the first part of the ventricle to

Text continued on p. 670

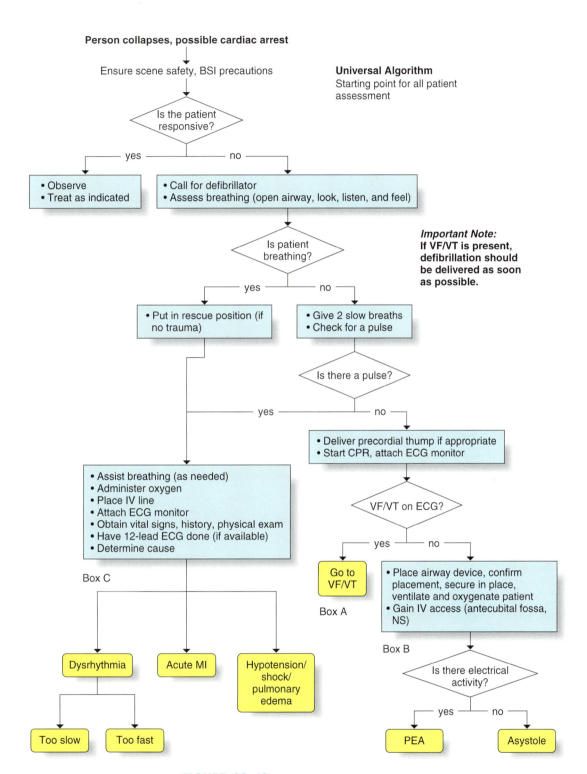

Person collapses, possible cardiac arrest

Ensure scene safety, BSI precautions

Universal Algorithm
Starting point for all patient assessment

Is the patient responsive?

yes — no

- Observe
- Treat as indicated

- Call for defibrillator
- Assess breathing (open airway, look, listen, and feel)

Important Note:
If VF/VT is present, defibrillation should be delivered as soon as possible.

Is patient breathing?

yes — no

- Put in rescue position (if no trauma)

- Give 2 slow breaths
- Check for a pulse

Is there a pulse?

yes — no

- Deliver precordial thump if appropriate
- Start CPR, attach ECG monitor

- Assist breathing (as needed)
- Administer oxygen
- Place IV line
- Attach ECG monitor
- Obtain vital signs, history, physical exam
- Have 12-lead ECG done (if available)
- Determine cause

Box C

VF/VT on ECG?

yes — no

Go to VF/VT

Box A

- Place airway device, confirm placement, secure in place, ventilate and oxygenate patient
- Gain IV access (antecubital fossa, NS)

Box B

Dysrhythmia

Acute MI

Hypotension/ shock/ pulmonary edema

Is there electrical activity?

yes — no

Too slow

Too fast

PEA

Asystole

FIGURE 23-43 ▲ Universal algorithm.

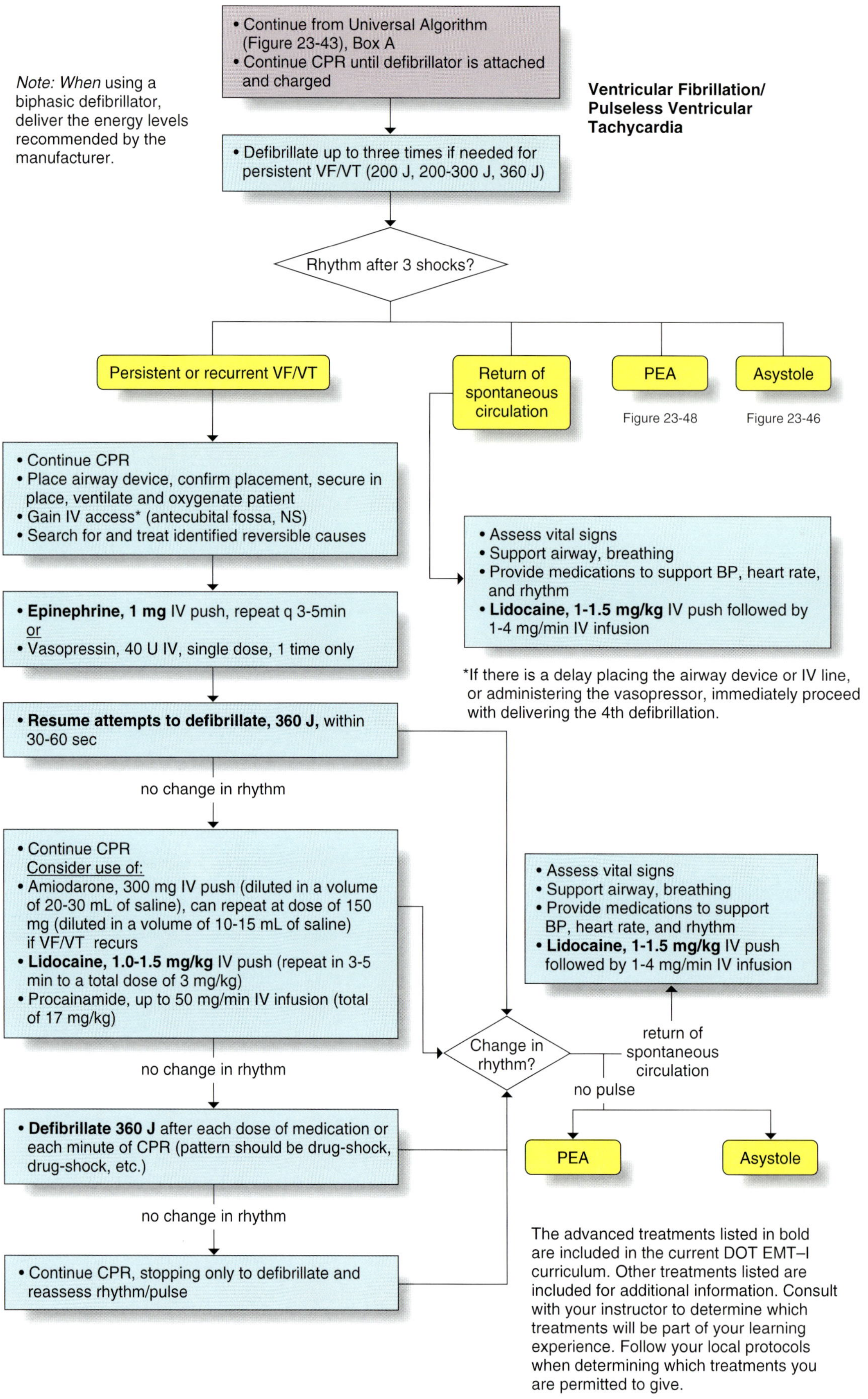

Note: When using a biphasic defibrillator, deliver the energy levels recommended by the manufacturer.

Ventricular Fibrillation/ Pulseless Ventricular Tachycardia

- Continue from Universal Algorithm (Figure 23-43), Box A
- Continue CPR until defibrillator is attached and charged

- Defibrillate up to three times if needed for persistent VF/VT (200 J, 200-300 J, 360 J)

Rhythm after 3 shocks?

Persistent or recurrent VF/VT

Return of spontaneous circulation

PEA — Figure 23-48

Asystole — Figure 23-46

- Continue CPR
- Place airway device, confirm placement, secure in place, ventilate and oxygenate patient
- Gain IV access* (antecubital fossa, NS)
- Search for and treat identified reversible causes

- Assess vital signs
- Support airway, breathing
- Provide medications to support BP, heart rate, and rhythm
- **Lidocaine, 1-1.5 mg/kg** IV push followed by 1-4 mg/min IV infusion

- **Epinephrine, 1 mg** IV push, repeat q 3-5min
or
- Vasopressin, 40 U IV, single dose, 1 time only

*If there is a delay placing the airway device or IV line, or administering the vasopressor, immediately proceed with delivering the 4th defibrillation.

- **Resume attempts to defibrillate, 360 J,** within 30-60 sec

no change in rhythm

- Continue CPR
Consider use of:
- Amiodarone, 300 mg IV push (diluted in a volume of 20-30 mL of saline), can repeat at dose of 150 mg (diluted in a volume of 10-15 mL of saline) if VF/VT recurs
- **Lidocaine, 1.0-1.5 mg/kg** IV push (repeat in 3-5 min to a total dose of 3 mg/kg)
- Procainamide, up to 50 mg/min IV infusion (total of 17 mg/kg)

- Assess vital signs
- Support airway, breathing
- Provide medications to support BP, heart rate, and rhythm
- **Lidocaine, 1-1.5 mg/kg** IV push followed by 1-4 mg/min IV infusion

no change in rhythm

Change in rhythm?

return of spontaneous circulation

no pulse

- **Defibrillate 360 J** after each dose of medication or each minute of CPR (pattern should be drug-shock, drug-shock, etc.)

PEA

Asystole

no change in rhythm

- Continue CPR, stopping only to defibrillate and reassess rhythm/pulse

The advanced treatments listed in bold are included in the current DOT EMT–I curriculum. Other treatments listed are included for additional information. Consult with your instructor to determine which treatments will be part of your learning experience. Follow your local protocols when determining which treatments you are permitted to give.

FIGURE 23-44 ▲ Ventricular fibrillation/pulseless ventricular tachycardia algorithm.

TABLE 23-21

Ventricular Fibrillation

CAUSES	ECG FINDINGS*	SIGNIFICANCE

Most commonly associated with significant cardiovascular system disease
May be precipitated by premature ventricular complexes, R-on-T phenomenon (rarely), or sustained ventricular tachycardia (VT)
Other causes:
  Myocardial ischemia
  Acute myocardial infarction
  Third-degree AV block with a slow ventricular escape rhythm
  Cardiomyopathy
  Digitalis toxicity
  Hypoxia
  Acidosis
  Electrolyte imbalance (hypokalemia, hyperkalemia, near-drowning)
  Electrical injury
  Drug overdose or toxicity (cocaine, tricyclic)
	Rhythm is totally chaotic
	No coordinated ventricular complexes are present; unsynchronized ventricular impulses occur at rates between 300 and 500 beats per minute
	No discernible P waves
	No PR intervals
	No discernible QRS complexes
		Ventricular fibrillation (VF) causes the heart muscle to wiggle, much like a handful of worms, rather than contracting efficiently
		Within 10 sec, the amount of blood pumped by the heart is essentially zero, causing all life-supporting physiological functions to cease because of lack of circulating blood flow
		If the patient is not promptly treated (with defibrillation), death occurs
		VF is the most common cause of prehospital cardiac arrest in adults

MANAGEMENT

Treatment includes prompt initiation of CPR and defibrillation. Defibrillate up to three times if needed for persistent VF/VT (200, 200-300, and 360 J) as soon as possible. Next, endotracheal intubation and placement of an IV line for normal saline infusion should be initiated (Figure 23-44).

Next, if allowed by local protocols, administer epinephrine (1.0 mg IV push every 3-5 min) or vasopressin (40 units by IV infusion). Then repeat defibrillation, and administer lidocaine (1-1.5 mg/kg IV push; repeat in 3-5 min to a total of 3 mg/kg) or amiodarone (300 mg IV push, diluted in a volume of 20-30 mL of saline). Amiodarone administration may be repeated at a dose of 150 mg (diluted in a volume of 10-15 mL of saline) if VF/VT recurs. Optional medications that may be used to treat this condition are shown in Figure 23-44.

Defibrillate at 360 J after each dose of medication or each minute of CPR (pattern should be drug-shock, drug-shock, etc.).

Continue CPR, stopping only to defibrillate and reassess rhythm.

If the rhythm is successfully converted to an effective electromechanical rhythm (with a pulse and good perfusion), assess vital signs, support airway and breathing, provide medications to support blood pressure and heart rate and rhythm, and administer lidocaine (1-1.5 mg/kg IV push followed by 1-4 mg/min IV infusion) or an infusion of the antidysrhythmic that was effective in restoring circulation.

*Bold type indicates key characteristic(s) identifying dysrhythmia.

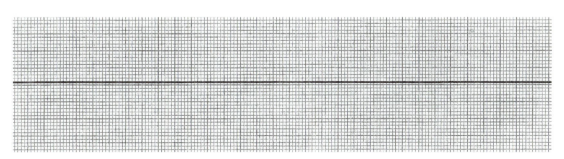

FIGURE 23-45 ▲ Ventricular asystole. (From Sanders MJ: *Mosby's paramedic textbook,* ed 2, St Louis, 2000, Mosby.)

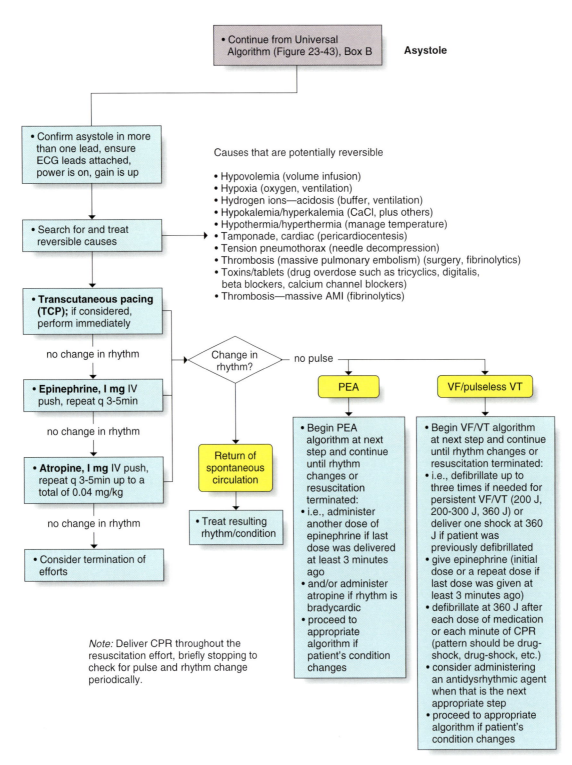

FIGURE 23-46 ▲ Asystole algorithm.

TABLE 23-22

Asystole

CAUSES	ECG FINDINGS	SIGNIFICANCE
May be the primary event in cardiac arrest May also occur in complete heart block when there is no functional escape pacemaker Usually associated with global myocardial ischemia or necrosis and often follows ventricular tachycardia (VT), ventricular fibrillation (VF), pulseless electrical activity (PEA), or an agonal escape rhythm in the dying heart	There is no electrical activity, only a flat line	Produces complete cessation of cardiac output Is a terminal rhythm; once a person has become asystolic, the chances of recovery are extremely low Some use the term *ventricular standstill* to differentiate conditions where the atria continue to beat but the ventricles have stopped from complete asystole (Although academically correct, this situation is rare and is not discussed here.) An ominous dysrhythmia, often representing a confirmation of death, in which the prognosis for resuscitation is dismal

MANAGEMENT

Treatment of asystole includes prompt initiation of CPR, high-concentration oxygen, endotracheal intubation, and placement of an IV line (Figure 23-46).

If permitted by local protocols, administer epinephrine (1.0 mg IV push every 3-5 min), followed by atropine (1 mg IV push every 3-5 min to a total of 0.04 mg/kg).

Continue CPR throughout the resuscitation effort, stopping periodically to reassess for a change in the rhythm and to check for the presence of a pulse.

Provide prompt transport.

Typically, transcutaneous pacing offers little benefit in asystole—follow local protocols.

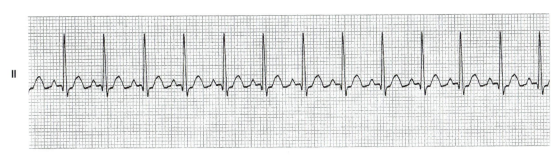

FIGURE 23-47 ▲ Pulseless electrical activity may be seen with any type of ECG rhythm.

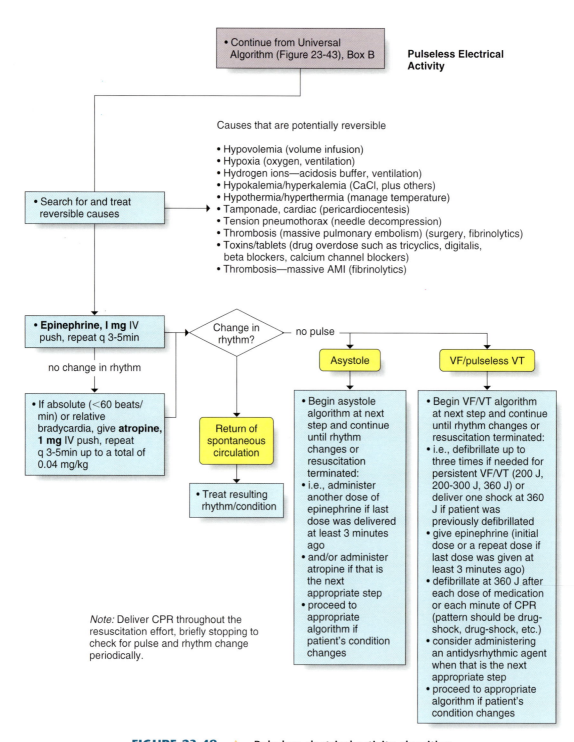

- Continue from Universal Algorithm (Figure 23-43), Box B

Pulseless Electrical Activity

Causes that are potentially reversible

- Hypovolemia (volume infusion)
- Hypoxia (oxygen, ventilation)
- Hydrogen ions—acidosis buffer, ventilation)
- Hypokalemia/hyperkalemia (CaCl, plus others)
- Hypothermia/hyperthermia (manage temperature)
- Tamponade, cardiac (pericardiocentesis)
- Tension pneumothorax (needle decompression)
- Thrombosis (massive pulmonary embolism) (surgery, fibrinolytics)
- Toxins/tablets (drug overdose such as tricyclics, digitalis, beta blockers, calcium channel blockers)
- Thrombosis—massive AMI (fibrinolytics)

- Search for and treat reversible causes

- **Epinephrine, I mg** IV push, repeat q 3-5min

no change in rhythm

- If absolute (<60 beats/min) or relative bradycardia, give **atropine, 1 mg** IV push, repeat q 3-5min up to a total of 0.04 mg/kg

Change in rhythm?

Return of spontaneous circulation

- Treat resulting rhythm/condition

no pulse

Asystole

VF/pulseless VT

- Begin asystole algorithm at next step and continue until rhythm changes or resuscitation terminated:
- i.e., administer another dose of epinephrine if last dose was delivered at least 3 minutes ago
- and/or administer atropine if that is the next appropriate step
- proceed to appropriate algorithm if patient's condition changes

- Begin VF/VT algorithm at next step and continue until rhythm changes or resuscitation terminated:
- i.e., defibrillate up to three times if needed for persistent VF/VT (200 J, 200-300 J, 360 J) or deliver one shock at 360 J if patient was previously defibrillated
- give epinephrine (initial dose or a repeat dose if last dose was given at least 3 minutes ago)
- defibrillate at 360 J after each dose of medication or each minute of CPR (pattern should be drug-shock, drug-shock, etc.)
- consider administering an antidysrhythmic agent when that is the next appropriate step
- proceed to appropriate algorithm if patient's condition changes

Note: Deliver CPR throughout the resuscitation effort, briefly stopping to check for pulse and rhythm change periodically.

FIGURE 23-48 ▲ Pulseless electrical activity algorithm.

TABLE 23-23

Pulseless Electrical Activity

CAUSES	ECG FINDINGS	SIGNIFICANCE
Often associated with severe underlying heart disease, but the following reversible causes should always be considered: Hypovolemia (most common) Tension pneumothorax Hypoxia Pericardial tamponade	Rhythm may be regular or irregular Rate may be fast, normal, or slow P waves may be present or absent, depending on the origin of the rhythm PR intervals may be present or absent, depending on the origin of the rhythm QRS complexes may be normal width (less than 0.12 sec) or wide and bizarre, depending on the origin of the rhythm	May appear as sinus rhythm, sinus tachycardia, idioventricular rhythm, or other rhythms Includes electromechanical dissociation (EMD), pseudo-EMD, idioventricular rhythms, ventricular escape rhythms, bradyasystolic rhythms, or postdefibrillation idioventricular rhythms

MANAGEMENT

Treatment of pulseless electrical activity (PEA) includes prompt initiation of CPR, high-concentration oxygen, endotracheal intubation, placement of an IV line, and prompt transport (Figure 23-48).

Some protocols allow the EMT–I to administer epinephrine (1.0 mg IV push every 3-5 min).

In bradycardic PEA, atropine may be administered (1 mg IV push every 3-5 min to a total of 0.04 mg/kg).

Continue CPR throughout the resuscitation effort, stopping periodically to reassess for a change in the rhythm and to check for the presence of a pulse.

In consideration of the possible causes, many experts recommend a fluid bolus, in addition to CPR and drugs (epinephrine and atropine), as part of the initial treatment for PEA. Follow local protocols.

TABLE 23-24

Dysrhythmias That Are Disorders of Conduction

TYPES OF DYSRHYTHMIAS	COMMON FEATURES
AV blocks (heart blocks) Disturbances of ventricular conduction Pulseless electrical activity Preexcitation syndromes	Degree of block does not directly reflect clinical severity Always consider specific rates of the atria and ventricles Always look at the patient, not just the ECG strip (This is true for *any* dysrhythmia.)

TABLE 23-25

First-Degree Atrioventricular Block

CAUSES	ECG FINDINGS*	SIGNIFICANCE
May occur for no apparent reason Sometimes associated with other conditions: Myocardial ischemia Acute myocardial infarction Increased vagal (parasympathetic) tone Digitalis toxicity	Rhythm is usually regular; depends on the underlying rhythm Rate is that of the underlying rhythm P waves are normal; one precedes each QRS complex **PR interval is constant and greater than 0.20 sec** QRS complexes are within normal limits (less than 0.12 sec)	Little or no clinical significance because all impulses are conducted to the ventricles Usually asymptomatic May progress to higher-degree block, especially in the face of inferior myocardial infarction

MANAGEMENT

There is no definitive management.

* Bold type indicates key characteristic(s) identifying dysrhythmia.

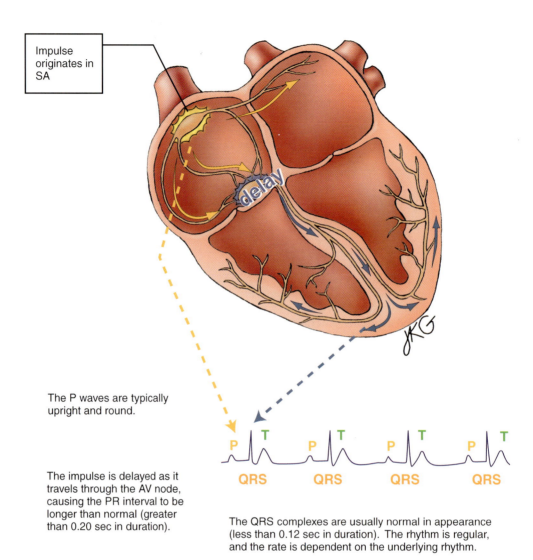

Impulse originates in SA

delay

The P waves are typically upright and round.

The impulse is delayed as it travels through the AV node, causing the PR interval to be longer than normal (greater than 0.20 sec in duration).

The QRS complexes are usually normal in appearance (less than 0.12 sec in duration). The rhythm is regular, and the rate is dependent on the underlying rhythm.

FIGURE 23-49 ▲ First-degree atrioventricular block.

be depolarized is the left side of the interventricular septum. The impulse passes through the septum to the other side. Then the right and left ventricles are stimulated simultaneously (Figure 23-55, p. 676).

Possible sites of block within the ventricular conduction include the following:

- *Right bundle branch*—Called a right bundle branch block (RBBB).
- *Left bundle branch*—Called a left bundle branch block (LBBB).
- *Left anterior fascicle*—Called a left anterior fascicular block (LAFB); also called a left anterior hemiblock (LAHB).
- *Left posterior fascicle*—Called a left posterior fascicular block (LPFB); also called a left posterior hemiblock (LPHB).

In addition, there may be any combination of these blocks.

▶ NOTE: LAHB, LPHB, and combination blocks are complex, potentially confusing, and beyond the necessary scope of knowledge of most out-of-hospital providers. For these reasons, they are given only cursory mention.

Whenever the normal path of ventricular conduction is blocked, the portion of myocardium supplied by the blocked "wire" receives its electrical stimulation from other parts of the normal conduction system. This occurs, however, only *after* they have stimulated the myocardium they normally "serve." The results are as follows (Figure 23-56, p. 676):

- An abnormal QRS configuration, reflecting abnormal ventricular conduction of the impulse (Often, the

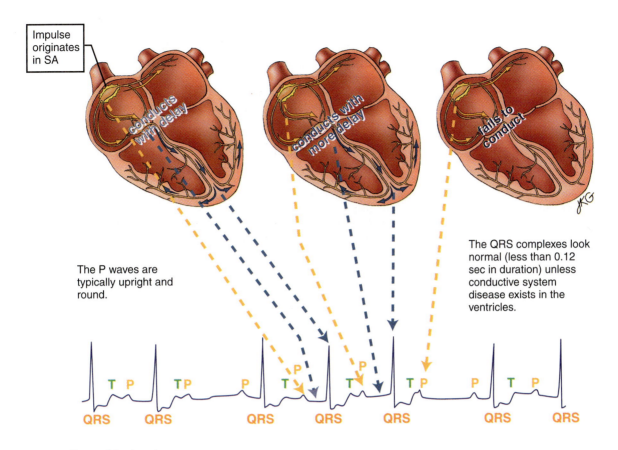

Impulse originates in SA

The P waves are typically upright and round.

The QRS complexes look normal (less than 0.12 sec in duration) unless conductive system disease exists in the ventricles.

Some of the impulses are blocked as they travel through the AV node. This results in there being more P waves than QRS complexes.

The rhythm is described as regularly irregular or patterned irregular as the cycle repeats itself over and over again. The atrial rate is normal, whereas ventricular rate is slower than normal.

The PR intervals of the conducted impulses are progressively longer in duration until finally an impulse is blocked.

FIGURE 23-50 ▲ Second-degree atrioventricular block, type I.

QRS complex is described as "biphasic," consisting of two separate R waves. These are often referred to as the R and R¹ (R-prime) waves.

- Widening of the QRS complex (sometimes visible only in specific leads), reflecting a delay in complete depolarization of the ventricle

A simplified, but often accurate, approach to recognizing bundle branch blocks using the MCL_1 lead is as follows:

- Is the QRS complex wide (less than 0.12 second)? If so, consider that a bundle branch may be present.
- Is the QRS complex mostly upright or mostly downward?
- Is the QRS biphasic?

Depending on the answers to these questions, the following conclusions can often be made:

- The presence of R and R¹ waves in a wide, upright QRS complex in lead MCL_1 strongly favors an ECG diagnosis of right bundle branch block.
- The presence of a wide, biphasic, downward QRS complex in lead MCL_1 strongly favors an ECG diagnosis of left bundle branch block.

The hemiblocks (LAHB, LPHB) involve a block of conduction in one of the left fascicles. LAHB is far more common. Although the ECG appearance of the hemiblocks differs somewhat from that of bundle branch blocks, the principles are similar; the normal conduction pathway is blocked. The affected myocardium receives its electrical innervation "retrograde" from the remaining intact parts of the conduction system. Since smaller areas are involved, the width of the entire QRS complex is usually not affected, but its configuration is.

Text continued on p. 676

TABLE 23-26

Second-Degree Atrioventricular Block, type I

CAUSES	ECG FINDINGS*	SIGNIFICANCE

Often occurs in acute my-ocardial infarction or acute myocarditis
Other causes include:
  Increased vagal tone
  Ischemia
  Acute cardiac disease
  Drug toxicity (digitalis, propranolol, verapamil)
  Head injury
  Electrolyte imbalance
	Ventricular rhythm is irregular with "grouped beating"; appears as a pattern (cycle seems to occur over and over again)
	Atrial rate is that of the underlying rhythm; ventricular rate is slightly less than atrial rate (slower than normal)
	P waves are upright and uniform; there are more P waves than QRS complexes, since some of the QRS complexes are blocked
	PR interval gets progressively longer until a P wave fails to conduct, resulting in a "dropped" QRS complex; after the blocked beat, the cycle starts all over again
	QRS complexes are within normal limits (less than 0.12 sec)
	P-P interval is constant; R-R interval decreases until a QRS complex is dropped
		By itself, is transient and re-versible but may progress to more serious blocks
		If dropped beats occur fre-quently, the patient may show signs and symptoms of decreased cardiac output

MANAGEMENT

If patient is asymptomatic, no specific treatment is needed.

Patients who are symptomatic (chest pain, hypotension, etc.) should receive high-concentration oxygen, an IV in-fusion of normal saline administered at a TKO rate, and prompt treatment.

If patient is symptomatic, consider atropine and transcutaneous pacing.

* Bold type indicates key characteristic(s) identifying dysrhythmia.

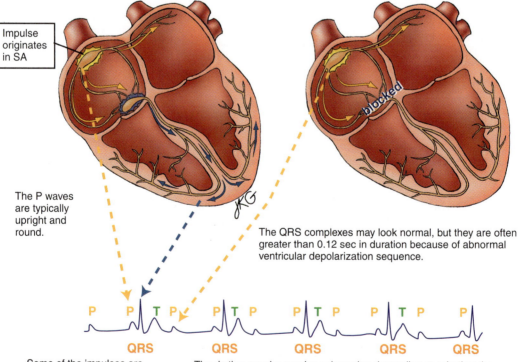

Impulse originates in SA

blocked

The P waves are typically upright and round.

The QRS complexes may look normal, but they are often greater than 0.12 sec in duration because of abnormal ventricular depolarization sequence.

Some of the impulses are blocked as they travel through the AV node. This results in there being more P waves than QRS complexes.

The PR intervals of the conducted impulses are the same duration (length).

The rhythm may be regular or irregular, depending on whether the conduction ratio is constant or varied. The atrial rate is normal, whereas the ventricular rate is slower than normal.

FIGURE 23-51 ▲ Second-degree atrioventricular block, type II.

TABLE 23-27

Second-Degree Atrioventricular Block, type II

CAUSES	ECG FINDINGS*	SIGNIFICANCE
Usually associated with acute myocardial infarction and septal necrosis Normally does not result solely from increased parasympathetic tone or drug toxicity	Rhythm is typically regular; will be irregular if the conduction ratio (number of P waves to each QRS complex) varies Atrial rate is that of underlying rhythm; ventricular rate is less than atrial rate **P waves are upright and uniform; some are not followed by QRS complexes (there are more P waves than QRS complexes)** AV conduction ratio may be fixed or may vary **PR interval is constant for conducted beats;** may be normal or prolonged QRS complexes may be within normal limits (less than 0.12 sec) or wide	A serious dysrhythmia is usually considered malignant in the emergency setting Slow ventricular rates may result in signs and symptoms of hypoperfusion May progress to a more severe heart block and even to ventricular asystole

MANAGEMENT

Patients who are symptomatic (chest pain, hypotension, etc.) should receive high-concentration oxygen, an IV infusion of normal saline administered at a TKO rate, and prompt treatment.

Atropine is no longer recommended in the treatment of Mobitz type II AV block or in third-degree block with new wide-QRS complexes.

Consider epinephrine (follow local protocols).

Consider transcutaneous pacing.

Immediate transport is indicated.

* Bold type indicates key characteristic(s) identifying dysrhythmia.

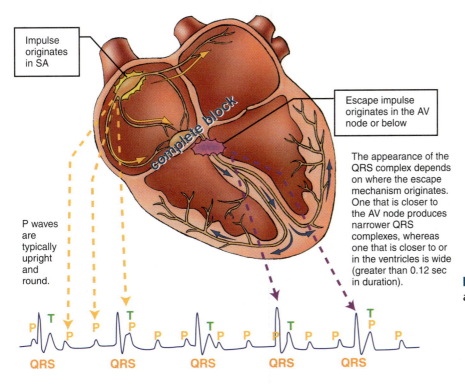

Impulse originates in SA

Escape impulse originates in the AV node or below

complete block

The appearance of the QRS complex depends on where the escape mechanism originates. One that is closer to the AV node produces narrower QRS complexes, whereas one that is closer to or in the ventricles is wide (greater than 0.12 sec in duration).

P waves are typically upright and round.

FIGURE 23-52 ▲ Third-degree atrioventricular block.

All of the impulses are blocked from traveling through the AV node. This results in there being two separate pacemaker sites.

Because the atrial rate is faster than the ventricular rate, there are more P waves than QRS complexes.

The PR intervals are absent, as there is no relationship between the atrial impulses and ventricular impulses.

The atrial and ventricular rhythms are regular, but because the atria and ventricular impulses are occurring at different rates, it appears the P waves "march through the QRS complexes." The atrial rate is normal, whereas the ventricular rate is typically less than 60 beats per minute.

TABLE 23-28

Third-Degree Heart Block

CAUSES	ECG FINDINGS*	SIGNIFICANCE
Increased vagal tone (which may produce a transient AV dissociation) Septal necrosis Acute myocarditis Digitalis, beta blocker, or calcium channel blocker toxicity Electrolyte imbalance May also occur in older adults from chronic degenerative changes in the conduction system	Atrial rate is that of the underlying rhythm; ventricular rate depends on the escape focus (40-60 beats per minute, junctional; greater than 40 beats per minute, ventricular) Atrial and ventricular rhythms are regular but independent of each other QRS complexes are normal if escape focus is junctional; widened if escape focus is ventricular P waves are present and normal, unrelated to QRS complexes; more P waves than QRS complexes **There is no relationship between the P waves and QRS complexes; "the P waves appear to march right through the QRS complexes"**	Severe bradycardia and decreased cardiac output may occur because of the slow ventricular rate and asynchronous action of the atria and ventricles May be associated with wide QRS complexes (ominous sign) Is potentially lethal; patients with this rhythm are often hemodynamically unstable

MANAGEMENT

Patients who are symptomatic (chest pain, hypotension, etc.) should receive high-concentration oxygen, an IV infusion of normal saline administered at a TKO rate, and prompt treatment.

Atropine *is no longer recommended* in the treatment of Mobitz type II AV block or third-degree block with new wide QRS complexes.

Consider epinephrine (follow local protocols).

Consider immediate transcutaneous pacing.

Immediate transport is indicated.

* Bold type indicates key characteristic(s) identifying dysrhythmia.

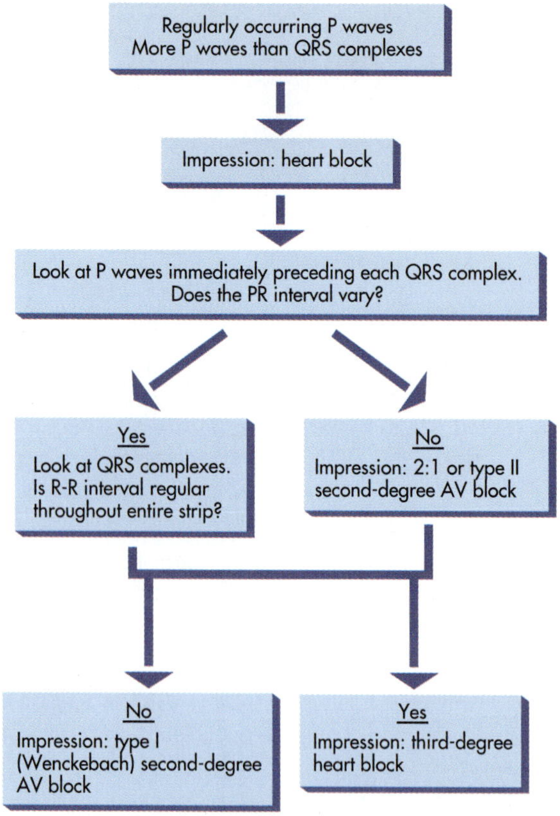

FIGURE 23-53 ▲ Identifying heart blocks.

Regularly occurring P waves
More P waves than QRS complexes
↓
Impression: heart block
↓
Look at P waves immediately preceding each QRS complex. Does the PR interval vary?

Yes → Look at QRS complexes. Is R-R interval regular throughout entire strip?

No → Impression: 2:1 or type II second-degree AV block

No → Impression: type I (Wenckebach) second-degree AV block

Yes → Impression: third-degree heart block

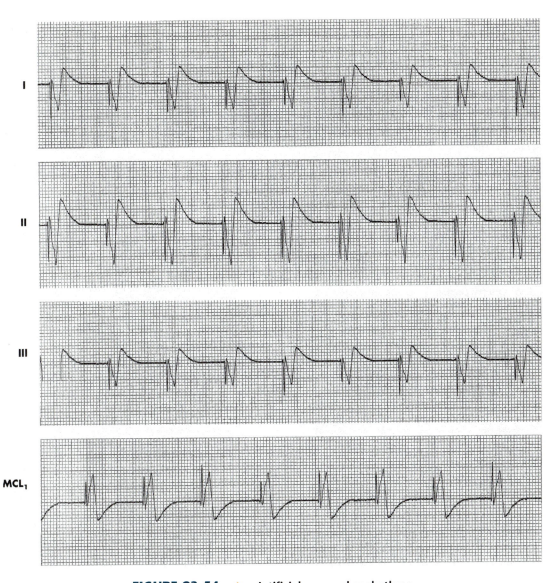

FIGURE 23-54 ▲ Artificial pacemaker rhythms.

TABLE 23-29

Artificial Pacemaker Rhythm

CAUSES	ECG FINDINGS	SIGNIFICANCE
There are numerous types of modern pacemakers. Here, we discuss only the ventricular pacemaker with the lead positioned in the right ventricle. It may fire continuously (asynchronous mode) or only when the patient's heart rate drops below a preset limit (demand mode).	Varies according to pacer settings; usually 60-80 beats per minute If paced, QRS is wide and bizarre, resembling a premature ventricular complex; preceded by a pacemaker spike; normal QRS in unpaced beats With normal pacer function, a wide QRS should follow each pacing spike P waves may be present or absent and are unrelated to pacing spikes and paced QRS complexes PR interval depends on underlying rhythm	Pacemaker spikes followed by a wide QRS indicate normal pacer capture; if there is no QRS after a pacing spike, no ventricular contraction occurs No specific treatment if pacer function is normal Pacemaker failure is a *true emergency* Consider immediate transcutaneous pacing

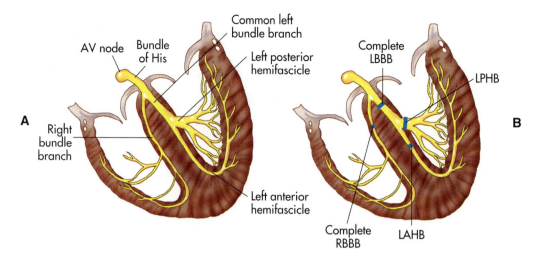

FIGURE 23-55 ▲ **A,** Simplified illustration showing the major divisions of the ventricular conduction system. After passing through the atrioventricular (AV) node and the bundle of His, the electrical impulse is carried to the right and common left bundle branches. The latter structure divides into the left anterior and posterior hemifascicles. **B,** Possible sites of block and the conduction deficits that may be produced. *LBBB,* Left bundle branch block; *RBBB,* right bundle branch block; *LAHB,* left anterior hemiblock; *LPHB,* left posterior hemiblock. (From Grauer K: *Practical guide to ECG interpretation,* St Louis, 1992, Mosby.)

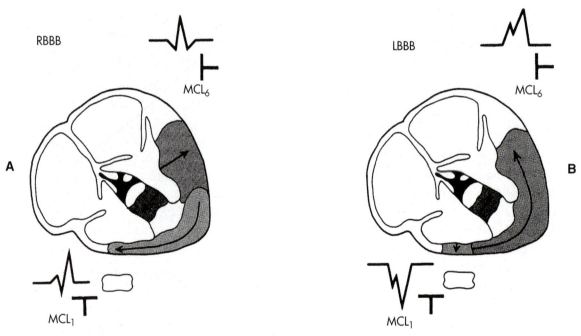

FIGURE 23-56 ▲ **A,** Right bundle branch block. **B,** Left bundle branch block. (From *JEMS,* pp 42-43, May 1990.)

In the normal ECG the QRS complex is mostly upright in leads I and II. In LAHB the direction of "current flow" within the myocardium changes so that the "wave" goes *away* from lead II, causing it to be mostly downward (Figure 23-57). Similarly, in LPHB the direction of "current flow" within the myocardium changes so that the "wave" goes *away* from lead I, causing it to be mostly downward (Figure 23-58).

Patients with any type of ventricular conduction block, and especially those with a combination, are at high risk of developing complete heart block. Depending on local protocols, standby transcutaneous

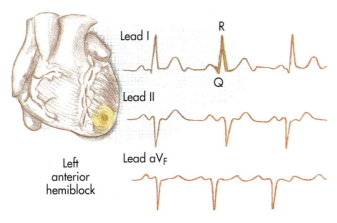

FIGURE 23-57 ▲ Left anterior hemiblock. (From Sanders MJ: *Mosby's paramedic textbook*, ed 2, St Louis, 2000, Mosby.)

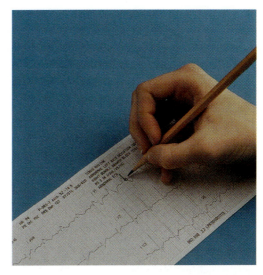

FIGURE 23-58 ▲ To distinguish left bundle branch block from right bundle branch block, find the J point of the QRS complex, draw a line backward into the QRS complex, and fill in the triangle created by this line and the last portion of the QRS complex. The direction in which the triangle points distinguishes the two types of blocks. (From Sanders MJ: *Mosby's paramedic textbook*, ed 2, St Louis, 2000, Mosby.)

pacing (TCP) should be considered for these individuals, especially in the face of acute myocardial ischemia.

Preexcitation Syndromes—Preexcitation syndromes involve the presence of abnormal conduction pathways (called *accessory conduction pathways*) between the atria and the ventricles. These pathways bypass the AV node and bundle of His, allowing atrial impulses to depolarize the ventricles earlier than usual. The most common preexcitation syndrome is the *Wolff-Parkinson-White (WPW)* syndrome. It occurs in 3 out of every 1000 people.

In WPW syndrome an accessory pathway (the *bundle of Kent*) connects the atrium to the ventricles, bypassing the AV node. Unless a tachycardia is present, WPW syndrome is usually of no significance. ECG features include (Figure 23-59) the following:

- Normal rate; regular rhythm
- QRS widened with slurring of the initial portion (*delta wave*)
- Normal P waves
- Shorter than normal (usually) PR interval (greater than 0.12 second)

Patients with WPW syndrome are susceptible to PSVT with rapid ventricular responses. Often the QRS complex is widened during tachycardia because of retrograde conduction via the accessory pathway. Drugs such as digitalis and verapamil are *contraindicated* in wide–QRS complex tachycardia for two reasons:

- If the patient really has VT, they are ineffective.
- If the patient has PSVT, WPW syndrome, and aberrant conduction (causing the wide QRS), they further block the AV node. This accelerates conduction even more down the faster accessory pathway and worsens the situation.

CAVEATS REGARDING TREATMENT

In treating any dysrhythmia, always remember these major points:

	Normal conduction	WPW
A		or Delta
B		Delta or

FIGURE 23-59 ▲ Characteristic findings in Wolff-Parkinson-White (WPW) syndrome (short PR interval, QRS widening, and delta wave) compared with normal conduction. **A,** Usual appearance of WPW syndrome in leads where the QRS complex is predominantly upright. **B,** Appearance of WPW syndrome; the QRS complex is predominantly negative. (From Grauer K: *Practical guide to ECG interpretation*, St Louis, 1992, Mosby.)

- Always look at the patient, as well as at the ECG strip.
- If the patient displays serious signs and symptoms, especially if the ventricular rate is greater than 150 beats per minute, prepare for immediate cardioversion.
- If the QRS complex is wide, treat the rhythm as VT until proven otherwise. Give lidocaine or amiodarone (follow local protocols) instead of adenosine or verapamil.

Generally:

- Lidocaine or amiodarone (follow local protocols) are first-line drugs for presumed VT. Although studies are limited, many experts currently favor amiodarone.
- Adenosine or procainamide (follow local protocols) are the initial choices for uncertain or presumed supraventricular tachycardia.
- Amiodarone or procainamide is now recommended over lidocaine and adenosine for the initial treatment of hemodynamically stable wide-complex tachycardia.
- Flutter waves may be difficult to identify when there is a 2:1 ratio of atrial to ventricular complexes. Suspect 2:1 flutter when the rhythm is regular and the ventricular rate is 150 beats per minute.
- An irregularly irregular supraventricular rhythm is *atrial fibrillation* until proven otherwise.
- Always consider digitalis toxicity with atrial fibrillation and a slow, *regular* ventricular response. The QRS complex may be normal or wide.

Always look for a pacer in an unconscious patient. In persons with pacemakers, remember:

- Pacemaker spikes indicate only that a pacemaker is discharging. They provide *no* information regarding ventricular contraction or perfusion.
- Treat all dysrhythmias as usual.
- Treat ventricular irritability with lidocaine or amiodarone (according to local protocols); do not worry about suppressing ventricular response to the pacer.
- Defibrillate in the usual manner.
- Use TCP in the usual manner.

Mobitz type II with 2:1 AV block is often difficult to distinguish from the generally more benign condition, Mobitz type I with 2:1 AV block (Wenckebach). Features indicating a Mobitz type II block include the following:

- Normal PR interval during conducted beats
- Wide QRS complex (less than 0.12 second)
- Inadequate escape rate

Features indicating a Wenckebach block include the following:

- Prolonged PR interval during conducted beats
- Narrow QRS complex
- Adequate escape rate

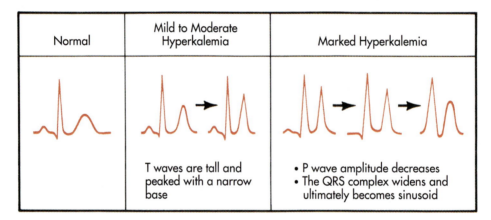

FIGURE 23-60 ▲ ECG changes suggestive of hyperkalemia.

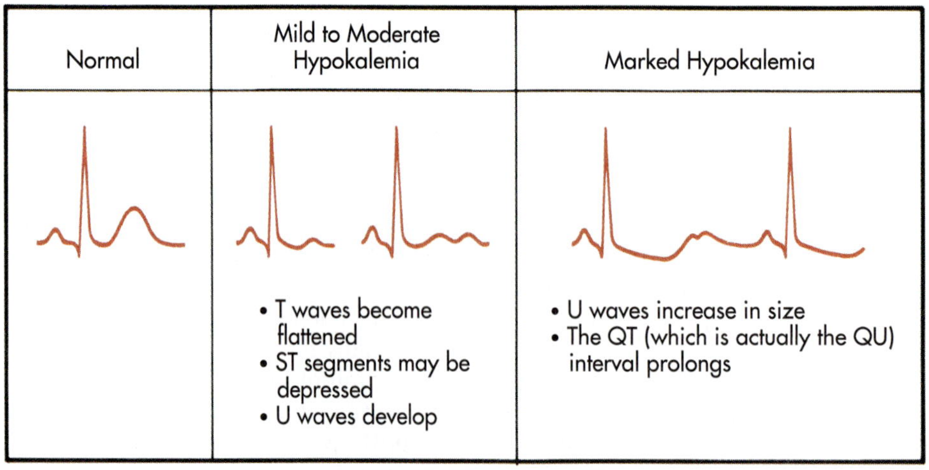

FIGURE 23-61 ▲ ECG changes suggestive of hypokalemia.

ELECTROCARDIOGRAM CHANGES DUE TO ELECTROLYTE IMBALANCES

The most immediately life-threatening electrolyte imbalances involve those of potassium. Levels that are too high (**hyperkalemia**) or too low (**hypokalemia**) may rapidly result in serious cardiac dysrhythmias. Physical signs of hyperkalemia include weakness, paralysis, and respiratory failure. Often ECG changes are present first:

- Peaked T waves (tenting)
- Flattened P waves
- Prolonged PR interval (first-degree AV block)
- Widened QRS complex
- Deepened S waves and merging of S and T waves
- Idioventricular rhythm
- Sine wave–appearing ECG
- VF and cardiac arrest

Of these, tenting of T waves is the most prominent early ECG sign (Figure 23-60).

Symptoms of hypokalemia include weakness, fatigue, paralysis, respiratory difficulty, constipation, and leg cramps. The following are suggestive ECG changes (Figure 23-61):

- U waves
- T-wave flattening
- ST-segment changes (nonspecific)
- Prolongation of the QT interval
- Dysrhythmias
- Pulseless electrical activity (PEA) or asystole

ELECTROCARDIOGRAM CHANGES DUE TO HYPOTHERMIA

There are no specific ECG changes associated with hypothermia. In the past, some texts described "J waves" or Osborne waves. However, recent data suggest that these are nonspecific and seen only rarely. The most common ECG changes involve dysrhythmias:

- Early hypothermia results in sinus tachycardia as a result of release of epinephrine.
- Moderate to severe hypothermia leads to bradydysrhythmias, including atrial fibrillation with a slow ventricular response.
- Severe hypothermia often results in refractory VF or asystole.

MANAGEMENT OF THE PATIENT WITH CARDIAC DYSRHYTHMIAS

General Management

The most accurate clinical approach to a patient with cardiac dysrhythmias involves careful attention to the adequacy of the airway, breathing, and circulation. Rather than being concerned with "naming" the rhythm, determine first if the patient is stable; look at the patient's perfusion status, as well as vital signs. Then decide if the patient is symptomatic (e.g., has chest pain, shortness of breath, dizziness). This information is vital for patient management using recommended algorithms of the American Heart Association (see p. 688).

Mechanical Interventions
VAGAL MANEUVERS

Vagal maneuvers stimulate the parasympathetic nervous system and may be tried in order to terminate PSVT in hemodynamically stable patients. Attempt vagal maneuvers only with medical control authorization. Have an IV line and ECG monitoring in place before beginning. The three commonly used vagal maneuvers, in order of their preference, are as follows:

1. *Valsalva maneuver*—Have the patient take in a deep breath and "bear down" as if to have a bowel movement. This results in forced expiration against a closed glottis and vagal nerve stimulation. Repeat the maneuver if it is unsuccessful initially.
2. *Ice-water maneuver*—Also known as the "cold pressor test," this maneuver involves having the patient hold his or her breath and then immerse the face briefly into ice water. The vagus nerve is stimulated because of the mammalian diving reflex. *Do not* perform this test if ischemic heart disease is present or suspected.
3. *Unilateral carotid sinus pressure*—Always auscultate both carotid arteries for a bruit (pulse-related "whooshing" sound) before performing this test. If a bruit is present, if the carotid pulses are not equal bilaterally, or if the patient has a history of cerebrovascular disease, *do not* perform this test. To proceed with the test, use your index and middle fingers placed over the carotid artery on the neck, just below the angle of the jaw. Compress gently while massaging the area. Maintain pressure for no longer than 5 to 10 seconds. Stop immediately if bradycardia or heart block develops, or if the tachycardia breaks. Only compress one side at a time. Repeat the procedure once in 2 to 3 minutes if it is ineffective initially.

STIMULATION

Direct physical or verbal stimulation may be effective temporarily in improving a patient's condition.

PRECORDIAL THUMP

Historically, the precordial thump was indicated in witnessed VF and pulseless VT. It is not specifically discussed, pro or con, in the latest American Heart Association recommendations. If used appropriately, this technique may be lifesaving. Follow local protocols.

COUGH

"Cough CPR" has been shown to be highly effective in maintaining cardiac output during specific resuscitation situations:

- Monitored cardiac arrest
- Arrest recognized before loss of consciousness

These situations are present only for the first 10 to 15 seconds of a cardiac arrest. Instruct the patient to cough forcefully and repetitively as frequently as possible.

Pharmacological Interventions

EMT–Is may be called on to administer or assist a paramedic-level provider in the administration of medications. Always follow local protocols when handling or assisting in the handling of any medication. Drugs commonly used in the treatment of dysrhythmias and cardiac arrest are summarized here.

ADENOSINE

Adenosine depresses AV node and SA node activity. It is effective in terminating PSVT. Its half-life is less than 5 seconds. The initial dose is a 6-mg rapid IV bolus followed by a 20-mL normal saline flush. If there is no response in 1 to 2 minutes, a 12-mg dose should be administered in the same manner. Adenosine should be used only when a supraventricular origin for a tachycardia is strongly suspected. Side effects include flushing, bradycardia, and rarely, cardiac arrest due to asystole.

AMIODARONE

Amiodarone is a complex drug with multiple effects. It is useful for both atrial and ventricular arrhythmias. It is preferred over other antidysrhythmic agents in patients with severely impaired heart function. Indications include the following:

- Ventricular rate control of rapid atrial dysrhythmias when digitalis is ineffective
- After defibrillation and epinephrine in cardiac arrest with persistent VT or VF
- Hemodynamically stable VT and wide–QRS complex tachycardia of uncertain origin
- Control of rapid ventricular rate due to accessory pathway conduction in preexcitation syndromes

In nonarrest situations 150 mg is given intravenously over 10 minutes, followed by a 1 mg/min infusion for 6 hours. In cardiac arrest due to pulseless VT or VF, 300 mg is given by IV push (diluted in a volume of 20 to 30 mL of saline); another 150 mg (diluted in a volume of 10 to 15 mL of saline) can be given if VF/VT recurs. Major side effects include hypotension and bradycardia.

ATROPINE

Atropine blocks discharge from the parasympathetic nervous system, leading to an increase in the heart rate. Indications include the following:

- Hemodynamically significant bradycardias
- Asystole

The initial dose of atropine is 0.5 to 1.0 mg IV push, unless the patient is in cardiac arrest; then the initial dose is 1.0 mg given intravenously. Doses of atropine may be repeated every 3 to 5 minutes to a maximum dose of 0.04 mg/kg (approximately 3 mg in the average 70-kg person). Atropine may also be administered endotracheally at 2 to 2.5 mg. Atropine is *relatively contraindicated* in type II AV block and third-degree block with new wide QRS complexes. Under these circumstances, atropine may cause paradoxical *slowing* of the heart rate.

CALCIUM CHANNEL BLOCKERS (VERAPAMIL)

Verapamil is a calcium channel blocker that slows conduction and increases refractoriness in the AV node. This may terminate many PSVTs, as well as control the ventricular response rate in patients with atrial fibrillation, atrial flutter, and MAT. The initial dose is 2.5 to 5 mg given intravenously over 2 minutes. Repeat doses of 5 to 10 mg may be given every 15 to 30 minutes to a maximum dose of 20 mg. Verapamil should be given only to persons with narrow–QRS complex tachycardia or dysrhythmias known with certainty to be supraventricular in origin. The drug is contraindicated in tachycardias resulting from preexcitation syndromes.

EPINEPHRINE

Epinephrine, or adrenaline, is the most common drug used in treatment of cardiac arrest. It is indicated in all types of arrest (VF, pulseless VT, asystole, PEA) and in many life-threatening dysrhythmias. Administration of epinephrine raises the aortic diastolic pressure. The coronary artery perfusion pressure is the difference between the aortic diastolic pressure and the central venous pressure. Thus epinephrine increases coronary perfusion pressure and increases a patient's chances of resuscitation from a cardiac arrest.

During a cardiac arrest, epinephrine usually is given intravenously, although it also may be administered via an endotracheal tube. In an adult the initial IV dose is 1 mg. Repeat doses are given every 3 to 5 minutes, depending on the patient's response. Current American Heart Association guidelines allow for much flexibility in the amount of epinephrine given in repeat doses, so local protocols should be followed.

▶ NOTE: High-dose epinephrine (up to 0.2 mg/kg given intravenously) in cardiac arrest is acceptable but not recommended because there is a lack of efficacy data.

LIDOCAINE

Lidocaine is an antidysrhythmic drug that is administered to treat ventricular dysrhythmias (frequent PVCs, VT, VF). It stabilizes the cardiac membrane and decreases the frequency of rhythm problems. Because of a lack of supportive evidence (that shows it is effective in terminating ventricular dysrhythmias), yet no evidence of significant harm, lidocaine is currently considered acceptable for the following:

- VF/pulseless VT that persists after defibrillation and administration of epinephrine
- Control of hemodynamically compromising PVCs
- Hemodynamically stable VT

In cardiac arrest, the *first* treatment of cardiac rhythm problems is defibrillation. Next is the placement of an endotracheal tube, placement of an IV line, and administration of epinephrine. Lidocaine (or other drugs) is then used only when electrical shock fails or following successful defibrillation, to prevent recurrence. In a cardiac arrest, administration of lidocaine may increase the chances of the heart responding to subsequent electrical shocks.

In cardiac arrest, the dose of lidocaine is 1 to 1.5 mg/kg IV push. This dose may be repeated every 3 to 5 minutes to a maximum of 3 mg/kg. In frequent PVCs and VT with a pulse associated with MI, lidocaine may be given at a dose of 1 to 1.5 mg/kg and repeated in 0.5 to 0.75 mg/kg boluses every 5 to 10 minutes to a maximum of 3 mg/kg. A maintenance infusion of lidocaine at a dose of 1-4 mg/min should be delivered following successful conversion of VF or pulseless VT. This maintenance infusion may also be used to maintain therapeutic levels of lidocaine when given in the treatment of PVCs and VT with a pulse.

▶ NOTE: Current American Heart Association recommendations state that lidocaine remains a second choice behind amiodarone and procainamide in many circumstances. Follow local protocols.

PROCAINAMIDE

Procainamide suppresses both atrial and ventricular dysrhythmias. Acceptable uses include the following:

- Pharmacological conversion of supraventricular dysrhythmias, such as atrial fibrillation and atrial flutter, to sinus rhythm
- Rapid ventricular rate control in tachycardias associated with preexcitation syndromes
- Wide-complex tachycardias of uncertain origin (ventricular versus supraventricular)

The drug is given as an infusion of 20 mg/min until the dysrhythmia is suppressed, hypotension occurs, the QRS complex is prolonged by 50% from its original duration, or a total of 17 mg/kg has been given. In urgent situations, up to 50 mg/min may be given. The currently recommended dose rate in refractory VF is 30 mg/min. The use of procainamide is avoided in persons with known QT prolongation (or torsade de pointes).

VASOPRESSIN

Vasopressin is a naturally occurring antidiuretic hormone. In high doses it acts as a powerful vasoconstrictor by direct stimulation of specific nonautonomic receptors. Some data indicate that vasopressin has a stronger beneficial effect on resuscitation after cardiac arrest than does epinephrine. Currently, it is considered as an alternative to epinephrine for the treatment of adult shock–refractory VF. Although less supportive data exist, this drug may also be beneficial in treatment of the following:

- Asystole
- PEA
- Vasodilatory shock

Vasopressin is given intravenously in a one-time dose of 40 units. If there is no response, the use of epinephrine is started or resumed as described earlier.

SUMMARY POINTS

Generally speaking:

- Lidocaine or amiodarone (follow local protocols) are first-line drugs for presumed VT with a pulse. Although studies are limited, many experts currently favor amiodarone.
- Adenosine or procainamide (follow local protocols) are the initial choices for presumed supraventricular tachycardia.
- Amiodarone or procainamide are now recommended over lidocaine and adenosine for the initial treatment of hemodynamically stable wide-complex tachycardia.

Defibrillation

Defibrillation is the delivery of an electrical shock to the heart in an attempt to terminate life-threatening rhythm disturbances such as VF or pulseless VT. By depolarizing a certain mass ("critical mass") of myocardium, it may restore an effective rhythm. Defibrillation also is referred to as unsynchronized countershock or asynchronous cardioversion.

Synchronized cardioversion is a *different* procedure, requiring a specific switch to be set on the defibrillator. The shock is automatically delivered during a portion of the cardiac cycle where the heart is not susceptible to the development of worse ventricular dysrhythmias (pulseless VT or VF).

Successful defibrillation depends on a number of factors, including the duration of time from the onset of fibrillation, transthoracic resistance, energy output, and paddle placement. The paddles must make good contact with the skin, and adequate conductive gel, paste, or pads must be present. The operator should apply approximately 25 pounds of firm arm pressure to the paddles to optimize defibrillation.

The earlier that defibrillation is done following the onset of VF, the more likely it is to be successful. Survival rates after VF cardiac arrest decrease 7% to 10% with every minute of delay to defibrillation. In cases of witnessed VF (or VT without a pulse) in which a defibrillator is immediately available, defibrillation should be done before initiating CPR.

Resistance to passage of the countershock caused by the tissues of the chest is referred to as transthoracic resistance. The greater the transthoracic resistance, the less energy delivered to the heart. Factors that influence transthoracic resistance include delivered energy, electrode size, interface between the chest wall and the electrodes, the number and time interval between previous shocks, pressure applied to the electrodes, the phase of the patient's ventilation, and the distance between electrodes.

▶ NOTE: "Traditional" defibrillators, both manual and automated, have used a single type of electrical waveform. This forms the basis for the recommendation of gradually increasing energy (200, 300, and 360 joules [J]). Recently, biphasic waveform defibrillators have been approved by the Food and Drug Administration (FDA), although their use is not yet widespread. Since the waveform is different, a lower energy setting (150 to 175 J) appears to be as effective without escalating doses. The current American Heart Association position is that there is insufficient evidence to warrant recommending one type of defibrillator over another. The most important thing is that the patient be defibrillated by some type of device and as soon as possible.

CLINICAL NOTES

Persons with refractory dysrhythmias may have an automated internal defibrillator or cardioverter device placed surgically. These use a minicomputer to determine the presence of life-threatening dysrhythmias and automatically deliver a shock to terminate the dysrhythmia.

AUTOMATED EXTERNAL DEFIBRILLATION

Because the early treatment of VF is crucial, several manufacturers have developed automated external defibrillators (AEDs). EMT–Is do *not* need to be able to interpret cardiac rhythms to use an AED. Once properly attached to the patient, these devices automatically analyze the heart rhythm and electronically determine if VF is present. If so, they either will automatically defibrillate the patient or advise the operator to push a button, causing the machine to defibrillate the patient.

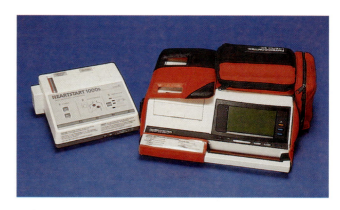

FIGURE 23-62 ▲ Automated external defibrillators can be either fully automatic *(left)* or semiautomatic *(right)*.

Types of Automated External Defibrillators— There are two types of AEDs (Figure 23-62):
* *Fully automatic defibrillators*—These devices analyze the patient's cardiac rhythm, decide whether or not defibrillation is warranted, and automatically (after warning the operator) deliver a shock when appropriate.
* *Semiautomatic defibrillators*—Also called shock advisory defibrillators, these devices analyze the patient's rhythm and decide if a shock is warranted. If so, they advise the operator of this fact. A button must be pushed before the device will deliver a defibrillatory shock to the patient.

Each model operates differently. The manufacturer's instructions should be followed for the use of each device.

Protocol for Automated External Defibrillation—The guidelines given here are generic in nature, because each device operates differently. EMT-Is *must* be familiar with the operating features of their particular AED.

The following basic steps apply to the use of any AED:
1. Recognize that the patient is in cardiac arrest.
2. Prepare and attach the defibrillator pads or electrodes.
3. Turn on the AED.
4. Push the "analyze" button on the AED.
5. Deliver the shock if indicated. The device either will automatically deliver a shock or will instruct the operator (via audible and visible signals) to "shock."

Many patients with cardiac arrest in the prehospital setting will have VF. If paramedic-level care is not immediately available, the *most* important thing the EMT–I can do is to attach the AED and analyze the rhythm. If two or more EMT–Is are present, one should apply and operate the AED. The second EMT–I should perform CPR. If only one EMT–I is present, he or she should first verify cardiac arrest, then immediately apply the AED. Defibrillation should *not* be delayed to set up oxygen, IV lines, mechanical CPR devices, or other forms of care. Ideally, these preparations should proceed at the same time if sufficient personnel are available.

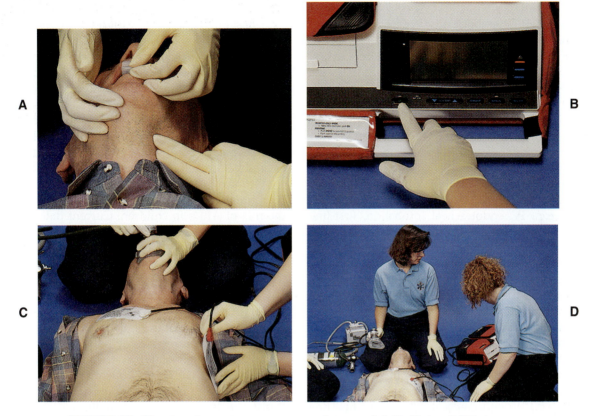

FIGURE 23-63 ▲ Operating an automated external defibrillator (AED). **A,** Perform an initial assessment to confirm cardiac arrest. **B,** Activate the device. **C,** Attach the electrodes and pads to the patient with the white electrode just below the clavicle and to the right of the sternum. The red electrode pad should be placed on the lower chest in the anterior axillary line. **D,** If the AED advises to shock, loudly say, "Stand clear," and push the "shock" button. Deliver the number of shocks indicated, up to three.

The EMT–I's first goal when providing care for a patient with cardiac arrest is to use the AED to quickly analyze for the presence of a dysrhythmia that is treatable by an electrical shock. The following steps are taken once it has been determined that a patient is in cardiac arrest (Figure 23-63, *A*):

1. Place the AED close to the patient's left ear. If possible, perform all defibrillation from the patient's left side. Some EMS systems have adopted different operator and device positions with equal success. Follow local protocols.
2. Turn on the power by either pressing the "power switch" or lifting up the monitor screen. At this point, the recording device is automatically activated (Figure 23-63, *B*).
3. Open the adhesive defibrillation pads, and attach them first to the cables and then to the patient's chest. Place one pad (right, or sternal) to the right of the sternum with the top edge at the bottom of the clavicle. Place the other pad (left, or apex) in the lower left chest in the anterior axillary line (Figure 23-63, *C*).

4. As soon as the pads are attached, stop CPR.
5. Push the "analyze" button. Most devices take between 5 and 15 seconds to interpret the rhythm. *Do not* touch or move the patient during the analysis phase (Figure 23-63, *D*).
6. If VF or pulseless VT is present, the device will note that a shock is indicated. Depending on the model, this notification may consist of a written message on the display screen, an audible alarm, a voice-synthesized statement, or a combination of these. At this point, immediately and loudly say, "Stand clear," so that no one is in contact with the patient when the shock is delivered.
7. If no shock is indicated, the patient does not have an electrically treatable rhythm. Check the pulse, and if the patient remains pulseless, continue CPR and transport to the hospital.
8. Administer drug therapy according to local protocols and medical control.
9. Automated devices will charge the capacitors and deliver a shock shortly after they have analyzed the rhythm to be VF or pulseless VT. A semiautomatic

model will advise to push the "shock" button to deliver a shock. The shock produces a sudden contraction of the patient's muscles.

10. *Do not* restart CPR or check for a pulse after the first shock is delivered. Instead, immediately press the "analyze" control. If the patient remains in a shockable rhythm, the device will again indicate that a shock is indicated. If indicated, proceed with delivery of a second shock.

11. If no shock is indicated, the patient does not have an electrically treatable rhythm. Check the pulse; if the patient remains pulseless, continue CPR, provide advanced life support according to local protocols (e.g., IV, endotracheal intubation, first-line cardiac drugs), and transport to the hospital.

12. Following the second shock, *do not* resume CPR or check for a pulse. Instead, immediately press the "analyze" control. If the patient remains in a shockable rhythm, the device will again indicate that a shock is indicated. If indicated, proceed with delivery of a third shock.

13. If no shock is indicated, the patient does not have an electrically treatable rhythm. Check the pulse; if the patient remains pulseless, continue CPR, provide advanced life support according to local protocols (e.g., IV, endotracheal intubation, first-line cardiac drugs), and transport to the hospital.

14. Use 200 J for the first shock, 200 to 300 J for the second shock, and up to 360 J for the third shock. Most currently available units will automatically set the required energy level.

15. Following the third shock, immediately perform CPR for 1 minute. After 1 minute of CPR, check for a pulse. If a pulse is present, monitor the patient, provide care as indicated, and transport to the hospital as soon as possible.

16. If the patient does not have a pulse following the third shock, provide advanced life support according to local protocols (e.g., IV, endotracheal intubation, first-line cardiac drugs). After 1 minute of CPR, immediately press the "analyze" button. Repeat sets of up to three "stacked" shocks, followed by 1 minute of CPR, as indicated. Follow the same guidelines as previously listed for the first series of shocks.

17. If a patient who initially develops a perfusing rhythm following defibrillation then rearrests, start the analysis sequence again from the top of the algorithm.

To summarize, in the absence of paramedic-level care, the EMT–I who has an AED and is trained to use it should do the following:

1. Immediately apply the device to the patient in apparent cardiac arrest.

2. Always shock in sets of not more than three, as advised by the AED. If the first or second shock is successful, it is *not* necessary to give all three shocks.

3. Following the initial assessment, touch the patient's chest only to perform CPR for 1 minute.

4. Continue to shock in sets of up to three, as advised, followed by 1 minute of CPR (and the provision of appropriate advanced life-support problems) until the device confirms that no shock is indicated.

Precautions for Automated External Defibrillation—Defibrillators do not discriminate; both the patient *and* the EMT–I can be shocked if these devices are used inappropriately. The area must be cleared before delivery of a shock.

According to the latest American Heart Association recommendations, further studies are needed to define the role of AEDs in children. Current data support attempted use in children who are older than 8 years of age and weigh more than 25 kg.

MANUAL DEFIBRILLATION

Performing Manual Defibrillation—Before defibrillation, place defibrillation pads on the patient's chest or apply conductive gel to the paddles. Resistance is very high if the metal electrodes are bare. All surfaces of the paddles should be touching the patient's skin. Push down with 20 to 25 pounds of firm arm pressure. Resistance is also lower when the patient's phase of ventilation is at full expiration.

For defibrillation of VF and pulseless VT, use up to three successive shocks at 200, 200 to 300, and 360 J, respectively. Use 360 J for subsequent shocks, which also may be delivered in sets of three. These "stacked shocks" are thought to decrease transthoracic resistance. In children an initial dose of 2 J/kg is used. If repeat shocks are necessary, the defibrillator is set at 4 J/kg.

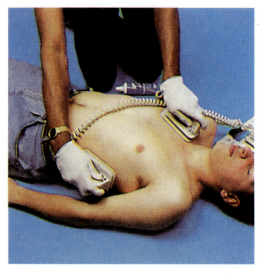

FIGURE 23-64 ▲ Standard placement of defibrillator paddles calls for one paddle to be placed to the right of the upper sternum and the other to the left of the nipple in the midaxillary line.

Two commonly used positions for paddle placement are the standard and anterior-posterior positions. Standard placement calls for one defibrillator paddle to be placed to the right of the upper sternum just below the right clavicle and the other to be placed just to the left of the nipple in the midaxillary line (Figure 23-64). With anterior-posterior placement, one paddle is positioned anteriorly, just to the left of the sternal border, and the other is positioned behind the heart.

The following is the procedure for defibrillating a patient:

1. Prepare the equipment, and bare the patient's chest.
2. Apply gel pads to the patient's chest or conductive gel to the defibrillator paddles (Figure 23-65, A).
3. Select the appropriate energy level, and charge the defibrillator (Figure 23-65, B).
4. Apply the paddles to the correct locations on the chest with approximately 25 pounds of firm arm pressure (Figure 23-65, C).
5. Reverify the dysrhythmia.
6. Instruct everyone to "stand clear," and make sure not to come in contact with the patient. Look in both directions to verify that no one is touching the patient or the stretcher (Figure 23-65, D).
7. Depress the buttons on both paddles simultaneously to deliver the shock.
8. Observe the rhythm after the defibrillation.
9. If the rhythm changes, or following three sequential shocks, check the carotid pulse.
10. *Do not* stop to check the pulse between defibrillatory shocks if the monitor still shows VF.

If the patient has an automatic implantable cardioverter defibrillator or an implanted pacemaker, defibrillator paddles or self-adhesive electrodes should be placed at least 5 inches from the device. The location of these devices can be identified by a visible scar on the chest or abdominal wall, as well as by palpation.

If the patient has a nitroglycerin patch in place, it should be removed before defibrillation. The electrical current can cause the patch to explode and burn the patient.

> **HELPFUL HINT**
> • Remove nitroglycerin patches before performing defibrillation.

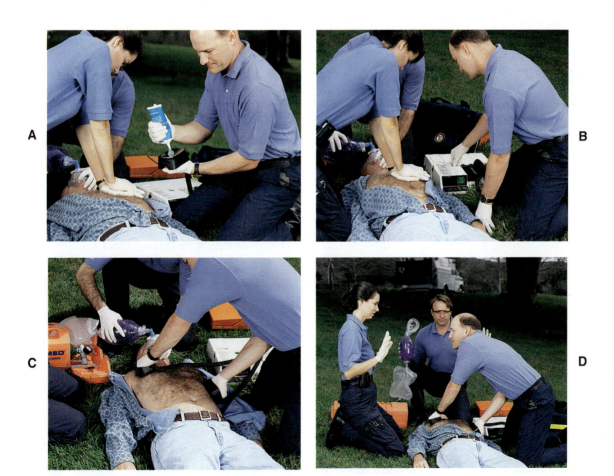

FIGURE 23-65 ▲ **A,** Apply gel pads to the patient's chest or conductive gel to the defibrillator paddles. **B,** Select the appropriate energy level, and charge the defibrillator. **C,** Apply the paddles to the correct locations on the chest with firm arm pressure. **D,** Say, "Stand clear," and verify that no one is touching the patient.

Safety and Operational Considerations—The following additional precautions should be taken when defibrillating a patient:

- On an ongoing basis, check the batteries and defibrillator unit for proper operation.
- Make sure the electrode pads, if used, have not expired. Otherwise, they may be dried out.
- Make sure that the paddles are clean from the last use.
- If using conductive gel or paste, make certain that the paddles are adequately coated.
- Make sure everyone is clear of the patient, including the operator, before delivering the countershock. Loudly say, "Stand clear," and look around before discharging the defibrillator.
- Use extreme caution when defibrillating patients who are wet or in contact with metal. If you are unable to move them, be certain that no one else, including the operator, is in contact with the moisture or metal.
- Double-check the rhythm before delivering a countershock to ensure that the patient has not reverted to another rhythm.
- Make sure the synchronized mode is turned off when defibrillating a patient with VF.
- If the rhythm changes, or following three sequential shocks, check the carotid pulse.

Cardiac Pacing

HISTORY

Transcutaneous pacing (TCP) was initially described in 1952. Because of severe patient discomfort, it fell into disfavor rapidly after its initial introduction and was replaced by transvenous pacing. In recent years, new designs have evolved for transcutaneous pacers, leading to a resurgence of their popularity. Newer devices also allow for the simultaneous monitoring of the patient's cardiac rhythm and pacing.

DESIGN

A typical TCP device consists of three parts: the electrode pads, a cardiac monitor, and the "pacing box" itself. The pads typically are large, gel-coated adhesive devices that are applied on the chest in an anterior-posterior orientation. These are then connected to the pacemaker.

The pacemaker "box" typically contains input and output ports and a control panel. Standard ECG leads are placed on the patient and connected to the pacer input port. These sense the patient's underlying rhythm. The skin electrode pads are connected to the output port, through which the pacing current, if necessary, is delivered.

The panel consists of several controls. These vary from device to device but generally include the following:

- *Power switch*—Determines if the pacing and sensing functions of the device are operable.
- *Type of pacing (mode)*—Determines whether pacing is demand pacing (pacing only as needed) or asynchro-

nous (continuous) pacing. Most devices allow the operator to choose between these two modes.

- *Pacing rate*—Determines the rate of electrical pacing; usually ranges from 40 to 180 stimuli per minute.
- *Sensitivity*—Determines how large a QRS complex must be generated by the patient's own heart rhythm in order for the pacemaker, in the demand mode, to sense ("notice") this and suppress firing a paced impulse.
- *Output*—Determines in milliamps (mA) the amount of pacing current delivered to the patient through the electrode pads.

Other controls may be present on devices with built-in monitors, such as QRS height, etc. Integrated defibrillator/pacemaker combination devices are also available whereby both functions are physically contained within the same device (Figure 23-66).

GENERAL USES OF TRANSCUTANEOUS PACING

TCP appears to be very helpful in treating patients with nonarrest but symptomatic bradydysrhythmias, such as complete heart block or sinus bradycardia. The incidence of both electrical and mechanical capture (the pacer generates both an ECG complex and a palpable pulse) in asystole or bradycardic PEA is uncommon. Since success in cardiac arrest situations is low even when the device is applied early, it is the symptomatic bradycardic patient who may benefit the most.

Advantages of TCP over other forms of cardiac pacing in the field include the following:

- It may be applied within a few minutes.
- Minimal training is required to use the devices.
- It is highly portable; it can be used in just about any field situation, including before extrication.
- It is highly effective in nonarrest situations, such as in the hemodynamically compromised bradycardic patient (where atropine may be contraindicated, such as with Mobitz type II heart block).

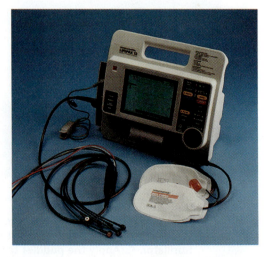

FIGURE 23-66 ▲ Life Defense Plus defibrillator-pacer. (Courtesy Matrix Medical Inc., Orchard Park, NY.)

DRAWBACKS TO TRANSCUTANEOUS PACING

There are a few drawbacks to TCP; these include the following:

- Difficult capture in certain patients, depending on chest wall resistance
- Patient discomfort
- Expense and cost

INDICATIONS FOR TRANSCUTANEOUS PACING

The principal indications for TCP are symptomatic bradycardia, heart block not responsive to atropine (or where atropine is contraindicated), pacemaker failure, and asystole (many question the efficacy of pacing in cardiac arrest). TCP is generally ineffective in PEA unless the underlying cause is corrected first. It is contraindicated in patients with open wounds or burns on the chest and in patients who are in a wet environment.

PROCEDURE FOR TRANSCUTANEOUS PACING

The procedure for using TCP is as follows:

1. Gather the required equipment.
2. Explain the procedure to the patient.
3. Connect the patient to a cardiac monitor, and obtain a rhythm strip.
4. Obtain baseline vital signs.
5. Apply the pacing electrodes (avoid large muscle masses) (Figure 23-67).
6. Attach the pacing cable and the pacing "box."
7. Select the pacing mode.
8. Select the pacing rate (usually 70 to 80 beats per minute), and set the current (begin with 50 mA or as per local protocols).
9. Activate the pacemaker, observing the patient and the ECG.
10. Obtain rhythm strips as appropriate.
11. Continue monitoring the patient and anticipate further therapy.

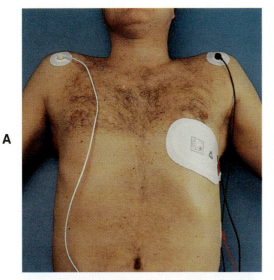

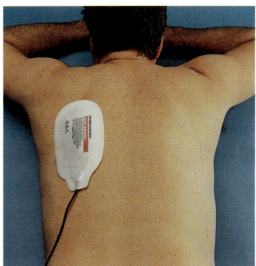

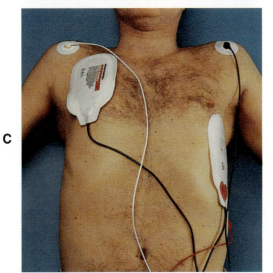

FIGURE 23-67 ▲ Proper electrode attachment for external pacing. **A** and **B**, Preferred anterior-posterior placement. **C**, Alternative anterior-anterior placement. (From Sanders MJ: *Mosby's paramedic textbook*, ed 2, St Louis, 2000, Mosby.)

▶ NOTE: TCP has been studied only to a limited degree in pediatric patients. Because of the extreme discomfort in children, its use is restricted to life-threatening situations where no other alternatives are available. Follow local protocols.

Specific Management of Nonarrest Dysrhythmias by the Algorithm Approach

Several treatments are common to all persons with nonarrest cardiac dysrhythmias, regardless of the type. These include the following:

- Careful assessment of the level of consciousness, airway, breathing, and circulation
- High-concentration oxygen
- IV access
- Consideration of aspirin administration if myocardial ischemia is present (follow local protocols)
- Management of ischemic pain (nitroglycerin, morphine)
- Judicious transport (avoid "hot" transport unless absolutely necessary) to the nearest appropriate facility
- Psychological support for both the patient and his or her family

Since the patient is not in cardiac arrest, problems such as VF, pulseless VT, asystole, and PEA are automatically excluded at this point. All that needs to be determined (rhythm-wise) is whether the patient's heart rate is normal, too fast (tachycardia), or too slow (bradycardia). The two extremes are separated in the discussion that follows. Clinically, the EMT–I must also decide whether the patient is stable. Unstable patients require more rapid treatment and transport than do those who are relatively stable. Remember, however, that *any* cardiac patient can always deteriorate at *any* time.

TACHYCARDIAS

The initial decision point in a nonarrested patient with tachycardia is stability; if the patient is unstable as a result of the increased heart rate, prepare for immediate cardioversion (follow local protocols). An EMT who is unable to perform cardioversion should transport the patient rapidly to the nearest appropriate medical facility.

If the patient is stable, determine whether the QRS complex is narrow (greater than 0.12 second) or wide (less than 0.12 second). This classification limits the diagnostic possibilities significantly:

- *Narrow QRS tachycardia*—Atrial fibrillation, atrial flutter, other narrow-complex tachycardia (e.g., PSVT)
- *Wide QRS tachycardia*—Stable monomorphic VT and/or polymorphic VT, or stable wide-complex tachycardia of unknown type

Although it is suggested that specific rhythm identification by means of a 12-lead ECG be done, this is not often possible in the field. As long as the patient is stable,

there is little urgency for a specific field diagnosis. Use ECG features on the rhythm strip and vagal maneuvers (if indicated) to differentiate among the four possibilities (atrial flutter/fibrillation, other narrow-complex tachycardia, VT, wide-complex tachycardia of unknown type).

Stable atrial fibrillation and atrial flutter rarely require acute treatment, other than careful attention to the airway, breathing, and circulation. Follow local protocols.

BRADYCARDIAS

The major decision, as usual, is patient stability. Unstable patients require immediate TCP. Remember that atropine is relatively contraindicated in type II second-degree (Mobitz II) AV block and third-degree AV block with new wide QRS complexes.

Cardiac Arrest: A Practical Approach

Once a person has gone into cardiac arrest, the clinical approach becomes extremely straightforward. There is no critical need to separate victims into VF, pulseless VT, PEA, or asystole. All cardiac arrest victims are in one of two possible rhythms: VF/VT rhythms or non-VF rhythms. Non-VF rhythms comprise asystole and PEA, which are treated alike.

In addition, all cardiac arrest victims receive the same three treatments:

- CPR
- Tracheal intubation
- Vasoconstrictors (e.g., epinephrine, vasopressin)

The *only* real difference is that patients with VF/VT rhythms receive defibrillation (and sometimes antidysrhythmics as well).

CHEST PAIN THAT MAY BE MYOCARDIAL IN ORIGIN

There are 12,200,000 people alive today who have a history of heart attack, angina pectoris (chest pain), or both. Twenty-seven percent of men and 14% of women will develop angina within 6 years after a recognized heart attack. Acutely, it is far more important to determine that chest pain may be due to myocardial ischemia, rather than determining the specific cause.

Definitions

Angina, also known as **angina pectoris,** is an intermittent attack of chest pain and related symptoms that is due to a reduction in blood flow to the heart muscle. Angina is brought on by exertion, emotional stress, or cold weather. The pain usually is relieved by rest or by administration of a medication that dilates the coronary arteries. Nitroglycerin is the most commonly used drug to treat angina.

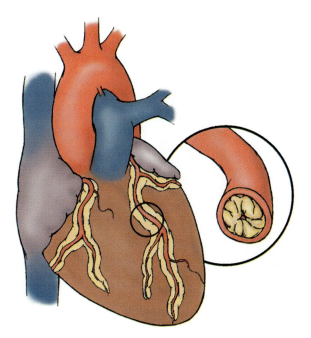

FIGURE 23-68 ▲ The narrowing of coronary arteries leads to decreased blood flow to the heart muscle.

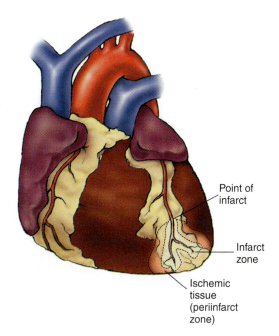

Point of infarct

Infarct zone

Ischemic tissue (periinfarct zone)

FIGURE 23-69 ▲ Acute myocardial infarction.

The heart muscle suffers from lack of oxygen (ischemia) when the coronary arteries have been narrowed by atherosclerotic plaque (Figure 23-68). Plaques consist of calcium, cholesterol, and connective tissue. The plaque reduces flow in the involved portion of the artery. Angina results when the heart needs more oxygen than can be provided through the partially occluded coronary arteries. The heart muscle senses this lack of oxygen and develops anginal pain. The pain goes away when the stress is decreased, and necessary oxygen supplies again flow to the myocardium.

Many cases of angina follow the pattern described; they come on with stress or exertion and are relieved by rest, nitroglycerin, or oxygen. This pattern of angina may persist for years in some patients and is called **stable angina. Unstable angina,** on the other hand, is angina that either is new in onset or differs from a patient's typical stable anginal pattern. For example, a patient may have been awakened during the night with pain, which has never happened previously. Or, he or she may have pain that now occurs while the patient is at rest. Either way, a change in previously stable angina is often a warning sign of an impending heart attack. Some classification systems also use the terms **progressive angina** (accelerating in frequency and duration) and **preinfarction angina** (pain at rest), although both are considered types of unstable angina.

A heart attack, also called acute **acute myocardial infarction (AMI),** is death of an area of heart muscle due to complete blockage of blood flow in a coronary artery. The area of myocardium supplied by that artery receives little or no oxygen and dies. Furthermore, myocardial tissue surrounding the infarcted area becomes ischemic,

and the size of the infarction can increase if the oxygen needs of the tissue are not met (Figure 23-69).

Heart attack is the leading cause of death in America. Every year, more than 1.5 million Americans suffer a heart attack. Many heart attack victims die before reaching a hospital. Typically, victims die of cardiac dysrhythmia.

The initial processes in angina and MI are similar—partial blockage of a coronary artery due to atherosclerotic plaque. MI occurs when the remaining open area (lumen) of the artery becomes occluded, usually as a result of a blood clot (thrombus) (Figure 23-70). A small number of patients develop occlusion as a result of spasm in the muscles of the arterial walls (Figure 23-71). An even smaller number of persons have coronary artery occlusion that is due to coronary artery trauma (chest trauma) or inflammation of the blood vessels (vasculitis).

When the coronary artery becomes completely occluded, blood flow to the area of the heart that the artery supplies is markedly reduced. The heart muscle suffers chemical changes that result in symptoms, as well as damage to the myocardium. Eventually, a portion of the involved myocardium dies and is replaced with scar tissue.

The most recent term for chest pain resulting from myocardial ischemia is **acute coronary ischemic syndromes.** This broad term implies that the clinician need not recognize the specific type of disease (e.g., stable angina versus AMI) but determine, *at a minimum,* that the patient is likely suffering from lack of oxygen to the myocardium. The next priority (after stabilizing the patient) is to decide whether or not the patient is a candidate for reperfusion therapy (thrombolysis, angioplasty [use of a "balloon" to open a blocked coronary artery]).

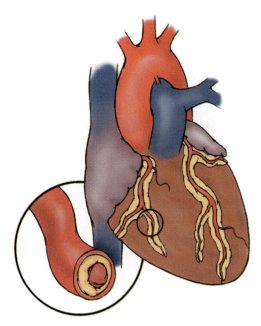

FIGURE 23-70 ▲ Myocardial infarction occurs when an artery supplying oxygen to the heart is blocked.

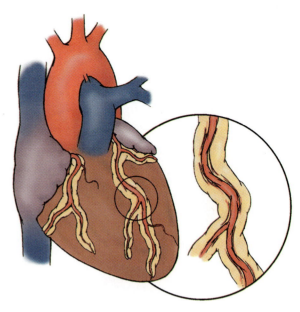

FIGURE 23-71 ▲ Rarely, spasms in the muscles of arterial walls cause blockage of the artery.

CLINICAL NOTES

The fact that most patients with MI have occlusion of the artery by a blood clot forms the basis for treatment with chemical agents that break up the clot and restore flow. These agents are called thrombolytic drugs. They have their greatest benefit when administered within 4 hours of the onset of pain. Transport of these patients to the hospital should not be unnecessarily delayed. This 4-hour period is often called the "window of opportunity" for thrombolytic therapy (Figure 23-72).

Other Causes of Chest Pain

Numerous diseases other than myocardial ischemia may result in chest pain. Although the signs and symptoms may be similar to acute myocardial ischemia, often the clinical differences will be apparent. Of course, if the EMT–I is uncertain, the safest approach is to assume that the patient has acute myocardial ischemia. Nonischemic causes of chest pain include the following:

- *Aneurysm*—An aneurysm is an abnormal dilation of the aorta that usually occurs in the abdominal portion. Occasionally, aneurysms may form in the chest. If they leak or impair circulation through the coronary arteries, chest pain may result (Figure 23-73).
- *Aortic dissection*—Aortic dissection occurs when a sudden tear occurs in the wall of the aorta, allowing a column of blood to enter. Portions of the vessel are essentially stripped apart, driven by the force of the

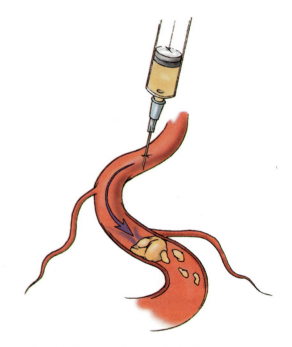

FIGURE 23-72 ▲ Thrombolytic drugs act to dissolve blood clots.

aortic blood pressure. Severe tearing-like pain is often present and may radiate between the shoulder blades (Figure 23-74).

- *Blunt trauma, chest wall irritation (costochondritis, tumors), or chest muscle irritation*—An irritation of the rib cartilage that connects to the rib or sternum, costochondritis pain usually is sharp and worsened with either deep inspiration or movement. Point tenderness over the area is common. Patients with this ail-

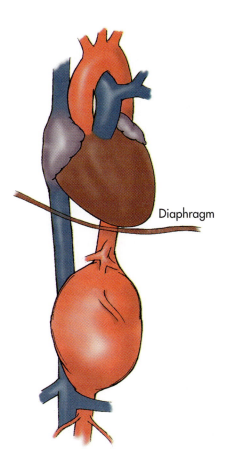

FIGURE 23-73 ▲ An abdominal aortic aneurysm is a saclike widening in the abdominal portion of the aorta.

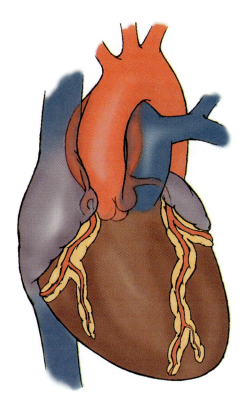

FIGURE 23-74 ▲ Dissecting thoracic aortic aneurysms are the result of blood entering a tear in the intimal lining of the vessel.

ment tend to hyperventilate, leading to subjective complaints of shortness of breath. Reproduction of the patient's exact symptoms by palpation over the tender area is diagnostic. Muscle strain is an injury caused by improper use or overuse of a muscle that results in pain, especially when performing movements that rely on the impaired muscle. Strain of chest wall muscles can lead to pain that, at times, may mimic that of MI. The correct diagnosis usually is evident when particular movements using the injured muscle lead to aggravation of the pain.

- *Cholecystitis*—Cholecystitis is inflammation of the gallbladder, located in the right upper quadrant. Although the pain is usually well localized, it may lead to more diffuse chest and epigastric discomfort that can be confused with acute myocardial ischemia.
- *Esophageal and gastrointestinal diseases*—These diseases include *esophageal spasm* and *peptic ulcer disease.* Esophageal spasm consists of violent contractions of the smooth muscle that makes up the esophagus, often resulting in severe substernal pain that may mimic MI. Diagnosis of this entity is particularly important in the differential diagnosis of chest pain, because esophageal spasm, as well as cardiac pain, may be relieved by nitroglycerin ad-

ministration. Peptic ulcer disease is an erosion in the lining of any portion of the gastrointestinal tract. Ulcers are most commonly located in either the stomach or the duodenum (located immediately distal to the stomach). Pain is often relieved by eating or by taking antacids. Complications of peptic ulcer disease include bleeding and perforation, with release of gastrointestinal tract contents into the abdominal cavity. At times, the epigastric discomfort of ulcer disease may mimic that of MI.

- *Herpes zoster (shingles)*—Caused by the same virus that causes chickenpox (varicella), herpes zoster affects skin nerves, leading to a skin rash that follows dermatomes (nerve distribution patterns). Before eruption of the rash, patients may have sharp, band-like pain over the affected area.
- *Hiatal hernia*—Technically termed esophageal reflux, heartburn is a painful burning sensation in the epigastrium and substernal area that may mimic cardiac pain. It usually occurs in the presence of a hiatal hernia that decreases the tension in the lower esophagus, allowing backflow of stomach acid into the esophagus. Irritation in the esophagus is due to the backflow of acidic stomach contents. Reflux is commonly relieved with the administration of antacids.

• *Pancreatitis*—Pancreatitis, an inflammation of the pancreas, results in pain that is located in the posterior epigastric region. Pain from pancreatitis is usually sharp and radiates to the back. Since it is often accompanied by nausea, vomiting, and diaphoresis, it may mimic the pain of acute myocardial ischemic syndromes.

• *Pericarditis*—Pericarditis, an inflammation of the membranous sac that surrounds the heart (the pericardium), results in substernal pain that is often aggravated with movement, especially assuming the recumbent position. Causes of pericarditis include infection (usually viral), connective tissue disease, and MI. It is unusual, although possible, for acute pericarditis to accompany acute MI. More commonly, however, pericarditis in conjunction with MI develops several days later.

• *Pleurisy*—Pleurisy, an inflammation of the pleura (lining of the chest cavity), leads to chest pain, especially on inspiration, and occasionally shortness of breath. Pleurisy usually is due to some type of infection. It is unusual, although possible, that pain from this illness may resemble that of acute MI.

• *Pneumothorax*—Pneumothorax is partial or complete collapse of the lung, associated with the presence of air in the pleural space (located between the lung and chest wall). The symptoms come on suddenly and are accompanied by shortness of breath. Ninety percent of patients with pneumothorax present with chest pain that is often described as sharp or pulling and usually pleuritic in nature.

• *Pulmonary embolism*—A pulmonary embolism is an acute blockage of one of the pulmonary arteries by a blood clot (Figure 23-75). This leads to lung dysfunction and improper oxygenation of the arterial blood. Death may result. The most common source of the clot is a thrombus in one of the large pelvic or leg veins. The pain is pleuritic (worsens with inspiration), and shortness of breath is often present (see p. 696 for further discussion on this topic).

• *Respiratory infections*—Pneumonia is an inflammation of the lungs, usually related to some type of bacterial or viral infection. The patient commonly has a cough, fever, chills, and sometimes, shortness of breath. Chest pain that is sharp and worsened with deep inspiration is common in some types of pneumonia because of concomitant pleuritic irritation. Similar pain may occur during *bronchitis*, inflammation of the bronchial tubes without lung involvement.

Remember that many of these conditions may still be life threatening (e.g., pneumothorax), even though they do not result from acute myocardial ischemia (Box 23-5).

Initial Assessment Findings

Persons with acute myocardial ischemia often exhibit anxiety and restlessness. This is due to catecholamine (epinephrine) release from a combination of fear, pain, and the disease process itself. Patients may also feel weak and fatigued. New-onset weakness is a common presenting sign in diabetic patients of all ages and in older persons. Although less common, near-syncope or vertigo may occur. The most common reasons are associated dysrhythmias or decreased cardiac output.

Although the respiratory rate is often increased somewhat, true dyspnea is unusual unless the patient has associated CHF or pulmonary edema. The quality of the peripheral pulses may vary, depending on the patient's condition. Often the skin is diaphoretic, although this finding, along with temperature and color, vary from patient to patient.

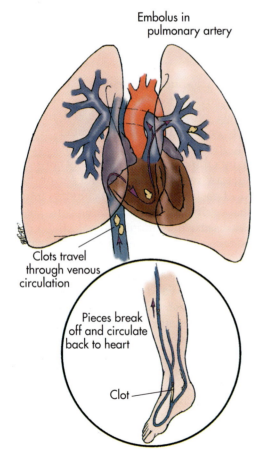

Embolus in pulmonary artery

Clots travel through venous circulation

Pieces break off and circulate back to heart

Clot

FIGURE 23-75 ▲ Pulmonary embolism is the blockage of a pulmonary artery by foreign matter.

BOX 23-5

POTENTIALLY LIFE-THREATENING CAUSES OF NONCARDIAC CHEST PAIN

• Aortic aneurysm
• Aortic dissection
• Pancreatitis
• Pericarditis
• Pneumothorax
• Pulmonary embolism

Focused History

Although patients often complain of chest pain, many use words other than *pain*. Words that are commonly used include *discomfort, pressure, aching,* and *heaviness*. Some describe a weight on the chest. Typically, pain is fairly sudden in onset. It is usually in the midchest region, below (behind) the sternum (substernal, retrosternal). Many persons have discomfort in the epigastric region and refer to it as "indigestion," rather than pain. Atypical symptoms are common, especially in diabetics and older persons. These may include weakness, fatigue, shortness of breath, or arm pain. In stable angina, symptoms are usually short-lived (3 to 15 minutes) and are usually relieved by rest and/or medication (nitroglycerin). The pain of MI usually lasts longer and may be unrelieved by rest or medications.

CLINICAL NOTES

Denial of pain is common in acute myocardial ischemia. In other words, the patient tries to minimize the significance or presence of the symptom. The most common indication of this is when the patient continually touches his or her chest, as if uncomfortable, but comments that "it really doesn't hurt that much." This scenario commonly suggests acute myocardial ischemia.

The *most important* part of the history in a person with chest pain is to determine whether or not the discomfort is pleuritic—worsened with inspiration or movement. Typical pain from acute myocardial ischemia is nonpleuritic. If a patient's chest pain is nonpleuritic in nature, the EMT–I should assume that it is due to acute myocardial ischemia until proven otherwise. On the other hand, just because the pain is pleuritic or has a pleuritic component does *not* exclude acute myocardial ischemia. It just makes it less likely.

CLINICAL NOTES

If a patient's chest pain is nonpleuritic in nature, assume that it is due to acute myocardial ischemia until proven otherwise.

Other major features to note during the focused history include the following:
- Determine if the pain began during exertion. Exertional chest pain is more likely to be angina, although work and exercise are both known causes of acute MI. Pain that comes on while the patient is at rest or that wakes him or her up at night indicates unstable angina or acute MI.
- Also ask if the patient has had other episodes of discomfort similar to the present one. Just because the

current bout of pain is similar to others in the past, however, does not make it any less potentially worrisome. On the other hand, *worsening of pain*, as compared with a previous episode, strongly suggests a more serious condition than the previous bout.
- Determine whether the patient has been taking aspirin for prevention of either stroke or acute MI.
- Determine whether the patient has taken any medications, either chronically or recently, for chest pain. Ask particularly about nitroglycerin (Figure 23-76), borrowed medications, over-the-counter preparations, and herbal preparations.
- Always reconfirm whether or not the patient has allergies to any medications.

Detailed Physical Examination

As usual, ensure the adequacy of the airway, breathing, and circulation first. Depending on the patient's condition, the lungs may be clear or sound congested. Often the patient's blood is elevated initially because of catecholamine release.

Management Considerations

Place the patient in a position of comfort. According to local protocols, consider administration of oxygen, aspirin, nitroglycerin, and morphine (Figure 23-77). Monitor the ECG rhythm strip, and obtain a 12-lead ECG if mandated by local protocols. Determine whether the patient is a candidate for reperfusion therapy according to local protocol criteria. If so, transport him or her in a safe, yet rapid, fashion to the nearest appropriate facility. Otherwise, if

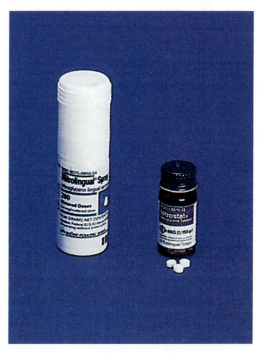

FIGURE 23-76 ▲ Nitroglycerin can be found in several forms, including sublingual tablets and spray.

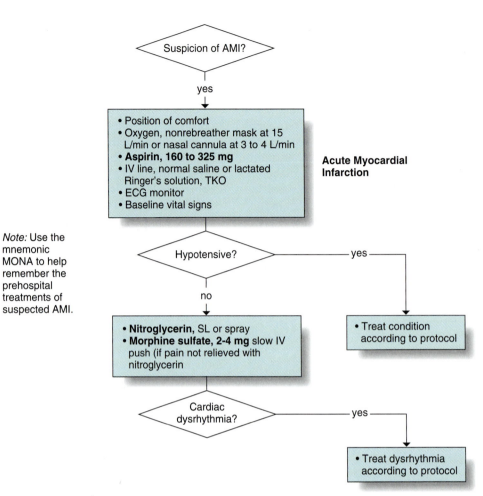

Note: Use the mnemonic MONA to help remember the prehospital treatments of suspected AMI.

FIGURE 23-77 ▲ **Treatment for acute myocardial infarction.**

the patient is stable and not a candidate for reperfusion therapy, most experts currently recommend less urgent transportation (no lights and siren). As always, appropriate psychological support for the patient, family, and significant others, as well as communication and transfer of vital data to the receiving facility, is necessary.

▶ NOTE: Current recommendations of the American Heart Association are that EMS personnel perform immediate assessment and treatment, including MONA (morphine, oxygen, nitroglycerin, aspirin), an initial 12-lead ECG (where feasible in an EMS system), and a review for fibrinolytic therapy indications and contraindications (according to local protocols). Selected EMS systems may actually administer thrombolytic drugs in the field. Although this is appropriate under certain circumstances, the subject of thrombolytic drug therapy is beyond the intended scope of this chapter. Follow local protocols.

CONGESTIVE HEART FAILURE AND ACUTE PULMONARY EDEMA

Congestive heart failure (CHF) is circulatory congestion due to inadequate flow of blood. It is caused by heart muscle damage that reduces the heart's ability to function as a pump. As a result of inadequate pumping,

blood backs up in the tissues. CHF varies from mild to severe and may be chronic or acute in onset. Acute pulmonary edema is a form of severe CHF (see Acute Pulmonary Edema).

Causes

All forms of CHF result from the heart's inability to function as a pump. The most common cause is coronary artery disease, with or without acute MI. Other causes of CHF include the following:
- Cardiomyopathy, a disease of the heart muscle
- Drugs that adversely affect the ability of the heart to pump
- Hypertension
- Thyroid disease
- Heart valve disease

Right-Sided Versus Left-Sided Congestive Heart Failure

There are two types of CHF: right-sided and left-sided. To understand the differences, the EMT–I should think of the right and left sides of the heart as separate pumps with the lungs located in between (Figure 23-78). With

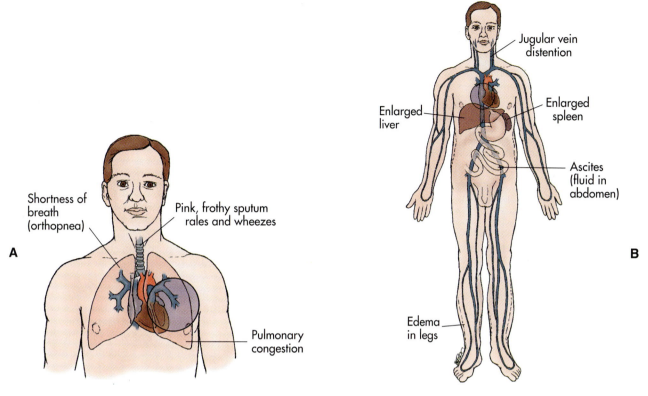

FIGURE 23-78 ▲ Congestive heart failure (CHF). **A,** Left-sided CHF results in a buildup of fluids in the lungs. **B,** Right-sided CHF results in a backup of blood in the vascular system.

left-sided CHF, the pumping capability of the left ventricle is decreased. Fluid backs up into the lungs, causing pulmonary congestion. In its worst form, the lungs fill with large amounts of fluid, resulting in pulmonary edema. The signs and symptoms of left-sided CHF include the following:

- Shortness of breath
- Pink, frothy sputum
- Audible abnormal breath sounds (rales and wheezes)

In *right-sided CHF* the pumping capacity of the right ventricle is impaired. Typically, this condition results from increased resistance to flow through the lungs, which is caused by left-sided failure. Blood draining into the right side of the heart backs up in the vascular system, resulting in the following conditions:

- Swelling (edema) of the extremities and lower back
- Abdominal swelling (ascites)
- Swelling of the liver and spleen
- Distention of the neck veins

Most patients with CHF have primarily left-sided symptoms, although in more severe cases, both left- and right-sided failure are present.

Assessment

The symptoms of CHF may be chronic, new in onset, or an acute worsening of a long-standing problem.

Patients are usually short of breath. The patient may be in marked respiratory distress, especially if acute pulmonary edema (see Acute Pulmonary Edema) occurs. In addition, any of the following may be present:

- Diaphoresis
- Restlessness, anxiety
- Shortness of breath (At night the patient may wake up unable to breathe; this symptom is called paroxysmal nocturnal dyspnea. Patients also may complain of orthopnea, or worsening of shortness of breath when lying down. The patient may state [if asked] that he or she sleeps sitting up or uses a number of pillows when sleeping to prevent shortness of breath at night.)
- Distended neck veins
- Swollen, edematous legs
- Weakness, fatigue
- Tachycardia
- Chest pain (may be present if CHF occurs with acute MI)
- Cyanosis
- Increased systolic blood pressure (Most patients with acute CHF have elevated blood pressure. Patients with acute pulmonary edema and hypotension are "priority" patients who may rapidly deteriorate and develop respiratory or cardiac arrest.)

Emergency Care

Emergency care for the patient with CHF includes the following (Figure 23-79):

- Keep the patient in a sitting position with the legs below the level of the heart if possible. Most patients naturally assume this posture.
- Maintain a patent airway. If frothy secretions are present, suction as necessary.
- Use oxygen as required. The preferred route of administration is high-flow oxygen by mask if tolerated by the patient. Patients with acute pulmonary edema may not accept a face mask because it worsens the smothering sensation. In these cases, use a nasal cannula at 6 to 8 L/min.
- Be prepared to assist ventilation and possibly intubate if necessary, according to local protocols.
- Start an IV line of normal saline at a TKO drip rate.
- Monitor cardiac rhythm if permitted by local protocols. Dysrhythmias especially are likely in the face of acute pulmonary edema.
- Monitor the vital signs and apply pulse oximetry frequently, at least every 5 minutes, if available.

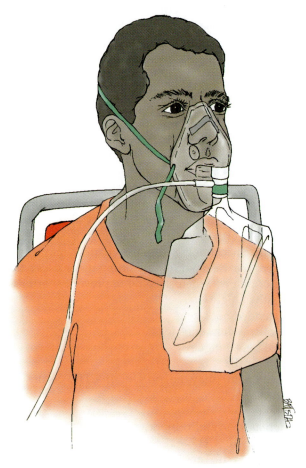

FIGURE 23-79 ▲ **Position the patient with congestive heart failure in a sitting position, and provide oxygen as required.**

PULMONARY EMBOLISM

Pulmonary embolism is common, potentially lethal, and highly underdiagnosed. It is the third most common cause of death in the United States, with approximately 650,000 cases occurring annually. Of these, 10% of patients die within 1 hour of the event. Among survivors, the diagnosis is missed in two out of three cases. In most cases the obstruction is due to a piece of a blood clot that has broken away from a pelvic or deep leg vein and traveled through the venous system to the heart and then to the lungs. As the clot passes through progressively smaller and smaller branches of the pulmonary circulation, it becomes lodged and blockage occurs. The lung tissue supplied by the blocked artery becomes ischemic. If circulation to the lung is sufficiently compromised, the affected area dies. Other causes of obstruction include fat, amniotic fluid, air, tumor tissue, and other foreign matter.

Pulmonary emboli may be small or large. Large pulmonary emboli occlude major branches of the pulmonary arteries. When these occur, the heart is forced to pump blood against very high pressures, resulting in acute right-sided heart failure (acute cor pulmonale).

Risks for pulmonary embolism include the following:

- Sedentary lifestyle (Pulmonary embolism is common in hospitalized patients and in those who have completed long automobile or airplane trips.)
- Obesity
- Thrombophlebitis (inflammation of the veins)
- Use of oral contraceptives (birth control pills)
- Fracture of a long bone (femur, humerus) (The source of emboli is fat released from the bone marrow.)
- Pregnancy (Amniotic fluid embolism may occur during delivery. It is often fatal.)
- Surgery (Patients may remain in the same position on the operating table for several hours, leading to blood clot formation in the veins of the pelvis and legs.)
- Blood disease (Rare blood disorders, such as polycythemia vera, can make a patient's blood more likely to clot.)

Patients with massive pulmonary emboli often suffer cardiac arrest or a syncopal spell as the first symptom of the illness. Patients with smaller emboli may have the following signs and symptoms:

- Sudden, unexplained onset of chest pain that increases in intensity with a deep breath (pleuritic chest pain; may be localized to the area of the chest overlying the involved lung tissue)
- Respiratory distress and shortness of breath (The patient's respiratory rate is almost always increased; the patient may hyperventilate.)
- Wheezing or coughing up of blood (hemoptysis)
- Anxiety
- Shock
- Hypotension

- If permitted by local protocols, assist the patient in taking his or her own nitroglycerin if the systolic blood pressure is greater than 100 mm Hg.

Acute Pulmonary Edema

Acute pulmonary edema (APE) is the rapid filling of both alveolar and interstitial lung tissue with fluid from the capillary beds. APE is a common complication of myocardial ischemia, whether or not acute MI has also occurred. In the face of MI, APE is associated with nearly an 80% mortality. By itself, recurrent episodes of APE result in a mortality rate that parallels the degree of underlying coronary artery disease, which is impossible to determine without invasive studies. APE may also lead to acute respiratory failure and death.

CLINICAL NOTES

Acute pulmonary edema (APE) is a form of acute, severe congestive heart failure (CHF). All CHF, however, is *not* APE. The degree of severity of CHF varies from mild to severe. Some patients with severe CHF have APE, but only a small percentage.

PATHOPHYSIOLOGY

The *cardiac output,* or amount of blood pumped per unit by the left ventricle, is related to many factors. The most important are as follows:
- **Preload**—The workload (amount of blood) that the ventricle has to pump. This is estimated by the left ventricular filling pressure, also known as the hydrostatic or pulmonary artery wedge pressure.
- **Afterload**—The resistance against which the ventricle has to pump its workload. Afterload is measured by the resistance in the vascular tree (primarily arterial) distant to the heart, also known as the systemic vascular resistance.

In APE the left-sided filling pressure (hydrostatic pressure) increases markedly and rapidly as a result of

sudden decreased pumping efficacy of the left ventricle. Decreased left ventricular contractility occurs as a result of ischemia, often simply underlying severe coronary artery disease and *not* AMI. The elevated pressure is transferred from the left atrium back into the lungs. This leads to a sudden leak of fluid from the pulmonary capillaries into both the interstitial tissue and the alveoli, resulting in APE (Figure 23-80). Changes in systemic vascular resistance do not usually play a significant role in the acute generation of pulmonary edema.

Chronic CHF, on the other hand, is often a more progressive condition that is also secondary to myocardial ischemia. Hydrostatic pressures increase less rapidly than during APE. As a result, fluid accumulation in the lungs begins in the interstitium and ultimately, in lieu of adequate treatment, progresses to include the alveoli over a period of time. The time of CHF progression varies markedly from patient to patient.

CLINICAL ASSESSMENT

Symptoms of gradually increasing shortness of breath, orthopnea (shortness of breath only with lying down), and waking up short of breath at night (paroxysmal nocturnal dyspnea) are suggestive of chronic CHF (see earlier discussion), *not* APE. Persons with APE often exhibit the following:
- There may be acute onset of severe shortness of breath. Often, a person is relatively well until APE "strikes." The onset has been likened to someone turning a "pulmonary edema switch."
- There may be diaphoresis, tachycardia, or anxiety.
- Patients may have a cough productive of pink, frothy sputum. This pink color comes from rupture of small alveolar blood vessels as a result of the markedly elevated hydrostatic pressures.
- There may be extraneous lung sounds; often wheezes are audible even without a stethoscope.
- Cyanosis is a late finding; severe hypoxia is unusual early in APE. As a result, most patients will benefit from nasal oxygen alone (see Treatment).
- Most patients are hypertensive initially as a result of a massive epinephrine outpouring. Persons with APE who have an initial systolic blood pressure greater than 150 mm Hg have been shown to have a markedly increased mortality rate.
- Cardiac dysrhythmias may or may not be present.

On the other hand, findings of *chronic CHF* are less common in APE unless the patient is one of few who have simply progressed from simple CHF to APE. The following findings are more compatible with chronic CHF than with APE, especially if the patient was relatively well before the acute onset of symptoms:
- *Jugular venous distention*—Present in only 60% of persons with APE but very common (less than 90%) in persons with significant chronic CHF due to fluid retention.

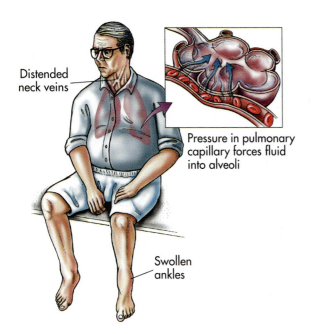

Distended
neck veins

Pressure in pulmonary
capillary forces fluid
into alveoli

Swollen
ankles

FIGURE 23-80 ▲ **Dyspnea results from pulmonary hypertension, causing fluids from the circulatory system to be driven into the alveoli. This fluid widens the gap between the alveolar-capillary membrane, making diffusion of oxygen and carbon dioxide less efficient. (From American College of Emergency Physicians; Pons PT, Cason D, chief editors: *Paramedic field care: a complaint-based approach,* St Louis, 1997, Mosby for ACEP.)**

- *Peripheral edema*—Unusual in APE unless the patient also has preexisting chronic CHF. Edema takes time to accumulate in the legs. The same is true for ascites. Both peripheral edema and ascites are findings of *chronic* CHF, not of APE. Their presence, of course, does not exclude APE, but it is not necessary to suspect the diagnosis.
- *Abnormal heart sounds*—The presence of a third heart sound (S_3 gallop rhythm) is present in less than 40% of persons with APE. It is more common (70%) in those with chronic CHF.

TREATMENT

APE is a life-threatening condition that typically follows one of two potential courses:
- *Rapid improvement with treatment*—Fortunately, this group encompasses the majority of patients. They tend to improve, often dramatically, with a few simple pharmacological interventions (e.g., oxygen, morphine, furosemide, and nitroglycerin).
- *Rapid deterioration regardless of treatment*—These individuals comprise the minority of patients. Despite appropriate initial drug therapy, they continue to deteriorate in terms of respiratory problems and vital signs. Even despite intubation, they may progress rapidly to severe cardiogenic shock and death.

Remember, most APE patients fall into one of these "extreme" groups. Very few patient responses are in between. Either patients get better rapidly (within 5 to 20 minutes), or they get worse rapidly, requiring intubation and ventilation. These individuals often die, despite the best and most timely interventions.

Typical APE-specific management includes the following (follow local protocols):
- *Oxygen*—Although some treatment protocols mandate high-concentration oxygen via face mask, the constricting nature of the mask worsens anxiety in many people. As a result, they either remove the mask or, if forced to keep it on, become considerably more anxious. Anxiety increases blood epinephrine levels and forces the acutely failing heart to work harder. The end result is harmful to the patient. Many experts currently recommend using nasal cannula oxygen at 3 to 4 L/min, pending the results of pharmacological interventions. A newer mask technique, nasal BiPAP (biphasic positive airway pressure) is being tried in the field but as of this writing is neither widely available nor considered a standard of care.
- **Nitroglycerin**—Either spray, sublingual tablets, or IV infusion forms will vasodilate and reduce the preload. This decreases the amount of work the failing heart must perform and increases cardiac output. Most EMS systems use systolic blood pressure levels of less than 100 to 110 mm Hg as a cutoff for safe administration of nitroglycerin (Figure 23-81).
- **Furosemide**—Furosemide (Lasix) acts initially as a vasodilator, decreasing the preload. In addition to this and its action as a diuretic, the drug has been shown to increase lymphatic flow from the lungs (efferent lymphatic flow), thus *reducing* the amount of pulmonary edema fluid. No other diuretic agent has been shown to do this in humans.
- **Morphine**—Morphine is a narcotic agent with many unique beneficial effects in APE. It acts on the central nervous system to reduce patients' anxiety. This leads to a decrease in epinephrine release, decreasing the workload on the failing heart. In addition, morphine also causes vasodilation (mostly via a central effect on the brain), leading to decreased preload and increased cardiac output.

CLINICAL NOTES

Some EMS protocols include the use of inhaled *bronchodilators*, such as albuterol, in persons with either APE or a possible combination of APE and COPD. Medical science supports the use of bronchodilators in APE; limited data suggest that some persons with APE have true bronchospasm.

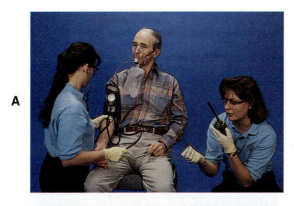
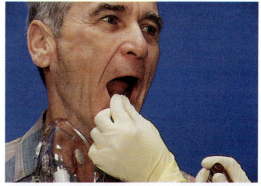
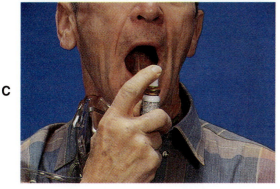
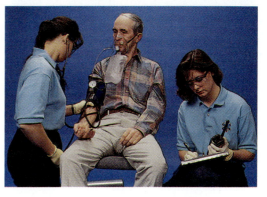

FIGURE 23-81 ▲ Administration of nitroglycerin. **A,** Obtain the appropriate order from medical direction. Reconfirm that the systolic blood pressure is above 100 mm Hg. Check the expiration date of the nitroglycerin on the bottle. Do not give the medication if it is expired. **B** and **C,** Direct the patient to lift his or her tongue, and place one tablet or spray one dose of medication under the tongue. If actually placing the pill or spray, be certain to wear gloves. Without gloves some of the medications may be absorbed via the skin. Do not shake the nitroglycerin spray before administration because this will result in an incorrect dose being given to the patient. **D,** Reassess the patient's blood pressure and symptoms, particularly the cessation or continuance of chest pain.

CLINICAL NOTES

Angiotensin converting enzyme (ACE) block-ers inhibit a specific enzyme in the renin-angiotensin system that tends to cause vasoconstriction, sodium, and water retention. Several preliminary studies suggest that these drugs (e.g., captopril, 12.5 to 25 mg given intravenously or sublingually) may offer additional benefit to furosemide, nitroglycerin, and morphine. ACE blockers are not considered a standard of care and are not usually approved for acute use by EMT–Is. Their use, however, is likely to become commonplace before the next curriculum revision.

HYPERTENSIVE EMERGENCIES

A **hypertensive emergency** is a sudden increase in the systolic blood pressure, the diastolic blood pressure, or both, which causes acute problems of the central nervous system, the heart, or the kidneys. Hypertensive emergencies can be life threatening. A delay in therapy can lead to stroke, AMI, pulmonary edema, or death.

Causes

The most common cause of a hypertensive emergency is an acute worsening of chronic hypertension. Often patients have suddenly stopped taking their blood pressure medicines. Other causes include the following:
- Drugs (Ingestion of cocaine is a common cause of hypertensive emergency.)
- Amphetamines ("speed") and thyroid medicine toxicity
- Acute heart failure
- Pregnancy-induced hypertension (eclampsia or toxemia of pregnancy)
- Acute kidney infection or abnormal kidney function
- Dissecting thoracic aortic aneurysm

• Intracranial event, such as stroke, head trauma, or brain hemorrhage (Almost all acute intracranial events are associated with a period of severe hypertension.)

Pathophysiology

Normally, the flow of blood within the brain is kept within a narrow range, regardless of the patient's blood pressure. This property is known as cerebral autoregulation. When a hypertensive emergency occurs, the brain's ability to maintain cerebral autoregulation is lost. As the blood pressure rises, so does the blood flow in the brain. As cerebral blood flow rises, the intracranial pressure increases, leading to symptoms of headache, drowsiness, vomiting, and visual disturbance.

The elevated blood pressure also places a stress on the heart and kidneys. As the blood pressure rises, so does the resistance against which the heart must pump blood. This increase in blood pressure places a strain on the myocardium, which may result in angina or MI. Similarly, increased vascular resistance interferes with blood flow through the kidneys, resulting in possible kidney failure.

Assessment

Patients with hypertensive emergency have markedly elevated blood pressure. Generally, the systolic pressure is greater than 250 mm Hg, and the diastolic pressure is greater than 120 mm Hg. However, these are not rigid criteria. Patients may have significant symptoms at lower readings. Local protocols should be followed. The following signs and symptoms may be present in hypertensive emergency:

• Severe headache or dizziness

CLINICAL NOTES

Assume that any patient with the sudden onset of a severe headache may have intracranial bleeding. Be especially concerned if a patient complains of headache accompanied by dizziness or vomiting, or if it is the worst headache a patient has ever had.

• Decreased level of responsiveness (The likelihood that an unresponsive patient with a significantly elevated blood pressure has an intracranial hemorrhage is quite high.)
• Visual disturbances, such as blurred or double vision (The pupils may be unequal. Slowly reactive, pinpoint pupils in a hypertensive patient with an altered level of responsiveness indicate an intracranial hemorrhage.)
• Nausea or vomiting
• Chest pain, shortness of breath

• Nosebleed (often results from elevated blood pressure whether or not a hypertensive emergency is present)

HELPFUL HINT

• Spontaneous nosebleeds (epistaxis) in hypertensive patients may be difficult to stop. Bleeding tends to recur in these patients. These patients need evaluation in the hospital even if the bleeding has stopped by the time EMS providers arrive.

Emergency Care

Emergency care for a patient with a suspected hypertensive emergency includes the following:

• Maintain a patent airway and administer high-concentration oxygen.
• Start an IV line of normal saline at a TKO rate.
• Monitor the cardiac rhythm if permitted by local protocols.
• Monitor the vital signs and pulse oximetry frequently, at least every 5 minutes.
• Provide safe transportation to the nearest appropriate facility.
• Provide appropriate psychological support for the patient, family, and significant others.
• Communicate vital patient data to the receiving institution.

NOTE: In the past, some EMS systems advocated treatment of hypertensive emergencies with drugs such as nitroglycerin or nifedipine. Nifedipine (Procardia) is now considered *contraindicated* in hypertensive emergencies because of the risk of brain- and life-threatening hypotension. Many experts now recommend only the use of nitroglycerin in hypertensive emergencies when the transport time is prolonged or when the patient has an intracerebral bleed (which is nearly impossible to determine in the field).

CARDIOGENIC SHOCK

Cardiogenic shock is caused by profound failure of the cardiac muscle, primarily the left ventricle. When greater than 40% of the left ventricle is nonfunctional, the heart loses its ability to efficiently pump blood into the systemic circulation. The mortality rate for cardiogenic shock is 50% to 80%. Cardiogenic shock can be caused by several factors, including the following:

• Severe MI
• Severe heart failure
• Cardiac valve muscle (papillary muscle) rupture
• Trauma causing excessive pressure on the heart (e.g., cardiac tamponade or tension pneumothorax)

Assessment

Along with the general signs and symptoms of shock, patients in cardiogenic shock may experience severe respiratory distress caused by backup of fluid from the right side of the heart into the lungs. Patients also may have chest pain if there has been an associated AMI.

Signs and symptoms of cardiogenic shock include the following:

- Abnormal mental status due to decreased flow of blood and oxygen to the brain
- Collapse of peripheral veins
- Cold, clammy skin
- Rapid, shallow respirations
- Rapid, thready pulse
- Lowered oxygen saturation on pulse oximetry

The blood pressure may be high, normal, or low. Patients with preexisting hypertension (high blood pressure) may have a near-normal blood pressure even in moderately severe cardiogenic shock. EMT–Is should *not* rely on hypotension as a definitive indicator of shock.

> ❗ **HELPFUL HINT**
> • Hypotension is not a definitive indicator of shock.

Emergency Care

The care for a patient with suspected cardiogenic shock includes the following:

- Call for more advanced cardiac response personnel if available and appropriate.
- Secure and maintain a patent airway. Perform endotracheal intubation if necessary, according to local protocols.
- Administer high-concentration oxygen.
- Start an IV line of normal saline at a TKO rate, and give a 250- to 500-mL fluid challenge if called for by medical direction or local protocols.
- Monitor the vital signs. Apply pulse oximetry frequently.
- Monitor at least every 5 minutes, if available.
- Provide safe transportation to the nearest appropriate facility.
- Provide appropriate psychological support for the patient, family, and significant others.
- Communicate vital patient data to the receiving institution.

▶ NOTE: The latest American Heart Association protocols for cardiogenic shock differentiate three causes:

- *Volume problems*—If hypovolemia is present, give fluids.
- *Pump problems*—Refers to decreased contractility of the heart muscle; other than a fluid bolus (according to local protocols), various pressor drugs (designed to increase the cardiac output and blood pressure) are indicated. If pressor drugs are necessary, they can be administered only by paramedics or hospital personnel, since these drugs are not within the standard practice of the EMT–I.
- *Rate problems*—If the heart rate is too slow, follow the protocols for bradycardia (see p. 639). If the heart rate is too fast, follow the protocols for tachycardia (see p. 648).

CARDIAC ARREST
Precipitating Causes

The causes of cardiac arrest, in general, vary markedly between the trauma patient and the medical patient. In addition, the age of the patient makes a significant difference. The most common causes of cardiac arrest in a trauma victim are as follows:

- Severe chest injury (aortic rupture, tension pneumothorax, pericardial tamponade)
- Bleeding (ruptured liver, ruptured aorta, ruptured spleen)
- Central nervous system injury (major head trauma)

In an adult medical patient the most common underlying cause of cardiac arrest is myocardial ischemia due to coronary artery disease, resulting in a fatal dysrhythmia (e.g., VF). Other, less common causes include electrolyte abnormalities (such as from drugs or chronic renal disease), hypothermia, drug overdose, large pulmonary emboli, central nervous system hemorrhage, and occult gastrointestinal bleeding. Causes of cardiac arrest in the adult vary little between younger and older adults (geriatric patients).

In children, however, the primary cause of medical cardiac arrest is a primary *respiratory* event. Coronary artery disease is unusual in children, although congenital heart problems may result in dysrhythmias and cardiac arrest.

An approach to the various cardiac dysrhythmias is discussed earlier in this chapter and is not repeated here in detail. The information presented here summarizes the general approach to a patient in cardiac arrest, as well as several ethical and medical-legal aspects.

Initial Assessment

Initial assessment mandates rapid recognition of an unresponsive patient who is apneic and pulseless. Once cardiac arrest is confirmed, the next step is to rapidly identify the rhythm. In essence, the possibilities in an arrested patient are either VF/VT or non–VF/VT (asystole, PEA).

Focused History

The keys to survival following cardiac arrest are early institution of CPR, prompt defibrillation, and prompt advanced cardiac life support (ACLS). CPR is a key link in the chain of survival. Especially in out-of-hospital cardiac arrest, CPR often makes the difference between patient survival and death. Also, the earlier CPR is administered, the better. Bystander CPR (BCPR) has consistently improved patient outcome in all but one study. In that particular study, the authors claimed that their EMS units arrived so rapidly (within 5 minutes) that any effect of BCPR was negated unless patients had PEA.

In many individuals, CPR appears to prolong the duration of VF, "buying" time until a defibrillator can be brought to the patient. CPR may triple a patient's chances of surviving out-of-hospital cardiac arrest from VF. Of course, CPR alone has a minimal effect if early defibrillation cannot be provided. However, CPR remains extremely important, even with prompt defibrillation.

The following should be determined and documented as part of the focused history:
- Whether the arrest was witnessed (either by bystanders or EMS personnel)
- The time from patient discovery to initiation of CPR
- The time from patient discovery to activation of the EMS system
- The patient's past medical history

Management: General Principles

Recent international agreement among experts in cardiac resuscitation has resulted in a specific set of terms:
- **Resuscitation**—Efforts are made to return spontaneous pulse and breathing to the patient in full cardiac arrest.
- **Return of spontaneous circulation (ROSC)**—The patient is resuscitated to the point of having a pulse without CPR. There may or may not be a return of spontaneous respirations. In addition, the patient may or may not go on to survive.
- **Survival**—The patient is successfully resuscitated and lives to hospital discharge. Most recent studies include the fact that the patient is neurologically intact—capable of relatively independent functioning outside of the hospital.

Indications for not initiating resuscitation in a victim of cardiac arrest vary. However, the following are applicable to most situations:
- Where there are signs of obvious death (rigor, fixed lividity, decapitation)
- As per local laws and protocols (e.g., advanced directives)

Although prompt defibrillation of VF/VT is the *single most important* skill that the EMS provider can offer a patient in cardiac arrest, the EMT–I should always be prepared, according to local protocols, to provide the following:
- Airway and ventilatory support (bag-valve ventilation, endotracheal intubation)
- Circulatory support (CPR, defibrillation, IV therapy)
- Pharmacological interventions (e.g., oxygen, epinephrine, lidocaine)
- Safe transportation to the nearest appropriate facility
- Appropriate psychological support for the patient, family, and significant others
- Communication of vital patient data to the receiving institution

Termination of Resuscitation

The EMT–I should always be familiar with local protocols regarding the termination of resuscitation efforts. The following are widely acceptable criteria for field termination of resuscitation:
- The patient is 18 years or older.
- The arrest is presumed to be cardiac in origin and not associated with a condition potentially responsive to hospital treatment (e.g., hypothermia, drug overdose, toxicological exposure).
- Endotracheal intubation has been successfully accomplished and maintained.
- Standard basic and advanced cardiac life support measures have been applied throughout the resuscitative effort.
- On-scene advanced life support (ALS) resuscitation efforts have been sustained for 25 minutes, or the patient remains in asystole through four rounds of appropriate ALS drugs.
- The patient has a cardiac rhythm of asystole or agonal rhythm (little or no effective electrical activity) at the time the decision to terminate is made, and this rhythm persists until the arrest is actually terminated.
- Victims of blunt trauma are in arrest, and their presenting rhythm is asystole or they develop asystole while the EMS provider is at the scene.

Some criteria by which patients may be excluded from prehospital termination of resuscitation protocols (i.e., the resuscitation efforts are continued) are as follows:
- A patient under the age of 18
- An etiology for which specific in-hospital treatment may be beneficial
- Persistent or recurrent ventricular tachycardia or fibrillation
- Transient return of a pulse
- Signs of neurological viability
- Arrest witnessed by EMS personnel
- Opposition of family or other responsible party to termination of resuscitation

The following factors are generally not considered to be helpful as to including or excluding a patient from prehospital termination of resuscitation protocols. In these cases, consultation with on-line medical control may be necessary:
- Patient age (e.g., geriatric patient)
- Time of collapse before EMS arrival
- Presence of a nonofficial do-not-resuscitate (DNR) order
- Quality-of-life valuations

Procedures for Field Termination of Resuscitation

As usual, always follow local protocols. Within these guidelines, typical procedures often include the following:

- *Direct communication with on-line medical direction*—Factors that must be communicated include the following:
  - The baseline medical condition of the patient
  - Known etiological factors (e.g., the patient was in hospice care and expected to die soon)
  - Therapy rendered
  - The fact that the family was present and appraised of the situation (Always communicate and document any resistance or uncertainty on the part of the family.)
  - Continuous documentation, including ECG rhythm strips
- *Mandatory review after the event*—Some EMS agencies mandate review and offer counseling for providers after dealing with field death. This may involve trained personnel within the agency itself or outside counselors. It may be difficult for EMS providers to terminate field resuscitation efforts, even according to specific well-established protocols. For this reason, many feel that appropriate support and counseling should be readily available.
- *Involvement of law enforcement*—Depending on the situation, local law enforcement personnel and, often, the medical examiner (coroner) must become involved in field termination of resuscitation efforts. Protocols should determine, in advance, how EMS providers deal with the following:
  - On-scene determination as to whether the event and/or patient requires assignment of the patient to the medical examiner (coroner)
  - Who communicates with the attending physician to sign the death certificate (In many localities this involves either a mortician or the medical examiner.)
- Cases where there is suspicion concerning the nature of the death or where the attending physician refuses or hesitates to sign the death certificate
- No attending physician identified (In these cases the patient is often assigned to the medical examiner.)

SUMMARY

Important points to remember from this chapter include the following:

- Cardiovascular disease is a common cause of medical problems. The most common symptom of cardiac disease is chest pain. During the initial patient assessment, the EMT–I should immediately determine if the patient has a pulse. If the patient is in cardiac arrest, cardiopulmonary resuscitation (CPR) should be started. In patients over 12 years of age and weighing more than 90 pounds, an automatic external defibrillator (AED) also should be applied.
- If the patient is responsive, the EMT–I should take an appropriate history. If the patient complains of cardiac pain and has previously prescribed nitroglycerin, the EMT–I may assist in the administration of this drug. The EMT–I must follow local protocols and obtain permission from medical control before giving any drug.
- Angina is an attack of chest pain and related symptoms that is due to a lack of oxygen in the heart muscle. Various stresses may produce myocardial ischemia, including exercise, cold, and emotion. The underlying lesion in angina, as well as in MI, is an atherosclerotic plaque that narrows the lumen of the coronary artery.
- Patients with angina complain of substernal chest pain. The discomfort may radiate to the epigastrium,

---

CASE HISTORY FOLLOW-UP ■■■

After starting the IV line and completing the history and physical examination, EMT–I Adams contacts medical direction for orders:

"MedCom, this is Metro 24. We have a 73-year-old male with chest pain and shortness of breath. The onset was approximately 30 minutes before our arrival, and the patient had taken two nitro [nitroglycerin] tabs SL [sublingually] without relief. The pain is squeezing, in the left anterior retrosternal region, and radiates to his left arm.

"His past medical history includes acute MI 2 months ago and several recent episodes of CHF that required emergency transportation and ICU hospitalization. He also has a past medical history of emphysema and uses a bronchodilator.

"He is responsive, alert, and oriented and in moderate distress. His vital signs are pulse 86 and irregular, respirations 26 and labored, with posterior-inferior bilateral crackles; BP is 156/96. He had central cyanosis on arrival; however, his color has improved with high-flow oxygen administration via nonrebreather mask.

"His ECG rhythm is normal sinus rhythm with approximately 9 PVCs per minute and pulse deficits. His pulse oxygen reading is 88%.

"We started an IV of normal saline and are running it at a TKO rate. Do you have any further orders?"

Medical direction responds:

"Metro 24, check the date of expiration of his nitro, and you can go ahead and give him one of yours. Contact us if his condition changes; we'll be waiting for you."

The oxygen, nitroglycerin, and reassuring care the EMT–Is provide for Mr. Molino give him some symptomatic relief.

arms, jaw, teeth, or neck. Other symptoms such as diaphoresis, shortness of breath, and nausea may be present. Anginal pain goes away with rest or with the administration of nitroglycerin.

- A heart attack (or acute myocardial infarction [AMI]) occurs when the blood flow through a coronary artery is completely blocked. A thrombus occludes an artery whose lumen has already been narrowed by an atherosclerotic plaque. Cigarette smoking is the major risk factor for the development of AMI. The pain of AMI typically lasts more than 15 minutes. Patients often look pale and ill. It is common for heart attack victims to deny the severity of their illness. Elderly patients may not complain of chest pain; they are more likely to simply have weakness or shortness of breath. Complications of AMI include cardiac arrest, congestive heart failure (CHF), and cardiogenic shock.

- Cardiogenic shock occurs when more than 40% of the myocardium is unable to effectively pump blood. The most common cause is AMI, although other conditions, such as a ruptured valve, also may lead to shock. The blood pressure may be high, low, or normal. The EMT–I should *not* rely on the presence of hypotension to make a diagnosis of cardiogenic shock.

- The EMT–I should care for patients suspected of experiencing AMI with high-concentration oxygen, placement of an IV line, monitoring of the electrocardiographic (ECG) rhythm, and transport in as calm and quiet a manner as possible. "Emergency mode" transport should not be used unless the patient's condition deteriorates. If the patient is in cardiogenic shock, an IV fluid bolus should be administered if mandated by local protocols.

- CHF is circulatory congestion due to inadequate flow of blood. CHF is caused by heart muscle damage. The most severe form is acute pulmonary edema. The most common cause of CHF is coronary artery disease. Both right-sided and left-sided CHF may occur.

- Patients with CHF have shortness of breath that is worse on lying down (orthopnea) and that may awaken the patient at night (paroxysmal nocturnal dyspnea). Diaphoresis, cyanosis, and edema also may be present. Distention of the neck veins and hypertension are common. Hypotension in a patient with acute pulmonary edema is a serious sign, and these patients tend to deteriorate rapidly.

- A hypertensive emergency is a sudden increase in the blood pressure, which results in functional disturbances of the central nervous system, heart, or kidneys. Without proper care, life-threatening complications can occur. The most common cause is an acute exacerbation of chronic hypertension. The EMT–I should consider ingestion of cocaine as a cause for hypertensive crisis in a young patient.

- Patients with hypertensive crisis have markedly elevated blood pressure. Dizziness and headache may be present. If there is an alteration in the patient's level of responsiveness and pupillary abnormalities are present, the EMT–I should assume that the patient has an intracranial hemorrhage.
- The ECG is a graphic representation of the electrical activity of the heart and consists of a P wave (atrial depolarization), PR segment (delay of the electrical impulse at the AV node so blood may pass from the atria to the ventricles), QRS complex (ventricular depolarization), ST segment, and T wave (ventricular repolarization). Lead II is the most commonly used monitoring lead in the prehospital setting.
- Cardiac dysrhythmias that commonly occur during cardiac arrest include ventricular fibrillation (VF), ventricular tachycardia (VT), and pulseless electrical activity (PEA). VF and pulseless VT are treated by administration of electrical shock defibrillation. The EMT–I may administer this shock manually or via an AED. In either case, local protocols should be followed regarding indications for defibrillator use. The EMT–I should always adhere to recommended safety precautions. Defibrillators do not discriminate—they can shock the EMT–I, as well as the patient.

- An EMT–I may be called on to administer or to assist in the administration of cardiac drugs, especially during a cardiac arrest. Epinephrine is the most commonly used cardiac drug; it is indicated in all forms of cardiac arrest and works by improving the coronary artery perfusion. Lidocaine is an antidysrhythmic agent used in the treatment of significant ventricular dysrhythmias as a result of AMI or myocardial ischemia. Amiodarone is a newer agent that is also indicated for ventricular dysrhythmias. (Local protocols should be followed.) Atropine is given in an attempt to reverse excess parasympathetic nervous system tone that may perpetuate bradycardia or asystole.
- Field termination of resuscitation efforts is becoming more and more widespread. The EMT–I should be aware of specific local protocols for inclusion and exclusion of patients. Grief counseling should be readily available for EMS providers when necessary.

REFERENCE

1. American Heart Association: *2000 heart and stroke statistical update*, Dallas, 1999, The Association.

24

Diabetic Emergencies

Key Terms

▪▪▪ CASE HISTORY

It is a warm Friday afternoon, and you are just finishing inventorying all the equipment and supplies on your ambulance. The only thing found to be lower in number than required is the number of 4 × 4 dressings. You plan to contact the supply officer today and have some brought out. Just as you and your partner finish signing the inventory sheet, the emergency phone rings. The dispatcher hurriedly tells you to respond to the corner of E. Sixth and Pearl Street for a male who is acting "crazy." Apparently, police are at the scene and calling for EMS.

You and your partner quickly move to the ambulance. Just as you climb into the driver's seat, you remember that the back door of the patient module is still open. You quickly climb out of the cab and go to the back of the ambulance to shut the door. As you continue your response to the scene, motorists seem to be taking their time moving out of your way. Some are even coming to complete stops right in front of you instead of pulling off to the right. It aggravates you a bit, but you keep remembering the talk your chief had with all the members of your shift about not letting little things like that bother you. Besides, you are close to the end of your shift, and you have the next 3 days off.

As you pull up to the scene, you see the police car positioned behind a blue sedan that is parked on the sidewalk. The driver is in the car behind the steering wheel. He is waving his arms frantically and shouting. One police officer is standing next to the open driver's side door while the other is standing next to the passenger's side door. You quickly park the ambulance and pull out the cot. You put your jump kit and oxygen unit on the cot and move it next to the blue sedan. One police officer tells you the patient was driving his car erratically and then pulled onto the sidewalk, where they stopped him. They turned off the car engine and removed the ignition keys to prevent the man from driving off.

You approach the 35-year-old man, who is extremely disoriented and very apprehensive. Just as you reach for his arm to feel for a pulse and take a blood pressure, he shouts a flurry of obscenities at you. The police officer holds him by the shoulder to keep him from moving. You notice he is wearing a medical alert bracelet. It identifies him as having diabetes. Your partner now moves next to you and begins conversing with the patient in an attempt to gather a history. Meanwhile, you are able to hold his arm long enough to identify that he has cool, pale, diaphoretic skin. He also has a strong pulse at a rate of 126 beats per minute.

You pull out your glucometer and use a lancet to pierce his finger to get a blood sample. Surprisingly, the patient offers little resistance. He has an initial blood glucose reading of 40. Your partner begins administering oral glucose to the patient while you set up a macrodrip administration set with a 1000 mL bag of normal saline and clear the line of air.

The patient's mental status improves a bit, and he is now more cooperative. As you apply the tourniquet above his elbow, you can see that he has a huge vein that runs along the lateral aspect of his forearm. You clean the site with povidone-iodine and wipe it with an alcohol wipe. Your partner hands you an 18-gauge catheter-over-needle. You are inclined to use a 16-gauge catheter-over-needle device, but you do not want to aggravate the patient any more than you have to. Just as you penetrate the skin with the needle, the patient jerks his arm backward. You were prepared for this type of reaction from the patient, so you held onto his arm tightly to prevent too much movement. You tell the patient to relax while you quickly pass the needle into the vein. You get an immediate flashback, so you advance the catheter into the vein and quickly release the tourniquet, letting it fall to the ground. While holding the hub of the catheter tight against his arm and tourniquetting the distal end of the catheter with your little finger, you use your other hand to place the used needle into a "sharps" container that has been positioned on the ground beside you.

Next, you attach the intravenous (IV) administration set tubing to the hub of the IV catheter and secure the two in place with a commercial device. Your partner now hands you a prefilled syringe of 50% dextrose (D_{50}) that he pulled out of the drug box and assembled. You use an alcohol wipe to clean the medication administration port of the IV line closest to the IV site, and then pull the protective cap off the needle and insert it into the port. You pinch off the IV line above the port to prevent the D_{50} from back flowing through the IV administration set tubing, and begin delivering the medication. Because the medication is so thick, it goes in slowly. By the time you finish pushing all the medication, your hand aches.

LEARNING OBJECTIVES

CHAPTER GOAL
Upon completion of this chapter, the EMT-Intermediate will be able to use assessment findings to formulate a field impression and implement a treatment plan for the patient with a diabetic emergency.

Cognitive Objectives
As an EMT-Intermediate you should be able to do the following:

- Describe the pathophysiology of diabetes mellitus.
- Describe the effects of decreased or increased levels of insulin on the body.
- Discuss the management of diabetic emergencies.
- Discuss the pathophysiology of hypoglycemia.
- Recognize the signs and symptoms of the patient with hypoglycemia.
- Describe the management of a hypoglycemic patient.
- Integrate the pathophysiological principles and assessment findings to formulate a field impression and implement a treatment plan for the patient with hypoglycemia.
- Discuss the pathophysiology of hyperglycemia.
- Describe the mechanism of ketone body formation and its relationship to ketoacidosis.
- Recognize the signs and symptoms of the patient with hyperglycemia.
- Describe the management of a hyperglycemic patient.
- Differentiate between diabetic emergencies on the basis of assessment and history.

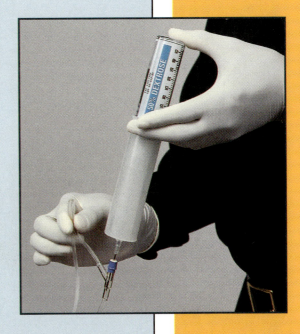

DIABETES AND INSULIN

Diabetes **mellitus** is a chronic disease of the endocrine system caused by a decrease in the secretion or activity of the hormone **insulin.** Insulin is released from the pancreas and, together with epinephrine and glucagon, regulates the blood sugar **(glucose)** level (Figure 24-1). Insulin moves glucose molecules from the blood into the cells, where they are stored (Figure 24-2). In addition, insulin prevents the breakdown of fat tissue in the body. Glucagon and epinephrine have the opposite effects, raising the blood sugar level. They are often called **counterregulatory hormones** (Figure 24-3) Table 24-1.

Persons with diabetes do not produce enough insulin to regulate the blood sugar level. Because of a hormonal imbalance, the blood sugar level may become too high (hyperglycemia) or too low (hypoglycemia). Either condition can result in potentially life-threatening problems.

When a person's insulin supply is insufficient, a state of cell starvation results. Although cells use glucose as their primary "food source," they will turn to fat, and then to muscle, if insulin lack prevents the inward movement of glucose. When the body metabolizes fats, ketones and ketoacids result. This occurs in any malnourished patient,

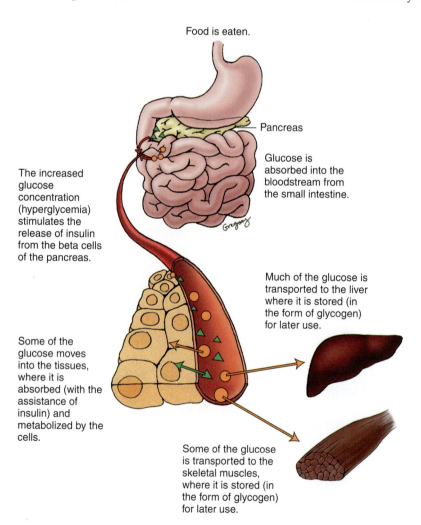

Food is eaten.

Pancreas

Glucose is absorbed into the bloodstream from the small intestine.

The increased glucose concentration (hyperglycemia) stimulates the release of insulin from the beta cells of the pancreas.

Much of the glucose is transported to the liver where it is stored (in the form of glycogen) for later use.

Some of the glucose moves into the tissues, where it is absorbed (with the assistance of insulin) and metabolized by the cells.

Some of the glucose is transported to the skeletal muscles, where it is stored (in the form of glycogen) for later use.

FIGURE 24-1 ▲ Secretion of insulin.

TABLE 24-1

Effects of Insulin and Glucagon on Target Tissues

TARGET TISSUE	RESPONSE TO INSULIN	RESPONSE TO GLUCAGON
Skeletal muscle, cardiac muscle, cartilage, bone, fibroblasts, leukocytes, and mammary glands	Increased glucose uptake and glycogen synthesis; increased uptake of certain amino acids	Little effect
Liver	Increased glycogen synthesis; increased use of glucose for energy (glycolysis)	Causes rapid increase in the breakdown of glycogen to glucose (glycogenolysis) and release of glucose into the blood Increased formation of glucose (gluconeogenesis) from amino acids and, to some degree, from fats Increased metabolism of fatty acids, resulting in increased ketones in the blood
Adipose cells	Increased glucose uptake, glycogen synthesis, fat synthesis, and fatty acid uptake; increased glycolysis	High concentrations cause breakdown of fats (lipolysis); probably unimportant under most conditions
Nervous system	Little effect except to increase glucose uptake in the satiety center	No effect

From Seely R: *Anatomy and physiology*, ed 2, St Louis, 1992, Mosby.

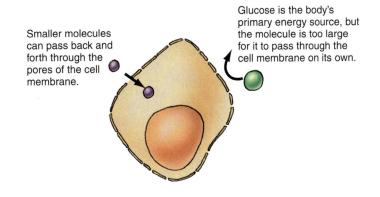

Smaller molecules can pass back and forth through the pores of the cell membrane.

Glucose is the body's primary energy source, but the molecule is too large for it to pass through the cell membrane on its own.

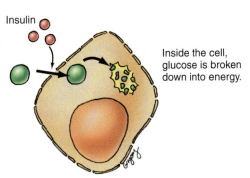

Insulin

Insulin secreted from the beta cells of the pancreas makes the glucose molecule lipid soluble, thereby allowing it to pass through the cell membrane.

Inside the cell, glucose is broken down into energy.

The movement of glucose across the cell membrane occurs through a process referred to as facilitated diffusion. This is a passive process that occurs without the expenditure of energy.

FIGURE 24-2 ▲ Movement of glucose into the cell.

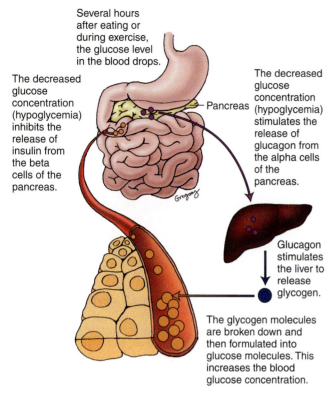

Several hours after eating or during exercise, the glucose level in the blood drops.

The decreased glucose concentration (hypoglycemia) inhibits the release of insulin from the beta cells of the pancreas.

Pancreas

The decreased glucose concentration (hypoglycemia) stimulates the release of glucagon from the alpha cells of the pancreas.

Glucagon stimulates the liver to release glycogen.

The glycogen molecules are broken down and then formulated into glucose molecules. This increases the blood glucose concentration.

FIGURE 24-3 ▲ **Glucagon secretion.**

not just in patients with diabetes. The difference in patients with diabetes is that the counterregulatory hormones are also affected. Excess ketone accumulation upsets the acid-base balance in the body, and acidosis develops (see Hyperglycemia and Diabetic Ketoacidosis).

Glucose is the sole source of oxidative metabolism (nutrition) for the central nervous system. When the blood sugar level falls significantly, altered states of consciousness or loss of consciousness may occur. Prolonged hypoglycemia (lasting longer than 20 to 30 minutes) may lead to permanent brain cell damage.

CLASSIFICATION OF DIABETES

Diabetes is often classified according to whether or not exogenous insulin injections are required for life:

- **Type 1 diabetes**—Insulin dependent; patients typically have disease onset at a younger age, are prone to diabetic ketoacidosis (DKA), and require insulin injections to live.
- **Type 2 diabetes**—Non–insulin dependent; usually, the onset of type 2 diabetes is after the teenage years. Although DKA may develop in any diabetic patient, patients with type 2 diabetes are less prone. Although they may require insulin injections for optimal regulation of blood sugar levels and prevention of complications, exogenous insulin is not necessary to maintain life.

▶ FINGERSTICK BLOOD SUGAR DETERMINATION
Measurement of the blood sugar level is usually done in a hospital laboratory. A useful measurement of the blood sugar level in the field involves using chemically treated paper strips or a battery-operated glucose monitoring system (glucometer) exposed to a drop of blood obtained by a fingerstick (Figure 24-4). Fingerstick measurements of the blood sugar level may be done easily in the field. Perform this test whenever necessary to aid in your assessment and treatment of patients.

To properly perform a **fingerstick blood sugar** determination:

1. Use either the index or middle finger.
2. Clean the fingertip with an alcohol swab.
3. Gently squeeze the finger at the joint below the fingertip.
4. At the same time, use either a small needle or special fingerstick lancet to pierce the skin of the fingertip. The tip should not go in deeper than 1 to 2 mm. Do this in a rapid "in and out" fashion. Do not leave the lancet or needle in place or twist it around.
5. Immediately remove the lancet or needle.
6. Using a gloved hand, gently squeeze the fingertip to express a drop of blood from the wound.
7. Turn the glucometer on. Then insert the test strip into the appropriate location on the device.
8. Apply the blood sample. It must be placed directly onto the designated location of the test strip (this varies according to the manufacturer).
9. Results will be displayed on the readout within 15 to 45 seconds.

If a known diabetic patient has an altered level of consciousness or neurological symptoms and a fingerstick blood sugar test is not readily available, assume that the blood sugar level is low and provide care accordingly.

COMPLICATIONS OF DIABETES MELLITUS

In addition to hyperglycemia or hypoglycemia, diabetic patients may have several chronic complications, including the following (Figure 24-5):

- *Eye disease*—Diabetic retinopathy (disease of the retina) causes bleeding in the vitreous humor of the eye and may lead to blindness.
- *Kidney disease*—Diabetic nephropathy (disease of the kidney) leads to abnormal function and may lead to complete renal failure. Diabetes is a leading cause of chronic renal failure, leading to the need for hemodialysis to maintain life.
- *Nerve disease*—Diabetic neuropathy (nerve disease) causes chronic pain and decreased sensation, especially in the lower extremities. As a result, many persons with diabetes develop severe foot

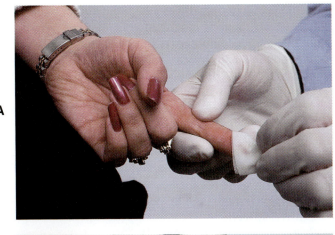

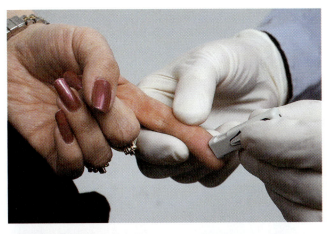

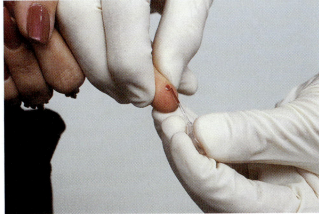

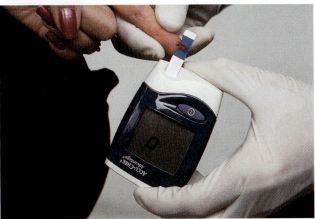

A

B

C

D

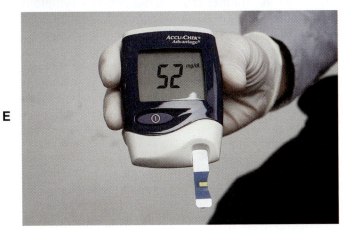

E

FIGURE 24-4 ▲ Dextrose evaluation using a glucometer. **A,** Clean the finger with an alcohol wipe. **B,** Use a lancet to pierce the finger. **C,** Use a pipette to obtain a blood sample (not needed for all situations or types of glucometers). **D,** Obtain a blood sample. **E,** Blood glucose reading.

infections from relatively minor injuries because they are unaware of the problem until it is far advanced. Diabetic neuropathy may also cause persons with diabetes to have atypical symptoms from common diseases, such as appendicitis and myocardial infarction.

- *Increased risk of cardiovascular disease*—Persons with either type 1 or type 2 diabetes have an increased risk of developing heart and vascular disease. In addition, they develop heart and vascular disease at a younger age than persons who do not have diabetes.

Strokes or heart attacks are relatively common in diabetic persons in their thirties—always consider the possibility of myocardial infarction in any patient with diabetes with new-onset weakness and fatigue, especially if hypoglycemia is not present.

HYPOGLYCEMIA

Hypoglycemia is an abnormally low blood sugar level. This condition is sometimes called insulin shock. However, these patients are rarely in shock. Since cir-

Retinopathy   Nephropathy

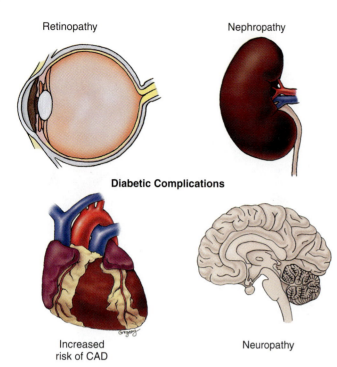

Diabetic Complications

Increased   Neuropathy
risk of CAD

FIGURE 24-5 ▲ Complications of diabetes. *CAD,* Coronary artery disease.

cumstances other than insulin overdose lead to low blood sugar, the preferred term is *hypoglycemia.*

Causes

Hypoglycemia occurs as a result of an imbalance in the amounts of insulin and glucose. Causes of hypoglycemia include the following:

- Medications (insulin, oral diabetic medications)
- Excessive exercise (causes too rapid absorption of insulin)
- Endocrine diseases
- Alcohol consumption
- Poor diet
- Hypothermia (severe cold exposure, p. 780)
- Liver disease

Hypoglycemia in a diabetic patient is most commonly caused by the patient taking his or her insulin and not eating enough food. Insulin forces sugar into the cells. Because of the lack of an inadequate dietary intake, insufficient sugar remains in the blood to maintain homeostasis. Low levels of blood sugar interfere with the function of the central nervous system.

Patient Assessment

Hypoglycemia generally develops rapidly, over a few minutes to a few hours. Normally, the counterregulatory hormones epinephrine and glucagon are secreted in response to hypoglycemia, causing early symptoms. However, in long-standing diabetes this "early warning

system" is absent, usually as a result of autonomic nervous system diabetic neuropathy. In that case the patient's presenting symptom of hypoglycemia is an alteration in the level of consciousness.

The signs and symptoms of mild to moderate hypoglycemia include the following:

- Shakiness, weakness
- Diaphoresis
- Rapid pulse and respiratory rate

Persons with more severe hypoglycemia often exhibit the following:

- Altered level of consciousness (The patient may appear intoxicated.)
- Slurred speech
- Neurological deficit (unusual)
- Seizures (unusual in adults; more common in children)

Severe hypoglycemia causes a marked alteration in the level of consciousness. Although seizures are unusual in adults, they may occur. The patient is often unconscious. Differentiating hypoglycemia from a stroke may be impossible, since hypoglycemia can cause paralysis and altered levels of consciousness. Always consider the possibility of a blood sugar abnormality in any patient with neurological complaints. Check the fingerstick blood sugar determination if that test is available.

Hypoglycemia, by itself, does not usually result in hypotension. Another cause of the patient's symptoms should be looked for if hypotension is present.

HELPFUL HINT

- *Always* ask the diabetic patient, "Did you eat today? Did you take your insulin (or other diabetic medication) today?"

Emergency Care

The care for a patient with known or suspected hypoglycemia includes the following:

- Control the airway, and assist breathing as necessary. Patients with an altered level of consciousness may have partial airway obstruction.
- Give oxygen by nasal cannula at a rate of 3 to 4 L/min.
- Monitor the electrocardiogram (ECG).
- If the patient is conscious, give orange juice with two packets of sugar dissolved in it. Alternatively, have the patient take a dose of oral glucose solution, corn syrup, or candy (Figure 24-6).

HELPFUL HINT

- Do not use diet drinks, Sweet and Low, aspartame (NutraSweet), or other sugar substitutes. These products will be of no help, since they do not contain sugar.

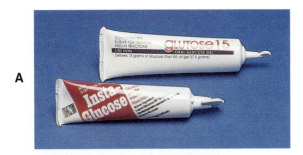

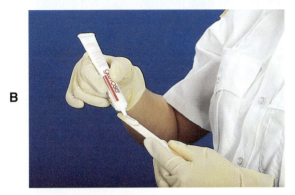

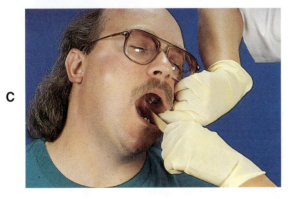

FIGURE 24-6 ▲ **A,** Instant glucose administration.
B, Applying instant glucose to a tongue blade.
C, Administering the instant glucose.

- Unless the symptoms are extremely mild, start an intravenous (IV) line; draw blood *before* giving any fluid or sugar (D_{50}).
- If permitted by local protocols, administer one ampule of D_{50}, or 50% dextrose (25 g of dextrose in 50 mL water), intravenously if the measured blood sugar is less than 60 mg% (Figure 24-7). If you are unable to measure blood sugar in the field, follow local protocols regarding the administration of IV D_{50}.

▶ WARNING: Watch out for unexpectedly violent, but involuntary, behavior as the patient wakes up following administration of sugar. Only a few persons with diabetes will have this, but it is impossible to predict ahead of time which ones.

- If you are unable to start an IV line through which to give 50% dextrose (D_{50}), place liquid glucose or glucose paste into the patient's mouth. Try to place it

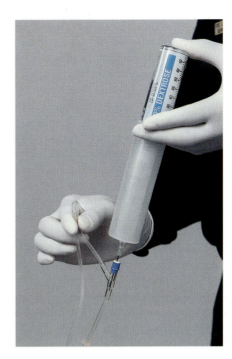

FIGURE 24-7 ▲ Administration of 50% dextrose.

HELPFUL HINT

- Follow your local protocols regarding administering liquid glucose or glucose paste into the mouth of an unconscious patient.

onto the inner cheeks. Oral glucose is contraindicated if the patient is unconscious and has no gag reflex.
- If you are in doubt as to whether the conscious patient has hypoglycemia or hyperglycemia (DKA), always assume that the patient is hypoglycemic and give sugar. Never give a diabetic patient insulin in the field.
- Transport the patient to the appropriate hospital for further evaluation and treatment.
- Provide appropriate psychological support. Patients may be embarrassed by their actions when hypoglycemic, especially if they showed a violent reaction on awakening following administration of D_{50}.

HYPERGLYCEMIA AND DIABETIC KETOACIDOSIS

Hyperglycemia is an elevation of the blood sugar level above normal. The most common cause of hyperglycemia is diabetes. **Diabetic ketoacidosis (DKA)** is a metabolic condition consisting of hyperglycemia, dehydration, and the accumulation of abnormal compounds, called ketones and ketoacids, in the body.

Causes of Diabetic Ketoacidosis

DKA occurs when a diabetic person has inadequate insulin circulating in the blood to properly control the blood sugar level. In addition, an excess of epinephrine and glucagon (counterregulatory hormones) is present. The reasons for this excess are unknown.

The patient's blood sugar level rises significantly, and the fatty tissue breaks down. The body forms compounds called **ketones** and **ketoacids** from the fat tissue. These substances change the acid-base balance in the body, harming the patient. The elevated blood sugar level causes the patient to urinate more frequently than usual, leading to dehydration and loss of body chemicals (particularly potassium) (Figure 24-8).

The most common reason why a diabetic person develops DKA is an infection. This stress results in an increased insulin requirement in the body. Unless the diabetic person recognizes the need to increase the daily dose of insulin when sick, metabolism and the regulation of the blood sugar level become abnormal (Box 24-1).

The term *diabetic coma* has been used in the past for DKA, but many patients with DKA are not in a coma. However, many patients with hypoglycemia or insulin shock are in a coma but are not in shock. Because of the confusing terms, the preferred terminology is *hypoglycemia* for low blood sugar and *hyperglycemia* for high blood sugar. Some patients with hyperglycemia will have DKA, although many will not. Distinguishing between hyperglycemia alone and DKA in the field is difficult.

> Many persons have hyperglycemia, but only a few of these have concomitant DKA. For DKA to develop, there must also be an abnormality in the body's production of the counterregulatory hormones (e.g., epinephrine, glucagon) that normally counterbalance the effects of insulin. Do not assume that a person has DKA just because the blood sugar level is elevated. Persons with DKA appear sick and dehydrated—the actual level of blood sugar elevation may not be impressive. Remember, treat the patient, not the number!

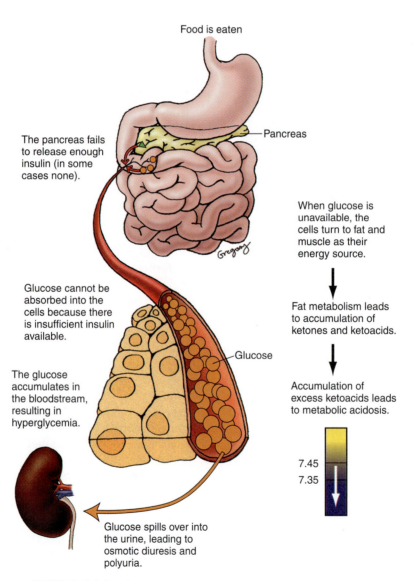

Food is eaten

The pancreas fails to release enough insulin (in some cases none).

Pancreas

Glucose cannot be absorbed into the cells because there is insufficient insulin available.

Glucose

The glucose accumulates in the bloodstream, resulting in hyperglycemia.

Glucose spills over into the urine, leading to osmotic diuresis and polyuria.

When glucose is unavailable, the cells turn to fat and muscle as their energy source.

Fat metabolism leads to accumulation of ketones and ketoacids.

Accumulation of excess ketoacids leads to metabolic acidosis.

7.45
7.35

FIGURE 24-8 ▲ Pathophysiology and diabetic ketoacidosis.

BOX 24-1

COMMON CAUSES OF DIABETIC KETOACIDOSIS

- Too small *insulin* dose
- Failure to take *insulin*
- Infection
- Increased stress (trauma, surgery)
- Increased dietary intake
- Decreased metabolic rate
- Other, less common predisposing factors, including significant emotional stress, alcohol consumption (often associated with hypoglycemia), and pregnancy

From Sanders MJ: *Mosby's paramedic textbook*, ed 2, St Louis, 2000, Mosby.

Patient Assessment

DKA has a relatively slow onset. Patients with DKA have symptoms that become worse over a matter of hours to days. Hypoglycemia, on the other hand, tends to progress rapidly (minutes to hours). The signs and symptoms of DKA are as follows:

- Weakness
- Nausea and vomiting
- Abdominal pain
- Frequent urination
- Thirst
- Rapid, deep, sighing respirations (**Kussmaul respirations**)
- Alterations in the level of consciousness
- A fruity, acetone-like odor to the breath
- Normal or mildly decreased blood pressure
- Rapid, weak pulse

The acetone-like odor described in DKA is not always present. Not all people can detect this odor even when it is. Do not rely on the breath odor to suspect DKA.

Emergency Care

The care for a patient with suspected hyperglycemia or DKA includes the following:

- Maintain the airway; assist breathing as necessary.
- Give high-concentration oxygen.
- Monitor the ECG.
- Start an IV line. Many of these patients are significantly dehydrated. Give a fluid bolus according to local protocols. Many systems administer 500 to 1000 mL of normal saline or lactated Ringer's solution as rapidly as possible.
- Watch carefully for shock, and care for the patient accordingly.
- Give nothing by mouth. An exception to this rule is when the patient is conscious and you are not certain whether a person has hypoglycemia or hyper-

glycemia. If you are unable to check the fingerstick blood sugar, always assume that hypoglycemia is present and give sugar. Never give a diabetic patient insulin in the field.

- Transport the patient to the appropriate hospital as soon as possible.
- Provide ongoing psychological support.

HELPFUL HINT

- If a diabetic emergency is present and the patient has an altered level of consciousness or neurological symptoms and you are unable to check the blood sugar, *assume* that he or she has a low blood sugar level, and provide care accordingly.

HYPERGLYCEMIC HYPEROSMOLAR NONKETOTIC COMA

Hyperglycemic hyperosmolar nonketotic coma (HHNC) refers to a state where the blood sugar is markedly elevated but no acidosis or accumulation of ketones is present. Although the exact pathophysiology is not yet known, a relative insulin deficiency is present. As a result, high levels of glucose in the cerebrospinal fluid lead to dehydration of the brain and decreased levels of consciousness (Figure 24-9). It is a relatively common cause of hyperglycemia and marked alterations in the level of consciousness, especially in the geriatric patient.

Persons with HHNC are typically over 60 years of age. Their underlying health is poor; often these persons are in a nursing home or other assisted-living setting. HHNC is precipitated by infection, extreme cold, or dehydration. The typical history is that of gradual deterioration in mental status over 4 or 5 days.

Other signs and symptoms include the following:

- Altered mental status (The patient may be unconscious or may appear to have had a stroke.)
- Evidence of dehydration, including poor skin turgor and furrowed tongue
- Kussmaul respirations and fruity breath odor (present in DKA) are conspicuously *absent* in HHNC.

The treatment for patients with HHNC is the same as that described earlier for DKA.

GENERAL MANAGEMENT OF ANY DIABETIC EMERGENCY

Determining the exact nature of a diabetic emergency is difficult, even in the hospital. The EMT–Intermediate's (EMT–I's) responsibility is to provide care based on clinical assessment rather than a specific diagnosis. Always pay close attention to maintenance of the ABCs (airway, breathing, and circulation). Measurement of the fingerstick blood sugar, if possible, provides valuable infor-

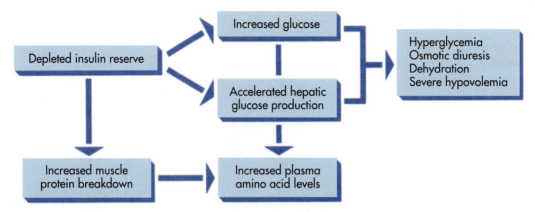

FIGURE 24-9 ▲ Pathophysiology of hyperglycemic hyperosmolar nonketotic coma. (From Sanders MJ: *Mosby's paramedic textbook,* ed 2, St Louis, 2000, Mosby.)

TABLE 24-2

Differential Considerations in Diabetic Emergencies

FINDINGS	HYPOGLYCEMIA	HYPERGLYCEMIA	HHNC
History			
Food intake	Insufficient	Excessive	Excessive
Insulin dosage	Excessive	Insufficient	Insufficient
Onset	Rapid	Gradual	Gradual
Infection	Uncommon	Common	Common
Gastrointestinal tract			
Thirst	Absent	Intense	Intense
Hunger	Intense	Absent	Intense
Vomiting	Uncommon	Common	Uncommon
Respiratory system			
Breathing	Normal or rapid	Deep or rapid	Shallow/rapid
Breath odor	Normal	Acetone smell	Normal
Cardiovascular system			
Blood pressure	Normal	Low	Low
Pulse	Normal, rapid, or full	Rapid or weak	Rapid or weak
Skin	Pale or moist	Warm or dry	Warm or dry
Nervous system			
Headache	Present	Absent	Absent
Consciousness	Irritability	Restless	Irritable
	Seizure or coma	Coma (rare)	Seizure or coma
Urine			
Sugar level	Absent	Present	Present
Acetone level	Usually absent	Usually present	Absent
Serum glucose levels	Less than 60 m/dL	Greater than 300 mg/dL	More than 600 mg/dL
Treatment response	Immediate (after glucose) (NOTE: If the hypo-glycemic episode is pro-longed or severe, the re-sponse may be delayed and may require more than one dose.)	Gradual (within 6-12 hr after medication and fluid replacement)	Gradual (within 6-12 hr after medication and fluid replacement)

From Clark F et al: *Pharmacological basis of nursing,* ed 4, St Louis, 1993, Mosby.
HHNC, Hyperglycemic hyperosmolar nonketotic coma.

mation. In addition, the following should be determined (Table 24-2):

- History:
  - Has the patient's insulin dosage changed recently?
  - Has the patient had a recent infection?
  - Has the patient suffered any psychological stress?
  - Has the patient had a change in the frequency of urination?
- Physical assessment:
  - Altered mental status
  - Abnormal respiratory pattern (Kussmaul respirations; p. 231)
  - Tachycardia
  - Hypotension
  - Fruity breath odor
  - Skin color and temperature
  - Hydration status

The following general guidelines should be followed when dealing with any type of suspected diabetic emergency:

- Manage the airway with supplemental oxygen and assisted ventilation, including endotracheal intubation, when necessary.
- According to local protocols, draw blood before giving any medication or IV fluid; determine a fingerstick blood sugar reading if possible.
- Monitor vital signs and the ECG.
- Administer 50% dextrose (D_{50}) according to local protocols.

CASE HISTORY FOLLOW-UP ■ ■ ■

Shortly after you administer the D_{50}, the patient becomes alert and oriented. It turns out that he dropped his family off at a local restaurant and was parking his car when he became disoriented and drove away. The police officers have another patrol car drive over to pick the family up to bring them to the scene. The patient says he feels fine now and does not want to go to the hospital. After several minutes of talking to him, you are able to persuade him to go. You recheck his blood glucose level. This time it is 104.

SUMMARY

Important points to remember from this chapter include the following:

- Diabetes is a disease of the endocrine system resulting from a lack of insulin. Insulin regulates the blood sugar level. Abnormal levels of insulin may result in either hypoglycemia or hyperglycemia. The EMT–I should always ask patients if they are diabetic and if they took their insulin (or other diabetic medication).
- Hypoglycemia is a state of low blood sugar. There are many causes of hypoglycemia. Most commonly, diabetic patients take their insulin and eat improperly. Symptoms develop rapidly and vary from shakiness to unconsciousness. It may be impossible to distinguish hypoglycemia from hyperglycemia, alcohol intoxication, or stroke.
- To care for the conscious hypoglycemic patient, sugar should be given in any of the following forms: orange juice with two added packets of sugar, glucose solution, candy, or corn syrup. The EMT–I should care for the unconscious patient according to local protocols. Some EMS systems allow EMT–Is to place a sugar solution into the mouth of an unconscious diabetic person.
- Hyperglycemia is an elevation of the blood sugar level. Diabetic ketoacidosis (DKA) is an abnormal metabolic condition resulting in hyperglycemia and the accumulation of ketones and ketoacids in the blood. The patient with DKA is severely ill and dehydrated. Care should be provided for shock, if present, and the patient transported to the nearest appropriate hospital as soon as possible.

25

Allergic Reactions

Key Terms

Allergen

Allergic Reaction

Anaphylaxis

Antibody

Antigen

Diphenhydramine

Epinephrine

Histamine

IgE

Mast Cell

■■■ CASE HISTORY

The crew of Medic 4 is at their station finishing lunch when suddenly the tone alert goes off and the dispatcher announces they have a call for a "female short of breath" at the far end of their response district. The dishes are thrown into the sink, and the crew hurries to the ambulance. After an 8-minute response, the ambulance pulls up to the address given by the dispatcher. A fire engine first responder company is already at the scene. The EMT–Is pull the oxygen unit, jump kit, drug box, and electrocardiogram (ECG) monitor out of the ambulance and carry them to the house. A fire lieutenant meets the EMT–Is at the front door of the duplex house and says, "She's inside. It looks like she's having an allergic reaction."

The EMT–Is find the 27-year-old patient crouched down on the floor next to her dining room table. One of the first responders is finishing taking her blood pressure, and the other two are setting up the oxygen unit. The first responder who took the blood pressure reports, "The patient has a respiratory rate of 22, a pulse rate of 120, a blood pressure of 106/72, and warm, flushed skin."

As one of the EMT–Is auscultates the lung sounds, the other applies the finger clip of the pulse oximetry unit to the patient's finger. The patient's husband, who is visibly upset, states, "We were eating dinner that we got from this takeout restaurant down the street when she started complaining that she itched all over. Then she said she couldn't breathe." Auscultation of the chest reveals bilateral wheezing, and the pulse oximetry shows an SaO_2 of 90%. Both EMT–Is note there is swelling about the patient's face, particularly around the eyes. One of the first responders tells the EMT–Is, "She's also complaining of abdominal cramps." On being questioned, the husband tells the EMT–Is that the patient is allergic to seafood.

One of the EMT–Is sets up a 1000-mL bag of normal saline and a macrodrip administration set and clears the line of air while the other attaches the patient to the ECG monitor. "Looks like sinus tachycardia with some PVCs [premature ventricular complexes]," reports the one EMT–I. The intravenous (IV) line is quickly established in the patient's right forearm, and a venous blood sample is drawn. "Go ahead and start a breathing treatment while I get some 1:1000 epi ready," the senior EMT–I directs.

CHAPTER GOAL

Upon completion of this chapter, the EMT–Intermediate will be able to use assessment findings to formulate a field impression and implement a treatment plan for the patient with an allergic or anaphylactic reaction.

Cognitive Objectives

As an EMT–Intermediate you should be able to do the following:

- Define allergic reaction, anaphylaxis, allergen, antigen, and antibody.
- Summarize the pathophysiology of anaphylaxis.
- Integrate the pathophysiological principles of anaphylaxis into the clinical presentation and treatment of a patient.
- Describe the common methods of entry of substances into the body.
- List common antigens most frequently associated with anaphylaxis.
- Recognize the signs and symptoms related to anaphylaxis.
- Describe physical manifestations in anaphylaxis.
- Correlate abnormal findings in assessment with the clinical significance in the patient with anaphylaxis.
- Differentiate between the various treatment and pharmacological interventions used in the management of anaphylaxis.
- Develop a treatment plan based on field impression in the patient with allergic reaction and anaphylaxis.

Affective Objectives
- None identified for this chapter.

Psychomotor Objectives
- None identified for this chapter.

ALLERGIC REACTIONS AND ANAPHYLAXIS

The terms *allergic reaction* and *anaphylaxis* are often used interchangeably. There are differences between them, but these are not absolute. **Allergic reactions** result from exposure to *any* substance to which an individual is sensitive ("allergic"). The generic term for *any* substance to which a person is allergic (sensitive) is an **allergen.** These terms apply despite the specific mechanism or manifestation of a persons' hypersensitivity (excessive sensitivity). Several pathophysiological mechanisms may cause allergic reactions. The symptoms and signs may include rashes, itchiness, a burning sensation of the skin, difficulty breathing, or hypotension.

Anaphylaxis is a specific type of allergic reaction caused by the interaction of an allergen, called an **antigen,** and one kind of **antibody.** Five types of antibodies are formed by the immune system and reside on the surface of **mast cells,** a type of white blood cell. Antibodies

Allergic reactions result from exposure to *any* substance to which an individual is sensitive.

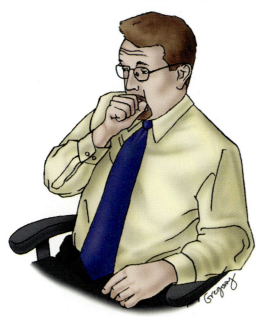

Anaphylaxis is a specific type of allergic reaction caused by the interaction of an allergen, called an **antigen,** and one kind of **antibody.**

FIGURE 25-1 ▲ **Allergic reactions and anaphylaxis.**

(also called "immunoglobulins") are abbreviated as *Ig,* followed by a letter (Figure 25-1):

- IgG   • IgE
- IgA   • IgD
- IgM

IgE antibody is the only one involved in an anaphylactic reaction. Other allergic reactions may involve antibodies (e.g., reaction to intravenous [IV] x-ray contrast dye involves IgM and IgG) but are not properly called anaphylaxis. Fortunately, these are unusual, and the clinical approach is the same, despite which antibody is involved (Box 25-1).

Spectrum of Severity

Many people incorrectly think of anaphylaxis as being only an extremely severe allergic reaction. Airway edema, difficulty breathing, and vascular collapse leading to shock occur in some patients. However, IgE-mediated reactions more commonly lead to less severe findings (e.g., hives, wheezing, mouth swelling). *Either* response (low grade or severe) can occur quickly and may lead to serious illness or death if the patient is not cared for immediately (Box 25-2).

PATHOPHYSIOLOGY

Antibodies respond to antigens. When an antigen to which one is sensitive enters the body (e.g., ingestion, injection, inhalation, absorption), it is attacked by an antibody.

▶ *Allergic reaction* is a generic term for *any* signs and symptoms that occur when a person is exposed to an allergen—*anything* he or she is sensitive to, *despite* the patient's response. *Anaphylaxis* is a specific term for an allergic reaction caused by the interaction of an allergen, called an antigen, and an IgE antibody. The severity of the symptoms ranges from progressive hives to cardiac arrest. All anaphylactic reactions are allergic reactions, but not all allergic reactions result in anaphylaxis.

▶ Although not technically correct, the terms *antigen* and *allergen* refer to the same thing in anaphylaxis—a foreign substance to which the patient is sensitive.

Antibodies function to destroy foreign substances. In the case of anaphylaxis, however, the IgE antibody does not destroy the antigen. Instead, the reaction between the antigen and the IgE antibody triggers a series of events. Chemical mediators are released, leading to symptoms ranging from hives to cardiac arrest. Mast cells release mediators after antigen and IgE antibodies have reacted on the cells' surface (Figure 25-2).

Histamine release occurs first. Several types of substances are released from mast cells during anaphylactic reactions. The most important of these is **histamine.** Release of histamine causes the following responses:

- Bronchospasm, which can cause airway compromise
- Vasodilation, which may be severe enough to result in shock
- Leaking of fluid from vessels that is due to a change in permeability

Histamine stimulates the release of additional mediators. Histamine also stimulates the manufacture and release of other chemical mediators from mast cells. Together, these substances result in an unpredictable spiral of events ranging from mild to extreme and sometimes causing death (Figure 25-3).

The biphasic (early and late) anaphylactic response is common. One in five persons has a biphasic anaphylactic response—recurrence of some type of symptoms 4 to 6 hours later. Typically, the initial symptoms have resolved completely and there is a symptom-free period before the onset of the late-phase reaction. It is nearly impossible to predict which patients will also develop a late reaction. In addition, the symptoms of the early and late reactions may be different. For example, a patient's early reaction might consist simply of progressive hives. The late-phase reaction, if it occurs, may result in shock. Assume that all patients with early-phase anaphylactic reactions, no matter how mild, are at risk for a late reaction that may be life threatening. Act accordingly by ensuring patient follow-up (Figure 25-4).

BOX 25-1

CLASSES OF IMMUNOGLOBULINS

IgG

IgG accounts for 70% to 75% of antibodies in normal serum. IgG is most abundant in blood but is also found in lymph, cerebrospinal, synovial, and peritoneal fluid and breast milk. It is the major antibody involved in secondary immune responses and the only antitoxin antibody developed. IgG is also the only immunoglobulin that crosses the placenta, providing temporary immunity in neonates.

IgM

IgM accounts for approximately 5% to 10% of antibodies in normal serum and is the dominant antibody in ABO incompatibilities. IgM triggers the increased production of IgG in acute infections and the complement fixation required for an effective antibody response.

IgA

IgA accounts for approximately 15% of antibodies in normal serum. This immunoglobulin is found in blood, secretions such as tears and saliva, and the respiratory tract, stomach, and accessory organs. IgA combines with a protein in the mucosa and defends body surfaces against invading microorganisms.

IgE

IgE accounts for less than 1% of antibodies in normal serum. It is found in some tissues and on the surface membranes of basophils and mast cells; it is responsible for immediate hypersensitivity reactions.

IgD

IgD accounts for less than 1% of antibodies in normal serum. Its precise biological function is unknown.

From Sanders, MJ: *Mosby's paramedic textbook,* ed 2, St Louis, 2000, Mosby.

BOX 25-2

SIGNS AND SYMPTOMS OF ANAPHYLAXIS

UPPER AIRWAY
- Hoarseness
- Stridor
- Laryngeal or epiglottic edema
- Rhinorrhea

LOWER AIRWAY
- Bronchospasm
- Increased mucus production
- Accessory muscle use
- Wheezing
- Decreased breath sounds

CARDIOVASCULAR SYSTEM
- Tachycardia
- Hypotension
- Dysrhythmias
- Chest tightness

GASTROINTESTINAL SYSTEM
- Nausea
- Vomiting
- Abdominal cramps
- Diarrhea

NEUROLOGICAL SYSTEM
- Anxiety

- Dizziness
- Syncope
- Weakness
- Headache
- Seizure
- Coma

CUTANEOUS SYSTEM
- Angioedema
- Urticaria
- Pruritus
- Erythema
- Edema
- Tearing of the eyes

From Sanders, MJ: *Mosby's paramedic textbook,* ed 2, St Louis, 2000, Mosby.

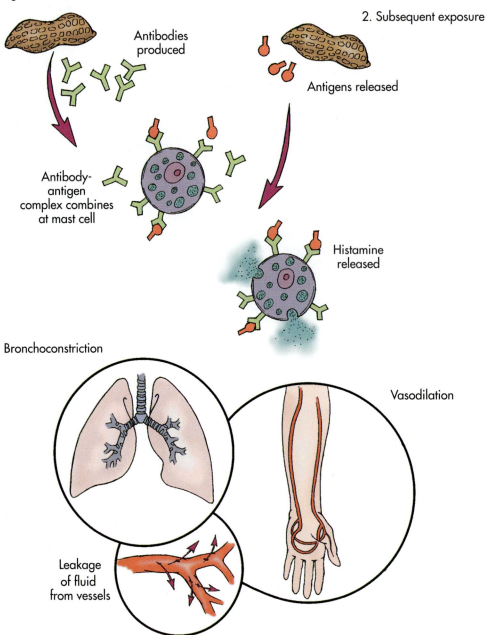

1. Allergic substance intake

Antibodies produced

2. Subsequent exposure

Antigens released

Antibody-antigen complex combines at mast cell

Histamine released

Bronchoconstriction

Vasodilation

Leakage of fluid from vessels

FIGURE 25-2 ▲ **The pathophysiological events of allergic reactions and anaphylaxis in the body.**

Common Allergens and Routes of Exposure

Common allergens include drugs, insects, foods, and animal hair. They may enter the body through many channels (Figure 25-5):
- *Skin contact*—Poison ivy, skin creams, cosmetics, detergents
- *Injections*—Medications such as penicillin, insect bites and stings

- *Inhalation*—Molds, pollen, perfumes
- *Ingestion*—Foods, chocolate, shellfish, peanuts

> ▶ Latex allergy is a *major* problem for both health care providers and patients alike. It is not just latex gloves and condoms that have caused the problem. Most medical devices (airways, oxygen tubing, bandages, tape, catheters, etc.) contain latex. Depending on the patient's sensitivity, the result may range from nothing, to hives, to fatal anaphylaxis. Nearly 20% of health care providers from varied fields and an unknown number of patients are susceptible. All EMS systems should have latex-free alternatives. ▲

ASSESSMENT

History

Unless there is a recent obvious insect sting, many cases of allergic reaction or anaphylaxis will not have any apparent cause. Ask the patient about the following:
- Recent insect sting or bite
- History of food or drug allergy
- Foods recently ingested
- Medications taken (name, dosage, when taken before reaction)
- New cosmetics, soaps, clothing, etc.

Determine if there is a history of other significant medical conditions:
- Identify current medications.
- Get a list of medications to bring to the hospital.

The largest concentrations of mast cells are in the skin, the respiratory tract, and the gastrointestinal tract. The most common symptoms of IgE-mediated reactions are hives, wheezing, and abdominal pain. The severity varies unpredictably. Not all described signs and symptoms are present every time.

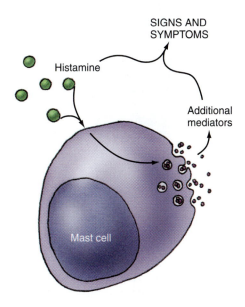

Histamine also stimulates the manufacture and release of other chemical mediators from mast cells. Together, these substances result in an unpredictable spiral of events ranging from mild to extreme, sometimes causing death.

FIGURE 25-3 ▲ **Histamine stimulates release of other mediators.**

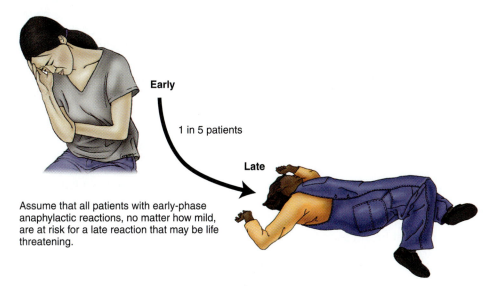

Assume that all patients with early-phase anaphylactic reactions, no matter how mild, are at risk for a late reaction that may be life threatening.

FIGURE 25-4 ▲ **Early and late signs of anaphylaxis.**

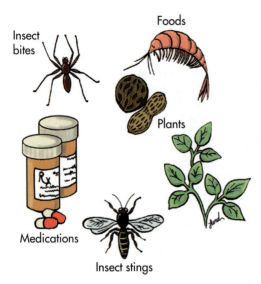

FIGURE 25-5 ▲ Common allergens to the human body. (Stacy Lund from Stoy W: *Mosby's EMT–Basic textbook,* St Louis, 1996, Mosby.)

Signs and Symptoms of Anaphylactic Shock

The signs and symptoms of anaphylactic shock differ somewhat from other forms of shock and may develop rapidly or gradually. Anaphylactic shock presents a special challenge, since profound airway compromise can develop quickly.

Signs and symptoms include the following (Figure 25-6):

- A sense of uneasiness or agitation (This is often the first symptom noticed by the patient.)
- Swelling of the soft tissues such as the hands, tongue, and pharynx (Patients may feel as if their tongue is swelling and their throat closing.)

> **CLINICAL NOTES**
>
> Listen for stridor in the upper airway, and look for associated signs of respiratory distress. Observe for pharyngeal edema. The uvula and soft palate may be swollen. Occasionally, the tongue may become so edematous that the airway is completely occluded.

- Skin flushing and hives (Figure 25-7)
- Coughing, sneezing
- Wheezing due to spasms of the upper and lower airway, rales, rhonchi, or absent breath sounds
- Tingling, burning, or itching skin
- Abdominal pain
- Tachycardia
- Weak, thready pulse
- Profound hypotension (late sign)

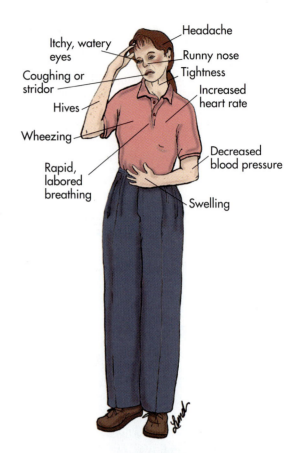

Itchy, watery eyes
Headache
Coughing or stridor
Runny nose
Tightness
Hives
Increased heart rate
Wheezing
Rapid, labored breathing
Decreased blood pressure
Swelling

FIGURE 25-6 ▲ Signs and symptoms of anaphylactic shock. (Stacy Lund from Stoy W: *Mosby's EMT–Basic textbook,* St Louis, 1996, Mosby.)

> **CLINICAL NOTES**
>
> The typical rash consists of raised lesions called urticaria or "hives." They may be widely scattered or noted only in some localized areas. They may come and go rapidly. Hives are *not* necessary for a patient to have anaphylaxis. Sometimes the patient's skin is red and swollen throughout the body. Do not assume that just because there are no obvious and distinct hives, anaphylaxis cannot be present.

> **CLINICAL NOTES**
>
> Wheezing may be either grossly audible or detectable only by auscultation.

- Confusion
- Decreased level of consciousness
- Weakness
- Profuse diaphoresis
- Retraction of intercostal spaces and accessory muscle use

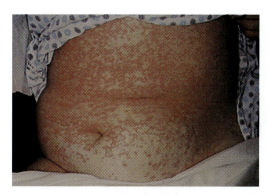

FIGURE 25-7 ▲ Skin flushing and hives. (Courtesy Gary Quick, MD; from Sanders MJ: *Mosby's paramedic textbook,* St Louis, 1994, Mosby.)

- Deep or shallow, labored respirations
- Diaphoresis
- Cyanosis
- Anxiety, depressed level of consciousness
- Peripheral edema

MANAGEMENT

Mild Allergic Reactions (Anaphylaxis)

The care for a patient with an allergic reaction is generally supportive in nature. Diphenhydramine (Benadryl), 25 mg administered by slow IV push or intramuscularly, is appropriate if permitted by local protocols and in the following situations:

- Vital signs are normal.
- There are no respiratory symptoms.
- The only manifestations of the reaction are itching, rash, and/or swelling on the outside of the body.

Diphenhydramine (Benadryl) is an antihistamine that blocks the effects of histamine. It probably has other effects against some of the other mediators as well. By itself, however, it may be inadequate in progressive reactions.

Some experts argue that progressive hives, by themselves, should be treated by low-dose epinephrine (0.1 to 0.2 mg of 1:1000 solution given subcutaneously) *and* diphenhydramine. The basis for this recommendation is the fact that several mediators are released in addition to histamine. Diphenhydramine is an antihistamine and may not effectively suppress actions of the other mediators. Follow local protocols.

Moderate and Severe Allergic Reactions (Anaphylaxis)

The care for a patient with a more severe reaction includes the following:

- Aggressive airway management

- Ventilatory support
- Oxygen therapy
- Circulatory support
- Administer epinephrine (1:1000), 0.1 to 0.5 cc, subcutaneously if:
  - Wheezing or stridor is present.
  - Edema of the pharynx, soft palate, or tongue is observed.
  - Manifestations of vascular compromise are noted (such as hypotension; confusion; weak, thready pulse; or tachycardia).

Epinephrine stimulates alpha and beta receptors of the sympathetic nervous system. This blocks multiple effects of anaphylactic mediators. In addition, it stabilizes mast cells, preventing the further release of mediators.

 Epinephrine may be administered via an autoinjector (Epi-Pen). In an adult 0.3 mg is administered via the intramuscular route. Remember, it requires a moderate to large amount of force to activate one of these devices. The manufacturer has "trainers" available—it would be helpful to become familiar with the amount of force required to properly use the Epi-Pen before giving it to a patient (Figure 25-8).

HELPFUL HINT

The definitive treatment for anaphylaxis is epinephrine. It vasoconstricts, has a positive inotropic action (the heart beats harder), bronchodilates, and directly counteracts released mediators. If you are trained to administer subcutaneous epinephrine, you should do so. Some patients may have their own physician-prescribed epinephrine for use in anaphylaxis. Even if you are not allowed to give drugs, you can help a patient self-administer the drug. Anaphylactic shock can be a life-threatening emergency where minutes can make the difference between life and death.

Anaphylaxis and Hemodynamic Compromise (Shock)

The care for a patient in anaphylactic shock includes the following:

- Provide continual reassurance to the patient.
- Ensure an adequate airway.
- Perform endotracheal intubation and administer high-concentration oxygen in any of the following situations:
  - The patient is unable to maintain an airway.
  - Ventilatory assistance is needed.
  - Respiratory distress is severe.
  - Cyanosis is present.
  - Significant hypotension (blood pressure <70 mm Hg systolic) is present.

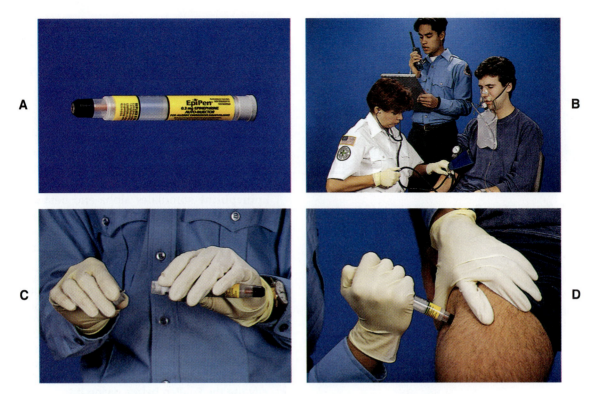

FIGURE 25-8 ▲ **A,** Epinephrine autoinjector. **B,** Obtain permission from on-line medical director or follow standing orders to use autoinjector. **C,** Remove safety cap on the autoinjector. **D,** Place the tip of the autoinjector at a 90° angle against the lateral portion of the patient's thigh midway between the waist and knee. (Vincent Knaus from Stoy W: *Mosby's EMT–Basic textbook,* St Louis, 1996, Mosby.)

- Apply electrocardiogram (ECG) electrodes, and provide continuous monitoring if permitted by local protocols.
- If the patient is experiencing an allergic reaction but breathing adequately, administer high-concentration oxygen, 10 to 15 L (85% to 100%) by nonrebreather mask. Use a nasal cannula delivering a 44% concentration of oxygen (flow rate of 6 L/ min) if the patient is afraid of or agitated by the oxygen mask.
- Establish an IV line, using a large-bore cannula.
  - Use normal saline or lactated Ringer's solution with a macrodrip administration set.
  - Draw bloods if time permits.
  - If blood pressure is less than 90 mm Hg systolic, run the IV line wide open, reassessing vital signs after each 300 cc.
  - If BP is greater than 90 mm Hg systolic, run the IV line TKO ("to keep open").
- Administer epinephrine, 1:1000, 0.1 to 0.5 cc of 1:1000 solution subcutaneously; repeat, if necessary, two or more times at 10- to 20-minute intervals. If the patient has his own autoinjector (Epi-Pen), you may help in giving the injection. Repeat every 5 to 10 minutes if the patient's response to treatment is inadequate. Always follow local protocols.
- If wheezing or stridor is present, administer a nebulized bronchodilator treatment with medications such as albuterol (Proventil, Ventolin) or isoetharine (Bronkosol) by nebulizer if permitted by local protocols. Both albuterol and isoetharine reverse bronchospasm.
  - With albuterol, add the solution to 2.5 ml of normal saline, place in the nebulizer device, and deliver with a flow rate of 4 to 6 L/min.
  - With isoetharine, place the solution (2.0-mL prefilled container of 0.25%) in the nebulizer device and deliver it with a flow rate of 4 to 6 L/min.
  - Position the patient in a position of comfort.
  - In some areas these drugs come in prepackaged ampules and do not need to be mixed in saline; follow local protocols.
- Identify "priority" patients, and make an appropriate transport/backup decision.
- Move the patient to the ambulance or squad on a stair chair or cot. Do not walk the patient to the vehicle.
- Place the patient in a position of comfort based on his or her physiological needs.
- Transport the patient rapidly to the nearest appropriate medical facility.
- Continue to reassess the patient's vital signs and response to treatment.
- In cases of bee stings, examine the sting site. If the stinger is still present, do not grasp it between your fingers or with a hemostat, tweezers, or any

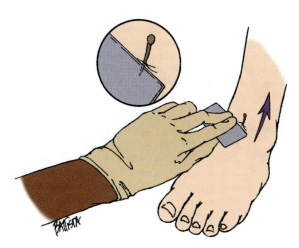

FIGURE 25-9 ▲ Removing a stinger.

kind of grasping device. Take a flat object, such as a tongue depressor, and scrape flat along the skin to remove the venom sac with or without the stinger (Figure 25-9).

CASE HISTORY FOLLOW-UP ■ ■ ■

The patient responds favorably to the treatment. So far, she has received oxygen at 15 L/min via nonrebreather mask, an IV infusion of normal saline delivered at a TKO rate, 0.3 cc of 1:1000 epinephrine subcutaneously, and an albuterol breathing treatment. Reassessment by the EMT–Is reveals that the patient has a respiratory rate of 16, a pulse rate of 110, a blood pressure of 136/90, and warm, dry skin. Auscultation of her chest reveals the lung sounds are now clear bilaterally. The ECG monitor reveals sinus tachycardia without ectopy, and the pulse oximetry shows an SaO_2 of 94%.

The first responder personnel and EMT–Is lift the patient onto the cot and move her to the back of the ambulance. On the way to the hospital, the patient tells the senior EMT–I, "As nice as he was trying to be . . . getting dinner and all for me, I don't think I am going to let my husband order the food anymore." The EMT–I, with a big grin, quips back, "I sure understand that!"

SUMMARY

Important points to remember from this chapter include the following:

- Allergic reactions result from exposure to any substance to which an individual is sensitive ("allergic"). The generic term for any substance to which a person is allergic (sensitive) is an allergen.

- Anaphylaxis is a specific type of allergic reaction caused by the interaction of an allergen, called an antigen, and IgE antibody. This interaction leads to the release of histamine from mast cells. Histamine stimulates the secretion of additional chemical mediators, and a potentially vicious circle follows.

- The spectrum of symptoms that may occur because of an anaphylactic reaction ranges from hives to shock.

- Since most mast cells are localized in the skin, respiratory tract, and gastrointestinal tract, many patients have hives or swelling, wheezing, and abdominal discomfort. The presence of hives is not mandatory to reach a field impression that a patient has anaphylaxis.

- Either response (low grade or severe) can occur quickly and may lead to serious illness or death if the patient is not cared for immediately.

- One in five patients has late-phase symptoms, which may differ completely from the initial presentation. It is impossible to identify "late-phase reactors" in advance—the EMT–I must act accordingly by ensuring medical follow-up care.

- All patients require careful attention to the ABCs (airway, breathing, and circulation). Antihistamines (diphenhydramine [Benadryl]) and epinephrine may be used for mild reactions, depending on local protocols.

- For more severe reactions, aggressive IV fluid administration and definitive airway management may be required. Epinephrine is nearly always administered under these circumstances. Nebulized bronchodilators may be helpful as well.

26

Poisoning and Overdose Emergencies

...CASE HISTORY

The crew of Fire Rescue 1452, consisting of EMT–Is Morant and Stokes and EMT–I student Parley, have finished putting the squad back in order after completing an emergency call. They are pulling out of the hospital emergency department parking lot when the dispatch center advises them to "respond to 12345 Sierra Lane, Apartment 6, for a 32-year-old female, possible drug overdose." After a relatively short trip, the ambulance pulls up to the address given by the dispatcher. A man meets the crew at the front door of the apartment building and says, in broken English, that his wife has taken an overdose of drugs.

As the crew enters the apartment, they see three small children standing in the living room. The children and husband are all very upset and concerned about the patient, a 32-year-old woman who is lying on the couch. EMT–I Morant begins to assess the patient while EMT–I Stokes obtains a history. EMT–I student Parley prepares to hook the patient up to oxygen.

As EMT–I Morant assesses the patient, he finds that she is unresponsive to verbal or painful stimuli. Her respiratory rate is only 8 breaths per minute, and her breath sounds are clear bilaterally. The pulse is strong and regular at the wrist, but the rate is slightly elevated at 105 beats per minute. Her pupils are pinpoint, blood glucose is 100, blood pressure is 106/82, and the electrocardiogram (ECG) shows sinus tachycardia.

Through questioning of the husband, EMT–I Stokes discovers that the patient has a history of substance abuse but that she has been "clean" for almost a year. Apparently, though, when the husband and children returned home after a movie, they found her like this.

LEARNING OBJECTIVES ✓

CHAPTER GOAL
Upon completion of this chapter, the EMT-Intermediate will be able to use assessment findings to formulate a field impression and implement a treatment plan for the patient with a toxic exposure.

Cognitive Objectives
As an EMT-Intermediate you should be able to do the following:
- Identify appropriate personal protective equipment and scene safety awareness concerns in dealing with toxicological emergencies.
- Identify the appropriate situations in which additional non-EMS resources need to be contacted.
- Review the routes of entry of toxic substances into the body.

- Discuss the role of the Poison Control Center in the United States.
- List the toxic substances that are specific to your region.
- Identify the need for rapid intervention and transport of the patient with a toxic substance emergency.
- Review the management of toxic substances.
- Differentiate between the various treatments and pharmacological interventions in the management of the most common poisonings by inhalation, ingestion, absorption, and injection.
- Integrate pathophysiological principles and the assessment findings to formulate a field impression and implement a treatment plan for patients with the most common poisonings by inhalation, ingestion, absorption, and injection.
- Review poisoning by overdose.
- Review the signs and symptoms related to the most common poisonings by overdose.
- Correlate abnormal assessment findings with their clinical significance in patients with the most common poisonings by overdose.
- Differentiate between the various treatments and pharmacological interventions in the management of the most common poisonings by overdose.
- Integrate pathophysiological principles and the assessment findings to formulate a field impression and implement a treatment plan for patients with the most common poisonings by overdose.

Affective Objectives
As an EMT–Intermediate you should be able to do the following:
- Appreciate the psychological needs of victims of drug abuse or overdose.

Psychomotor Objectives
- None identified for this chapter.

GENERAL TOXICOLOGY, ASSESSMENT, AND MANAGEMENT

Poisonings, or *"toxicological emergencies,"* involve the ingestion, inhalation, absorption, or injection (generically summarized here as "exposure") of any harmful substance. Nearly one half of poisonings involve prescription drugs. Many poisonings are unintentional but preventable. Poisonings are most common among children younger than 10 years old. In adults most poisonings are suicide attempts or drug abuse.

There is a difference between the terms *poisoning* and *overdose*:
- **Poisoning** connotes exposure to a substance that is generally only harmful and has no usual beneficial effects (e.g., cyanide).
- **Overdose** suggests excessive exposure to a substance that has normal treatment uses (e.g., aspirin). In excess, harm results.

Since the approach for the EMT–Intermediate (EMT–I) is similar in both cases, these differences are pointed out only when they affect clinical assessment or management.

Types of Toxicological Emergencies

There are three generic types of toxicological emergencies:
1. **Unintentional poisoning**—Poisonings where there is no intent by any individual to poison or hurt someone include the following:
   - **Dosage errors**—These may be an error by the prescribing physician, treating EMS provider, nurse, physician assistant, or pharmacist. Patients or their families may

also be responsible for errors. By definition, there is no intent to harm.

- **Idiosyncratic reactions**—These are untoward side effects that are unpredictable and different from those common to any particular drug. For example, nitroglycerin may cause hypotension; this potential side effect is well known and does not usually come as a surprise. On the other hand, nitroglycerin is expected to improve many cases of ischemic chest pain. An isolated patient who develops *worse chest pain* and *shortness of breath* following nitroglycerin has had an idiosyncratic reaction.
- **Childhood poisoning**—Unless harmful intent is present, most childhood poisonings are the result of caregiver inattention and innate childhood curiosity. Accidental (unintentional) childhood poisonings make up the greatest number of calls to regional Poison Control Centers each year in the United States.
- **Environmental exposures**—Many exposures to toxins occur without intent and without warning. Examples include carbon monoxide in a school with inadequate ventilation, chemical exposure when driving near a freshly sprayed crop field, and smoke inhalation in persons living downwind from a large fire in progress.
- **Occupational exposures**—Small amounts of potentially toxic chemicals seep into the air and are inhaled by workers every day. As a rule, they are not harmful or special precautions are routine (e.g., respirator masks). Accidental occupational exposure is usually the result of an unforseen leak or explosion, resulting in the spread of toxic materials absorbed by unprotected workers.
- *Neglect and abuse*—There is a fine line between "accidental" neglect and criminal neglect and abuse. Leaving children inside a running car with the windows open in a closed garage while a parent answers the phone is accidental neglect. Exposing children to known toxins, such as cigarette smoke, is deliberate neglect and abuse.
2. *Drug and alcohol abuse*—Also referred to as **substance abuse,** often intentional, is responsible for millions of dollars in injury and illness each year. The costs, both emotional and financial, are magnified by loss of productive work time and property damage.
3. *Intentional poisoning or overdose*—An intentional poisoning or drug overdose is usually the result of one of the following:
   - *Chemical warfare*—The Gulf War during the last century brought the realities of chemical agent warfare to widespread public awareness. Incidents of national and international terrorism further exacerbated fears. Many public safety offices have assumed that chemical weapons are likely to play a role in the future and have planned accordingly.
   - *Assault or homicide*—Historically, the use of poison to commit homicide dates to pre-Biblical days. Some personal defensive devices, such as pepper spray, are used not only for self-protection but also to assault and rob individuals.
   - *Suicide attempts*—Deliberate exposure to either a known poisonous agent or an excess amount of a therapeutic drug is considered a suicide attempt.

Provider Safety and Resources Identification

As in *any* scenario, *scene size-up comes first.* Virtually no toxin discriminates between the patient and EMS providers—all are potential victims. Immediately assess the need for personal protective equipment. Do not enter the scene until doing so is safe. As in any toxic exposure, it may be necessary to enlist the assistance of special hazardous materials teams to extricate, remove, and detoxify the patient before providing care.

Appropriate equipment includes, but is not limited to, the following:
- Airway protection (respirations, self-contained breathing apparatus [SCBA] packs)
- Body surface absorption protection suits and isolation
- Specialized equipment

Additional resources that may be needed should be identified early. These include the following:
- Hazardous materials teams
- Police
- Fire department
- Specialized rescue services

Follow local protocols regarding decontamination of personnel, equipment, and the environment before going back into service.

Use of Poison Control Centers

Regional Poison Control Centers (PCCs) are found throughout the United States. Most have a toll-free number that is easily accessible by cellular phone. Although protocols differ, many EMS systems require or encourage EMT–Is to contact the PCC, either directly or via medical control. Experts agree that the PCC is the most reliable and up-to-date source of information on the assessment and treatment of toxicological emergencies.

Routes of Absorption

There are four routes by which poisons are introduced into the human body (Figure 26-1):
- **Ingestion**—A poison may enter the body by the mouth and be absorbed by the gastrointestinal tract. Ingestion is the most common poisoning route.

Examples include eating poisonous mushrooms or a deliberate overdose of sleeping pills.

- **Inhalation**—Toxic fumes or gases may be inhaled into the lungs. The material may damage the lungs or be absorbed into the blood, leading to systemic toxicity. Carbon monoxide poisoning is an example of inhalation exposure.
- **Absorption**—Substances may pass through the skin into the bloodstream. Many chemicals dissolve easily in the fat of the skin. These materials are the most likely to cause poisoning by absorption. Pesticides and agricultural chemicals are often absorbed this way.
- **Injection**—Toxic material may be injected by needles or insect stingers.

Geographically Specific Toxicological Emergencies

Some types of poisoning, such as prescription drugs, are common everywhere. Other exposure potentials are geographically specific. These include many possibilities, such as the following:

- *Venomous snakes*—Although several types of snakes are common throughout the United States (rattle-snakes), some live in specific climates (e.g., the coral snake in the South, especially Florida).
- *Spiders*—Brown recluse spiders, black widow spiders.
- *Marine animals*—Jellyfish, Portuguese man-of-war, lionfish.
- *Manufacturing industries*—Chemical plants, gasoline refineries.
- *Transportation industries*—Railroad routes, interstate highways.

Grouping of Toxicologically Similar Agents

The key approach to any toxicological emergency is self-protection and maintenance of the ABCs (airway, breathing, and circulation). Specific antidotes play a role at times, but attention to the basics is even more important. Several groups of drugs present with similar clinical patterns of toxicity. These syndromes are sometimes called **toxidromes.** They are useful for remembering the assessment and management of toxicological emergencies but do not consider how or why the toxin has been introduced into the body. In addition to specific treatments, always consider the route of entry.

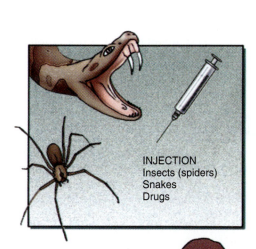
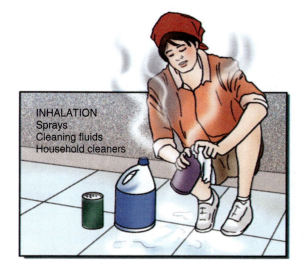
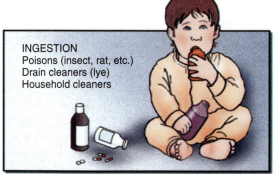
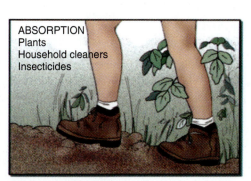

FIGURE 26-1 ▲ **Four routes of how poisons are introduced into the body.** (From McSwain NE et al: *The basic EMT: comprehensive prehospital patient care,* St Louis, 1997, Mosby.)

GENERAL PRINCIPLES OF TOXICOLOGICAL EMERGENCIES

Patient Assessment

When caring for a patient who is the victim of poisoning, try to gather information about the event:
* What was taken
* How much was ingested
* When the poisoning occurred
* What, if anything, has been done for the patient

Patients may state that they took a poison. If the patient is a child, the parent may be able to identify the substance involved. Always bring any containers, pills, syringes, and pill bottles to the hospital with the patient. If the patient vomits, try to collect the vomitus in a plastic bag and bring it to the hospital for analysis.

Signs and symptoms of poisoning vary, depending on the particular substance involved. They may include the following:
* Burning and tearing of the eyes
* Respiratory distress, wheezing, chest pain
* Cyanosis
* Nausea, vomiting, diarrhea
* Excessive sweating or salivation
* Weakness
* Headache, dizziness, seizures
* Altered level of consciousness (ranging from hyperactivity to coma)
* Pain, burning, or itching of the skin
* Burns or stains around the mouth

Physical findings may help identify the poison involved (Boxes 26-1 to 26-3):
* *Pulse*—Tachycardia suggests stimulant ingestion; bradycardia may be caused by various heart medications and by pesticide poisoning.
* *Respiratory rate*—Isolated increases in the respiratory rate, especially in children, suggest the possibility of aspirin toxicity (which causes hyperventilation). Depressed respirations occur from narcotics, sedatives, and carbon monoxide poisoning.
* *Temperature*—Body temperature is elevated with poisoning by aspirin and stimulants; it is lowered (hypothermia) with poisoning by alcohol, sedatives, narcotics, and pesticides.
* *Blood pressure*—The blood pressure may be decreased if the patient took depressant or narcotic agents. It is often elevated if the patient took cocaine or amphetamines.

Poisonings may affect several body systems. Indications of poisoning may be apparent during the focused examination:
* *Respiratory system*—Many poisonings cause respiratory depression and partial airway obstruction. Inhaled toxins may cause respiratory distress and wheezing.
* *Cardiovascular system*—Some poisonings can cause irregular heart rhythm, chest pain, shock, and cardiac arrest.
* *Neurological system*—Poisonings may result in changes in the pupil size. Narcotics usually cause constricted pupils, whereas stimulants result in pupillary dilation.

Care of the Poisoned Patient

Control of airway, breathing, and circulation is the first concern in management of poisoning incidents. The care for a patient with any type of poisoning includes the following:
* Assess and maintain the airway; follow the vital signs and pulse oximetry frequently.
* Place the patient on a cardiac monitor.

BOX 26-1

COMMON ACID AND ALKALI SUBSTANCES

ACIDS
Hydrochloric acid
  Metal cleaners
  Swimming pool cleaners
  Toilet bowel cleaners
Sulfuric acid
  Battery acid
  Toilet bowl cleaners
Phenol
Acetic acid
Bleach disinfectants

ALKALIS
Sodium or potassium
  hydroxide (lye)
  Washing powders
  Pain removers
Drainpipe and toilet
  bowel cleaners
Disk (button)
  batteries
Bleach
Ammonia
  Metal cleaners or
    polishes
  Hair dyes and tints
  Jewelry cleaners

From Sanders MJ: *Mosby's paramedic textbook*, ed 2, St Louis, 2000, Mosby.

BOX 26-2

CLINICAL FEATURES OF HYDROCARBON INGESTION

IMMEDIATE: UP TO 6 HOURS
Gastrointestinal system
Mucous membrane
  hyperemia
Irritation
Abdominal pain
Nausea and vomiting
Belching
Respiratory system
Cough and choking
Inspiratory stridor
Tachypnea
Cyanosis
Dyspnea
Neurological system
Lethargy
Coma
Seizures

Systemic factors
Fever
Malaise

DELAYED: DAYS TO WEEKS
Gastrointestinal system
Diarrhea
Hepatic toxicity
Respiratory system
Bacterial pneumonia
Dyspnea
Sputum production
Atelectasis
Pulmonary edema
Systemic factors
Spontaneous
  hemorrhage
Hemolytic and
  aplastic anemias

- Position the patient to prevent aspiration (left lateral decubitus position, head down).
- Give high-concentration oxygen by mask. If the patient is vomiting, give oxygen by nasal cannula (3 to 4 L/min). If the patient is unconscious, consider endotracheal intubation, according to local protocols.
- Use a pneumatic antishock garment (PASG) as necessary, according to local protocols.
- If the patient is uncooperative, violent, or suicidal, restrain according to local guidelines. Be sure to document the need for restraints in the run report. Do not be a hero—call for police assistance with violent patients.
- Notify the hospital of the suspected substances involved.

After providing life-maintaining care, consult the local PCC or your medical control center for specific advice. Depending on the patient's condition, this may be done en route to the hospital. Bring all suspected material and containers to the hospital.

Ingested Poisons

Care for these patients as recommended by the PCC or medical control. Some EMS systems advise giving syrup of ipecac to induce vomiting. However, syrup of ipecac is not universally accepted. Follow local protocols regarding the use of ipecac. Do not induce vomiting if the patient is having seizures or if ingestion of acid, lye, or petroleum products is suspected. Also, do not induce vomiting if the patient has a decreased level of consciousness or may lose consciousness. Do not delay transport to wait for ipecac to take effect.

Some protocols advise the administration of activated charcoal to absorb the poison. Do not give charcoal until ipecac has caused vomiting. Otherwise, the charcoal will absorb the ipecac, and vomiting will not occur (Figure 26-2).

▶ SYRUP OF IPECAC

Syrup of **ipecac** is a drug that produces vomiting by irritating the lining of the stomach. It is used to empty the stomach in certain cases of poisoning. Some Poison Control Centers recommend that ipecac be limited to home use, when the patient does not require hospital evaluation.

The preferred method of care in the hospital is activated charcoal and/or gastric lavage. Gastric lavage involves placing a tube into the stomach through which fluids are given to dilute and rinse the stomach contents. The liquid is then removed through the gastric tube by suction.

Activated charcoal, in addition to absorbing and neutralizing many poisons, serves as a marker to show when a poison has passed through the digestive tract. Cathartic drugs, such as magnesium citrate, are also sometimes given to speed the passage of substances through the digestive system.

The dosage of syrup of ipecac is 30 mL for adults and 15 mL for children. It is given by mouth, followed by several glasses of water. Syrup of ipecac should not be given to children younger than 9 months old.

Do not induce vomiting in the following situations:
- The patient is comatose or has an altered level of consciousness.
- The patient is seizing or has a history of seizures.
- The patient is in the third trimester of pregnancy.
- The patient has a history of cardiac problems.
- The patient has ingested corrosives, such as strong acids or alkali.
- The patient has ingested petroleum products.
- The patient has ingested iodine, silver nitrate, or strychnine.

BOX 26-3

COMMON POISONOUS PLANTS, TREES, AND SHRUBS

HOUSE PLANTS	Jessamine
Dieffenbachia	Rhododendron
Hyacinth	Wisteria
Narcissus	
Mistletoe	*OTHER PLANTS*
Oleander	Buttercups
Poinsettia	Jack-in-the-pulpit
	Mayapple
FLOWER-GARDEN	Nightshade
PLANTS	Water and poison
Daffodil	hemlock
Foxglove	
Iris	*TREES AND SHRUBS*
Larkspur	Elderberry
Lily of the valley	Oaks
	Wild and cultivated
ORNAMENTAL PLANTS	cherries
Azaleas	
Daphne	

From Sanders MJ: *Mosby's paramedic textbook*, ed 2, St Louis, 2000, Mosby.

Inhaled Poisons

Inhaled poisons may be odorless and colorless. When caring for a victim of inhalation poisoning, survey the scene to make sure that approaching the patient is safe. Waiting for respirators or other specialized equipment before caring for the patient may be necessary.

Care begins by removing the patient from the source of exposure:
- Move the patient to an area outside or with freely circulating air.
- Suspect carbon monoxide poisoning in all victims of fire (see Carbon Monoxide Poisoning; Figure 26-3).
- Help breathing as necessary, and provide high-concentration oxygen by mask.
- Keep the patient at rest, and transport to the hospital as soon as possible.

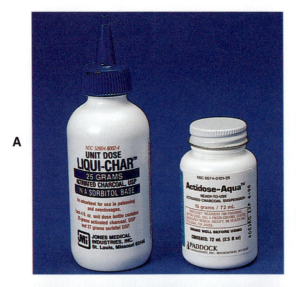

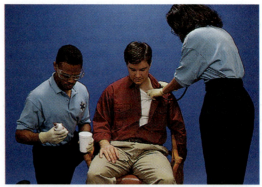

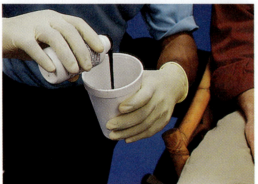

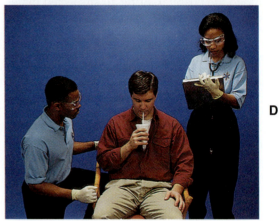

FIGURE 26-2 ▲ Administering activated charcoal to a poisoned patient. **A,** Various types of activated charcoal. **B,** Shake the container to suspend the medication in the fluid. **C,** Pour the liquid into a container. **D,** Have the patient drink the full dose.

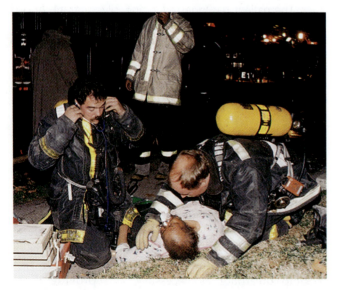

FIGURE 26-3 ▲ Carbon monoxide poisoning is a serious possibility with fire victims. (William Greenblatt from Stoy W: *Mosby's EMT–Basic textbook,* St Louis, 1996, Mosby.)

Absorbed Poisons

The care for a patient with absorbed poisoning involves reducing the contact of the toxic material on the patient's skin:

- Brush off any visible chemical.
- Flush the affected area with large amounts of water.
- Remove contaminated clothing while flushing.
- Protect yourself from exposure to the poison.

CHOLINERGICS

Common Causative Agents

Cholinergic agents lead to stimulation of the parasympathetic nervous system. They prevent the breakdown of **acetylcholine,** the major cholinergic neurotransmitter, by acetylcholinesterase. These agents are sometimes called **anticholinesterases.** Pesticides (organophosphates, carbamates) and nerve gas agents (sarin, soman) are the most common exposures. These agents are readily ab-

BOX 26-4

SIGNS AND SYMPTOMS OF CHOLINERGIC AGENT POISONING

CARDIOVASCULAR SYSTEM	Defecation	Convulsions
Bradycardia	Increased bowel sounds	Respiratory depression
Variable blood pressure		
(usually hypotensive)	**VISION**	**MUSCULOSKELETAL SYSTEM**
	Miosis	Fasciculations
RESPIRATORY SYSTEM	Rapidly changing pupil size	Flaccid paralysis
Rhinorrhea	Lacrimation	
Bronchoconstriction	Blurred vision	**SKIN**
Wheezing		Diaphoresis
Dyspnea	**CENTRAL NERVOUS SYSTEM**	
	Anxiety	**OTHER**
GASTROINTESTINAL SYSTEM	Dizziness	Salivation
Cramps	Coma	Urination
Emesis		

From Sanders MJ: *Mosby's paramedic textbook,* ed 2, St Louis, 2000, Mosby.

sorbed through the skin—always ensure scene safety before approaching the patient or area.

Assessment Findings

Patient complaints depend on the agent, route of exposure, duration of exposure, and strength of exposure. Early symptoms include headache, dizziness, weakness, and nausea. These are nondescript and may be unaccompanied by more severe findings. Making the association between cholinergic agent exposure and symptoms may be difficult (Box 26-4).

More severe symptoms have been called the **SLUDGE** syndrome:

- **S** —Salivation
- **L** —Lacrimation
- **U** —Urination
- **D** —Defecation
- **G** —Gastrointestinal cramping
- **E** —Emesis

In addition, patients may demonstrate the following:

- Bradycardia
- Wheezing, bronchoconstriction
- Myosis (small pupils)
- Coma
- Convulsions

Management

Some cholinergic agents, such as nerve gas, are extremely toxic and penetrate the skin easily. Always ensure your own safety before attempting to provide patient care. Use appropriately trained and equipped hazardous materials teams as necessary, especially to help in patient and rescuer decontamination. As usual, maintenance of airway, breathing, and circulation is cardinal. Depending on local protocols, certain pharmacological interventions may be warranted:

- **Atropine**—Directly blocks the parasympathetic nervous system from further stimulation by acetylcholine that cannot be degraded. High total doses (5 to 15 mg given intravenously) are often required. These are much greater than those used in cardiac patients (usual maximum of 3 mg total). In military or prehospital populations, prefilled automatic injectors are available. By itself, atropine is only weakly effective against nerve agents.
- **Pralidoxime (2-PAM chloride)**—Specifically reactivates acetylcholinesterase, acting as an antidote to cholinergic agents. In the military or prehospital setting it is often provided in automatic injectors, along with atropine.
- **Diazepam**—Benzodiazepines, such as diazepam, may be helpful for seizures and severe muscle cramps and tremors. Follow local protocols.
- **Activated charcoal**—If there has been an oral ingestion, this agent should always be considered (according to local protocols). These too are supplied in autoinjectors for easy administration.

Provide psychological support and transport the patient by the most appropriate mode to the most appropriate health care facility.

ANTICHOLINERGICS

Common Causative Agents

Anticholinergic drugs block the parasympathetic nervous system. They are often called **vagolytic** agents and include atropine, **ipratropium,** and many other medications. Many **antihistamines, antispasmodics** (for abdominal cramps), and tricyclic antidepressant drugs have anticholinergic actions, especially when taken in excess (e.g., deliberate overdose). Several over-the-counter cold and allergy preparations also contain antihistamines.

TABLE 26-1

Acronyms SLUDGE Versus ANTI-SLUDGE

SLUDGE	ANTI-SLUDGE
Salivation	Lack of salivation; dry mouth and skin
Lacrimation	Lack of lacrimation
Urination	Difficulty urinating; bladder distention
Defecation	Constipation
Gastrointestinal cramping	No cramping, but nausea may be present
Emesis	Emesis not present

Assessment Findings

Patient complaints depend on the agent, route of exposure, duration of exposure, and strength of exposure. Since the effects of anticholinergic agents are opposite those of the cholinergics, the clinical acronym is **ANTI-SLUDGE** (Table 26-1).

The usual description of patients with anticholinergic poisoning is "red, hot, hyper, and mad." The skin is red because patients are warm (unable to sweat). Tachycardia and tachypnea are often present as a result of the parasympathetic inhibition (unopposed sympathetic stimulation). Especially in larger doses, anticholinergics induce a temporary psychotic state (thus the patient is "mad").

Management

Always ensure your own safety before attempting to provide patient care. As usual, maintenance of airway, breathing, and circulation is cardinal. Specific pharmacological interventions (e.g., physostigmine) are available to counteract anticholinergic drug toxicity but are rarely used. These antidotes are more dangerous than the anticholinergics themselves. Supportive treatment is best. If the patient has a gag reflex and its administration is permitted by local protocols, activated charcoal may be helpful. Provide psychological support and transport the patient by the most appropriate mode to the most appropriate health care facility.

NARCOTICS/OPIATES

Common Causative Agents

Narcotics/opiates are central nervous system and respiratory depressants, even when used therapeutically as analgesics. They include heroin, morphine, codeine, meperidine, propoxyphene, fentanyl, and **hydrocodone.**

Assessment Findings

Findings depend on the agent, the routes of exposure (oral, intravenous [IV]), and the dose of drug taken. Common signs are as follows:

- Euphoria
- Hypotension
- Respiratory depression
- Respiratory arrest
- Nausea
- Pinpoint pupils
- Seizures
- Coma

In addition, needle track marks and drug paraphernalia may be found in cases of IV heroin abuse and overdose.

Management

Always ensure your own safety before attempting to provide patient care. As usual, maintenance of airway, breathing, and circulation is cardinal. Depending on local protocols, certain pharmacological interventions may be warranted.

Naloxone (Narcan) specifically antagonizes narcotic-opiate drugs. It may also precipitate acute withdrawal syndromes and unpredictable behavior. Many experts suggest that doses be carefully titrated. Adequate respiratory levels must be restored without precipitating acute withdrawal. In addition, a patient who is completely awakened may choose to refuse care. The duration of action of IV naloxone is 1.5 hours, but many narcotic-opiate agents last 3 to 4 hours. Thus toxicity may recur later. An easy way to avoid both the problem of naloxone wearing off before the drug wears off and violent awakenings is to give the drug intramuscularly. A dose of 2 mg given intramuscularly is effective in most patients; they awaken in a smoother fashion, are less likely to be violent, and have 4 to 6 hours of sustained protection (naloxone given intravascularly persists much longer than naloxone given intramuscularly). As always, follow local protocols. Another specific narcotic-opiate antagonist (nalmefene) is commercially available. It is more expensive and offers no advantage over intramuscular naloxone.

If the patient has a gag reflex and its administration is permitted by local protocols, activated charcoal may be helpful.

Provide psychological support and transport the patient by the most appropriate mode to the most appropriate health care facility.

TOXIC GAS INHALATION

Categories of Toxic Gases

There are three categories of toxic gases that an EMT–I may have to deal with (Tables 26-2 and 26-3):

- **Inert gases**—These gases generally cause no direct tissue toxicity. Inhalation displaces oxygen, and injury or death occurs because of asphyxiation. Common inert gas inhalations include carbon dioxide and the fuel gases (e.g., methane, ethane,

TABLE 26-2

Categories of Toxic Gases

CATEGORY	GASES
INERT GASES—DEATH BY ASPHYXIATION	Carbon dioxide Fuel gases: methane, ethane, propane, acetylene
IRRITANTS	Ammonia (more H_2O soluble) Formaldehyde Chloramine Chlorine Nitrous dioxide Phosgene (less H_2O soluble)

SYSTEMIC TOXINS	Gases that interfere with oxygen transport and delivery
	   Carbon monoxide
	   Cyanide
	   Hydrogen
	Aromatic and halogenated hydrocarbons
	   Carbon tetrachloride
	   Benzene
	   Toluene

propane, acetylene). Inhalation of fuel gases in an attempt to get high ("gas huffing") is also popular in some areas. Aberrant mental status, seizures, and cardiac dysrhythmias are more likely to occur with inhalation than with asphyxiation.

- **Irritant gases**—These gases cause direct irritation to tissues. They are inhaled into the lungs to a variable degree, depending on their water solubility. Gases that are highly water soluble (e.g., ammonia and chlorine) dissolve in the saliva and irritate the mucus membranes of the mouth, nose, and pharynx. They tend to do less damage to the lungs. On the other hand, agents that are less water soluble (e.g., nitrous dioxide, phosgene) pass harmlessly through the upper airway, depositing in the bronchioles and alveoli. Here, they cause severe destruction of lung tissue.
- **Systemic toxins**—These gases poison the cells, leading to severe dysfunction. Agents such as carbon monoxide, cyanide, and hydrogen interfere with oxygen transport and delivery, resulting in immediate toxicity. The aromatic and halogenated hydrocarbons (e.g., carbon tetrachloride, benzene, and toluene) cause more chronic types of damage, especially to the liver and kidneys. They are not discussed further here.

Sources of Toxic Gases

Accidents and fires are the most common sources of toxic gas. Tank car rollovers, semitrailer accidents, and other types of road crashes may result in the release of toxic chemicals. Leaking chemical storage tanks are also a hazard. The by-products of combustion from a fire are often poisonous—many common plastics give off cyanide when they burn. Carbon monoxide is universal

in a fire. Home heaters and space heaters serve as sources of carbon monoxide when they fail to operate properly. Finally, the products of chemical reactions, such as in the production of silo gas, may result in toxic gas formation.

Pathophysiology

Several factors determine the effects of gas inhalation on the patient:

- *Water solubility*—If the gas is highly water soluble, it is absorbed into the saliva and remains in the upper airway; injury to the lungs and alveoli is uncommon. If the gas is not absorbed in the saliva, it travels further into the respiratory system, causing alveolar injury.
- *Depth and rate of breathing*—The amount of gas absorbed may be affected by how fast and deep the patient is breathing. The effects of these parameters vary significantly from gas to gas.
- *Smell*—Some gases, such as hydrogen sulfide, rapidly cause olfactory fatigue; this means that over time, the patient is no longer able to smell and avoid them. On the other hand, certain gases (e.g., cyanide) have discernible odors, leading to rapid detection. Carbon monoxide has no odor; it may not be known that it is in the atmosphere.
- *Concentration of the gas*—Whether the concentration of the gas is strong or weak is significant.
- *Length of exposure*—How long the person is exposed to the gas is significant.
- *Differences in host susceptibility*—Certain individuals are more sensitive to toxic gas inhalation than others.

TABLE 26-3

Clinical Features of Toxic Gases and Fumes

CLASS OF TOXIN	TOXIN	SOURCE	CLINICAL FEATURES	MANAGEMENT
Simple asphyxiants	Propane Methane Carbon dioxide Inert gases (nitrogen, argon)	Cooking gas Cooking gas All fires Industry (especially welding)	Displacement of normal air and lower fractional inspired oxygen concentration; symptoms of hypoxemia without airway irritation	Remove patient from source; give oxygen
Chemical asphyxiants	Carbon monoxide	Fires	Formation of carboxyhemoglobin; inhibition of oxygen transport (Headache is earliest symptom.)	Give 100% oxygen
	Hydrocyanic acid	Industry, burning plastics, furniture, fabrics	Highly toxic cellular asphyxiant	Use cyanide antidote
	Hydrogen sulfide	Liquid manure pits, decaying organic materials	Highly toxic cellular asphyxiant similar to cyanide; sudden collapse; ability to smell characteristic odor of rotten eggs; rapid fatigue	Use sodium nitrite for cyanide (makes sulmethemoglobin); *do not* use thiosulfate
Irritants High solubility in water	Chlorine gas Hydrochloric acid	Industry, swimming pool chemicals, bleach mixed with acid at home	Early onset of lacrimination, sore throat, stridor, tracheobronchitis; with heavy exposure, pulmonary edema in 2-6 hr	Use humidified oxygen, bronchodilators, and airway management
	Ammonia	Industry, burning fabrics		
Low solubility in water	Nitrogen dioxide	Burning cellulose, fabrics Grain silos (acrid red gas)	Sweet "electric" smell; delayed onset (12-24 hr) of tracheobronchitis, pneumonitis, and pulmonary edema; late chronic bronchitis	Give oxygen: observe for 24-48 hours; give steroids (controversial)
	Ozone	Inert gas arc welding, industry		
	Phosgone	Burning of chlorinated organic material		
Allergenic	Toluene diisocyanate	Manufacture of polyurethanes	Reactive bronchoconstriction; possible long-term effects (chronic obstructive pulmonary disease) in susceptible persons	Use bronchodilators
Metal fumes	Zinc Copper Tin Teflon	Welding (especially galvanized metal welding)	"Metal fumes fever"; chills, fever, myalgias, headache, nonproductive cough, leukocytosis 4-8 hr after exposure	Self-limited (12-24 hr)
	Arsine	Burning arsenic-containing ores, electronics industry	Highly toxic effect; hemolysis, pulmonary edema, renal failure; chronic arsenic toxicity	Exchange transfusion use dimercaprol (BAL) for chronic arsenic toxicity only
	Mercury Lead	Industry, welding	See specific metals	

From Ho MT: *Current emergency diagnosis and treatment,* ed 3, Norwalk, Conn, 1990, Appleton & Lange.

- *Smoking habits*—Cigarette smokers have a lower resistance to toxic gas inhalation. This may be a result of a decrease in the lungs' ability to clear waste products.

In addition to these factors, underlying lung disease, such as cardiopulmonary obstructive disease (COPD) (Chapter 22), will play a role in how severely the patient is affected by gas inhalation.

Clinical Presentation

Anoxia-causing gases typically result in sudden death without significant warning symptoms. Sometimes a headache will precede sudden loss of consciousness. Gases that cause metabolic problems, such as cyanide, typically act in one of two fashions. In large doses (e.g., a gas chamber during a prison execution), sudden death results. Even immediate medical treatment would have no effect. In cases where the EMT–I may have a chance to provide care, the effects come on over several minutes to hours.

Irritant gases have three distinct periods of effects: immediate, delayed, and chronic. The immediate reaction occurs within 1 to 2 hours following inhalation. It consists of an irritant reaction resulting in laryngotracheobronchitis and bronchospasm. Persons who inhale carbon monoxide may suffer acute myocardial infarction (MI) or pulmonary embolus. The delayed reaction occurs 6 to 24 hours later. It consists of laryngeal edema, hoarseness, inspiratory stridor, and noncardiogenic pulmonary edema. Although complete recovery is usually the rule, chronic problems such as recurrent pneumonia and other severe lung disease can occur (Box 26-5).

Management

The most important rule in treating toxic inhalations is to protect yourself. Remove the victim from the area, if possible, before providing emergency care. Use appropriately trained and equipped hazardous materials teams as necessary, especially to help in patient and rescuer decontamination. Provide the following care:

- High-concentration oxygen; intubate if necessary
- Placement of an IV line
- Nebulized bronchodilators according to medical control
- Prompt transport to the nearest appropriate medical facility

CARBON MONOXIDE POISONING

Carbon monoxide is a colorless, odorless, flavorless, and nonirritating gas that is a common source of poisoning. Carbon monoxide is a product of incomplete combustion of carbon-containing substances. Poisoning by carbon monoxide is the major cause of industrial deaths and deaths caused by fire. Sources of carbon monoxide gas around the home include barbecues, automobiles, and improperly ventilated heating systems. Gas heaters are among the most common source of domestic carbon monoxide exposure.

Pathophysiology

Carbon monoxide binds strongly with hemoglobin in red blood cells, producing a compound called **carboxyhemoglobin**. The strength of hemoglobin's bond with carbon dioxide is greater than that with oxygen. As a result, the hemoglobin molecule is unable to carry oxygen. Perfusion may be severely impaired. Carboxyhemoglobin also directly affects the cellular energy transport system, leading to cell death (Figure 26-4).

Assessment Findings

Suspect carbon monoxide poisoning in any patient exposed to fire or smoke, or found in a closed space, particularly if several people in the same location have the same poisoning symptoms. The signs and symptoms of carbon monoxide poisoning include the following (Box 26-6):

- Malaise, weakness, headache
- Confusion, dizziness
- Nausea, shortness of breath
- Drowsiness
- Unconsciousness that may occur without warning
- Chest pain (Persons with carbon monoxide poisoning may develop an acute myocardial infarction or pulmonary embolism.)

BOX 26-5

CLINICAL PRESENTATION OF IRRITANT GAS EXPOSURE

IMMEDIATE (WITHIN 1 TO 2 HOURS)
Irritant reactions (laryngotracheobronchitis)
Red, inflamed mucous membranes
Eye and nasal irritation
Bronchorrhea, cough
Sore throat
Bronchospastic reaction (dyspnea, chest tightness, wheezing)

DELAYED (6 TO 24 HOURS)
Laryngeal edema
Hoarseness
Inspiratory stridor
Lump in throat
Noncardiogenic pulmonary edema

CHRONIC: COMPLETE RECOVERY USUALLY THE RULE
Late problems
Bronchiectasis
Bronchiolitis obliterans (prevent with steroids)
Interstitial fibrosis

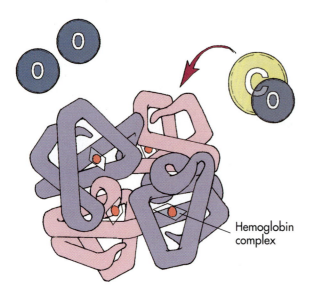

Hemoglobin
complex

FIGURE 26-4 ▲ Carbon monoxide has a stronger attraction to hemoglobin than does oxygen. When carbon monoxide enters the body, it binds with hemoglobin, causing a decrease in the delivery of oxygen to tissue.

- Cherry red skin and mucous membranes (This is a late sign and is actually rarely seen. The absence of cherry red skin does not rule out carbon monoxide poisoning.)
- Abnormal lung sounds (rales, rhonchi)
- Seizures
- Blisters on the skin

HELPFUL HINT

Pulse oximetry readings may be inaccurate in cases of carbon monoxide poisoning. Oxygen saturation (SaO_2) readings may be falsely high.

HELPFUL HINT

Since carbon monoxide is odorless, colorless, and flavorless, protect yourself before entering a potentially hazardous environment.

Management

The most important rule in treating toxic inhalations is to protect yourself. Remove the victim from the area, if possible, before providing emergency care. Use appropriately trained and equipped hazardous materials teams as necessary, especially to help in patient and rescuer decontamination. Provide the following care:

- Immediately remove the patient to fresh air.
- Secure the airway; ventilate as necessary.
- Give high-concentration oxygen; intubate if necessary.
- Place an IV line.

BOX 26-6

DIAGNOSIS OF CARBON MONOXIDE POISONING

SYMPTOMS
Malaise, weakness, headache
Confusion, dizziness
Nausea, shortness of breath
Unconscious (can occur without premonitory symptoms)
Symptoms of myocardial infarction, pulmonary embolism

PHYSICAL
Cherry red skin, mucous membrane (rare)
Rales, rhonchi (if pulmonary edema present)
Retinal hemorrhages
Seizures
Bullae, blisters

LABORATORY
ECG (ischemic ST-T changes, infarction, atrial dysrhythmias)
Carboxyhemoglobin level (Normal does not exclude diagnosis!)
Arterial blood gases (difference in measured vital signs; calculated percent saturation, PO_2 usually normal)
Complete blood count, "lytes," cardiac enzymes

- Care for life-threatening injuries.
- Make the patient comfortable, and transport to the hospital when possible.
- If the patient is unconscious, combative, or hallucinating, consider transporting the patient to a specialty center with a hyperbaric chamber. Follow local protocols.

HELPFUL HINT

Hyperbaric oxygen is sometimes used to treat severe carbon monoxide poisoning. Extremely high concentrations of oxygen can be given in a pressurized vault—the hyperbaric chamber. At a pressure equal to 3 atmospheres (atm), enough oxygen can be carried in the bloodstream to maintain perfusion without the need for hemoglobin. At these high pressures the oxygen displaces carbon monoxide on the hemoglobin molecule, allowing the poisonous gas to be eliminated through the lungs.

TRICYCLIC ANTIDEPRESSANTS
Common Causative Agents

The **tricyclic antidepressants (TCAs)** are commonly prescribed for many medical conditions, including depression. Other uses include bed-wetting, panic disorder, migraine headache, Tourette's syndrome, and attention deficit hyperactivity disorder. Common agents include amitriptyline (Elavil), amoxapine (Asendin), clomipramine (Anafranil), doxepin (Sinequan, Adepin), imipramine (Tofranil), and nortriptyline (Aventyl, Pamelor).

Pharmacology and Pharmacokinetics

TCAs block the reuptake of norepinephrine and serotonin in the brain. They also have diverse effects on the autonomic nervous system and cardiac conduction system. Although specific effects vary somewhat from agent to agent, most have some anticholinergic and cardiac membrane actions. Dry mouth and heat intolerance are common side effects. Persons taking these drugs are more likely to present with heat-related injuries, such as heat exhaustion or heat stroke (see Chapter 29). Minor prolongation of the QT interval is common; if significant, the patient may develop ventricular tachydysrhythmias (e.g., torsade de pointes, an atypical ventricular tachycardia). At toxic levels, TCAs also cause widening of the QRS complex.

TCAs are particularly dangerous in a deliberate overdose situation because their therapeutic-toxicity ratio is low—the number of pills in a typical 1-month prescription is more than enough to be fatal. In addition, the onset of toxicity may be rapid—the patient may be coherent at one moment and unconscious or seizing (without warning) the next.

Assessment Findings

Findings vary, depending on the drug taken, the dose, and the time since ingestion. Many suicide attempts also involve other agents, especially alcohol. Early findings of toxicity are as follows:
- Dry mouth
- Confusion
- Hallucinations

These findings are primarily due to the anticholinergic effects of the tricyclics. More serious findings may develop rapidly:
- Delirium
- Respiratory depression
- Hypotension
- Hyperthermia
- Seizures
- Coma

Management

Always ensure your own safety first before attempting to provide patient care. As usual, maintenance of airway, breathing, and circulation is cardinal. Remember that patients with tricyclic overdose may deteriorate

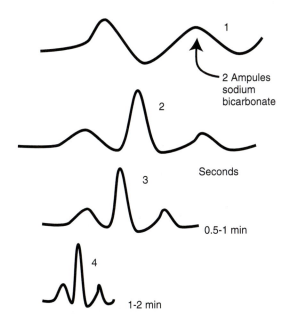

FIGURE 26-5 ▲ Narrowing of the QRS complex in tricarboxylic acid poisoning after sodium bicarbonate administration.

rapidly. According to local protocols, administer oxygen and start an IV line.

Depending on local protocols, certain pharmacological interventions may be warranted:
- **Sodium bicarbonate**—One to two ampules given intravenously, followed by one ampule dissolved in a liter of normal saline drip is commonplace. Bicarbonate directly affects the binding of TCAs to protein, immediately reducing cardiac membrane toxicity. Narrowing of the QRS complex usually appears on the cardiac monitor within seconds (Figure 26-5).
- **Activated charcoal**—Although it is helpful in reducing toxicity, the fact that persons with TCA ingestion may suddenly become unconscious or seize contraindicates the use of oral charcoal in many patients. If permitted by local protocols, instillation of activated charcoal via nasogastric tube may be beneficial.
- **Diazepam**—If permitted by local protocols, IV diazepam is beneficial if seizures develop, although sodium bicarbonate may have similar effects and is safer.

Provide psychological support and transport the patient by the most appropriate mode to the most appropriate health care facility. If patients initially refuse transportation and an intentional overdose is suspected, consult local protocols. Often, "tincture of time" provides the solution when the patient who has initially refused care suddenly seizes or loses consciousness. At this point, consider providing care under the "emergency care" implied consent provisions discussed in Chapter 3. Always follow local protocols and legal advisor recommendations.

BITES AND STINGS

Common Causative Agents

Many bites or stings are painful. Some are potentially dangerous. Treatment of allergic reactions to bites or stings is discussed in Chapter 25. Common offending organisms include hymenoptera (e.g., bees, wasps), spiders, other arthropods (ants, scorpions), snakes, and marine animals (Figures 26-6 to 26-11).

Assessment Findings

Findings depend on the organism involved. Allergic reactions may develop from any bite or sting. Large ma- rine animal bites may cause significant bleeding, infec- tion, and shock (Boxes 26-7 and 26-8).

Management

Always ensure your own safety before attempting to provide patient care. Use appropriately trained and equipped teams as necessary, especially to help in pa- tient rescue. As usual, maintenance of airway, breathing, and circulation is cardinal. Generally, unless anaphylaxis is present, no certain pharmacological interventions are warranted.

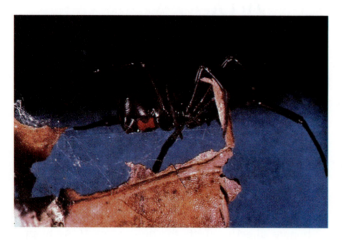

FIGURE 26-6 ▲ Black widow spider. (Courtesy Saint Louis Zoo, St Louis.)

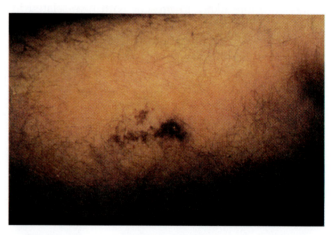

FIGURE 26-8 ▲ Brown recluse spider bite at approx- imately 6 hours, with a central hemorrhagic vesicle and gravitational pattern spread of venom. (Courtesy Paul Auerbach and Riley Rees.)

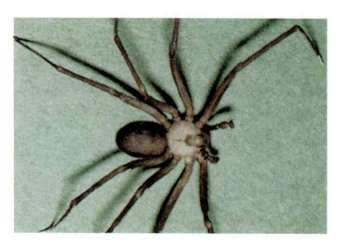

FIGURE 26-7 ▲ Brown recluse spider. (Courtesy Indiana University Medical Center.)

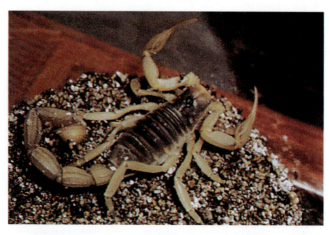

FIGURE 26-9 ▲ Giant hairy scorpion commonly found in the deserts of the American Southwest. (Courtesy R David Gaban.)

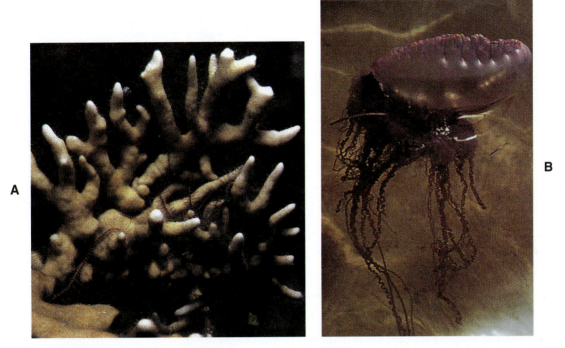

FIGURE 26-10 ▲ Coelenterates. **A**, Fire coral. **B**, Atlantic Portuguese Man-of-war. (**A**, Photo by Paul Auerbach; **B**, Photo by Norbert Wu.)

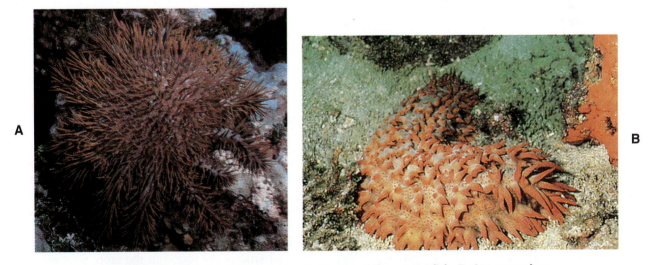

FIGURE 26-11 ▲ Echinoderms. **A**, Crown-of-thorns starfish. **B**, Sea cucumber with extended tentacles. (Photos by Paul Auerbach.)

BOX 26-7

TYPES OF REACTIONS TO VENOMS

LOCAL REACTION
- Marked and prolonged edema at the sting site
- Possible involvement of one or more neighboring joints
- Possible occurrence in the mouth or throat, producing airway obstruction
- Severe local reactions that may increase the likelihood of future systemic reactions (controversial)
- Symptoms that usually subside within 24 hours

TOXIC REACTION*
- Gastrointestinal disturbances:
  Vomiting
  Diarrhea
  Lightheadedness
- Other symptoms:
  Syncope (common finding)
  Headache
  Fever
  Involuntary muscle spasms
  Edema without urticaria
  Convulsions (rare)
- Symptoms that usually subside within 48 hours

SYSTEMIC (ANAPHYLACTIC) REACTION†
- Reactions that can progress to death within minutes

- Immediate symptoms:
  Itching eyes or generalized itching
  Facial flushing
  Generalized urticaria
- Subsequent symptoms:
  Respiratory failure, cardiovascular collapse, or both
  Hypotension
  Chest or throat constriction or both
  Wheezing
  Dyspnea
  Cyanosis
  Nausea and vomiting
  Chills and fever
  Laryngeal stridor
  Shock
  Loss of consciousness
  Loss of bowel or bladder control
  Bloody and frothy sputum production

DELAYED REACTION‡
- Serum sickness symptoms:
  Fever
  Malaise
  Headache
  Urticaria
  Polyarthritis

From Sanders MJ: *Mosby's paramedic textbook,* ed 2, St Louis, 2000, Mosby.
*Should be considered with a history of 10 or more stings.
†May occur in response to single or multiple stings.
‡Usually occurs 10 to 14 days after a sting.

BOX 26-8

SIGNS AND SYMPTOMS OF SCORPION ENVENOMATION

- Hyperesthesia at the site of the bite
- Pain, tingling, and a burning sensation radiating along the nerves at the location of the bite
- SLUDGE: salivation, lacrimation, urination, defecation, gastrointestinal distress, and emesis
- Initial bradycardia followed by tachycardia
- Cardiac dysrhythmias
- Muscle twitching
- Convulsions
- Roving eye movements (cranial nerve dysfunction)
- Temporary blindness

From Sanders MJ: *Mosby's paramedic textbook,* ed 2, St Louis, 2000, Mosby.

SNAKEBITES

Common Snakes in the United States

There are more than 7000 venomous snakebites annually in the United States. Most of these are from rattlesnakes. The severity varies widely from puncture wounds to death. Despite many species of snakes in the United States, only two families are of great concern: coral snakes (elapids) and vipers.

Coral snakes are found in the more Southern states from Arizona to Florida. They are brightly colored with alternating black, white (or yellow), and red bands that encircle the entire body. Their nasal area is totally black. These features distinguish them from several nonpoisonous snakes with similar markings. The old adage may be helpful: "Red on yellow will kill a fellow; red on black, venom lack." They may be up to 3 feet in length (Figure 26-12).

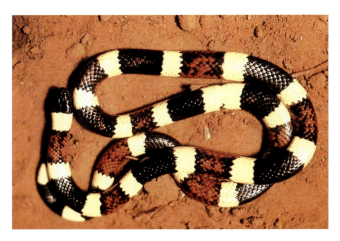

FIGURE 26-12 ▲ Coral snake. (Courtesy Saint Louis Zoo, St Louis.)

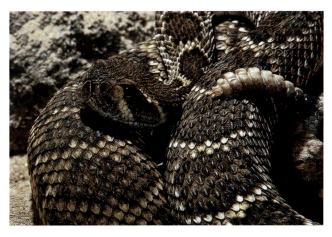

FIGURE 26-13 ▲ Pit viper. (Courtesy Saint Louis Zoo, St Louis.)

Vipers include the cottonmouth, copperhead, massasauga, pigmy rattlesnake, and the "true" rattlesnakes (Figure 26-13). Most are widely distributed across the United States, with the cottonmouth being limited to the southeastern states and Texas. These reptiles characteristically have a triangular head, vertically slit pupils, heavy bodies, and movable folding upper fangs. The famed rattle is lacking on copperheads and cottonmouths. The skins of these animals may be very attractive. In fact, 30% to 40% of rattlesnake bite victims each year are engaged in collecting or marketing the snakes when they are bitten. Although uncommon, there are reported cases of persons being "bitten" by removed snake heads preserved for several weeks (Figure 26-13).

Snake Venoms

Snake venoms have several physiological properties: **neurotoxicity** (paresthesias, paralysis, neuromuscular transmission disturbances), **hemotoxicity** (coagulant, anticoagulant, hemolytic, platelet problems), and **cardiotoxicity** (decreased cardiac output and blood pressure). In addition, enzymes in the venom lead to tissue destruction. Most venoms are a complex mixture of proteins with mixed effects.

Coral Snakebite

ASSESSMENT FINDINGS

Fang marks from the coral snake may be difficult to find, and initially there may be no pain around the wound. The venom is primarily neurotoxic. Although these bites are rarely fatal, the following may be observed:

- Euphoria, drowsiness, nausea, vomiting
- Increased salivation, mostly from a decreased ability to swallow
- Paresthesias, headache

- Ptosis (droopy eyelid), blurred vision
- Shortness of breath, abnormal reflexes
- Generalized paralysis

MANAGEMENT

As for treatment, incision, suction, and ice are ill-advised. Unless the animal is a Sonoran coral snake, for which no antivenin, exists, early administration of antivenin is recommended. It should be repeated later if symptoms of envenomation actually occur. This should all be done in consultation with the regional PCC.

Pit Viper Bites

ASSESSMENT FINDINGS

Clinically, diagnosing pit viper bites is somewhat easier because there will usually be a visible puncture wound, often oozing blood. Despite this, 20% of patients with a true fang mark will show no evidence of envenomation. This may relate to the size of the snake or the interval between attacks; if the snake has just struck, the "poison sacs" may have not adequately "recharged" for a bite to envenomate.

Signs and symptoms of **envenomation** may include any or all of the following (Box 26-9):

- Rapidly occurring pain and numbness locally near the bite (If a limb was bitten, the pain and numbness may travel proximally.)
- Early edema traveling up the extremity (Despite what is often massive swelling, arterial compromise is rare. The fluid that pours into the tissues with this edema may account for some hypotension a patient may have.)
- Local ecchymoses initially, which then spreads and leads to a bluish hue around the bite area
- Local blebs filled with hemorrhagic transudate

SIGNS AND SYMPTOMS OF PIT VIPER ENVENOMATION

MILD ENVENOMATION
Presence of one or more fang marks
Local swelling and pain
Lack of systemic symptoms

MODERATE ENVENOMATION
Presence of one or more fang marks
Pain and edema beyond the site
Systemic signs and symptoms:
   Weakness
   Diaphoresis
   Nausea and vomiting
   Paresthesias

SEVERE ENVENOMATION
Presence of one or more fang marks
Massive edema
Subcutaneous ecchymosis
Severe systemic symptoms
Shock

From Sanders MJ: *Mosby's paramedic textbook,* ed 2, St Louis, 2000, Mosby.

- Signs of lymphangitis/lymphadenitis (red streaking up and down the extremity, swollen/tender lymph nodes)
- Paresthesias, muscle fasciculations, generalized weakness
- Unresponsive hypotension, petechiae, conjunctival hemorrhage, and bleeding (This constellation of findings suggests widespread coagulopathy.)

In addition, an abnormal electrocardiogram (ECG) (nonspecific finding) is present in 26% of patients.

The severity of envenomation is a continuum. Anywhere from 10% to 25% of patients bitten are *not* envenomated. Severity is classified as follows:

- *Minimal*—Local manifestations, no systemic signs, no laboratory abnormalities.
- *Moderate*—Manifestations beyond the immediate bite area, significant systemic signs/symptoms, decreased fibrinogen and platelets, signs of hemoconcentration (elevated hematocrit and sodium levels).
- *Severe*—Manifestations throughout the extremity or body part, serious systemic signs and symptoms (e.g., hypotension), marked and widespread laboratory abnormalities.

MANAGEMENT

The general treatment of viper bites is as follows:
- Provide basic life support as needed.
- Administer high-concentration oxygen.
- Give IV normal saline, according to local protocols.
- Minimize the patient's activity (if possible).
- Remove jewelry or tight-fitting clothes.
- Observe and mark with a pen any border of advancing edema (at least every 15 minutes).
- Immobilize the affected part.
- Monitor pulses and sensation distal to the envenomation site.
- Provide local wound care as you would for any other contaminated wound.
- Follow your local protocols.

Antivenin treatment of viper bites has its greatest effect if given within 4 hours. It should be reserved for life-threatening envenomations, since the risk of serious hypersensitivity reactions, including anaphylaxis to the horse serum used, is high. This is *not* recommended for field use.

"Pearls" to Remember Regarding Snakebites

Keep the following in mind when caring for victims of poisonous snakebites:
- Do not chill or apply ice to the wound—severe tissue damage can occur.
- Do not apply a tourniquet; if others have applied one before your arrival, place a less constricting band more proximal, and with an IV line in place, slowly remove the original tourniquet.
- Do not use steroids or antihistamines except in a severe hypersensitivity reaction.
- Early work suggesting the potential benefit of electrical current therapy for snakebites has not proved to be useful.

CASE HISTORY FOLLOW-UP ■ ■ ■

EMT–I Morant pulls out the bag-valve-mask device and begins ventilating the patient. The EMT–I student attaches an oxygen line to the bag-valve-mask and sets the flow rate to 15 L/min. EMT–I Morant then turns the task of ventilating the patient over to the EMT–I student. "Here, take over while I get some naloxone out of the drug box."

EMT–I Stokes attaches a 1000 mL bag of normal saline to a macrodrip administration set and clears the line of air. "Do you think we should intubate her?" EMT–I Stokes asks as he applies the tourniquet to the patient's arm. EMT–I Morant responds, "I think we should wait and see if she responds to the naloxone. I don't want her fighting the tube if we put it in and she wakes up."

The IV line is placed with ease, and EMT–I Morant begins to slowly deliver 2 mg of naloxone. After about half the naloxone has been delivered, the patient starts to wake up, moving her arms and legs. "I'm going to hold off delivering the rest of this until we see she needs it," remarks EMT–I Morant. "I don't want her fighting us all the way to the hospital."

EMT–I Stokes reassesses the patient's vital signs to find she is breathing on her own at a rate of 12 breaths per minute; she has a pulse rate of 100 beats per minute, and her blood pressure is now 126/80. They continue delivering oxygen and transport her to the hospital, where she undergoes further treatment.

SUMMARY

Important points to remember from this chapter include the following:

- Poisoning is the ingestion, inhalation, absorption, or injection of any harmful substance (generically summarized here as "exposure").
- Nearly one half of poisonings involve prescription drugs.
- Many poisonings are unintentional but preventable.
- Practically speaking, poisoning connotes exposure to a substance that is generally only harmful and has no usual beneficial effects (e.g., cyanide). Overdose suggests excessive exposure to a substance that has normal treatment uses (e.g., aspirin). In excess, harm results.
- There are three generic classes of toxicological emergencies: unintentional poisoning, drug and alcohol abuse, and intentional poisoning or overdose.

- There is virtually no toxin that discriminates between the patient and EMS providers. The EMT–I should immediately assess the need for personal protective equipment and should not enter the scene until doing so is safe.
- As in any toxic exposure, enlisting the assistance of special hazardous materials teams to extricate may be necessary to remove and detoxify the patient before providing care.
- Although protocols differ, many EMS systems require or encourage EMT–Is to contact the Poison Control Center (PCC), either directly or via medical control. Experts agree that the PCC is the most reliable and up-to-date source of information on the assessment and treatment of toxicological emergencies.
- There are four routes by which poisons or toxins are introduced into the body: ingestion, inhalation, absorption, and injection.
- Possible exposures may vary from one geographical area to another.
- Often, groups of agents with similar clinical presentations are grouped together as "toxidromes." Common toxidromes are cholinergic agents, anticholinergic agents, narcotics/opiates, toxic gas inhalation, tricyclic antidepressant overdose, and bites/stings (including snakebites).
- A careful history is helpful in determining the clinical approach. Assessment findings vary widely, depending on the agent involved. Indications of poisoning may be apparent during the focused examination:
  - *Respiratory system*—Many poisonings cause respiratory depression and partial airway obstruction. Inhaled toxins may cause respiratory distress and wheezing.
  - *Cardiovascular system*—Some poisonings can cause irregular heart rhythm, chest pain, shock, and cardiac arrest.
  - *Neurological system*—Poisonings may result in changes in the pupil size. Narcotics usually cause constricted pupils, whereas stimulants result in pupillary dilation.
- Control of airway, breathing, and circulation is the first concern in poisoning management.
- Depending on the agent, specific antidotes may be available, such as atropine and 2-PAM chloride for cholinergic agent poisoning or overdose.
- Local protocols should be followed regarding naloxone, activated charcoal, ipecac, atropine, sodium bicarbonate, diazepam, and any other pharmacological agents.

27

Neurological Emergencies

> ...**CASE HISTORY**
>
> EMT–Is Stevens and Perez have been dispatched to a "man down" at a nearby park. En route, the EMT–Is are advised that a passerby witnessed a possible heart attack and called 9-1-1 via her cell phone. An emergency medical dispatcher is on-line with the caller and is instructing her on how to position the patient, open his airway, and assess his breathing and circulation. The EMT–Is advise medical direction of the call and their 4-minute estimated time of arrival to the scene.
>
> On arrival, the EMT–Is find a large group of onlookers being contained by park security personnel. One of the security officers, a trained first responder, is kneeling next to the patient and maintaining his open airway. He advises the EMT–Is that the patient is unresponsive and has shallow respirations and a rapid pulse. Another officer tells the EMT–Is that the man is a "regular" at the park. The patient is presumably homeless and often has to be removed from the park by law enforcement personnel.
>
> The middle-aged patient is pale and extremely diaphoretic. Per protocol, EMT–I Perez administers high-concentration oxygen and assists the patient's respirations while EMT–I Stevens begins the initial assessment. The physical examination is unremarkable, and the patient's vital signs are stable. The patient's ECG reveals a borderline sinus tachycardia. EMT–I Stevens makes radio contact with on-line medical direction and gives the hospital an initial patient report. Based on his general impression of the patient, EMT–I Perez requests an order for naloxone (Narcan) to rule out or reverse a possible narcotic depression.
>
> The emergency department physician denies EMT–I Perez's request. Based on information provided in the radio report and the lack of available patient history, the physician instructs EMT–I Stevens to measure the patient's blood sugar to rule out hypoglycemia. Using a glucometer, the patient's serum glucose is measured dangerously low at 58 mg/dL. An IV is initiated, and 1 amp of 50% dextrose is administered. Immediately, the patient's respiratory status improves, and he begins to respond appropriately to verbal stimuli. The patient is packaged and made ready for transport to the emergency department.
>
> The EMT–Is deliver the patient to the hospital and give a brief report to the emergency department nurse who will be assuming his care. The EMT–Is complete the necessary paperwork and replenish their supplies. Before leaving the hospital to return to service, the emergency department physician advises the EMT-Is that this call should be reviewed during a critique session as part of continuing education.

LEARNING OBJECTIVES

CHAPTER GOAL

Upon completion of this chapter, the EMT–Intermediate will be able to use assessment findings to formulate a field impression and implement a treatment plan for the patient with a neurological emergency.

Cognitive Objectives

As an EMT–Intermediate you should be able to do the following:

- Discuss the general pathophysiology of nontraumatic neurological emergencies.
- Discuss the general assessment findings associated with nontraumatic neurological emergencies.
- Identify the need for rapid intervention and transport of the patient with nontraumatic emergencies.
- Discuss the management of nontraumatic neurological emergencies.
- Discuss the pathophysiology of coma and altered mental status.
- Discuss the assessment findings associated with coma and altered mental status.
- Discuss the management of coma and altered mental status.
- Discuss the pathophysiology of seizures.
- Discuss the assessment findings associated with seizures.
- Describe and differentiate the major types of seizures.
- List the most common causes of seizures.
- Discuss the pathophysiology of syncope/weakness.
- Discuss the assessment findings associated with syncope/weakness.
- Discuss the management of syncope/weakness.
- Discuss the pathophysiology of headache.
- Discuss the assessment findings associated with headache.
- Discuss the management of headache.
- Discuss the pathophysiology of stroke.
- Describe the causes of stroke.
- Discuss the assessment findings associated with stroke.
- Discuss the management of stroke.
- Define the term *stroke*.
- Recognize the signs and symptoms related to stroke.
- Discuss the pathophysiology of a transient ischemic attack (TIA).
- Discuss the assessment findings associated with a TIA.
- Discuss the management of a TIA.
- Define the term *transient ischemic attack*.
- Recognize the signs and symptoms related to a transient ischemic attack.
- Differentiate among neurological emergencies on the basis of assessment findings.
- Correlate abnormal assessment findings with the clinical significance in the patient with neurological complaints.
- Develop a patient management plan based on field impression in the patient with neurological emergencies.

Key Terms
—cont'd

Hemorrhagic Stroke

Idiopathic Seizure

Ischemic Penumbra

Lorazepam

Meningitis

Migraine Headache

Motor Control

Multiple Sclerosis (MS)

Naloxone

Neuroprotective Agents

Parkinson's Disease

Petit Mal Seizures

Photophobia

Postictal State

Seizure

Sensation

Simple Partial Seizures

Status Epilepticus

Stroke

Syncope

Systemic Lupus Erythematosus (SLE, Lupus)

Thrombolytic Stroke

Tonic-Clonic Seizure Movements

Transient Ischemic Attacks (TIAs)

Vasculitis

Vertigo

VINDICATE

Affective Objectives
As an EMT–Intermediate you should be able to do the following:
- Characterize the feelings of a patient who regains consciousness among strangers.
- Develop ways to convey empathy to patients with limited ability to communicate.

Psychomotor Objectives
As an EMT–Intermediate you should be able to do the following:
- Perform an appropriate assessment of a patient with a nontraumatic neurological emergency.

GENERAL NERVOUS SYSTEM PATHOPHYSIOLOGY, ASSESSMENT, AND MANAGEMENT

Anatomy and Physiology Review

Most serious neurological problems involve the central nervous system (CNS)—brain and spinal cord. These alterations affect one or more of the main CNS functions:

- **Cognitive systems**—These systems, which maintain alertness, awareness, and a normal wakeful state ("consciousness"), are controlled by several areas of the brain, including the cerebral cortex and the *reticular activating system (RAS).*
- **Cerebral homeostasis**—Homeostasis in the body means balance. A major goal of cerebral homeostasis is to maintain brain perfusion and oxygenation despite fluctuations in the mean arterial blood pressure. The brain does this via the process of **cerebral autoregulation.** Within a wide range of mean arterial blood pressures, cerebral blood flow remains constant. This is due to opening and closing of prearteriolar and postarteriolar sphincters, much as a farmer would open or close irrigation gates in a field to keep the crops appropriately watered. Thus cerebral blood flow remains the same even if the arterial pressure varies considerably.
- **Motor control**—Alterations in the motor control systems result in a variety of conditions ranging from localized random movements (tics) to generalized seizures, and from weakness to generalized paralysis.
- **Sensation**—Alterations in sensory systems (e.g., loss of feeling in an area) commonly accompany other abnormalities, such as weakness or paralysis.

Types of Central Nervous System Disorders

Many conditions can lead to CNS disorders. One helpful mnemonic to remember disease categories, in general, is **VINDICATE,** which is explained in Figure 27-1.

This mnemonic can be applied to CNS disorders as follows:

- *Vascular*—Cerebrovascular diseases involve the circulation to the brain and spinal cord. The most common is stroke—an abrupt decrease in blood flow to a part of the CNS due to disruption in the circulatory supply. Migraine headache results from an abnormality of the cerebrovascular circulation.
- *Infectious*—Infections of the CNS and surrounding meninges may be life threatening. Many, such as bacterial meningitis, are also *highly contagious.* EMT–Is must always protect themselves first before caring for any patient. CNS infections may present with a wide range of symptoms, including altered mental status, headache, and neurological changes. The following are the most common:
  - **Meningitis**—Inflammation of the membranes surrounding the brain (the meninges) and the cerebrospinal fluid (CSF). Brain tissue is not directly involved. The more severe form is caused by bacteria (bacterial meningitis). Viral meningitis is more common and usually milder. Patients present with headache, fever, malaise, and stiff neck. Neurological abnormalities are not common.
  - **Encephalitis**—Infection of the brain tissue itself. Encephalitis can be caused by any biological organism, although viruses are the most common. Recently an increased incidence of human immunodeficiency virus (HIV) infection has resulted in atypical forms of encephalitis (e.g., herpes

▶ Loss of cerebral autoregulation occurs in many neurological conditions (e.g., stroke, seizure, head trauma, CNS infection). The result is that the only remaining way for the body to keep the brain perfused adequately is to elevate the blood pressure. Thus the normal body response to many neurological problems (due to loss of cerebral autoregulation) is *normal responsive hypertension.* This is common in the first 24 to 48 hours and generally is not of specific concern unless the patient has intracerebral bleeding or is worsening because of increasing blood pressure.

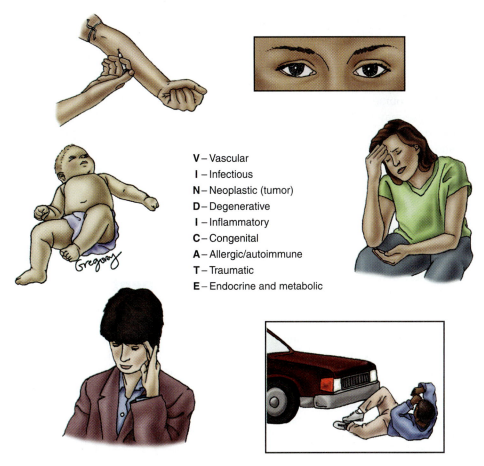

V – Vascular
I – Infectious
N – Neoplastic (tumor)
D – Degenerative
I – Inflammatory
C – Congenital
A – Allergic/autoimmune
T – Traumatic
E – Endocrine and metabolic

FIGURE 27-1 ▲ **VINDICATE is helpful for remembering the cause of many diseases.**

viruses, tuberculosis, HIV encephalitis). Patients complain of severe headache, nausea, vomiting, weakness, and malaise. They may have alterations in their level of consciousness. Neurological abnormalities, especially of the cranial nerves (e.g., pupillary responses) are far more common than in meningitis.

- **Brain abscess**—A localized collection of pus and debris within the brain. Brain abscess may occur from primary brain infection but is more commonly a result of organisms spread from other locations. Probably the most common source of infection seen in emergency care is **bacterial endocarditis**—infection of the lining of one or more heart valves. This disease is a life-threatening complication of intravenous (IV) drug abuse. As a result, small clumps of bacteria break off from the valve leaflet and flow to the brain, lungs, liver, and kidneys. Once they reach the smaller vessels, they multiply and initiate localized infection. Patients may present with new-onset neurological abnormalities. Often, seizures are the first symptom.

- *Neoplastic*—Many common tumors metastasize to the brain (e.g., from the lung, breast, prostate, colon). Primary tumors of the brain itself are responsible for

one out of five new-onset seizures in persons over 21 years of age. New-onset neurological defects in any person with a history of cancer are due to metastasis to the brain or spinal cord until proven otherwise.

> ▶ A devastating neurological presentation of breast cancer is spinal cord compression, with complete paralysis below the involved level. Often this occurs in a patient who has survived her initial disease and is doing well. Symptoms progress rapidly, with localized severe back pain, followed by progressive weakness, then paralysis. Sensory function is not affected as severely.

- *Degenerative*—This category encompasses many conditions. The common denominator is progressive deterioration of a portion or portions of the CNS. Some more common conditions are as follows:

- **Alzheimer's disease**—Progressive and premature deterioration in cognitive function and also motor control. Patients often have confusion, memory failure, disorientation, restlessness, speech disturbances, and hallucinations. The disease usually begins in later middle life and occurs with equal frequency in men and women. The cause is still unknown.

- **Multiple sclerosis (MS)**—Disease resulting from spotty destruction of the myelin coat of CNS tissue. MS typically comes on in the teenage years and follows a highly variable course. Patients with previously unknown disease may present to the EMT–I with new-onset seizures or weakness, or because of trauma from a sudden loss of motor coordination.
- **Parkinson's disease**—Progressive degenerative brain condition resulting in a tremor, progressive loss of motor control, and speech difficulty. Patients may present to the EMT–I because of the disease itself or with complications to an anti-Parkinsonian drug.
- *Inflammatory*—Although infection is a common cause of inflammation anywhere in the body, many inflammatory conditions may affect the CNS without infection. The following are common inflammatory conditions that may affect the CNS:
  - **Rheumatoid arthritis (RA)**—Typically thought of as a joint problem, RA has systemic effects in some persons. Any organ system may be affected.
  - **Systemic lupus erythematosus (SLE, lupus)**—SLE is a common inflammatory condition that is more common in young women. It occurs as a result of the development of antibodies by the body's own immune system against itself. This is termed an autoimmune disease. The result is a process of recurrent inflammation, pain, and tissue damage. Lupus cerebritis (inflammation of the cerebral lobes) is a common cause of both headache and altered level of consciousness in young women. It may be deadly.
- *Congenital*—Rupture of a congenital (present at birth) aneurysm of a cerebral vessel is the most common cause of spontaneous intracerebral hemorrhage in a young person.
- *Allergic and autoimmune*—Lupus cerebritis, described under Systemic Lupus Erythematosus, is an autoimmune inflammatory condition that may be life threatening. Severe allergic reactions, such as anaphylactic shock, may result in enough cerebral hypoperfusion to cause permanent brain damage, neurological defects, or seizures.
- *Traumatic*—Although common, head trauma is discussed separately in Chapter 19.
- *Endocrine and metabolic*—Virtually any glandular abnormality or abnormal laboratory value (e.g., sodium, potassium, PO_2, PCO_2, pH, blood sugar [glucose]) may result in neurological symptoms ranging from seizures to weakness to coma. In the prehospital setting, hypoxia and hypoglycemia are common and easily cared for.

Assessment Findings

History and physical findings for specific conditions are discussed in the following sections. Box 27-1 and

Table 27-1 summarize the main areas to evaluate in any patient with a neurological emergency:

Management

Part of acute management is ongoing assessment. Pay careful attention to the ABCs (airway, breathing, and circulation). Assess the blood glucose level in any patient with a neurological emergency; treat hypoglycemia according to local protocols. Table 27-2 summarizes general patient management techniques for neurological emergencies:

CEREBRAL ISCHEMIC SYNDROMES: STROKE AND TRANSIENT ISCHEMIC ATTACK

Cerebral ischemic syndromes are the result of disrupted circulation to the brain. These syndromes are differentiated by the causes and duration of disruption. Temporary disturbances are called transient ischemic attacks (TIAs) and do not result in permanent injury. More profound and often permanent damage occurs following stroke, which may be due to either hemorrhage (intracranial bleeding) or occlusion (thrombosis or embolus) (Figure 27-2).

Stroke

A **stroke,** or cerebrovascular accident (CVA), is a condition that results from disruption of circulation to the brain, causing ischemia and damage to brain tissue. Neurological symptoms persist longer than 24 hours. Recovery of function, to varying degrees, takes place over a period of weeks to months.

TYPES OF STROKES

There are two types of strokes: occlusive and hemorrhagic. About three out of four strokes are occlusive, caused by blockage in a blood vessel that is due to either an atherosclerotic plaque (thrombosis—**thrombotic stroke**) or an embolus—**embolic stroke.** The most common source of emboli is the heart. **Hemorrhagic strokes**

TABLE 27-1

Physical Evaluation for Neurological Emergencies

AREA	SPECIFIC COMMENTS
General appearance	The first impression of how sick the patient appears is very important.
Level of consciousness: Mood Thought Perceptions Judgment Memory and attention	Some patients show cognitive dysfunction only when asked to do challenging tasks, such as "Start at 100 and count backward by sevens (100, 93, 86, 79, etc.)."
Speech	Abnormal speech patterns may be chronic; try to learn if there have been any recent changes.
Skin	A splotchy, nonblanching rash (looks like bruising or "purpura") may be present in bacterial meningitis.
Posture and gait	Determine if there have been any recent changes.
Vital signs: Hypertension Hypotension Heart rate Ventilation rate Temperature	Remember, an initial period of hypertension may be "normal" in a patient because of loss of cerebral autoregulation. Pay close attention to the patient's airway—persons with neurological problems tend to hypoventilate even though they may "look good."
Head and neck: Facial expression Eyes—position, alignment Pupils Mouth—breath odors	Do not assume that patients are "just intoxicated" because their breath smells of alcohol. This finding is also common in patients with diabetes. Ketones have a similar odor on the breath. If the pupils are unequal, assume that a serious condition is present until proven otherwise.
Thorax and lungs	Persons with neurological emergencies tend to hypoventilate. Carbon dioxide retention and hypoxia are common. Monitor the patient carefully, administer oxygen, and control the airway as necessary.
Cardiovascular: Heart rate Cardiac rhythm ECG monitoring	Neurological disturbances can cause a variety of cardiac abnormalities, including ECG changes that mimic acute myocardial infarction and dysrhythmias.
Nervous system (motor system): Muscle tone Muscle strength Coordination	Look for *symmetry* while performing the neurological examination. Marked differences between right and left sides of the body are probably abnormal. Of course, being *symmetrically abnormal* is possible as well.

are caused by bleeding into the brain tissue secondary to rupture of a weakened blood vessel. This may be due to a congenital defect (e.g., aneurysm, vascular malformation) or to underlying hypertension (intracerebral bleeding). Whatever the underlying anatomy, the result is ischemic brain tissue (Figure 27-3).

PATHOPHYSIOLOGY AND THROMBOLYTIC THERAPY ("CLOT BUSTERS")

When part of the brain becomes hypoxic, some tissue dies (infarcts). There is usually an area of potentially viable, but ischemic, tissue surrounding the infarct zone. This has been termed the **ischemic penumbra.**

Ischemia leads to the production of toxic substances by the brain and body. Over time, the combination may lead to death of further brain tissue. Studies have shown that restoration of arterial blood flow within 3 hours following occlusion in thrombotic stroke improve a patient's neurological outcome. Unfortunately, few patients qualify for "clot buster" thrombolytic therapy for the following reasons:

- The time frame is very limited; current thrombolytic drugs must be given within a "window" of 30 hours from the onset of symptoms.
- Most cases of thrombotic stroke (the type necessary to receive thrombolysis) occur during sleep; patients wake up in the morning with neurological deficits.

TABLE 27-2

Management of Neurological Emergencies

AREA MANAGEMENT	SPECIFIC COMMENTS

Airway and ventilatory support:
  Oxygen
  Positioning
  Assisted ventilation
  Suction
  Advanced airway devices, if necessary
	Always assume that patients with neurological problems hypoventilate and are hypoxic until proven otherwise.
	Studies have shown that even patients "who look good" may have significant abnormalities on formal blood gas analysis.

Circulatory support:
  Venous access
  Draw blood for analysis at the hospital
	The consensus regarding fluids in neurological emergencies is to use a low flow rate of normal saline or lactated Ringer's solution rather than D_5W. Follow local protocols.
	Prehospital blood specimens are helpful in determining if a patient is a candidate for thrombolytic therapy in stroke.

Pharmacological interventions:
  Dextrose 50%
  Naloxone (Narcan)
  Diazepam (Valium)
	Administer dextrose, according to protocol, for suspected hypoglycemia.
	Some protocols mandate both naloxone and dextrose in unconscious persons (the "coma cocktail") or those with significantly altered mental status.
	In case of refractory seizures, diazepam may be helpful.

Nonpharmacological interventions:
  Positioning
  Spinal precautions
	Always consider the possibility of a spinal injury in a patient with neurological symptoms.
	Spinal immobilization is *not* beneficial in persons with nontraumatic neurological emergencies.

Transport considerations:
  Appropriate mode
  Appropriate facility
	For a suspected acute stroke, follow any special "code stroke" protocols for thrombolytic therapy candidates.

Psychological support and communication	Remember that patients may understand persons talking to them even when they appear unable to respond.

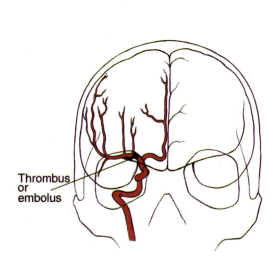

FIGURE 27-2 ▲ Causes/types of strokes. Thrombosis or embolus. A stroke due to thrombosis occurs when, as a result of the loss of the smooth inner surface, clots form at the site of arterial sclerosis. A stroke due to an embolus occurs when a small clot from the heart or central vessel comes loose and travels to a vessel within the brain that is smaller than the clot, where it becomes lodged. (From Henry MC, Stapleton ER: *EMT prehospital care*, ed 2, Philadelphia, 1997, WB Saunders.)

Thrombus or embolus

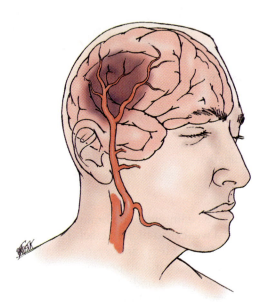

FIGURE 27-3 ▲ A hemorrhagic stroke results from a rupture of a vessel within the brain. The symptoms of the hemorrhagic stroke tend to be more abrupt and more severe than the other types of stroke.

- Health care providers must assume that in patients who wake up with symptoms, the stroke began shortly after they went to sleep. Since most people sleep more than 3 hours, few will qualify for thrombolytic therapy.
- Recent studies have shown that despite widespread public information campaigns by health care professionals, including EMS services, the mean time from the onset of symptoms to emergency department presentation is still 5.7 hours—outside the "window of opportunity."

Despite what initially might be discouraging statistics, the push for early identification and transport of potential stroke victims is not in vain. Even if a person does not qualify for thrombolytic therapy, other therapies aimed at restoring cerebral homeostasis (oxygenation, blood sugar control, fluids) are still beneficial. Specific drugs **(neuroprotective agents)** will likely become available in the future to counteract some deleterious substances produced in stroke. Clearly, "time is brain," just as "time is muscle" in cardiac thrombolysis for myocardial infarction.

RISK FACTORS

Certain characteristics increase a person's chances of developing a stroke. The risk factors for stroke are similar to those for cardiovascular disease:

- Age (increases with age)
- Gender (more common among males)
- Race (more common among African-Americans)
- Hypertension
- Cigarette smoking
- Cardiac dysrhythmias (increases risk of embolus)
- Birth control pills (increases blood clotting)
- Alcohol consumption
- Elevated blood cholesterol levels
- Glue sniffing
- Cocaine use

Some factors—such as age, gender, and race—cannot be modified. For those who have these factors, it is even more important to control those risks that can be modified.

> **HELPFUL HINT**
> - The use of cocaine is becoming the most common cause of stroke in young persons.

PATIENT ASSESSMENT

Patients with a stroke may have gradual or rapid onset of neurological symptoms. Patients may wake up in the morning with a deficit, or the symptoms may appear suddenly while they are already awake (see also Box 27-1).

The most common finding is paralysis. Usually, one complete side of the body is affected (Figure 27-4, *A*). This is called **hemiplegia.** Because nerve fibers cross

sides in the brainstem, damage to one side of the brain affects the opposite side of the body.

Facial droop—sagging muscles beneath the eye and cheek, and asymmetrical movement of the mouth—may be present on one side of the face (Figure 27-4, *B*). The victim may have other neurological deficits, such as impaired language or speech and decreased sensation. The acute onset of slurred speech or hemiplegia is considered to be due to a stroke (occlusive or hemorrhagic) until proven otherwise.

A method of identifying a patient experiencing a stroke is the *Prehospital Stroke Scale.* It was developed in Cincinnati and evaluates three key physical findings: facial droop, arm drift, and speech (Box 27-2). Use of this scale assists in the assessment and provides specific information that can be conveyed to the hospital, alerting them of a patient being transported to their facility who is likely experiencing a stroke.

Other signs and symptoms of stroke include the following:

- Seizures
- Dizziness
- Loss of consciousness
- Stiff neck, headache
- Altered level of consciousness
- Airway problems and hypoventilation
- Cardiac dysrhythmias
- Nausea, vomiting
- Pupillary abnormalities

Most stroke patients have an elevated blood pressure. A systolic blood pressure less than 100 mm Hg is unusual. If the patient is hypotensive, suspect shock and provide care accordingly. Pinpoint pupils in a patient with an altered level of consciousness suggest drug overdose or intracranial bleeding.

> **HELPFUL HINT**
> - If the unconscious patient is hypotensive, consider drugs or shock as possible causes.

> **HELPFUL HINT**
> - Pinpoint pupils are a common finding in certain drug overdoses. Determining the exact cause of pinpoint pupils is less important than supporting the airway, breathing, and circulation.

MANAGEMENT

The care for a patient with stroke includes the following:

- Establish and maintain the airway. Support ventilation as needed.

> **HELPFUL HINT**
> - Airway problems are common in stroke; maintain the patency of the airway and provide oxygen.

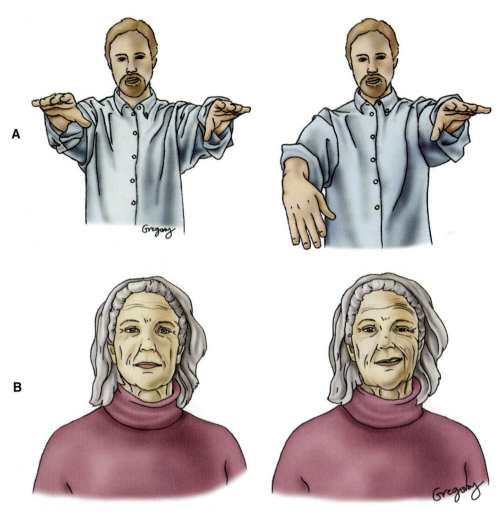

FIGURE 27-4 ▲ **A,** Arm drift. **B,** Right-sided facial droop and change in appearance after the patient is told to "look up and smile and show your teeth."

BOX 27-2

THE CINCINNATI PREHOSPITAL STROKE SCALE

FACIAL DROOP (have patient show teeth or smile):
- Normal—both sides of face move equally well
- Abnormal—one side of face does not move as well as the other side

ARM DRIFT (patient closes eyes and holds both arms out):
- Normal—both arms move the same or both arms do not move at all (other findings, such as pronator grip, may be helpful)
- Abnormal—one arm does not move or one arm drifts down compared with the other

SPEECH (have the patient say "you can't teach an old dog new tricks"):
- Normal—patient uses correct words with no slurring
- Abnormal—patient slurs words, uses inappropriate words, *or* is unable to speak

From Sanders MJ: *Mosby's paramedic textbook,* ed 2, St Louis, 2000, Mosby.

- Give high-concentration oxygen by mask (15 L/min flow rate).
- Consider endotracheal intubation if the patient is unable to manage the airway.
- Give nothing by mouth; be prepared for vomiting.
- Reassure patients. Talk to them even if they are not able to respond. Unconscious persons may still be able to hear.
- Start an IV line.
- Place the patient on a cardiac monitor.
- If the patient is unconscious, measure the blood glucose. Consider the use of 50% dextrose (D_{50}) intravenously (if the patient is hypoglycemic) and/or naloxone (see Coma and Altered Level of Consciousness) according to local protocols.

Transient Ischemic Attack

Transient ischemic attacks (TIAs), sometimes called "mini-strokes," are strokelike neurological deficits that completely resolve within minutes to hours. People who have TIAs are at an increased risk for a stroke. In the field, distinguishing a TIA from a stroke may be impos-

▶ There are many similarities between diseases of the cardiovascular system and those of the nervous system. Stroke is like a "heart attack" of the brain. TIA is like "unstable angina" of the brain.

sible. The patient care is identical. At times, a person's symptoms and signs will have completely resolved by the time the EMT–I arrives; however, recommending evaluation at a hospital is still appropriate.

SEIZURES AND EPILEPSY

A **seizure (convulsion)** is a sudden episode of abnormal brain cell electrical activity resulting in a period of atypical muscular activity or abnormal behavior. Seizures spontaneously recurring over a span of years are termed **epilepsy.** Up to 6% of the population will experience at least one seizure at some stage of life. Three out of four patients with epilepsy have their first seizure before 20 years of age.

Types of Seizures

There are four types of seizures:

- **Generalized major motor seizures**—These involve jerking movements of the entire body as the muscles rapidly contract and relax—called **tonic-clonic seizure movements.** The victim may become incontinent of urine and feces. Generalized seizures, sometimes called grand mal seizures, usually last 2 to 5 minutes.
- **Focal motor seizures**—These involve abnormal movements of part of the body, such as the arm and hand. Sometimes they are called **simple partial seizures.** The movements may spread to involve the entire body (generalized seizure) or remain focal. Focal seizures generally last 1 to 2 minutes.
- **Behavioral seizures**—These involve a brief "absence" spell or other abnormal behavior. The victim may make purposeless movements, such as smacking the lips and picking at his or her clothes. In children these absence spells are called **petit mal seizures.** In adults these events are usually due to temporal lobe epilepsy, named for the lobe of the brain in which they originate. These are often called psychomotor or **complex-partial seizures.**
- **Status epilepticus**—A series of seizures without an interval of wakefulness between them.

Causes of Seizures

Seizures are not a disease, but a symptom of an underlying abnormality. Seizures may be **idiopathic** (no demonstrable cause) or secondary (due to a brain lesion or metabolic abnormality). CNS causes of secondary seizures include the following:

- Infection (meningitis, brain abscess, encephalitis)
- Fever (Convulsions from fever [febrile convulsion] occur in children. Fever by itself is an uncommon cause of seizures in adults.)
- Trauma (Immediately following head trauma, seizures can occur from damage to brain tissue. Late-onset seizures may be caused by the formation of scar tissue in the brain.)
- Stroke
- Tumor (One out of five patients over age 21 with new-onset seizures has a brain tumor as the cause.)

Causes of seizures not directly involving the CNS include the following:

- Failure to take prescribed antiseizure medications (This is the most common cause of seizures in many patients.)
- Metabolic abnormalities, including blood chemistry imbalance (low sodium, high calcium, low blood sugar), too much acid in the blood, and hypoxia
- Drug or alcohol withdrawal
- Overdose of drugs (especially tricyclic antidepressants or cocaine)
- Hypertensive emergency
- Liver or kidney failure

Patient Assessment

Often, the information available at the scene is minimal. The patient is of little help because of postseizure amnesia (see discussion on the postictal state on the following page). Bystanders may not provide an accurate description of events. The mnemonic **FACTS** describes some historical information that should be gathered:

- **F**—Focus; was there a single initiating movement or simply generalized body involvement from the onset of the seizure?
- **A**—Activity; what movements took place during the event?
- **C**—Color; did the patient become cyanotic during the seizure? *C* also stands for cocaine, a common cause of seizures in young individuals. Always ask patients if they took drugs, herbal stimulants, or over-the-counter "stay alert" preparations. These may also cause seizures.
- **T**—Time; how long did the seizure last?
- **S**—Secondary information; what was the patient doing before the seizure? Was there an aura? Did incontinence occur? Did the patient bite his or her mouth or tongue? Is there a history of seizures? Is the patient taking antiseizure medications?

Before a seizure, some patients will notice the presence of an **aura.** An aura is a warning sign that consists of seeing, hearing, or smelling something unusual before losing consciousness. A few patients may relate that they "feel as though they are about to have a seizure." These patients should be observed carefully, with appropriate care provided if a seizure occurs.

Most generalized seizures follow a typical pattern:
- An aura may occur.
- The patient develops a glassy-eyed stare and becomes unresponsive.
- Unconsciousness rapidly develops.
- Alternating tonic-clonic muscle movements of the entire body occur.
- The patient may hold his or her breath and become cyanotic.
- The patient may drool, foam at the mouth, or vomit.
- The patient may become incontinent of urine or feces.
- Generally, the seizure lasts less than 5 minutes.

Following a seizure, the patient is usually in a **postictal state.** This is a period of decreased level of consciousness after a generalized seizure. As patients gradually wake up, they may look at the person providing care but cannot respond.

Generally, the postictal period lasts less than 30 minutes. At times, patients may have a prolonged postictal period that may mimic coma. When patients are completely awake and lucid, they generally do not remember the seizure. If a patient develops another seizure before becoming lucid, he or she is in status epilepticus.

A patient's behavior during the postictal period may be unusual. Most patients are disoriented. Some become violent. Be alert for violent postictal behavior and be prepared to restrain the patient as necessary. Remember, patients with violent postictal behavior are not aware of what they are doing.

HELPFUL HINT

Watch for violent postictal behavior.

HELPFUL HINT

Some patients will have a neurological deficit following a seizure. This deficit is called Todd's postictal paralysis and lasts up to 2 hours. This may appear identical to a stroke. A small number of patients actually suffer injury to the head or spine during the seizure. If cervical spine tenderness or neurological deficit is present, assume that spinal injury has occurred and immobilize the patient.

Management

Witnessing a seizure can be extremely disturbing for bystanders, relatives, and health care providers. It is important to maintain a calm, concerned, and professional attitude toward the patient. If the patient is a child, the family may be hysterical. Calm and reassure them, but do not compromise patient care.

The care for a seizure patient includes the following:
- Give high-concentration oxygen by mask.
- Maintain the airway as best as possible. Many patients with seizures develop transient airway obstruction during the seizure. If the obstruction is due to a muscle spasm, it will not respond to standard airway procedures.
- Do not insert airways, or bite bars between the teeth of a seizing patient. Doing so would likely damage the patient's teeth and your fingers.
- Assist ventilation as required during the postictal state.
- Be prepared to suction the patient during the seizure. It is common for the mouth to become full of secretions and vomitus. Suction this material using a rigid-tip device without forcing the suction catheter between the patient's teeth.
- Do not restrain the patient. The seizure cannot be stopped by restraining muscle movements. The best approach is to let the seizure take its course. Place a pillow, rolled blanket, or other padding material beneath the patient's head to help prevent injury.
- Start an IV line. This may be difficult during the seizure; wait until the seizure movements have lessened.
- Place the patient on a cardiac monitor; sometimes life-threatening arrhythmias (dysrhythmias) can cause seizures because of decreased blood flow to the brain.
- Keep alert for violent postictal behavior.
- Check oxygen saturation via the pulse oximeter.
- Transport the patient in the coma position following a seizure.

HELPFUL HINT

Many patients fail to take antiseizure medication regularly. Some are compliant with medications but need to have the dosage adjusted. Transport all patients who have had seizures to the hospital for evaluation.

- If cervical spine tenderness or neurological deficit is present, assume that spinal injury has occurred and immobilize the patient.
- Some patients may have bitten their mouth or tongue during the seizure. Care for these wounds as you would for any other open wound.

Specific Pharmacological Therapy (Benzodiazepine Sedatives)

If permitted by local protocols, administration of the drug **diazepam** (Valium) in small IV doses may break status epilepticus. Some EMS systems use a related agent, **lorazepam** (Ativan). Both are **benzodiazepine** sedative agents. The most common serious side effect is

> ▶ Flumazenil (Romazicon) is a specific benzodiazepine antagonist. Although it may help some sedative effects induced by diazepam or lorazepam, its effect on respiratory depression is small. In addition, the drug has been shown to precipitate status epilepticus, especially in patients with a tricyclic antidepressant overdose (see discussion in Chapter 26). Most experts believe that this drug has no role in prehospital care. ▲

respiratory depression. This is rare if small doses are given and the patient's breathing is carefully observed. Common doses in adults are as follows:

- Diazepam, 2 mg given intravenously every 5 to 10 minutes to a maximum dose of 20 mg. Diazepam has a serum half-life of 36 hours but lasts in the CNS less than 30 minutes.
- Lorazepam, 1 mg given intravenously every 5 to 10 minutes to a maximum dose of 5 mg. The serum half-life of lorazepam is short (6 to 8 hours), but its duration of CNS depressant action is 1.5 to 2.0 hours.

COMA AND ALTERED LEVEL OF CONSCIOUSNESS

Coma is a state of unconsciousness characterized by the absence of spontaneous eye movements, response to painful stimuli, and vocalization. The comatose person cannot be aroused. Rather than simply calling the patient "comatose," it is better to describe the patient's status—for example, "unconscious and unresponsive to pain and verbal stimulus" or "conscious and alert" (see discussion of the AVPU mnemonic in Chapter 11).

> **HELPFUL HINT**
>
> • Maintaining consciousness requires the normal function and interaction of at least one of the two cerebral hemispheres, as well as the ascending reticular activating system (ARAS). The ARAS consists of nervous tissue connections running from the brainstem to the thalamus. Dysfunction of the ARAS or the cerebral hemispheres can produce coma.

Causes of Coma

Coma is no more than an extreme alteration of mental status (unresponsiveness); the causes, assessment, and management approaches are similar. *Coma* includes *any* significant alteration of mental status. Causes of coma originating from within the brain include the following:

- Intracranial bleeding

- Stroke
- Tumor
- Infection (meningitis, encephalitis)
- Seizure (see discussion of postictal state, on the previous page).

Causes of coma arising outside the nervous system include the following:

- Blood chemistry abnormalities, including high sodium (hypernatremia), low sodium (hyponatremia), high calcium (hypercalcemia), low sugar (hypoglycemia), and high sugar (hyperglycemia)
- Hypertensive emergency
- Kidney or liver failure
- Abnormalities of the endocrine glands, including underactive thyroid (hypothyroidism), underactive adrenal gland (Addison's disease), and pituitary gland failure
- Vitamin deficiencies
- Drugs (Alcohol, narcotics, and depressant drugs ["downers," antidepressants, tranquilizers] are the most common cause of a drug-induced coma.)
- Psychiatric problems (catatonia)

> **HELPFUL HINT**
>
> • Use the AEIOU-TIPS mnemonic to remember the causes of coma:
> **A** —Acidosis, alcohol
> **E** —Epilepsy
> **I** —Infection
> **O** —Overdose
> **U** —Uremia (kidney failure)
> **T** —Trauma
> **I** —Insulin
> **P** —Psychosis
> **S** —Shock, stroke

Patient Assessment

The following information should be gathered regarding the comatose patient:

- When was the patient last well?
- How did the symptoms progress?
- Did any symptoms precede the onset of coma, such as seizures, confusion, or trauma?
- Are there any pill bottles, syringes, or strange odors present that may give a clue to drug intoxication? Any medications, syringes, or other suspected drug paraphernalia recovered at the scene should be brought to the hospital with the patient.

Patients in coma are unconscious and exhibit no response to stimuli. Pay attention to the following findings:

- Abnormal breathing (Hypoventilation is common. Monitor the vital signs and pulse oximetry reading frequently.)
- Evidence of trauma (Suspect a spinal injury until proven otherwise.)

- Abnormal pupil response.
- Evidence of drug abuse, such as needle tracks.
- Abnormal blood pressure (An elevated blood pressure suggests that some type of intracranial event may be responsible for the coma. Hypotension suggests drug intoxication or shock.)

Management

The care for a comatose patient includes the following:
- Establish and maintain the airway including endotracheal intubation, as necessary. Assist breathing, if necessary.
- Give high-concentration oxygen via mask or bag-valve device.
- If a spinal injury is likely, immobilize appropriately.
- Monitor the vital signs frequently.
- Transport the patient either supine or in the coma position.
- Be prepared for vomiting and airway problems.
- If allowed by local protocols and there is no evidence of eye injury, remove contact lenses.
- Remember that the comatose patient is totally dependent on you. Avoid causing injury or aggravating preexisting problems.
- Start an IV line; infuse normal saline or lactated Ringer's solution TKO ("to keep open") rate or employ a heparin lock.
- Do a blood sugar determination (fingerstick), if possible.

> **ADMINISTRATION OF IV DEXTROSE (D$_{50}$)**
> An ampule of 50% dextrose (D$_{50}$) contains 25 g of dextrose dissolved in 50 mL of sterile water. This agent is indicated for persons with altered levels of consciousness due to hypoglycemia. In many systems a blood glucose reading is done before administration of D$_{50}$. In others, administration of this agent is routine in the treatment of unconscious persons. Follow local protocols.
>
> IV dextrose is highly acidic and very concentrated. Given improperly, it could result in severe tissue damage. Follow these guidelines:
> - Administer via a large-bore catheter in a large vein, if possible.
> - Double-check the patency of the IV line before administering D$_{50}$.
> - Keep the injection site and the area above it as visible as possible.
> - Infuse into a fast-flowing IV line instead of pinching the tubing above the injection port; depend on flow, not pressure, to administer D$_{50}$.
> - Administer D$_{50}$ slowly; 2 minutes is considered a minimum by many.

> **NALOXONE**
> The drug **naloxone** (Narcan) antagonizes the depressant actions of narcotics (e.g., morphine, heroin, Demerol, Dilaudid, and codeine). It does this by affecting the place in the brain where these drugs bind. Narcotics are usually reversed within 5 to 10 minutes following IV administration of naloxone; reversal is somewhat slower if naloxone is given intramuscularly. The effect lasts about 90 minutes. Patients respond differently to the administration of naloxone. Persons who have overdosed on propoxyphene (Darvon) may require large doses of naloxone to respond.
>
> Many EMS systems recommend that providers give only enough naloxone to increase the respiratory rate to acceptable levels. Large doses of naloxone may cause the patient to suffer acute narcotic withdrawal. Besides becoming violent, the patient may then refuse further treatment. Most narcotics remain in the body for at least 3 to 4 hours. Since naloxone wears off after 90 minutes, the patient could become symptomatic again. Some systems have changed their protocols, giving naloxone (2 mg) intramuscularly instead of intravenously. Large scientific studies are not yet available, but limited anecdotal experience suggests that the drug lasts longer when give via the IM route.

- If permitted by local protocols, administer one ampule (25 g) of D$_{50}$ intravenously if the measured blood glucose is less than 60 mg%. If you are unable to measure blood sugar in the field, follow local protocols regarding the administration of IV D$_{50}$.
- Give naloxone intravenously if there is no response to dextrose; use the dose recommended in your protocols. The best route and dose of naloxone are not agreed on. Many EMS systems start with 0.8 mg given intravenously; others titrate the dose, based on the patient's respirations, whereas still others simply give 2.0 mg intravenously.
- Monitor cardiac rhythm.
- Apparently unconscious patients may still be able to hear and understand persons talking to them. Although the patient is unable to respond, continue to reassure him or her.

Syncope and Weakness

Syncope is a partial or complete loss of consciousness from which the patient has recovered. There are many causes (Figure 27-5). The most important management consideration is to monitor the patient for a cardiac dysrhythmia. When persons faint, they often have jerking movements ("myoclonal jerks") secondary to transient cerebral hypoperfusion. Many laypersons assume that this was a seizure (Table 27-3).

Localized or generalized weakness differs, from a diagnostic point of view, from seizures, coma, or syncope.

Causes vary from depression to severe metabolic disturbance to drug reaction. Unless there is postictal paralysis (see earlier discussion), weakness does not typically accompany a seizure.

HEADACHE

Headache means head pain for any reason. Although most headaches result from minor ailments (such as fever, anxiety, or tension), some are due to potentially serious conditions:

- Brain tumors
- Intracranial bleeding
- Hypertensive emergency
- Meningitis
- Poisoning

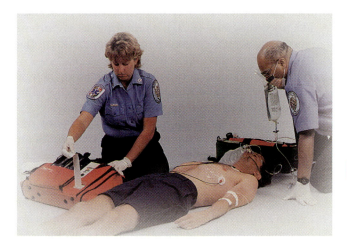

FIGURE 27-5 ▲ It is important to monitor the patient experiencing syncope for cardiac dysrhythmias. (From American College of Emergency Physicians; Pons PT, Cason D, chief editors: *Paramedic field care: a complaint-based approach,* St Louis, 1998, Mosby for ACEP.)

Pathophysiology

Brain tissue itself has no pain receptors. Therefore all headaches result from irritation or stretching of nearby structures (e.g., meninges, paraspinal muscles). Two general categories of headaches are as follows:

- *Vascular*—Involving the cerebrovascular circulation. Migraine headache results from alternating constriction and vasodilation of cerebral vessels. Some rheumatic and autoimmune diseases (e.g., lupus, rheumatoid arthritis) cause inflammation of intracerebral vessels and headache **(vasculitis).** Stroke may also result in a vascular headache.
- *Nonvascular*—Not involving the cerebrovascular circulation. The most common causes are infection (meningitis), mass lesion (tumor), and muscle spasm.

Patient Assessment

The location of head pain varies, depending on the cause. The onset of pain may be gradual or rapid. In addition to pain, other symptoms may be present:

- Visual disturbances, such as blurred vision
- Nausea, vomiting
- **Vertigo** (spinning of the room)
- Stiffness of the neck

> ▶ Consider the rapid onset of a severe headache to be due to intracranial bleeding until proven otherwise. Patients often state that it is the worst headache of their life. If you suspect that the patient has an intracranial hemorrhage, transport immediately to the nearest appropriate hospital.

- Neurological deficit, such as hemiplegia
- Elevated blood pressure

TABLE 27-3

Differentiating Characteristics of Syncope and Seizure

CHARACTERISTICS	SYNCOPE	SEIZURE
Position	The seizure usually starts in a standing position.	The seizure may start in any position.
Warning	There is usually a warning period of lightheadedness.	There is little or no warning.
Level of consciousness	The patient usually regains consciousness immediately on becoming supine; fatigue, confusion, and headache last less than 15 minutes.	The patient may remain unconscious for minutes to hours; fatigue, confusion, and headache last longer than 15 minutes.
Clonic-tonic activity	Clonic movements (if present) are of short duration.	Tonic-clonic movements occur during the unconscious state.
ECG analysis	Bradycardia is caused by increased vagal tone associated with syncope.	Tachycardia is caused by muscular contraction associated with seizure activity.

From Sanders MJ: *Mosby's paramedic textbook,* St Louis, 1994, Mosby.

- Unequal or pinpoint pupils
- Eye pain with bright light **(photophobia)**

Management

Assume that any patient with a headache severe enough to activate the EMS system has a dangerous condition. Provide the following care:

- Monitor the airway, breathing, and circulation carefully.
- Prepare for vomiting.
- Reduce bright lights.
- Place an ice pack to the head over the area of pain.
- Give oxygen (2 to 4 L/min) via nasal cannula.

CASE HISTORY FOLLOW-UP ■■■

En route back to the base, the EMT–Is discuss how important it is to keep an open mind and to consider "all the possibilities" when assessing and managing an unresponsive patient. EMT–I Perez realizes that his assessment was tainted by the park officer's report that the patient was indigent. And he was hasty in concluding that a drug overdose was the most likely cause of the patient's condition. Although drug use was a possibility, it should not have been his initial assumption. He learned in class that in cases of coma of unknown origin, naloxone (Narcan) should be considered only after hypoglycemia is ruled out. Administering the narcotic antagonist would have delayed the delivery of the lifesaving glucose. The medical direction physician is right—this will be a good call to critique in a continuing education class.

SUMMARY

Important points to remember from this chapter include the following:

- Most neurological emergencies affect one or more of the major CNS functions: cognitive systems, cerebral homeostasis (autoregulation), motor control, and sensation. The mnemonic VINDICATE (see text) is helpful for remembering the various conditions that may lead to disease.
- The most important observation to make in persons with neurological emergencies is airway assessment. Despite appearing "okay," many patients hypoventilate and are hypoxic. The EMT–I should always assume this to be the case, until proven otherwise, and treat accordingly.
- Many persons are relatively hypertensive as a result of loss of cerebral autoregulation; acutely lowering their blood pressure may worsen cerebral ischemia.
- Electrocardiogram (ECG) monitoring is important, since neurological problems commonly cause cardiac dysrhythmias and other changes.
- Whenever possible, a blood glucose reading should be obtained and abnormal levels managed according to local protocols.
- Cerebral ischemic syndromes are the result of disrupted circulation to the brain. These syndromes are differentiated by the causes and duration of disruption. Temporary disturbances are called transient ischemic attacks (TIAs) and do not result in permanent injury. Persons who have had a TIA may be symptom free on arrival of the EMS. Since TIA is a sign of an impending stroke, they still require hospital evaluation.

- More profound and often permanent damage occurs following stroke, which may be due to either hemorrhage (intracranial bleeding) or occlusion (thrombosis or embolus). Prompt recognition of stroke patients is important because some will be candidates for thrombolytic therapy, and whether or not thrombolysis is used, "time is brain."

- A seizure is a sudden episode of abnormal brain cell electrical activity resulting in a period of atypical muscular activity or abnormal behavior. Generalized seizures are the most likely type to come to EMS attention. A seizure is a sign of an underlying abnormality in most cases. Also, easily treatable causes—hypoglycemia, hypoxia, hypovolemia, cardiac dysrhythmia—should be excluded. If permitted by local protocols, a benzodiazepine drug (diazepam, lorazepam) can be used to suppress recurrent seizures.

- Coma is a state of unconsciousness characterized by the absence of spontaneous eye movements, response to painful stimuli, and vocalization. The comatose person cannot be aroused. Coma is no more than an extreme alteration of mental status (unresponsiveness); the causes, assessment, and management approaches are similar. As used in this chapter, *coma* includes *any* significant alteration of mental status.

- Careful attention should always be given to the airway and the patient's breathing; persons with an altered level of consciousness are often hypoxic and hypoventilate, despite a relatively normal appearance. The EMT–I should administer naloxone and dextrose according to local protocols.

- Although most headaches result from minor ailments (such as fever, anxiety, or tension), some are due to potentially serious conditions (e.g., intracranial bleeding, brain tumor). Patients often state that headache due to intracranial bleeding is the worst headache of their life.

- The EMT–I should consider the rapid onset of a severe headache to be due to intracranial bleeding until proven otherwise and transport the patient with a suspected intracranial hemorrhage immediately to the nearest appropriate hospital.

28

Nontraumatic Abdominal Emergencies

Key Terms

■■■ CASE HISTORY

It is 2:30 PM on a Sunday afternoon, and EMT–Is Churchill and Wertz are washing the outside of their ambulance. It has been a slow shift so far. Just as they finish drying it off, the dispatch center gives them a call over the radio. They are to respond to the home of a 69-year-old female who is reportedly "throwing up blood." On their arrival, they find the woman, Mrs. Chandler, sitting at the dining room table; she is slumped over, with her head and arms resting on the table, moaning in discomfort. Their initial assessment reveals that the patient is alert; has cool, pale, diaphoretic skin; a blood pressure of 94/60; a pulse rate of 120 beats per minute; and respiratory rate of 20 breaths per minute. The pulse oximetry reading is 84%.

"Why did you call for the ambulance today?" asks EMT–I Churchill.

Mrs. Chandler answers, "Well, I've had diarrhea this morning, and it looked dark. You know, kind of like coffee grounds. Now that didn't bother me too much, but then I got this real bad pain in my stomach and threw up bright red blood. It had some clots in it, so that worried me a bit. I thought I better call you folks."

EMT–I Wertz pulls out the oxygen unit and a nonrebreather mask while EMT–I Churchill palpates Mrs. Chandler's abdomen. It is soft without mass, but his palpation reveals lower abdominal pain. According to Mrs. Chandler, she has a history of heart and respiratory problems for which she takes theophylline, quinidine, and verapamil (Calan). Also, last Monday she began taking indomethacin (Indocin). Further questioning reveals that Mrs. Chandler is allergic to meperidine (Demerol).

"We need to get her into a supine position before we do anything else," EMT–I Chandler remarks as he goes out to the ambulance to get the cot. While he is gone, EMT–I Wertz sets up an intravenous (IV) line using a 1000 mL bag of normal saline and a macrodrip administration set. Once they get Mrs. Chandler into a supine position on the cot, EMT–I Wertz applies the tourniquet to her left arm, just above the elbow. Mrs. Chander remarks, "I really don't like lying on my back like this. Can you sit me up?"

EMT–I Wertz replies, "We are going to keep you flat for just a few minutes. It helps get blood to your brain, and it makes it easier for us to start the IV."

Mrs. Chandler responds in an agitated tone, "So you think that's my problem? I'm not getting enough blood to my brain?"

Noting the inflection in Mrs. Chandler's voice, EMT–I Wertz gently responds, "No, Mrs. Chandler, it's just that when you lose blood like this, you don't get as much to your vital organs, like your brain. Lying flat helps treat that. Once we get some IV fluids in you, it will help improve your blood circulation, and we can sit you up some."

As EMT–I Wertz lifts the patient's arm and looks at the patient's veins, she can see they are a bit small and fragile. "Great," she thinks to herself, "this lady is already irritated with us, and now I may have to stick her more than once. She's really going to like us."

EMT–I Wertz uses a 20-gauge catheter-over-needle to penetrate the skin. But as she pushes against the vein with the tip of the needle, it starts to wiggle. "Uhh oh," she thinks to herself, "I'd better pull the skin a bit tighter to hold the vein in place."

She then pushes the needle into the vein. It wiggles a bit, but she is able to get it in without passing the needle through the other side of the vein. Advancing the needle slightly, she then gently slips the catheter into the vein. EMT–I Chandler remarks, "Looks like your streak is intact." He is referring to the 50 IV lines in a row that EMT–I Wertz has successfully started.

Key Terms
—cont'd

Ruptured Viscus

Upper Gastrointestinal (GI) Bleeding

Urinary Stones

Urinary Tract Infection

LEARNING OBJECTIVES

CHAPTER GOAL
Upon completion of this chapter, the EMT-Intermediate will be able to use assessment findings to formulate a field impression and implement a treatment plan for the patient with nontraumatic abdominal pain.

Cognitive Objectives
As an EMT-Intermediate you should be able to do the following:
- Discuss the pathophysiology of nontraumatic abdominal emergencies.
- Discuss the signs and symptoms of nontraumatic acute abdominal pain.
- Discuss the signs and symptoms of peritoneal inflammation relative to acute abdominal pain.
- Describe the questioning technique and specific questions the EMT–I should ask when gathering a focused history from a patient with nontraumatic abdominal pain.
- Describe the technique for performing a comprehensive physical examination on a patient with nontraumatic abdominal pain.
- Recognize the signs and symptoms of nontraumatic abdominal pain.
- Describe the management of the patient with nontraumatic abdominal pain.
- Describe the common causes of gastrointestinal bleeding.
- Describe the proper care for a patient with gastrointestinal bleeding.

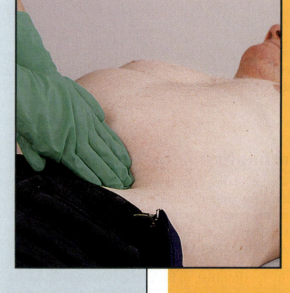

Affective Objectives
As an EMT-Intermediate you should be able to do the following:
- Understand the potential fears a patient experiences during a gastrointestinal bleeding episode.

Psychomotor Objectives
As an EMT-Intermediate you should be able to do the following:
- Demonstrate a focused physical examination on a patient with nontraumatic abdominal pain.
- Demonstrate a focused physical examination on a patient with gastrointestinal bleeding.

INTRODUCTION

The term **acute abdomen** refers to acute abdominal pain *not* due to injury. See Chapter 15 for information on abdominal injuries.

The approach of the EMT–Intermediate (EMT–I) toward the patient with acute nontraumatic abdominal pain is as follows:

- Start by asking, does this patient have a life-threatening condition, including severe pain or shock? If so, rapidly provide necessary care and transport the patient as a "priority."
- If the patient does not have a life-threatening illness, care for the patient and transport him or her to the nearest appropriate hospital.

It is *not* necessary for the EMT–I to make a diagnosis in the field. The signs and symptoms of many abdominal conditions are similar. It may be impossible to determine in the field if the situation is potentially life threatening or not. It should always be assumed that a serious condition may be present until proven otherwise.

ANATOMY AND PHYSIOLOGY REVIEW

The **abdominal cavity** extends from the diaphragm to the pelvic bones and contains the organs of digestion, the organs of the urinary and reproductive tracts, the vertebral column, and major blood vessels. The abdomen is divided into four quadrants by two perpendicular lines intersecting at the umbilicus (Figures 28-1 and 28-2).

ABDOMINAL PAIN

Pathophysiology and Causes

There are numerous mechanisms, both systemic and within the abdomen itself, that may result in acute abdominal pain. Common abdominal causes include the following:

- *Bacterial contamination*—This is usually caused by infection in the bowel, the surrounding peritoneal cavity **(peritonitis)**, or both.
- *Chemical irritation*—This is usually due to leakage of bile or some other body substance (e.g., blood) into the wrong space, often the peritoneal cavity.
- *Peritoneal inflammation*—This may be due to bacterial contamination, chemical irritation, or direct trauma.
- *Bleeding*—Bleeding anywhere in the gastrointestinal (GI) tract may result in painful cramping; if blood seeps into the peritoneal cavity, peritoneal inflammation will result.
- *Obstruction*—Any factor that slows or blocks the movement of digestive contents through the bowel results in distention and pain.

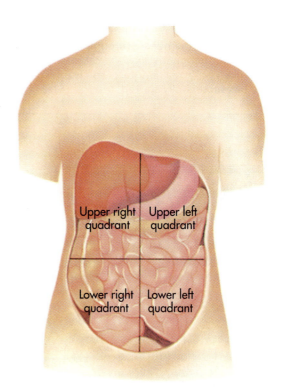

FIGURE 28-1 ▲ Abdominal quadrants of the abdomen. (From Sanders MJ: *Mosby's paramedic textbook,* ed 2, St Louis, 2000, Mosby.)

There are many diseases that may cause acute abdominal pain. Four diseases are immediately life threatening:

- *Acute myocardial infarction*—The pain of acute myocardial infarction may occur anywhere from the umbilicus upward (see Chapter 23).
- *Ruptured abdominal aortic aneurysm*—An **abdominal aortic aneurysm** is an outpouching of the abdominal portion of the aorta due to atherosclerosis. Aneurysm formation weakens the wall of the artery; if the aneurysm ruptures, severe abdominal and back pain, as well as shock, result. The patient may easily bleed to death.
- *Ruptured ectopic pregnancy*—An **ectopic pregnancy** occurs when the fertilized egg implants outside the uterus. Internal structures may rupture, causing severe internal bleeding. The patient has abdominal pain, vaginal bleeding, and shock (see Chapters 31 and 32).
- **Ruptured viscus**—*Viscus* is a general term for any hollow organ. The most common viscus to rupture is the duodenum, usually because of a peptic ulcer. The patient develops the sudden onset of sharp epigastric pain and shock. The abdomen is rigid.

Other common causes of acute abdominal pain that are not usually life threatening include the following:

- **Peptic ulcer disease**—Erosions in the lining of the GI tract. Ulcers result from excess acid production by the stomach, often in combination with bacterial in-

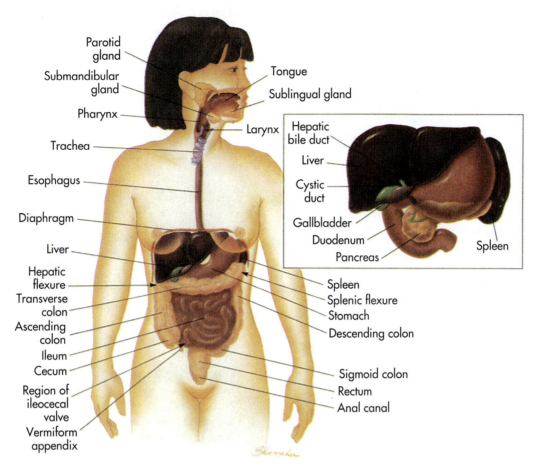

FIGURE 28-2 ▲ Location of digestive organs. (From Thibodeau G: *Structure and function of the body,* ed 11, St Louis, 2000, Mosby.)

fection, and are associated with stress, cigarette smoking, and the intake of certain drugs (steroids and antiinflammatory agents). Symptoms include gnawing upper abdominal pain and nausea that is often relieved with food or antacids.

- **Gastritis**—Inflammation of the lining of the stomach resulting from drugs, alcohol, or infection. Gastritis is characterized by loss of appetite, nausea, vomiting, and epigastric discomfort after eating. The pain may be relieved with antacids.
- **Pneumonia**—Infection and inflammation of the tissues of the lungs. Pneumonia of the lower lobes of the lungs can cause upper abdominal pain.
- **Pancreatitis**—Inflammation of the pancreas due to either stones that block the ducts or alcohol. The pain is epigastric and radiates straight through to the patient's back. Nausea and vomiting are common.
- **Kidney stones** *(nephrolithiasis)*—Kidney stones are small, rocklike structures that are formed in the kidney. The passage of a stone down the urinary tract causes severe, intermittent pain. The discomfort starts in the flank and radiates to the abdomen and groin. Nausea and vomiting are common. Kidney

failure, acute or chronic, is unlikely to result in significant abdominal pain if no other pathology is present. Urinary tract infection (UTI) or kidney infection (pyelonephritis) may cause severe abdominal pain.

- **Pelvic inflammatory disease (PID)**—Inflammation of the female internal genitalia, usually due to sexually transmitted disease. The patient complains of lower abdominal pain. She may have vaginal discharge, fever, and chills.
- **Appendicitis** *(inflammation of the appendix)*—Inflammation resulting from obstruction of the lumen of the appendix. The patient initially has pain around the umbilicus that then localizes to the right lower quadrant. Loss of appetite (anorexia) is common. Rupture of the appendix can result in peritonitis, an inflammation of the abdominal cavity.
- **Cholecystitis** *(gallbladder attack)*—Occlusion of the gallbladder duct, leading to inflammation and pain. The pain is usually intermittent, located in the right upper quadrant, and accompanied by nausea. Pain may radiate to the posterior scapula or right shoulder. Attacks are often self-limited and may be brought on with the ingestion of fatty foods.

- **Pyelonephritis** (*kidney infection*)—Infection that causes flank pain, which may radiate to the abdomen. The patient has discomfort with urination, nausea, and vomiting.
- **Diverticulitis**—Infection of diverticula—small, saclike outpouchings in the intestine. Infection of these leads to cramplike abdominal pain in the left lower quadrant. Diverticulitis may be accompanied by fever, diarrhea, or constipation.
- **Bowel obstruction**—A blockage of the intestinal tract. The symptoms include cramping pain, vomiting, abdominal tenderness, and distention of the abdomen.

Nonabdominal causes include sickle cell anemia crisis, black widow spider bite, diabetic ketoacidosis (Chapter 24), and anaphylactic shock.

HELPFUL HINT

- Consider any woman with abdominal pain who is capable of ovulation to have an ectopic pregnancy until proven otherwise.

HELPFUL HINT

- Consider any patient with right lower quadrant abdominal pain to have appendicitis until proven otherwise (Box 28-1).

Patient Assessment
INITIAL ASSESSMENT

As with any patient, initial assessment consists of evaluating the ABCs (airway, breathing, and circulation), as well as disability, and determining the patient's chief complaint.

HISTORY

Patients with an acute abdominal condition complain of localized or diffuse pain. The abdominal organs have nerve receptors for pressure, but not for pain. Often, abdominal discomfort is vaguely located and referred to other parts of the body. Conditions that originate in the abdomen can cause pain in distant locations, such as the neck, shoulder, chest, or flank (Figure 28-3). Always ask the patient about recent weight loss and when his or her last meal was.

Other symptoms of an acute abdomen include the following:
- Nausea, vomiting
- Changes in bowel habits (diarrhea, constipation, stool color or consistency)
- Decreased appetite
- Chills, fever
- Painful urination
- Blood in the urine, stool, or vomitus
- Vaginal bleeding or discharge

BOX 28-1

LOCATION OF ABDOMINAL PAIN AND POSSIBLE ORIGINS

RIGHT UPPER QUADRANT
Cholecystitis
Hepatitis
Pancreatitis
Perforated ulcer
Renal pain (right)

LEFT UPPER QUADRANT
Pancreatitis
Gastritis
Renal pain (left)

RIGHT LOWER QUADRANT
Appendicitis
Abdominal aortic dissection or rupture
Ruptured ectopic pregnancy
Ovarian cyst (right)
Pelvic inflammatory disease
Urinary calculus
Hernia
Ovarian or testicular torsion

LEFT LOWER QUADRANT
Diverticulitis
Abdominal aortic dissection or rupture
Ruptured ectopic pregnancy
Ovarian cyst (left)
Pelvic inflammatory disease
Urinary calculus
Hernia
Ovarian or testicular torsion

EPIGASTRIC PAIN
Gastritis
Esophagitis
Pancreatitis
Cholecystitis
Abdominal aortic aneurysm
Myocardial ischemia

DIFFUSE PAIN
Intestinal obstruction
Perforation
Generalized peritonitis

From Sanders MJ: *Mosby's paramedic textbook*, ed 2, St Louis, 2000, Mosby.

- Vaginal bleeding in a woman of childbearing years is assumed to be due to ectopic pregnancy until proven otherwise. Do not perform a vaginal examination in the prehospital setting.

- Cough (if pneumonia is present)
- Chest pains, shortness of breath (in myocardial infarction)

FOCUSED PHYSICAL EXAMINATION

On examination, evaluate for the following:
- *General appearance*—Patients with acute abdominal conditions may be lying extremely still (any movement worsens the pain) or writhing in pain (common with kidney stones and gallbladder attacks).
- *Abdominal tenderness and guarding to palpation*—The abdomen may be soft, rigid, or distended. There may be localized or diffuse tenderness to palpation. **Rigidity** means that the abdomen feels rigid to palpation. **Guarding** is voluntary or involuntary resistance to touch. The patient may lie on the back or side with the knees drawn toward the chest.
- *Pulsating mass in the abdomen*—This suggests an abdominal aortic aneurysm. Always check distal pulses bilaterally in all patients with abdominal pain.
Also evaluate for signs of shock (Chapter 16) and fever.

Management and Treatment

The care for a patient with acute abdominal pain includes the following (Box 28-2):
- Maintain the airway. Give high-flow oxygen and assist breathing if necessary.
- Allow the patient to lie in a comfortable position.

BOX 28-2

SUMMARY OF EMERGENCY CARE FOR ACUTE ABDOMINAL PAIN

1. High-concentration oxygen administration
2. Adequate intravenous access with a crystalloid solution (Application of the pneumatic antishock garment for the treatment of shock with acute abdominal pain is controversial and should be authorized by medical direction.)
3. Electrocardiogram monitoring
4. Rapid and gentle transport to an appropriate medical facility

From Sanders MJ: *Mosby's paramedic textbook,* ed 2, St Louis, 2000, Mosby.

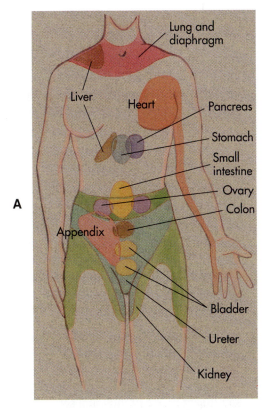
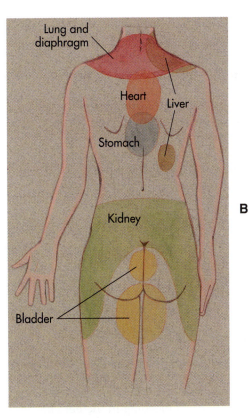

FIGURE 28-3 ▲ Referred pain. **A,** Anterior view. **B,** Posterior view. (From Sanders MJ: *Mosby's paramedic textbook,* ed 2, St Louis, 2000, Mosby.)

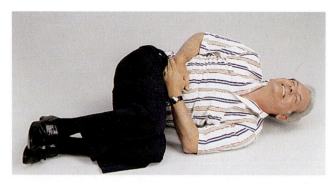

FIGURE 28-4 ▲ Often, the most comfortable position for a patient experiencing acute abdominal pain is flat on the back (or on the side) with the knees drawn up to the chest.

Often the best position is flat on the back (or on the side) with the knees drawn up (Figure 28-4).
- Do not give anything by mouth.
- Start an intravenous (IV) line; if the patient appears dehydrated or is hypotensive, give a fluid bolus as per local protocols. The usual dose is 500 to 1000 cc of normal saline or lactated Ringer's solution given intravenously as rapidly as possible. Avoid interventions that can mask signs and symptoms, such as pain medications.

▶ NOTE: Administration of pain medications to persons with an acute abdomen is controversial—follow local protocols or medical control directions.

- Place the patient on a cardiac monitor, and care for shock if present. Use a pneumatic antishock garment (PASG) if necessary, according to local protocols.
- Be prepared for vomiting. Have suction equipment available.
- Always consider the possibility of acute myocardial infarction in a patient with abdominal pain, especially if the location is epigastric.
- Transport patients in a gentle but rapid fashion. Maintain a calm, caring, and competent attitude, and keep the patient informed of your actions.

GASTROINTESTINAL BLEEDING

GI bleeding refers to hemorrhage anywhere in the GI tract (from the mouth to the anus) that is due to a lesion of the mucosa (lining). GI bleeding accounts for 1% to 2% of hospital admissions in the United States.

Approach to Gastrointestinal Bleeding

GI bleeding can rapidly result in life-threatening hypovolemic shock (Chapter 16). The chances of determining the exact cause of GI bleeding in the field are slim. Rather than being concerned with the cause, evaluate the following:

- Is the patient's airway open? Airway obstruction due to vomiting of blood is common.
- Is the patient in shock?
- Is active bleeding present?

Causes

Causes of GI bleeding are divided into upper and lower sources. **Upper gastrointestinal (GI) bleeding** originates anywhere in the GI tract from the mouth to the duodenum. Most commonly, the patient vomits blood, but if the bleeding rate is sufficient, blood will be passed via the rectum as well. Because of the action of gastric fluids, vomited blood usually has the appearance of coffee grounds.

Lower gastrointestinal (GI) bleeding results from bleeding due to a lesion of the GI tract below the level of the duodenum. Blood from these lesions always passes rectally and may appear as bright red blood passing from the rectum or as red-streaked or tarry-looking stool.

Common causes of upper GI bleeding include the following:
- Peptic ulcer disease
- Gastritis
- **Esophageal varices**—Dilation of veins of the esophagus due to liver disease. This is a common cause of upper GI bleeding in alcoholic patients.
- **Esophagitis**—Irritation of the esophagus, similar to that which occurs in gastritis.

Common causes of lower GI bleeding include the following:
- Diverticulosis—Diverticula may become inflamed (leading to diverticulitis) or may bleed.
- *Tumors, hemorrhoids, polyps*—These commonly result in lower GI bleeding, but usually the bleeding is not significant in the prehospital setting.

All patients with rectal bleeding are considered high risk. Monitor and care for shock.

Patient Assessment

Patients may report use of aspirin, alcohol, or antiinflammatory agents such as ibuprofen. The patient may vomit blood, either bright red or coffee-ground vomitus. Blood passed by the rectum may be bright red or appear as dark, tarry stool. During assessment, pay special attention to the following:

- Airway patency
- Signs and symptoms of shock
- Abdominal pain
- Fever

CLINICAL NOTES

Hematochezia is the presence of bright red blood in the stool. **Melena** is black, tarry stool caused by digested blood passing slowly through the GI tract.

CLINICAL NOTES

Hematemesis is the vomiting of blood. Coffee-ground vomitus has the appearance of coffee grounds. The appearance is due to digestion of the blood by stomach acid.

CLINICAL NOTES

More than 80% of patients with upper GI bleeding have fever. The reason for this is unclear.

Emergency Care

The care for a patient with GI bleeding includes the following:

- Maintain control of the airway.
- Give high-concentration mask oxygen. If the patient is nauseated or vomiting, use nasal cannula (3 to 4 L/min).
- Assist breathing as necessary.
- Care for shock if present. Patients with GI bleeding are at a high risk for shock. Use PASG as needed, as per local protocols.
- Start an IV line; if the patient appears dehydrated or is hypotensive, give a fluid bolus as per local protocols. The usual dose is 500 to 1000 mL of normal saline or lactated Ringer's solution given intravenously as rapidly as possible; follow local protocols.
- Anticipate vomiting and be prepared to suction the patient.
- Give nothing by mouth.

- Assume that any patient with ongoing GI bleeding has a significant, potentially life-threatening lesion, and provide care accordingly.

CASE HISTORY FOLLOW-UP ▪▪▪

The administration of oxygen and the IV infusion help Mrs. Chandler's condition. Her blood pressure improves to 110/70, her pulse rate slows to 100 beats per minute, and her respiratory rate is 14 breaths per minute. At her request, Mrs. Chandler is elevated to a semisitting position. A recheck by EMT–I Wertz reveals that there is no change in Mrs. Chandler's blood pressure. On the way to the hospital, Mrs. Chandler's electrocardiogram (ECG) rhythm starts to wander from the top to the bottom of the ECG screen. EMT–I Wertz determines that the problem is a loose electrode. She fixes the problem by applying a new electrode.

SUMMARY

Important points to remember from this chapter include the following:

- The term *acute abdomen* refers to acute abdominal pain *not* caused by injury. It is *not* necessary for the EMT–I to make a diagnosis in the field. The signs and symptoms of many abdominal conditions are similar. A serious condition should always be assumed to be present until proven otherwise. The following is a prudent approach:
  - Does the patient have a life-threatening condition, including severe pain or shock? If so, provide necessary care and transport as soon as possible.
  - If the patient does not have a life-threatening condition, care for the patient and transport him or her to the nearest appropriate hospital.
- Common causes for abdominal pain include bacterial contamination, chemical irritation, peritoneal inflammation, bleeding, and obstruction. Any of these may be caused by a variety of illnesses, some originating outside of the abdominal cavity (e.g., myocardial infarction, pneumonia, diabetic ketoacidosis). Of all potential causes for the acute abdomen, four are potentially acutely life threatening:
  - Myocardial infarction
  - Ruptured abdominal aortic aneurysm
  - Ruptured ectopic pregnancy
  - Rupture of a hollow viscus (organ)
- Numerous other conditions may lead to an acute abdomen. Common causes include the following:
  - Peptic ulcer disease
  - Gastritis
  - Pancreatitis
  - Kidney stones
  - Appendicitis
  - Cholecystitis

- Urinary tract infection
- Bowel obstruction
- Metabolic abnormalities (e.g., diabetic ketoacidosis)
- Black widow spider bite
- As with any patient, initial assessment consists of evaluating the airway, breathing, and circulation, as well as disability, and determining the patient's chief complaint. The patient should always be asked about recent weight loss and when his or her last meal was. In addition to the standard OPQRST questions, the patient should be asked about the following:
  - Nausea or vomiting
  - Changes in the bowel habits and stool
  - Difficulty or discomfort during urination
  - Chest pains, "indigestion pain"
- During the focused physical examination, the EMT–I should pay particular attention to palpation of the abdomen. Rigidity means that the abdomen feels rigid to palpation. Guarding is voluntary or invol-

untary resistance to touch. Signs of shock may be present.

- Regarding care, careful attention to the ABCs (airway, breathing, and circulation) is essential. An IV line should be established according to local protocols. Use of a pneumatic antishock garment (PASG) may be lifesaving in cases of ruptured abdominal aortic aneurysm or ectopic pregnancy. As a general rule, the EMT–I should avoid administering pain medications unless directed to do so by medical control or local protocols. Gentle, but prompt, transportation to the appropriate medical facility is warranted.

- Gastrointestinal (GI) bleeding, either upper or lower, may result from a number of lesions. It is difficult, if not impossible, to determine the exact cause in the field. Most important is management of the airway, breathing, and circulation, since the biggest risk is hemorrhagic shock. Rapid transport to the appropriate facility is warranted.

29 Environmental Emergencies

Key Terms

Acclimatization

Acute Mountain Sickness (AMS)

Afterdrop Phenomenon

Air Embolism

The "Bends"

Classic Heat Stroke

Cold Diuresis

Compensated Hypothermia

Conduction

Convection

Core Body Temperature (CBT)

Decompression Sickness

Drowning

"Dry" Drowning

Environmental Emergency

Environmental Illness

Evaporation

Exertional Heat Stroke

Frostbite

Heat Cramps

Heat Stroke

Heat Exhaustion

...CASE HISTORY

It is a brutally hot Friday afternoon in mid-July, and EMT–Is Jones and Daily are working for a hospital-based emergency medical service. The temperature is just above 100° F with a humidity of close to 80%. The workload is exhausting. Many of the emergencies they respond to are heat related. EMT–I Jones has been sweating heavily all day long. He has been trying to stay hydrated by drinking lots of water and remaining inside in the air-conditioning whenever possible. As he works to resuscitate a patient suffering from cardiac arrest, he begins to feel very fatigued. He assists his fellow team members with resuscitating and delivering the patient to the hospital before he feels too tired to continue any longer. One of the nurses notices his pale color and heavy sweating and suggests that he lie down while she checks his vital signs. His uniform is soaked with sweat. She reports to the physician treating EMT–I Jones that his blood pressure is 76/58, pulse rate is 130, and temperature is 38.3° C (101° F). She tells EMT–I Jones that he is experiencing heat exhaustion and starts an intravenous (IV) infusion of lactated Ringer's solution.

LEARNING OBJECTIVES ☑

CHAPTER GOAL
Upon completion of this chapter, the EMT-Intermediate will be able to use assessment findings to formulate a field impression and implement a treatment plan for the patient with an environmentally induced or exacerbated emergency.

Cognitive Objectives
As an EMT-Intermediate you should be able to do the following:
- Define *environmental emergency*.
- Identify risk factors that predispose persons to environmental emergencies.
- Identify environmental factors that may cause illness or exacerbate a preexisting illness.
- Identify environmental factors that may complicate treatment or transport decisions.
- List the principal types of environmental illnesses.

- Identify normal, critically high, and critically low body temperatures.
- Describe several methods of temperature monitoring.
- Describe the body's compensatory process for overheating.
- Describe the body's compensatory process for excess heat loss.
- List the common forms of heat and cold disorders.
- List the common predisposing factors associated with heat and cold disorders.
- List the common preventive measures associated with heat and cold disorders.
- Define heat illness.
- Identify signs and symptoms of heat illness.
- List the predisposing factors for heat illness.
- List measures to prevent heat illness.
- Relate symptomatic findings to the commonly used terms: *heat cramps, heat exhaustion,* and *heat stroke.*
- Discuss how one may differentiate between fever and heat stroke.
- Discuss the role of fluid therapy in the treatment of heat disorders.
- Differentiate among the various treatments and interventions in the management of heat disorders.
- Integrate the pathophysiological principles and the assessment findings to formulate a field impression and implement a treatment plan for the patient who has dehydration, heat exhaustion, or heat stroke.
- Define the term *hypothermia.*
- List predisposing factors for hypothermia.
- List measures to prevent hypothermia.
- Identify differences between mild and severe hypothermia.
- Describe differences between chronic and acute hypothermia.
- List signs and symptoms of hypothermia.
- Correlate abnormal assessment findings with their clinical significance in the patient with hypothermia.
- Discuss the impact of severe hypothermia on standard basic life support (BLS) and advanced cardiac life support (ACLS) algorithms and transport considerations.
- Integrate pathophysiological principles and assessment findings to formulate a field impression and implement a treatment plan for the patient who has either mild or severe hypothermia.
- Define the term *near-drowning.*
- List signs and symptoms of near-drowning.
- Discuss the complications and protective role of hypothermia in the context of near-drowning.
- Correlate the abnormal assessment findings with the clinical significance in the victim of near-drowning.
- Differentiate among the various treatments and interventions in the management of near-drowning.
- Integrate pathophysiological principles and assessment findings to formulate a field impression and implement a treatment plan for the victim of near-drowning.
- Integrate pathophysiological principles regarding the patient affected by an environmental emergency.
- Differentiate between environmental emergencies on the basis of assessment findings.

- Correlate abnormal findings in the assessment with the clinical significance in the patient affected by an environmental emergency.
- Develop a patient management plan based on the field impression of the patient affected by an environmental emergency.
- Recall and integrate into practice specific patient assessment and management techniques for particular locale-specific emergencies (e.g., diving accidents, altitude emergencies).

Affective Objectives
- None identified for this chapter.

Psychomotor Objectives
- None identified for this chapter.

INTRODUCTION

An **environmental emergency** is a medical condition caused or exacerbated by weather, terrain, atmospheric pressure, or other local factors. Examples include heat stroke, hypothermia, and frostbite. By themselves, environmental emergencies may be life threatening. They may also aggravate other medical or traumatic conditions. For example, trauma patients who are hypothermic have a worse outcome (because of excess bleeding) than those who are normothermic.

Risk Factors

As with any condition, certain preexisting factors make environmental emergencies more dangerous. These include the following:

- *Age*—Persons at the extremes of age (small children, geriatric patients) are at greater risk for environmental emergencies. Small children have a large body surface area, especially of the head, and very limited ability to compensate for acute major changes in temperature. Older patients lose their ability to internally regulate their temperature and are more susceptible to temperature extremes. They get colder or warmer quicker and with less awareness than younger individuals.
- *General health*—Anyone who has a serious underlying medical condition (e.g., heart failure, cancer), especially if he or she is undernourished, is more susceptible to environmental influences.
- *Fatigue*—When people are tired, they may not exercise appropriate judgment in potentially dangerous environmental situations (i.e., staying outside in the heat too long). In addition, fatigue may upset the body's normal regulatory mechanisms, making the person more likely to suffer harm.
- *Predisposing medical conditions*—Although any person in poor general health is more susceptible to environmental emergencies, particularly risky conditions include diabetes (decreased sensation in the extremities), congestive heart failure (alterations of autonomic nervous system function), and thyroid disease (excess or abnormally low sensitivity to heat or cold).

- *Medications*—Both prescription and over-the-counter medications may predispose persons to environmental injury, especially heat. Many common medications (e.g., antihistamines, psychotropic drugs [tricyclic antidepressants]) have anticholinergic (vagus nerve blocking) side effects. The result is an impaired ability to sweat and dissipate heat. Heat intolerance is a common side effect of these drugs, whether they be prescription or over-the-counter drugs. A careful medication history (particularly in regard over-the-counter and herbal/natural remedies) should always be obtained in any patient with an environmental emergency.

CLINICAL NOTES

Many common over-the-counter medications have anticholinergic side effects, predisposing patients to heat illness. This includes most antihistamines, cold remedies, and allergy preparations.

Environmental Factors

Although factors related to climate, season, weather, atmosphere, and terrain are important considerations, *anyone* can suffer an environmental emergency under the right conditions. For example, heat exhaustion is relatively common in fishermen off the coast of Alaska. The reason—the engine room of the boat is confined, hot, and humid. This sounds paradoxical at first (given the climate of Alaska), but it really does make sense. Or, consider the elderly patient who falls onto a tile floor and is rendered unconscious. Regardless of the ambient temperature, the person will quickly lose body heat to the tile, resulting in hypothermia. Finally, consider the effect of the wind chill factor—have you ever gotten out of a swimming pool on a hot but very windy day? Magnify the chill you feel, and hypothermia is inevitable. Do not exclude the possibility of an environmental emergency just because the ambient conditions do not seem to initially "fit the picture."

Types of Environmental Illnesses

Environmental illnesses are those caused by the patient's surroundings or environment. Generally, environmental illnesses can be divided into two categories, systemic and localized. Regarding emergency care, systemic problems are more potentially harmful than are localized ones. These include cold illness (hypothermia) and heat illness (heat cramps, heat exhaustion, heat stroke). Examples of localized environmental injuries are frostbite and sunburn (see Chapter 17 for sunburn).

PATHOPHYSIOLOGY, ASSESSMENT, AND MANAGEMENT

Homeostasis

Homeostasis is the normal state of balance. In terms of body temperature, this means that various body factors interact to maintain the body temperature at or near 37° C (98.6° F). "Normal" temperature usually refers to the core, or inner, body temperature. **Core body temperature (CBT)** is most accurately measured by a rectal temperature or by

---

CLINICAL NOTES

Palpated skin temperature (cool, warm, hot) is important yet does not always correlate with measured core temperature.

BOX 29-1

HYPERTHERMIC AND HYPOTHERMIC COMPENSATION

HYPERTHERMIC COMPENSATION
Increased heat loss
Vasodilation of skin vessels
Sweating
Decreased heat production
Decreased muscle tone and voluntary activity
Decreased hormone secretion
Decreased appetite

HYPOTHERMIC COMPENSATION
Decreased heat loss
Peripheral vasoconstriction
Reduction of surface area by body position (or clothing)
Piloerection (not effective in humans)
Increased heat production
Shivering
Increased voluntary activity
Increased hormone secretion
Increased appetite

From Sanders MJ: *Mosby's paramedic textbook*, ed 2, St Louis, 2000, Mosby.

---

measuring immediately the temperature of freshly voided urine. Other methods of temperature measurement (oral, axillary, tympanic) are less accurate. Tactile measurement (touching the skin) is notoriously unreliable, although palpable skin temperature is important to note.

CLINICAL NOTES

To accurately measure the temperature in a hypothermic patient, you must use a special thermometer that reads low temperature values properly.

Thermolysis

Thermolysis refers to normal bodily means of heat loss and gain (Box 29-1). Heat is generated by muscular activity and through metabolic reactions in the body. As the body temperature increases, changes occur in each organ system. If an individual gradually exposes himself or herself to a hot environment, the body acclimates, or becomes used to the heat. Heat is dissipated from the body by four mechanisms (Figure 29-1):

Radiation—Transmission of heat through space (e.g., warmth from a radiant heater or fireplace).

Conduction—Transmission of heat from warmer to cooler objects in direct contact (e.g., touching a cold surface, lying on a cold floor).

Convection—Transfer of heat by circulation of heated particles (e.g., wind chill, cold water exposure, or cooling soup by blowing on it) (Table 29-1).

Evaporation—Loss of heat at the surface from vaporization of liquid (e.g., sweating, spraying water mist on the body to keep cool while sunbathing).

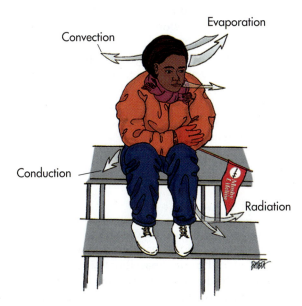

FIGURE 29-1 ▲ The four mechanisms of heat dissipation: radiation, conduction, convection, and evaporation.

TABLE 29-1

Cooling Power of Wind on Exposed Flesh Expressed as an Equivalent Temperature (Under Calm Conditions)

ESTIMATED WIND SPEED (IN MPH)	ACTUAL THERMOMETER READING (°F)											
	50	40	30	20	10	0	−10	−20	−30	−40	−50	−60
	EQUIVALENT CHILL TEMPERATURE (°F)											
Calm	50	40	30	20	10	0	−10	−20	−30	−40	−50	−60
5	48	37	27	16	6	−5	−15	−26	−36	−47	−57	−68
10	40	28	16	4	−9	−24	−33	−46	−58	−70	−83	−95
15	36	22	9	−5	−18	−32	−45	−58	−72	−85	−99	−112
20	32	18	4	−10	−25	−39	−53	−67	−82	−96	−110	−124
25	30	16	0	−15	−29	−44	−59	−74	−88	−104	−118	−133
30	28	13	−2	−18	−33	−48	−63	−79	−94	−109	−125	−140
35	27	11	−4	−21	−35	−51	−62	−82	−98	−113	−129	−145
40	26	10	−6	−21	−37	−53	−69	−85	−100	−116	−132	−148

(Wind speeds greater than 40 mph have little additional effect.)	Little danger. In <5 hr with dry skin. Maximum danger. is false sense of security.			Increasing danger. Danger from freezing of exposed flesh within 1 min.			Great danger. Flesh may freeze within 30 sec.					
Trenchfoot and immersion foot can occur at any point on this chart.												

From Sheehy S: *Emergency nursing*, ed 3, St Louis, 1992, Mosby.
Measure local temperature and wind speed if possible. If not, *estimate.* Enter table at closest 5° F interval along the top and with appropriate wind speed along left side. Intersection gives approximate equivalent chill temperature (i.e., the temperature that would cause the same rate of cooling under calm conditions). Note that regardless of cooling rate, a person does not cool below the actual air temperature unless wet.

Heat is also lost during respiration; the majority of this loss is thought to be due to evaporation.

In humans, conduction is not a major mechanism of heat loss unless the clothing is removed and the individual lies on a cool surface. Convection is also hindered by clothing. At room temperature, 75% of heat dissipation is by radiation and convection. Evaporation, the loss of moisture from the lungs (during respiration) and skin, accounts for about 25% of heat loss.

As the ambient temperature approaches body temperature, radiation is no longer effective to dissipate heat. The body may actually pick up heat by conduction and convection. At high temperatures, evaporation becomes the only effective method of heat dissipation. High humidity seriously impairs heat dissipation, since evaporation occurs slowly.

HEAT DISORDERS

General Concepts

Heat illness is defined as increased CBT due to inadequate thermolysis. Most heat injury syndromes occur in individuals who are unacclimated. Signs of thermolysis include diaphoresis, increased skin temperature, and flushing. Signs of thermolytic inadequacy are an altered mentation or level of consciousness. Findings of dehydration often accompany thermolytic inadequacy.

As noted earlier, extremes of age markedly increase a person's sensitivity to both heat and cold. Underlying diabetes often leads to autonomic neuropathy. This interferes with heat regulation by affecting vasodilation and perspiration. Medications, especially antihistamines, also impair the body's ability to sweat and eliminate heat (Box 29-2).

Relevant contributing factors are the length and intensity of exposure. Ambient environmental conditions (humidity, wind) also play a significant role, whether the person is inside or outside.

It is essential that all persons exposed to warm environments maintain adequate fluid intake, regardless of thirst. Thirst is a poor indicator of dehydration, especially if the ambient temperature is not terribly warm (e.g., racing in an indoor swimming pool).

Persons who are acclimatized (used) to warm temperatures are less likely to suffer heat illness. Proper **acclimatization** requires at least a week of gradually increasing heat exposure. This results in increased sweat production (perspiration) but with a lower sodium (salt) concentration than usual. The result is an increase in fluid volume in the body.

Three types of heat-related syndromes can develop: heat cramps, heat exhaustion, and heat stroke.

Heat Cramps

Heat cramps are cramps or pains in the muscles, especially of the abdomen and lower extremities, that occur in a hot environment. They are due to dehydration and overexertion. Heat cramps are the most common of the heat injury syndromes. They do not usually lead to heat exhaustion or heat stroke.

The cause of heat cramps is excessive loss of salt and water in the sweat. Cramps usually occur in the young, unacclimatized individual who engages in exercise or heavy labor in hot climates and sweats profusely. Often, victims fail to drink adequate water.

Signs and symptoms of heat cramps include the following:

- Muscle twitching, followed by painful spasms, especially involving the lower extremities and abdomen
- Nausea and vomiting
- Weakness
- Diaphoresis

The care for a patient with heat cramps includes the following:

- Remove the patient to a cool environment.
- If permitted by local protocols, massage the affected muscles.
- If the patient is completely conscious, give sips of cool water. Avoid liquids that are extremely cold, salty, or sweet. This may cause nausea or vomiting.
- Start an intravenous (IV) line; a fluid bolus of 500 to 1000 mL of normal saline (10 mL/kg) will often decrease pain. Follow local protocols.
- *Do not* give the patient salt pills.
- Provide high-concentration oxygen by face mask (15 L/min flow).
- Transport the patient to the hospital.

CLINICAL NOTES

Although heat cramps do not necessarily lead to heat exhaustion, some patients have both. Assume that the patient is dehydrated, and treat accordingly.

Heat Exhaustion

Heat exhaustion is a more severe loss of fluid and salt than occurs in heat cramps, usually following exertion in a hot, humid environment. Some patients simply develop dehydration without further signs or symptoms of heat exhaustion. Fluid replacement therapy is similar for dehydration with or without heat exhaustion.

There is a high incidence of heat exhaustion in young children, individuals taking diuretics, and the debilitated who are unable to maintain an adequate oral fluid intake or those having prolonged bouts of diarrhea.

Signs and symptoms of heat exhaustion include the following:

- Lack of skin coloration (pallor)
- Profuse sweating
- Hypotension, especially with positional changes
- Headache, often with weakness and fatigue
- Thirst
- Normal or slightly elevated temperature

The care for a patient with heat exhaustion includes the following:

- Remove the patient from the hot environment to a cool environment (into the shade if that is the only alternative).
- Give high-concentration oxygen by face mask (15 L/min flow).
- Do not give anything by mouth.
- Start an IV line; give a fluid bolus as per local protocols.
- Monitor the electrocardiogram (ECG).
- Transport the patient to the hospital as soon as possible.

Symptoms that do not resolve rapidly with rest and supine positioning are an indicator of impending heat stroke and must be treated aggressively.

Heat Stroke

Heat stroke, or sun stroke, a failure of the body's temperature regulation mechanisms, is an extreme medical emergency. Heat stroke develops when the body is no longer able to get rid of heat. Unlike the victim of heat exhaustion, the person with heat stroke sweats very little or not at all. Usually, the skin is hot, red, and dry. As heat accumulates, the body temperature can reach a dangerously high level.

Some patients with heat stroke may have 1 or 2 days of lethargy, fatigue, weakness, nausea, vomiting, and dizziness before developing full-blown heat stroke **(classic heat stroke).** Other cases develop rapidly. These victims become confused or irrational, followed by loss of consciousness within a period of minutes. This usually occurs during a period of exercise or heavy exertion and is termed **exertional heat stroke,** such as during a marathon on a hot day.

Any individual who develops loss of consciousness in a hot environment should be suspected of having heat stroke. Signs and symptoms of heat stroke include the following:

- Altered level of consciousness
- Increased body temperature

- Minimal or no sweating
- Collapse
- Signs and symptoms of shock
- Nausea and vomiting
- Shortness of breath

CLINICAL NOTES

Heat exhaustion rarely results in significant changes of mental status. If a patient has signs of thermolysis and an altered level of consciousness, always consider heat stroke.

CLINICAL NOTES

Remember, there are other causes of elevated body temperature and altered mental status (e.g., meningitis, acute hyperthyroidism ["thyroid storm"]).

Rapid cooling is vital for the victim of heat stroke. Time is extremely important. If the victim's body temperature is not quickly lowered, permanent brain damage may result.

The care for a patient with heat stroke includes the following:

- Place the patient in a cool environment, such as an air-conditioned ambulance, as soon as possible.
- Remove the patient's clothing.
- Cool the patient immediately by applying ice packs to the neck, axillae (armpits), wrists, and groin. Other alternative methods for patient cooling are cold water immersion or misting with lukewarm water and fanning the patient. Research has suggested that misting and fanning may be the most effective means of rapid cooling both in the field and in the emergency department. Ice packs and cold water immersion may produce reflex vasoconstriction and shivering because of their effect on peripheral thermoreceptors. Follow local protocols.
- Give high-concentration oxygen by mask.
- Start IV fluids (normal saline or lactated Ringer's solution) at 250 to 500 mL/hr.
- Monitor the ECG.
- Wrap the patient with wet sheets if there is good ambient airflow present. Do not postpone transport in order to cool the patient in the field.
- Transport the patient to the hospital as soon as possible. Use the air-conditioner in your ambulance, as well as any available fans, to cool the patient. Depending on local protocols, IV sedation may be helpful if the patient develops uncontrollable shivering.

Summary of Care for Heat Illness

Regardless of the syndrome, always consider the following when caring for victims of heat illness:

- Remove the patient from the environment as soon as possible.
- When necessary, use any of several available methods for active cooling. Misting and fanning appear to be the most efficient from a thermodynamic (the physics of heat) point of view—evaporation releases more energy than melting (ice bath) or iced peritoneal lavage. Many experts prefer tepid water for cooling because of the decreased risk of reflex vasoconstriction and shivering (increases body temperature).
- Consider oral fluid therapy. Avoid oral fluids if the patient has an altered level of consciousness. Otherwise, cool (not cold!) water or an electyrolyte replacement solution may be helpful. Follow local protocols. Salt tablets are irritating to the stomach and may cause hypernatremia (excessive sodium elevation), nausea, and vomiting. Do not use them unless specifically instructed to do so by medical control.
- Consider IV fluid therapy. Other than in extremely mild cases, persons with heat illness are dehydrated. Thus they will benefit from the administration of normal saline. Follow local protocols.

COLD DISORDERS: HYPOTHERMIA

Generalized **hypothermia** is a condition in which the CBT is less than 35° C (95° F) as a result of either decreased production of heat or increased heat loss from the body. This may occur with or without the presence of external cold stress. Patients lose heat by the mechanisms defined above (radiation, convection, evaporation, and conduction).

Causes and Predisposing Factors

The three primary causes of hypothermia are cold water immersion, cold weather exposure, and **urban hypothermia,** meaning that it occurs in people who are inside but lack appropriate thermoregulation. Cold water immersion is the principal cause of death following boating accidents. With the exception of wool, wet clothing loses 90% of its insulating value. Thus individuals whose clothing is soaked are effectively nude. Cold weather exposure runs a close second in terms of incidence. Finally, cold stress among the aged, intoxicated, or debilitated can cause fatal hypothermia (urban hypothermia).

Conditions that may contribute to hypothermia include alcohol, the use of central nervous system depressants (such as barbiturates or alcohol), infections, endocrine system diseases (e.g., hypothyroidism, malnutrition, hypoglycemia), brain dysfunction, and burns. Hypothermia may also occur while skiing, camping, or hiking.

CLINICAL NOTES

Severe infection (sepsis) may actually result in hypothermia when the body's fever-producing centers are overwhelmed. This finding is common in persons who are relatively immobile, such as in a nursing home.

CLINICAL NOTES

Even warm water that is less than body temperature can lead to heat loss. Hypothermia due to water immersion is *not* limited to cold water.

Predisposing factors to hypothermia include the following (Box 29-3):
- Any elderly person living alone, especially one with chronic disease or who has suffered a stroke
- People who are intoxicated with alcohol
- Children younger than 1 year old

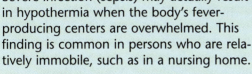

BOX 29-3

PREDISPOSING FACTORS FOR GENERALIZED HYPOTHERMIA

- Cold environments
- Immersion in water
- Age (elderly and the very young)
- Alcohol
- Shock
- Head or spinal cord injury
- Burns
- Generalized infection
- Diabetes
- Hypoglycemia
- Some medications and poisons

Stoy W: *Mosby's EMT-basic textbook,* St Louis, 1996, Mosby.

- Victims of submersion injury, especially in cold water
- Patients suffering head trauma, especially if the accident occurred outdoors
- Any patient with a history of trauma and subsequent blood loss with shock
- Getting lost or immobilized in cold weather, especially if the individual is wet

Many medications interfere with thermogenesis (heat production) and predispose the patient to hypothermia:
- Narcotics, phenothiazines, alcohol, and barbiturates
- Antiseizure medications
- Antihistamines and other allergy medications
- Antipsychotics, sedatives, and antidepressants
- Various pain medications, including aspirin, acetaminophen, and nonsteroidal antiinflammatory drugs (NSAIDs)

Note that some of these medications can also lead to heat intolerance (e.g., antihistamines, antipsychotics, phenothiazines).

Victims of hypothermia stop shivering when the body temperature is below 32.2° C (90° F). The severity of cold illness depends on the length and intensity of exposure, as well as on the ambient environmental conditions. Persons participating in outdoor activities should anticipate the possibility of hypothermia and prepare accordingly:
- By wearing proper clothing
- By getting proper rest
- By having adequate nutrition
- By limiting exposure time

Classification of Hypothermia

The severity of hypothermia is determined by the CBT and the presence of signs and symptoms (Table 29-2):
- **Mild hypothermia** is defined as the presence of signs and symptoms with a CBT greater than 32.2° C (90° F).
- **Severe hypothermia** is the presence of signs and symptoms with a CBT less than 32.2° C (90° F).
- **Compensated hypothermia** is the presence of signs and symptoms with a normal CBT. In this case the temperature is being maintained by the body's intrin-

TABLE 29-2

Vital Signs in Hypothermia

SIGN	EARLY HYPOTHERMIA	LATE HYPOTHERMIA
Pulse	Rapid	Slow and barely palpable, Irregular
Blood pressure	Normal	Low or absent
Breathing	Rapid	Shallow, slow, absent
Skin	Red	Pale, cyanotic, Stiff and hard
Pupils	Reactive	Sluggish

Stoy W: *Mosby's EMT-basic textbook,* St Louis, 1996, Mosby.

sic thermogenesis processes (metabolic processes that result in heat production). As energy stores (liver and muscle glycogen) are exhausted, the CBT will drop. The onset of hypothermia parallels the cause:

- *Acute onset*—Occurs rapidly, such as cold water immersion; without immediate rescue, chances of survival are low.
- *Subacute onset*—Comes on over minutes to hours, such as exposure during a winter hike. The prognosis may be better than with the acute onset form unless the patient is not rescued or treated for a long period of time.
- *Chronic onset*—The patient has been hypothermic for hours to days, depending on the circumstances. This often is due to urban hypothermia. An example is an elderly stroke victim who has fallen and is unable to move off of a tile floor.

Sometimes hypothermia is the primary cause of the patient's problem (e.g., cold water immersion). Other times, hypothermia is a sign of another disease (e.g., sepsis, hypoglycemia, hypothyroidism). The differentiation may be impossible in the field.

Signs and Symptoms

There is no reliable correlation between signs or symptoms and specific CBT. Common findings include the following:

- *Diminished coordination and psychomotor function*—Initially, patients lose fine motor control; as hypothermia progresses, their movements become slower and less coordinated.
- *Altered mentation*—As hypothermia progresses, the patient's level of consciousness decreases.
- *Cardiac irritability*—For years, J waves on the ECG have been described as a sign of hypothermia. This is no longer believed to be the case and should not be relied on. On the other hand, cardiac dysrhythmias commonly accompany hypothermia. Atrial fibrillation is the most common. As CBT continues to drop, bradydysrhythmias emerge. Ventricular fibrillation

may occur but is usually more common during the rewarming phase in a severely hypothermic patient (see later discussion).

Severe hypothermia mimics clinical death. It may be impossible to distinguish a patient who is still alive, but profoundly hypothermic, from the victim of a cardiac arrest. Patients who have been pronounced dead from hypothermia have actually awakened in the morgue.

Mental status and motor function changes caused by hypothermia are listed in Box 29-4.

Treatment

The first priority, after the ABCs (airway, breathing, and circulation), is to stop ongoing heat loss (Box 29-5):

- Remove the patient from the cold environment.
- If patients are wet, dry them as much as possible.
- Provide barriers from wind, vapor, and excessive moisture in the air.
- Insulate the patient.
  Specific care includes the following:
- Handle these patients gently. Rough handling may precipitate cardiac dysrhythmias.
- Perform cardiopulmonary resuscitation (CPR) as necessary. Check the pulse for 30 to 45 seconds before beginning chest compressions. Use normal chest compression and ventilation. Apply the automatic external defibrillator (AED) as per local protocols.
- Give high-concentration oxygen by mask (10 to 15 L/min).
- Give warm fluids if the patient is completely conscious. Observe the patient carefully to prevent aspiration. Do not give fluids before or during an air medical transport.
- Start an IV line. Hypothermic persons tend to be dehydrated. Cold stress causes peripheral vasoconstric-

---

BOX 29-4

MENTAL STATUS AND MOTOR FUNCTION CHANGES CAUSED BY HYPOTHERMIA

- Poor coordination
- Memory disturbances
- Reduced or absent sensation of touch
- Mood changes
- Joint or muscle pain
- Poor judgment (e.g., the patient may actually remove clothing)
- Less communicative
- Dizziness
- Speech difficulties

Stoy W: *Mosby's EMT-basic textbook,* St Louis, 1996, Mosby.

BOX 29-5

SUMMARY OF GENERAL PRINCIPLES FOR TREATING ALL HYPOTHERMIA PATIENTS

1. Remove the patient from the cold environment, and protect the patient from further heat loss.
2. Remove any wet clothing, and cover the patient with a blanket.
3. Handle the patient with extreme care. Avoid rough handling.
4. Administer high-flow oxygen. If possible, the oxygen should be warmed and humidified, using special equipment. If your EMS system warms and humidifies oxygen, follow your local protocols.
5. Do not allow the patient to eat or drink stimulants (chocolate, coffee, tea, etc.) or alcohol.
6. Do not massage the extremities.
7. Check for a pulse for 30 to 45 seconds before starting cardiopulmonary resuscitation (CPR).

Stoy W: *Mosby's EMT-basic textbook,* St Louis, 1996, Mosby.

tion and increased central volume. This results in a cold diuresis and hypovolemia in many patients. Consider a fluid bolus of 500 to 1000 cc normal saline or lactated Ringer's solution as rapidly as possible, if allowed by local protocols. IV fluids are especially helpful if they can be warmed to approximately 40° C (104° F) before administration.

- Care for other life-threatening injuries or conditions. Dress and protect frostbitten extremities.
- Remove wet clothing and maintain the patient in a warm, draft-free environment.
- Follow local protocols for rewarming. In some areas, rewarming is not attempted if the estimated time of arrival (ETA) to a hospital is less than 1 hour. Simply cover the patient with a blanket and transport him or her in a warm ambulance compartment to the hospital as soon as possible. Remove wet clothing before covering the patient.
- If local protocols include rewarming or if the ETA is greater than 1 hour, begin controlled rewarming with hot packs placed over the carotids, head, lateral thorax, and groin. Chemical hot packs can cause burns. Pad these with towels before placing them next to the skin.
- Administer warm (38.8° C to 40° C [102° F to 104° F]), moist oxygen to help prevent heat loss, if permitted by local protocols. There are several commercial devices available for this purpose.
- Warmed IV fluids (38.8° C to 40° C [102° F to 104° F]) serve the same purpose. The actual heat transferred to the patient is minimal, but such methods are crucial to prevent further heat loss.
- Warm water immersion and other methods (e.g., heat guns, lights) have little use in the out-of-hospital setting.
- Do not try to rewarm the patient's extremities. Active external rewarming causes reflex vasodilation and may lead to rewarming shock or afterdrop (Figure 29-2).

HELPFUL HINT

- Do *not* attempt to rewarm the extremities alone. This causes vasodilation of the arms and legs, resulting in a bolus of cold acidotic blood and waste products suddenly flowing into the central circulation. The patient's core temperature may actually decrease, this is called the **afterdrop phenomenon.** In addition, if the patient is somewhat dehydrated as a result of hypothermia **(cold diuresis),** then vasodilation will worsen intravascular volume status. The vasodilation and resultant hypotension that occurs with rewarming procedures, such as hot water immersion is called **rewarming shock.**

Advanced Cardiac Life Support Considerations

Cold may affect the potency of first-line cardiac drugs. Avoid these whenever possible until the patient is rewarmed—follow local protocols. There is no increased risk of inducing ventricular fibrillation (VF) from oro-tracheal or nasotracheal intubation as long as the patient is preoxygenated adequately. Rough handling, however, *can* induce VF.

The most common dysrhythmias in hypothermia-associated cardiac arrest are VF and asystole. The hypothermic heart is often resistant to defibrillation. The risks of VF are related to both the depth and the duration of hypothermia. It is generally impossible to electrically defibrillate a hypothermic heart that is colder than 30° C (86° F). Avoid lidocaine and procainamide in hypothermia, since they paradoxically lower the VF threshold, increasing resistance to defibrillation. VF often occurs as a patient is being rewarmed when the heart temperature rises above 30° C (86° F). Reasons for this are unknown.

The American Heart Association recommends that defibrillation be attempted as soon as possible. If a series of three consecutive shocks fails, continue CPR, aggressively rewarm the patient, and repeat defibrillation attempts periodically as the CBT rises.

Hypothermia and cardiac arrest in the face of near-drowning are common. Rapid lowering of the CBT during cold water immersion may protect the organs, especially the brain, during the period of anoxia. Following rescue, treat hypoxia first. Assume that all near-drowning patients are hypothermic until proven otherwise.

Transport

Gentle transportation is mandatory because of myocardial irritability. If the patient is in cardiac arrest, transport to a facility capable of performing cardiac bypass rewarming if possible, depending on local protocols.

NEAR-DROWNING

Drowning is defined as death due to asphyxiation during an immersion episode. It may occur with or without inhalation of the surrounding fluid. **Near-drowning** occurs when the process of drowning is interrupted or reversed—a submersion episode with at least transient recovery.

Causes

Causes of near-drowning are usually swimmer exhaustion, lack of skill, and panic. An acute medical incident during swimming (myocardial infarction, seizure, trauma) can result in acute incapacitation, leading to drowning. Hyperventilation in preparation for a long underwater swim can suppress the respiratory drive sufficiently to result in anoxia while submerged. Suicide attempts are a final way that near-drowning occurs. Often this is in association with jumping from a bridge or ledge, and multiple serious traumatic injuries are also present. Thus an immersion episode of unknown etiology warrants trauma management. Despite this, the single most important causative factor in adult drowning is the use of alcohol and mind-altering drugs. Studies have shown that anywhere from 35% to

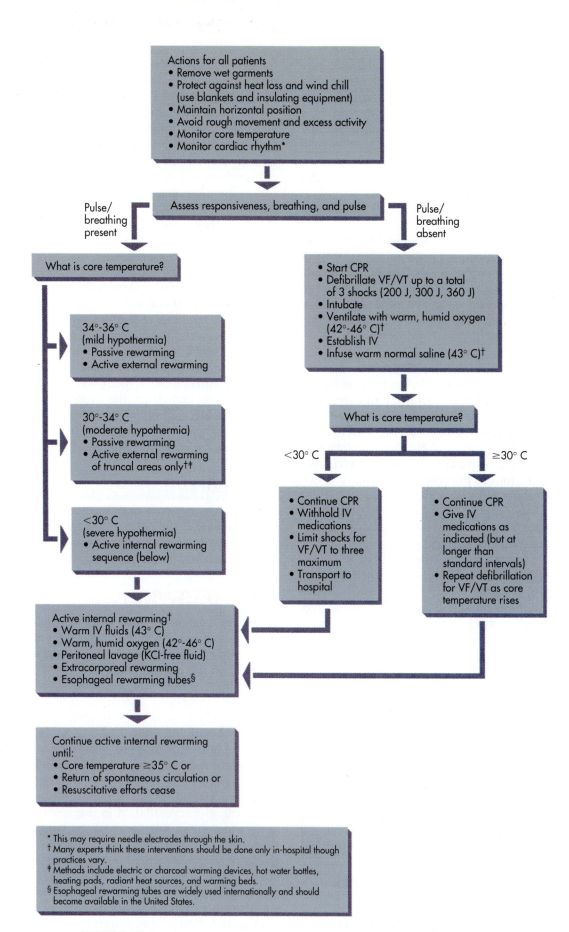

FIGURE 29-2 ▲ Algorithm for the treatment of hypothermia. (Reproduced with permission, CPR Issue of *JAMA* 268:2199-2275, 1992. Copyright © American Medical Association.)

75% of drowning victims have elevated blood alcohol levels.

Epidemiology

Affected individuals are often the very young or the aged. Males have a five to eight times greater incidence than females. Similarly, blacks have a three to five times greater frequency than do whites. The majority of drowning and near-drowning incidents *do not* occur in the ocean but rather in lakes, rivers, ponds, and back-yard pools. This is thought to be due to better surveillance and rescue techniques used by ocean lifeguards. Interestingly, many victims are competent swimmers; greater than 90% of incidents occur within 10 yards of shore, often in shallow water. Residential pools are a significant cause, especially in children, as are bathtubs. Spas and hot tubs are becoming increasingly more involved in drowning. This is likely because of their widespread popularity and the effects of alcohol use while bathing in them.

Types of Drowning

There are three types of drowning. **"Dry" drowning** encompasses 10% to 20% of victims. Here, asphyxiation is caused by anoxia as a result of laryngeal spasm, which prevents the entrance of water, as well as air, into the lungs. This leads to cerebral anoxia, edema, and unconsciousness. These victims have the best chance of survival. **"Wet" drowning** involves 80% to 90% of cases. In this type of drowning, the victim makes a violent respiratory effort and fluid fills the lungs. **Secondary drowning** is defined as the recurrence of respiratory distress (usually in the form of pulmonary edema or aspiration pneumonia) after successful recovery from the initial incident. It can occur from a few minutes to up to 4 days later (Figure 29-3).

Special Considerations for Care

Many immersion victims are hypothermic. Cold stimulation of the vagus nerve may lead to decreased heart rate and unconsciousness. This can lead to drowning and is potentiated by the presence of alcohol in the blood. On the positive side, cold may decrease cerebral metabolism and prolong survival.

Seawater Versus Freshwater Drowning

Differences between seawater and freshwater drowning have been overemphasized in the past and are based primarily on animal work. Although the end points are the same, the mechanisms of lung damage from seawater and freshwater near-drowning are very different. Seawater is hypertonic to blood (three to four times as

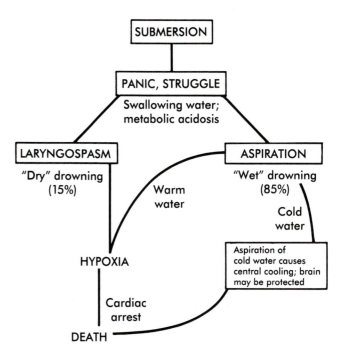

FIGURE 29-3 ▲ Progression of the drowning incident. (From Auerbach PS: *Management of wilderness and environmental emergencies,* ed 2, St Louis, 1989, Mosby.)

concentrated in electrolytes and other osmotically active particles); its presence in the lung causes the influx of hypotonic serum. This fills the alveoli and leads to a large shunt with profound hypoxemia (i.e., blood cannot exchange oxygen and carbon dioxide with filled alveoli, and they are bypassed).

Freshwater aspiration, on the other hand, leads to a washout of surfactant. This compound is required for the lung tissue to maintain its elasticity. Loss of surfactant results in collapse of alveoli with subsequent hypoxemia. Thus aspiration of either seawater or fresh water decreases pulmonary compliance and results in pulmonary edema and hypoxia (Figure 29-4).

Cerebral hypoxia often precipitates neurogenic pulmonary edema, worsening an already bad situation. The end points in near-drowning, no matter *what* type of water is involved, are metabolic acidosis, pulmonary edema, and aspiration injuries.

Patient Assessment

When examining victims of near-drowning, it is important to note that they may appear initially to be normal. Usual signs and symptoms of problems include the following:
- Progressive dyspnea
- Wheezing or other extraneous lung sounds
- Tachycardia
- Cyanosis
- Chest pains or mental confusion (may be present)
- Coma, respiratory, or cardiac arrest (can occur)

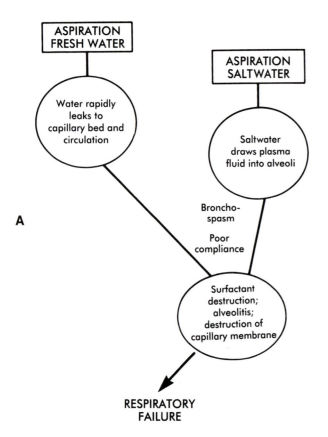

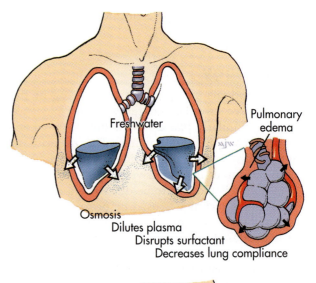

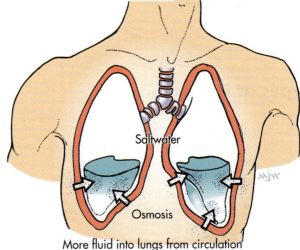

FIGURE 29-4 ▲ **A,** Pulmonary effects of water aspiration. **B,** The effects of fresh water and saltwater on the lungs. (**A,** From Auerbach PS: *Management of wilderness and environmental emergencies,* ed 2, St Louis, 1989, Mosby. **B,** From American College of Emergency Physicians; Pons PT, Cason D, chief editors: *Paramedic field care: a complaint-based approach,* St Louis, 1997, Mosby for ACEP.)

The temperature (which *must* be taken rectally at some point in time) may be high, low, or normal. This is because of either heat loss secondary to hypothermia or hyperpyrexia (increased temperature) due to hypothalamic injury (the hypothalamus is the portion of the brain that regulates temperature) from hypoxia.

Treatment

Mouth-to-mouth respirations may be given in the water after clearing the airway. Remove the victim from the water as soon as possible. If there is any possibility of neck injury (e.g., in a diving accident), stabilize the neck before removing the patient from the water (Figure 29-5). Start CPR if required. Perform the following measures:

- Administer high-flow oxygen (10 to 15 L/min by mask) *regardless* of the patient's condition.
- Perform ECG monitoring.
- For saltwater victims only: perform positional drainage of lungs (head-dependent position). This recommendation is somewhat controversial and not universally accepted. Follow local protocols.

- Start an IV infusion of normal saline or lacted Ringer's solution at a TKO ("to keep open") rate.
- Place the patient on a cardiac monitor.

Some have recommended the immediate application of a subdiaphragmatic thrust (the Heimlich maneuver) to all near-drowning patients. Although this is still controversial, the current recommendation of the American Heart Association is that this be used only if rescue breathing fails to successfully resuscitate the victim.

Complications

Several complications can occur following near-drowning. Persistent hypoxemia is common and usually multifactorial. Infection, especially pneumonia, may occur even several days later. Renal failure has been reported but is not overly common. The most bothersome complication is a persistent neurological deficit. The best predictor of severity is the time to the first spontaneous gasp following removal from the water. The shorter this period, the better the neurological prognosis. Patients

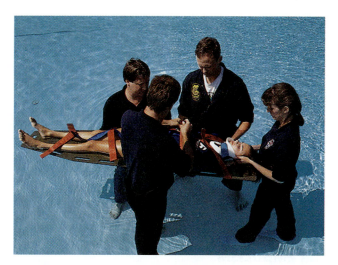

FIGURE 29-5 ▲ **Fully immobilize a conscious patient with a suspected spinal injury while the patient is still in the water.**

taking more than 1 hour for this to occur (if it does at all) have a bleak prognosis.

Pearls to Remember

The following "clinical pearls" must be kept in mind when dealing with near-drowning victims:

- Be prepared for vomiting at any time.
- Transport *all* submersion victims. Even if patients initially appear to be fine, they can deteriorate rapidly. Pulmonary edema is especially likely. Late deterioration occurs in about 1 out of 20 near-drowning victims. It usually occurs within 4 hours, but with saltwater immersion, latent periods of up to 46 hours have been reported.
- Beware of neck injuries—they often go unrecognized. It is best to treat any unconscious submersion victim with spinal immobilization.
- Hypothermic victims are not dead until they are "warm and dead." Follow local protocols.

LOCALE-SPECIFIC PROBLEMS

Diving Emergencies

Diving is gaining rapidly in popularity throughout the country. Because of the transportation conveniences of our society, it is also possible for individuals to have the rapid mobility necessary for some postdiving problems to occur (such as those caused by flying in an airplane shortly after diving). This section is not designed to be an extensive treatise on diving emergencies but rather a brief review of potential problems that may be seen by any EMT–I. The types of problems discussed are related to the breathing of compressed air underwater.

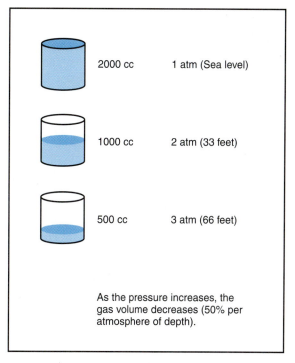

As the pressure increases, the gas volume decreases (50% per atmosphere of depth).

FIGURE 29-6 ▲ **Barotrauma. Boyle's law of gases as applied to diving.**

DIVING PHYSIOLOGY

When diving, an individual is exposed to atmospheric pressures greater than those on land. This results in contraction of the gases in the lungs. As a rough estimate, pressure increases about 1 pound per square inch (psi) with each 2 feet of depth. To compensate, pressurized (compressed) air must be taken in from *self*-contained *underwater breathing apparatus* **(scuba)** gear so that the lungs will not collapse. The events discussed here can occur with any source of compressed air used for breathing: scuba gear, a hose from the surface, a bucket, or air trapped in a submerged car.

The term *atmosphere (atm)* is used as an arbitrary unit of pressure. At sea level the pressure on the body is 1 atm. At 33 feet of water depth (34 feet in fresh water), it is 2 atm; at 66 feet it is 3 atm, etc. *Boyle's law* states that the volume of a gas varies inversely with the absolute pressure. In other words, as the pressure increases, the gas volume decreases. If a pair of lungs contains 2000 cc of air at sea level, this volume will decrease with descent to 1000 cc at 33 feet, 500 cc at 66 feet, etc. (Figure 29-6).

If a scuba tank is added to normal lungs at sea level, the volume of air in the lungs stays constant as the diver forcefully inhales supplemental air from the tank. Thus the volume in the lungs remains constant, regardless of depth (assuming proper breathing techniques).

If the diver ascends but forgets to exhale on the way up, the pressure will decrease with ascent and the volume of gas "trapped" (because of failure of exhalation) in the lungs will expand. Thus if a diver at 33 feet with a combined lung volume of 4000 cc ascends and fails to exhale, the total lung volume at sea level will be 8000 cc.

Other hazards are also associated with breath holding during diving. As one descends, more oxygen is made available to the tissue because of the increased pressure. At depths, one's breath-holding ability is markedly increased. With ascent, the drop in pressure of the tissue oxygen supply decreases sharply. This may lead to a sudden loss of consciousness, on surfacing, in a diver who has pushed limits at depths in terms of improper breathing. This has been called "shallow water blackout." Thus a cardinal rule of scuba diving is that a diver must never hold his or her breath while underwater

Henry's law states that at a constant temperature, the solubility of any gas in a liquid is almost directly proportional to the pressure of the liquid. The deeper one dives, the greater the pressure and the greater the soluble gas (i.e., nitrogen) that becomes dissolved in the blood and tissue fluids. The reverse occurs on ascent. It may take a much longer period of time for the gas to revaporize on ascent than it did to originally dissolve in the fluid.

GENERAL PRINCIPLES

It is extremely important to take an adequate history on any patient potentially suffering an emergency related to diving. The first question that must be asked is, Did the victim breathe compressed air underwater? Remember, this can occur with scuba gear, a surface hose, a bucket, or within a submerged car. Make certain the patient was not just snorkeling and that he or she is not really a victim of near-drowning.

CLINICAL NOTES

Always make certain the patient breathed compressed air underwater. If not, you may be dealing with a near-drowning victim.

A detailed history of the entire diving day is necessary. If the patient needs to be sent to a hyperbaric (de-compression) chamber, this information will be vital. The number of dives, depth of each, and bottom time are important. The type of equipment used, as well as the diver's activities, should be noted (hard work increases the risk of certain problems). Environmental factors, such as the type of water and the conditions, as well as the type of water entry, may be significant. It is useful to know if the diver was with a companion (who should then also be questioned) and exactly what type of gas mixture was being breathed. It also needs to be determined whether in-water recompression was attempted. Finally, it should be noted if the diver flew in an airplane or jogged before developing symptoms (Box 29-6).

AIR EMBOLISM

Air embolism is defined as the presence of air bubbles in the central circulation. It is the most serious of diving-related emergencies. The cause is breath holding on ascent with resultant expansion of air in the lungs. As the lung tissue expands, alveoli eventually rupture, resulting in the escape of air. Although it may occur, pneumothorax is not necessarily a consequence of alveolar rupture. Interstitial air occurs first and can track anywhere in the body, including the pleural space (pneumothorax), pericardial space (pneumomediastinum), and distant sites via the bloodstream (air embolus) (Box 29-7). Since divers most commonly ascend in a vertical position, bubbles of air in the bloodstream often travel to the brain. This can occur during an ascent from as little as 4 feet of water.

Air embolism may also occur in divers with lung infection, lung cysts, tumors, scar tissue, mucus plugs (asthma), and obstructive lung disease. These areas trap air that cannot be exhaled properly during ascent. Smokers, for unknown reasons, have an increased risk.

Signs and Symptoms—Signs and symptoms of air embolism include chest tightness and shortness of breath. Pink, frothy sputum may be noted coming from the nose and mouth. Vertigo, paresthesias, paralysis, seizures, and loss of consciousness may be noted in cerebral emboli. Findings tend to appear suddenly during or immediately after surfacing and may resemble a stroke. Signs and symptoms of tension pneumothorax may be present.

BOX 29-6

DIVING HISTORY

- Number of dives, depth, bottom time
- Type of equipment
- Diver's activities
- Environmental factors
- Type of water
- Type of water entry
- Companion
- Gas mixture
- In-water recompression
- Flew or jogged before developing symptoms

BOX 29-7

PATHOPHYSIOLOGY OF AIR EMBOLI

Breath holding on ascent leads to the following:
- Overexpansion of air in the lungs
- Air trapping (localized or generalized)
- Rupture of lung tissue
- Escape of air into the bronchial circulation, which then passes through the heart, entering the central circulation
- Pneumothorax (may or may not occur)

Treatment—The treatment of suspected air embolism is as follows:

- High-flow oxygen (mask, 10 to 15 L/min; 100% if possible). Beware of using positive-pressure devices with the possibility of an untreated pneumothorax.
- Emergency needle thoracostomy if tension pneumothorax is present. Follow local protocols.
- Trendelenberg position (feet elevated) with the patient on his or her left side (left lateral decubitus position). This traps air within the heart and prevents it from traveling to the brain, causing cerebral embolism.
- Recompression. This should be attempted as soon as possible. The National Diving Accident Network (DAN) provides a 24-hour number (919-684-8111) for assistance and referral. They will accept collect calls in an emergency situation.

NITROGEN NARCOSIS

Nitrogen narcosis, often referred to as **rapture of the depths,** is the development of an apathetic, slightly euphoric mental state resulting from the narcotic effect of dissolved nitrogen. This effect is analogous to excessive ethanol levels. The cause is Henry's law.

As the pressure increases (i.e., the depth of descent), so does the amount of dissolved nitrogen (which is normally 79% of room air). The greater the depth, the greater the amount of nitrogen dissolved and the greater the "high" achieved. Mild effects may be noted in depths of as little as 50 feet. This problem has been referred to as "martini's law": the mental effects of each 50 feet of descent, while breathing compressed air, are approximately equivalent to those of one dry martini. As depth increases, so does the severity of symptoms.

Patient Assessment—At 125 to 150 feet, narcosis usually begins; at 150 to 200 feet, the diver exhibits drowsiness and decreased mental functioning; at 200 to 250 feet, there is decreased strength and coordination; and at 300 feet, the diver is essentially "useless." At depths between 250 and 400 feet, unconsciousness and death can occur. Generally speaking, recreational divers should descend no deeper than 100 to 150 feet. Commercial divers often use a mixture of helium and oxygen, rather than nitrogen and oxygen (room air), enabling them to dive far deeper without the risk of nitrogen narcosis.

Treatment—The treatment of nitrogen narcosis involves gradual ascent to shallower water. Assistance from one's diving companion is usually necessary. *(One should never dive alone!)* This problem may be prevented by avoiding dives to excess depths.

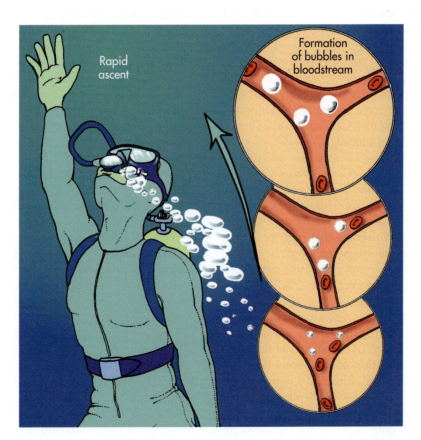

FIGURE 29-7 ▲ Rapid changes in atmospheric pressure result in decompression sickness. (From American College of Emergency Physicians; Pons PT, Cason D, chief editors: *Paramedic field care: a complaint-based approach,* St Louis, 1997, Mosby for ACEP.)

DECOMPRESSION SICKNESS

Decompression sickness is an illness occurring during or after ascent secondary to rapid release of nitrogen bubbles (Figure 29-7). Colloquially, it is called **the "bends."** The cause is a sudden decrease in environmental pressure from a too rapid ascent. This releases previously absorbed excess nitrogen from the tissues into the bloodstream in the form of bubbles.

Pathophysiology—Multiple factors appear to be responsible for the development of decompression sickness in one diver but not in another when both have had equal bottom times. Many believe that decompression sickness occurs when the tissues become "supersaturated" with inert gas, such as nitrogen. As pressure is reduced, these gases will leave via the lungs. This takes a while, however, and if the pressure changes too rapidly, the "unloading process" will fall behind. Thus the partial pressure of gas in the tissue far exceeds that of the ambient pressure, and supersaturation exists. Rapid pressure changes favor the formation of bubbles as tissue supersaturated with gas attempts to release it and equilibrate the pressure. Only small degrees of this can be tolerated.

The "coke bottle" analogy helps explain supersaturation. Before the bottle cap is removed, gases are dissolved quietly in solution. Removing the cap leads to a sudden drop in pressure and a state of supersaturation with resultant bubbling. Current research suggests that more may actually be involved than the physical occlusive effects of gas bubbles.

The microcirculation of the spinal cord venous plexus is especially favorable for the formation of gas bubbles. This may explain why patients with decompression sickness tend to have spinal cord symptoms that resolve with time; venous occlusion has a far better prognosis than does arterial blockage.

Most cases of decompression sickness are due to repetitive diving (i.e., more than one dive in a 12-hour period). It takes about 12 hours for a liquid to become completely desaturated of a gas. Thus cumulative effects occur when a diver enters the water more than one time within this period. Within the first hour of ascent, 85% of the signs and symptoms occur. Very few people develop new symptoms or initial symptoms more than 3 hours following ascent. However, up to 1% of patients may present later than 24 hours.

Patient Assessment—There are a variety of symptoms that may affect many organ systems. These result from both the physical effects of nitrogen bubbles in the lung tissues and the activation of numerous body inflammatory mechanisms (e.g., kinin and complement systems). These responses lead to a decrease in tissue perfusion and ischemia. A vicious circle can result, with decreased perfusion leading to tissue hypoxia and interstitial edema, which further decrease perfusion.

- A blotchy red rash on the torso may be present. The patient may complain of burning, prickly, or mottled skin (the "itches"). This is due to subcutaneous air.
- Pain in the legs or joints (the "bends") is present in 90% of cases. The most commonly involved joint is the shoulder, although multiple joints may be involved in serious cases. Recurrent pain is common.
- Dizziness (the "staggers"), vertigo, and visual or hearing abnormalities may be noted in up to 5% of patients.
- Paralysis occurs in 2% of victims; permanent sequelae are possible although uncommon. The development of spinal cord manifestations may be preceded by abdominal pain.
- Shortness of breath (the "chokes") may occur in up to 2% of patients. A fiery red pharynx (back of the throat) is noted, and there may be pleuritic chest pain and a nonproductive cough. Spinal cord symptoms commonly accompany this, warranting careful neurologic evaluation.
- Collapse is present in 0.5% to 1% of victims. Death, if it occurs, is usually from a cardiovascular cause. A delayed shock syndrome with pulmonary edema (adult respiratory distress syndrome) can occur 1 to 3 hours later.

Factors that increase the severity of the signs and symptoms include the following: extremes of water temperature, increasing age, and obesity. Fatigue, poor conditioning, alcohol ingestion, and heavy work during diving may also play a role. A previous case of decompression sickness may increase one's susceptibility to recurrence.

Treatment—The following are general recommendations; always adhere to local protocols:

- Contact DAN to arrange for immediate transportation to a decompression chamber.
- Provide total bed rest in the combined Trendelenberg and left lateral decubitus position. Transport and *keep* the patient in this position at all times.
- Administer 100% oxygen via mask.
- Start an IV infusion of normal saline at a TKO rate; increase as necessary for hypotension (which is common if the condition is severe). In serious cases, judicious fluid administration may help hemoconcentration. Do not use 5% dextrose in water (D_5W) alone (because of the possibility of increased intracranial pressure).
- Place the patient on a cardiac monitor.
- If a decompression chamber is not available, the patient can be monitored closely, following the steps outlined above. This is *not* recommended.
- Some experts recommend giving two aspirin (325 mg each) as an antiplatelet agent to conscious patients. There is no uniform consensus on this matter. Follow local protocols.

Pearls to Remember—Keep the following in mind:

- Any complaint of joint soreness (in the absence of obvious injury) 24 to 48 hours after a dive should be considered for decompression therapy. At a minimum, a diving medicine (hyperbaric medicine) consultation should be obtained.
- Decompression sickness can occur at depths of less than 33 feet. It is more likely if the diver has been below that depth with sufficient bottom time to permit

supersaturation of the body tissues with inert nitrogen gas. One should suspect air embolism in symptomatic divers who have been at depths of less than 33 feet and whose symptoms occur immediately after ascent.

- It is unwise to fly in an unpressurized aircraft for at least 24 hours following a dive. Commercial aircrafts pressurize their cabins to about 8000 feet. Thus exact waiting times vary, depending on the bottom time.
- If the patient needs to be evacuated by air, the pilot should be instructed to fly as close to the ground as safely possible (1000 feet is recommended). If the aircraft is pressurized, the cabin pressure should be kept as near to sea level as possible. It is best to use an airplane that is capable of cabin pressurization to 1 atm (Lear Jet or Hercules C 130). Be sure to bring the patient's equipment along to give to the hyperbaric medical experts.
- If paralysis involves both sides of the body (i.e., both hands, legs, etc.), suspect decompression trauma with a spinal cord syndrome. If loss of sensation or motion is unilateral, the odds favor an air embolus to the brain.
- Late recompression (even 10 days or more after the incident) of decompression sickness problems can be accomplished with relief of symptoms and morbidity. Long delays are common in the lay diving population because of the lack of recognition of symptoms and "wishful thinking" that symptoms will "go away."

"SQUEEZE" SYMPTOMS

"Squeeze" is defined as severe pain caused by compression of air trapped in hollow "chambers." The cause is breath holding on descent or air getting trapped in a hollow cavity. These symptoms occur when the outside pressure is greater than that inside the body.

Patient Assessment—Although not the most severe potential adverse effect of diving, "squeeze" symptoms are the most common. They may occur in these areas:

- *Ears, sinuses*—Pain is secondary to blocked eustachian tubes, sinus ostia (openings), or external ear canals. The trapped air is then compressed, with resultant painful bulging of the tympanic membrane (eardrum). This usually occurs early in the dive. Rupture of the eardrum can occur. If the diver is bareheaded, cold water can rush in, markedly affecting one's balance and leading to vertigo and nausea. Devastating circumstances may result.
- *Lungs, airways, and thoracic cavity*—Pain usually occur during "free diving" (diving without a compressed air source). This is rare because this practice is not common. If symptoms develop (crushing chest pain), they are often at great depths.
- *Teeth (cavities, dental abscesses)*—Hollow areas, such as cavities and abscesses, trap gas and may be subject to "squeeze" symptoms. This can result in excruciating pain and disorientation.

- *Added air spaces*—At times, severe bruising of the skin can occur because of face masks and wet suits. The eyes and eyelid linings are the most susceptible to damage, especially if only goggles, which have no method of pressure equalization, are used for anything but very shallow diving. A tight diving suit covering the external ear canal can result in "squeeze" of the external ear canal, with possible tympanic membrane rupture.
- *"Gut" squeeze*—This does not occur commonly because the structures of the gastrointestinal tract have supple walls that are easily compressed. Expansion within the gastrointestinal tract with ascent may lead to discomfort, however. Significant flatulence or diarrhea can occur at this time. This usually occurs in novice divers who swallow a lot of air or in those who ate heartily before diving.

Signs and symptoms include pain, edema, rupture, and bleeding, depending on the area involved.

Treatment—The treatment is gradual ascent to shallower depths, reassurance, and analgesics as needed. In the event of suspected rupture of the eardrum, medical evaluation should be performed promptly.

High-Altitude Illness

High-altitude illness occurs as a result of decreased atmospheric pressure, resulting in hypoxia. Many different activities may be associated with these syndromes, including mountain climbing, travel to higher elevations on vacation, and flying in unpressurized aircraft. The most common altitude syndromes are acute mountain sickness (AMS), high-altitude pulmonary edema (HAPE), and high-altitude cerebral edema (HACE). Emergency care is similar for all forms and includes the following:

- Maintenance of airway, breathing, and circulation
- Descent to a lower altitude
- Appropriate transport to the appropriate facility for further evaluation (Box 29-8)

ACUTE MOUNTAIN SICKNESS

Acute mountain sickness (AMS) occurs after rapid ascent by an unacclimatized person to altitudes in excess of 8000 feet. Symptoms usually develop within 4 to 6 hours of reaching altitude and may last 3 to 4 days. They include the following:

- Dizziness
- Headache
- Irritability
- Breathlessness
- Euphoria

Older persons and those with underlying cardiac or respiratory disorders may suffer pulmonary edema or heart failure. If AMS becomes severe, the victim may experience an altered level of consciousness and impaired judgment. Coma often follows.

BOX 29-8

SIGNS AND SYMPTOMS OF HIGH-ALTITUDE ILLNESS

ACUTE MOUNTAIN SICKNESS (AMS)

Headache (most common symptom) attributed to subacute cerebral edema or to spasm or dilation of cerebral blood vessels secondary to hypocapnia or hypoxia

Malaise	Irritability
Anorexia	Impaired memory
Vomiting	Dyspnea on exertion
Dizziness	

HIGH-ALTITUDE PULMONARY EDEMA (HAPE)

Shortness of breath	Generalized weakness
Dyspnea	Lethargy
Cough (with or without frothy sputum)	Disorientation

HIGH-ALTITUDE CEREBRAL EDEMA

Headache	Drowsiness
Ataxia	Stupor
Confusion	Coma
Hallucinations	

Sanders MJ: *Mosby's paramedic textbook,* ed 2, St Louis, 2000, Mosby.

HIGH-ALTITUDE PULMONARY EDEMA

High-altitude pulmonary edema (HAPE) results from increased pulmonary artery pressures that develop in response to hypoxia. This leads to the release of various vasoactive substances that increase alveolar permeability. Fluid leaks into the alveoli, and pulmonary edema occurs. Symptoms often begin 24 to 72 hours after exposure. At times, they are preceded by exertion. They include the following:

- Shortness of breath
- Rapid respiratory rate (tachypnea)
- Cyanosis

HIGH-ALTITUDE CEREBRAL EDEMA

High-altitude cerebral edema (HACE) is due to increased intracranial pressure and is the most severe form of acute high-altitude illness. Patients have signs of AMS and a progressively worsening level of consciousness. Progression from mild AMS to HACE and unconsciousness usually takes 1 to 3 days. This progression may occur, however, within hours of altitude exposure. Not all patients with AMS progress to HACE; it is currently impossible to predict who will. There is much overlap between HACE and severe AMS—it is not necessary to distinguish the difference. HACE rapidly progresses to coma and death without treatment. Thus the patient must be appropriately transported to an appropriate facility as soon as possible.

LOCAL COLD INJURIES: FROSTBITE

Frostbite is the formation of ice crystals within the tissues. These crystals damage the blood vessels and other tissues. Eventually, frostbitten tissues may die. The worst tissue damage occurs when an area freezes, thaws, and then refreezes. **Trench foot** is a condition resembling frostbite that historically affected the feet of soldiers who kept their feet in wet socks and shoes for long periods. Evaluation and treatment are similar.

Patient Assessment

The signs and symptoms of frostbite depend on the stage at which the patient is seen:

- Initially the frostbitten extremity appears waxy, yellowish white, or bluish white (Figure 29-8).
- Whether the skin of a frostbite victim feels soft or firm to frozen depends on the severity of injury. In severe frostbite the area is hard to the touch, cold, and insensitive to pain.
- With rewarming, the extremity becomes flushed with a red to purple-burgundy color.
- Swelling appears within hours of thawing and may persist for days to weeks.
- Following thawing, fluid-filled blisters may form.
- After 9 to 15 days, a black, hard scar will form over the frostbitten area.
- If tissue death occurs, the area will appear moist and weeping with pus (Figure 29-9).

Generally, there is an initial cold sensation that subsides, leading to numbness. The patient may say that the affected area feels "like a stump." This feeling is due to lack of oxygen. Following thawing, there is severe, throbbing pain. This pain may last for several weeks. There may also be tingling and burning secondary to nerve damage that lasts for 3 to 4 weeks. Pain following thawing tends to be severe, requiring strong medications for relief.

Other symptoms may develop up to 4 years later. These consist of cold feet, excess sweating, and numbness. The symptoms are worse in the winter. Patients who have had one bout of frostbite develop an exaggerated response to cold and are therefore more susceptible to another episode.

Treatment

The care for a patient with frostbite includes the following:

- Rule out the presence of other significant injuries or illnesses such as total-body hypothermia, fractures, or bleeding.
- If the patient has total-body hypothermia, do not care for a frostbitten extremity until the body's core temperature is normal.
- Transport the patient to the hospital as soon as possible.
- Protect the involved site by covering it and handling it gently.

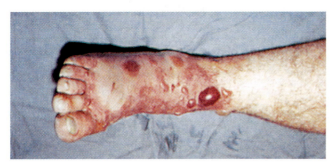

FIGURE 29-8 ▲ Edema and blister formation 24 hours after frostbite injury in an area covered by a tightly fitted boot. (From Auerbach PS: *Wilderness medicine,* ed 4, St Louis, 2001, Mosby.)

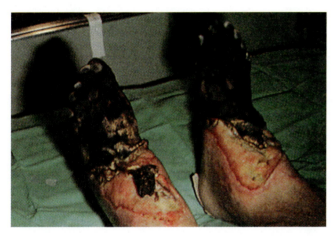

FIGURE 29-9 ▲ Gangrenous necrosis 6 weeks after a frostbite injury. (From Auerbach PS: *Wilderness medicine,* ed 4, St Louis, 2001, Mosby.)

- Do not break any blisters. Cover them with dry, sterile dressings.
- Do not allow the patient to smoke. This constricts blood vessels and aggravates hypoxemia to the involved area.
- Do not rewarm frostbite in the field. An exception is if a limb is frozen to an object that cannot be moved.

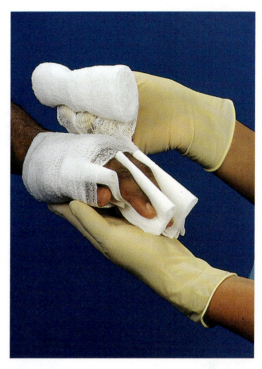

FIGURE 29-10 ▲ Place dressings between the fingers affected by local cold injury. (Stoy W: *Mosby's EMT-basic textbook,* St Louis, 1996, Mosby.)

In this case, warm the area just enough to move the patient.
- Do not rub a frostbitten area, especially with ice or snow. This can cause severe tissue damage (Figure 29-10).

SUMMARY

Important points to remember from this chapter include the following:
- The environment has a significant impact on the human body and its metabolism. The body maintains homeostasis within a fairly wide range of temperature and pressure. Disease occurs when heat gain or loss exceeds the body's capacity to compensate *or* pressure changes exceed the body's capacity to compensate.
- Features common to different environmental emergencies include the following:
  - Abnormal core body temperatures
  - Signs of metabolic decompensation (e.g., failure to sweat, loss of shivering)
  - Development of shock in late disease
- Based on these principles, management in the field is primarily aimed at stabilization of the patient:
  - Removal of the abnormal environmental influence
  - Support of metabolic decompensation (e.g., airway control, IV fluids)
  - Appropriate and timely transport to the appropriate treatment facility

30

Behavioral Emergencies and Substance Abuse

Key Terms

Abnormal Behavior

Alcohol Abuse

Alcohol Withdrawal Seizures

Alcoholism

Behavior

Behavioral Emergency

Body Language

Delirium Tremens (DTs)

Depressants

Depression

Drug Abuse

Drug Addiction

Drug Misuse

Drug Withdrawal

Drugs

Hallucinogens

Maladaptive Behavior

Narcotics

Neurosis

Psychosis

Shakes

Stimulants

Suicide

Suicide Attempt

Suicide Gesture

Volatile Chemicals

▪▪▪ CASE HISTORY

EMT–Is Keegan and Bravo are dispatched to 2135 Sunrise Drive at 5:17 PM for a "possible overdose, 17-year-old female." They arrive in 12 minutes and are directed to a second-floor bedroom by the patient's mother.

The mother says, "I came home from work and found her lying in bed. I couldn't wake her up; that's when I called 9-1-1."

EMT–I Bravo begins the initial assessment and treatment for the unresponsive teenager while EMT–I Keegan continues to ask the patient's mother questions and takes a quick look around the bedroom for clues to the patient's condition.

"Has anything like this ever happened before?" EMT–I Keegan asks.

"No. Never," the mother responds.

"Does she have any medical conditions that require a doctor's care?" EMT–I Keegan asks.

"No."

"Is she a diabetic?"

"No."

"Is she allergic to anything?"

"Penicillin. But she isn't ill. She hasn't needed any medications."

EMT–I Bravo has placed the patient in the left lateral recumbent position and applied oxygen and the electrocardiogram (ECG) monitor. He is preparing to start an intravenous (IV) line of normal saline solution. EMT–I Keegan notes that the pulse oximetry shows 92% saturation.

EMT–I Keegan takes a look at the patient's dresser and notices two empty pill bottles, and then she sees a handwritten note next to them:

Dear Mommy and Daddy,

I'm sorry. I love you. Please don't be too mad at me. I can't tell you everything.

Love,

Susie

LEARNING OBJECTIVES ✓

CHAPTER GOAL

Upon completion of this chapter, the EMT-Intermediate will be able to use assessment findings to form a field impression and implement a management plan for patients with behavioral or drug abuse emergencies.

Cognitive Objectives

As an EMT-Intermediate you should be able to do the following:

- Distinguish between normal and abnormal behavior.
- Discuss the pathophysiology of behavioral emergencies.
- Define the terms *active listening, anxiety, behavior, behavioral emergency, body language, confusion, depression,* and *overt behavior.*
- Discuss appropriate measures to ensure the safety of the patient, EMT–I, and others.
- Identify techniques for a physical assessment on a patient with behavioral problems.
- Describe therapeutic interviewing techniques for gathering information from a patient with a behavioral emergency.
- List factors that may indicate a patient is at increased risk for suicide.
- Describe methods for managing patients with behavioral emergencies.
- Describe circumstances in which relatives, bystanders, and others should be removed from the scene.
- Describe medical-legal considerations for managing a patient with a behavioral emergency.
- List situations in which an EMT–I is expected to transport a patient against his or her will.
- Describe methods of restraint that may be necessary in managing a patient with a behavioral emergency.
- Identify four conditions that may mimic alcohol or substance abuse.
- Describe alcohol withdrawal syndrome.
- Identify five major classes of abused drugs.
- Describe the care given to patients suspected of alcohol or drug abuse.
- Formulate a field impression based on the assessment findings.
- Develop a patient management plan based on the field impression.

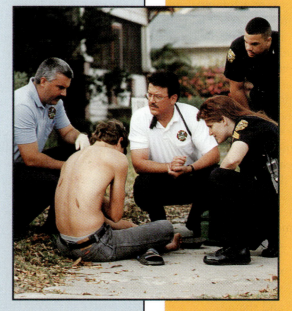

Affective Objectives

As an EMT-Intermediate you should be able to do the following:

- Advocate for empathetic and respectful treatment for individuals experiencing behavioral or drug abuse emergencies.

Psychomotor Objectives

As an EMT-Intermediate you should be able to do the following:

- Demonstrate safe techniques for managing and restraining a violent patient.

BEHAVIORAL EMERGENCIES

Definitions of Behavior and Behavioral Emergency

Behavior is defined as how a person acts. There is disagreement over what constitutes "normal" behavior, since no clear definition or ideal model exists. Ideas of normal also vary widely by culture, ethnic group, and acceptance by society.

Similar confusion applies to use of the term **abnormal behavior.** This type of behavior consists of actions that deviate from society's norms and expectations. Typically, the behavior interferes with a person's well-being and ability to function, although the individual may not be aware of it. Sometimes, but not always, abnormal behavior is harmful to the patient or other people. A more practical term for abnormal behavior is **maladaptive behavior,** which indicates that a person is unable to properly adapt to various challenging circumstances.

The term **behavioral emergencies** covers a broad range of behavioral and psychiatric disorders of varying severity. In general, this term refers to a group of disorders characterized by abnormal or maladaptive behavior. There is a disturbance in normal mental function that may be caused by emotion, physiological conditions, or a combination of conditions. Regardless of the cause, the result is undesirable consequences.

Behavioral emergencies are situations where patients feel they have lost control of their lives. In some cases patients may not be aware of this loss of control—these patients tend to be more severely emotionally compromised and may in fact have serious psychiatric illness. These situations are challenging in all areas of medical practice, especially in the prehospital setting. Behavioral emergencies incapacitate more people than all other health problems combined.

Dealing with these situations presents a challenge to health care providers. A major reason is the prevalence of several common misconceptions about behavioral emergencies, including the following:

- Abnormal behavior is always bizarre.
- All mental patients are unstable and dangerous.
- Mental disorders are incurable.
- Having a mental disorder is cause for embarrassment and shame.

None of these are uniformly correct in any given patient, although some may be partially applicable under specific circumstances.

Causes

There are several potential causes for behavioral emergencies. These may be organized into three categories:

1. *Biological/organic*—Any of a number of diseases may result in acute or chronic (permanent) behavioral abnormalities (Box 30-1). Some of these conditions are acquired (e.g., brain damage following head injury), and some are hereditary (e.g., some metabolic problems).

   Various toxins and drugs account for a significant proportion of acute behavioral emergencies. Drugs, especially cocaine, can induce behavioral problems, either acutely or as a chronic problem. Hallucinogens, such as lysergic acid (LSD) or phencyclidine (PCP), may significantly distort reality, resulting in a behavioral emergency.

   Many psychiatric disorders have been shown to have a biochemical basis; some are known to have genetic tendencies as well. Any of these may result in behavioral emergencies. Often persons with chronic disease have acute worsening of their condition. This may be due to a lack of medications, to a need for different medications, or to a life event, such as loss of a relative.

   In addition to presenting as psychiatric problems, several medical conditions can present as behavioral disorders. These include diabetes, stroke, and hypoxia.

2. *Psychosocial*—These problems may arise as a result of childhood trauma (mental, physical, or both), lack of adequate parenting, or a dysfunctional family structure.

3. *Sociocultural*—Life events may also lead to a behavioral emergency, either as a direct response or by precipitating an underlying abnormal behavioral tendency. These factors include the following:
   - Environmental violence (e.g., living in a war zone)
   - Death of a loved one
   - Economic or employment problems
   - Prejudice and discrimination

Assessment

During the scene size-up, the major responsibility of the EMT–Intermediate (EMT–I) is to determine whether a violent or potentially unsafe situation exists. This is the time to call for additional resources, such as from public safety personnel. *Do not* become a victim. In the absence of obvious danger, observe the scene for information to use in patient assessment and care, such as the following:

- Signs of violence
- Evidence of substance abuse
- Environmental conditions

Follow these guidelines when performing the initial assessment (Box 30-2):

- Limit the number of people around the patient, isolating the patient if necessary.
- Always stay alert to potential danger.
- Determine the presence of life-threatening medical conditions by rapid assessment of the ABCs (airway, breathing, and circulation), followed by rapid intervention, if necessary.
- Observe the overt behavior of the patient, as well as **body language** (nonverbal gestures, posture, or evidence of rage, elation, hostility, depression, fear, anger, anxiety, or confusion).

Follow these guidelines when performing the focused history and physical examination:

- Approach the patient slowly and purposefully.
- Avoid threatening actions, statements, and questions.
- Respect the patient's territory—allow at least 3 to 4 feet of personal space between you and the patient whenever possible.
- Limit physical touch to necessary procedures (e.g., shaking hands, obtaining vital signs).
- Remove the patient from the crisis or disturbing situation, if possible.
- Center your questions around the immediate problem.
- Establish rapport with the patient using "therapeutic interviewing techniques"—those that calm the patient

BOX 30-1

COMMON MEDICAL CONDITIONS PRESENTING AS BEHAVIORAL DISORDERS

METABOLIC DISORDERS
Glucose, sodium, calcium, or magnesium imbalance
Acid-base imbalance
Acute hypoxia
Renal failure
Hepatic failure

ENDOCRINE DISORDERS
Thyroid disease
Parathyroid disease
Adrenal hormone imbalance

INFECTIOUS DISEASES
Encephalitis
Meningitis
Brain abscess
Severe systemic infection

TRAUMA
Concussion
Intracranial hematoma (especially subdural hematoma)

CARDIOVASCULAR DISORDERS
Cardiac dysrhythmia
Hypotension
Transient ischemic attack
Cerebrovascular accident (or stroke)
Hypertensive encephalopathy

NEOPLASTIC DISEASES
Central nervous system tumors or metastases

DEGENERATIVE DISEASES
Dementia of the Alzheimer's type
Other dementias

DRUG ABUSE
Alcohol
Barbiturates
Sedative-hypnotics
Amphetamines and other stimulants
Hallucinogens

DRUG REACTIONS
Beta-adrenergic blockers
Antihypertensives
Cardiac drugs
Bronchodilators
Beta-adrenergic agonists
Anticonvulsants

From Sanders MJ: *Mosby's paramedic textbook*, ed 2, St Louis, 2000, Mosby.

BOX 30-2

TEN USEFUL INTERVIEWING SKILLS FOR BEHAVIORAL EMERGENCIES

1. Listen to the patient in a caring, concerned, and receptive manner. Be aware of nonverbal communications such as eye contact, facial expression, and posture, which can reassure the patient that you are responding with empathy.
2. Elicit feelings, as well as facts, to help develop a more accurate impression of the patient. If the patient is anxious, encourage him or her to share information relevant to that feeling.
3. Respond to the patient's feelings by acknowledging and labeling them (e.g., "You seem angry"). This may help validate and legitimize the patient's intense and sometimes overwhelming feelings.
4. Correct cognitive misconceptions or distortions. If a distorted sense of reality is producing fear or anxiety, offer a simple and correct explanation.
5. Provide information on the nature of the intervention or the care the patient can expect after arrival at the hospital.
6. Offer honest and realistic reassurance and support. Providing this support helps calm the patient and establishes rapport.
7. Ask effective questions. When seeking immediate information, ask closed-ended questions such as "Are you thinking of hurting yourself?" and "What medicines did you take?" More open-ended questions are appropriate after identifying problems that require immediate attention; such questions permit the individual to develop answers that usually help the paramedic completely understand the problem.
8. Avoid questions that may lead the person to say things he or she did not intend.
9. Structure the interview to develop a pattern rather than permitting a natural flow of information. Chronologically reported histories or sequences of events usually permit more complete understanding of the patient's problem (particularly causal relationships) and help the patient to organize thoughts. Keep the patient's responses focused by comments such as "What happened next?" and "Was that before or after what you were just telling me about?"
10. Conclude the interview. After obtaining relevant information, encourage the patient to describe other important events or feelings.

From Bassuk E et al: *Behavioral emergencies: a field guide for EMTs and paramedics*, Boston, 1983, Little, Brown.

and encourage him or her to cooperate. Therapeutic interviewing techniques include the following:
- Engage in active listening.
- Be supportive and empathetic.
- Limit interruptions.

- Avoid threatening actions, statements, and questions.
- Evaluate the patient's potential for suicide. Factors increasing a person's suicidal risk include the following (Box 30-3):
- Recent depression

- Recent loss of family or friend (e.g., death, divorce)
- Financial setbacks
- Drug use (including alcohol)
- Having a detailed plan to commit suicide

During assessment of the patient, pay particular attention to the following:

- *General appearance, hygiene, and dress*—Some persons with behavioral problems (both organic and psychiatric) exhibit an abnormal lack of regard for their own personal hygiene.
- *Motor activity*—Many behavioral emergencies are associated with abnormal motor activity. Note if the patient appears "hyper" or abnormally lethargic. Always consider the possibility of drug intoxication, pain, blood sugar abnormality, or hypoxia when abnormal motor activity is present.
- *Physical complaints*—These may indicate underlying or concomitant organic disease.
- *Intellectual function*—Orientation, memory, concentration, and judgment should be evaluated. This may require use of some type of a "mini-mental examination" consisting of simple questions and mathematical calculations. Several variants of these have been studied in the medical literature; consult with your physician advisor for recommendations.
- *Thought content*—Note disordered thoughts (thoughts that seem illogical), delusions, hallucinations, unusual worries, fears, and any suicide threat or threat of injury to others.
- *Language*—Patients with behavioral problems often speak either much faster or far slower than normal. Note the speech pattern and content. Garbled or unintelligible speech, unless the patient is actively hallucinating, is more likely to be due to an organic illness (e.g., stroke) than to a psychiatric problem.
- *Mood*—What is the patient's level of alertness? Does he or she appear to be distracted (possibly hallucinating)?

Management Considerations

Although people often go through emotional "ups and downs," a behavioral emergency occurs when the patient is unable to handle the situation emotionally. Often, the patient perceives the situation as threatening or dangerous to his or her well-being.

The reaction to crisis varies from individual to individual. Once someone feels that he or she has "lost control" or has lost his or her support system (e.g., spouse, children, job), the world appears to "crash in." Some persons withdraw; some become excessively active. The patient may become depressed or violent. When violent tendencies develop, these may be directed either at the patient himself or herself, such as in a suicide attempt, or at others.

Management of behavioral emergencies consists, first, of maintaining scene and personal safety. If the scene is safe, the next task is to build good rapport with the pa-

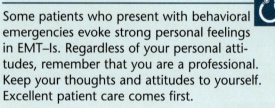

BOX 30-3

RISK FACTORS OF SUICIDE

- Patients more than 40 years of age, widowed or divorced, alcoholic, or depressed
- Patients who have spoken of taking their own lives
- Patients with a previous history of self-destructive behavior
- Patients with recently diagnosed serious illness
- Patients in an environment where there is an unusual gathering of destructive articles (e.g., guns or large amounts of pills)
- Patients who have recently lost a loved one
- Patients who were recently arrested or imprisoned
- Patients who have lost their job

From Stoy W: *Mosby's EMT-Basic textbook,* St Louis, 1996, Mosby.

CLINICAL NOTES

Some patients who present with behavioral emergencies evoke strong personal feelings in EMT–Is. Regardless of your personal attitudes, remember that you are a professional. Keep your thoughts and attitudes to yourself. Excellent patient care comes first.

tient. Speak in a calm, even voice, and exhibit a willingness to listen to the patient. Be honest—most people can easily detect a "snow job." Describe everything you intend to do, step-by-step, to the patient. Avoid any sudden moves.

In the unrestrained patient, follow these guidelines to minimize the chances of a violent situation developing:

- Have physical assistance nearby. In the field this may be your partner, additional personnel, or law enforcement. Maintain an open exit for both you and the patient. If there is an open exit for both of you, the patient will be calmer and you will be safer. Do *not* attempt the initial contact with a person who has a behavioral emergency in the back of a closed ambulance compartment alone (Figure 30-1).
- Allow the patient to "ventilate," expressing anger and frustration verbally instead of physically.
- Form an alliance with the patient—try to understand how the patient is feeling. You do not need to agree. For example, if a patient says, "FBI agents are following me," you might make a comment such as "That would bother me; how do you feel?"
- Avoid eye contact; looking someone directly in the eye is often taken as a challenge or threat.

If the situation escalates, you have a choice—either regain control, or leave. If you are trapped, try to keep talking to the patient until help can arrive. Otherwise, get away from the patient as quickly as possible, and summon assistance.

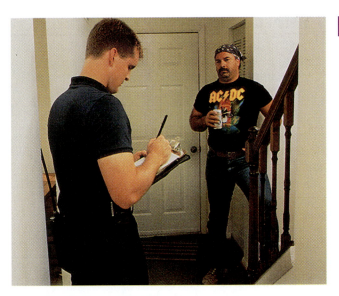

FIGURE 30-1 ▲ Do not allow any participant in a dispute to position himself or herself between you and the door or exit route. (From Krebs: *When violence erupts*, St Louis, 1990, Mosby.)

BOX 30-4

SIGNS OF POTENTIAL PATIENT VIOLENCE

- Sitting on edge of seat, as if ready to move
- Clenched fists
- Yelling and using profanity
- Standing or moving toward EMT
- Throwing things
- Holding onto a potentially dangerous object
- Any behavior that makes the EMT uneasy

From Stoy W: *Mosby's EMT-Basic textbook*, St Louis, 1996, Mosby.

Although an apparently calm patient sometimes becomes rapidly out of control, avoid placing yourself in a situation where a patient may become violent unless you are trained and have adequate backup immediately available. It is impossible to list every single behavior that might be a warning of things going bad. Rely on your judgment, experience, and "gut feelings." Situations with the potential for a patient's developing violent behavior, as well as guidelines for dealing with these situations, include the following (Box 30-4):

- A patient who is pacing back and forth, unable to keep one position for more than a couple of seconds. Ask the patient, once, to be seated. If this fails and you are uncomfortable, leave.
- A patient who appears to get more and more angry as he or she speaks. This behavior may simply be a reflection of the patient venting. If there is excessive body language, such as a red face or the patient starts to swing his or her arms, you have a choice—try to talk with the patient, stating, "Man, you're really upset" or "I know you're upset, but you need to let yourself chill out just a bit," or leave. If talking to the patient does not work, or if you feel uncomfortable, leave.
- A patient who is starting to act out, such as thrashing out with the arms, hitting the wall, or throwing things. You may be the next target. There is no room for negotiation here; get away from the person as soon as possible. If there are any obvious weapons (e.g., knives, guns, baseball bats), leave immediately.
- A patient who is bragging about how tough he or she is, telling stories of "how many cops it took to hold me the last time." The easiest way to deal with this sort of behavior is to agree with the patient—"I'm on

your side; I'm not going to mess with you." If the patient begins implying that you would make an easy target—"I could whip you with one hand"—you have to make a choice. Agree with the patient ("I'm sure you could") and continue the interview, or leave.

- Any domestic violence–related situation, particularly where the alleged perpetrator is still present. It is unwise to enter a scene involving domestic violence without appropriate law enforcement backup on-scene and available. Separate the involved parties as soon as possible. Ideally, this role belongs to law enforcement personnel, not the EMT–I. These scenes are very dangerous and should not be entered until fighting parties are separated.
- Any patient who is suspected of being intoxicated or on "drugs." The potential for violence varies from person to person, but the mere presence of substance abuse makes violent behavior more likely to occur.
- A patient who persistently complains about your EMS system or service received in the past. Statistically speaking, unhappy patients are more likely to become violent, whether or not they are in the midst of a behavioral emergency.

Men are more likely than women to exhibit violent behavior. Do not let your guard down, however, if dealing with a female patient. Similarly, do not be misled by the patient's age—persons of all ages can get violent.

Legal Issues

Generally, EMT–Is are expected to act in a calm manner but never jeopardize their own safety. Each state, and sometimes locality, has specific regulations for handling apparently behaviorally challenged individuals, including patients who exhibit self-destructive behavior. EMT–Is are responsible for following both state laws and local protocols regarding treatment of persons with mental illness, as well as those with temporarily impaired mental status (e.g., alcohol intoxication, drug overdose). Be aware of local facilities and procedures for the following:

- Psychiatric evaluation and hospitalization

- Alcohol and drug detoxification
- Crisis intervention

As a general rule, patients should be transported against their will in the following situations:

- They present a threat to themselves or others.
- It is ordered by medical direction.

The process should be implemented with the assistance of law enforcement authorities, if at all possible. Using restraints should be in accordance with local protocols. A number of different types of restraints are available (e.g., leather or Velcro wrist and ankle restraints, full jacket restraints, handcuffs) (Figure 30-2). Principles for using restraints are listed in Box 30-5. Important documentation involving the use of restraints and other patient care is described in Box 30-6.

Common Field Situations and Behavioral Problems

NEUROSIS AND PSYCHOSIS

A **neurosis** is an abnormal anxiety reaction to a perceived fear. There is no basis in reality for that fear (e.g., a fear of heights so strong that it prevents a person from leaving the first floor of any building). To some degree, just about everyone has some type of neurotic fear at one time or another. This does *not* mean that a person is

> **HELPFUL HINT**
>
> - Some EMS providers carry handcuffs for use as restraints. There are many well-documented cases of nerve injury to the wrist and hands caused by improperly applied handcuffs, even by experienced law enforcement personnel. Unless you are properly authorized and trained in their use, avoid handcuffs.

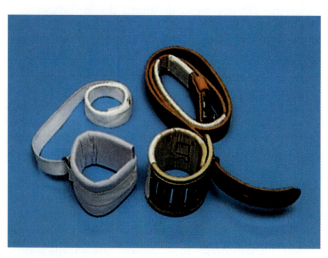

FIGURE 30-2 ▲ Example of restraints. (From Sanders MJ: *Mosby's paramedic textbook*, St Louis, 1994, Mosby.)

> **HELPFUL HINT**
>
> - Several deaths have been reported in EMS patients as a result of postural asphyxia. Improper positioning, especially face down on a stretcher or gurney, may be fatal.

insane or crazy. Most people cope with their fears. Again, a behavioral emergency occurs only when a person is *unable* to cope. A patient with a **psychosis**, on the other hand, has no concept whatsoever of reality. The person truly believes an unreal situation or condition is real. Often the psychotic person hears voices.

> **BOX 30-5**
>
> ### RESTRAINING A PATIENT
>
> 1. Have adequate help, including police assistance if possible.
> 2. Have a plan of action.
> 3. Use only necessary force.
> 4. Stay beyond patient's range of motion.
> 5. Act quickly.
> 6. Talk to the patient.
> 7. Work with another EMT or personnel, deciding in advance how each of you will restrain a limb, and approach together.
> 8. Secure limbs with approved equipment, such as restraints.
> 9. It may be necessary to turn the patient face down on the stretcher.
> 10. You may cover the patient's face with a surgical or oxygen mask if the patient is spitting or biting.
> 11. Reassess the situation frequently, including the patient's vital signs and physical status.
> 12. Document all your and the patient's actions.
>
> From Stoy W: *Mosby's EMT-Basic textbook*, St Louis, 1996, Mosby.

> **BOX 30-6**
>
> ### IMPORTANT DOCUMENTATION FOR BEHAVIORAL EMERGENCIES
>
> - Document the position in which the patient was found.
> - Document any aggressive or abnormal action produced by the patient.
> - Document anything unusual the patient says, in direct quotations if possible.
> - Document every aspect of assessment and the findings in detail.
> - Document any restraining procedures used and assessment findings before and after their use.
> - Document any persons assisting or witnessing the treatment and transport of the patient.
>
> From Stoy W: *Mosby's EMT-Basic textbook*, St Louis, 1996, Mosby.

In drug-induced psychosis, hallucinogens or stimulant agents cause the patient to lose touch with reality. Often, the person develops hyperactive, and often dangerous, behavior. The best way to deal with hallucinations is the "talk-down" technique—gently calming and reassuring the patient that everything is okay.

DEPRESSION

Depression is a common reaction to major life stresses. Several signs and symptoms may suggest that a person is depressed:

- An unkempt appearance. It appears as though the patient does not care about anything.
- Speech that is different from usual. Persons who are depressed may not speak, or they may reply in short, monotone phrases. They lack any spark or enthusiasm in their speech and actions.
- Frequent crying bouts. These often appear to have no precipitant.
- Abnormally increased or decreased appetite. Significant weight gain or loss is common.
- Sleep disturbances. Often, depressed persons fall asleep without a problem, only to wake within a couple of hours. They are then unable to fall asleep again the rest of the night. Sometimes depressed persons have an increased desire to sleep to avoid feeling depressed.

Depression may present as another disease. Elderly persons commonly appear to have organic illness (e.g., cardiac or respiratory conditions) when, in reality, they are severely depressed.

Your primary responsibility as an EMT–I is to provide a safe and caring environment for these patients. Respect their feelings and communicate to them that you care. Arrange for a mental health specialist or social worker to evaluate the patient if possible (depending on local community's resources and local protocols). Otherwise, turn to the nearest appropriate facility for assistance.

SUICIDAL PATIENTS

Suicide is the intentional taking of one's life. It is a significant cause of death in the United States, especially in young males (ages 15 to 35) and the elderly (both sexes). A **suicide gesture** is something done by a person whose intention is to ask for help, rather than to die. The person performs the deed in a potentially reversible way, such as taking a few aspirin tablets or a small handful of pills. Unfortunately, small amounts of certain medications can be very poisonous. Persons with suicidal gestures need to be treated as poisoning patients, with careful attention paid to the behavioral emergency. Sometimes, people intend to kill themselves, take pills, and then change their minds.

A **suicide attempt** is made by a patient who has a true desire to die. Often the person has planned the event; he or she has purchased a gun, or driven far out of town, or gotten a double refill of a prescription medication.

Whether the situation encountered is an actual suicide attempt or a gesture, do not discount the patient's emotional state in any way. Directly ask the patient, "Were you trying to kill yourself," or "Did you want to die?" Many persons are not aware of what resources are available to them for help, but they are aware that people at the hospital do know. A suicide gesture is the patient's way of seeking help.

The following factors increase the risk that a person is suicidal:

- Male sex
- Age less than 19 or greater than 45
- The presence of depression or hopelessness
- Previous suicide attempts or psychiatric care
- Excessive alcohol or drug use
- Loss of rational thinking
- A patient who is separated, widowed, or divorced
- An organized or well-thought-out attempt, such as use of a firearm, a "life-threatening" presentation, or leaving a suicide note
- Lack of a good support system (e.g., family, friends, job, religious affiliation)
- Stated intent to try again in the future to commit suicide
- A major life event (e.g., recent divorce, buying or selling a house, recent loss of job, death of spouse or other loved ones).

Many states require that a person who has threatened or attempted suicide be evaluated by a mental health professional. Follow local laws and protocols regarding transporting persons who do not wish to go to the hospital. Otherwise, transport the patient to the hospital and provide as gentle and nonthreatening an environment as possible. Do not make any judgmental comments, pro or con, regarding what the patient did, regardless of your personal feelings. Professionalism is paramount—and the patient comes first.

SUBSTANCE ABUSE
Alcohol Abuse

Alcohol is a drug, and it can be lethal. **Alcohol abuse** is defined as medical, behavioral, or social problems related to excessive alcohol consumption. Alcohol abuse is not the same as **alcoholism,** which is a chronic condition characterized by dependence on alcohol, as well as a pattern of abnormal behaviors. Alcohol abuse has no socioeconomic boundaries. Similar percentages of alcohol-related problems are found in high-income areas and in lower-income areas.

Alcohol tends to potentiate or increase the strength of many drugs, especially sleeping pills and other depressants. Ingestion of alcohol in combination with other drugs can be fatal.

PATIENT ASSESSMENT

Signs and symptoms of alcohol intoxication are often multiple and include the following:

- Odor of alcohol on the breath
- Unsteady gait
- Slurred, loud, and inappropriate speech
- Nausea, vomiting
- Flushed face
- Altered level of consciousness
- Abnormal behavior, ranging from elation to violence
- Injuries, often from unexplained sources

    Additional signs seen with severe alcohol intoxication include the following:

- Hallucinations
- Hypotension
- Slow or labored respirations
- Marked dehydration
- Seizures
- Unconsciousness or coma

    Conditions That May Mimic Alcohol Intoxication—Other life-threatening illnesses can mimic alcohol intoxication. Even patients who have alcohol on the breath and appear intoxicated can have other, more serious problems. Do not get "tunnel vision." Consider the possibility of the following conditions in any patient who appears to be intoxicated:

- Drug abuse
- Brain tumor
- Hypoglycemia (Chapter 24)
- Meningitis (Chapter 27)
- Head injury
- Stroke (Chapter 27)
- Postictal state (Chapter 27)
- Diabetic ketoacidosis (Chapter 24)
- Hypoxia (Chapter 8)

EMERGENCY CARE

The care for a patient with alcohol intoxication includes the following:

- Maintain the airway; assist breathing if necessary. Be prepared to suction.
- Give high-concentration oxygen, if the patient permits it. If you suspect trauma, stabilize and immobilize the cervical spine.
- Check for hypoglycemia using a fingerstick blood sugar test.

- Attempt to build rapport and trust with the patient.
- If permitted by local protocols, restrain the patient as necessary for the patient's protection, as well as your own safety.
- Summon police or other assistance when necessary if the patient is uncooperative, agitated, or combative. Remember, in this and all other types of cases, that the purpose of obtaining help from law enforcement is to protect both yourself *and* the patient.

- Transport severely intoxicated patients. It is possible that another illness may be present. Severely intoxicated patients are a danger both to themselves and to others. These patients should be evaluated medically and observed for a period of time in the emergency department.

ALCOHOL WITHDRAWAL SYNDROMES

When a patient abruptly stops drinking alcohol, especially after a prolonged period of intoxication, the body can experience alcohol withdrawal syndromes. These reactions include the following:

Shakes—These occur within 24 hours of drinking cessation. The patient is shaky and tremulous, and has a mild sleep disturbance. The eyes are bloodshot, and the blood pressure is elevated. Although these patients are often uncomfortable, this condition by itself is not dangerous. Care for these patients as described earlier in the previous column, and transport to the hospital for further evaluation and care.

Alcohol withdrawal seizures—The patient may have grand mal (generalized) seizures within 24 to 48 hours of stopping drinking. One third of these patients will progress to having delirium tremens (DTs). Care for these patients as you would for any patient with a seizure (Chapter 27).

Delirium tremens (DTs)—This is a severe state of delirium, hallucinations, and autonomic nervous system hyperactivity (fever, tachycardia, hypertension). DTs is a serious condition; up to 15% of patients die from associated problems. Symptoms may begin from 12 to 48 hours after the last ingestion of alcohol. Restrain the patient as necessary for the patient's own protection, as well as yours. Care for any related conditions, and transport the patient to the hospital. Notify the emergency department in advance that you are transporting a violent patient. Get law enforcement personnel involved as per local protocols.

Antabuse or Antabuse-like reactions can be a threat to life. Patients have nausea, vomiting, palpitations, anxiety, hypotension, and flushing. Shock and cardiovascular collapse can develop. If you suspect this type of reaction in a patient, administer oxygen, start a large-bore IV line of normal saline, protect the airway, place the patient on a cardiac monitor, care for shock, and transport the patient to the hospital immediately.

Drug Abuse

Drugs are substances taken by mouth; injected into a muscle, the skin, a blood vessel, or a body cavity; or placed on the skin (topical) to treat or prevent a disease or condition. Drugs may be ethical (manufactured by a legitimate pharmaceutical company for the purpose of treating certain medical problems) or illicit (manufactured—usually illegally—solely for the purpose of abuse). Sometimes, ethical drugs (also known as "ethical pharmaceuticals") are used for illicit purposes. For example, certain pain medications are sold on the street "to get high."

Drug misuse is the intentional or accidental use of a medication for a medical purpose other than what it was intended, or in a dose different from that prescribed (e.g., taking penicillin tablets left over from a previous sore throat for an ear infection). Failure to take prescribed medication is also a form of drug misuse. This is called poor patient compliance and is common.

Drug abuse is the use of a drug for a nontherapeutic effect, especially one for which it was not prescribed or intended. The most common reason is to "get high." The exact meaning of this term differs from person to person. To some, "getting high" means escaping reality; to others, it may mean hallucinations. Often the term *substance abuse* is used, instead of drug abuse, to include alcohol and marijuana. In this same category are various substances that are taken as drugs that were not "intended" to be used as such (e.g., glue sniffing, gas huffing).

Drug addiction is a condition characterized by an overwhelming desire to continue taking a drug to which one has become "hooked" through repeated consumption because it produces a particular effect. True addiction is both a psychological and a physical event—the patient has both a physical and a psychological craving for the drug, as well as for the effect. Drug dependence is a psychological craving for or a psychological reliance on a chemical agent, resulting from abuse or addiction. Drug dependence is a psychological problem, not a physical one.

Drug withdrawal is a set of signs and symptoms that develop in a person following abrupt cessation of taking a drug. Most often, the individual has developed a dependence or addiction to the drug. The most dangerous drug withdrawal reactions occur in persons who are addicted—both physically *and* psychologically to a particular drug. Classic examples include alcohol withdrawal seizures and DTs (previous column). Psychological withdrawal, although severe, is often not life threatening.

Withdrawal syndromes can also result from the sudden stoppage of several prescription medications that are not considered "addictive" by most criteria. For example, if a person suddenly stops taking certain antihypertensive drugs, he or she can develop a rebound hypertensive emergency (Chapter 27). Persons who stop taking beta blockers, a type of heart medicine, abruptly may develop myocardial infarction (Chapter 27).

Drug abuse is a significant problem in the United States, as well as a leading cause of trauma, heart attacks, and strokes. Illicit drugs are taken by various routes: inhalation, oral ingestion, or injection. Persons may take drugs to "get high" or during a suicide attempt.

> **HELPFUL HINT**
>
> - Drug abuse (especially abuse of alcohol, marijuana, and cocaine) has been shown to play a significant role in homicide, suicide, and unintentional trauma (such as falls or motor vehicle accidents).

DRUGS OF ABUSE

There are five classes of drugs of abuse. The classes, representative agents, and common symptoms of intoxication are as follows:

- **Stimulants**—These drugs, also known as "uppers," stimulate the central nervous system. Cocaine is the most widely abused drug in this category. Other drugs include amphetamines (speed), caffeine, and thyroid medication. "Ice" is a highly concentrated form of amphetamine that lasts 12 to 24 hours. Symptoms of stimulant intoxication include hyperactivity, euphoria, tachycardia, hypertension, dilated pupils, diaphoresis, sleeplessness, seizures, and disorientation. Cocaine causes hypertensive crises, seizures, myocardial infarction, and stroke.
- **Depressants**—These drugs, also known as "downers," depress the central nervous system. Marijuana is the best-known drug. Others include barbiturates, sleeping pills, tranquilizers, and antidepressant pills. Symptoms of depressant intoxication include sluggishness, poor coordination, slurred speech, decreased respiration or respiratory arrest, and impaired memory and judgment.
- **Hallucinogens**—These drugs induce a sense of euphoria and hallucinations. Lysergic acid diethylamide (LSD) is the best-known agent. Others include mescaline, psilocybin, and phencyclidine (PCP, or angel dust). PCP may result in suicidal and extremely violent behavior. Often, several people may be required to restrain a violent patient who is under the influence of PCP. Hallucinogen ingestion leads to hallucinations, unpredictable behavior, tachypnea, nausea, dilated pupils, increased pulse, and blood pressure.
- **Narcotics**—This category includes heroin, morphine, methadone, meperidine (Demerol) hydromorphone (Dilaudid), pentazocine (Talwin), codeine, hydrocodone (Vicodin), and propoxyphene (Darvon). Ingestion of these agents may result in drowsiness, impaired coordination, sweating, respiratory depression, constricted pupils, shock, convulsions, and coma. Respiratory and cardiac arrest are possible.

- **Volatile chemicals**—This category includes aerosols (paint spray, hair spray, industrial chemicals), glue, and gasoline. Patients who inhale or otherwise ingest these compounds may have the following symptoms: altered level of consciousness, swollen mucous membranes of the mouth and nose, increased pulse and respiratory rates, respiratory distress (particularly with gasoline inhalation, such as during siphoning), and nausea.

> **HELPFUL HINT**
>
> - Any drug, prescription or otherwise, may be abused. Nitroglycerin and amyl nitrate ("poppers") are used to treat heart pain (Chapter 23). These agents have also become popular as street drugs because they cause a warm, flushed feeling that is said to be especially good during sex. The anesthetic gas nitrous oxide ("laughing gas") is abused in a similar fashion.

PATIENT ASSESSMENT

In addition to the signs and symptoms of substance abuse, keep the following principles in mind:

- Expect the history to be unreliable. If possible, determine what substances were taken, when were they taken, how they were taken, how much was taken, and if any care has been started.
- Attempt to assess if the patient is suicidal. Ask, "Did you want to hurt yourself?" Record the patient's answer in the run report. This is essential, particularly if you need to restrain a suicidal patient to prevent the patient from doing further harm to himself or herself.
- Expect a mixed intoxication. Many ingestions, especially if a suicide attempt is involved, are a mixture of alcohol and other drugs.
- Expect the unexpected. Violent behavior is common in many patients who are taking drugs.
- Ineffective street treatments for drug withdrawal or overdose include ice immersion, placing an ice bag on the groin, IV milk, and IV saline (saltwater). These are often used by drug abusers in the hopes of avoiding having to call an ambulance. These findings in the history or physical assessment may help in determining whether to suspect drug abuse.

EMERGENCY CARE

The care for a patient with drug abuse–related problems includes the following:

- Maintain the airway and assist breathing as necessary.
- Monitor the patient carefully for deterioration in respiratory status.
- Give oxygen by nasal cannula (3 to 4 L/min), nonrebreather mask (10 to 15 L/min), or as per local protocols.
- Watch for vomiting.
- Be prepared to suction.

EMT–I Keegan sees that the bottles had contained 20 barbiturate and 30 acetaminophen tablets. "Do you know how many pills were left in these bottles? she asks the patient's mother. "It will help us determine how many she may have taken."

"I had about five of the Seconal left. The bottle of Tylenol was nearly new. Only two or three pills would have been missing," her mother says.

"Do you know when she took them?" she asks.

"No. I got home from work about 5:00 and started dinner. She usually gets home around 3:45, but I found out from a neighbor that she hadn't gone to school today. She could have taken them any time."

EMT–I Bravo says, "Her pulse is 136 and strong, respirations are 32, and her blood pressure is 136/84. She's responding to a sternal rub with groaning and withdrawing from pain."

EMT–I Keegan calls medical direction for physician's orders and is instructed to "transport only."

It looks as though the patient has a good chance to recover. When EMT–I Keegan checks with the hospital 3 days later, however, they tell her that the patient died the day before. She asks her service medical director about the case at the next continuing education program. "Why wouldn't she have made it if her vital signs weren't that bad?" she asks.

The medical director answers, "Well, acetaminophen is one of the safest drugs on the market if it's used appropriately. However, taken with alcohol or other drugs that affect the liver, or even in moderate overdoses, the effects can be lethal, as you saw here. Also, the effects of the poisoning are insidious. That is, they don't appear to be too bad at first, but once the liver damage is done, the patient is doomed. Patients often appear to improve for a few days and will look like they're out of the woods, for a while. We treated her aggressively here. We evacuated her stomach with a gastric lavage and administered Mucomyst, an antidote, as well as Mazicon. Her death was a tragedy."

- Notify law enforcement officials and the Poison Control Center as required by local protocols.
- Consult with the local Poison Control Center or emergency department physician to determine whether syrup of ipecac should be given to induce vomiting or if activated charcoal should be given. Many EMS physicians no longer prescribe ipecac for use in the field or hospital. Activated charcoal and gastric lavage (usually in the hospital) are becoming the treatments of choice. Give ipecac only on the advise of the Poison Control Center or medical control.
- Give dextrose (D_{50}) if indicated by fingerstick blood glucose results.
- Give naloxone if advised by medical control or the Poison Control Center.
- Monitor the ECG.
- Place an IV line.
- Monitor for shock and provide care as appropriate.
- Restrain the patient as necessary to prevent the patient from injuring himself or herself or others. Follow local protocols for holding a suicidal patient against the patient's will. Do not try to be a hero; get help from the police if necessary.
- Do not be judgmental.

SUMMARY

Important points to remember from this chapter include the following:
- Behavioral emergencies involve situations where patients feel that they have, in some way, lost control of their life. The patient may or may not be violent. In many instances medical problems or substance abuse may contribute to the patient's behavior. The EMT–I *must* be aware of local procedures for dealing with patients who have acute behavioral problems.
- The cardinal principle in dealing with a behavioral emergency is to try to build good rapport with the patient. EMT–Is should always try to allow themselves an exit if the situation escalates. They should never place themselves in a potentially violent situation without appropriate backup.
- Alcohol abuse includes the medical, behavioral, or social problems related to alcohol consumption. Patients who are intoxicated exhibit inappropriate behavior and abnormal coordination. Severe intoxication may lead to hypotension, respiratory depression, seizures, and coma.
- The EMT–I must always be alert to life-threatening conditions that can mimic alcohol intoxication. Severely intoxicated persons should be transported to the hospital for evaluation and observation.
- Abrupt cessation of alcohol can cause withdrawal symptoms: the shakes, seizures, or delirium tremens (DTs). Reactions to Antabuse can be life threatening. These patients should be transported to the hospital as soon as possible.
- Drug abuse is a common problem. There are five categories of drugs of abuse: stimulants, depressants, hallucinogens, narcotics, and volatile chemicals.
- The history in any drug abuse patient is usually unreliable.
- An attempt should be made to determine whether the patient has tried to commit suicide. Assistance should be obtained from law enforcement personnel, according to local protocols.
- The airway should be watched carefully in any patient who has ingested drugs. These patients tend to develop respiratory depression quickly.

31 Gynecological Emergencies

....CASE HISTORY

Shortly after beginning their shift, EMT–Is Walsh and Delaney are requested to respond to Middlefield Drive for a 22-year-old female complaining of vaginal bleeding. On arrival, they note the patient to be pale and diaphoretic. A moderate amount of blood is present on the bed. Examination of her abdomen reveals diffuse tenderness that is greatest in the lower aspect of the left lower quadrant. She states she does not know if she is pregnant but is worried because her normal menses is 6 weeks late. Her past gynecological history includes two normal pregnancies, pelvic inflammatory disease, and pelvic surgery to resolve a large ovarian cyst.

Her vital signs include a pulse of 140, blood pressure of 88/52, and respiratory rate of 24.

What is the potential etiology of her abdominal pain and bleeding? What aspects of her history support the working diagnosis? What interventions are needed at this time? What considerations must be made in selecting a transport destination?

LEARNING OBJECTIVES

CHAPTER GOAL
Upon completion of this chapter, the EMT-Intermediate will be able to use assessment findings to formulate a field impression and implement the management plan for the patient experiencing a gynecological emergency.

Cognitive Objectives
As an EMT-Intermediate you should be able to do the following:

- Review the anatomic structures and physiology of the female reproductive system.
- Describe how to assess a patient with a gynecological complaint.
- Explain how to recognize a gynecological emergency.
- Describe the general care for any patient experiencing a gynecological emergency.
- Describe the pathophysiology, assessment, and management of specific gynecological emergencies, including pelvic inflammatory disease, ruptured ovarian cyst, ectopic pregnancy, and vaginal bleeding.

- Describe the general findings and management of the sexually assaulted patient.

Affective Objectives
As an EMT–Intermediate you should be able to do the following:
- Value the importance of maintaining a patient's modesty and privacy while obtaining necessary information.
- Defend the need to provide care for a victim of sexual assault while still preventing destruction of crime scene information.
- Serve as a role model for other EMS providers when discussing or caring for patients with gynecological emergencies.

Psychomotor Objectives
As an EMT–Intermediate you should be able to do the following:
- Demonstrate how to assess a patient with a gynecological complaint.
- Demonstrate how to provide care for a patient with vaginal bleeding or abdominal pain.
- Demonstrate how to provide care for a victim of sexual assault.

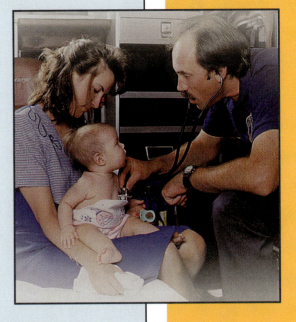

INTRODUCTION

Although normally associated with the celebration of pregnancy and new life, the internal organs related to fertility and childbearing can be associated with a number of significant emergencies. These include the following:
- Multiple types of infection, either chronic or acute
- Significant hemorrhage associated with bleeding not only from the uterus but also from the fallopian tubes and ovaries
- Ectopic pregnancy

Ectopic pregnancy poses a particular risk, with the growing pregnancy potentially causing the fallopian tube to rupture, leading to massive internal bleeding. This gynecological emergency can lead to maternal death if not recognized and treated appropriately. As in any case of infection or hemorrhage, if it is not identified at the right time or is not treated correctly, there can be significant morbidity and mortality that will ultimately affect maternal well-being.

ANATOMY AND PHYSIOLOGY REVIEW

A woman's fertility is under tight hormonal regulation. Each month, the levels of certain hormones rise and fall, stimulating development of the woman's eggs in the ovaries, as well as thickening of the inner lining of the uterus (also known as the endometrium) (Figure 31-1). If an egg is fertilized by sperm and implants within the endometrium, the pregnancy begins and the woman typically has no further menses. If no egg is fertilized, the normal hormonal regulation causes the inner lining of the endometrium to shed and normal menses ensues. Menses occurs approximately every 28 days in most women, although it can vary. The first day of menstruation is typically considered the first day of the cycle, which lasts generally from 3 to 7 days.

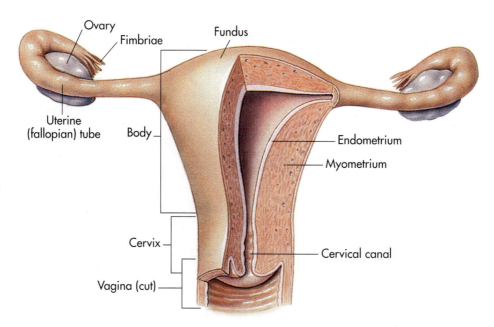

FIGURE 31-1 ▲ The female reproductive system. (From Thibodeau GA: *Structure and function of the body*, St Louis, 1992, Mosby.)

✖ **Menstrual Cycle** • Vaginal bleeding that typically occurs every 28 days when an egg does not implant in the uterus.

✖ **Uterus** • The muscular pelvic structure that protects and nourishes the fetus during development and contracts to facilitate delivery.

As a result of hormonal stimulation, at approximately the fourteenth day of the **menstrual cycle,** an egg is released from the ovary, where it travels down the fallopian tube to the **uterus.** Typically, it is implanted in the uterus after it is fertilized. If it is not fertilized, the egg is shed with the normal menstrual flow.

Menarche is the very first menstrual cycle that the female experiences. This typically occurs at age 12 years but can occur anywhere between the ages of 8 and 14 years. It is common that the first few periods after menarche are irregular regarding the length of days of bleeding, heaviness of bleeding, and associated cramps. Menopause occurs anywhere between 35 and 60 years of age. At menopause there is no further menstrual bleeding. The menstrual cycles leading up to menopause can be quite different from normal menstrual cycles. At times the flow may be particularly heavy, and other times the flow may be very light. It is not uncommon during the months preceding menopause for the woman to notice much longer delays in the start of when she would expect a normal period.

As mentioned earlier, once a properly fertilized egg implants in the endometrium and the pregnancy starts, there should be no further bleeding, or menses, until well after the pregnancy is completed. There are a number of other reasons why a woman may not be having her normal menses. In addition to the period approach-ing menopause, birth control pills, malnutrition, and other endocrine disorders may cause significant delays or the absence of normal menses.

ASSESSMENT

As with any patient the EMT–Intermediate (EMT–I) is called on to evaluate, assessment should start with the initial assessment of the ABCs (airway, breathing, and circulation). Although not typically associated with the high acuity of critical trauma or cardiac emergencies, acute gynecological emergencies can result in significant hemorrhage or overwhelming infection that can cause shock and be life threatening.

The organs of fertility located in the pelvis are close to other abdominal organs. Women complaining of acute abdominal pain or other abdominal emergency may actually have a gynecological problem. Assessment of any woman with a possible disorder of the bladder,

HELPFUL HINT

● Many adolescents are very uncomfortable discussing their gynecological history with anyone, let alone an unknown EMT–I during a crisis. Some questions or aspects of the examination may need to be conducted without the parents being present or possibly even delayed until the patient can be taken to the hospital. If the patient is reluctant to share information, pursue only questions that are pertinent to the immediate assessment and stabilization, delaying other questions until a more private setting can be arranged.

urinary tract, gastrointestinal tract, or other abdominal organs should also consider the possibility of a gynecological origin. A woman's gynecological history, as well as the current gynecological emergency, is of a very sensitive nature. The presence of a female EMS member during the history, evaluation, and treatment may make the patient feel more comfortable and may facilitate a more accurate exchange of information.

History of the Present Illness

Gynecological emergencies can have the same signs and symptoms as emergencies involving other abdominal organs. Questions that are asked should be broad enough to gather information regarding the current function or dysfunction of other abdominal organs. These types of questions should include the following:
- Is there any pain or cramping?
- Is there any radiation of the pain?
- When did the pain or cramping start?
- Is there any vaginal bleeding or vaginal discharge?
- Is there any nausea, vomiting, or change in appetite?
- Is there any fever? Is there any diaphoresis or sweating?
- Has the patient experienced any change in her normal bowel habits, including any diarrhea or constipation?
- Is there any frequency of urination, pain with urination, or blood noted during urination?

STREET WISE

Many illnesses or diseases can present with severe abdominal pain. Your role as an EMT–I is not to make an immediate diagnosis, but to recognize signs and symptoms that may fit disease patterns, keeping in mind that the definitive diagnosis will be made after a thorough assessment in the emergency department.

Another challenging aspect of prehospital patient evaluation is determining the nature or cause of abdominal pain. As mentioned earlier, abdominal pain can be of gynecological origin, but it can also be intestinal, hepatic, or genitourinary in origin. Specific questions must elicit as much information about the pain or discomfort as possible. These include the following:
- Is the pain associated with the onset of the menstrual cycle or menstrual bleeding? *Pain with menses is called dysmenorrhea.*
- What types of activities make the pain worse? Is the pain increased with ambulation or activity? Is it increased with bowel movements? Does the patient complain of pain with intercourse? *Pain with intercourse is referred to as dyspareunia.*
- What sorts of activities make the pain better? Is the pain improved with rest, sitting, or lying in a certain position?

- Has the patient ever had pain of a similar nature in the past? How long ago did the pain occur, and what was the etiology of the pain at that time?

Part of the rapid comprehensive prehospital evaluation includes placing the patient's current medical emergency in the context of her normal state of health. It is important to inquire about preexisting conditions or chronic ongoing medical problems that could contribute to or worsen the current symptoms.

As it becomes clear that the current problem is gynecological in origin, specific questions regarding any vaginal bleeding or discharge must be asked. It is important to remember that women routinely have vaginal bleeding associated with their menses and that any change in the frequency or volume must be related to the pattern of their normal cycle.
- When did the bleeding first start? Has the bleeding been intermittent or constant?
- How heavy is the bleeding in relation to normal periods? How many pads per hour is she using?

Women may also complain of vaginal discharge other than vaginal bleeding. This can be attributed to multiple types of infections or may be physiological. Questions regarding the vaginal discharge should include the following:
- What is the color and odor of the discharge?
- How heavy is the discharge?
- Has the patient attempted any self-therapy to correct the discharge?

At this point in the history taking, it is important to recognize that many of the patient's past medical and gynecological events may contribute to the emergency. The past gynecological history primarily revolves around any infections, surgeries, and history of normal menses. This information can be gathered by asking the following questions:
- When was the patient's last period?
- Are the periods regular?
- How many days do they normally last?
- Are there normally any associated abdominal pains or cramps with the menses?
- Has the patient had any recent gynecological infections, including yeast infections, that have required any antibiotic or antifungal use? It is important to recognize that many women treat vaginal discharges as yeast infections and may attempt therapy with over-the-counter preparations long before seeking formal medical attention.
- Has the patient ever been diagnosed with an ectopic, or tubal, pregnancy? Although historically these have been treated with surgery, there are now pharmacological therapies available. The EMT–I may encounter patients who are currently diagnosed with an ectopic pregnancy who are undergoing therapy and may still be at risk for bleeding or complications.
- Has the patient ever had to have a cesarean section or other adjunct to facilitate delivery because of

excessive fetal size, maternal body size, or other complications?

- Has the patient had any abdominal or pelvic surgeries? Specifically, has the patient had any surgeries on her uterus, a hysterectomy, a tubal ligation, any surgeries for infections, or any ectopic pregnancies?

At this point, the woman should be asked about past pregnancies. It is important to recognize and inquire about *all* pregnancies regardless of ultimate outcome. Many women hesitate or neglect to discuss specific information concerning miscarriages, elective or spontaneous abortions, and even children conceived out of wedlock. These are sensitive issues for some women, and the EMT–I should attempt to show as much compassion and empathy as possible during the evaluation.

❌ Gravida • Refers to a woman's total number of pregnancies.

❌ Para • Refers to a woman's total number of live births.

> **❗ HELPFUL HINT**
>
> - A woman's obstetrical history can easily be relayed using the terms **gravida** ("G") and **para** ("P"). A 47-year-old woman who is G5P2 has had five pregnancies and two live births.

Special Concerns Regarding the Gynecological Patient

For the vast majority of patients the EMT–I will encounter, the physical examination is a fairly straightforward and routine part of the entire assessment. This is not always the case with the patient experiencing an acute gynecological emergency or who is the victim of sexual assault. In these patients the EMT–I may need to ask very direct questions regarding the patient's sexual history. In rare instances and with the woman's specific permission, the EMT–I may need to view the woman's pelvic area to conduct an appropriate examination. There are several points that should be considered in order to facilitate the evaluation and treatment of these unique patients:

- *Professional behavior*—Gynecological emergencies are typically emotionally trying for patients. They have the potential to be embarrassing as well. The attitude of the EMT–I will help establish trust and support that the patient may desperately need. As public servants, EMT–Is should avoid categorizing or passing judgment on these patients, using their skills as medical care providers to assist these patients as much as possible.
- *Privacy and modesty*—Every precaution should be taken to protect the modesty and privacy of patients undergoing an acute gynecological emergency. The EMT–I should immediately take charge of the scene and limit the number of personnel who have access

to the patient. Moving the patient into the ambulance or a private room will further help ensure her privacy. Taking these steps will also help establish levels of trust between the patient and the care providers. During the examination it may be necessary to not remove certain clothing in order to protect the patient's modesty, or at least the patient should be covered with a blanket or sheet at all times.

- *Pain*—Another crucial consideration is that the patient may be experiencing significant physical pain in addition to emotional stress. Steps should be undertaken to make the patient as comfortable as possible, and consideration should be given to administering analgesics.

> **STREET WISE** ✳
>
> Many gynecological emergencies, including sexual assaults, are often high-profile situations. As an EMT–I, your duty to maintain the patient's privacy continues even after the patient is taken to the hospital. This includes avoiding any discussion of the nature of the patient's emergency, patient evaluation, or treatment in the ambulance or at the hospital. It may even be necessary to limit the access of other departmental personnel to the patient care record or other run documents.

General Examination

As with any patient, the initial examination should consist of a focused, initial assessment that evaluates the patient for any immediate life-threatening hemorrhage or physiological derangement. For the patient experiencing an acute gynecological emergency, this typically consists of obtaining an initial set of vital signs, observing the general level of consciousness, and assessing the type and amount of vaginal bleeding.

VITAL SIGNS

- *Blood pressure*—Hypotension in the patient experiencing an acute gynecological emergency is most commonly due to either internal hemorrhage in the pelvis

> **STREET WISE** ✳
>
> Try to obtain orthostatic vital signs in the field before initiating intravenous fluid resuscitation. This will allow the emergency department staff to have a clearer understanding of what the hydration status of the patient was before EMS interventions.

or external bleeding from the vagina. Hypotension can also be due to overwhelming infection that may be of gynecological origin.

- *Pulse*—Tachycardia can be attributed to dehydration, blood loss resulting in anemia, infection (including sepsis), pain, or anxiety.
- *Respiratory rate*—Any increased respiratory rate can be seen with gynecological infections, pain, anemia, or increased emotional states.

OTHER INITIAL ASSESSMENT

- *Skin*—Examination of the skin can provide significantly useful clinical information. Cyanosis may indicate severe anemia or respiratory insufficiency. Pallor in the patient may also indicate anemia and can be seen in hypotensive states. Warm and flush skin may indicate overwhelming infection and fever. Any lacerations, abrasions, or ecchymosis should be noted.
- *Genitourinary examination*—In some cases, vaginal bleeding or discharge can be indirectly noted on the patient's clothing, bed, or chair. The color and quantity of any bleeding should be noted, as well as the presence of any clots or other tissue that may be present. It is uncommon for EMT–Is to perform a genitourinary examination in cases other than childbirth. If a direct examination is performed, it must be by specific request of the patient and with an appropriate chaperone.
- *Abdomen*—The initial evaluation of the abdomen should be simple observation to see if the abdomen appears distended or whether it is flat and normal in shape. Palpation of the abdomen should be performed to identify any obvious masses or areas of tenderness. Guarding may be present when the patient has either voluntary or involuntary tightening of the abdominal wall muscles. This is in response to significant irritation and inflammation within the abdominal cavity. Rebound tenderness is also a sign of significant intraabdominal inflammation. This is elicited by slowly pressing down at a specific point on the abdomen and then quickly releasing. If the patient has significant pain following the release of pressure, this is considered a positive rebound tenderness test.

GENERAL MANAGEMENT

There are many serious medical problems that present with severe abdominal pain. Specific diagnoses are difficult to determine in the field, so the potential for a life-threatening emergency must always be considered. While performing the initial assessment on the patient, the EMT–I should determine any airway or breathing problems, as well as evaluate the circulatory status of the patient. In most patients with a gynecological emergency, oxygen therapy consists of a nasal cannula with

low-flow oxygen if the patient has normal vital signs. If vital signs are abnormal, oxygen therapy may involve the use of a nonrebreather mask with high-flow oxygen. Use of bag-valve-mask–assisted ventilations should be considered if respiratory efforts are inadequate. Hypoventilation in the gynecological patient is typically due to profound shock from hemorrhage or overwhelming infection.

Circulation

Although many women with mild to moderate vaginal bleeding or pelvic pain do not require intravenous (IV) access, placement of an IV line should be considered in any patient who has derangement of her physiological vital signs. If the vaginal bleeding is excessive, or if the patient has tachycardia, hypotension, or unusually severe pain, a large-bore IV line should be established and IV fluids initiated. Serial sets of vital signs should be obtained to assess the patient for response to therapy. Placing the patient in the Trendelenburg position may help improve vital organ perfusion if shock is present.

Medications

In general, analgesics are not recommended until the patient has had a thorough and proper medical evaluation in the emergency department. Prehospital use of medications like morphine or meperidine may mask significant abdominal pain or complaints that help guide the physician in determining a correct diagnosis. In addition, the use of analgesics risks lowering the blood pressure in some patients. This may be a particular detriment to patients who are already experiencing shock.

> **HELPFUL HINT**
>
> - Always consider pregnancy as a possible diagnosis any time a woman of childbearing age complains of abdominal pain or vaginal bleeding. There are occasions where women may take a pregnancy to term and still not believe they are pregnant. This may be due to the patient's body size, emotional state, or other factors. Have the necessary equipment for immediate newborn delivery when evaluating a patient with pelvic pain or vaginal bleeding.

SPECIFIC GYNECOLOGICAL EMERGENCIES

Acute abdominal pain in a woman can have several causes of gynecological origin. Examples include pelvic inflammatory disease, ruptured ovarian cyst, and ectopic pregnancy.

Pelvic Inflammatory Disease

✖ **Pelvic Inflammatory Disease (PID)** • Infection involving the pelvic structures, including the uterus and fallopian tubes.

Pelvic inflammatory disease (PID) results from either acute or chronic infection involving the pelvic structures. Bacteria can enter the woman's pelvis through the vagina and then move through the uterus into other pelvic organs, including the uterus, fallopian tubes, and ovaries. The infection can also involve specific support structures for the pelvic organs and even progress through the abdomen to involve areas such as the liver. The patient with PID commonly complains of fever, lower abdominal pain, vaginal discharge, and pain with intercourse (dyspareunia). Typically, there is intense pain with minimal palpation, abdominal guarding, and difficulty lying completely supine. Complications from PID include overwhelming sepsis and damage to pelvic structures, resulting in infertility or increased risk of future ectopic pregnancy.

Ruptured Ovarian Cyst

✖ **Ruptured Ovarian Cyst** • An often painful condition that occurs when a large cyst or ovary ruptures.

During the menstrual cycle, hormonal stimulation causes follicles on the ovaries to enlarge during the midcycle phase. Large follicles are generally considered cysts, and the presence of the cyst itself may cause pain. Rupture of an ovarian cyst can cause severe intense lower abdominal pain that is typically located on one side of the abdomen. Some **ruptured ovarian cysts** are associated with significant hemorrhage into the pelvis, and the patient may become hypotensive.

Ectopic Pregnancy

✖ **Ectopic Pregnancy** • The implantation of a fertilized egg outside of the uterus, usually in the fallopian tubes.

The incidence of **ectopic pregnancy** (Figure 31-2) is rising in the United States and is currently about 1 in 200 diagnosed pregnancies. Ectopic pregnancy should be considered in any female of reproductive age with lower abdominal pain. Certain factors increase the risk of an ectopic pregnancy:

- Previous abdominal surgery with adhesion formation
- Pelvic infections, or PID
- Tubal ligation
- Use of an intrauterine device (IUD)

The most common site for an ectopic pregnancy is within the fallopian tube. As the pregnancy progresses, bleeding can occur, along with lower abdominal cramping. If there is tubal rupture, massive bleeding can occur in the pelvis and the patient may present with shock.

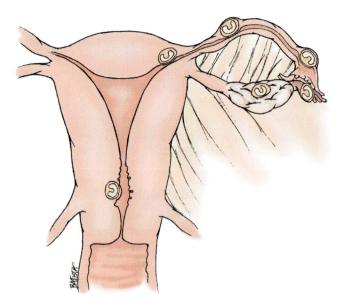

FIGURE 31-2 ▲ A pregnancy is considered ectopic if the embryo implants itself outside the uterus. This situation can be life threatening to the mother.

✖ **Miscarriage** • The spontaneous demise of a pregnancy.

Although pelvic pain and vaginal bleeding are commonly seen with ectopic pregnancy, these signs and symptoms are also encountered during the early stages of a miscarriage or threatened abortion. It should not be assumed that these symptoms are necessarily due to a **miscarriage;** rather, the woman should be treated for the possibility of a life-threatening ectopic pregnancy until she has had a proper gynecological examination at the hospital.

Suspicion of ectopic pregnancy should be high on the diagnostic problem list in a patient who has lower abdominal or pelvic pain, a missed or late period, vaginal bleeding, any signs of shock, and a history of risk factors for ectopic pregnancy.

Specific management of the patient with a potential ectopic pregnancy includes routine evaluation and monitoring, the establishment of two large-bore IV lines, and placement of the patient in the Trendelenburg position if she is hypotensive. The patient should be transported to a facility able to provide emergency gynecological surgical intervention.

Vaginal Bleeding

Although vaginal bleeding is part of the normal physiological process for most women, there are times when vaginal bleeding can signify a more acute medical emergency. It should never be assumed that vaginal bleeding is just the woman's normal period. Other, more serious or life-threatening conditions must be considered and the proper assessments and intervention undertaken. The significant causes of vaginal bleeding that must be considered include miscarriage and placenta previa or abruptio placentae.

MISCARRIAGE

Miscarriages are also called threatened abortions or spontaneous abortions. Although some women have unusual vaginal bleeding in the first or second trimester of an otherwise healthy pregnancy, bleeding may also be associated with the early phases of a miscarriage. Important historical information that should be gathered includes prior episodes of miscarriage and any known bleeding problems. A number of medical conditions predispose women to an increased incidence of miscarriage. If possible, the EMT–I should also collect and transport any large clots or apparent tissue for review at the hospital.

CLINICAL NOTES

It is crucial to recognize the need for emotional support of the woman who may be experiencing a miscarriage. Most women experience significant emotional attachment to the pregnancy, and this may impact your interactions with the patient. In these situations it is important to be as straightforward with the patient as possible. It is improper to comment on the overall health of the pregnancy; however, it is appropriate to help her direct her questions to the staff at the receiving facility.

PLACENTA PREVIA AND ABRUPTIO PLACENTAE

Placenta previa and abruptio placentae can cause significant bleeding in the third trimester of pregnancy. (Chapter 32 address both of these conditions in detail.) Both conditions can cause significant complications for the health of the pregnancy, as well as blood loss from the mother. They are acute obstetrical emergencies, and the patient should be transported rapidly to the emergency department.

OTHER CAUSES OF VAGINAL BLEEDING

Vaginal bleeding can range in intensity from light spotting to heavier bleeding and may be associated with the following:
- Onset of labor
- Infectious processes within the vagina or within the uterus
- Localized trauma to the vaginal wall from intercourse or other instrumentation
- Traumatic processes that injure the internal structures of the pelvis and abdomen

ASSESSMENT AND MANAGEMENT

The specific history of the patient with vaginal bleeding includes the time the vaginal bleeding started, the volume of vaginal bleeding (frequently measured in the number of sanitary pads the patient uses per hour), and any previous history of similar unusual vaginal bleeding. The woman's ability to compensate for the vaginal bleeding must be adequately assessed. Orthostatic vital signs should be obtained, and ongoing evaluations conducted during transport.

In general, the management of the woman with vaginal bleeding in the prehospital setting consists of observation only. A count of the number of sanitary pads the patient has used, as well as other towels or clothing that are soaked with blood, may help facilitate determining the volume and rate of bleeding. The EMT–I should not pack any dressing in the vagina in an attempt to tamponade or slow the bleeding.

If the patient is experiencing shock, a second IV line should be established (if this has not already been done), and additional fluid resuscitation undertaken. Placing the patient in the Trendelenburg position with the head down and feet elevated facilitates blood flow to the central nervous system and vital organs.

Abdominal or Perineal Trauma

✖ **Straddle Injury** • Trauma to the perineal area, typically from a fall with the legs abducted.

Vaginal bleeding may also be related to trauma that the patient has suffered. Common injuries that may cause vaginal bleeding include the following:
- *Straddle injuries*—A **straddle injury** occurs when the female falls or strikes an object with both legs abducted, causing significant trauma or laceration to the perineal area.
- *Blunt trauma to the lower abdomen*—Although most commonly seen from motor vehicle crashes, blunt trauma can also result from physical assault of the patient or from falls.
- *Foreign bodies*—Whether inserted voluntarily or in conjunction with an assault, foreign bodies may cause significant vaginal hemorrhage. No attempts should be made to remove the foreign body until the patient has arrived at the emergency department.

STREET WISE

Some women may attempt to abort a pregnancy through unusual means. Significant laceration and injury can occur to the vaginal wall, as well as to the cervix and uterus. Hemorrhage may be severe, and the patient should be assessed for shock.

ASSESSMENT AND MANAGEMENT

As with any patient with vaginal bleeding, the assessment should include the heart rate, blood pressure, orthostatic vital signs, and general neurological responsiveness. Management is directed toward supportive care, continuous monitoring, and IV fluids. In general, no attempts should be made to pack the vagina in an attempt to tamponade the bleeding unless directed by local medical control.

Sexual Assault

✖ **Sexual Assault** • Any assault crime that involve the genitalia of either party.

Victims of **sexual assault** can be among the most challenging patients EMT–Is can encounter and require an immense amount of professionalism, respect for the patient, and empathy for the circumstances the patient has suffered. The patient has undergone severe emotional stress, as well as possible physical injuries. Numerous responses may be expressed by the patient, including severe agitation, anxiety, withdrawal, or the entering of a catatonic state.

When approaching the sexual assault patient, the EMT–I should assume a very clear posture of being gentle and nonthreatening. Rather than having the course of action dictated to her, the patient should be given choices and allowed to have input into the decisions. Questions regarding the patient's past sexual history or sexual practices should be avoided, as well as any actions that may provoke guilt in the patient. It is acceptable to simply ask the patient, "Do you want to tell me what happened to you?" and use subsequent information for the history of present illness. *It is critical to note the role of EMS as an advocate for the patient. Every effort should be made to protect the patient's privacy and to provide her with the most comforting environment possible.*

ASSESSMENT AND MANAGEMENT

After requesting the patient's permission to conduct an examination, the EMT–I should perform a brief initial assessment, including vital signs and general neurological state. The genitalia should be examined only at the patient's request; this step is typically performed by the staff at the receiving facility.

Management techniques include the following:

- Ensure that the environment is safe and quiet, and that it provides as much psychological support as possible for the patient. Ask permission to ask questions and examine the patient. Empower the patient to make as many decisions as she can.
- Although the role of EMS is to be a patient advocate, remember that a crime has been committed:
  - If the patient has already removed her clothing, ask her to place it in a paper bag. Always wear gloves when handling clothing, and avoid touching any of the clothing as much as possible. If the patient is still in the clothes she was wearing at the time of the assault, request that she not change her clothes but bring a change of clothes with her to the receiving facility
  - In addition to requesting that the patient not change her clothes, ask her not to bathe, urinate, or perform any other cleansing of her body.
  - Unless absolutely necessary, do not cleanse traumatic injuries until proper documentation has been obtained at the hospital.
  - Attempt to preserve the crime scene as much as possible by not disturbing any weapons or other objects at the scene. Ideally, local law enforcement should arrive at the scene before EMS transport; immediate transport is not required as long as the patient is otherwise physically stable.

STREET WISE

Become familiar with the local resources available for the sexual assault patient. In some locations, certain hospitals are designated as the primary destination for the sexual assault patient and are therefore equipped with specialized examination tools, specially trained personnel, and social support staff. Some regions may also have implemented sexual assault centers or teams not associated with hospitals. Discussions with local medical control should help determine the general destination for patients who are victims of a sexual assault.

Any patient with abnormal vital signs or evidence of head injury or any other trauma should be transported to a medical facility able to provide trauma care.

CASE HISTORY FOLLOW-UP ■■■

Although there are numerous etiologies for abdominal pain and bleeding, this woman most likely has a ruptured ectopic pregnancy. The past history of pelvic surgery and pelvic infections raises the risk of ectopic pregnancy. As in this case, ectopic pregnancies may occur before a woman has seen an obstetrician, and she may not even know that she is pregnant. Immediate interventions include high-flow oxygen, the establishment of two IV lines, and placement of the patient in the Trendelenburg position. The patient should be transported to a facility that can perform rapid gynecological examination and surgery.

SUMMARY

Important points to remember from this chapter include the following:

- Acute gynecological emergencies represent a spectrum of diseases that range from benign to clearly life threatening.
- Abdominal pain can result from a variety of causes. Specific to the gynecological structures are pelvic inflammatory disease, ruptured ovarian cysts, and ectopic pregnancies.
- Although vaginal bleeding is typically associated with normal menses, it can also be seen in ectopic pregnancies, bleeding disorders, miscarriages, placenta previa, and abruptio placentae.
- The EMT–I should be prepared to interact with and evaluate a woman who is the victim of sexual assault. Many hospitals and local social service agencies have specific resources for these patients.

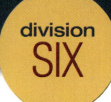

SPECIAL CONSIDERATIONS

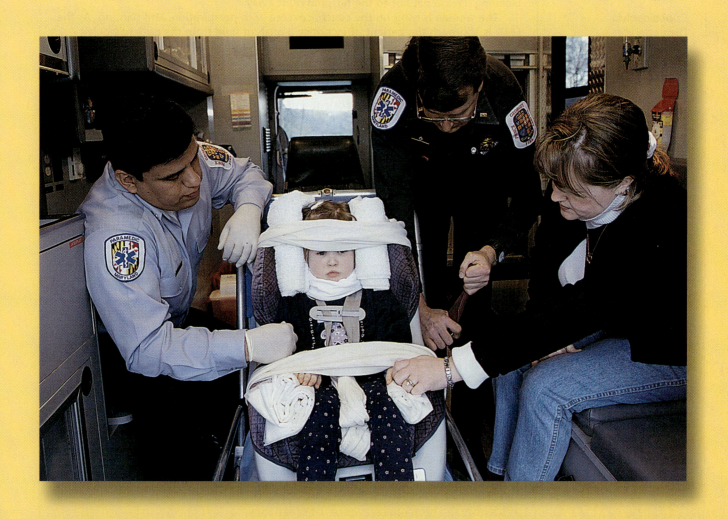

32

Obstetrical Emergencies

▪▪▪ CASE HISTORY

At 10:00 PM, EMT–Is Bradley and Miller respond to a 28-year-old female reported to be "in labor." On arrival, a very anxious husband and four small children meet them at the door. As they enter the house, her husband says, "She's seven-and-a-half months, and she's bleeding. Please get her to the hospital right away."

The woman is lying on the couch, covered with perspiration, and panting. As the EMT–Is approach the patient, they notice a gush of fluid from the patient's pelvic area, and she turns and screams, "The baby is coming NOW!"

The husband reports that his wife delivered two of their children early. The woman states that her labor started about 4 hours ago but progressed rapidly in the last 20 minutes. Her contractions are 1 to 2 minutes apart.

EMT–I Bradley looks at the patient and sees that she is crying and afraid. "We're going to take good care of you and your baby," he says, in a confident and supportive voice. He then asks the woman for permission to examine her. While EMT–I Miller is assessing vital signs, EMT–I Bradley examines the woman to find obvious crowning of the newborn. Her pulse (heart rate) is 124, respirations are 24 between contractions, and blood pressure is 94/76. Her respirations are easy and quiet. EMT–I Miller places her on oxygen while Bradley opens the obstetrics kit and positions the sterile pads under the patient's buttocks and covers her belly. "We're going to deliver the baby right here," EMT–I Bradley tells her.

LEARNING OBJECTIVES

CHAPTER GOAL
Upon completion of this chapter, the EMT-Intermediate will be able to apply and utilize the assessment findings to formulate and implement a treatment plan for normal and abnormal labor.

Cognitive Objectives
As an EMT-Intermediate you should be able to do the following:
- Review the anatomical structures and physiology of the reproductive system.
- Identify the normal occurrences of pregnancy.
- Describe how to assess an obstetrical patient.
- Identify the stages of labor and the role the EMT–I plays in each stage.
- Differentiate between normal and abnormal delivery.

- Identify and describe the complications associated with labor and delivery.
- Identify predelivery emergencies.
- Describe the management of a patient with a predelivery emergency.
- Describe indications of an imminent delivery.
- State the steps in preparing the mother for delivery.
- Describe the steps involved in delivering the newborn.
- Describe the indications and procedure for cutting the umbilical cord.
- Discuss the steps involved in delivery of the placenta.
- Describe the care of the mother after the delivery.
- Describe the procedures involved with handling the following:
  - Abnormal deliveries
  - Complications of pregnancy
  - Complications of labor
- Describe the significance of meconium being present in the amniotic fluid.
- Describe special considerations surrounding the delivery of a premature newborn.

Affective Objectives
As an EMT–Intermediate you should be able to do the following:
- Advocate the need for treating two patients (mother and newborn).
- Understand the importance of maintaining a patient's modesty throughout the assessment and intervention stages.
- Value the importance of body substance isolation.

Psychomotor Objectives
As an EMT–Intermediate you should be able to do the following:
- Assess an obstetrical patient.
- Care for a patient with excessive vaginal bleeding.
- Care for a patient with severe abdominal pain.
- Prepare the mother and equipment for delivery.
- Assist in normal cephalic delivery of the fetus.
- Deliver the placenta.
- Care for the mother and newborn after delivery.
- Know the interventions needed in abnormal deliveries.

INTRODUCTION

Pregnancy typically is a joyful time for the expectant mother. The vast majority of pregnancies complete to term with only occasional minor complications. The delivery of the newborn is a very natural process. The role of the EMT–Intermediate (EMT–I) during normal and uncomplicated deliveries is simply to provide supportive care to the mother and the newborn. The EMT–I can provide significant assistance in recognizing and intervening when a complication of pregnancy or abnormal delivery is encountered.

The EMT–I must recognize that labor and delivery are very personal and intimate events for the mother and the family. Every effort should be made to protect the mother's privacy during this process. It is also critical to realize that throughout the process, there are two patients to care for: the mother and the child.

Anatomy

An EMT–I should be familiar with the structures of the female reproductive system, as follows (see Figure 31-1):

- **Ovaries**—A walnut-sized pair of glands located on each side of the uterus in the upper pelvic cavity. The ovaries produce mature ova (eggs) and secrete primarily female sexual hormones (estrogen and progesterone).
- **Fallopian tubes**—A pair of muscular tubes that extend from the uterus into the pelvic cavity. Each tube has a funnel-shaped open end, which is close to an ovary. The tubes provide a passageway for the transport of sperm to the ova and transport the ova back to the uterus by wavelike, muscular contractions.
- **Uterus**—A hollow, muscular organ shaped like an inverted pear located in the pelvic cavity between the urinary bladder and the rectum. The uterus is divided into three parts: the fundus, the body, and the cervix. The inner lining of the uterus, the endometrium, serves as the site of implantation of the fertilized egg, as well as the organ of menstruation. During pregnancy, the fetus develops within the uterus.
- **Cervix**—The inferior, narrow portion of the uterus that opens into the vagina. During labor, the cervix will thin out (efface) and dilate to allow the fetus and placenta to pass into the birth canal or vagina.
- **Vagina**—The birth canal or passageway between the uterus and the external genitalia or perineum. The vagina is the female sex organ that receives the penis during intercourse. It also provides a passageway for menstrual flow and for the fetus during delivery.
- **Perineum**—The external female genital region between the urinary opening (urethra) and the anus or rectal opening. This area includes the external female genitalia and the opening of the vagina. The labia are structures that protect the vaginal and urethral openings.

During pregnancy, certain organs or structures develop that are not present in the non-pregnant state. They are as follows (Figure 32-1):

- **Placenta**—A disk-shaped spongy organ that develops in the uterus during pregnancy. The placenta exchanges oxygen and nourishment from mother to fetus and transfers waste products, including fetal carbon dioxide, from the fetus to the mother's bloodstream via blood vessels in the umbilical cord. It also manufactures hormones (estrogen and progesterone) that not only prevent menses, but also influence anatomical changes within the mother in preparation for childbirth. When the placenta passes from the vagina following delivery of the newborn, it is sometimes referred to as the afterbirth.

- **Umbilical cord**—The attachment between the fetus and the placenta. The umbilical cord contains two arteries and one vein, and provides continuous blood flow from mother to fetus and from fetus to mother. The blood, oxygen, and nourishment to the fetus from the mother are carried via the umbilical vein. The arteries carry deoxygenated blood from the fetus back to the placenta.

- **Amniotic sac**—Protective membranous sac that insulates and protects the fetus during pregnancy. The sac contains 500 to 1000 milliliters (mL) of amniotic fluid after the twentieth week of pregnancy. The fluid is normally clear in color and rupture of the membranes will typically cause a clear watery discharge. Together, the sac and fluid protect the fetus while in the uterus.

- **Fetus**—The unborn child.

✖ **Menarche** • The onset of menstruation in a female.

✖ **Menopause** • The point at which a woman stops menstruating.

Physiology

Each month the uterus is stimulated by hormones to develop a thickened inner lining or endometrium. If sperm fertilizes an egg, it is implanted in the uterus and nourished by this lining and pregnancy begins. If no

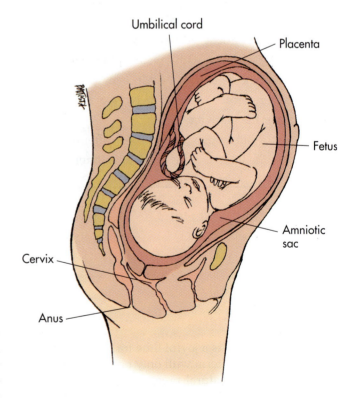

FIGURE 32-1   ▲   **The female anatomy during pregnancy.** (Kimberly Battista from Stoy W: *Mosby's EMT-Basic textbook*, St Louis, 1996, Mosby.)

egg is fertilized, the uterus sheds the lining, which is composed of cells and blood. This process is known as the *menstrual cycle* or *menstrual period.*

The onset of menstruation, or **menarche,** usually occurs in girls between the ages of 8 and 14. The average **menstrual cycle** lasts 28 days, but there is a great deal of individual variation. The onset of menstrual flow is counted as the first day of the cycle. Menstruation generally lasts for 3 to 7 days.

Under the influence of hormonal changes, an ovary releases an egg on approximately the 14th day of the cycle. This process is known as *ovulation.* The egg then travels down the fallopian tube toward the uterus, where it will be implanted if it is fertilized. If not fertilized, the egg will be shed with the menstrual flow.

Generally, between the ages of 35 and 60 years, the menstrual cycle and a woman's reproductive years come to an end. This process, known as **menopause,** may occur gradually or suddenly. When menopause occurs, the woman will no longer have a menstrual period.

Fetal growth and development is an extremely complex process. The following developmental points are important:

- At the completion of the third month (13th week) of pregnancy:
  - Fetal gender can be determined
  - Heart is beating
  - Every structure found at birth is present
- At the completion of the fifth month (21st week) of pregnancy:
  - Fetal heartbeat can be heard with simple abdominal ultrasound
  - "Quickening" occurs, which is the noticing of fetal movement
- At the completion of the sixth month (24th week) of pregnancy:
  - Chances of survival increase if birth is premature
- At the completion of the ninth month (40th week) of pregnancy:
  - Considered "at term"

Overview of Normal Pregnancy

Pregnancy and childbirth are natural conditions (Box 32-1). Full-term pregnancies last approximately 280 days (40 weeks) from the first day of the woman's last menstrual period (LMP) until delivery. Although pregnancy is a common condition, every woman may experience the changes of pregnancy in a different way. The most common signs and symptoms of early pregnancy include the following:

- Missed or late menstrual period
- Nausea and vomiting (although typically referred to as "morning sickness," nausea and vomiting may occur at any time of the day)
- Breast tenderness and enlargement
- Frequent urination

Pregnancy leads to significant changes in nearly all body systems. These alterations in physiology from the nonpregnant state become important in cases of illness or injury (Figure 32-2).

Respiratory System

Pregnant women will develop an increased respiratory rate and depth. During the fourth to fifth month of pregnancy the fetus begins to take up increased space in the abdominal cavity and will compromise the ability of the diaphragm to flatten completely. The expectant mother will become tachypneic to compensate for this decreased volume of the thoracic cavity. As a result of the increased respiratory rate, a respiratory alkalosis develops.

Cardiovascular System

The cardiovascular system is significantly affected during pregnancy. An increase in the total blood volume of 40% to 50% occurs, which is referred to as hypervolemia of pregnancy. There is a proportionately greater increase in the amount of plasma than in red blood cells (RBCs), resulting in a dilution in the concentration of RBCs. This condition results in physiological anemia. In addition, there is an increase in the number of white blood cells and in cardiac output during pregnancy. The expectant mother also is prone to developing blood clots in her legs.

Vital Signs

The normal range for vital signs changes during pregnancy. The resting heart rate (HR) typically increases 10 to 20 beats per minute and the normal blood pressure (BP) drops 10 to 15 mm Hg from nonpregnant levels.

BOX 32-1

SPECIFIC OBSTETRICAL TERMINOLOGY

Antepartum—Before delivery
Postpartum—After delivery
Prenatal—Occurring before birth
Natal—Connected with the birth
Gravida (or "G")—Total number of pregnancies
Para (or "P")—Total number of pregnancies carried to term
Primipara (or "primip")—A woman who is pregnant with or delivering her first child
Multiparous—A women who has given birth multiple times
Gestation—The age, typically in weeks, of the fetus
Expected date of confinement (EDC)—Due date calculated from first day of last normal menses or by ultrasound examination of the fetus.

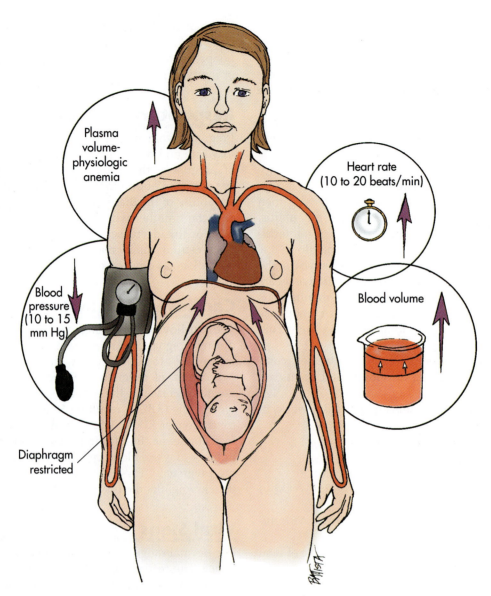

FIGURE 32-2 ▲ **Physiological changes observed.**

Gastrointestinal System

There tends to be decreased motility of the gastrointestinal tract and upward displacement of the diaphragm during pregnancy. Both result in a decrease in the movement of foodstuffs through the gastrointestinal tract. For this reason, an increased risk of vomiting and aspiration occurs in the later stages of pregnancy. Heartburn is common.

Urinary System

The bladder is displaced anteriorly and superiorly in pregnancy and is very vulnerable to penetrating or blunt trauma. Due to an increased cardiac output, the pregnant woman makes more urine, which leads to increased frequency of urination. The risk of urinary tract infections also increases during pregnancy.

Minor and Common Problems With Pregnancy

Pregnancy is divided into three trimesters, each lasting approximately 13 weeks. During each trimester, the patient may experience any of a number of minor but common problems. Although bothersome, these complaints are not often dangerous to either mother or fetus and may include the following:

1. First trimester
   - Frequent urination
   - Nausea and vomiting
   - Breast pain/tingling/tenderness
   - Weakness and fatigue
2. Second trimester
   - Constipation
   - Heartburn
   - Leg cramps

3. Third trimester
- Hemorrhoids
- Varicose veins
- Leg cramps
- Braxton-Hicks contractions (painless irregular uterine contractions)

CLINICAL NOTES

The abbreviations G, P, and A are commonly used in relaying obstetrical histories. *Gravida (G)* refers to the total number of pregnancies, including the current pregnancy. *Para (P)* refers to the number of previous live births. The total number of **miscarriages (spontaneous abortions)** or elective abortions is abbreviated with an *A*. The patient's last normal menstrual period is often abbreviated as *LNMP* or *LMP* and is indicated by the date of onset of the flow of the most recent menses. For example, if a woman's last normal menses started on April 16, the LMP is 4/16. Furthermore, if she had four previous full-term pregnancies and two spontaneous miscarriages, and is again currently pregnant, then her obstetrical history can be reported as *G7P4A2 with LMP 4/16*.

ASSESSMENT OF THE OBSTETRICAL PATIENT

Patient assessment always begins with scene size-up and initial assessment. The EMT–I should correct any life-threatening conditions before proceeding into the focused history and physical examination. Remember to follow all body substance isolation (BSI) procedures during each patient encounter.

Female patients with various complaints may have a dysfunction of the urinary tract, the gastrointestinal tract, or any of the reproductive organs. An accurate gynecological and obstetrical history is essential to the assessment of all female patients. Whenever possible, another woman should be present during patient evaluations that involve the examination of the genitalia or sexual history taking.

History of Present Illness

Gathering a quick and complete history of the patient's current condition will assist the EMT–I in building a correct working diagnosis and treatment plan. In addition to asking the normal SAMPLE information (see

STREET WISE

Many patients feel uncomfortable speaking candidly about genital or urinary conditions. Adolescents may be particularly reluctant to discuss these conditions honestly while their parents are present. If the patient seems uncomfortable or embarrassed, the EMT–I should ask only those questions that are necessary for immediate care and make every effort to ask the questions in as private a setting as possible. As a health care provider, the EMT–I's professional demeanor will increase the patient's comfort level. A more complete history may be obtained at the hospital.

Chapter 9), the following additional specific questions should be asked:
1. Does the mother have pertinent medical history, including:
   - Diabetes
   - Heart disease
   - Hypertension or hypotension
   - Seizures
2. What is the current health of the mother?
3. Have there been any recent illnesses, fever, or injuries?
4. What is the level of prenatal care?
5. Does the mother use any illicit drugs, alcohol, or tobacco?

These questions can help the EMT–I identify women with pregnancies prone to developing complications and anticipate difficult deliveries.

Specific questions regarding the current pregnancy include the following:
1. What was the first day of the LMP?
2. Has the obstetrician informed the mother of the anticipated delivery date, also known as expected date of confinement?
3. How many previous pregnancies and term deliveries?
4. Any previous complications with any prior pregnancies or deliveries?
5. Are there any known complications of the current pregnancy, such as gestational diabetes, multiple gestations, or preeclampsia?
6. Are there any expected difficulties with this delivery (e.g., large fetus or abnormal position)?
7. When did the contractions start, and how far apart are they?
8. Is there any pain that is different than the contractions?
9. Is there any vaginal bleeding or discharge?
10. If bleeding still continues, note the amount, color and duration of bleeding.

Substance Abuse History

Many substances may be harmful and may also alter the growth and development of the fetus during pregnancy. Commonly abused substances include cigarettes, alcohol, and drugs.

Knowing potential toxins that the fetus is exposed to during pregnancy may help the EMT–I anticipate delivery of a newborn that will need aggressive resuscitation or other special needs.

Physical Examination

Physical examination of the pregnant female should include the normal primary examination that ensures that the ABCs are intact. Some obstetrical emergencies can be associated with profound shock; therefore assessing the patient for hypotension and tachycardia is critical. Another unique aspect of evaluating and treating the pregnant female is the importance placed on protecting the patient's modesty and privacy throughout all stages of the examination.

Vital signs should be obtained in all cases. Palpation of the uterus may help indicate when a contraction is starting, but this may be difficult in patients who are obese.

Visual inspection of the genital area should be performed to assess for vaginal bleeding or discharge. It is also important to note if the newborn's head is clearly visible, which is also called **crowning.**

General Management

Specific management of a newborn delivery and unusual problems are discussed later in this chapter, but certain basic management techniques should be employed with all obstetrical patients, as follows:

- *Oxygen*—Oxygen should be delivered to all pregnant females, especially if labor has started. The fetus extracts oxygen from the maternal circulation and undergoes significant stress during delivery. Providing supplemental oxygenation may be beneficial to the fetus.
- *Intravenous (IV) fluids*—Each pregnant patient should have a large-bore IV line established. Even though the female expands her blood volume during pregnancy, there can be significant blood loss associated with delivery and fluid resuscitation may be needed. If signs of hypotension or unusually heavy blood loss are present, a second IV line should be considered.
- *Positioning*—At approximately 24 weeks of pregnancy, the enlarging uterus can exert enough pressure on the inferior vena cava to restrict blood flow returning to the heart, causing hypotension in the mother and potential hypoperfusion of the placenta and the fetus. This is known as *supine hypotensive syndrome.* Positioning the mother in the left lateral recumbent position will move the uterus off the vena cava and promote more normal blood flow (Figure 32-3).

STREET WISE

The inferior vena cava lies just to the right of midline. Transporting the pregnant patient tilted to the left will displace the gravid uterus off the vena cava and prevent supine hypotensive syndrome.

Complications of Pregnancy

Various medical and surgical conditions may arise during pregnancy. Many of these are related to the physiological changes noted previously.

Diabetes

Women with preexisting diabetes mellitus may experience unpredictable swings in blood sugar levels. Insulin therapy must be closely monitored and adjusted for periods of increased or decreased food intake.

Women with no history of diabetes may also develop gestational diabetes and be prone to episodes of high blood sugar levels. Almost all women are screened early in pregnancy for gestational diabetes.

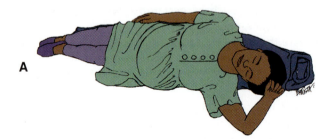
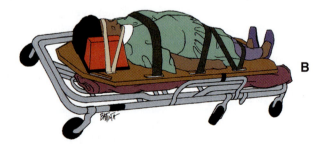

FIGURE 32-3 ▲ **A,** Transport a pregnant patient on her left side to reduce pressure placed on her circulatory system by the fetus. **B,** If a pregnant patient is immobilized on a long board, tilt the board on her left side. (Kimberly Battista from Stoy W: *Mosby's EMT-Basic textbook,* St Louis, 1996, Mosby.)

Most women can manage gestational diabetes with diet and exercise, although some may need to take doses of insulin or alter their diet to maintain a proper blood sugar level. Risk factors for gestational diabetes include obesity, a family history of diabetes, having given birth previously to a very large newborn, a stillbirth, a child with a birth defect, and having too much amniotic fluid (polyhydramnios).

Ectopic Pregnancy

Ectopic pregnancy refers to a pregnancy located outside of the uterus. This poses a significant risk to the mother from rupture of the fallopian tube and subsequent hemorrhage. In ectopic pregnancies the fertilized egg typically implants in the fallopian tube. As the pregnancy grows, pressure on the tube can lead to rupture, significant bleeding, and shock. Maternal risk factors for ectopic pregnancy include the following:

- Previous abdominal surgery and fibrous adhesion bands within the lower abdomen
- Pelvic infection
- Tubal ligation
- Use of an intrauterine device to prevent fertilization

Suspicion should be raised for an ectopic pregnancy in any woman with known pregnancy or missed menses who complains of abdominal pain or vaginal bleeding or shows signs of hypotension and shock. Treatment involves establishing IV lines and beginning fluid resuscitation. The patient should be transported to a facility equipped to evaluate and manage this potential surgical emergency. Ectopic pregnancy is also discussed in Chapter 31.

Supine Hypotensive Syndrome

As the uterus enlarges, at approximately 20 weeks gestation, its weight may compress the inferior vena cava when the mother is in a supine position, creating hypotension and restriction of blood flow to the placenta, or **supine hypotensive syndrome.** Although easily relieved, this situation can be fatal to the fetus if uncorrected.

The easiest treatment is prevention, specifically, keeping the pregnant woman positioned on her left side rather than in a supine position. In pregnant trauma victims, the EMT–I should apply immobilizing devices as he or she normally would, using caution to not compress the uterus with straps. Once the patient is immobilized, the backboard should be tilted to place the patient with her left side down. A turnout coat, blankets, or other suitable objects can be placed under the board on the mother's right side to keep the board tilted to her left.

Appendicitis

Although appendicitis is common in patients of all ages and both genders, it occurs in one out of every 1000 pregnancies. The appendix normally is located in the right lower quadrant of the abdomen. Pregnancy causes many organs, including the appendix, to be displaced superiorly. Appendicitis is more difficult to assess during pregnancy, especially in the last two trimesters, partially due to this anatomical change. The inflamed appendix is two to three times more likely to rupture in the pregnant patient. The EMT–I should care for the pregnant patient as he or she would any patient presenting with abdominal pain. The EMT–I should give her nothing by mouth, administer oxygen, consider an IV line, and transport the patient with her left side down per local protocols.

Preeclampsia and Eclampsia

Preeclampsia is an abnormal state during pregnancy characterized by hypertension and fluid retention. **Eclampsia** is defined as the occurrence of seizures in addition to the syndrome of preeclampsia. Eclampsia peaks during the third trimester and is life threatening to both the mother and fetus. Both preeclampsia and eclampsia may occur up to 1 week after delivery.

Situations in which the patient is more likely to have pregnancy-induced hypertension or preeclampsia include the following:

- First-time pregnancy in a woman under 20 years or over 35 years of age
- Multiple gestation (twins)
- Preexisting hypertension
- Diabetes mellitus
- Family history of preeclampsia or eclampsia
- Previous pregnancies with preeclampsia or eclampsia

Signs and symptoms of preeclampsia/eclampsia include the following:

- *Elevated blood pressure*—In mild cases, the patient's BP is approximately 140/90 mm Hg; in severe cases, it may be as high as 160/110 mm Hg. The EMT–I should not rely solely on the presence of hypertension, however, because preeclampsia may exist without elevated BP. In general, an acute rise in the systolic BP by 20 and diastolic BP by 10 is associated with preeclampsia.
- *Fluid signs*—Puffiness around the eyes, face, and swelling of fingers and feet. The EMT–I should listen for rales in the lungs
- *Excessive weight gain*—Most experts consider the following to be abnormal:
  - Greater than 3 pounds (lb) per month during the second trimester
  - Greater than 1 lb per week during the third trimester
  - A sudden weight gain of 4 to 4.5 lb per week anytime during the pregnancy
- *Headache*—A transient headache indicates a mild case, whereas a very severe headache may indicate severe preeclampsia.
- Visual disturbances (blurring/double vision)

- Irritability or change in mental status
- Epigastric abdominal pain
- Protein in the urine (tested at hospital or doctor's office)
- Decreased urine output

The onset of seizures or coma heralds eclampsia, which requires emergency treatment. Any patient with seizures during pregnancy or labor, or soon after delivery must be suspected of having eclampsia.

To care for the patient with preeclampsia or eclampsia, the EMT–I should do the following:

- Ensure that the airway, breathing, and circulation intact.
- Administer oxygen by nonrebreather mask at 10 to 15 liters (L)/min.
- Start an IV line per protocol.
- Place the patient on her left side and transport.
- Protect the airway and the patient from injury.
- If seizures occur, use medications to stop the seizure and control the BP as recommended by local protocol and medical direction:
  - Valium (diazepam), 5 to 10 mg IV
  - Magnesium sulfate ($MgSO_4$) up to 4 gm IV
- Avoid emergency lights or siren during transport as they may precipitate seizures. Try to minimize stimulation as much as possible.
- Notify the receiving hospital of the patient's status and the estimated time of arrival (ETA).

Pregnancy-induced hypertension is a problem in approximately 5% of all pregnant women in the United States. *Pregnancy-induced hypertension* is defined as a rise in systolic BP of 30 mm Hg or a rise in diastolic BP of 15 mm Hg above the woman's normal baseline values. If the patient's baseline BP is not known, a BP of 140/90 is also considered hypertension during pregnancy. Pregnancy-induced hypertension alone is not considered life threatening.

Trauma During Pregnancy

A call to care for a pregnant trauma patient creates fear and anxiety in many emergency care providers. Pregnancy can complicate patient assessment and cause an alteration in vital signs. No matter how minimal trauma may appear, a physician should evaluate all pregnant patients who experience blunt or penetrating trauma.

Due to the physiological changes previously noted, the pregnant woman has an increased HR and lower BP. Therefore changes in vital signs may be difficult to interpret. In addition, the increased blood volume of pregnancy may allow greater blood loss to occur before signs or symptoms of shock develop. By the time the EMT–I even notices a change in vital signs, the pregnant patient may have lost 35% of her circulating blood volume. Maternal hypovolemia will decrease blood flow to the uterus and reduce oxygen delivery to the fetus. The fetus may suffer harm before the EMT–I notices signs and symptoms of decreased perfusion in the mother.

To provide general prehospital care for the pregnant trauma patient, the EMT–I should do the following:

- Assess the airway, breathing, and circulation.
- Administer oxygen by nonrebreather mask at 10 to 15 L/min.
- Provide IV fluid resuscitation as per local protocols.
- Provide spinal immobilization. Immobilize a pregnant trauma patient as any other patient, and then tilt the board and patient on the left side.
- Transport the pregnant trauma patient to the closest appropriate medical facility. Keep in mind that this facility should have trauma, obstetrics, gynecological, and neonatal intensive care unit capabilities.
- Reassure the patient.
- Notify the receiving hospital of the patient's injuries and ETA.

Placenta Previa • An abnormal positioning of the placenta low in the uterus.

Abruptio Placenta • The premature detachment of the placenta.

Third Trimester Bleeding and Abdominal Pain

Vaginal bleeding in the third, or last, trimester indicates a serious and potentially life-threatening emergency for both the mother and fetus. The three common causes of third-trimester hemorrhage are noted in the following pages. Prehospital care for these conditions is the same regardless of the suspected condition.

Placenta Previa

Placenta previa is the abnormal positioning of the placenta within the uterus that occurs in approximately 1 in 300 births. If the placenta implants low in the uterus, it will be the presenting part. At the onset of labor, with the dilation of the cervix, the placenta will begin to detach. Once the placenta delivers or begins to separate, the fetus will not receive oxygen or nutrients. Predisposing factors include multiple pregnancies, rapid succession of pregnancies, mothers over age 35 years, and previous history of placenta previa. *Typically, the patient presents with profuse, painless bright red bleeding from the vagina.* The uterus may be soft or may develop contractions (Figure 32-4).

Abruptio Placenta

Abruptio placenta is the premature detachment of a normally situated placenta. This detachment may be complete or partial and can occur in any stage of pregnancy but is usually a third-trimester complication. Signs and symptoms of abruptio placentae include the following:

- Sudden onset of severe and constant lower abdominal pain
- Dark vaginal bleeding (Bleeding may occur behind the placenta with no obvious external bleeding. Visible blood loss should NOT be used as a guide for internal blood loss in this condition.)
- Soft, tender, or contracting uterus
- Shock

Risk factors for developing abruptio placenta include a history of preeclampsia (at least 25% of cases), chronic hypertension, multiple pregnancies, previous abruptio placenta, motor vehicle trauma, or cocaine use (Figure 32-5).

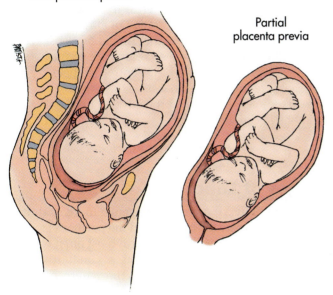

Total placenta previa

Partial placenta previa

FIGURE 32-4 ▲ **Placenta previa is an abnormal positioning of the placenta low in the uterus.**

> ❗ **HELPFUL HINT**
>
> To differentiate placenta previa from abruptio placenta, the EMT–I should look for painless bleeding in placenta previa or uterine pain and tenderness with less obvious bleeding in abruptio placenta.

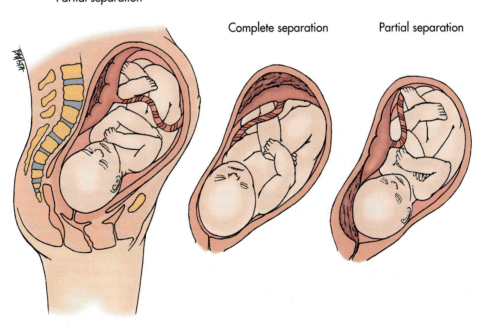

Partial separation

Complete separation

Partial separation

FIGURE 32-5 ▲ **Abruptio placenta is a premature detachment of an otherwise normal placenta.**

Uterine Rupture

Uterine rupture occurs most commonly after the onset of labor. The patient will complain of severe abdominal pain, which may appear to be the onset of normal labor or a severe contraction. Contractions will then cease as the uterus ruptures. This condition has a high mortality rate for both mother and fetus. Risk factors for developing uterine rupture include a history of uterine surgery (including Cesarean section), trauma, prolonged or obstructed labor, and an abnormal fetal presentation.

Signs and symptoms of uterine rupture include the following:
- Continuous severe abdominal pain
- Minimal vaginal bleeding
- Tearing sensation in abdomen
- Nausea
- Shock
- Easily palpable fetus in abdomen

General Care During the Third Trimester

It is often difficult to distinguish between the possible complications encountered late in pregnancy. To provide care for any patient who is in her third trimester of pregnancy and complains of either abdominal pain or bleeding, the EMT–I should do the following:
- Administer oxygen by nonrebreather mask at 10 to 15 L/min.
- Continuously monitor the patient's vital signs.
- Place the patient on her left side.
- Provide resuscitation per local protocol.
- Provide rapid, gentle transport to the closest appropriate hospital with obstetrical and neonatal care.
- Notify receiving hospital to alert the obstetrics staff and inform them of the ETA.
- Reassure the patient.

LABOR AND DELIVERY

Labor

Labor is defined as rhythmic contractions that occur with increasing frequency and forcefulness. The discomfort may be experienced in the abdomen or the lower back. The contraction interval is measured from the beginning of one contraction to the beginning of the next. As labor progresses, the contractions usually become stronger and closer together, lasting 30 to 60 seconds and occurring every 2 to 3 minutes.

> **CLINICAL NOTES**
>
> Braxton-Hicks contractions are benign uterine contractions that occur intermittently throughout the last trimester. They are generally painless and may be relieved by walking.

> **CLINICAL NOTES**
>
> Any labor that begins before term (38 weeks) is considered preterm labor. Physiological derangements in the mother or anatomical abnormalities within the uterus can both increase the likelihood of preterm labor. Premature rupture of the membranes will also stimulate the uterus and contractions will begin. The greatest risk of preterm labor is early delivery of the fetus before adequate development to support life outside of the uterus. Treatment should involve the administration of intravenous fluids and oxygen. The mother should be transported to a hospital that can resuscitate premature newborns. Local medical control can help determine the facilities that have this capacity, which usually involve a hospital with a neonatal intensive care unit.

Stages of Labor

Labor and delivery are natural events. In general, the EMT–I only assists the mother and the newborn as necessary. In fact, prehospital childbirth most often will be "unexpected" rather than "emergency" childbirth.

Labor occurs in three stages. The length of each stage of labor varies from patient to patient and from pregnancy to pregnancy. Most often, the second stage of labor will be approximately one half as long as the first stage (Figure 32-6).

The stages of labor are as follows:
1. First stage (dilation)
   - Beginning of regular contractions to complete dilation of the cervix (10 cm)
   - Contractions may occur at intervals of 10 to 15 minutes
   - Effacement occurs (thinning and shortening of the cervix)
   - On average, may last 12.5 hours in a primipara female and only 7 hours in a multipara female
2. Second stage (expulsion)
   - Complete cervical dilation to delivery of the newborn
   - Contractions may occur every 2 to 3 minutes and last 60 seconds
   - Amniotic sac typically will rupture in this stage
   - Urge to push increases
   - Crowning and then delivery occurs
   - Averages 80 minutes in primipara, and only 30 minutes in a multipara female
3. Third stage
   - Delivery of newborn to delivery of the placenta
   - Averages 5 to 20 minutes

Patients in labor may experience any or all of the following signs or symptoms:

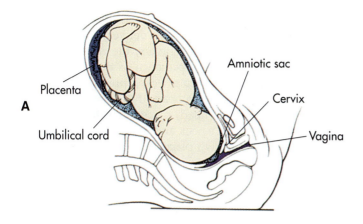

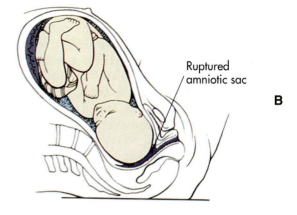

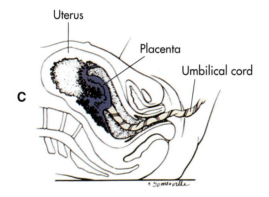

FIGURE 32-6 ▲ Stages of labor. **A,** The fetus moves into the birth canal. **B,** The cervix completes dilation. **C,** The placenta separates from the uterus. (From Sanders M: *Mosby's paramedic textbook,* St Louis, 1994, Mosby.)

- *Ruptured membranes (or breaking of the "water")*—This usually occurs spontaneously and is characterized by a gush or slow leak of fluid. The amniotic fluid is usually clear but may be tinged with meconium. The patient may not be aware of this rupture. Occasionally, the patient's membranes may not rupture until the actual delivery.
- *Contractions*—Contracting of the uterine muscle that occurs when the fetus begins to move into the birth canal. Contractions are timed from the beginning of one contraction to the beginning of the next.
- *Bloody "show"*—The passage of a mucus, a blood-tinged discharge that is often referred to as a *mucus plug;* usually occurs in early labor.
- *Pain*—Abdominal pain, back pain, or both. Labor is very painful and is very hard work. Every patient's pain tolerance varies. Each stage of labor brings a greater awareness of stronger, longer contractions to the patient.
- *Transition*—Occurs close to delivery. The patient may panic and be "out of control" with overwhelming contractions. Expect a very irritable patient attempting rapid breathing exercises. Most patients cannot speak through contractions at this point of labor.
- *Urge to push*—Either to have a bowel movement or to simply push the newborn out. Occurs close to delivery.
- *Crowning*—The appearance of the newborn's head bulging at the perineum shortly before delivery. Marks the beginning of the final stage of labor (Figure 32-7).

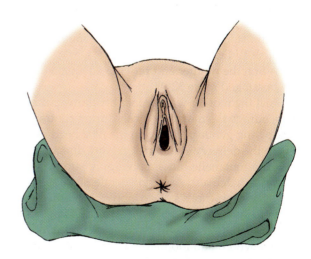

FIGURE 32-7 ▲ Crowning, when the fetus's head bulges at the perineum, marks the final stage of labor and imminent delivery. (From Kimberly Battista from Stoy W: *Mosby's EMT-Basic textbook,* St Louis, 1996, Mosby.)

Delivery is imminent when a woman with her first pregnancy has the urge to move her bowels, the "water" has broken, and crowning is present. It is important that the EMT–I identifies and prepares for an imminent delivery. Often transportation to the hospital is delayed when delivery is imminent.

If delivery is imminent, it will be obvious simply by examination of the external genitalia. The EMT–I should assess for the likelihood of delivery using the previously mentioned guides. If the patient is at the pushing stage, she should be encouraged to push during the contractions and to relax in between contractions. The EMT–I should provide as much assistance and support to the mother as possible. If birth is not imminent, as noted by the absence of crowning or contractions not occurring every 2 to 3 minutes, the mother should be placed on her left side (if tolerated) and transported to the hospital.

If birth is imminent, the patient should be placed in a semireclining position on the stretcher or a firm, comfortable surface. The stretcher is preferred because the patient can be moved rapidly. The EMT–I should be sure to help protect the privacy of the patient. Many times the patient will have a spouse or "coach" with her. Allowing a significant other to remain with the patient can be very helpful (Box 32-2 and Figure 32-8).

Delivery of the Newborn

1. Ensure adequate space and privacy for delivery.
2. Prepare the equipment, including mask, goggles, and gloves needed for BSI, as follows:
   * Warm clean towels to dry and then wrap newborn
   * Umbilical cord clamps (2)
   * Scalpel or sterile scissors to cut umbilical cord
   * Bulb syringe to suction newborn's mouth and nose
3. Administer high flow oxygen to the mother and establish IV line.
4. Position the mother and provide adequate draping if possible (Figure 32-9).
5. Assist the mother with proper breathing patterns.
6. Encourage the mother to push during contractions.
7. Applying gentle pressure on the fetal head can best help the delivery. Avoid placing any direct pressure on the fontanelle but simply apply support to the head as it delivers. Applying gentle, steady pressure over the newborn's head and the mother's perineum can prevent an explosive delivery. A slow, controlled delivery will avoid or minimize injury to the newborn and mother.

8. Manually rupture, if necessary, the amniotic sac if it is still intact in this stage of the delivery.
9. As the newborn's head delivers, the next critical step is to check for the presence of the umbilical cord around the newborn's neck. If present, slip the cord over the newborn's head. If the cord will not slip easily over the head, place some fingers between the newborn's neck and the cord, and if necessary, clamp it in two places and cut the cord between the clamps (Figure 32-10).
10. Suction the newborn's mouth first and then the nose. Positioning the newborn's head slightly lower than the rest of the body may allow retained fluids in the airway to drain into the oropharynx to be suctioned (Figure 32-11).
11. Support the head while the head rotates and the shoulders and torso deliver.
12. Clamp the umbilical cord (Figure 32-12).
    * Place the first clamp 4 inches from the newborn's umbilicus.
    * Then place the second clamp farther from the newborn, at 6 inches from the umbilicus.
    * Cut the cord between the two clamps.
13. Evaluate and support the newborn.
14. Record the time of delivery and initial APGAR score (Table 32-1 and Figure 32-13).

Delivery of the Placenta

The placenta will deliver almost spontaneously 5 to 20 minutes after the newborn is delivered. The mother may feel another urge to push just prior to placental delivery. Although continuous gentle tension on the umbilical cord may facilitate placental delivery, the EMT–Is first priorities are caring for the newborn and evaluating the hemodynamics of the mother. Transportation should not be delayed while waiting for the placenta to deliver. If delivered, the placenta should be placed in a plastic bag or other clean container (Figure 32-14).

BOX 32-2

SUMMARY OF SIGNS OF IMMINENT DELIVERY

Frequent contractions, typically less than 2 minutes apart
Intense maternal urge to push
Crowning of the presenting part of the newborn
NOTE: As a general rule, mulitparous mothers will progress through labor much more rapidly than primiparous mothers do.

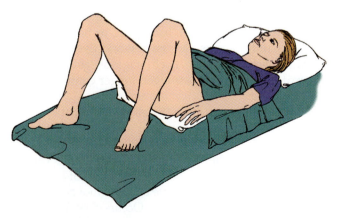

FIGURE 32-8 ▲ If birth is imminent, position the patient in semireclining position. (Kimberly Battista from Stoy W: *Mosby's EMT-Basic textbook,* St Louis, 1996, Mosby.)

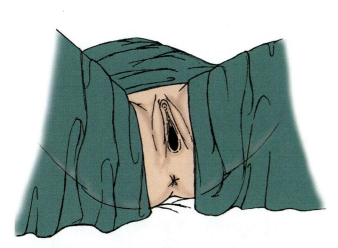

FIGURE 32-9 ▲ Prepare necessary equipment before birth including warm towels, sheets, or other linens to create a sterile field for delivery. (Kimberly Battista from Stoy W: *Mosby's EMT-Basic textbook,* St Louis, 1996, Mosby.)

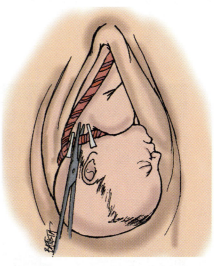

FIGURE 32-10 ▲ If the cord cannot be removed from the newborn's neck, clamp it in two places and cut between the clamps. (From Kimberly Battista from Stoy W: *Mosby's EMT-Basic textbook,* St Louis, 1996, Mosby.)

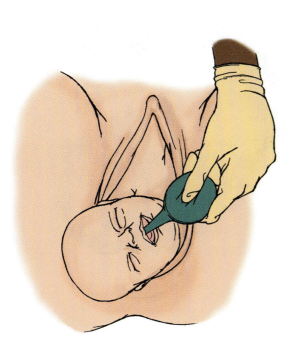

FIGURE 32-11 ▲ Suction the newborn's airway to open the passages and encourage breathing. This is especially important if meconium is present. (Kimberly Battista from Stoy W: *Mosby's EMT-Basic textbook,* St Louis, 1996, Mosby.)

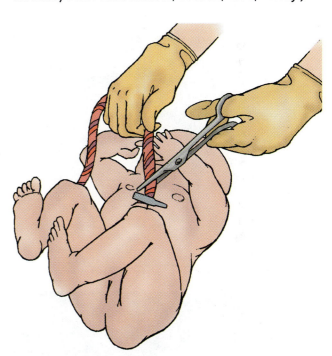

FIGURE 32-12 ▲ Leaving approximately 4 inches of cord for the newborn, clamp the cord in two places and cut between the clamps. (Kimberly Battista from Stoy W: *Mosby's EMT-Basic textbook,* St Louis, 1996, Mosby.)

TABLE 32-1

APGAR Scoring System

SIGN	0	1	2
Appearance	Blue, pale	Body pink, blue extremities	Completely pink
Pulse rate (heart rate)	Absent	<100 beats/min	>100 beats/min
Grimace (irritability)	No response	Grimace	Cough, sneeze, cry
Activity (muscle tone)	Limp	Some flexion	Active motion
Respirations (respiratory effort)	Absent	Slow, irregular	Good, crying

From Aehlert B: *Pediatric advanced life support guide,* St Louis, 1994, Mosby.

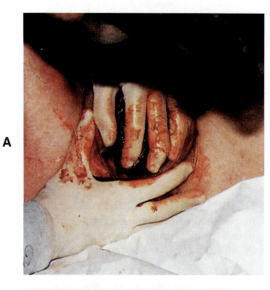

A

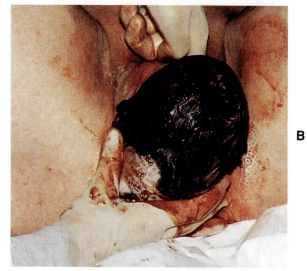

B

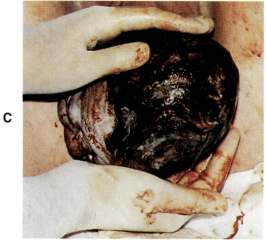

C

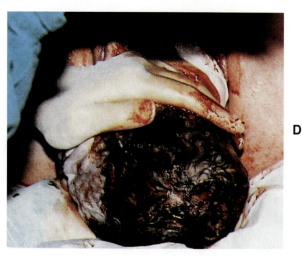

D

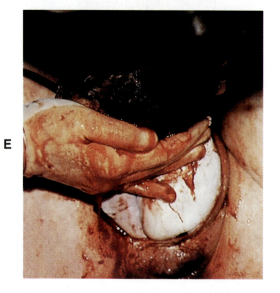

E

FIGURE 32-13 ▲ Stages of a normal delivery.
A, Apply gentle, steady pressure over the newborn's
head and mother's perineum. **B,** Examine the newborn's
neck for the umbilical cord. **C,** Support the newborn's
head as it turns. **D,** Guide the newborn's head downward
for delivery of the shoulder. **E,** Guide the newborn's head
upward to deliver the second shoulder. (From Azzawa A:
Colour atlas of childbirth and obstetric techniques, London,
1991, Wolfe Medical Publishers.)

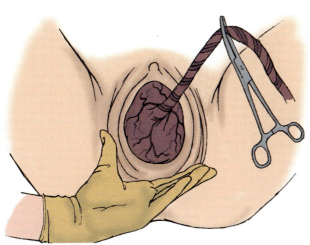

FIGURE 32-14 ▲ Delivery of the placenta will usually occur within 20 minutes after delivery of the newborn. (Kimberly Battista from Stoy W: *Mosby's EMT-Basic textbook,* St Louis, 1996, Mosby.)

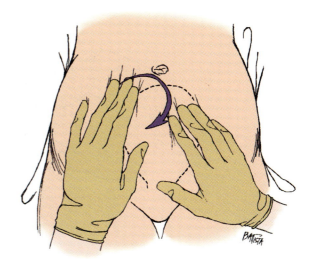

FIGURE 32-15 ▲ If postpartum bleeding is excessive, manage the bleeding by massaging the mother's abdomen.

CLINICAL NOTES

If the membranes have ruptured, the EMT–I should observe the color of the fluid. If the fluid is not clear, the EMT–I is dealing with a "meconium newborn." Meconium is a fetal waste substance produced by the newborn in distress. If the newborn aspirates during delivery, he or she may experience severe respiratory damage. Thick, dark meconium increases the potential severity of aspiration. The newborn's airway must be suctioned *before* its first breath to prevent meconium aspiration. After deep suctioning of the newborn, the mother should be encouraged to push and deliver the newborn's shoulders.

HELPFUL HINT

The EMT–I may need to remove thick meconium from the airway before the newborn's first breath. Performing direct laryngoscopy with a laryngoscope and suctioning below the vocal cords may avoid serious complications. Check with local medical control regarding newborn endotracheal suctioning protocols.

Postpartum Care of the Mother

The mother will have a moderate amount of postpartum bleeding. To reduce bleeding, the EMT–I should place the dry, warm newborn with the mother and encourage the mother to breastfeed the newborn. This will reduce the bleeding by constricting the uterus.

Massaging the uterus may also help control postpartum hemorrhage (Figure 32-15). This is accomplished by palpating the lower abdomen in a circular fashion in the area between the pubis and umbilicus. The EMT–I then should apply a maternity sanitary napkin and cold pack to the mother's perineal area. If heavy bleeding continues, establish a second IV line and administer a fluid bolus.

Newborn Care

After the newborn is delivered, the EMT–I should begin to stimulate breathing by drying the newborn and rubbing the spine (Figure 32-16). Because the newborn is wet and has a large surface area, it is very important to preserve warmth. The newborn will begin to cry and achieve a normal skin color. The EMT–I should record the newborn's APGAR scores (evaluate the newborn's HR, respiratory rate, muscle tone, reflex irritability, and color) (see Table 32-1) at 1 and 5 minutes after delivery. Until the umbilical cord is cut, the newborn should remain level with the mother's vaginal area. After the umbilical cord stops pulsating, usually 20 to 30 seconds after delivery, the cord should be clamped in two places. Place the first clamp on the umbilical cord 4 inches from the newborn, then place the second clamp 6 inches from the newborn. Using a sterile knife or scissors (provided in commercial obstetrical kits), the EMT–I should cut the cord between the clamps (see Figure 32-12).

CARE OF THE NEWBORN IN DISTRESS

Unfortunately, there are times when it becomes necessary to resuscitate a newborn. Complications can develop during the pregnancy, labor, or delivery. Assessment of the newborn actually begins before delivery, with an

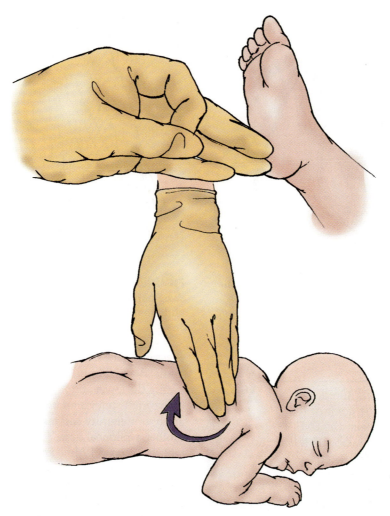

FIGURE 32-16 ▲ **If necessary, stimulate the newborn by flicking the foot or rubbing the back.**

accurate history. A mother at risk may have had problems with the pregnancy, prenatal care, or previous deliveries. Once the newborn is delivered, assessment begins immediately. Normal vital signs for the newborn are a pulse (HR) of 160 beats per minute; BP of 80; respirations at 40. It is typically very difficult to measure a manual BP on a newborn in the prehospital setting.

❗ HELPFUL HINT

> • In most instances, basic life support, including warming and stimulation, is all that is necessary to successfully resuscitate the newborn.

The newborn should be positioned on his or her back with the head slightly lower than the rest of the body. Suction the mouth first, then the nose, with a bulb syringe device for up to 15 seconds and then evaluate the newborn. If the newborn still does not cry, he or she should be stimulated by gently rubbing the soles of the feet or the back. There is no need to spank the newborn.

The newborn should be dried thoroughly, and any wet towels should be discarded. The rubbing action used to dry the newborn provides stimulation and allows the newborn to be kept warm until arrival at the hospital. Using a different towel, wrap the newborn to keep him or her as warm as possible. Cover the head with a blanket, towel or hat to prevent heat loss. Clamp the cord after it stops pulsating. After cutting the cord as described previously, place the newborn against the mother's skin for warming.

If the newborn does not respond within 30 seconds to these techniques, position the newborn with his or her head in a sniffing position. A rolled towel can be placed under the newborn's shoulders to promote good positioning, but avoid hyperextending the head, because this may cause airway collapse. Administer oxygen by holding a mask near the newborn's face until his or her condition improves (skin color goes from cyanotic to pink).

If the newborn still is unresponsive, he or she should be ventilated by bag-valve-mask with 100% oxygen at a rate of 40 to 60 breaths per minute. When using an oropharyn-

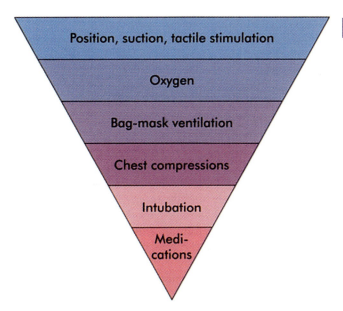

FIGURE 32-17 ▲ **Pyramid represents the relative frequencies of newborn resuscitative measures.**

SUMMARY OF HIGH-RISK DELIVERIES

The following prehospital childbirth situations are "priority" conditions:
- **Uncontrolled predelivery or postpartum bleeding from the mother**
- **Breech presentation**
- **Prolapsed cord**
- **Limb presentation**
- **Cephalopelvic disproportion**
- **Severe abdominal pain with rigidity (other than labor)**
- **Any time more than drying and stimulation are needed to resuscitate a newborn**

geal airway, ensure that the correct size is used. During insertion, the airway should not be rotated at a 180-degree angle as is done for adults because it may cause damage to the newborn's mouth and tongue. Instead, use a tongue depressor to hold the tongue in place while inserting the airway. If the newborn starts breathing on his or her own, the respiratory rate, as well as depth and HR should be assessed. If the HR remains below 100 beats per minute, ventilations should be continued with 100% oxygen. If the newborn's HR is absent or below 60 beats per minute, initiate cardiopulmonary resuscitation (CPR). At this point, advanced life-saving intervention is necessary. Notify the receiving emergency department to be ready for a newborn resuscitation (Figure 32-17).

HELPFUL HINT
- Cardiac arrest in the most newborns is usually secondary to respiratory failure.

Guidelines for Newborn Resuscitation

After the newborn has been dried and suctioned, if respirations are inadequate or the HR is below 100 beats per minute, the EMT–I should do the following:

1. Properly position the newborn. Quickly provide blow-by oxygen near the newborn's mouth and nose. Do not aim directly at the face or eyes.
2. Begin bag-valve-mask resuscitation with 100% oxygen at a rate of 40 to 60 breaths per minute.
3. If the HR is absent or below 60 beats per minute, begin CPR. CPR should also be provided if the HR is between 60 and 80 but does not increase even with

30 seconds of positive-pressure ventilation and supplemental oxygen.
4. Newborns most often experience cardiopulmonary arrest due to hypoxia. For this reason, initial therapy consists of ventilation and oxygenation. However, when these measures do not resolve the problem, IV fluids and medications including atropine, epinephrine, lidocaine, and naloxone may be administered. Fluid therapy should consist of 10 mL/kilogram (kg) of saline or lactated Ringer's solution given by syringe over a 5- to 10-minute period.
5. Transport in "priority" mode to the closest appropriate hospital. Notify them in advance that a newborn requiring resuscitation will be arriving.

▶ NOTE: It is imperative that the newborn be kept warm during resuscitation and transportation. The EMT–I should make sure the newborn is well wrapped and has a head cover. The ambulance should be warm enough to be uncomfortably hot for the EMT–Is.

Abnormal Presentations and Multiple Births

An abnormal presentation is when the first body part passing through the cervix is not the newborn's head. Multiple births are often complicated by abnormal presentations such as breech births (Box 32-3).

Multiple Births

Twins occur in 1 in 90 live births. Multiple births are given special consideration by prehospital providers because the newborns are generally smaller in size than a single newborn. In addition, multiple-birth newborns are premature almost 40% of the time, and they are small because the uterus sometimes cannot expand to hold two or more full-size newborns. Lower birthweight newborns have difficulty regulating body temperature. The newborn will exhaust all efforts in keeping warm and probably will not succeed alone. The newborn will depend on the EMT–I's efforts to survive.

To provide care for the woman with suspected multiple births, the EMT–I should do the following:

- Obtain an accurate history to determine if the mother is carrying more than one newborn.
- If, after delivery of one newborn, the abdomen remains unusually large, suspect multiple births.
- Follow normal delivery procedures for each birth.
- With multiple births, there may be a shared placenta or a placenta for each newborn.
- Follow the same resuscitation procedures for newborns in distress with special attention to warming procedures.
- Be prepared to treat postpartum hemorrhage after multiple-birth deliveries.

Breech Presentation

Breech presentation includes any delivery in which the buttocks or feet present first rather than the head of the newborn (Figure 32-18). Breech deliveries make up only 3% to 4% of all deliveries. Preterm deliveries, however, are breech 20% to 30% of the time. Newborns in breech presentation have an increased risk for birth trauma. To provide care for the woman and newborn in breech presentation, the EMT–I should do the following:

- Do not try to push the newborn back in.
- Encourage the mother to push during the contractions.
- Do not attempt to pull the newborn out.
- Allow the newborn's legs and trunk to deliver to the level of the umbilicus. Support the trunk by wrapping a towel around the body and supporting it on an arm.
- Extract an approximately 6-inch loop of umbilical cord.
- Rotate the neonate for anterior-posterior shoulder positioning.

- Apply gentle traction until axilla visible.
- Guide newborn upward and deliver posterior shoulder.
- Guide newborn downward and deliver anterior shoulder.
- Ease the head out avoiding excessive manipulation.

If the newborn does not deliver within 3 minutes or begins to breathe before the head is delivered, put a gloved hand in the vagina. Turn the newborn to face the mother's back and conduct the following:

- Form a ∨ with the fingers on either side of newborn's nose and mouth. Gently guide the newborn's head out by lifting the body slightly anteriorly (Figure 32-19).
- If the newborn's head does not deliver within 3 minutes, transport the mother either with her buttocks elevated or in a knee-chest position while maintaining the ∨.
- Administer oxygen by nonrebreather mask at 10 to 15 L/min.
- Start an IV line in the mother.
- If delivery occurs, be prepared to resuscitate the newborn.
- Notify the receiving hospital to prepare personnel and equipment.

Prolapsed Cord

A **prolapsed cord** is a condition in which the umbilical cord is the presenting part during delivery. It occurs in 1 out of 200 pregnancies. This condition is an emergency complication of delivery, because the cord may be compressed between the newborn and the mother's pelvis,

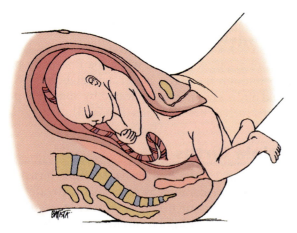

FIGURE 32-18 ▲ Breech presentation is a delivery in which the newborn's head is delivered last. (Kimberly Battista from Stoy W: *Mosby's EMT-Basic textbook,* St Louis, 1996, Mosby.)

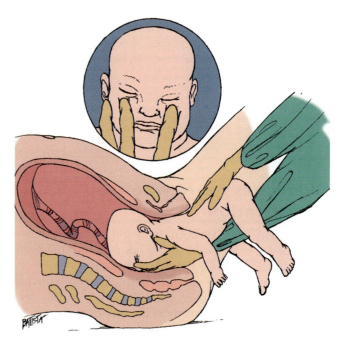

FIGURE 32-19 ▲ Manage the breech presentation with a ∨ shape around the nose and mouth. (From Kimberly Battista from Stoy W: *Mosby's EMT-Basic textbook,* St Louis, 1996, Mosby.)

cutting off fetal circulation before delivery. Breech presentation, preterm deliveries, large fetuses, and multiple gestations increase the likelihood of a prolapsed umbilical cord (Figure 32-20).

To care for the woman and the newborn with a prolapsed cord, the EMT–I should do the following:

- Elevate the newborn off the cord by inserting a gloved hand in the vagina and pushing up on the newborn's head.
- Monitor for pulsations in the cord. A pulsating cord indicates a viable newborn.
- Position the mother in a knee-to-chest or Trendelenberg position (Figure 32-21). If unable to do so, place her supine with the hips elevated.
- Ask the mother to pant during contractions and to not bear down.
- Transport rapidly but carefully. Notify the receiving hospital as early as possible.

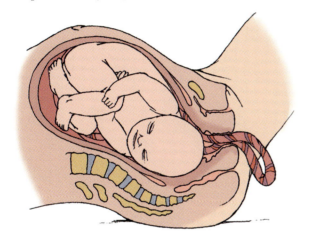

FIGURE 32-20 ▲ Prolapsed cord presents an emergency to the newborn because the cord may be compressed. (Kimberly Battista from Stoy W: *Mosby's EMT-Basic textbook,* St Louis, 1996, Mosby.)

- *Do not push the cord back in under any circumstances.*
- Cover the exposed cord with a warm, moist gauze or cloth pad.
- Administer oxygen to the mother by nonrebreather mask at 10 to 15 L/min.
- Establish IV access in the mother.

Limb Presentation

Limb presentation occurs when an arm or a leg is the presenting part during delivery (Figure 32-22). Again, this situation often is complicated by preterm delivery. There is little the EMT–I can do for this condition, other than providing care for the woman and newborn. Take the following steps:

- Transport the patient to the hospital.
- Do not attempt delivery in the prehospital setting.
- Administer oxygen to the mother by nonrebreather mask at 10 to 15 L/min.
- Establish an IV line in the mother.
- Notify and transport the patient to a hospital with the capacity to perform emergent cesarean section.

Cephalopelvic Disproportion

Cephalopelvic disproportion occurs when the relative size of the fetus in respect to the pelvis may compromise a normal delivery. The fetus may be abnormally large, as in a woman with diabetes or a past-due delivery. The pelvis may also be unusually small, an aspect most often seen in primiparous women. Cephalopelvic disproportion may be occurring when there is lack of expected progress through the stages of delivery. Contractions may be unusually prolonged as well. Treatment consists of high-flow oxygen, IV line, and rapid transport to a hospital with the capacity to perform an emergent cesarean section.

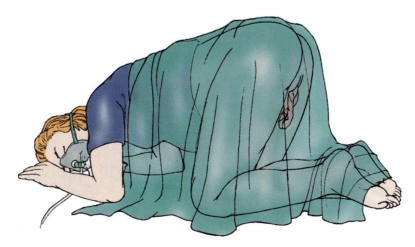

FIGURE 32-21 ▲ If presented with a prolapsed cord, transport the mother in the head and torso down position.

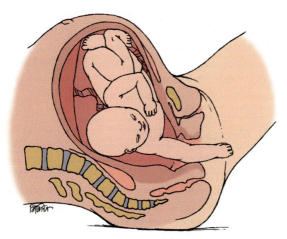

FIGURE 32-22 ▲ Limb presentation is a condition in which an arm or leg is the presenting part. (Kimberly Battista from Stoy W: *Mosby's EMT-Basic textbook,* St Louis, 1996, Mosby.)

CLINICAL NOTES

Women can have significant bleeding following delivery. Hemorrhage more than 500 mL immediately after delivery should be concerning to the EMT–I caring for the patient. Postpartum hemorrhage may be due to the following:

- Vaginal or cervical tears and lacerations
- Retained placenta
- Bleeding or clotting disorders

Therapy consists of uterine massage, considering establishing a second IV line and administering a fluid bolus.

CASE HISTORY FOLLOW-UP ■■■

EMT–I Bradley supports the newborn's head as it presents in a downward orientation on the next contraction and immediately suctions the mouth and nose with a rubber bulb aspirator. He notes that there is no meconium staining or odor.

As the patient contracts again, EMT–I Bradley is able to support the newborn's chest and right arm. The patient breathes with heavy puffing breaths and screams with each contraction, and the newborn fully delivers. It is a girl, purple and covered with white pasty fluid. EMT–I Bradley immediately dries the newborn off with a clean towel, wraps her in the warm, dry blanket, and places her on her mother's belly. She is not moving yet.

EMT–I Bradley suctions the newborn's mouth and nose again, and then rubs his fingertips gently on her spine to stimulate her. Finally, she begins to move.

SUMMARY

- One of the most satisfying aspects of prehospital care is being able to assist a woman with the unexpected delivery of her newborn child. The EMT–I can provide significant psychological and physical support throughout the birthing process.
- Rapid suctioning and assessment of the newborn will further contribute to this typically joyful process.
- Although uncommon, significant complications can occur throughout pregnancy and in the various stages of labor, including breech presentations, prolapsed umbilical cord, limb presentation, uterine rupture, placenta previa, and abruptio placenta.
- The EMT–I must be able to rapidly identify these conditions when they occur, make every possible prehospital intervention, and rapidly transport the mother and child to the hospital.

33 Neonatal Resuscitation

Key Terms

- Acrocyanosis
- Bronchopulmonary Dysplasia (BPD)
- Central Cyanosis
- Hyaline Membrane Disease (HMD)
- Infant
- Meconium
- Meconium Aspiration Syndrome (MAS)
- Neonate
- Newborn
- Peripheral Cyanosis
- Premature or Preterm Newborn
- Primary Apnea
- Respiratory Distress Syndrome (RDA)
- Secondary Apnea
- Sepsis
- Septicemia
- Surfactant

...CASE HISTORY

EMT–Is Jensen and Williams provide emergency medical services in a small, rural town. They are dispatched to a house for a "woman in labor." On arrival, they see a woman running toward them, and she is screaming, "The baby's coming now! She's not due for another 2 months!" The EMT–Is grab the childbirth kit and the pediatric bag and enter the house. In a back bedroom is a 16-year-old girl complaining of abdominal cramps. The head is crowning.

LEARNING OBJECTIVES

CHAPTER GOAL
Upon completion of this chapter, the EMT-Intermediate will be able to utilize assessment findings to formulate a field impression and implement the treatment plan for the resuscitation of a neonatal patient.

Cognitive Objectives
As an EMT-Intermediate you should be able to do the following:
- Define the terms newborn, neonate, and infant.
- Identify important antepartum factors that can affect childbirth.
- Identify important intrapartum factors that can cause the newborn to be high risk.
- Identify the factors that lead to premature birth and low–birth-weight newborns.
- Distinguish between primary and secondary apnea.
- Discuss pulmonary perfusion and asphyxia.
- Identify the primary signs utilized for evaluating a newborn during resuscitation.
- Formulate an appropriate treatment plan for providing initial care to a newborn.
- Determine when ventilatory assistance is appropriate for a newborn.
- Determine when chest compressions are appropriate for a newborn.
- Determine when endotracheal intubation is appropriate for a newborn.

- Determine when vascular access is indicated for a newborn.
- Determine when blow-by oxygen delivery is appropriate for a newborn.
- Discuss the initial steps in resuscitation of a newborn.
- Discuss the effects of maternal narcotic usage on the newborn.
- Discuss appropriate transport guidelines for a newborn.
- Determine appropriate receiving facilities for low- and high-risk newborns.
- Describe the epidemiology, including the incidence, morbidity/mortality, risk factors, and prevention strategies for meconium aspiration.
- Discuss the pathophysiology of meconium aspiration.
- Discuss the assessment findings associated with meconium aspiration.
- Discuss the management/treatment plan for meconium aspiration.
- Describe the epidemiology, including the incidence, morbidity/mortality, and risk factors for premature newborns.
- Discuss the pathophysiology of premature newborns.
- Discuss the assessment findings associated with premature newborns.
- Discuss the management/treatment plan for premature newborns.

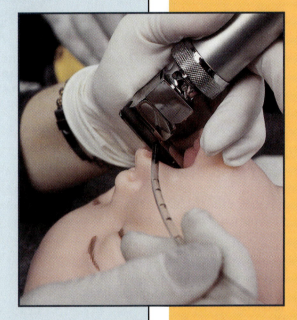

Affective Objectives
- None identified for this chapter.

Psychomotor Objectives
As an EMT-Intermediate you should be able to do the following:
- Demonstrate preparation of a newborn resuscitation area.
- Demonstrate appropriate assessment technique for examining a newborn.
- Demonstrate appropriate assisted ventilations for a newborn.
- Demonstrate appropriate endotracheal intubation technique for a newborn.
- Demonstrate appropriate meconium aspiration suctioning technique for a newborn.
- Demonstrate appropriate insertion of an orogastric tube.
- Demonstrate appropriate chest compression and ventilation technique for a newborn.
- Demonstrate appropriate techniques to improve or eliminate endotracheal intubation complications.
- Demonstrate vascular access cannulation techniques for a newborn.
- Demonstrate the initial steps in resuscitation of a newborn.
- Demonstrate blow-by oxygen delivery for a newborn.

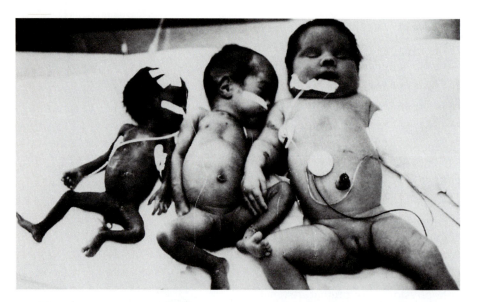

FIGURE 33-1 ▲ Three newborns, left to right, of the same gestational age, weighing 600, 1400, and 2750 g, respectively. Their associated risks of mortality are more than 50%, 10%, and less than 4%, respectively. (From Korones SG: *High-risk newborn infants: the basis for intensive nursing care*, ed 4, St Louis, 1986, Mosby.)

TABLE 33-1

Risk Factors Before and During Birth

BEFORE BIRTH (ANTEPARTUM)	DURING BIRTH (INTRAPARTUM)
Multiple gestation (e.g., twins, triplets, and so on)	Premature labor
Inadequate prenatal care	Meconium-stained amniotic fluid
Mother's age <16 or >35	Rupture of membranes >24 hours before delivery
History of perinatal morbidity or mortality	Use of narcotics within 4 hours of delivery
Post-term gestation	Abnormal presentation
Drugs and/or prescribed medications	Prolonged labor or precipitous delivery
Toxemia	Prolapsed cord
Hypertension	Bleeding
Diabetes	

INTRODUCTION

A **newborn** is a recently born baby and is considered a newborn during the first few hours of life. A **neonate** is a baby during the first 28 days of life. After that time, the baby is referred to as an **infant**.

INCIDENCE

Approximately 6% of all deliveries require some type of life support. The incidence of complications increases as the newborn's birthweight decreases (Figure 33-1).

RISK FACTORS

Various risk factors may be present in the mother that will affect the delivery of the child. These factors can occur before birth or during the actual delivery process. See Table 33-1 for specific risk factors.

The high-risk newborn, regardless of gestational age or birthweight, has a greater-than-average chance of morbidity or mortality because of conditions or circumstances associated with birth and the adjustment to existence outside of the uterus. The high-risk period encompasses human growth and development from the time of viability (gestational age at which survival outside the uterus is believed to be possible or as early as 23 weeks of gestation) up to 28 days after birth. It includes threats to life and health that occur during the prenatal, perinatal, and postnatal periods.

Assessment and prompt intervention in life-threatening prenatal emergencies often make the difference between a favorable outcome and a lifetime of disability. The EMT–Intermediate (EMT–I) should be familiar with the characteristics of newborns and recognize the significance of serious deviations from expected observa-

TABLE 33-2

Classification of High-Risk Neonates

CLASSIFICATION	TERM	DEFINITION
Size	Low–birth-weight (LBW) neonate	Neonate whose birth-weight is less than 2500 grams (g), regardless of gestational age
	Moderately-low–birth-weight (MLBW) neonate	Neonate whose birth-weight is 1501 to 2500 g
	Very-low–birth-weight (VLBW) neonate	Neonate whose birth-weight is less than 1500 g
	Extremely-low–birth-weight (ELBW) neonate	Neonate whose birth-weight is less than 1000 g
Gestational age	Premature (preterm) neonate	Neonate born before completion of 37 weeks gestation, regardless of birth-weight
	Full-term neonate	Neonate born between the beginning of 38 weeks and the completion of 42 weeks of gestation, regardless of birth-weight
	Postmature (postterm) neonate	Newborn born after 42 weeks of gestation, regardless of birth-weight
Mortality	Live birth	Birth in which the neonate manifests any heartbeat, breathes or displays voluntary movement, regardless of gestational age
	Fetal death	Death of the fetus after 20 weeks of gestation and before delivery, with absence of any signs of life after birth
	Neonatal death	Death that occurs in the first 27 days of life
		Early neonatal death occurs in the first week of life
		Late neonatal death occurs at 7 to 27 days
	Perinatal mortality	Describes the total number of fetal and early neonatal deaths per 1000 live births
	Postnatal death	Death that occurs at 28 days to 1 year

tions. When the need for specialized care can be anticipated and planned for, the probability of successful outcome is increased.

High-risk newborns are most often classified according to birth-weight, gestational age, and neonatal outcome instead of pathophysiological problems. See Table 33-2 for classifications of high-risk neonates.

The leading cause of death in the neonatal period is associated with newborns who are born at low birthweight. These babies are 20 times more likely to die within the first month of life than are newborns that have weights greater than 2500 grams (g). Consequently, the lowest perinatal mortality is found in the newborn who weighs between 3000 and 4000 g and whose gestational age is more than 36 weeks. The less the newborn's gestational age at birth, the greater is the mortality risk, especially if he or she is less than 32 weeks of gestation.

Factors contributing to high infant mortality rates include a number of intrauterine events that eventually result in low birth-weight. They are as follows:

- Decreased placental perfusion, often occurring as a result of pregnancy-induced hypertension

- Infection (significant cause of low birth-weight among black neonates)
- Maternal complications of pregnancy
- Lack of prenatal care, especially among younger women and those who live at or below the poverty level
- Complications involving the placenta, cord, and membranes

There is a higher incidence of prematurity and low birth-weight in newborns born to teenagers. It is difficult to determine if this is a result of the developmental stage of the mother or a reflection of multiple factors associated with teenage pregnancies, including poor nutrition, lower socioeconomic status, ongoing disease, and late or no prenatal care. First birth, immaturity, illegitimacy, and the young age of the mother can create a cumulative effect that places the teenager and the newborn in a possible high-risk situation.

Another potential risk to the newborn is narcotic use by the mother. The child may have respiratory depression after delivery because of ongoing drug use by the mother.

ADJUSTMENT TO EXTRAUTERINE LIFE

To prepare for what can go wrong during the birth of a newborn, it is important to understand fetal adjustment to extrauterine life. This transition from fetal or placental circulation to independent respiration is the most profound physiological change the newborn will make. Anything that interferes with this transition or increases asphyxia (i.e., a condition of hypoxemia, hypercapnia, and acidosis) will affect fetal adjustment.

Respiratory System

The onset of breathing is the most critical and immediate physiological change required of the newborn. The stimuli that help initiate respiration are primarily chemical and thermal. Chemical factors are low oxygen, high carbon dioxide, and low pH. These factors initiate impulses that excite the respiratory center in the medulla. As the fetus leaves a warm environment and enters a cooler atmosphere, the primary thermal stimulus is the sudden chilling that occurs. Sensory impulses in the skin are excited with the abrupt change in temperature, and these impulses transmit to the respiratory center.

The initial entry of air into the lungs is opposed by the surface tension of the fluid that filled the fetal lungs and alveoli. However, the pulmonary capillaries and lymphatic vessels remove fetal lung fluid. Some fluid is also removed during the normal forces of labor and delivery.

As the chest emerges from the birth canal, fluid is squeezed from the lungs through the nose and mouth. Following complete emergence of the neonate's chest, a brisk recoil of the thorax occurs. Air enters the upper airway to replace the lost fluid. In the alveoli, the surface tension of the fluid is reduced by surfactant, a substance produced by the alveolar epithelium that coats the alveolar surface.

Circulatory System

Circulatory changes occur gradually and are the result of pressure changes in the lungs, heart, and major vessels. The transition from fetal circulation to postnatal circulation involves the functional closure of the fetal shunts: the foramen ovale and the ductus arteriosus. See Figure 33-2 for these changes in circulation at birth.

Once the lungs are expanded, the inspired oxygen dilates the pulmonary vessels, which decreases pulmonary vascular resistance and consequently increases pulmonary blood flow. As the lungs receive blood, the pressure in the right atrium, right ventricle, and pulmonary arteries decreases. At the same time, there is a progressive rise in systemic vascular resistance from the increased volume of blood through the placenta at cord clamping. This action increases the pressure in the left

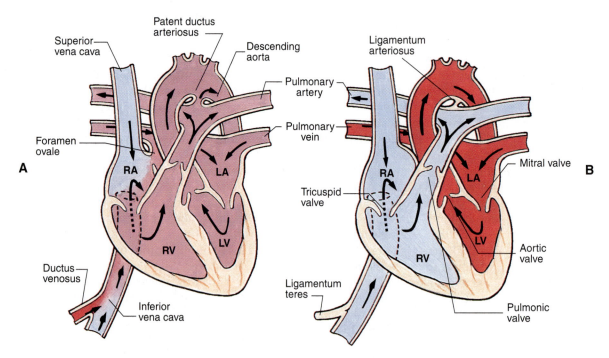

FIGURE 33-2 ▲ Changes in circulation at birth. **A,** Prenatal circulation. **B,** Postnatal circulation. Arrows indicate direction of blood flow. Although four pulmonary veins enter the LA, for simplicity this diagram shows only two. *RA,* Right atrium; *LA,* left atrium; *RV,* right ventricle; *LV,* left ventricle. (From Wong D: *Whaley and Wong's nursing care of infants and children,* ed 6, St Louis, 1999, Mosby.)

side of the heart. Since blood flows from an area of high pressure to one of low pressure, the circulation of blood through the fetal shunts is reversed.

The most important factor controlling ductal closure is the increased oxygen concentration of the blood. The foramen ovale closes functionally at or soon after birth from compression of the two portions of the atrial septum. The ductus arteriosus is closed functionally by the fourth day of life. Failure of the ducts to close results in various types of congenital heart defects.

Thermoregulation

Next to establishing respiration, heat regulation is most critical to the newborn's survival. Several factors predispose the newborn to excessive heat loss (Table 33-3).

Hemopoietic System

The blood volume of the newborn depends on the amount of placental transfer of blood. A full-term newborn has a blood volume of about 80 to 85 milliliters (mL)/kilogram (kg) of body weight. Immediately after birth, the total blood volume averages 300 mL. Depending on how long the newborn is attached to the placenta, as much as 100 mL can be added to the blood volume.

CARE OF THE NEWBORN IN DISTRESS

There are times when it becomes necessary to resuscitate a newborn. Complications can develop during the pregnancy, labor, or delivery. Assessment of the newborn actually begins before delivery, with an accurate history. A mother at risk may have had problems regarding the pregnancy, prenatal care, and/or previous deliveries.

The majority of newborns who are full term will not require any advanced life support intervention. The process of drying the newborn, warming the newborn,

and clearing the airway are usually the only actions that will be needed. See Chapter 32 for typical delivery and atypical presentations.

> **❗ HELPFUL HINT**
>
> ● In most instances, basic life support, including warming and stimulation, is all that is necessary to successfully resuscitate the newborn.

ASSESSMENT AND MANAGEMENT OF THE AIRWAY

As the head is delivered, suction the mouth first, then the nose with a bulb syringe device for up to 15 seconds at a time. If the newborn delivers quickly, it may be difficult to suction and support the rest of the body. As the body delivers, position the newborn on his or her back with the head slightly lower than the rest of the body. If not previously done, suction the newborn's mouth and nose at this point. Nasal suctioning is a stimulus to breathe.

Dry the newborn's head, face, and body thoroughly, and discard any wet towels. The rubbing action taken to dry the newborn provides stimulation. It also allows the newborn to be kept warm until arrival at the hospital. Using a different towel, the EMT–I should wrap the newborn to keep him or her as warm as possible. The head should be covered with a blanket, towel, or hat to prevent heat loss through the head.

Breathing

Quickly evaluate the newborn's breathing. If the newborn is not breathing and still does not cry, he or she should be stimulated by gently rubbing the soles of the feet or the back. There is no need to spank the newborn.

Remember that the newborn is extremely sensitive to hypoxia. In addition, hypoxemia will result in permanent brain damage. Every effort must be made to make sure the newborn stays well oxygenated.

TABLE 33-3

Factors Causing Excessive Newborn Heat Loss

FACTOR	RESULT	DISCUSSION
Large surface area	Facilitates heat loss to the environment	Neonate produces only two thirds as much heat as an adult but loses twice as much heat per unit area
Thin layer of subcutaneous fat	Negatively affects the conservation of body heat	Core body temperature is about 1° F higher than surface body temperature and causes a heat transfer from a higher to lower temperature
Mechanism for producing heat	Cannot shiver	Cannot increase heat production like a child or adult

Apnea occurs when the newborn is not visibly breathing. **Primary apnea** can be reversed by touching and stimulating the newborn as when drying the newborn. Suctioning should also stimulate breathing. **Secondary apnea** will not reverse with simple stimulation techniques and requires assisted ventilation.

Clamp the cord after it stops pulsating and inspect it for blood loss. After cutting the cord, place the newborn against the mother's skin for warming. If the newborn does not respond within 30 seconds to these techniques, he or she should be positioned with the head in a sniffing position. A rolled towel can be placed under the newborn's shoulders to promote good positioning, but the EMT–I should avoid hyperextending the head because this action may cause airway collapse. Oxygen is administered by holding a mask near the newborn's face until his or her condition improves (skin color goes from cyanotic to pink).

If breathing is absent, inadequate, or irregular, ventilate the newborn with a bag-valve-mask device with 100% oxygen at a rate of 40 to 60 breaths per minute. If the newborn starts breathing on his or her own, the respiratory rate and depth, as well as the heart rate (HR) should be assessed.

Oropharyngeal airways are rarely used in newborns. If used, ensure that the correct size is used. During insertion, the airway should not be rotated at a 180-degree angle, as is done for adults, because it may cause damage to the newborn's mouth and tongue. Instead, use a tongue depressor to hold the tongue in place while inserting the airway.

Evaluation of Heart Rate

> **HELPFUL HINT**
> - Cardiac arrest in most newborns is usually secondary to respiratory failure

The newborn who is crying and active will have an adequate heart rate. Auscultate for a heartbeat at the apex of the heart. If the HR is below 100 beats per minute, ventilate with 100% oxygen even if breathing is already present. Newborns will be bradycardic from hypoxia and will increase their HR after ventilation. If the newborn's pulse is absent or below 60 beats per minute, initiate cardiopulmonary resuscitation (CPR).

Evaluation of Color

Look at the color of the newborn. Cyanosis may be present until the newborn has begun to breathe air. This color is normal immediately after birth. If **central cyanosis** (bluish color to the trunk and face) persists after stimulation and breathing has started, oxygen is necessary. Hypoxia is present in this case and will not resolve without additional oxygen.

Many newborns will have **acrocyanosis** or **peripheral cyanosis** (bluish color to the hands and feet) for up to 48 hours after birth. This condition does not require any additional therapy.

Additional Treatment

Newborns most often experience cardiopulmonary arrest due to hypoxia. For this reason, initial therapy consists of ventilation and oxygenation. However, when these measures do not resolve the problem, intubation; intravenous (IV) fluids; and medications, including atropine, epinephrine, lidocaine, and naloxone, may be administered. Fluid therapy should consist of 10 mL/kg of saline or lactated Ringer's solution given by syringe over a 5- to 10-minute period.

Most newborns have one or two possible IV sites on each arm and foot and four to eight sites on the scalp. Since superficial veins of the scalp have no valves, they can be infused in either direction. The temporal and forehead areas are suitable and do not interfere with side-to-side head movements. Scalp veins have little subcutaneous tissue to obscure visualization of the vein, and there are no joints to interfere with movement.

The use of a scalp vein site may require shaving the area around the site to better visualize the vein and provide a smoother surface on which to tape the tubing. Check with medical direction about this procedure. Shaving off a portion of the newborn's hair is very upsetting to the parents and may cause more anxiety in an already tense situation.

A rubber band slipped onto the head from brow to the back of the head will usually work well as a tourniquet. However, if the vessel is visible, a tourniquet may not be necessary in some newborns.

A regular tourniquet may be used on an extremity. Remember that although using a tourniquet makes the veins more visible and provides a more rapid blood return, the added venous pressure may cause fragile veins to "blow" when punctured, resulting in a hematoma. See Chapter 34 for more advanced life support procedures. Endotracheal intubation, vascular access, and pharmacological interventions are described.

Figure 33-3 describes methods to be used in newborn resuscitations. Figure 33-4 reviews guidelines for newborn resuscitation.

MECONIUM-STAINED AMNIOTIC FLUID

Meconium is a thick, greenish black material that is normally expelled from the intestine shortly after birth and provides evidence of patency of the GI tract. If the fetus is subjected to intrauterine stress that causes the anal sphincter to relax (e.g., fetal asphyxia), meconium passes into the amniotic fluid. The fluid will appear light green to thick green, depending on the amount of meconium mixed in it.

Meconium aspiration syndrome (MAS) occurs when the fetus or newborn inhales the thick, sticky meconium. Once the meconium is swallowed or inhaled by the fetus, any gasping activity may cause the sticky and tenacious material to be aspirated into the lower airways. The net results are partial airway obstruction, air trapping, and hyperinflation of the lungs distal to the obstruction. As the newborn struggles to take in more air (air hunger), even more meconium may be aspirated. Hyperinflation, hypoxemia, and acidemia result in increased pulmonary vascular resistance.

Newborns who have released meconium in utero for some time before birth are stained from green meconium stools. Those with more recent meconium passage may not be stained. Tachypnea, hypoxia, and a depressed mental state may be present at birth. They develop expiratory grunting, nasal flaring, and retractions similar to those experienced by newborns with respiratory distress syndrome.

Severe meconium aspiration progresses very rapidly to respiratory failure. These newborns exhibit profound respiratory distress with gasping, ineffective ventilations, marked cyanosis and pallor, and hypotonia.

The EMT–I can prevent meconium aspiration by vigorous suctioning of the hypopharynx before delivery of the shoulders. Suctioning the trachea in newborns with thick, particulate meconium is performed by direct visualization and laryngoscopy using an endotracheal tube. A meconium aspirator may also be used whenever available. Resuscitation is initiated and maintained until the newborn is stabilized.

When attempting to remove the meconium, the EMT–I should NOT use his or her mouth to directly suction the endotracheal tube or the catheter. This procedure does not provide any real advantage over mechanical suction techniques, and there is great risk to the EMT–I performing the suctioning.

If the meconium is thin and of a "pea-soup" consistency and the newborn is active and without respiratory distress, suction the mouth and nose only while performing standard newborn care. This newborn more than likely will not require suctioning of the lower airway.

PREMATURE OR PRETERM NEWBORNS

Prematurity places newborns at risk for neonatal complications (i.e., respiratory distress syndrome) as well as other high-risk factors (e.g., congenital anomalies in association with prematurity). A **premature** or **preterm newborn** is born before completion of 37 weeks gestation, regardless of birth-weight.

In many instances, the actual cause of prematurity is not known. The incidence is lowest in the middle to high socioeconomic classes, in which pregnant women are generally in good health, are well nourished, and receive prompt and comprehensive prenatal care. The incidence is highest in the lower socioeconomic class, in which a combination of circumstances is present. Other factors, such as multiple pregnancies, pregnancy-induced hypertension, and placental problems that interrupt the usual course of gestation before completion of fetal development are responsible for a large number of preterm births.

The outlook for preterm births is mostly related to the state of physiological and anatomical immaturity of the various organs and systems at the time of birth. Full-term newborns have advanced to a state of maturity sufficient to allow a successful transition to the extrauterine environment. Those born prematurely must make the same adjustments but with functional immaturity proportional to the stage of development reached at the time of birth.

Preterm newborns are born before their lungs are fully prepared to serve as efficient organs for gas exchange. This reason appears to be a critical factor in the development of respiratory distress. These newborns are also born with numerous underdeveloped and many uninflatable alveoli.

Preterm newborns also have less surfactant available. **Surfactant** acts much like a detergent in water in that it reduces the surface tension of fluids that line the alveoli and respiratory passages. This action causes uniform expansion and maintenance of lung expansion at low intraalveolar pressure. Immature development of these functions produces consequences that seriously compromise respiratory efficiency. Deficient surfactant production causes unequal inflation of alveoli on inspiration and the collapse of alveoli at the end of expiration. Without surfactant, newborns are unable to keep their lungs inflated and therefore exert a great

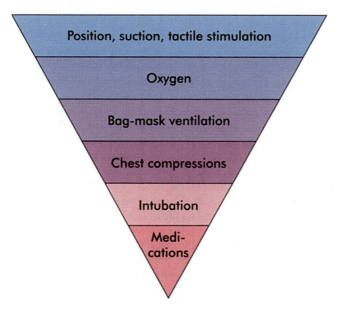

FIGURE 33-3 ▲ **Pyramid represents actions taken during newborn resuscitation (starting at the top).**

CLINICAL EVALUATION

PRETERM   TERM

Posture—The preterm newborn lies in a "relaxed attitude," limbs more extended; the body size is small, and the head may appear somewhat larger in proportion to the body size. The term newborn has more subcutaneous fat tissue and rests in a more flexed attitude.

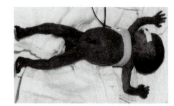 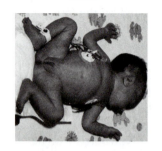

A

Ear—The preterm newborn's ear cartilages are poorly developed, and the ear may fold easily; the hair is fine and feathery, and lanugo may cover the back and face. The mature newborn's ear cartilages are well formed, and the hair is more likely to form firm, separate strands.

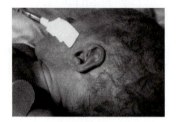 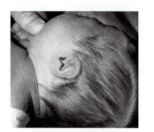

B

Sole—The sole of the foot of the preterm newborn appears more turgid and may have only fine wrinkles. The mature newborn's sole (foot) is well and deeply creased.

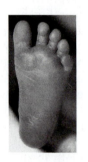 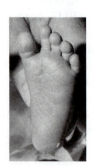

C

NEUROLOGIC EVALUATION

PRETERM   TERM

Grasp reflex—The preterm newborn's grasp is weak; the term newborn's grasp is strong, allowing the infant to be lifted up from the mattress.

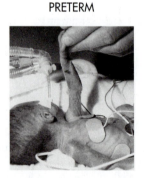 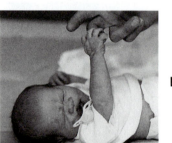

D

FIGURE 33-4 ▲ **A,** *Posture*—The preterm newborn lies in a "relaxed state," with limbs more extended; the body size is small, and the head may appear somewhat larger in proportion to the body size. The full-term newborn has more subcutaneous fat tissue and rests in a more flexed position. **B,** *Ear*—The preterm newborn's ear cartilages are poorly developed, and the ear may fold easily; the hair is fine and feathery, and lanugo may cover the back and face. The mature newborn's ear cartilages are well formed, and the hair is more likely to form fine, separate strands. **C,** *Sole*—The soles of the foot of the preterm newborn may only have fine wrinkles. The mature newborn's sole (foot) is well and deeply creased. **D,** *Grasp reflex*—The preterm newborn's grasp is weak; the full-term newborn's grasp is strong, allowing the newborn to be lifted up from the mattress. (From Wong D: *Whaley and Wong's nursing care of infants and children,* ed 6, St Louis, 1999, Mosby.)

deal of effort to reexpand the alveoli with each breath. This process causes more oxygen to be used than what is taken in, which rapidly leads to exhaustion. With increasing exhaustion, they are able to open fewer and fewer alveoli.

Preterm newborns have distinct characteristics at various stages of development, with the degree of immaturity determining the physical features. They are very small and appear scrawny because they lack or have only minimal subcutaneous fat deposits. They have a proportionately large head in relation to the body. The skin is bright pink; possibly translucent, depending on the degree of immaturity; smooth; shiny; and with small blood vessels clearly visible underneath the thin epidermis. The ear cartilage is soft and pliable, and the soles and palms have minimal creases resulting in a smooth appearance. The bones of the skull and the ribs feel soft, and the eyes may be closed. See Box 33-1 for a comparison of preterm and full-term newborns.

Preterm newborns are inactive and listless. Reflex activity is only partially developed so that sucking is absent, weak, or ineffectual. Swallow, gag, and cough reflexes are absent or weak. They are unable to maintain body temperature and have increased susceptibility to infection. A pliable thorax, immature lung tissue, and an immature regulatory center are often present.

Once the premature newborn is born, attempt resuscitation as previously discussed. Keep the mother and family informed throughout the resuscitation. Explain what is being done and why the newborn requires further support at the hospital.

If no signs of life exist and the newborn is dead, allow the family time to grieve. Follow local protocols for pronouncement of death and transport of the newborn to the morgue.

If the newborn is alive, prepare to transport him or her to a facility with special services for preterm newborns whenever possible. If initial transport to that type of facility is not feasible, the newborn may need to be taken to one hospital for stabilization and then transferred to a tertiary facility with a neonatal intensive care unit (NICU).

OTHER NEONATAL EMERGENCIES

Apnea of Prematurity

Apnea of prematurity (AOP) is common in the preterm newborn and is rarely observed in full-term newborns. Almost all apparently healthy newborns less than 30 weeks gestational age and about one third of newborns less than 32 weeks gestational age have apneic spells. Characteristically, preterm newborns are periodic breathers in that there are short periods of no visible or audible respirations. Apnea is primarily an extension of this periodic breathing and can be defined as a lapse of

---

BOX 33-1

GUIDELINES FOR NEWBORN RESUSCITATION

After the newborn has been dried and suctioned, if respirations are inadequate or the heart rate (HR) is below 100 beats per minute, the EMT–I should do the following:

1. Properly position the newborn. Quickly provide blow-by oxygen near the newborn's mouth and nose. Do not aim directly at the face or eyes.
2. Begin bag-valve-mask ventilation with 100% oxygen at a rate of 40 to 60 breaths per minute.
3. If the pulse is absent or below 60 beats per minute, begin cardiopulmonary resuscitation (CPR). CPR should also be provided if the heart rate is between 60 and 80 but does not increase even with 30 seconds of positive-pressure ventilation and supplemental oxygen.
   - Newborns most often experience cardiopulmonary arrest due to hypoxia. For this reason, initial therapy consists of ventilation and oxygenation. However, when these measures do not resolve the problem, intubation, intravenous fluids, and medications including atropine, epinephrine, lidocaine, and naloxone may be administered. Fluid therapy should consist of 10 milliliters/kilogram of saline or lactated Ringer's solution given by syringe over a 5- to 10-minute period. See Chapter 32 for more advanced life support procedures. Endotracheal intubation, vascular access, and pharmacological interventions are described.
4. Transport in "priority" mode to the closest appropriate hospital. Notify the receiving facility in advance that a newborn requiring resuscitation will be arriving.

NOTE: It is imperative that the newborn be kept warm during resuscitation and transportation. Make sure the newborn is well wrapped and has a head cover. The ambulance should be warm enough to be uncomfortably hot for the EMT–Is.

---

spontaneous breathing for 20 or more seconds, which may or may not be followed by bradycardia and color change.

Apnea in newborns is further classified according to origin as follows:

- *Central apnea*—Absence of diaphragmatic and other respiratory muscle function that causes a lack of respiratory effort
- *Obstructive apnea*—Air flow ceases, yet chest and/or abdominal wall movement is present
- *Mixed apnea*—A combination of central and obstructive apnea
- *Periodic breathing*—Regular respirations for up to 20 seconds with subsequent apneic periods that last no longer than 10 seconds and occur three times in succession

Many of these newborns may be on aminophylline, theophylline, or caffeine at home to reduce the spells of apnea-bradycardia. Theophylline and caffeine act as central nervous system stimulants to breathing. These babies have their serum drug levels measured regularly and must be closely observed for symptoms of toxicity, as in the following:

- Tachycardia at rest (greater than 180 to 190 beats per minute)
- Vomiting
- Irritability
- Restlessness
- Dysrhythmias
- Jitteriness
- Gastritis (hemorrhagic)

Assess and treat airway, breathing, and circulation. Connect the newborn to a cardiac monitor to assess the cardiac rhythm for bradycardia related to hypoxia.

Respiratory Distress Syndrome

Respiratory distress is a name applied to respiratory dysfunction in newborns and is primarily a disease related to developmental delay in lung maturation. Other terms are **respiratory distress syndrome (RDS)** and **hyaline membrane disease (HMD).** This severe lung disorder is responsible for more newborn deaths than any other disease and also carries the highest risk in terms of long-term respiratory and neurological complications. It is seen almost exclusively in preterm newborns.

Newborns with RDS can develop respiratory distress either acutely or over a period of hours. This time frame depends on the acuity of pulmonary immaturity, associated illness factors, and gestational maturity.

Assess and treat airway, breathing, and circulation. Connect the newborn to a cardiac monitor to assess the cardiac rhythm for bradycardia related to hypoxia.

Bronchopulmonary Dysplasia

Bronchopulmonary dysplasia (BPD) is also known as chronic lung disease in the newborn. It is a pathological process that may develop in the lungs of newborns, primarily extremely low–birth-weight and very low–birth-weight newborns with RDS. It may also develop in newborns with meconium aspiration syndrome, persistent hypertension, pneumonia, and cyanotic heart disease.

BPD is caused by therapies used to treat lung disease as with the following:

- Exposure to high oxygen concentrations
- Use of positive-pressure ventilation (CPAP or positive end-expiratory pressure [PEEP])
- Endotracheal intubation
- Prolonged use of these therapies
- Fluid overload
- Patent ductus arteriosus

The reported incidence of this disorder in survivors of RDS is between 20% and 30%. Newborns who survive are at risk for frequent hospitalization because of their borderline respiratory reserve, hyperactive airway, and increased susceptibility to respiratory infection.

These newborns may eventually be discharged to home where they continue to be on oxygen therapy, ranging from a nasal cannula to a tracheostomy. They also have an increased risk of infection and can be threatened by even a minor illness due to their minimum respiratory reserve.

A significant proportion of deaths occur after discharge from the hospital. Emergency medical services may be requested if the parents are unable to resuscitate the newborn or infant.

Assess and treat airway, breathing, and circulation. Connect the newborn or infant to a cardiac monitor to assess the cardiac rhythm for bradycardia due to hypoxia. Resuscitate as needed.

Sepsis

Infants are highly susceptible to infection as a result of their diminished immunity. **Sepsis** or **septicemia** is a generalized bacterial infection in the bloodstream that occurs in infants. Because of the infant's poor response to infectious agents, there is usually no local inflammatory reaction at the portal of entry to signal an infection. Instead, the resulting signs and symptoms tend to be vague and nonspecific, potentially delaying diagnosis and treatment. A high-risk infant has a four times greater chance of developing septicemia than does the normal infant.

The parent may explain that the infant is not progressing well or that he or she just does not "look right." Other clinical signs that may indicate possible sepsis are listed in Box 33-2.

Assess and treat airway, breathing, and circulation. Connect the infant to a cardiac monitor to assess the cardiac rhythm for bradycardia related to hypoxia. Decrease any additional physiological or environmental stress (e.g., keep the newborn warm and provide comfort). Observe for signs of complications including meningitis and septic shock, a severe complication caused by toxins in the bloodstream.

TRANSPORT

The EMT–I may be involved in the transfer of a newborn from an outlying hospital to a tertiary facility. Some tertiary hospitals have neonatal intensive care units (NICU) for critically ill newborns and neonates. These units provide three prescribed levels of care with special equipment, skilled personnel, and ancillary services concentrated in a centralized institution:

- *Level I facility*—Provides management of normal maternal and newborn care but can identify high-

BOX 33-2

MANIFESTATIONS OBSERVED IN NEONATAL SEPSIS

GENERAL SIGNS
Newborn generally "not doing well"
Poor temperature control: hypothermia, hyperthermia (rare)

CIRCULATORY SYSTEM
Pallor, cyanosis, or mottling
Cold, clammy skin
Hypotension
Edema
Irregular heartbeat: bradycardia, tachycardia

RESPIRATORY SYSTEM
Irregular respirations, apnea, or tachypnea
Cyanosis
Grunting
Dyspnea
Retractions

CENTRAL NERVOUS SYSTEM
Diminished activity: lethargy, hyporeflexia, coma
Increased activity: irritability, tremors, seizures
Full fontanelle
Increased or decreased tone
Abnormal eye movements

GASTROINTESTINAL SYSTEM
Poor feeding
Vomiting
Diarrhea or decreased stooling
Abdominal distention
Hepatomegaly
Hemoccult-positive stools

HEMATOPOIETIC SYSTEM
Jaundice
Pallor
Petechiae, ecchymosis
Splenomegaly

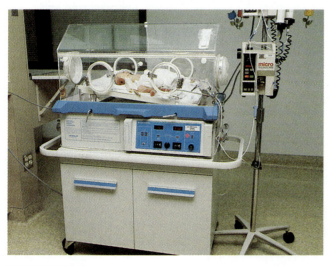

FIGURE 33-5 ▲ Newborn in incubator. (From Wong D: *Whaley and Wong's nursing care of infants and children,* ed 6, St Louis, 1999, Mosby.)

risk pregnancies and/or high-risk newborns early and implement emergency care in the event of complications
● *Level II facility*—Provides a full range of maternity and newborn care and is equipped to manage the majority of maternal and neonatal complications, depending on the resources available
● *Level III facility*—Offers the full range of maternal and newborn services of a level II facility and has the capacity to provide care for the most complex neonatal complications; at least one full-time neonatologist is on the staff

During the transport, several members of the transport team may be on board the ambulance or helicopter. They may include a neonatologist or fellow in neonatology, a respiratory therapist, and one or more nurses. Since the newborn will be transported in an incubator, detailed preparation must be made in whatever vehicle is used to accommodate the incubator (Figure 33-5).

EMT–I Jensen quickly assesses the situation and sees that the newborn is about to be born. He prepares the childbirth kit as his partner, EMT–I Williams, prepares the mother and gets a quick set of vitals on her. She is in charge of the first patient, the mother. EMT–I Jensen is in charge of the second, the baby about to be born.

The head delivers, and he suctions the mouth and nose. There is no sign of meconium. The remainder of the newborn delivers quickly, and he immediately begins to dry a newborn boy. He positions him on his back with his head slightly lower than the rest of his body. There are no signs of respiration.

EMT–I Jensen tells the mother that she has a son, and she asks why he is not crying. He explains that he is still cleaning him off. EMT–I Williams talks with the medical command physician at the local hospital and tells her the newborn is alive but premature with potential respiratory distress.

The newborn begins to initiate shallow breaths on his own as EMT–I Jensen finishes drying him. Heart rate (HR) is 80. He wraps him in a clean, dry towel and prepares to ventilate him at 100% oxygen with a bag-valve-mask device, since his respiratory rate is shallow and his HR is only 80. The newborn's APGAR score at 1 minute is 3.

Sign	Assessment	Value
Appearance	Blue and pale	0
Pulse rate	<100	1
Grimace	No response	0
Activity	Some flexion	1
Respirations	Slow and irregular	1

EMT–I Jensen continues ventilations, and the newborn starts to move around. He still has peripheral cyanosis, and his trunk and face are now pink. HR is now 118. He begins to have a weak cry.

The cord has stopped pulsating. It is short because of the prematurity of the newborn. EMT–I Jensen clamps it in two places and then cuts it. He updates the mother as she hears the newborn begin to cry. His APGAR score at 5 minutes is 7.

Sign	Assessment	Value
Appearance	Body pink; extremities blue	1
Pulse rate	>100	2
Grimace	Grimace	1
Activity	Some flexion	1
Respirations	Crying weakly	2

EMT–I Jensen stops ventilations and administers blow-by oxygen. He places the newborn on his mother's abdomen and continues to monitor his airway, breathing, HR, and skin color.

EMT–I Williams states that the placenta has delivered and the mother is ready for transport. The two EMT–Is transfer the mother and newborn into the back of the ambulance. The mother of the 16-year-old girl is secured in the front passenger seat. The heater inside the vehicle has been turned on to provide extra warmth for the newborn.

En route, EMT–I Williams contacts the medical command physician at the receiving hospital. She says to bring the newborn to the local hospital, and the staff will have the neonatal transport team en route by air by the estimated time of arrival.

Transport time to the hospital is approximately 30 minutes. The mother is doing well, and EMT–I Jensen continues to assess the newborn throughout the trip. He notices the newborn's body is very relaxed and floppy. His head is large, and his body size is small.

From conversations with the mother, EMT–I Jensen estimates that the newborn is approximately 32 weeks gestation. The mother's prenatal care has been sporadic, and her diet has been suboptimal. She denies any drug use or cigarette smoking. She only found out she was pregnant about 2 months ago.

A report is provided to the physicians and nurses on arrival at the hospital. EMT–I Jensen is still there finishing the trip report when the neonatal transport team arrives by helicopter. They move the newborn to an incubator and leave the hospital. He says goodbye to the mother and grandmother and wishes them good luck. Two weeks later, he contacts the family and finds out that the newborn is still in the NICU and is doing well.

SUMMARY

- Premature newborns have an increased risk of respiratory distress, hypothermia, and head and brain injury. In addition to low birth-weight, various risk factors may affect the need for resuscitation.
- At birth, newborns make three major physiological adaptations necessary for survival:
  - Emptying fluids from their lungs and beginning ventilation
  - Changing their circulatory patterns
  - Maintaining body temperature
- The priorities of neonatal resuscitation are prevent heat loss, clear the airway by positioning and suctioning, provide tactile stimulation and initial breathing if necessary, and further evaluate the newborn.
- If the newborn's condition gets worse or fails to improve after oxygenation and continued ventilation, endotracheal intubation and drug administration may be required. Medications used most frequently include epinephrine, volume expanders, and naloxone.
- Complications during the post resuscitation phase include endotracheal position change to include dislodgement, tube occlusion by mucus or meconium, and pneumothorax.

- Maintain body temperature, oxygen administration, and ventilatory support of the newborn during transport.
- Advanced life support may be required for respiratory disorders (e.g., apnea, respiratory distress, and cyanosis), cardiovascular disorders (e.g., bradycardia and cardiac arrest), gastrointestinal disorders (e.g., vomiting and diarrhea), seizures, fever, hypothermia, and hypoglycemia.
- The EMT–I should be aware of the normal feelings and reactions of parents, siblings, other family members, and caregivers while providing emergency care to an ill or injured child.

WEBSITES WITH ADDITIONAL INFORMATION

American Academy of Pediatrics: http://www.aap.org
American College of Emergency Physicians: http://www.acep.org
Center for Pediatric Emergency Medicine: http://www.cpem.org
Emergency Medical Services for Children: http://www.ems-c.org

34

Pediatric Emergencies

Key Terms

Apnea

Broselow Tape

Child Abuse

Child Maltreatment

Croup Epiglottis

Family-Centered Care

Ketogenic Diet

Laryngotracheo–
bronchitis

Neglect

Respiratory Arrest

Respiratory Distress

Respiratory Failure

Shaken Baby
Syndrome

Status Asthmaticus

Sudden Infant Death
Syndrome (SIDS)

Vagus Nerve
Stimulator (VNS)

...CASE HISTORY

Finally, after a series of busy 24-hour shifts at the fire department, EMT–I Ward is on a much-deserved "four day." The kids are in bed, and EMT–I Ward and her husband are enjoying a quiet evening at home watching an old movie on TV. On the way to the kitchen to get some popcorn, EMT–I Ward hears her youngest child call out to her. She goes to his room and finds him sitting upright in his bed, struggling to breathe. She sees that classic tripod position that he uses whenever it is a "bad" attack. He is wheezing, his color is not good, and he is telling his mother that he "can't catch his breath." EMT–I Ward attempts to calm him while her husband gets the inhaler. She tells her son to breathe slowly and deeply, but he is doing everything he can to move air in and out.

EMT–I Ward administers one inhalation of her son's prescribed albuterol; but, as usual, there is little response. The inhalers just are not doing much good these days. He is still using accessory muscles to breathe, and his color is not improving. Quietly, she tells her husband to call the ambulance. EMT–I Ward recalls his last attack and the trouble they had reversing his bronchospasm. Her son spent 2 days in the pediatric intensive care unit, and she had been afraid he would not recover.

Within minutes, the Wards' quiet evening at home becomes a busy emergency medical service (EMS) scene. An ambulance, a fire truck, and two police cars are parked out front. EMT–I Ward's husband asks the neighbors to stay with the other children while they are both at the hospital. EMT–I Ward tells the EMS team that this is her child's third asthma attack in several weeks and that the last one required hospitalization. She states that he has had one dose of albuterol and that his medication includes corticosteroids to help reduce his inflammatory response. She helps them apply an oxygen mask to her son, and she quickly carries him to the ambulance.

LEARNING OBJECTIVES

CHAPTER GOAL
Upon completion of this chapter, the EMT-Intermediate will be able to use assessment findings to formulate a field impression and implement the treatment plan for a pediatric patient.

Cognitive Objectives
As an EMT-Intermediate you should be able to do the following:
- Outline differences in adult and pediatric anatomy and physiology.
- Identify the growth and developmental characteristics of infants and children.

- Identify the common responses of families to acute illness and injury of an infant or child.
- Describe techniques for successful interaction with families of acutely ill or injured infants and children.
- Describe techniques for successful assessment of infants and children.
- Discuss pediatric patient assessment.
- Describe the primary causes of altered level of consciousness in infants and children.
- Describe the epidemiology, including the incidence, morbidity/mortality, risk factors, and prevention strategies for respiratory distress/failure in infants and children.
- Define respiratory distress and respiratory failure.
- Discuss the pathophysiology of respiratory distress/failure in infants and children.
- Discuss the assessment findings associated with respiratory distress/failure in infants and children.
- Identify the major classifications of pediatric cardiac rhythms.
- Discuss the appropriate equipment used to obtain pediatric vital signs.
- Identify normal vital sign values for the various pediatric age groups.
- Describe techniques for successful treatment of infants and children.
- Discuss the management/treatment plan for respiratory distress/failure in infants and children.
- Determine appropriate airway adjuncts and discuss complications of improper use in infants and children.
- Discuss appropriate endotracheal (ET) intubation equipment for infants and children.
- Identify the type of ET tube used in children less than eight years of age.
- Identify complications of improper ET intubation procedure in infants and children.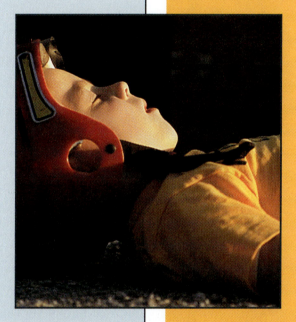
- Discuss appropriate ventilation devices and complications of improper use in infants and children.
- List the indications for gastric decompression for infants and children.
- Discuss the appropriate equipment for vascular access in infants and children.
- Identify complications of vascular access for infants and children.
- Discuss age-appropriate vascular access sites for infants and children.
- Describe the epidemiology (e.g., incidence, morbidity/mortality, risk factors, and prevention strategies) and pathophysiology for cardiac dysrhythmias in infants and children.
- Discuss the primary causes of cardiopulmonary arrest in infants and children.
- Integrate advanced life support (ALS) skills with basic cardiac life support for infants and children.
- Discuss basic cardiac life support (e.g., cardiopulmonary resuscitation [CPR]) guidelines for infants and children.
- Identify appropriate parameters for performing infant and child CPR.

Continued

- Discuss the assessment findings and management/treatment plan associated with cardiac dysrhythmias in infants and children.
- Differentiate between upper and lower airway obstruction.
- Describe the epidemiology, including the incidence, morbidity/mortality, risk factors, and prevention strategies for hypoperfusion in infants and children.
- Discuss the pathophysiology of hypoperfusion in infants and children.
- Discuss the common causes and evaluate the severity of hypoperfusion in infants and children.
- Discuss the assessment findings associated with hypoperfusion in infants and children.
- Discuss the management/treatment plan for hypoperfusion in infants and children.
- Describe the epidemiology, including the incidence, morbidity/mortality, risk factors, and prevention strategies for neurological emergencies in infants and children.
- Discuss the pathophysiology of neurological emergencies in infants and children.
- Discuss the assessment findings associated with neurological emergencies in infants and children.
- Discuss the management/treatment plan for neurological emergencies in infants and children.
- Describe the treatment of an infant or child in status epilepticus.
- Identify the signs and symptoms of meningitis in the infant or child.
- Identify common poisons ingested by children.
- Describe the epidemiology, including the incidence, morbidity/mortality, risk factors and prevention strategies for trauma in infants and children.
- Identify methods/mechanisms that prevent injuries to infants and children.
- Discuss the pathophysiology of trauma in infants and children.
- Identify common lethal mechanisms of injury in infants and children.
- Discuss anatomical features of children that predispose or protect them from certain injuries.
- Discuss the assessment findings associated with trauma in infants and children.
- Discuss the management/treatment plan for trauma in infants and children.
- Discuss fluid management and shock treatment for infant and child trauma patients.

- Describe aspects of infant and child airway management that are affected by potential cervical spine injury.
- Identify infant and child trauma patients who require spinal immobilization.
- Describe the process for pediatric immobilization.
- Describe treatment for a child with hypothermia.
- Define water rescue, submersion, and drowning.
- Define sudden infant death syndrome.
- Describe the epidemiology, including the incidence, morbidity/mortality, risk factors, and prevention strategies for infants with sudden infant death syndrome (SIDS).
- Discuss the pathophysiology of SIDS in infants.
- Discuss the assessment findings associated with SIDS.
- Discuss the management/treatment plan for SIDS.
- Discuss the parent/caregiver responses to the death of an infant or child.
- Define child abuse and child neglect.
- Describe the epidemiology, including the incidence, morbidity/mortality, risk factors, and prevention strategies for abuse and neglect in infants and children.
- Discuss the pathophysiology of abuse and neglect in infants and children.
- Discuss the assessment findings associated with abuse and neglect in infants and children.
- Discuss the management/treatment plan for abuse and neglect in infants and children.
- Recognize examples of cognitive and physical disabilities.
- Identify family issues encountered when working with children who have special health care needs.
- Determine when pain management and sedation are appropriate for infants and children.
- Discuss appropriate transport guidelines for infants and children.
- Discuss appropriate receiving facilities for low- and high-risk infants and children.

Affective Objectives
As an EMT–Intermediate you should be able to do the following:
- Demonstrate and advocate appropriate interactions with the infant/child that conveys an understanding of their developmental stage.
- Recognize the emotional dependence of the infant/child on his or her parent/guardian.

LEARNING OBJECTIVES—cont'd

- Recognize the emotional impact of infant/child injuries and illnesses on the parent/guardian.
- Recognize and appreciate the physical and emotional difficulties associated with separation of the parent/guardian/caregiver of a child with special health care needs.
- Demonstrate the ability to provide reassurance, empathy, and compassion for the parent/guardian.
- Demonstrate the ability to provide family-centered care.

Psychomotor Objectives
As an EMT-Intermediate you should be able to do the following:
- Demonstrate the appropriate approach for treating infants and children.
- Demonstrate appropriate intervention techniques with families of acutely ill or injured infants and children.
- Demonstrate an appropriate assessment for different developmental age groups.
- Demonstrate appropriate techniques for measuring pediatric vital signs.
- Demonstrate the use of a length-based resuscitation device for determining equipment sizes, drug doses, and other pertinent information for a pediatric patient.
- Demonstrate the techniques/procedures for treating infants and children with respiratory distress.
- Demonstrate proper technique for administering blow-by oxygen to infants and children.
- Demonstrate the proper use of a pediatric nonrebreather oxygen mask.
- Demonstrate appropriate use of airway adjuncts with infants and children.
- Demonstrate appropriate use of ventilation devices for infants and children.
- Demonstrate ET intubation procedures in infants and children.

- Demonstrate appropriate treatment/management of intubation complications for infants and children.
- Demonstrate proper placement of a gastric tube in infants and children.
- Demonstrate appropriate technique for insertion of peripheral intravenous (IV) catheters for infants and children.
- Demonstrate appropriate techniques for administration of intramuscular, subcutaneous, rectal, ET, and oral medication for infants and children.
- Demonstrate appropriate techniques for insertion of an intraosseous line for infants and children.
- Demonstrate age appropriate interventions for infants and children with an obstructed airway.
- Demonstrate appropriate airway control maneuvers for infant and child trauma patients.
- Demonstrate appropriate treatment of infants and children requiring advanced airway and breathing control.
- Demonstrate appropriate immobilization techniques for infant and child trauma patients.
- Demonstrate treatment of infants and children with head injuries.
- Demonstrate appropriate treatment of infants and children with chest injuries.
- Demonstrate appropriate treatment of infants and children with abdominal injuries.
- Demonstrate appropriate treatment of infants and children with extremity injuries.
- Demonstrate appropriate treatment of infants and children with burns.
- Demonstrate appropriate parent/caregiver interviewing techniques for infant and child death situations.
- Demonstrate proper infant cardiopulmonary resuscitation.
- Demonstrate proper child CPR.
- Demonstrate proper techniques for performing infant and child defibrillation and synchronized cardioversion.

INTRODUCTION

Pediatric emergencies represent a unique challenge for the EMT–Intermediate. Many calls involving pediatric patients can be quite intimidating or stressful for the EMT–I because of previous experience, his or her own children, or a lack of confidence in assessing and treating this population. In addition, the infant, child, or adolescent is involved as the primary patient yet the family, caregiver, school nurse, or child care provider may also be at the scene of the illness or injury and may want to be involved in the child's treatment. Last, being involved in a situation in which a child dies can be emotionally draining. This chapter will address many pediatric issues to give the EMT–I a better understanding of the knowledge and skills needed to treat these patients.

THE PEDIATRIC PATIENT

Epidemiology

In rural and urban areas, approximately 10% of all emergency medical services (EMS) treatment is for children under 14 years of age. Children between 5 and 14 years of age are most commonly seen because of trauma. Medical illness is the most frequent reason given for children less than 5 years of age. In children less than 2 years of age, serious illness, including cardiopulmonary arrest is most common.

It is critical that the EMT–Intermediate (EMT–I) be trained to deal with emergencies involving infants and young children. Once trained, the prehospital provider must maintain those skills, particularly in areas where pediatric field experience is limited. In many instances, the majority of pediatric patients seen are not in severe distress. However, a critically ill pediatric patient can present at any time. Workshops, continuing education programs, and other clinical opportunities must be made available to EMS personnel to enhance the level of care rendered to pediatric patients.

Anatomical Differences

Infants and children are anatomically different from adults. The term *infant* is used to refer to those individuals under the age of 1 year, whereas the term *child* is used to refer to those individuals from age 1 to 8 years. More specific classifications are listed in Box 34-1. Remember that these are only guidelines. The patient's weight is the key to providing treatment. See Table 34-1 for a summary of anatomical differences.

AIRWAY

Occlusion of the upper airway is one of the major causes of pediatric death in the prehospital setting when not appropriately managed. Therefore it is important for the EMT–I to be aware of the significant anatomical differences between adult and pediatric airways. First, the overall size of the pediatric airway is smaller. Therefore the airway of an infant or child is more likely to become occluded by foreign bodies, blood, vomit, or loose teeth. Secondly, a child less than 8 years of age has a larger tongue in comparison to the size of the mouth, a large and floppy epiglottis, and an airway that is narrowest at the cricoid cartilage (see Chapter 9). Lastly, the tonsils and adenoids (found in the posterior aspect of the pharynx) also may affect the patency of the airway. The weak muscles of the neck also may lead to obstruction, due to their inability to hold the various anatomic structures clear of the airway.

The location of the vocal cords in a child is also different than in an adult. A child's cords sit more superior and anterior on the cervical spine than an adult. In infants the cords are located at approximately the first (or second) cervical vertebra. As the child grows, the cords begin to move downward closer to the level of the third vertebra.

INTERNAL ORGANS

In infants and children, the internal organs are larger in proportion to body size. The skeletal structure is smaller, so the internal organs are basically "packed" into a smaller space. Because of this relationship, there is a higher incidence of internal injuries to infants and children. The organ that is most often injured is the liver. This difference in size and structure explains why multisystem injuries occur more often in childhood than in adulthood.

HEAD, NECK, AND BONES

Because the head of an infant and young child is so large, many childhood accidents usually involve a head injury. Cervical injuries can occur more easily because the head is large and heavy, exerting more pressure on the cervical spine. In medical situations the child may complain of a sore, stiff, or swollen neck.

Infants also have fontanelles, or soft spots, on the tops of their heads. Fontanelles are spaces between the bones of the infant's cranium that are covered by a

---

BOX 34-1

PEDIATRIC CLASSIFICATIONS

Neonate—Birth to 1 month
Young infant—1 to 5 months
Infant—6 to 12 months
Toddler—1 to 3 years
Preschooler—3 to 5 years
School age—6 to 12 years
Adolescent—12 to 15 years

tough membrane. The diamond-shaped, anterior fontanelle can be palpated until approximately 18 to 24 months of age. The posterior or triangular-shaped fontanelle usually closes approximately 2 months after birth. These fontanelles bulge with any increase in intracranial pressure and are depressed when dehydration is present. The EMT–I should gently palpate the fontanelles during the infant's assessment (Figure 34-1).

Children's bones are different as well. They are softer and have less calcium and fewer other minerals as compared with an adult. Therefore an injury to the child's bone can be a "bending" of the bone without an actual break. Similarly, a child's ribs are more pliable and can withstand more force. They are injured less frequently than are an adult's. The result is that the underlying lung can be injured without an overlying rib fracture.

TABLE 34-1

Summary of Anatomical Differences in Pediatric Patients

AREA	ADULT	PEDIATRIC DIFFERENCE	PEDIATRIC CONSIDERATIONS
Airway	Diameter of trachea is approximately 20 mm. Tongue size is relative to size of mouth. Epiglottis is firm. Muscles in neck are firm.	Lumen of trachea is approximately 4 mm; narrowest part of the laryngeal airway is the cricoid cartilage. In children less than 8 years, tongue is larger compared with the size of the mouth. Epiglottis is large and floppy. Muscles of neck are weak in infants and younger children.	Smaller tracheal opening can occlude more easily. Tongue can easily occlude the airway due to its large size. Epiglottis may be source of airway occlusion. Weak muscles may lead to obstruction due to their inability to adequately support the various anatomic structures.
Internal organs	Size of organs are proportionate to body size. Skeletal structure is full grown.	Internal organs are larger in proportion to body size. Skeletal structure is smaller; hence internal organs are "packed" into smaller space.	Internal organs are larger in proportion to body size. Skeletal structure is smaller; hence internal organs are "packed" into smaller space.
Head and neck	Both are proportionate to size of body. There are no open areas along the skull.	Infants and toddlers have large and heavy heads and necks in comparison to body. Infants have fontanelles on top of head.	Infants and children are more prone to head and cervical injuries because of large and heavy head. Fontanelles bulge with any increase in intracranial pressure and may be depressed when dehydration is present.
Bones	Adults have fully grown bones, but they may be weak in geriatric patients due to osteoporosis. Ribs are fully grown but may be weak in geriatric patients due to osteoporosis.	Bones are softer with less calcium and fewer other minerals. Ribs more pliable and can withstand more force.	Injury to child's bone may be a bending instead of actual break. Ribs are injured less frequently; underlying lung can be easily injured without overlying rib fractures.
Nervous system	Adults have mature nervous systems.	Infants and children have immature nervous systems. Nerves are not well insulated, and reflexes are less developed.	Infant or child does not know how to move out of the way when an object suddenly comes at them, so there is increased risk for injury.

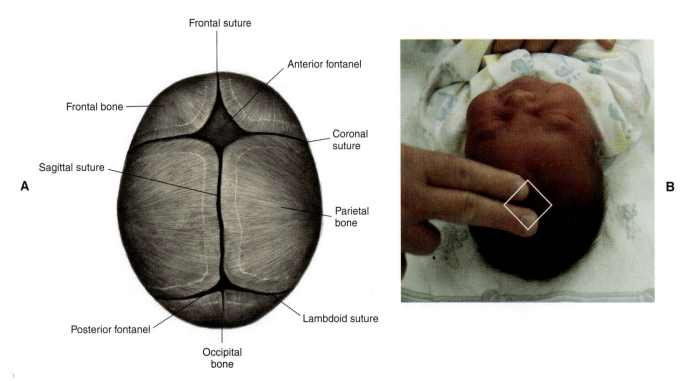

FIGURE 34-1 ▲ **A,** Location of sutures and fontanelles. **B,** Palpating anterior fontanelle. (From Wong DL: *Whaley and Wong's nursing care of infants and children,* ed 6, St Louis, 1999, Mosby.)

NERVOUS SYSTEM

The child's control of the nervous system is also immature. Their nerves are not well insulated, and their reflexes are less developed. An infant or child really does not know how to move out of the way when an object suddenly comes at him or her.

Approaching the Pediatric Patient

Children can present unique challenges to the EMT–I simply due to age and level of language comprehension. This section reviews the stages that children go through as they grow and how the EMT–I should handle each stage. The EMT–I should incorporate this information into his or her assessment and treatment of pediatric patients. See Box 34-2 for approach strategies to use with each developmental stage of the pediatric patient.

The psychological aspect of injury and illness in the pediatric patient should be considered. Most children do not have the ability to understand what is occurring around them. They may be aware that something is hurting them or is painful. They become fearful of voices with which they are not familiar or the tones of those voices. If the psychological aspect is not taken into account in the prehospital setting, the pediatric patient may experience significant psychological scarring in future years. The goal for all patients is care of the total person.

The parents of the injured child also must be considered as part of the child's psychological environment.

The parents must know what is happening. They often require psychological assistance in dealing with their injured or ill child. They may feel responsible for the child receiving the injuries or that there was something they did or did not do to cause the injury. In dealing with parents, many EMT–Is have found the following to be helpful.

First, the EMT–I must remember that he or she is the authority at the scene, and patient care is the top priority. Parents can be the greatest allies or represent the greatest obstruction. If the parents are calm, the EMT–I should make eye contact and have them assist with the care of their child. However, if the parents are not able to control their emotions, others should be sought at the scene to assist with the parents. The EMT–I should always keep the parents informed.

Finally, the EMT–I should not forget to take into account his or her own personal psychological well-being. The stress of the job is tremendous, and being exposed to pediatric illness and/or injury can be devastating. Pediatric emergencies are ranked among the highest in creating stress for the healthcare provider. The EMT–I should be sure to seek assistance from peers or even professional help should he or she be confronted with a particularly stressful situation. The EMT–I is important as well.

Before interacting with the child, the EMT–I should ask the following questions:
- What is the child's chronological age and/or approximate weight?

BOX 34-2

DEVELOPMENTAL STAGES AND APPROACH STRATEGIES FOR PEDIATRIC PATIENTS

INFANTS

Major Fear:
- Separation and strangers

Approach Strategies:
- Provide consistent caretakers.
- Decrease parent's anxiety (transmitted to infant).
- Minimize separation from parents/caregivers.

TODDLERS

Major Fear:
- Separation and loss of control

Characteristics of Thinking:
- Primitive
- Inability to recognize views of others
- Little concept of body integrity

Approach Strategies:
- Keep explanations simple.
- Choose words carefully.
- Let toddler play with equipment (stethoscope).
- Minimize separation from parents/caregivers.

PRESCHOOLERS

Major Fears:
- Bodily injury and mutilation
- Loss of control
- The unknown and the dark
- Being left alone

Characteristics of Thinking:
- Highly literal interpretation of words
- Inability to abstract
- Primitive ideas about their bodies (fear all blood will "leakout" if bandage removed)

Approach Strategies:
- Keep explanations simple and concise.
- Choose words carefully.
- Emphasize that a procedure will help the child be more healthy.
- Be honest.

SCHOOL-AGE CHILDREN

Major Fears:
- Loss of control
- Bodily injury and mutilation
- Failure to live up to expectation of others
- Death

Characteristics of Thinking:
- Vague or false ideas about physical illness, body structure, and function
- Ability to listen attentively without always comprehending
- Reluctance to ask questions about something they think are expected to know
- Increased awareness of significant illness, potential hazards of treatment, lifelong consequences of injury, and the meaning of death

Approach Strategies:
- Approach child to explain what is understood.
- Provide as many choices as possible to increase the child's sense of control.
- Assure the child that he or she has not done anything wrong and that necessary procedures are not punishment.
- Anticipate and answer questions regarding long-term consequences (such as what the scar will look like, how long activities may be restricted, etc.).

ADOLESCENTS

Major Fears:
- Loss of control
- Altered body image
- Separation from peer group

Characteristics of Thinking:
- Ability to think abstractly
- Tendency toward hyperresponsiveness to pain (reactions not always in proportion to event)
- Minimal understanding of the structure and workings of the body

Approach Strategies:
- When appropriate, allow adolescents to be part of decision making about their care.
- Give information sensitively.
- Express how important their compliance and cooperation are to their treatment.
- Be honest about consequences.
- Use or teach coping mechanisms such as relaxation, deep breathing, and self-comforting talk.

From McSwain NE Jr et al: *The basic EMT: comprehensive prehospital patient care,* ed 2, St Louis, 2001, Mosby.

- What is the child's level of language comprehension? (NOTE: It may not always match the age.)
- Is someone present whom the child knows and/or trusts (e.g., parents, older siblings, caregivers, or teachers) who can be with the child to offer emotional support?
- Does anyone know the child's medical history or other information that may be helpful to the EMT–I (e.g., details of the accident, type of seizure activity)?
- Are there any special circumstances present (e.g., language barrier, physical or mental disabilities, special equipment)?

To adequately care for children, it is also essential to have equipment specific to the pediatric population. The EMT–I should work with personnel in the ambulance service, as well as the medical director, to ensure access to the appropriate pediatric equipment.

Family-Centered Care

Family-centered care is a philosophy that involves the parent or other family member in the care of the pediatric patient. The family is a vital component of the care team and should be trusted when they describe what happened to their child. Whenever possible, they should be included in the treatment process.

The EMT–I may see many different emotions when dealing with families of an ill or injured infant or child. Some parents may be extremely upset or feel guilty that their child was injured. Others may seem oblivious to what happened and may be in shock. Still others may show little to no emotion or inappropriate responses (e.g., such as blaming their child for the injury).

In families that are not intact, parents may be fighting with one another over the child. Custody battles may intensify during a child's illness or injury. In abusive situations, the family may seem distant to the child.

Do not assume that a calm parent is a noncaring parent. Some children with special health care needs are hospitalized, transported by ambulance, or are critically ill quite often. The parents may have adapted their coping skills so that they remain concerned yet calm.

Family members should be allowed to assist in providing treatment if they prefer to do so and are psychologically able. If the family is overwhelmed, significantly stressed or abusive, the EMT–I may need to be more assertive. However, the EMT–I should not simply take over as the medical professional and push the family aside.

GENERAL PEDIATRIC ASSESSMENT
Scene Survey

Before the child is assessed, the EMT–I must determine if the scene is safe and what potential mechanism of injury or illness exists. Observation of the interaction between the child and a parent or caregiver is also important. Use the following list as a guide:

- Are there any weapons or dangerous animals in the environment?
- Are any pills, household chemicals, or medicine bottles near the child?
- In what position is the child found?
- What is the interaction between the parent/caregiver and the child? Do the history and injuries match? Is the parent concerned, angry, or indifferent?

Initial Assessment

There are several components to the initial assessment. They include the pediatric assessment triangle, the actual physical examination to assess ABCs, and a decision regarding transport.

Pediatric Assessment Triangle

There are three components to the pediatric assessment triangle (PAT):
- Appearance (mental status and muscle tone)
- Work of breathing (respiratory rate and effort)
- Circulation (skin signs and color)

Assessment of these components should be completed in approximately the first 30 to 60 seconds and will give the EMT–I a first impression of the status of the child. It provides valuable information and can help determine if a life-threatening condition exists. Most EMT–Is already ascertain this general impression when they first approach a child. It should be done for every pediatric patient.

APPEARANCE

The initial appearance of the child before any physical examination is done can give information about the child's mental status, respiratory status, and how well the brain is being perfused. An 18-month-old child who has pink skin or mucous membranes, is crying, clinging to his father, and afraid of the EMT–I has a patent airway, good respiratory effort, adequate circulation, and an appropriate response to strangers. Another child of the same age who is pale, is not crying, does not maintain any eye contact, is limp, and does not express any fear toward the EMT–I is potentially very ill. Remember, however, that the child who does not initially look ill may in fact be ill or injured without any current signs of distress.

WORK OF BREATHING

Evaluating how hard the child is working to breathe will quickly reveal the child's ability to oxygenate and ventilate. The infant with retractions of the chest or nasal flaring should immediately signal the EMT–I to suspect a respiratory problem. These signs indicate that the infant is using accessory muscles and is therefore working hard to try to breathe. An older child sitting upright and leaning slightly forward on his or her hands with the neck extended forward (tripod position) is an indication that accessory muscles are being used to breathe. The child who is sitting forward in a sniffing position indicates an upper airway obstruction.

CIRCULATION

Circulation to the skin can reflect the child's cardiovascular status. The child with cool, mottled extremities may be in shock and only perfusing vital organs. The child with pale skin or mucous membranes may also be in shock but may still be compensating for it. Any cyanosis must be treated immediately. The only exception is cyanotic hands and feet in the newborn or an infant less than two months old. This cyanosis may simply indicate that the infant is cold.

Initial Triage Decision

At this point, the EMT–I should initially decide if the child is urgently in need of treatment. If so, a rapid airway, breathing, and circulation (ABCs) assessment, treatment, and transport should be done. If the child's condition is not urgent, the EMT–I can proceed with a focused history and a detailed physical examination.

PHYSICAL EXAMINATION TO ASSESS VITAL FUNCTIONS (RAPID ABC ASSESSMENT)

The intent of the initial examination is to detect any life-threatening injuries and treat them. If the child's condition is not urgent, the focused history and detailed examination will provide a more detailed accounting of the patient's condition.

LEVEL OF CONSCIOUSNESS

A brief neurological examination should permit the classification of the child's level of consciousness. The EMT–I should use the acronym AVPU to determine if the pediatric patient is as follows:

A	Alert
V	Responsive to verbal stimuli
P	Responsive to painful stimuli
U	Unresponsive

These results should be adjusted based on the child's age and baseline mental status, if known. The child's level of consciousness may be depressed due to a head injury, respiratory failure, a postictal period after a seizure, and so forth.

AIRWAY

If the child's airway is patent, it was more than likely obvious during the PAT. Make sure that there is adequate chest rise with each breath. If an obstruction is present, the child may present with abnormal airway sounds such as stridor or wheezing. Gurgling usually indicates some type of liquid in the airway such as blood or mucus.

BREATHING

Respiratory distress in a pediatric patient can be a life-threatening event by itself. For this reason, prompt assessment of the child's respiratory status should be accomplished immediately. According to the American Heart Association (AHA), approximately 90% of pediatric cardiopulmonary arrests start as respiratory problems. Early identification and intervention is the best way to *prevent* pediatric cardiac arrest and can significantly enhance the child's future quality of life. Once the pediatric patient arrests, the prognosis is poor.

Respiratory distress is a condition of hypoxia whereby the work of breathing is increased. The infant or child tries to compensate to maintain oxygenation and ventilation by increasing the work of breathing to make up for the decrease in gas exchange. **Respiratory failure** is defined as the inability of the respiratory apparatus to maintain adequate oxygenation of the blood, with or without carbon dioxide retention. This process involves pulmonary dysfunction that generally results in impaired alveolar gas exchange, which can lead to hypoxemia and/or hypercarbia. **Respiratory arrest** is the cessation of respiration. **Apnea** is absence of airflow (breathing) for more than 15 seconds.

The first sign of respiratory distress in an infant is usually tachypnea. Other signs of respiratory distress that may be present in infants or children are increased respiratory rate and/or effort, diminished breath sounds, decreased level of responsiveness or response to parents or pain, poor skeletal muscle tone, and/or cyanosis.

As the child's respiratory effort increases, the following signs and symptoms may be present:
- Nasal flaring
- Intercostal, subcostal, and suprasternal inspiratory retractions
- Head bobbing
- Grunting
- Stridor
- Prolonged expiration

If an infant or child is acutely ill, a slow or irregular respiratory rate is a dismal sign. This sign usually indicates that the child's status is declining due to fatigue, central nervous system depression, or hypothermia. Many times the child will be tachypneic for a period of time, become fatigued from working so hard, and slow his or her rate of breathing. The EMT–I should not be fooled into thinking the child is improving because the respiratory rate drops. In reality, the child may progress to respiratory arrest and possibly cardiac arrest if not treated appropriately.

The EMT–I should briefly assess the neck for trauma, jugular venous distention, and tracheal deviation. The chest should be checked for deformities, contusions, abrasions, penetrations, paradoxical motion, accessory muscle usage, and intercostal retraction. With a stethoscope, the EMT–I should listen anteriorly, posteriorly, and under the arms along the midaxillary line to do an adequate assessment. The child should have equal breath sounds bilaterally. These sounds can be transmitted easily across the thorax because the child's chest wall is so thin. Therefore, it may be difficult to identify areas of decreased function on one side because the EMT–I will be able to hear sounds from the lung on the other side.

CIRCULATION

Many of the usual heart rates for infants and children show normal tachycardia. Sinus tachycardia also can occur as a result of stress due to hypovolemia, hypoxia, anxiety, fever, pain, increased carbon dioxide, or cardiac impairment.

Bradycardia usually occurs when the child can no longer maintain adequate tissue oxygenation. This condition is usually a precursor to cardiopulmonary arrest and should be treated quickly. Many times, proper oxygenation will cause the heart rate to rise, increasing the child's cardiac output.

Infants have short, chubby necks, which makes it extremely difficult to palpate the carotid artery. Therefore, the brachial artery should be palpated on the inside of the upper arm between the infant's elbow and shoulder (Figure 34-2). The carotid artery can be palpated for children older than 1 year of age (Figure 34-3). If a central pulse cannot be palpated, initiate cardiopulmonary resuscitation.

A peripheral pulse should also be palpated to determine the presence of distal circulation. Attempt to palpate a femoral pulse in infants and young children. A radial pulse may be used for older children. If the child has a carotid or brachial pulse yet no radial pulse, the child is hypotensive.

Assess the quality of the pulse. Is it rapid or slow? Does the pulse feel strong, or is it weak? Is a peripheral pulse even present?

Assess the color and temperature of the skin. Is the skin warm, cool, pale, or cyanotic? Is the child in a cold or hot environment? If so, these factors may affect the temperature of the skin without any underlying illness or injury.

Look for any signs of active hemorrhage. Obvious bleeding or swelling may indicate active bleeding.

VITAL SIGNS

The following vital signs should be assessed:
- Respiratory rate and quality
- Pulse rate and quality
- Blood pressure (not necessary in children less than 3 years of age)
- Pupil condition
- Skin color, temperature, and condition

To assess vital signs, the EMT–I must have the following equipment available:
- Pediatric stethoscope
- Adult stethoscope (for larger children and adolescents)
- Pediatric sphygmomanometer
- Adult sphygmomanometer (for larger children and adolescents)

Vital signs in infants and children vary with age. In addition, "normal" vital signs actually can vary from patient to patient. See Table 34-2 for a review of pediatric vital signs by age.

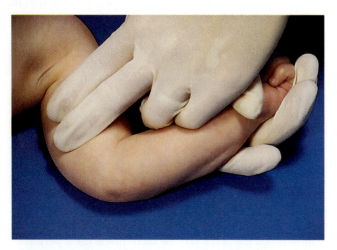

FIGURE 34-2 ▲ In infants, palpate the brachial artery for a pulse. (Vincent Knaus from Aehlert B: *Pediatric advanced life support,* St Louis, 1994, Mosby.)

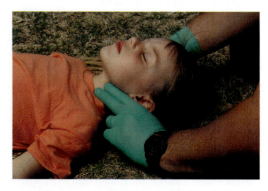

FIGURE 34-3 ▲ In children, palpate the carotid artery for a pulse. (Vincent Knaus from Aehlert B: *Pediatric advanced life support,* St Louis, 1994, Mosby.)

TABLE 34-2

Vital Signs—Normal Pediatric Values

HEIGHT AND WEIGHT RANGE FOR PEDIATRIC PATIENTS

| | | RANGE OF MEAN NORMS | |
GROUP	AGE	HEIGHT (AVERAGE)	WEIGHT (AVERAGE)
Newborn	Birth-6 weeks	51-63 cm	4-5 kg
Infant	7 weeks-1 year	56-80 cm	4-11 kg
Toddler	1-2 years	77-9 cm	11-14 kg
Preschool	2-6 years	91-122 cm	14-25 kg
School age	6-13 years	122-165 cm	25-63 kg
Adolescent	13-16 years	165-182 cm	62-80 kg

RESPIRATORY RATES FOR PEDIATRIC PATIENTS

GROUP	AGE	BREATHS/MIN	SUSPECT POSSIBLE ↓ MINUTE VOLUME AND NEED FOR VENTILATORY ASSIST WITH BVM
Newborn	Birth-6 weeks	30-50	↓30 or ↑50
Infant	7 weeks-1 year	20-30	↓20 or ↑30
Toddler	1-2 years	20-30	↓20 or ↑30
Preschool	2-6 years	20-30	↓20 or ↑30
School age	6-13 years	(12-20)-30	↓20 or ↑30
Adolescent	13-16 years	12-20	↓12 or ↑20

PULSE RATES FOR PEDIATRIC PATIENTS

GROUP	AGE	BEATS/MIN	ASSUME A SERIOUS PROBLEM EXISTS (BRADYCARDIA OR TACHYCARDIA)
Newborn	Birth-6 weeks	120-160	↓100 or ↑150
Infant	7 weeks-1 year	80-140	↓80 or ↑120
Toddler	1-2 years	80-130	↓60 or ↑110
Preschool	2-6 years	80-120	↓60 or ↑110
School age	6-13 years	(60-80)-100	↓60 or ↑100
Adolescent	13-16 years	60-100	↓60 or ↑100

BLOOD PRESSURE IN PEDIATRIC PATIENTS

GROUP	AGE	EXPECTED MEAN FOR BLOOD PRESSURE	LOWER LIMIT OF SYSTOLIC BP
Newborn	Birth-6 weeks	74-100 mm Hg 50-68 mm Hg	↓70 mm Hg
Infant	7 weeks-1 year	84-106 mm Hg 56-70 mm Hg	↓70 mm Hg
Toddler	1-2 years	98-106 mm Hg 50-70 mm Hg	↓70 mm Hg
Preschool	2-6 years	98-112 mm Hg 64-70 mm Hg	↓70 mm Hg
School age	6-13 years	104-124 mm Hg 64-80 mm Hg	↓80 mm Hg-90 mm Hg
Adolescent	13-16 years	118-132 mm Hg 70-82 mm Hg	↓80-90 mm Hg

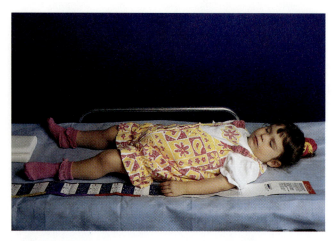

FIGURE 34-4 ▲ A Broselow resuscitation tape can be used to identify the proper range of vital signs for a pediatric patient. (Vincent Knaus from Aehlert B: *Pediatric advanced life support,* St Louis, 1994, Mosby.)

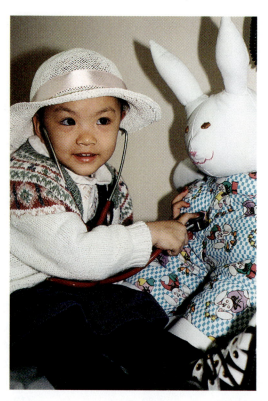

FIGURE 34-5 ▲ This child practices on a stuffed toy during the transition phase to see how the EMT–I will listen to her lungs. (From Wong DL: *Whaley and Wong's nursing care of infants and children,* ed 6, St Louis, 1999, Mosby.)

It may be difficult for the EMT–I to remember all of this information. A more practical method is to keep some type of reference material in the ambulance. The **Broselow tape,** a resuscitation tape developed by Broselow and colleagues, is an example of a tool that can be used (Figure 34-4).

Transition Phase

If the child's condition is not urgent (e.g., conscious and not acutely ill or injured), a brief transition phase can occur. During this time, the child can become familiar with the prehospital providers and the equipment being used. Depending on the child's age, allow him or her to touch the stethoscope, the blood pressure cuff, or whatever other equipment is appropriate (see Figure 34-5). This interaction will help ease the child's anxiety and build confidence in the provider of care.

Again, the seriousness of the child's condition dictates whether or not this phase is used. If the child is unconscious or acutely ill or injured, the EMT–I should proceed to the physical examination.

Focused History and Detailed Physical Examination

The focused history and detailed physical examination is a reexamination of the patient. All the components of the initial assessment should be included. However, this survey may be performed slowly so that a greater understanding of the patient's condition can be reached.

HISTORY

From whom do you elicit the history in a pediatric patient? Infants, toddlers, and preschoolers are unable to relate details so the EMT–I should obtain information from the parent, guardian, or caregiver. For the school-age child and young adolescent, information may be obtained from the parent, guardian, or school nurse. Some children may be able to explain certain items of their histories (e.g., allergies, use of an inhaler at school, medicine for epilepsy, and so on).

Older adolescents are capable of relating their own histories. Make every effort to question them alone about issues in which privacy is important: smoking, illegal drug or alcohol use, sexual activity, potential pregnancy, and so on.

The pneumonic SAMPLE is an excellent way to remember what questions to ask. It involves the following components:

S Signs and symptoms
- Evaluate signs of distress as appropriate for each age level.
- Evaluate symptoms relative to the chief complaint.
- If the infant or child is crying, are tears present?

A Allergies
- Has the child had a reaction to any medication? Does he or she have any other significant allergies?

M Medications
- Ask the parent or guardian if the child's immunizations are up-to-date.
- If the child is on medication, when was it last given? Has the child missed any doses today? Did the child vomit close to when the last medication was given?

- If the child has been given fever reducers, when was the last dose?

P Past medical history
- Ask the parent or guardian (if known) about the perinatal period. Was this child delivered on time, early, or late? If the child was premature, how many weeks gestation at delivery? Were there any problems during labor and delivery?
- Is the infant or child currently under the care of a physician? If so, how often does the child see his or her primary care physician?
- Are there any chronic illnesses present? Is any special equipment or assistive technology used?

L Last meal
- When did the child last have anything to eat or drink?
- For infants, include bottles and breast feeding.

E Events leading up to the current injury or illness
- Focus on events that may affect the current situation.
- When did the child's pain begin?
- When did he or she start to feel ill?
- When did the fever start?
- For infants and children still using diapers, how many wet diapers have there been in the last 24 hours?
- Has the child had frequent vomiting or diarrhea?
- Was there any recent head injury?

DETAILED PHYSICAL EXAMINATION

All body regions should be examined in detail. With infants and young children, start at the toes and work up to the head. For older children, start at the head and work down to the toes. See Chapter 10 for more information on the detailed physical examination.

CAPILLARY REFILL

Capillary refill also should be evaluated. The EMT–I should be aware that young children have poor collateral circulation, especially in a cold environment, so capillary refill may not provide an accurate assessment of perfusion (see Chapter 6).

PULSE OXIMETRY

Pulse oximetry provides continuous monitoring of a child's arterial oxygen saturation. It evaluates oxygenation and not the effectiveness of ventilation (elimination of carbon dioxide). It is quite useful as an adjunct, but the EMT–I should not rely solely on this tool. If the child's clinical status is questionable (e.g., tachypnea, cyanosis, decreased heart rate), yet the pulse oximeter reading is within normal limits, the EMT–I should rely on his or her assessment and treat the child for respiratory distress regardless of the number on the machine.

An infant sensor is used on the ear lobe and also can be applied to the nares, cheek at the corner of the mouth, or the tongue if the child is unresponsive. Adult sensors can be used around the hand or foot of an infant (see Figure 34-6). Regardless of what type of sensor is

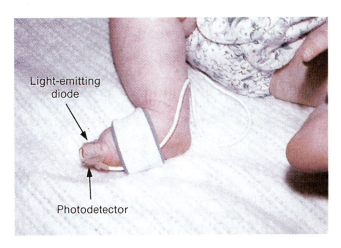

FIGURE 34-6 ▲ **Pulse oximeter sensor on great toe. Note that sensor is positioned with the light-emitting diode (LED) opposite the photodetector. The cord is secured to the foot with a self-adhering band (not tape) to minimize movement of the sensor. (From Wong DL: *Whaley and Wong's nursing care of infants and children,* ed 6, St Louis, 1999, Mosby.)**

used, the EMT–I should be familiar with the particular device available to him or her (see Chapter 10).

CARDIAC MONITOR

Cardiac monitoring may be necessary to further evaluate heart rate. Use pediatric electrodes for infants and young children. Adult electrodes may be used for larger children and adolescents. Make sure pediatric paddles are available for defibrillation if necessary.

ONGOING EXAMINATION

The following items should be monitored on an ongoing basis:
- Respiratory effort
- Color
- Mental status
- Pulse oximetry
- Vital signs
- Temperature

PROCEDURES AND EQUIPMENT FOR MANAGEMENT OF AIRWAY, BREATHING, AND CIRCULATION

If the child has a medical problem with no suspicion of trauma, allow him or her to assume a position of comfort. For infants and young children, allow the parent or caregiver to hold the child to decrease anxiety.

A child's airway must be managed in a specific manner to ensure its patency. Procedures with pediatric patients are relatively easy to perform. However, there must be attention to detail.

The appropriate method of opening the child's airway is to use the chin-lift or jaw-thrust maneuver. To perform this maneuver, the EMT–I places the fingers on the angle of the mandible and pulls gently anteriorly. This motion opens the airway, clears the tonsils and adenoids from obstructing the airway, and brings the tongue forward, allowing air to move more freely. Depending on the age and size of the child, a small blanket roll may be placed under the base of the neck or shoulders to assist in maintaining a sniffing position. If after performing these procedures the airway is still obstructed, suction may be needed to help clear the airway.

The tongue is the primary cause of airway obstruction in the infant or child. Two other potential causes are foreign objects and swelling from infections. If the tongue is the culprit, the head must be repositioned. Airway obstruction from an object is managed by first visualizing the object. If something is seen in the airway, it must be removed with the EMT–I's fingers or Magill forceps. If forceps are used, the EMT–I should be careful to avoid the adenoids and tonsils, because they are very vascular and may complicate the situation with bleeding if injured. If nothing is seen in the airway, the EMT–I should not blindly sweep the mouth because this may result in the object moving deeper into the airway.

If there is a foreign body obstruction, abdominal thrusts may be performed on older children but should never be performed on infants. Infants may benefit from back blows or chest thrusts. It is essential that the EMT–I maintain proficiency in basic cardiac life support and pay particular attention to those aspects of managing the pediatric airway.

A suction device may be more helpful in removing fluids that may be causing the obstruction. If an infant requires suction, a bulb syringe may prove to be more effective. Another means of suctioning infants is to wrap a piece of gauze around the finger and gently clear the pharynx. In older children, powered suction devices may be used but should be set on the lowest setting possible.

It is crucial that basic life support measures be initiated as soon as the need for airway management and/or ventilatory assistance is identified. Adequate artificial ventilation can buy critical minutes and also may be just enough to deter further respiratory and/or circulatory compromise.

Airway Adjuncts
OROPHARYNGEAL AIRWAY

An oropharyngeal airway can be used in an unresponsive infant or child to maintain a clear, unobstructed airway when there is no gag reflex. It is very important to select the proper size airway so that no harm is done to the child. The airway is measured the same as for the adult. The airway should reach from the corner of the mouth to the angle of the jaw (Figure 34-7, A).

Oropharyngeal airways come in many different sizes. The age of the child helps determine the size of the device. However, it is important to measure the airway to ensure a proper fit. If the EMT–I attempts to place an oropharyngeal airway that is too large in the mouth of an infant or child, vomiting or trauma to the soft tissues may occur. If an oropharyngeal airway that is too small is placed into the airway, it may fail to adequately open the airway and may push the tongue back causing an obstruction.

The best method of airway insertion is to depress the tongue with a tongue blade and insert the airway device over the blade (Figure 34-7, B). The EMT–I must be extremely careful not to lacerate or tear any of the anatomic structures. Correct positioning of the child's

A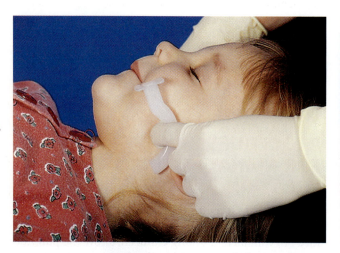

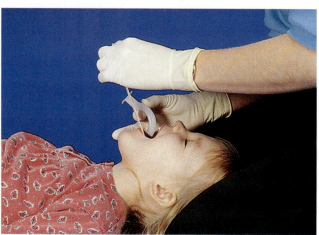 B

FIGURE 34-7 ▲ Using an oropharyngeal airway in a pediatric patient.
A, Measure the airway from the corner of the mouth to the angle of the jaw.
B, Using a tongue depressor to move the tongue, insert the airway right side up.
(Vincent Knaus from Stoy W: *Mosby's EMT-Basic textbook,* St Louis, 1996, Mosby.)

head must be maintained to ensure a patent airway once the device is in place.

NASOPHARYNGEAL AIRWAY

Again, it is important that the nasopharyngeal airway is the proper size. The EMT–I should measure the length of this airway from the tip of the patient's nose to the tragus (small extension of the outside cartilage of the ear anterior to the external opening) of the ear. He or she then lubricates the airway with a water-soluble substance and gently inserts it into one of the child's nares. This device may need to be suctioned to maintain patency.

If the properly sized nasopharyngeal airway is not available, a 3-mm endotracheal (ET) tube should be used as a substitute. The EMT–I should use the same measurement (from the tip of the nose to the tragus) and shorten the ET tube. The 15-mm attachment should be firmly reinserted so the tube does not go in past the nares (Figure 34-8).

SUCTION EQUIPMENT

If the child is crying, he or she swallows air and is prone to vomiting. Frequent suctioning may be necessary because of the presence of vomitus, saliva, mucus, blood, teeth, and so forth. A force greater than 120 mm Hg should not be used for an infant or child to avoid traumatizing the airway during the procedure.

Also, a flexible plastic catheter should be used whenever possible. A large-bore (tonsil-tip) catheter may be used for larger amounts or thicker material, but the EMT–I must be cautious not to be too vigorous. The EMT–I must not cause soft-tissue damage to the

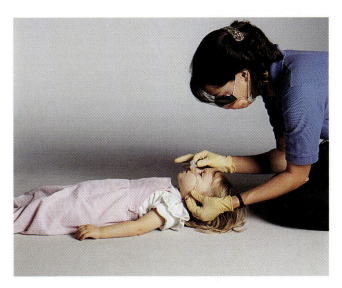

FIGURE 34-8 ▲ If necessary a 3 mm ET tube can be used as a substitute for a nasal airway in a pediatric patient.

oropharynx and increase the obstruction because of bleeding.

The heart rate should be monitored during suctioning. Irritation of the posterior pharynx, larynx, or trachea produces vagal stimulation, which in turn causes the heart rate to drop. If the heart rate decreases, the EMT–I should stop the procedure and hyperventilate the child with high-concentration oxygen.

Once basic life support skills have been performed on the infant or child, consideration should be given to more advanced procedures. The EMT–I must continue to reassess the patient to determine if these skills should be attempted at the scene, en route to the hospital, or not at all.

ENDOTRACHEAL INTUBATION

Once the decision has been made to initiate an advanced airway procedure, intubation remains the method of choice. This method provides the most effective airway control and allows direct ventilation of the lungs.

Indications—Indications for intubation of the child include the following:
1. Inadequate central nervous system control of ventilation
2. Functional or anatomic airway obstruction
3. Excessive work of breathing leading to fatigue
4. Need for high peak inspiratory pressure or positive end expiratory pressure to maintain effective alveolar gas exchange

Before intubating the infant or child, several considerations should be taken into account. First, the size of the ET tube should be determined. The easiest and quickest way to determine the appropriate size ET tube is to use the nostrils as a guide. Generally, but not always, the nares should accept the ET tube size that is to be placed into the trachea. If the tube is too small, it will not secure the airway. On the other hand, if the tube is too large, damage to the vocal cords may occur.

Several other methods may be useful when determining ET tube size for the pediatric patient. The EMT–I can look at the outside diameter of the patient's little finger or use the following formula for children older than 2 years of age:

$$\text{ET tube (in mm)} = \frac{\text{Age in years}}{4} + 4$$

Using the length (height) of the infant or child is actually more accurate than using the age. Resuscitation tapes help with this method. The EMT–I should keep in mind that calculations are often a difficult task to perform when a child is seriously ill and use whatever method best meets his or her needs.

Once the ET tube size has been selected, a handle and blade must be prepared. The laryngoscope handle for a pediatric patient has a smaller diameter and therefore uses smaller batteries, which allows for

TABLE 34-3

Endotracheal Tube Sizes in Infants and Children Less Than 8 Years of Age

AGE	INTERNAL DIAMETER OF TUBE IN MM	SUCTION CATHETERS*
Premature infant	2.5-3.0 uncuffed	5-6 French
Newborn (term)	3.0-3.5 uncuffed	6-8 French
6 months	3.5-4.0 uncuffed	8 French
1 year	4.0-4.5 uncuffed	8 French
2 years	4.5-5.0 uncuffed	8 French
4 years	5.0-5.5 uncuffed	10 French
6 years	5.5 uncuffed	10 French
8 years	6.0 cuffed or uncuffed	10 French
10 years	6.5 cuffed or uncuffed	12 French
12 years	7.0 cuffed	12 French
Adolescent	7.0, 8.0 cuffed	12 French
Adult woman	7.5-8.0 cuffed	12 French
Adult man	8.0-8.5 cuffed	14 French

From American Heart Association: *Pediatric advanced life support,* Dallas, Texas, 1997, The Association.
*Endotracheal tube selection for a child should be based on the child's size and not his or her age. Tubes one size larger and one size smaller should be allowed for individual variations.

greater control of the handle and more importantly, the blade. Using a pediatric handle will actually make the intubation easier.

The blade selection for intubation also is measured, and it is important to select the proper size blade. For intubation of infants and toddlers, a straight blade (or Miller blade) is recommended because it provides better visualization. For older children, a curved blade (or Macintosh blade) may be more helpful.

As a general rule, the ET tube sizes outlined in Table 34-3 should be used for pediatric intubation.

Procedure—To perform ET intubation in the pediatric patient, the EMT–I should do the following:

1. Begin artificial ventilations and provide high-concentration oxygen as soon as it is available. Suction the airway as necessary, and hyperventilate the child prior to the intubation attempt.
2. Assemble the laryngoscope and blade. Check the light to make sure it works and is tightly attached before attempting intubation. Also, a straight blade is easier to use in the child because it lifts up the epiglottis for easier visualization of the larynx.
3. Select the appropriate size tube (see Table 34-3). The AHA generally recommends a cuffed tube for children 8 to 10 years of age or older. Infants and children less than those ages can use uncuffed tubes because of their natural "cuffs" at the level of the cricoid cartilage.
4. Place the child's head in the sniffing position. If trauma is suspected, manually maintain a neutral position so that the head and neck are stabilized for each intubation attempt (Figure 34-9, *A*).
5. Hold the laryngoscope in the left hand, and insert it into the child's mouth from the right. Sweep the tongue to the left and move the blade into position.

Because the airway is shorter and the glottis higher than an adult's, the cords will appear quickly.

6. Lift the mandible and tongue until the glottis can be seen. Remember to keep the wrist straight and to avoid pressure on the mouth or teeth if present. If the cords are not visualized, slowly withdraw the blade and watch for the larynx to drop into view (Figure 34-9, *B*).
7. Using the right hand, insert the tube into the mouth through the glottic opening until it passes through the cords. Do not insert the tube through the groove in the laryngoscope blade, which may block the view of the cords. Continue to hold the tube in place (Figure 34-9, *C*).
8. Do not let intubation attempts last more than 30 seconds. If intubation is unsuccessful, hyperventilate the patient with a bag-valve-mask device before any subsequent attempts.
9. Once intubation is successful, ventilate the patient with a bag-valve-mask device. Listen for breath sounds in the upper and lower lung fields and over the epigastrium. Breath sounds alone may not adequately represent success due to easy transmission of sounds in the child's small chest, especially in the infant. Also look for rise and fall of the chest, as well as improvement in the child's or infant's color and/or heart rate (Figure 34-9, *D* and *E*).
10. After confirming placement of the tube, secure it to the face. Minimize movement of the head and neck so as not to dislodge the tube. Even after the tube has been secured, continue to manually stabilize it whenever possible.
11. Continue to reassess the child to ensure proper placement of the tube throughout transport.

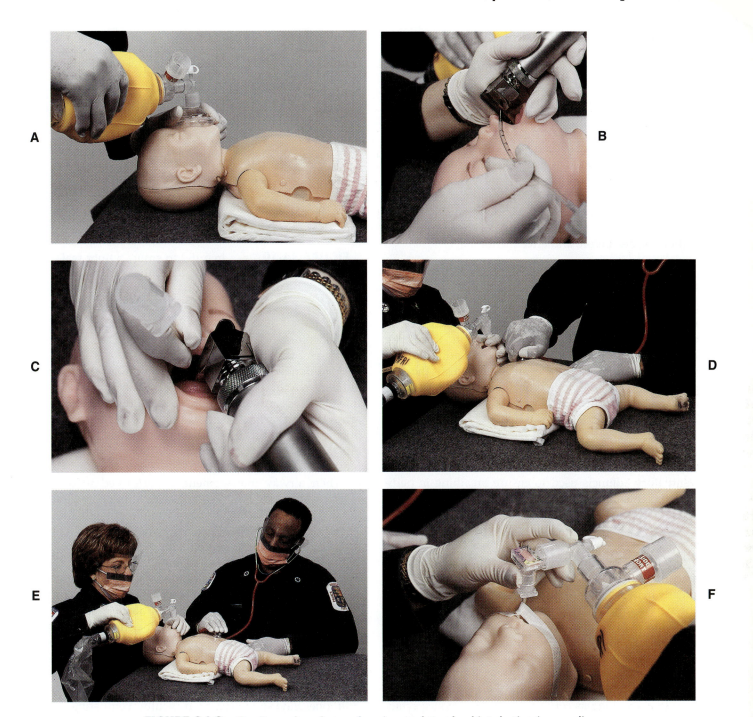

FIGURE 34-9 ▲ Procedure for performing endotracheal intubation in a pediatric patient. For specific steps, see text.

Considerations—Several items are important to remember when working with the airway of an infant or child. First, a child has a greater proportion of soft tissue in the oropharynx as well as a larger tongue. Extra care should be used when inserting the laryngoscope so as not to cause any trauma. Also, the EMT–I should be careful to sweep the tongue out of the way as completely as possible. Secondly, the larynx is higher in the pediatric patient than in the adult, and the epiglottis is not as firm. Visualization of the cords prior to intubation may therefore be more difficult. Thirdly, the cricoid cartilage is the narrowest part of the upper airway, and the structures are more flexible than in an adult. These differences may make correct tube placement even more of a challenge. With all of these points in mind, the EMT–I should not be tempted to extend the intubation attempt more than 30 seconds.

The child's or infant's heart rate should be monitored during the intubation procedure. If the laryngoscope is moved around excessively while inserting the ET tube, the vagal nerve may be stimulated, causing a marked decrease in the heart rate and a subsequent decrease in the blood pressure. Hypoxemia from prolonged intubation attempts also can decrease the heart rate. If the cardiac rate drops significantly at any time, the EMT–I should stop the procedure and provide high-concentration oxygen using a bag-valve-mask device.

Suction equipment should be readily available and in good working order. The child's airway may become obstructed with vomitus, blood, increased saliva, or mucus. The EMT–I should use a pediatric suction catheter to clear away the obstruction as quickly as possible and provide hyperventilation with high-concentration oxygen before and after suctioning.

END-TIDAL CARBON DIOXIDE DETECTOR

The end-tidal carbon dioxide detector can be used in children and is most effective in verifying correct ET tube placement in infants weighing more than 2 kg (Figure 34-9, *F*). It can, however, be misleading during the resuscitation phase of a pulseless arrest. The low reading in that situation is probably a result of low pulmonary blood flow, not placement of the tube in the esophagus.

Ventilatory Adjuncts

Ventilatory adjuncts used to ensure breathing in pediatric patients include the devices listed in the following sections.

BAG-VALVE-MASK VENTILATION

The proper use of the bag-valve-mask device will assist greatly in the survival of the infant or child. The mask of the system must be tightly secured and sealed to the patient's face. If it is difficult to obtain or maintain a seal around the patient's mouth and nose, it may be beneficial to invert the mask on the infant's or child's face (Figure 34-10).

The chin-lift maneuver should be performed when ventilating as long as cervical trauma is not suspected. The EMT–I should be careful not to push too hard on the soft tissue under the chin because this may move the tongue into an obstructing position.

The ventilation rate for infants and children is at least 20 breaths per minute. The EMT–I should be sure that the oxygen is attached to the bag-valve-mask device and is set to at least 15 L/min. A bag-valve-mask device that provides at least 450 mL of volume and is not equipped with a pop-off valve should be used on pediatric patients. The infant bag-valve-mask device previously carried by many ambulance services only provides approximately 250 mL and should NOT be used because it cannot give enough tidal volume and provide

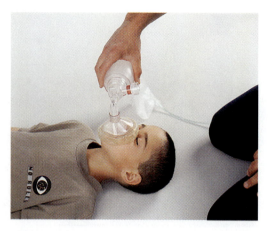

FIGURE 34-10 ▲ In order to ensure a tight seal during bag-valve-mask ventilations, the mask may be inverted on a child's face.

a longer time for inspiration. Many services have completly removed it from their vehicles.

For infants and young children, the EMT–I should not use an adult bag-valve-mask device with the intention of just giving smaller puffs. The child in respiratory arrest presents a very stressful situation, and the EMT–I may lose sight of the goal to give small breaths. Larger breaths will cause the lungs to overinflate, and a pneumothorax may result.

When airway management is performed in older children, it may be necessary to use the adult bag-valve-mask device to provide a larger volume of ventilation. The EMT–I should be extremely careful not to force high volumes of oxygen into the patient's airway.

Bag-valve-mask ventilation must be done with two hands: one to hold the mask on the face and maintain the head-tilt/chin-lift maneuver and one to squeeze the bag. When treating infants and toddlers, the EMT–I should support the mandible with the middle or ring finger. For older children, the fingertips of the third, fourth, and fifth fingers should be placed under the mandible to hold the jaw forward and extend the head (which accomplishes the jaw-thrust maneuver).

If one EMT–I is having difficulty ventilating the child, a two-person approach should be used. One EMT–I uses both hands to maintain the airway maneuver and mask seal on the face, while the second EMT–I performs the ventilation (Figure 34-11).

Maintenance of the head in a neutral, sniffing position without hyperextension is usually adequate for infants and toddlers. Hyperextension actually can occlude the infant's soft airway. Children more than two years of age do well with padding behind the head to displace the cervical spine anteriorly.

Obviously, if the EMT–I suspects a cervical spine injury, all airway maneuvers and ventilation should be done with the head in a neutral, in-line position. A

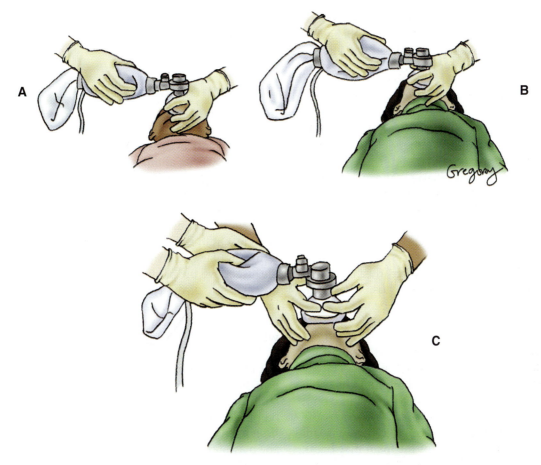

FIGURE 34-11 ▲ **A,** One provider ventilation of infant. **B,** One provider ventilation of child. **C,** Two rescuer ventilation of child.

trauma jaw-thrust or chin-lift maneuver without the head-tilt can be used to maintain airway patency.

The goal of the bag-valve-mask device is to achieve effective ventilation. If this goal is not achieved, the EMT–I should do the following:

- Make sure the tongue is not obstructing the airway.
- Reposition the head. Using a folded towel under the infant's or child's shoulders may help maintain the sniffing position.
- Make sure the mask is snug against the patient's face.
- Lift the jaw.
- Suction the airway.
- Check the bag-valve-mask device for damage.
- Provide an adequate source of oxygen.
- List the indications for gastric decompression for infants and children.

The EMT–I should watch for gastric distention, which is very common during bag-valve-mask ventilation. Appropriate suction should be readily available. If the infant or child is unresponsive, cricoid pressure (Sellick's maneuver) should be applied to minimize gastric inflation and passive regurgitation. This maneuver compresses the esophagus between the cricoid ring and

the cervical spine. The second EMT–I should apply this pressure with one fingertip in infants and the thumb and index finger in children. Excessive pressure should not be used because this can cause tracheal compression and obstruction in infants. Lastly, it is critical to use a child bag-valve-mask device, depending on the size of the pediatric patient (see Chapter 8).

Although it is recognized that there may not always be an abundance of personnel at the scene, it is crucial to the child's ongoing survival to provide adequate oxygenation and ventilation. If the EMT–I must request additional personnel, he or she should do so without unnecessarily delaying transport of the pediatric patient.

NEEDLE DECOMPRESSION

For those EMT–Is approved to perform the skill of needle decompression, it can be done on the infant or child if a tension pneumothorax is suspected. The same procedure is used as for the adult except that an 18- to 20-gauge over-the-needle catheter is used (see Chapter 8).

Communication with medical direction is essential for this procedure. In addition, routine skills reviews should be offered for those EMT–Is who do not have an opportunity to perform this skill regularly in the field.

Oxygen can be administered to pediatric patients via the nasal cannula and oxygen masks.

NASAL CANNULA

The EMT–I should use the pediatric size nasal cannula and insert the two plastic prongs into the child's nares. A flow rate of between 2 to 4 liters (L)/min should be used. Higher rates irritate the nasopharynx and do not substantially improve the child's oxygenation. If more oxygen is needed, the EMT–I should switch to a face mask.

OXYGEN MASKS

Children can use a simple partial rebreather or nonrebreather face mask, depending on the cause of their illness or injury. The pediatric size should be used to provide a proper fit on the child's face and adequate oxygen concentration. Many children, however, do not tolerate the face mask because they feel restricted or suffocated. The EMT–I may administer oxygen via the blow-by method by having the child or parent hold the mask in front of the child's face instead of directly on it (Figure 34-12). A paper cup may also be used so the child can pretend to drink and receive oxygen instead. Do not use foam cups, as pieces of the foam may break off and potentially be a choking hazard. If those techniques are not successful, consider holding the tubing pointed at the nose.

Intravenous Therapy

Intravenous (IV) access is of utmost importance in ill or injured children. The insertion of an IV line in a child is not an easy task even when the child appears to be cooperative. However, at times, venous access is necessary in the pediatric patient for drug and fluid administration.

Specific equipment and complications related to vascular access are explained in Chapter 6.

The sites for insertion should include the hands, the arms just at the elbow, or if the neck is accessible, an external jugular vein. Alternatively, the area inside the ankle just above the medial malleolus, near the ankle bone on each side of the patient, can be used. Scalp vein or lateral foot access may be permitted in some systems (Figure 34-13). Many times, local protocols dictate which pediatric IV sites can be used in prehospital care.

There are several instances when the EMT–I should not take the time or aggravate the child to start an IV line. First and foremost are traumatic situations. If the child has sustained a traumatic injury and is hemodynamically compromised, the EMT–I should not waste time at the scene trying to get that line started. He or she may start the line in the ambulance once en route to

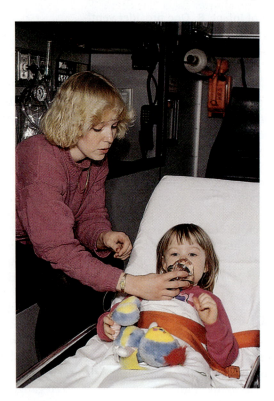

FIGURE 34-12 ▲ The parent can help with administering oxygen to an infant or child. (From Stoy WA and the Center for Emergency Medicine: *Mosby's EMT-Basic textbook,* St Louis, 1996, Mosby.)

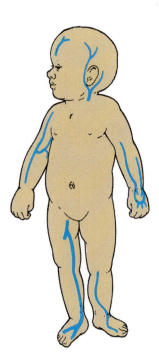

FIGURE 34-13 ▲ These superficial veins are used most often for IV infusion in infants and young children. (From Smith DF et al, eds: *Comprehensive child and family nursing skills,* St Louis, 1991, Mosby.)

the hospital. Most of the time, the EMT–I cannot catch up to the amount of blood the child is losing. Rather than delaying that child's access to definitive care, the EMT–I should provide good respiratory support and transport immediately.

Another instance when an IV line should not be started is the child with epiglottitis or some other form of severe respiratory distress. If an IV is attempted, the child usually will experience at least a fair amount of emotional distress. This crying and struggling can cause the child with epiglottitis to completely obstruct and the child in respiratory distress to get worse. In either case the EMT–I runs the risk of complete respiratory arrest if the child is too agitated. It may be safer to defer the IV line until the child is in a controlled setting in the emergency department. Be sure to refer to local protocols.

Intraosseous Infusion

In cases in which the child is in severe shock or cardiac arrest, consideration should be given to the use of intraosseous infusion if the EMT–I is approved to initiate this therapy. This technique is accomplished by inserting a needle into the long bone of the leg. Infusion of IV fluids into the marrow cavity of the bone can circulate to the heart in 20 seconds or less. The amount of fluid resuscitation with intraosseous infusion is comparable to IV therapy. Intraosseous infusion should be withheld as a last resource of fluid replacement.

This technique was used in the early 1900s to administer fluid and blood. It fell out of favor in the 1950s once disposable IV catheters became available. However, within the past decade, it again has become popular and is most effective in children 6 years of age and under.

This procedure should be used only in children who are unresponsive and only after all other attempts at peripheral cannulation have failed (e.g., situations such as cardiopulmonary arrest, shock from trauma, burns, sepsis, and so forth that lead to peripheral vascular collapse). Again, local protocol may mandate when an infusion can be attempted.

Medications and fluids can be given through this direct route. If a rapid fluid bolus or viscous drugs and/or solutions are to be given, they should be infused under pressure to overcome resistance. If drugs are given, they should be flushed with at least 5 mL of a sterile saline solution to make sure they reach the central circulation. Sterile technique is recommended during intraosseous infusion whenever possible.

To perform intraosseous infusion, the EMT–I should do the following:

1. Consult with medical direction before the procedure or follow local protocol.
2. Gather the necessary equipment: Betadine wipes, disposable gloves, adhesive tape, gauze 4 × 4s, a 10-mL syringe, a specialized intraosseous needle or a Jamshidi-type bone marrow aspiration needle, a microdrip or pediatric infusion set, and the IV fluid ordered (e.g., lactated Ringer's solution or normal saline).
3. Wash hands if possible and apply gloves.
4. Identify the preferred site at the anteromedial surface of the tibia, one to two finger-breadths below the tibial tuberosity (Figure 34-14, A). The bone marrow cavity under this flat area is very large, and the potential for injury to adjoining tissues is minimal.
5. Cleanse the skin over the insertion site with povidone iodine (Betadine).
6. Check the needle for proper alignment of bevels of outer needle and internal stylet.
7. Insert the needle perpendicular to the bone or angled away from the joint. Point it away from the epiphyseal plate (Figure 34-14, B).
8. Use a boring or twisting motion to advance the needle through the bone. A decrease in resistance will be felt when entering the bone marrow cavity. If bone marrow is aspirated, irrigate the needle to prevent obstruction.
9. Remove the stylet (Figure 34-14, C). The needle should remain upright without support.
10. Stabilize the needle. Connect the syringe filled with 10 mL of normal saline and slowly inject the fluid to verify placement. Note any increased resistance to injection, increase in circumference of the calf, or increased firmness of the tissue (Figure 34-14, D).
11. If there is no infiltration, remove the syringe and connect the infusion set and IV bag. Apply tape to the needle and tubing and wrap a bulky dressing (gauze 4 × 4s) around the needle for support (Figure 34-14, E).
12. If signs of infiltration are present, stop the infusion, remove the needle, and attempt the procedure again on the other leg.
13. Document the process in writing.
14. Reassess the patient, and provide an update to medical direction.

▶ NOTE: Spinal needles (short, wide-gauge needles with internal stylets) are not routinely recommended because they bend easily. They should be used only as a last resort. Regular hypodermic needles are NOT to be used.

Complications are uncommon but can be severe when they do occur, including tibial fracture, compartment syndrome, skin necrosis, and osteomyelitis. For the most part, this particular skill should be used only on critically ill infants and children until an alternate method of venous access can be obtained.

Fluid Administration

Fluid resuscitation therapy is recommended at 20 mL/kg of an isotonic, crystalloid solution (Figure

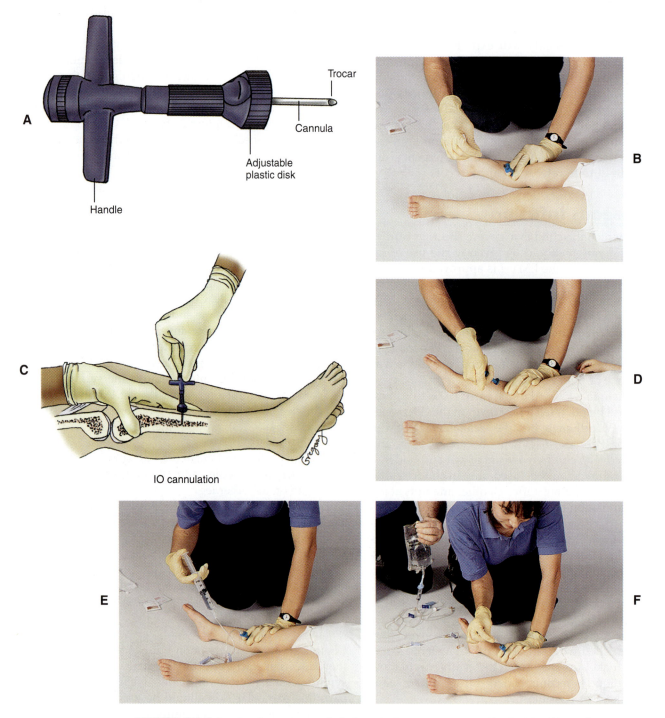

FIGURE 34-14   ▲   Intraosseous infusion. **A,** Intraosseous needle. **B,** Identify and cleanse the area of injection. **C,** Insert the needle perpendicular to the bone with a boring motion. **D,** Remove the stylet. **E,** Inject 10 mL of normal saline and look for infiltration. **F,** Connect the infusion.

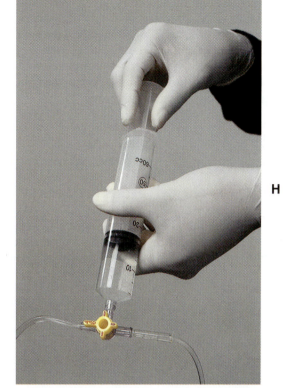

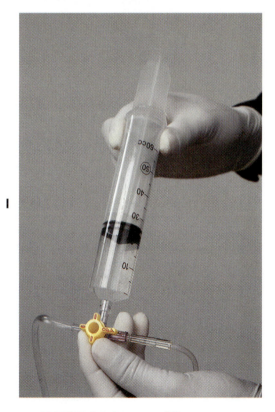

Securing IO needle in place

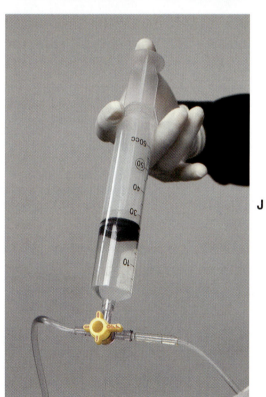

FIGURE 34-14, cont'd ▲ Intraosseous infusion. **G,** Secure intraosseous needle in place. **H** through **J,** fluid administration.

34-14, *H* to *J*). This solution should be given as rapidly as possible (in less than 20 minutes). Many times these boluses are given through a 35- to 50-mL syringe to facilitate rapid administration. Lactated Ringer's or normal saline can be used for this purpose. Large volumes of dextrose-containing solutions should not be used because the child may become hyperglycemic.

Frequent reassessments are necessary to determine the need for additional fluid boluses. If the signs of shock persist, another bolus of 20 mL/kg should be given. Additional boluses may be given, depending on the patient's overall clinical picture according to medical direction. If the child begins to develop signs of fluid overload such as rales, the boluses should be stopped.

TABLE 34-4

Most Commonly Used Drugs in Pediatric Advanced Life Support

DRUG	PEDIATRIC DOSAGE	REMARKS
Adenosine	0.1 mg/kg (up to 6 mg); 0.2 mg/kg for second dose; maximum single dose: 12 mg	Give a rapid intravenous (IV) bolus
Amiodarone	5 mg/kg; maximum dose 15 mg/kg/day	Give via rapid IV or IO bolus
Atropine sulfate	0.02 mg/kg IV/IO/TT* minimum dose: 0.1 mg; maximum single dose is 0.5 mg in a child and 1.0 mg in an adolescent	Give rapidly through IV line
Calcium chloride 10%	20 mg/kg IV/IO	Give via slow IV bolus
Dobutamine	2 to 20 μg/kg min	Titrate to desired effect
Dopamine	2 to 20 μg/kg/min	Titrate to desired effect; dose >15 μg/kg/min produce alpha-pressor effects
EPINEPHRINE		
For bradychardia	IV/IO: 0.01 mg/kg (1:10,000, 0.1 mL/kg TT: 0.1 mg/kg (1:1,000, 0.1 mL/kg)	
For asystolic or pulseless arrest	First dose: IV/IO: 0.01 mg/kg (1:10,000, 0.1 mL/kg) TT: 0.1 mg/kg (1:1,000, 0.1 mL/kg)	
	Subsequent doses: IV/IO/TT: 0.01 to 0.1 mg/kg (1:1,000, 0.1 mL/kg) Repeat every 3 to 5 min.	IV/IO doses as high as 0.2 mg/kg of 1:1,000 may be effective
Epinephrine infusion	Initial dose: 0.1 μg/kg/min	Titrate to desired effect (0.1 to 1.0 μg/kg/min).
Dextrose	0.5-1.0 g/kg IV/IO Maximum dose: 2 to 4 mL/kg of 25% solution 5% = 10 to 20 mL/kg 10% = 5 to 10 mL/kg 25% = 2 to 4 mL/kg (in large vein)	Use maximum concentration of 25% dextrose in water ($D_{25}W$) via a peripheral vein. If supplied as $D_{50}W$, dilute 1:1 with sterile water before administration. For infants, use $D_{10}W$ (dilute $D_{50}W$ 1:4 with sterile water).
Lidocaine	1 mg/kg IV/IO/TT	Titrate to desired effect.
Lidocaine infusion	20 to 50 μg/kg/min	
Magnesium sulfate	20 to 50 mg/kg maximum dose: 2 g	Administer over 10 to 20 min.
Naloxone	If $\leq$ 5 years of age or up to 20 kg, give 0.1 mg/kg IV. If >5 years of age to >20 kg, give 2 mg IV.	
Sodium bicarbonate	1 mEq/kg/dose	Infuse slowly and only if ventilation is adequate.

NOTE: For TT administration, dilute medication with normal saline to reach a volume of 3 to 5 mL. Follow the injection with several positive-pressure ventilations.
*IV: intravenous, IO: intraosseous, TT: tracheal tube.

Medications

The drugs most commonly used in pediatric advanced life support are outlined in Table 34-4.

PEDIATRIC RESUSCITATION

In infants and children, cardiac arrest usually results from hypoxemia and acidosis caused by respiratory insufficiency or shock. These conditions interfere with normal function of the sinoatrial and atrioventricular nodes and slow conduction through the normal conduction pathways. This reduction leads to dysrhythmias such as sinus bradycardia, sinus node arrest with a slow junctional or ventricular escape, and asystole. Life-threatening rhythm disturbances are rarely a primary event except in those situations of congenital heart disease or other anomalies. The utmost attention must be given to establishing and maintaining a patent airway, effective ventilation, adequate oxygenation, and circulatory stabilization.

Integrate advanced life support skills with basic cardiac life support skills for infants and children.

Figures 34-15 and 34-16 represent the two most common situations encountered during pediatric resuscitations. These algorithms are recommended by the AHA.

Asystole

Asystole is characterized as a flat line on the electrocardiogram monitor. Occasionally P waves are seen. Clinically, there is no pulse, spontaneous respirations are absent, and perfusion is poor.

To treat the child with asystole, the EMT–I should do the following:
- Continue cardiopulmonary resuscitation [CPR].
- Ventilate with a bag-valve-mask device equipped with a reservoir and supplied with 10 to 15 L of oxygen.
- Perform tracheal intubation using the appropriate tube.
- Establish an IV using normal saline (or lactated Ringer's solution).
- Administer epinephrine at an initial dose of 0.0 1 mg/kg (1:10,000) for the IV/intraosseous routes and 0.1 mg/kg (1:1,000) for the tracheal tube (TT) route.
- Repeat epinephrine at a dose of 0.01 to 0.1 mg/kg (1:1,000) for the IV/intraosseous (IO)/ET routes (doses up to 0.2 mg/kg of 1:1,000 may be effective) every 3 to 5 minutes.

Ventricular Fibrillation

Ventricular fibrillation is a chaotic-looking rhythm with waveforms that vary in size and shape and have no recognizable P waves, QRS complexes, or T waves. It rarely occurs in children unless there is the presence of congenital heart disease, acidosis, electrolyte imbalance (e.g., calcium, potassium, magnesium, or glucose imbalance), hypothermia, or drug toxicity (e.g., digitalis or tricyclic antidepressants).

To treat the child with ventricular fibrillation, the EMT–I should do the following:
- Continue CPR.
- Ventilate with a bag-valve-mask device equipped with a reservoir and supplied with 10 to 15 L of oxygen.
- Defibrillate up to three times, starting with 2 joules (J)/kg, then 2 to 4 J/kg, and then increasing the dose to 4 J/kg (maximum of 360 J) with subsequent shocks.
- Perform tracheal intubation using the appropriate size tube.
- Establish an IV using normal saline or lactated Ringer's solution.
- Administer epinephrine at an initial dose of 0.01 mg/kg (1:10,000) for the IV/IO routes and 0.1 mg/kg (1:1000) for the TT route. Use TT Route if there is any delay in getting the IV started.
- Repeat defibrillation at 4 J/kg 30 to 60 seconds after each medication administration. The pattern should be CPR-drug-shock (repeat) or CPR-drug-shock-shock-shock (repeat).
- Repeat epinephrine at a dose of 0.01 mg/kg (1:10,000) for the IV/IO routes. For tracheal tube administration, give 0.1 mg/kg (1:1,000).
- Consider administration of antidysrhythmics such as: Amiodarone 5 mg/kg bolus IV/IO *or* Lidocaine 1 mg/kg bolus IV/IO/TT.
- Identify and treat causes such as hypoxemia, hypovolemia, hypothermia, hyper/hypokalemia and metabolic disorders, tamponade, tension pneumothorax, toxins/poisions/drugs, and/or thromboembolism.

▶ NOTE: The EMT–I should open the airway and begin ventilations before defibrillating. However, the EMT–I should not delay defibrillation by attempts at IV insertion or intubation.

PEDIATRIC RESPIRATORY COMPROMISE

There are several illnesses that are usually seen primarily in children. Some of these illnesses may be life-threatening and must be recognized and treated in an appropriate manner.

For any of the respiratory illnesses, the EMT–I should note if there are any smokers around the child or residing in the house. Smoking can contribute to the severity of the illnesses.

Upper Airway Obstructions

Obstructions of the upper airway may be caused by foreign body aspirations, tonsillitis, croup, and the very rare yet dangerous epiglottitis.

FOREIGN BODY ASPIRATION

Toddlers and preschoolers are the most common victims of foreign body aspiration. However, it can occur at any age (see Chapter 8).

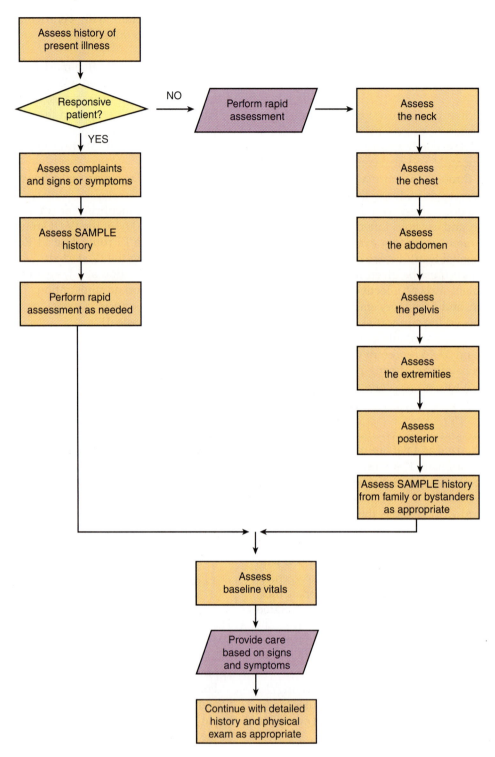

FIGURE 34-15 ▲ Bradycardia decision tree. (From Journal of the American Medical Association: *JAMA* 268:2199-2275, 1992.)

CROUP

Also known as **laryngotracheobronchitis, croup** is a respiratory illness that occurs in children between 3 months and 3 years of age. It is usually a viral infection that has a slow onset, usually after the child has had an upper respiratory infection and low fever. Inflammation of the larynx causes the primary symptoms.

Most commonly, the child will be hoarse with respiratory stridor and a characteristic "bark" in the form of a cough. The stridor is due to subglottic edema, and the

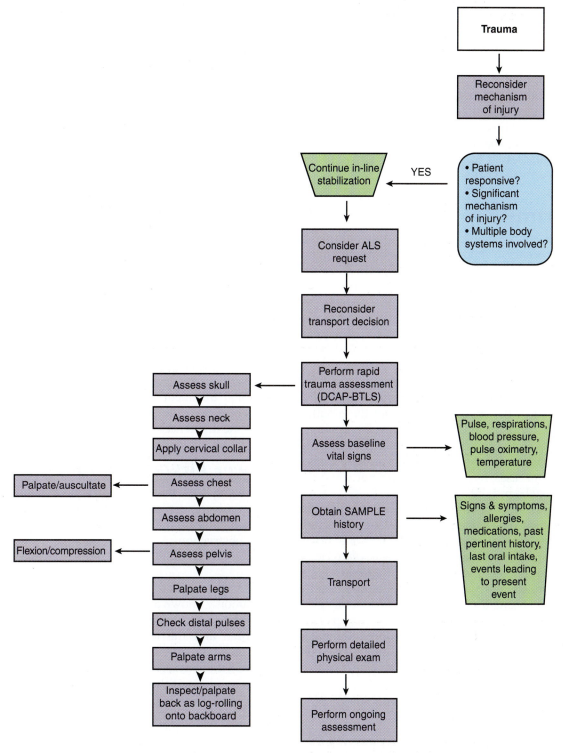

FIGURE 34-16 ▲ Asystole and pulseless electrical activity (PEA) arrest decision tree. (From *Journal of the American Medical Association: JAMA* 268:2199-2275, 1992.)

barking cough is from edema of the vocal cords. If the lower airways are involved, wheezing will be heard.

The emergency often occurs during the middle of the night. The child wakes up with a barking cough and may show signs of respiratory distress. The amount of swelling usually will dictate the severity of the situation. The EMT–I must be aware, however, that the child is at risk of complete airway obstruction from the narrowed diameter of the trachea. The patient often prefers to lie down.

High-concentration oxygen should be administered (cool and humidified when possible), and the patient should be transported in a comfortable position. If the patient is lying down, the EMT–I should be alert for airway compromise. Monitor vital signs, the cardiac rhythm, and the pulse oximeter, if used. Many times the outside environment (if air is cool and humid) during transfer from the home to the ambulance may cause an improvement in the child's condition. The patient should be reassessed frequently to detect any changes or signs of airway obstruction.

EPIGLOTTITIS

Epiglottitis is an inflammation of the epiglottis, which most often occurs in children from 3 to 7 years of age. It is caused by bacteria and progresses rapidly. It is a true emergency because the child can progress to complete airway obstruction and respiratory arrest if the epiglottis swells over the opening of the trachea. With current immunizations of infants against the bacteria *Haemophilus influenzae type B*, epiglottitis is quite rare yet still deserves a review.

The child with epiglottitis looks very ill, is quiet, and is doing everything possible just to keep breathing. The child will sit in the tripod position, and the mouth is usually open with the tongue protruding. Swallowing is very painful so the child may be drooling. In addition, the child usually will show signs of respiratory distress and, in severe cases, hypoxia. A muffled voice and stridor also may be present.

Every patient who has indications of epiglottitis should be treated as having a life-threatening condition. No attempts should be made to visualize the airway. Under no circumstances should anything be placed in the patient's mouth. Manipulation of the child's airway can lead to complete obstruction and respiratory arrest. All efforts should be made to keep the child comfortable and as calm as possible. To properly care for these patients, the EMT–I should not make them lie down. The parent should remain with the child at all times to alleviate fear and more importantly to keep the child from crying. If possible, the child should sit on the parent's lap.

The EMT–I should handle the child gently. Rough handling and stress could lead to a total airway obstruction. High-concentration, humidified oxygen should be given via either a mask or blow-by method, depending on what the child will tolerate. Administration of oxygen should not be delayed, however, while waiting for humidification. The EMT–I should monitor the child's vital signs, cardiac rhythm, and pulse oximeter if doing so does not further agitate the child.

The EMT–I should be prepared to ventilate using positive pressure through a bag-valve-mask device. He or she should be able to force enough oxygen past the obstruction to buy some time until arriving at the hospital. Needle cricothyrotomy may be ordered as a last resort, but this procedure is difficult to perform on small children. Intubation only should be done by those EMT–Is highly experienced in the skill and in an environment where an emergency cricothyrotomy or tracheostomy can be performed if the intubation is not successful. The patient should be transported to the nearest appropriate facility as soon as possible.

The EMT–I should communicate with medical direction so that everyone at the receiving facility is prepared. Optimal treatment includes intubation and IV antibiotics once the child reaches the hospital. Table 34-5 outlines the differences between croup and epiglottitis.

Lower Airway Obstructions

Wheezing is the most common abnormal airway sound when a lower airway obstruction occurs. Asthma and bronchiolitis are the most common causes of lower airway obstruction.

ASTHMA

Commonly known as asthma, reactive airway disease is considered the most common chronic illness among children and the leading cause of school absences. Children can have an acute asthma attack along with status asthmaticus, exhibiting the same signs and symptoms as adults, including wheezing.

TABLE 34-5

Differences Between Croup and Epiglottitis

CROUP	EPIGLOTTITIS
Usually caused by viral infection	Usually caused by bacterial infection
Usually occurs during late fall and early winter	No seasonal preference
Occurs in ages 3 months-3 years	Occurs in ages 3-7 years
Slow onset	Rapid onset
Patient will either lie down or sit up	Patient will sit upright in a tripod position
Barking cough present	No barking cough
No drooling	Pain on swallowing causing drooling
Temperature: 104° F	Temperature: 104° F

Status asthmaticus is a life-threatening situation in which an asthma attack is severe, prolonged, and cannot be broken with traditional bronchodilators. The child should be transported rapidly in a position most comfortable for him or her. The EMT–I should monitor the airway, cardiac rhythm, and pulse oximeter and be prepared to intubate and provide ventilation.

Sometimes the attack can be so severe that there is no wheezing because the child is not able to move air adequately. As with adult patients with asthma or status asthmaticus, this condition should be considered life threatening. Any first case of asthma must be dealt with as if it were status asthmaticus.

EMS may be requested because the child is having an episode of dyspnea and increased wheezing. Treatment is focused on opening the air passages to make the child breathe easier. The EMT–I should provide humidified oxygen (he or she should not wait for a humidifier if one is not immediately available) and monitor the child's vital signs, cardiac rhythm, and pulse oximeter. The EMT–I should communicate with medical direction, and follow local protocols concerning administration of drugs such as bronchodilators or epinephrine.

In severe cases, respiratory failure can occur. If the child has been struggling for a while, he or she finally may tire and stop breathing altogether. Equipment should be readily available to assist the child's ventilations and for intubation, if necessary. Circulatory support also may be necessary if the ventilatory support is not adequate.

When treating a child with asthma, the EMT–I should not be fooled by a cooperative, lethargic child who is not wheezing. This child's bronchioles may be so tight that he or she cannot move any air.

BRONCHIOLITIS

Bronchiolitis is an infection of the lower respiratory tract, which is most often caused by a virus. It usually affects children between the ages of 6 and 18 months. Usually the child has a mild fever, cough, and runny nose, which progress to respiratory distress. Edema and increased mucous secretions obstruct the bronchioles, and wheezing is sometimes present. The child is usually most comfortable in a sitting or semisitting po-

sition. This condition is different from asthma because it is caused by a virus, and bronchospasms may not always respond to medications.

The EMT–I should provide high-concentration, humidified oxygen (again, he or she should not wait for a humidifier if it is not readily available) and should transport the patient to the hospital for further evaluation. These patients often will benefit from vaporized or nebulized water. These patients also must be seen at a medical facility. The respiratory and cardiac status, as well as vital signs and pulse oximeter, should be monitored. The EMT–I should attempt to keep the child as calm as possible and maximize respiratory effect.

If respiratory distress increases, ventilatory support should be provided, including intubation if necessary. Medical direction should be contacted with an update. Sometimes epinephrine or an albuterol treatment through a nebulizer may decrease the respiratory symptoms. Table 34-6 lists the differences between asthma and bronchiolitis.

PNEUMONIA

Pneumonia is an infection of the lower airway and lung and is most common in infants, toddlers, and preschoolers. It may be caused by a bacteria or a virus.

Signs and symptoms of pneumonia in a pediatric patient include the following:
- Signs of respiratory distress or failure (depending on the involvement of the pneumonia)
- Grunting respirations secondary to air trapping and expiratory obstruction
- History of lower respiratory infectious symptoms
- Fever
- Poor eating habits
- Irritability or anxiousness
- Decreased breath sounds in the area where the pneumonia is located (more common in children greater than 1 year of age)
- Rales (more common in children greater than 1 year of age)
- Rhonchi (may be localized or diffuse)
- Pain in the chest

Treatment consists of airway and ventilatory support. Provide oxygen as tolerated by the child without

TABLE 34-6

Differences Between Asthma and Bronchiolitis

ASTHMA	BRONCHIOLITIS
Occurs at any age	Occurs between 6-18 months of age
Occurs in winter and spring	Can occur at any time
Response to allergy, exercise, or infection	Caused by a virus
Family history of asthma	Usually no history of asthma
Drugs reverse bronchospasm	Drugs may not always be effective

making him or her more anxious, thus increasing the work of breathing. Ventilate with a bag-valve-mask device if the child is in respiratory failure or arrest. Provide circulatory support if necessary with IV or intraosseous access. During transport, allow the child to assume a position of comfort and to remain with a parent or caregiver whenever possible.

COMMON PEDIATRIC MEDICAL EMERGENCIES

Shock

Shock is defined as an abnormal condition characterized by inadequate delivery of oxygen and is the body's response to poor perfusion (see Chapter 10).

A child's circulatory system is different than an adult's system and may lose up to 20% of its blood volume before showing any change in the child's appearance. The circulatory aspect of pediatric patients can best be evaluated by looking at the child's skin color and feeling the pulse. The skin of children is thinner than adults' skin. Therefore changes in color or temperature are very obvious.

Mottling of the skin or skin that appears to have two different colors is a very common finding in a child who has lost a significant amount of blood vol-

ume. Also, simultaneous palpation of the peripheral pulse and apical heart rate can provide clues regarding pediatric hypovolemia. The child who is in shock will have a rapid, thready peripheral pulse, indicating that there is not an adequate blood volume circulating to the extremities.

The two stages of shock in the pediatric patient are as follows:

1. In compensated shock, the child's blood pressure remains normal even though signs of inadequate tissue perfusion are seen. This stage happens early in the shock cycle and is usually reversible. Children tend to remain in this stage longer than adults as their bodies fight longer to compensate for the shock state.

2. In decompensated shock, the child is hypotensive and shows signs of inadequate tissue perfusion. Note that when children finally decompensate, it happens quickly and is often irreversible.

The leading cause of shock in children across the world is gastroenteritis with dehydration. This infection, along with diarrhea causing dehydration and the severe loss of fluid, can lead to hypovolemic shock.

Shock also can occur from partial-thickness and full-thickness burns, which damage the skin and allow fluid to escape through the burn surface (Figure 34-17). That fluid often enters extravascular tissue. Nevertheless, it is not available to the circulating volume, and the

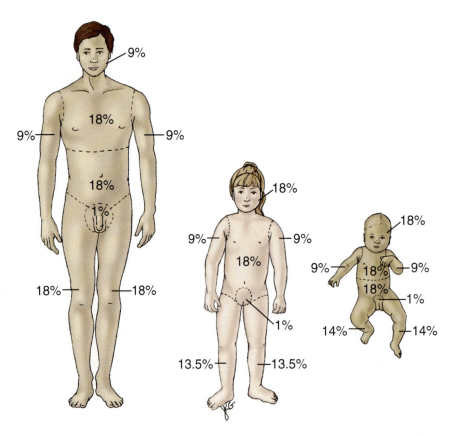

FIGURE 34-17 ▲ The pediatric rule of nines can be used to estimate the percentage of the body that is burned.

child's blood pressure drops. Blood loss associated with trauma is also a cause of hypovolemic shock.

> ### CLINICAL NOTES
>
> In children with a primary head injury who are also hypotensive, the EMT–I should always consider the possibility of some other source of bleeding. Only infants (with their open fontanelles) have enough space in their heads to accommodate enough blood to cause hypotension.

Other reasons for shock in the child are sepsis and anaphylaxis. The child with meningitis or some other type of infection can develop sepsis (systemic infection), which can lead to septic shock.

Signs of shock include the following:
- Altered level of responsiveness (confusion to irritability to lethargy to coma; make a note if the young child does not care if he or she is separated from the parent)
- Hyperventilation leading to respiratory failure
- Tachycardia
- Normotension progressing to hypotension
- Cool or cold, clammy skin
- Diminished peripheral pulses
- Prolonged capillary refill
- Oliguria (the EMT–I should ask if the child has urinated recently or how many diapers the child has wet within the last 24 hours)
- Acidosis

The treatment for shock in the pediatric patient is very similar to that for the adult patient. If bleeding is present, it should be controlled with direct pressure. When appropriate, the patient should be placed in the Trendelenburg position or the shock position.

The EMT–I should be aware, however, that the infant or child can compensate for shock longer than the adult. The patient will maintain an adequate blood pressure and appear stable only to "crash" very quickly and become hypotensive. Therefore, the EMT–I should not be misled and have a false sense of security based on blood pressure.

Dehydration

Vomiting, diarrhea, fever, burns, and poor fluid intake can contribute to a loss of body fluids. These symptoms can lead to dehydration, which poses a threat to the infant and child. The subsequent decrease in cardiac output from a smaller circulating volume can lead to renal failure, shock, and death if not treated properly.

A fever in a child can cause diaphoresis and tachycardia. If a viral gastrointestinal disorder is present, the child may be nauseated or have vomiting and/or diar-

rhea. These symptoms may cause the child to refuse food and fluids, which further jeopardizes the body's fluid balance. This cycle continues until the child is lethargic and in danger of circulatory collapse.

Infants and young children are particularly susceptible to this loss of fluid because a greater proportion of their bodies is composed of water. In addition, their fluid needs are higher. For example, 65% of an infant's total weight is water. If a toddler weighs 10 kg (22 lb), approximately 7 kg (14 lb) are made up of water alone (Figure 34-18).

During the assessment, signs and symptoms of dehydration should be noted (Table 34-7). The dehydration can be mild, moderate, or severe depending on what clinical signs are found during the assessment. In fact, the EMT–I simply may discover signs and symptoms of mild dehydration as he or she assesses the child for another chief complaint (e.g., the child who has had a febrile seizure).

The EMT–I should ask the parents/caregivers or child (if he or she is old enough and developmentally appropriate) specific questions about the child's history. How long has the child been ill? Was there any fever, vomiting, or diarrhea? If present, how high was the fever? How much or how often has the child vomited or had diarrhea? When did the child last have something to drink (by cup or bottle)? How many bottles has the infant taken within the past 24 hours? Is the child urinat-

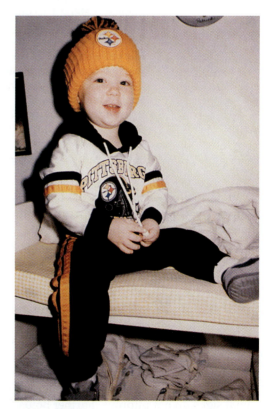

FIGURE 34-18 ▲ A toddler weighing 22 lb is approximately 14 lb of water.

TABLE 34-7

Dehydration Assessment

LEVEL	SIGNS AND SYMPTOMS	MANAGEMENT
Mild (5% loss of body weight)	Normal vital signs Alert Flat fontanelles Normal to slightly decreased skin turgor Dry mucous membranes Warm and pale skin Normal tears when crying Increased thirst Normal urine output	Supportive Child can usually take oral fluids Emergency medical services not usually requested
Moderate (5 to 10% loss of body weight)	Increased heart rate (HR) and respiratory rate (RR) Normal blood pressure (BP) Decreased peripheral pulses Capillary refill of 2 to 3 seconds Irritable Depressed fontanelles Decreased skin turgor Mucous membranes very dry Cool and pale skin Some tears when crying Sunken and darkened eyes Intense thirst Decreased urine output	Restore tissue perfusion and increase intravascular volume High-concentration oxygen Intravenous (IV) normal saline or lactated Ringer's solution Bolus of fluid at 20 mL/kg Transport Repeat bolus if no improvement
Extreme (>10% loss of body weight)	HR >130 beats/min Increased RR Systolic BP <80 No peripheral pulses Capillary refill >3 seconds Drowsy to comatose Sunken fontanelles Markedly decreased skin turgor Parched mucous membranes; no tears Cold, clammy, and cyanotic skin Sunken and soft eyes Intense thirst (if responsive) Decreased urine output	True emergency requiring rapid transport High-concentration oxygen IV of normal saline or lactated Ringer's solution en route ONLY Bolus of fluid at 20 mL/kg Repeat bolus if no improvement Consider intraosseous route for fluid resuscitation

From Wertz E: *Emergency care for children*, Albany, NY, 2001, Delmar Thomson Learning.

ing or wetting his or her diaper in the usual manner? How many diapers have been wet with urine or diarrhea within the past 24 hours? No special treatment is necessary if mild dehydration exists. It is important, however, to reassess the child in case the dehydration progresses.

In moderate to severe cases of dehydration, high-concentration oxygen should be provided. The child's vital signs and cardiac status should be monitored, and ventilations assisted, if necessary. If the patient is hypovolemic, the EMT–I should start an IV or intraosseous line, if indicated and necessary, of normal saline or lactated Ringer's solution, give a bolus of 20 mL/kg initially, and repeat this procedure in 5 minutes if the child's vital signs do not improve. Further boluses may be necessary to restore an adequate blood pressure and

subsequent tissue perfusion. The EMT–I should prepare for immediate transport and maintain contact with medical direction. CPR may be required.

Seizures/Epilepsy

Seizures account for approximately 8% of pediatric prehospital transports. In many children, seizures are a complication of a fever. In fact, approximately one out of every 20 children under the age of 7 years will have a seizure resulting from a fever. Seizures occur because of the rapid rise in temperature and not the final degree of the temperature.

Some children with epilepsy continue to have seizures on a regular basis despite aggressive medical

Modified from Wong D: *Whaley and Wong's nursing care of infants and children,* ed 6, St Louis, 1999, Mosby.
NOTE: A postictal period usually follows a generalized seizure.

BOX 34-3

INTERNATIONAL CLASSIFICATION OF EPILEPTIC SEIZURES

PARTIAL SEIZURES (ALSO CALLED FOCAL)
Simple partial seizures
No loss of consciousness or awareness
1. Motor signs limited to one side of the body (e.g., isolated jerking of part of the body).
   • Seizures may begin in a small part of the body, such as the corner of the mouth, a finger, or a toe, and then spread to other parts of the body
2. With sensory symptoms:
   • Sight (may be described as seeing flashing lights)
   • Smell
   • Sound (may be described as hearing buzzing sounds)
   • Taste (may have a metallic taste in mouth)
   • Touch (may be described as "pins and needles"
   • Emotions (may be described as feeling frightened or angry)
Complex partial seizures
Also called psychomotor or temporal lobe seizures; loss of awareness of surroundings
1. Person may stop whatever he or she is doing and begin doing some purposeless behavior such as:
   • Lip smacking
   • Picking at clothes
   • Wandering around room
   • Eye blinking or staring
2. Person may continue what he or she is doing but in an inappropriate manner
3. Aura may be followed by impairment of consciousness
4. Partial seizures may evolve to generalized seizures
5. Confusion follows the seizure

GENERALIZED SEIZURES
Absence seizures
1. Formerly called petit mall
2. Total loss of consciousness or awareness (no jerking or stiffening of the body)
3. Short periods of blinking, staring, or minor movements lasting a few seconds
Clonic seizures
Jerking muscle activity
Tonic seizures
Stiffening of the body
Tonic-clonic seizures
1. Formerly called grand mal
2. Total loss of consciousness with convulsions usually lasting 1 to 3 minutes
Myoclonic seizures
1. Single or multiple myoclonic jerks
2. Usually start or stop abruptly
Atonic seizures
1. Also called "drop attacks"
2. Unexpected lack of muscle tone
3. Body drops to the floor
Akinetic seizures
Lack of movement
Unclassified
1. Includes all seizure types that cannot be classified because of inadequate or incomplete data
2. Include some neonatal seizures such as rhythmic eye movements, chewing, and swimming movements

therapy. The seizures interfere with the daily lives of the child and his or her family and subsequently constitute a chronic problem. Also, the growth and development of the child may be affected, and injuries often result, at which time EMS may become involved.

Assessment of infants and children experiencing seizures includes thorough examinations. If no life-threatening instances are discovered, attention is then directed toward the seizure itself.

According to the International League Against Epilepsy, seizures are classified into several types (Box 34-3).

During the assessment of the child having a seizure, the EMT–I should make note of the following:
• Duration of the seizure
• Presence of any aura
• Level of responsiveness
• Part(s) of body involved
• Eye deviation and direction (if present)
• Postictal period (if present)
• Loss of bladder or bowel control, which can affect the older child's self-esteem

The EMT–I should find out if the child has a history of seizures and under what circumstances they usually occur. He or she also should determine what precipitated this recent event, if more than one seizure occurred, what medications may have been taken, and so forth.

If a seizure is witnessed, the child should be assisted gently to a lying position with the head turned to the side. In addition, the area should be cleared of hazardous items that might cause injury during the seizure activity. The EMT–I should **not** insert anything into the mouth if the patient's teeth are clenched. A nasal airway is an appropriate alternative adjunct for this situation, should follow local protocols and maintain contact with medical direction whenever possible.

Rectal diazepam is now available in a gel form (Diastat) and can be used much easier during seizure activity than trying to start an IV line and give IV drugs. It is recommended for children 2 years of age and older. It is supplied in prefilled syringes of 2.5, 5, and 10 mg with a pediatric length tip. It also is available in 10, 15, and 20 mg with an adult length tip for older children. The recommended doses are outlined in Table 34-8.

Status epilepticus is a continuous seizure lasting more than 30 minutes or a series of seizures in which the patient does not regain responsiveness. If this condition occurs, immediate intervention is necessary. Complications include aspiration of blood or vomit, hypoxia resulting in brain damage, long bone and spinal fractures, and severe dehydration. The EMT–I should maintain the child's airway and monitor cardiac activity. IV glucose (25% to 50%, depending on the size of the child) may be ordered to correct hypoglycemia from the prolonged seizure activity.

and the airway should be maintained and suctioned ONLY as necessary.

Ventilations should be assisted with a bag-valve-mask device if hypoventilation or apnea occur for a prolonged period. Short periods of apnea occur with most tonic-clonic seizures, and respirations then return at the completion of the seizure. The EMT–I should use common sense to decide if the infant or child must be ventilated.

If the seizure is due to a fever, attempts to reduce the fever may be appropriate, such as removing clothing, sponging the infant or child with 4 × 4s moistened with tepid water only, keeping the patient compartment cool, and so forth.

When the seizure has subsided, the EMT–I should reassure the child and the family. If a postictal period occurs, the EMT–I should continue to maintain the airway as necessary. For some seizures an IV line and administration of diazepam (Valium) or lorazepam (Ativan) may be required to stop the seizure activity. The EMT–I

Meningitis

Meningitis is defined as an inflammation of the membranes that surround the brain and spinal cord. It is caused by viruses, bacteria, or other microorganisms and may develop concurrently with viral illnesses such as mumps or chicken pox or a bacterial illness such as that seen with an ear infection. However, the child also may contract meningitis without any ongoing illness. The diagnosis is confirmed only after the infant or child

TABLE 34-8

Doses of Diazepam Rectal Gel (Diastat)

AGE	DOSE
2 to 3 years	0.5 mg/kg
6 to 11 years	0.3 mg/kg
12 years and older	0.2 mg/kg

has a lumbar puncture or "spinal tap" to collect cerebrospinal fluid for examination.

Bacterial meningitis is much more serious than viral or aseptic meningitis. The most common forms of bacterial meningitis are hemophilus meningitis (caused by *Haemophilus influenzae*), pneumococcal meningitis (caused by *Streptococcal pneumoniae*), and meningococcal meningitis (caused by *Neisseria meningitidis*). The first strain is much less common with the current *H. influenzae* type B vaccine routinely given to children. Meningococcal meningitis is the most life-threatening strain of the three.

In younger patients, signs and symptoms of meningitis may include the following:
- Fever
- Dehydration
- Disorientation or lethargy
- Bulging fontanelle
- Irritability (infant or child does not want to be touched or held)
- Loss of appetite
- Poor feeding (may be a sign in young infants)
- Vomiting
- Seizures
- Respiratory distress
- Cyanosis
- Rash

In the older child, in addition to the above signs and symptoms, the following may be present:
- Stiffness of the neck
- Kernig's sign (pain when extending the legs)
- Headache

As the bacteria or virus spreads, the child will become increasingly ill. In bacterial meningitis, cerebral edema can occur, which can lead to increased intracranial pressure with brain stem herniation.

Permanent complications, which occur in approximately 30% of children with bacterial meningitis, include hearing loss (most common), seizure disorders, developmental and cognitive delay (mental retardation), hydrocephalus, motor impairment, paralysis, and ataxia. Approximately 5% to 15% of children with bacterial meningitis die, depending on the type of bacteria involved.

Some patients with meningococcal meningitis develop meningococcemia, which occurs when the *N. meningitidis* bacteria invade the bloodstream (Figure 34-19). Symptoms may include a sudden onset of chills; muscular and joint pain; sore throat; headache; petechiae (a perfectly round, purplish red spot caused by intradermal or submucous hemorrhage); and severe exhaustion. Profound shock occurs as the peripheral circulation collapses, and it is fatal if not treated aggressively. Infants and children who survive may be left permanently disfigured by the loss of skin and parts of their limbs damaged by the bacteria.

Treatment focuses on maintaining the child's respiratory and circulatory efforts. The EMT–I should monitor vital signs and cardiac status, provide high-concentration oxygen, and assist ventilation as necessary. He or she also should start an IV of lactated Ringer's solution and infuse fluid in boluses of 20 mL/kg as necessary to treat shock. The child should be made as comfortable as possible and transported immediately if meningitis is suspected. The EMT–I should notify medical direction and frequently reassess the child, watching closely for any seizure activity.

> **! HELPFUL HINT**
> - Meningitis is considered a true emergency in infants and children.

In a suspected case of meningitis, the EMT–I must protect himself or herself. The Centers for Disease Control and Prevention (CDC) recommends using body substance isolation (BSI) precautions. Because meningitis is spread by respiratory secretions (e.g., mucus) and not droplet nuclei like tuberculosis, a specialized mask or respirator is not necessary. Any mask is appropriate as long as it provides a barrier that prevents contact with the patient's respiratory secretions.

If an exposure to bacterial (meningococcal) meningitis has occurred, the health care facility receiving the patient is required by law to notify emergency personnel involved in that patient's care. Prophylactic antibiotics usually are prescribed to prevent the spread of the dis-

> **! HELPFUL HINT**
> - For the EMT–I's own protection, he or she should talk with personnel at the receiving facility after the call is completed. The EMT–I should ask to be notified if the child is diagnosed with bacterial meningitis. In such a case, the EMT–I may be given medication to prevent contracting the disease.

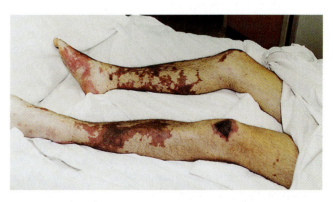

FIGURE 34-19 ▲ Petechiae on the lower extremities of a child with meningococcemia. (From Wong DL: *Whaley and Wong's nursing care of infants and children,* ed 6, St Louis, 1999, Mosby.)

ease. They should be taken exactly as prescribed, and the exposed individual should be monitored by a physician for development of meningitis symptoms.

Poisoning

Young children are at an extremely high risk for accidental poisonings because of their inquisitive nature. As the child grows older, poisoning may occur from drugs or alcohol as the child experiments with mind-altering substances. Poisoning is a preventable death.

Poison is defined as any substance that produces harmful physiologic or psychological effects. Children between the ages of 18 months to 3 years account for approximately 30% of all accidental ingestion of poisons. The most common types of poisons are as follows:

- Household products (e.g., petroleum-based agents, cleaning agents, cosmetics, lawn and garden supplies)
- Medications (prescription and nonprescription)
- Toxic plants (e.g., poinsettia plants during the holiday season)
- Contaminated foods (e.g., potato salad left out all day at a summer picnic)

Between school age and adolescence, the most common poisons are as follows:

- Alcohol
- Organic solvents (e.g., hydrocarbons and fluorocarbons, which are present in gasoline, typewriter correction fluid, and airplane glue)
- Mind-altering drugs (e.g., marijuana, hashish, LSD, PCP, mescaline)
- Narcotics (e.g., heroin, morphine)
- Central nervous system (CNS) depressants (e.g., barbiturates)
- CNS stimulants (e.g., amphetamines, cocaine, crack)

Treatment for the prehospital patient depends on the type of poison ingested.

PEDIATRIC TRAUMA

Children will present with a particular injury pattern and physiologic response to trauma. These responses depend on the child's size, level of maturation, and overall development. However, basic life support and adequate assessments are still critical to the child's survival.

Prevention

The most frightening fact about pediatric trauma is that 20% to 40% of the deaths that occur are preventable. Many EMS and trauma systems are now focusing more on trauma prevention. Educational activities, for example, are directed toward children and their families and may include such things as helmet safety, bike rodeos, seat belt use, proper use of car seats, swimming pool safety, spinal injury prevention programs, antiviolence campaigns, and so forth.

Unique Pediatric Characteristics of Trauma

Blunt trauma continues to be the most common pediatric mechanism of injury. However, penetrating injuries have increased to almost 15% of all injuries. Causes of pediatric injuries are categorized as follows from most to least common:

1. Falls (most frequent in children less than 5 years of age)
2. Vehicular-related trauma (leading cause of permanent brain injury and new cases of epilepsy)
3. Accidental injury (e.g., drowning, near drowning, burns, and so on)
4. Sports-related injury (e.g., football, hockey, baseball, and so on)
5. Assaults (abuse, "knife and gun club," and so on)

Children may not show many external signs of injury. Therefore it is important to expect multisystem injuries as opposed to single-system injuries until otherwise confirmed, which usually takes place once the child reaches the hospital.

The physical differences between children and adults include the following:

- The child is smaller than an adult and therefore prone to a wider range of injuries.
- A child has less body fat.
- The child's connective tissue is more elastic.
- The child's organs are much closer together. Therefore more organs can be injured when energy is transferred during a traumatic situation.
- The child's skeleton is not completely calcified and has many active growth centers. This difference makes the skeleton more resistant to injury so that a severe injury may exist to the underlying organs without any broken bones. Children can withstand a higher level of energy without signs of external injury.
- The child has a larger surface area and can lose heat more quickly.

The child's future growth and development may be adversely affected by the trauma and subsequent injuries. The injuries may heal, but the child may be left with life-long physical, mental, and/or psychologic disabilities. In addition, the costs for rehabilitation and subsequent care for these children can be staggering. The EMT–I directly influences not only the immediate survival of the child but also the long-term functioning of that child.

Assessment

Thorough initial and ongoing assessments are still performed on the pediatric patient, and it is even more critical for the EMT–I to recognize the potential for life-threatening injuries. Even if the child appears stable during assessment of the airway, breathing, and circulation, the EMT–I should go with his or her instincts if it is possible the child has sustained a substantial mechanism of injury. The EMT–I should initiate rapid transport to a pediatric trauma center if he or she believes the potential for decompensation exists.

If a life-threatening situation does not exist, the on-going assessment should be continued. The EMT–I should pay close attention to anything that possibly could cause permanent damage such as injuries resulting in paralysis or paresthesias. In addition, any isolated extremity injury may require hospital evaluation to determine if the growth plate has been damaged.

The three most common causes of death in the infant and child are the same as in the adult: hypoxia, overwhelming central nervous system trauma, and massive hemorrhage. If the EMT–I is not quick to recognize these conditions or the possibility of these life-threatening conditions, the child may have a life-long disability or not even survive the traumatic event.

Treatment

Pediatric trauma patients need to be managed according to their presenting signs and symptoms, as well as the mechanism of injury. Even if the child does not appear to be unstable, the EMT–I must continue to suspect a decline in the child's status based on the mechanism of his or her injury. Specific treatment modalities are discussed under each subsection below.

If the patient is hypovolemic, the EMT–I should start an IV of normal saline or lactated Ringer's solution, give a bolus of 20 mL/kg initially, and repeat this procedure in 5 minutes if the child's vital signs do not improve. Further boluses may be necessary to restore an adequate blood pressure and subsequent tissue perfusion. The EMT–I should prepare for immediate transport and maintain contact with medical direction. CPR may be required.

Remember that the blood loss from internal bleeding will not be adequately managed by normal saline or lactated Ringer's. This patient will need definitive care at a trauma center. DO NOT waste time trying to start an IV line for those children in shock or with a significant mechanism of injury that may indicate serious internal injury.

Head Trauma

Head injury is the most common cause of death in the pediatric patient because children tend to land on their heads after a fall. Closed head injuries often result and may range from a momentary loss of responsiveness to coma or death. Adequate assessment, resuscitation, and transport to a facility designed to manage pediatric trauma are critical.

It is crucial to initially manage the airway and provide ventilation and supplementary oxygenation in an attempt to prevent further damage and sustain neurologic function. If the child is unresponsive, ventilation should occur immediately by either bag-valve-mask

device or, optimally, ET intubation. Ventilation helps to adequately oxygenate the child. It is the most important intervention for the child with head trauma.

Even if the child only briefly has lost responsiveness, it is important for that child to be evaluated. Cerebral edema, hematoma formation, and hypoperfusion still may occur and serious secondary injury must be ruled out.

Remember that children up to approximately 14 months will have an open anterior fontanelle and sutures. The posterior fontanelle closes approximately two months after birth. Since the anterior opening allows for possible expansion of the brain, intracranial pressure may increase without the usual signs and symptoms.

Scalp lacerations can lead to a significant blood loss in children. Any lacerations to the head should be controlled as quickly as possible to minimize blood loss.

Spinal Trauma

The spine in the infant or child has not yet calcified, has more active growth centers, and is more flexible. Serious injury to the spinal cord can occur (e.g., pinching, stretching, bruising, tearing) without any signs of external injury. In fact, changes may not even be seen on a radiograph once the child is evaluated at the hospital. If the child has any signs of deficit or if the mechanism of injury was significant, serious injury should be suspected and adequate precautions taken.

CAUSES OF PEDIATRIC SPINAL TRAUMA

The large head of an infant or child together with a lack of neck muscle strength leads to greater stress on the cervical spine region. When an acceleration/deceleration mechanism occurs, there is increased momentum in that area leading to injury. In fact, 60% to 70% of pediatric neck fractures occur at C1 or C2.

Despite an increase in the use of car safety seats, the potential for injury to infants and young children still exists. Many parents buckle their infants into the seats and forget to secure the seats in the vehicles. If a motor vehicle collision occurs, the seat bounces around the inside compartment, which can result in injury to the child and/or other occupants of the vehicle.

Motor vehicles are also an origin of spinal trauma for older children. Many children, especially those between ages 4 and 10 years, ride completely unfastened, despite laws requiring them to be secured in the car. Some parents simply do not adhere to the law and do not serve as good role models themselves. For example, some parents who own a minivan or station wagon permit children to ride unrestrained in the cargo area. During a collision, these unrestrained children become projectiles and are susceptible to serious head, spinal, and other traumatic injury.

Children who do wear safety belts also may suffer spinal injury, but this injury usually is not nearly as great as that suffered by unrestrained children. Use of a lap belt may cause injury to the abdomen or lumbar spine, so it is important for the EMT–I to examine the placement of the belt on the child (Figure 34-20). Is it high on the abdomen, or was it secured across the pelvis? Also, in vehicles equipped with shoulder harnesses in the front and back seats, the shoulder strap sometimes falls across the smaller child's neck or face, contributing to a possible cervical spine injury.

Children riding on dirt bikes, all-terrain vehicles, or as passengers on a motorcycle also may suffer spinal trauma. The EMT–I should observe the mechanism of injury, the vehicle involved, and what type of safety equipment may or may not have been used.

Lastly, warm weather tends to mean more children are outside and are therefore prone to more injuries. Riding bicycles, skateboarding, playing kickball in the street, swimming, and so forth are all recreations during which serious injury may occur.

INITIAL ASSESSMENT

Initial evaluation of the scene and mechanism of injury is crucial to performing a good assessment on any patient. When called to an incident involving possible pediatric spinal trauma, it is especially important for the EMT–I to notice what type of equipment, if any, was being used at the time of the incident. Has the equipment (e.g., a bicycle) sustained any damage? Was the surface on which the child landed made of cement, grass, padded material, or dirt? If it was a bicycle accident, was the child wearing a helmet? If so, is the helmet still in place or was it knocked off the head upon impact? Was the helmet damaged? This information, if available, can tell the EMT–I a great deal about the injuries that may have occurred.

Particular attention should be paid to playgrounds and the equipment available to children. Many playgrounds now have cedar chips or some similar material on the ground under the equipment. This material provides a softer surface in the case of falls. It is important for the EMT–I to make note of this surface when evaluating the mechanism of injury and relay the information to personnel at the emergency department.

A thorough initial assessment with frequent reassessment is even more important in children. Infants and children can compensate for a serious injury longer than an adult because they usually are healthy before the trauma. However, they decompensate rapidly. Evaluation of the airway with special attention to the cervical spine in addition to assessment of breathing and circulation should be done first. Then the EMT–I should perform a quick neurological examination and expose the patient to complete the initial assessment. Once any life-threatening injuries have been ruled out, the EMT–I then can begin the ongoing assessment.

Children between the ages of 12 and 17 years actually have bodies with the same anatomical ratios as adults. Children 7 years of age and younger, however, are significantly different in their anatomic configurations. The most notable difference is the size of the head.

TREATMENT

When cervical spine trauma is suspected in the infant or child, all airway maneuvers must be accomplished with the head in a neutral, in-line position. One EMT–I must hold the head while the other provider inserts an oral or nasal airway, ventilates, or performs tracheal intubation.

The indications for pediatric immobilization are based on the same criteria used for adults: evaluation of the mechanism of injury, one or more injuries suggesting some type of violent interaction, or specific signs and symptoms indicative of spinal trauma such as numbness, tingling, and so forth. However, mechanism of injury should be a key determination for immobilization even if the patient is asymptomatic. If the EMT–I believes the child may have been exposed to a force great enough to cause violent or sudden movement of the spine, the child needs to be properly immobilized.

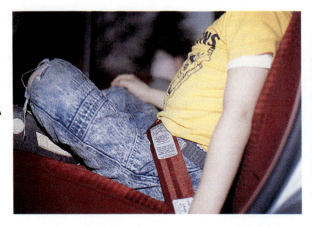 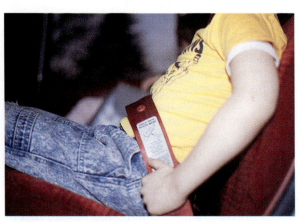

FIGURE 34-20 ▲ **A,** Correct and **B,** incorrect positions for lap belts on children. (From McSwain NE et al: *The basic EMT: comprehensive prehospital patient care,* ed 2, St Louis, 2001, Mosby.)

Once the possible existence of cervical and/or other spinal trauma has been identified, the EMT–I should begin treatment. The goal is to secure the child in a neutral, in-line position to a rigid board. Although this procedure may sound the same as that for an adult, the process used to achieve that goal is different for children.

To immobilize a pediatric patient, the EMT–I should do the following:

1. Ensure scene safety and quickly evaluate the mechanism of injury.
2. Approach the child and manually hold the head.
3. Bring the head into a neutral, in-line position. If any resistance is met or pain is elicited, stop any movement and immobilize the head in that position.
4. Perform an initial assessment to rule out any life-threatening injuries. If any are found, immediately begin treatment.
5. Apply a rigid cervical spine immobilization device to the neck ONLY IF IT FITS PROPERLY (Figure 34-21, *A*). If a properly-sized device is not available, use towels, washcloths, or other material to immobilize the head as best as possible (Figure 34-21, *B*).
6. If no life-threatening injuries are found, continue with the ongoing assessment.
7. Perform any treatments necessary (e.g., administer oxygen, immobilize fractures).
8. Logroll the child onto a rigid board and fasten the torso to the board (Figure 34-21, *C* and *D*). Towels may be used under the torso, depending on the age of the child, to bring the head and neck into a neutral, in-line position (to accommodate for a large occiput).
9. Secure the torso as appropriate.
10. Fasten the head securely to the board (Figure 34-21, *E* and *F*). Manual immobilization can be discontinued at this time.
11. Secure the board to the stretcher and reassess the patient.
12. Prepare to transport and perform any other treatments as necessary.

IMMOBILIZATION DEVICES

Regardless of the immobilization equipment used, some padding may still be necessary depending on the size of the child. The EMT–I should use his or her best judgment to pad the open areas before securing the torso to the board.

CHILD SAFETY SEATS

If the child is small and is found in an infant safety seat, chances are that the thoracic and lumbar spine may have been protected. However, the cervical spine is susceptible to maximum flexion, especially if the seat is not in the backward position, as recommended for infants.

Other safety seats accommodate a child until approximately 4 years of age or 40 lb. In these seats, the child

actually extends beyond the margin of the seat and may be susceptible to all types of trauma. Also, if the child's head is above the back of the seat (more common in older models), the head may be hyperextended during a rear-end collision.

If the child is critically injured or if the EMT–I anticipates deterioration, the safety seat should NOT be used for immobilization. Instead, the child should be gently extricated from the seat onto a rigid board. Short backboards work well for this. The EMT–I should maintain manual stabilization of the head and move the child as a unit onto the board. The child then can be secured as discussed below.

No EMT–I can be an expert on each child safety seat. In the event of a motor vehicle collision, he or she should do the following:

- When an infant or child is found in a safety seat, it can be used for immobilization only after a brief inspection. Has the seat sustained any major structural damage as a result of the accident? In other words, can it still effectively support immobilization? Can it be secured appropriately in the ambulance? If the answer to either of these questions is no, do not use the seat for immobilization.
- If the seat includes a protection plate over the child's chest, remove it so the patient's thoracic area is easily accessed. This removal permits adequate lung assessment and manual chest compressions if necessary.
- If a chest plate is not present, use the straps to secure the child in place whenever possible (Figure 34-22, *A*). Additional padding and/or cravats between the straps and the child or tightening of the straps may be needed.
- Small blankets, towels, and the like should be used as padding for all open areas around the child's body so the child does not move. Padding also should be placed around the head and neck if a properly sized rigid cervical spine immobilization device is not available (Figure 34-22, *B*). Use cravats or something equivalent around the head and arms to prevent forward movement (Figure 34-22, *C*).
- Once adequately immobilized, the patient and seat should be transferred to the ambulance. The seat then should be carefully secured to the stretcher or captain's seat so that it is not mobile during transport to the hospital (Figure 34-22, *D*).
- Remember, only take the time to immobilize the infant or child in the safety seat **if the patient is stable.** Do not waste precious time if the patient is seriously injured.
- If the child safety seat is not adequate for immobilization or the child is unstable, place the child safety seat on its back on a long backboard.
- Unstrap the child and slide him or her onto the long backboard. Slide the child out of the seat AS A UNIT. Do *NOT* pull on the child's head or neck. HINT: Use a padded board splint to keep the child's spine in a neutral, in-line position.

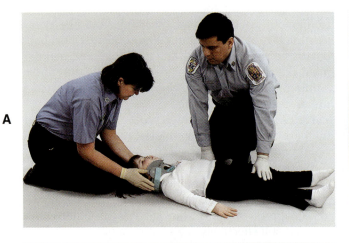

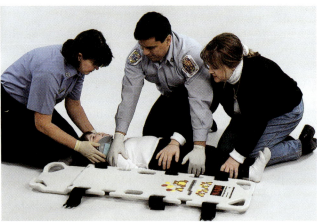

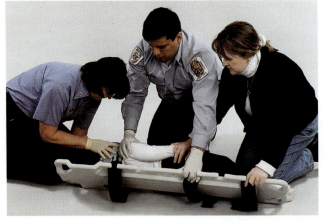

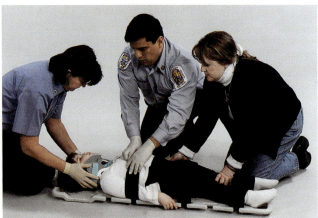

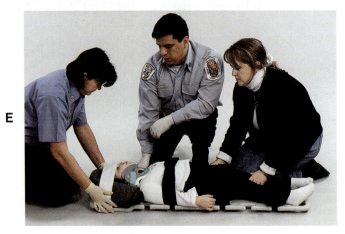

FIGURE 34-21 ▲ Immobilizing a pediatric patient. **A,** Apply a properly-sized rigid cervical collar. If a collar is not available, provide immobilization with other materials. **B, C** and **D,** Logroll the child onto a rigid board and fasten the torso to the board. **E,** Securely fasten the child's head to the board.

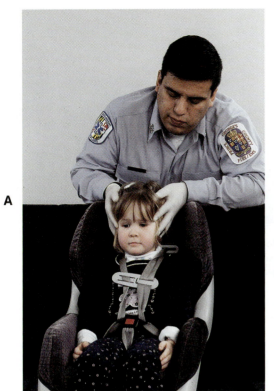

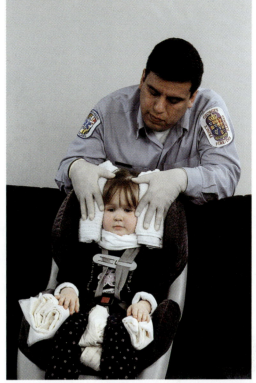

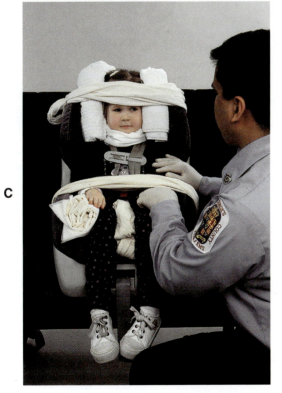

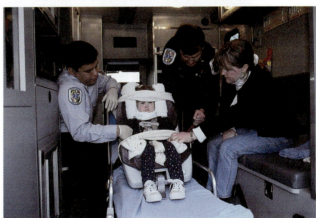

FIGURE 34-22 ▲ **A,** Manually stabilize the child's head and neck. Use the chest straps to secure the child in place whenever possible. **B-C,** Pad any open areas of the child seat so that the child cannot move, especially around the head and neck. **D,** Secure the safety seat in place for transport. *Continued*

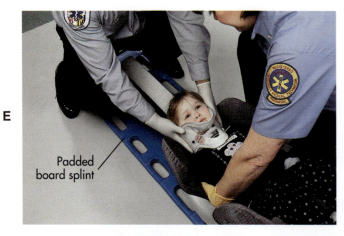

Padded board splint

E

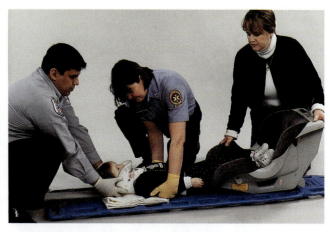

F

FIGURE 34-22, cont'd ▲ **E,** If the child safety seat is not adequate for immobilization or the child is unstable, place the seat on its back. Unstrap the child and slide him or her onto the long backboard. HINT: Use a padded board splint to keep the child's spine in a neutral, in-line position. **F,** Slide the child along the board, and remove the safety seat. Immobilize the child to the board.

CERVICAL SPINE IMMOBILIZATION DEVICES

A rigid cervical spine immobilization device is recommended for any patient who is suspected to have sustained a cervical spine injury. In pediatric patients, however, the EMT–I should make sure the device chosen does not hyperextend the child's neck because of improper sizing. If the device is too large, it should not be used. If an appropriate-size device is not available, the EMT–I should improvise as much as possible with padding to attempt to keep the neck immobilized. A cervical spine immobilization device alone is not adequate immobilization, therefore, manual stabilization must continue until the child is completely secured to a long backboard or equivalent device.

BACKBOARDS

A short or long backboard can be used for immobilization depending on the height of the child. If the short backboard is used to secure an infant, for example, it should be turned around so the head can be immobilized to the larger end.

Children have larger heads than adults and have less developed back muscles, which causes a natural flexion when the child is supine. The torso may need as much as 2 inches of padding to bring the spine into a neutral, in-line position. A flat blanket should be placed under the back from the upper margin of the pelvis and extended out to the left and right edges of the board. All open areas then should be additionally padded.

When the child has been strapped to the backboard, the EMT–I will notice open areas between the straps and the edge of the board. Additional padding is also necessary along the outside of the torso and around both sides of the legs so that the board can be tilted without any movement of the child from side to side (Figure 34-23).

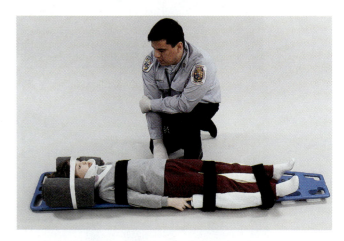

FIGURE 34-23 ▲ When immobilizing a child on a backboard, padding may be necessary under the shoulders, along the torso, and between the legs.

For a smaller child, cravats should be used instead of straps. One area of importance is across the pelvis because young children have abdomens that extend past the iliac crest of the pelvis. Abdominal excursion is a necessary part of ventilation through approximately seven years of age, and a strap could impede that process. Cravats also are advised instead of straps under the axillae. Big, wide straps can inhibit brachial circulation and actually cause more damage. If cravats are not available, tape may be used.

VEST DEVICES

Although in many parts of the country an adult vest device such as the Kendrick extrication device (KED) is used to immobilize children, this method is not recommended. Using a KED in a manner other than that for which it was intended has not been proven in the literature to be beneficial. For example, wrapping an adult

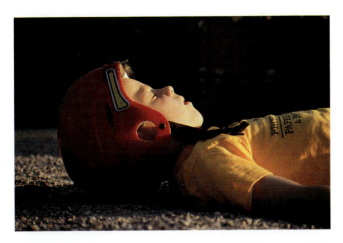

FIGURE 34-24 ▲ Helmets alone should be removed in pediatric patients.

vest device around the child like a papoose raises several concerns. One problem is that respiratory distress can occur if the thorax or abdomen is not permitted to expand adequately. Another concern is that in-line spinal immobilization is not achieved in many instances. More appropriate studies are needed before this method can be recommended.

HELMETS

Because children are now strongly encouraged to wear helmets during biking, skateboarding, and so on, chances are the EMT–I will be confronted with an injured child who is wearing a helmet. According to the American College of Surgeons Committee on Trauma, helmet removal is recommended so that vital functions can be assessed and immobilization can be maintained. They make no distinction between adults and children. In fact, it may be even more critical to remove a helmet in children to prevent increased flexion of the child's head from the helmet when placed in the supine position (Figure 34-24). Also, because cartilage in children may not be calcified, airway compromise can occur easily during hyperflexion.

Many children participate in sports in which a helmet is used in conjunction with other equipment (e.g., football helmet plus shoulder pads). The EMT–I should work with the athletic trainers in the area. In some situations, the helmet and additional equipment such as shoulder pads may need to be removed as a unit.

SPECIAL CONSIDERATIONS

When faced with a potential spinal injury in a child, the EMT–I should remember to rule out life-threatening injuries before turning his or her attention to full-body immobilization. Initial manual stabilization of the head and cervical spine should begin immediately during assessment of the airway. Further immobilization should not occur until adequate assessment and treatment have

been completed. When immobilization can be performed, the best possible equipment available should be selected.

Chest and Abdominal Trauma

The child's rib cage is extremely resilient, and the chest can suffer major internal injury without any bony fractures. Rib fractures that do occur are associated with a high mortality due to the amount of force required to break the ribs.

Flail segments are rare in children. If a flail segment is found without the corresponding mechanism of injury, suspect child abuse.

Internal chest injuries may not result in the usual signs and symptoms found in an adult. For instance, a child with a cardiac tamponade usually only has hypotension as a physical sign.

Tension pneumothorax in a child is poorly tolerated. This situation represents an immediate threat to the child's life.

The EMT–I should carefully observe for respiratory compromise and shock when treating a child with trauma to the chest and torso. He or she should evaluate the mechanism of injury and suspect injury even if the child appears to be fine. In addition, the child's cardiac rhythm should be monitored for signs associated with a cardiac contusion if present.

The EMT–I should assess for any signs of blunt trauma to the abdomen such as bruising (e.g., from a lap belt in a motor vehicle); unstable pelvis; abdominal distension, rigidity, or tenderness; or signs of unexplained levels of shock. Children less than 8 years of age also tend to be "belly breathers"; therefore respiratory distress also may be a sign of abdominal trauma.

The abdominal organs most commonly injured in a child are the liver, kidney, and spleen. There is minimal muscular protection, and the viscera is easily susceptible to injury.

Because the child's abdomen is small, take care to palpate only one quadrant at a time. If the child is conscious and complaining of pain in a certain area of the abdomen, palpate that area last.

If the child is crying, it may be difficult to perform an abdominal examination. Guarding and distention can be missed if the child is upset. A crying child, however, is usually one who is hemodynamically intact. The EMT–I should become concerned if the child suddenly quiets down and allows him or her to assess the abdomen.

The ideal treatment for chest and abdomen trauma in the child is the same as for an adult: definitive care at the hospital. The EMT–I should provide high-concentration oxygen, monitor vitals, make the child as comfortable as possible, and prepare for rapid transport to an appropriate facility. The EMT–I should not waste time in the field if chest or abdominal trauma is suspected in the pediatric patient even if the child appears to be stable. This patient can decompensate rapidly.

Hypothermia

Children are susceptible to hypothermia due to their large body surface area in comparison with their weight. In addition, their compensatory mechanisms such as shivering are not well developed. Newborns in particular can quickly become hypothermic because they have little subcutaneous fat.

Hypothermia is defined as a core body temperature below 95° F (35° C). It often occurs in children as a result of prolonged exposure to cold temperatures. Leaving the child uncovered in a cool environment during examination and treatment also can lead to hypothermia. Other causes include metabolic disorders (e.g., hypoglycemia), sepsis, and trauma or other brain disorders that interfere with the body's temperature regulating system. If alcohol and/or drugs have been ingested, the peripheral blood vessels dilate, and the body cannot conserve heat. Hypothermia often develops in such cases.

During the assessment, information about the incident should be obtained. How long was the child exposed to the cold, rain, or snow, and so on? Was the child submersed in water? What was the approximate temperature of the water? Is it known if the child ingested any alcohol or drugs? Does the child have a history of diabetes or an ongoing infection?

The EMT–I should look for specific signs and symptoms of hypothermia (Table 34-9). Hypothermia can be mild, moderate, or severe, depending on the temperature.

In addition, the EMT–I should look for areas of frostbite on the hands, fingers, feet, toes, ears, and nose. If the child complains of pain and a burning feeling, superficial frostbite probably has occurred. If there is no pain or feeling and the body part is blistered, a deeper injury may be present.

When treating the patient with hypothermia, the EMT–I should move him or her to a warmer environment as quickly as possible. If trauma is suspected, the child should be briefly immobilized before moving. All wet clothing should be removed and the child should be

TABLE 34-9

Signs and Symptoms of Hypothermia

TEMPERATURE	CHARACTERISTICS
95° F (35° C)	Increased respiratory rate and decreased intestinal motility
	Vigorous shivering
	May be conscious and alert
	Task performance often impaired
90° F (32° C)	May continue uncontrollable shivering or may begin to show muscular rigidity
	Decreased respiratory rate
	Atrial fibrillation
	May still be conscious but sensorium changes evident
	Impaired cognition, reasoning, and speech
	Loss of manual skills and dexterity
	Brief vasodilation that causes flushes and warm sensation and possible confusion
86° F (30° C)	Decreased cerebral blood flow
	May show increased blood pressure (may be difficult to obtain); tachycardia; and tachypnea
	May have supraventricular dysrhythmia, premature ventricular contractions (PCVs), and T-wave inversion
	Usually conscious, but a loss of consciousness is preceded by irritability
80° F (27° C)	Bradycardia and slowed respiratory rate; metabolic rate decreased by 50%
	Decreased oxygen uptake, carbon dioxide production
	Ventricular fibrillation
	Rigid extremities
77° F (25° C)	Hypotension
	Blood flow to kidneys reduced by 30%
68° F (20° C)	Unconscious
	Nonfunctioning reflexes
	Unresponsive pupils
	Respirations barely detectable or undetectable
	Extremities and trunk cold to touch
	Abnormal electrocardiogram
	Pulse may decrease to 4 beats/min, progressing to cardiac standstill
	Dead appearance
65° F (18° C)	Injury to peripheral tissue

From Wong DL: *Whaley and Wong's nursing care of infants and children,* ed 6, St Louis, 1999, Mosby.

wrapped in blankets. Once the blankets become wet, new, dry blankets should be applied. The head should be covered, especially in young children, to minimize further heat loss. If the child is responsive, the EMT–I may give warm liquids by mouth. Under no circumstances should the EMT–I allow anyone to give the child any form of alcohol to increase warmth (some people mistakenly believe a "hot toddy" will help the rewarming process).

If the hypothermia is moderate to severe, the first priority is maintenance of the airway. The EMT–I should provide high-concentration oxygen by face mask or ventilate with a bag-valve-mask device if necessary. If there is no pulse, he or she should begin chest compressions. The EMT–I should transport the child rapidly and continue CPR until arrival at the hospital. Resuscitation should not be discontinued until the child's temperature has returned to normal. At that time a decision can be made to stop or continue the resuscitation.

If a heart rate is present, the EMT–I should not provide any stimulation, including tracheal intubation, CPR, or suctioning. The goal is to prevent ventricular fibrillation from occurring. In addition, the EMT–I should not waste time attempting to start an IV. The patient should be handled gently when moving to prevent any lethal dysrhythmias. The EMT–I should continue with basic life support and rapidly transport to the hospital.

Heat packs may be used as long as they do not directly touch the skin. They should be placed under the axillae and in the groin area over the blanket. If frostbite has occurred, those affected extremities should be wrapped in a blanket. The EMT–I should not aggressively rub the part or expose it to dry heat, which may cause tissue damage.

Drowning

In the United States, drowning is the third leading preventable cause of pediatric deaths and results in approximately 2000 deaths annually. In about 5 to 20 percent of children hospitalized for a submersion event, severe, permanent brain damage occurs.

According to the 2000 Guidelines developed by the American Heart Association, the term *near drowning* is not to be used any longer. The proper terminology includes the following:
- Water rescue—This child may have had some distress in the water yet is alert. Coughing and other transient symptoms may be present, but they clear quickly. The child may not require any further evaluation or care.
- Submersion—This child had some swimming-related distress that required support in the field. He or she is usually transported to an emergency facility for further observation and treatment.
- Drowning—The event is considered fatal. The child is pronounced dead after a submersion incident at the scene of the attempted resuscitation, in the

Emergency Department, or in the hospital. The term *drowning-related death* is used if the child dies within 24 hours of the event. Until the drowning-related death occurs, the victim is called a *submersion victim*.

Most drowning events involving younger children occur in fresh water without proper adult supervision (e.g., bathtubs, buckets, swimming pools, lakes, toilets, fish tanks). Because children under 3 years of age have such large, heavy heads, they cannot get out of the water after falling head first into buckets, toilets, and so forth. In older children, drowning usually occurs after drug or alcohol use, swimming long distances, or boat accidents.

During the initial assessment, the EMT–I should focus on airway, breathing, and circulation. In many submersion cases, the child will be in cardiopulmonary arrest.

Treatment for these patients focuses on maintaining the respiratory and cardiac status. CPR should be initiated if appropriate. The EMT–I should remove wet clothing, wrap the child with blankets or towels, and use heat packs or other rewarming measures if the infant or child is hypothermic.

While the EMT–I is resuscitating the child, someone at the scene (e.g., police officer, additional prehospital personnel, fire department personnel) should gather more information about the incident. How long was the child under the water? Was the child found in warm or cold water? Was the water shallow or deep? Were there signs of breathing or a pulse on rescue? Was CPR started? If so, how quickly was it started after the child was removed from the water? Is there any other medical history available such as medications or seizure history?

Resuscitation should be attempted on children who have been submerged in cold water for a long period of time. If the child is very cold and has a heart rate, invasive procedures such as intubation should not be performed, because stimulation of the vagus nerve may cause asystole. Instead, bag-valve-mask ventilation with high-concentration oxygen should be provided.

The patient should be rapidly transported to a pediatric trauma center whenever possible or to a facility with the capability to provide intensive care services for pediatric patients.

OTHER PEDIATRIC PROBLEMS
Sudden Infant Death Syndrome

Sudden infant death syndrome (SIDS) is defined as the sudden death of an infant under 1 year of age that remains unexplained after a complete post-mortem examination which includes an investigation of the death scene and a review of the case history. SIDS is the third leading cause of death in children between the ages of 1 month and 1 year and claims the lives of approximately 3400 infants annually. Table 34-10 summarizes the major epidemiological characteristics of SIDS.

TABLE 34-10

Epidemiology of Sudden Infant Death Syndrome

FACTORS	OCCURRENCE
Incidence	1.4:1000 live births
Peak age	2 to 4 months; 95% occur by 6 months
Gender	Higher percentage of males affected
Time of death	During sleep
Time of year	Increased incidence in winter; peak in January
Racial	Greater incidence in Native Americans and blacks, followed by whites, Asians, and Hispanics
Socioeconomic	Increased occurrence in lower socioeconomic class
Birth	Higher incidence in the following: • Premature infants, especially infants of low birth weight • Multiple births* • Neonates with low APGAR scores • Infants with central nervous system disturbances and respiratory disorders such as bronchopulmonary dysplasia • Increasing birth order (subsequent siblings as opposed to firstborn child) • Infants with a recent history of illness
Sleep habits	Prone position Use of soft bedding Overheating (thermal stress) Possibly co-sleeping with adult
Feeding habits	Lower incidence in breast-fed infants
Siblings	May have greater incidence
Maternal	Young age Cigarette smoking, especially during pregnancy Substance abuse (heroin, methadone, cocaine)

From Wong DL: *Whaley and Wong's nursing care of infants and children,* ed 6, St Louis, 1999, Mosby.
*Although a rare event, simultaneous death of twins from sudden infant death syndrome can occur.

Certain groups of children are at increased risk for SIDS. These groups include the following:
• Infants with one or more episodes requiring cardiopulmonary resuscitation or vigorous stimulation to resume breathing
• Preterm infants who continue to have apnea at the time of hospital discharge
• Siblings of two or more previous victims of SIDS
• Infants with certain types of diseases or conditions that may affect their ability to breathe

The cause of SIDS is unknown even though various theories have been proposed. The most compelling hypothesis is that SIDS is related to a brainstem abnormality in the neurological regulation of cardiorespiratory control. Abnormalities include prolonged sleep apnea, increased frequency of brief inspiratory pauses, excessive periodic breathing, and impaired arousal responsiveness to increased carbon dioxide or decreased oxygen.

Another theory is that SIDS may be caused by rebreathing of carbon dioxide. Infants sleeping prone and/or with soft bedding may be unable to move their heads to the side, thus increasing the risk of suffocation and lethal rebreathing.

In the United States, mortality from SIDS has dramatically decreased since the American Academy of Pediatrics (AAP) initiated its Back to Sleep campaign in 1996. The AAP recommends that healthy infants be placed to sleep in the supine position.

Typically, the mother finds the child dead in the crib. By the time the EMT–I arrives at the house, one or both parents may be holding the infant or trying to resuscitate the baby.

Ask appropriate questions and do not overwhelm the parents with a detailed examination of their lives. If the infant is no longer in his or her bed, try to determine what the scene looked like when he or she was found. Remember that this recollection may be devastating for the parents to report.

The infant is usually found in a disheveled bed, with blankets over the head, and huddled into a corner. The infant may have been lying face down in secretions, suggesting that he or she bled to death. The hands may have been clutching the sheets, as if the infant was in distress before death.

On assessment, the mouth and nostrils are usually filled with frothy, blood-tinged fluid. Breathing and heart tones are absent. The diaper is wet and full of stool. Depending on how long the infant has been dead, there may be signs of dependent lividity.

If the parents are performing CPR, continue the resuscitation. Contact the medical control physician to determine if resuscitation should be stopped at the scene or continued through transport to a hospital. Follow local protocols.

If the infant is obviously dead, comfort the members of the family as much as possible. Do not give the impression of indicating that there was any wrongdoing, abuse, or neglect on the part of the parents. A compassionate, sensitive approach to the family during the very first few minutes can help spare them some of the overwhelming guilt and anguish that commonly follow this type of death.

Follow local protocols for the pronouncement of death. Remember that procedures vary from state to state. Involve law enforcement personnel to assist with transport to the morgue and funeral arrangements.

The loss of a child from SIDS presents several crises with which the parents must cope. In addition to grief and mourning for the death of their child, the parents must face a tragedy that was sudden, unexpected, and unexplained. The initial appearance of the baby combined with the shock of such an unexpected event adds to the horror that the parents must face. In addition, it is not uncommon for either parent to place blame on the other parent for the child's death.

The reaction of siblings must also be addressed. Young children may feel responsible for the infant's death, especially if they were jealous of the new baby.

The EMT–I must stress that SIDS cannot be predicted or prevented. Parents, siblings, and other family members at the scene need to understand that they were not responsible for the infant's death.

The family should be encouraged to reach out to organizations and/or support groups that may be available to help with long-term assistance. The American Sudden Infant Death Syndrome Institute has a website at http://www.sids.org that may provide helpful information.

The EMT–I should take advantage of critical incident stress management opportunities after being involved in this type of encounter. No matter how many years the EMT–I has been practicing, seeing a dead infant is never easy.

Child Abuse or Maltreatment

The broad term, **child maltreatment,** includes intentional physical abuse or neglect, emotional abuse or neglect, and sexual abuse of children, usually by adults. The Child Abuse Prevention and Treatment Act (CAPTA), as amended and reauthorized in October of 1996, defines **child abuse** as, at a minimum, any recent act or failure to act that results in imminent risk of serious harm, death, serious physical or emotional harm, sexual abuse, or exploitation of a child (i.e., person under the age of 18 unless the child protection law of the state in which the child resides specifies a younger age for cases not involving sexual abuse) by a parent or caretaker who is responsible for the child's welfare. **Neglect** is generally defined as the failure of a parent or

other person legally responsible for the child's welfare to provide for the child's basic needs and an adequate level of care.

Child abuse, also called *nonaccidental trauma,* happens to more than 1 million children in the United States annually. It involves the maltreatment of children by their parents, guardians, or other individuals responsible for their care. In 1995, approximately 52% of victims suffered neglect, 25% physical abuse, 13% sexual abuse, 5% emotional maltreatment, 3% medical neglect, and 14% other forms of maltreatment. Some children, in fact, suffer more than one type of maltreatment. More than half were 7 years of age or younger; and of these, 56% were younger than 4 years of age. Although the reporting of abuse has increased, it is still difficult to know how many cases actually are occurring each year, despite the fact that reporting is mandatory by law in all 50 states.

Certain factors can place families and children at a greater risk to abuse or be abused. Table 34-11 shows some of these risk factors for child maltreatment.

Child abuse can be divided into the following four major types:
- *Physical abuse*—Any injury intentionally delivered to the child by a caregiver. Activities include the infliction of physical injury as a result of punching, beating, kicking, biting, burning, shaking, or otherwise harming a child.
- *Sexual abuse*—Any sexual activity between a child and an older child or adult. Activities include fondling a child's genitals, intercourse, incest, rape, sodomy, exhibitionism, and commercial exploitation through prostitution or the production of pornographic materials.
- *Emotional or psychological abuse*—Behaviors inflicted on the child that are degrading, terrorizing, isolating, or rejecting. Activities include acts of omissions by parents or other caregivers that have caused, or could cause, serious behavioral, cognitive, emotional, or mental disorders.
- *Neglect*—Failure to meet the child's basic needs (e.g., food, clothing, shelter, medical care, safety). Activities include any failure to provide for the child's physical, educational, or emotional needs.

Emotional abuse is almost always present when other forms are identified. The assessment of child neglect requires consideration of cultural values and standards of care, as well as recognition that the failure to provide the necessities of life may be related to poverty.

As difficult as it may be, the most important role for the EMT–I in a suspected case of child abuse is to be nonjudgmental. The EMT–I must not accuse anyone of child abuse even though it may appear obvious to him or her. That type of approach may make the potential abuser angry and may even place the EMT–I in danger.

TABLE 34-11

Risk Factors for Child Maltreatment

CHILD CHARACTERISTICS	PARENTAL CHARACTERISTICS	ENVIRONMENTAL CHARACTERISTICS
Temperament ("easy" versus "difficult" child and how parent is able to deal with that behavioral style)	Negative relationship with own parents	Poverty and/or unemployment
Position of child in family	Received severe punishment as a child	Divorce or dysfunctional relationships
Illegitimate or unwanted	Difficulty controlling aggressive impulses (leading to free expression of violence on children)	Poverty
Additional physical needs if ill or physically/mentally disabled	Socially isolated; fewer supportive relationships	Alcoholism and/or drug addiction
Prematurity (due to lack of parent/child bonding in early infancy)	Teenage mothers	Increased exposure between children and parents (such as that which occurs in crowded living conditions)
Difficult pregnancy, labor, or delivery	Loneliness and isolation / Low self-esteem / Less adequate maternal functioning	Poor housing, frequent relocation

From Wong DL: *Whaley and Wong's nursing care of infants and children,* ed 6, St Louis, 1999, Mosby.

The EMT–I should focus on patient care yet be aware of the surroundings by objectively documenting where the child was found, the condition of the home, interactions with parents or family members, the condition of other children at the same location, and so forth. This information should be relayed to the physicians and nurses at the receiving facility. In some states, it is mandatory that EMTs report suspected child abuse or maltreatment. The EMT–I should consult confidentially with medical direction if he or she has any doubts.

Recognition of abuse and neglect requires a familiarity with both the physical and behavioral signs that suggest maltreatment. See Box 34-4 for clinical manifestations of potential child maltreatment and Box 34-5 for warning signs of abuse.

Shaken baby syndrome is a form of physical abuse that can cause fatal intracranial trauma without signs of external head injury. The EMT–I should suspect shaken baby syndrome in infants less than 1 year of age who present with subtle signs of a head injury (Box 34-6).

Treatment of the child who has been maltreated varies. If there are physical injuries, treat them as appropriate. For instance, a child who has been sexually abused may be treated as a victim of rape. A child who has been severely beaten should be treated as a trauma patient.

One goal is to protect the child from further abuse. All states and provinces in North America have laws for mandatory reporting of child maltreatment. The information is reported to the local authorities, and telephone numbers are usually listed under Child Abuse in the business white pages of the local telephone directory. The EMT–I can also contact the emergency child abuse hotline at 1-800-422-4453 (1-800-4-A-CHILD).

CHILDREN WITH SPECIAL HEALTH CARE NEEDS

The EMT–I does not need to have a degree in special education to treat "special" children. When responding to a scene involving an ill or injured child who also has a special health care need such as hearing impairment, mental retardation, tracheostomy, gastrostomy, cerebral palsy, or spina bifida, the EMT–I must think about how his or her assessment and treatment will change.

The term *special needs* indicates any condition with the potential to interfere with usual growth and development and can include physical disabilities, mental disabilities, chronic illnesses, or forms of technologic support. When specifically relating to children with special needs, the issues of growth, development, and education may surface. Therefore the EMT–I's treatment of these unique patients can have a profound effect on their future well being.

Various disabilities may be encountered in the pediatric patient. Only a handful are discussed here, but many others exist. The EMT–I should incorporate this knowledge into his or her overall patient management.

BOX 34-4

CLINICAL MANIFESTATIONS OF POTENTIAL CHILD MALTREATMENT

PHYSICAL NEGLECT
Suggestive physical findings
Failure to thrive
Signs of malnutrition, such as thin extremities, abdominal distention, lack of subcutaneous fat
Poor personal hygiene, especially of teeth
Unclean and/or inappropriate dress
Evidence of poor health care, such as nonimmunized status, untreated infections, frequent colds
Frequent injuries from lack of supervision
Suggestive behaviors
Dull and inactive; excessively passive or sleepy
Self-stimulatory behaviors, such as finger-sucking or rocking
Begging or stealing food
Absenteeism from school ⎫
Drug or alcohol addiction ⎬ in older child
Vandalism or shoplifting ⎭

EMOTIONAL ABUSE AND NEGLECT
Suggestive physical findings
Failure to thrive
Feeding disorders, such as rumination
Enuresis
Sleep disorders
Suggestive behaviors
Self-stimulatory behaviors such as biting, rocking, sucking
During infancy, lack of social smile and stranger anxiety
Withdrawal
Unusual fearfulness
Antisocial behavior, such as destructiveness, stealing, cruelty
Extremes of behavior, such as overcompliant and passive or aggressive and demanding
Lags in emotional and intellectual development, especially language
Suicide attempts

PHYSICAL ABUSE
Suggestive physical findings
Bruises and welts
  On face, lips, mouth, back, buttocks, thighs, or areas of torso
  Regular patterns descriptive of object used, such as belt buckle, hand, wire hanger, chain, wooden spoon, squeeze or pinch marks
  May be present in various stages of healing
Burns
  On soles of feet, palms of hands, back, or buttocks
  Patterns descriptive of object used, such as round cigar or cigarette burns, "glovelike" sharply demarcated areas from immersion in scalding water, rope burns on wrists or ankles from being bound, burns in the shape of an iron, radiator, or electric stove burner

Absence of "splash" marks and presence of symmetric burns
  Stun gun injury—lesions circular, fairly uniform (up to 0.5 cm), and paired approximately 5 cm apart (Frechette and Rimsza, 1992)
Fractures and dislocations
  Skull, nose, or facial structures
  Injury may denote type of abuse, such as spiral fracture or dislocation from twisting of an extremity or whiplash from shaking the child
  Multiple or old fractures in various stages of healing
Lacerations and abrasions
  On backs of arms, legs, torso, face, or external genitalia
  Unusual symptoms, such as abdominal swelling, pain, and vomiting from punching
  Descriptive marks such as from human bites or pulling out of hair
Chemical
  Unexplained repeated poisoning, especially drug overdose
  Unexplained sudden illness, such as hypoglycemia from insulin administration
Suggestive behaviors
Wariness of physical contact with adults
Apparent fear of parents or of going home
Lying very still while surveying environment
Inappropriate reaction to injury, such as failure to cry from pain
Lack of reaction to frightening events
Apprehensiveness when hearing other children cry
Indiscriminate friendliness and displays of affection
Superficial relationships
Acting-out behavior, such as aggression, to seek attention
Withdrawal behavior

SEXUAL ABUSE
Suggestive physical findings
Bruises, bleeding, lacerations or irritation of external genitalia, anus, mouth, or throat
Torn, stained, or bloody underclothing
Pain on urination or pain, swelling, and itching of genital area
Penile discharge
Sexually transmitted disease, nonspecific vaginitis, or venereal warts
Difficulty in walking or sitting
Unusual odor in the genital area
Recurrent urinary tract infections
Presence of sperm
Pregnancy in young adolescent

Continued

BOX 34-4

CLINICAL MANIFESTATIONS OF POTENTIAL CHILD MALTREATMENT—cont'd

SEXUAL ABUSE—cont'd
Suggestive behaviors
Sudden emergence of sexually related problems, including excessive or public masturbation, age-inappropriate sexual play, promiscuity, or overtly seductive behavior
Withdrawn behavior, excessive daydreaming
Preoccupation with fantasies, especially in play
Poor relationships with peers
Sudden changes, such as anxiety, loss or gain of weight, clinging behavior
In incestuous relationships, excessive anger at mother for not protecting daughter
Regressive behavior, such as bed-wetting or thumb-sucking

Sudden onset of phobias or fears, particularly fears of the dark, men, strangers, or particular settings or situations (e.g., undue fear of leaving the house or staying at the daycare center or the baby-sitter's house)
Running away from home
Substance abuse, particularly of alcohol or mood-elevating drugs
Profound and rapid personality changes, especially extreme depression, hostility, and aggression (often accompanied by social withdrawal)
Rapidly declining school performance
Suicidal attempts or ideation

From Wong DL: *Whaley and Wong's nursing care of infants and children,* ed 6, St Louis, 1999, Mosby.

BOX 34-5

WARNING SIGNS OF ABUSE

Physical evidence of abuse and/or neglect, including previous injuries
Conflicting stories about the "accident" or injury from the parents or others
Cause of injury blamed on sibling or other party
An injury inconsistent with the history, such as a concussion and broken arm from falling off a bed
History inconsistent with child's developmental level; such as a 6-month-old turning on the hot water
A complaint other than the one associated with signs of abuse (e.g., a chief complaint of a cold when there is evidence of first- and second-degree burns)
Inappropriate response of caregiver, such as an exaggerated or absent emotional response; refusal to sign for additional tests or to agree to necessary treatment; excessive delay in seeking treatment; absence of the parents for questioning
Inappropriate response of child such as little or no response to pain; fear of being touched; excessive or lack of separation anxiety; indiscriminate friendliness to strangers
Child's report of physical or sexual abuse
Previous reports of abuse in the family
Repeated visits to emergency facilities with injuries

From Wong DL: *Whaley and Wong's nursing care of infants and children,* ed 6, St Louis, 1999, Mosby.

BOX 34-6

PHYSICAL FINDINGS IN SHAKEN BABY SYNDROME

Retinal hemorrhages
Central nervous system (closed head) injury
Bleeding (subdural, epidural, subarachnoid, subgaleal)
Laceration
Contusion
Concussion
Bruises (facial, scalp, arms, abdomen, back)
Soft tissue swelling
Skull fracture(s)
Other fracture(s) (long bones, ribs, metaphyseal)
Abdominal injuries
Chest injuries
Hypotension
Tense fontanelle

From Brodeur AE, Monteleone JA: *Child maltreatment: a clinical guide and reference,* St Louis, 1994, GW Medical.

rhage, anoxia, inherited disorders, trauma, or other conditions that may damage the brain. The child usually is considered to have a learning disability, mental retardation, or some form of developmental delay.

In most circumstances, the actual physical examination is essentially unchanged. The most prominent differences will be in the child's level of understanding and ability to communicate. In addition, the EMT–I should direct questions in a positive light and focus on the child's abilities instead of his or her disabilities. The EMT–I should ask the parent or teacher what the child is able to do and what he or she understands.

Cognitive Disabilities

Cognitive disabilities involve some degree of impaired adaptation in learning, social adjustment, and/or maturation. They result from a variety of causes such as metabolic disorders, infections, intracranial hemor-

Respect should be the key ingredient to any modality involving the child with a cognitive disability. Approach the child in a manner consistent with his or her developmental level.

Regardless of what action is taken, the EMT–I should explain it even if it seems that the child does not understand. It is possible that the child may comprehend what the EMT–I is saying without registering any reaction. A short explanation of what the EMT–I is doing to the child also will go a long way to alleviate some of the fears on the part of the parents or caregiver.

Physical Disabilities

Physical disabilities involve some type of limitation of mobility and are caused by birth anomalies, spinal cord injuries, infections, disease processes, and so forth. Examples include hearing or vision impairments, cerebral palsy, spina bifida, and spinal cord injuries. During the assessment, it is important to determine, if possible, what type of disability was present before the emergency (e.g., Did the child previously have any paralysis of the lower extremities or is that a result of the present injury?).

Many children with physical disabilities use some type of adaptive device, such as a wheelchair, braces, crutches, or a combination of devices. Some children may use corrective splints at different times during the day or night. The EMT–I should ask the patient, parents, or caregivers to explain the device and use their knowledge to help assess and treat the child. Splints or braces also can serve as tools for immobilization if trauma is suspected. However, if circulation or breathing are impaired or major bleeding is present, these devices should be removed. If a wheelchair is used, make sure someone assumes responsibility for getting it back to the child's classroom, home, personal care facility, and so on.

Chronic Illnesses

Any disease, condition, or situation that extends for a prolonged period is considered chronic. Chronic illnesses include reactive airway disease (asthma), diabetes, epilepsy, terminal illnesses such as cancer or cystic fibrosis, children who are awaiting or who have had transplants, children with head or spinal cord injuries after rehabilitation, and children with congenital cardiac anomalies.

For example, it may be difficult to think of seizures alone as a disability. However, many children have multiple seizures that resist control despite aggressive medical and surgical therapy. The seizures interfere with the daily lives of these children and their families and subsequently constitute a chronic problem. Children's growth and development are often negatively affected by the number of seizures as well as the side effects of multiple medications.

Some children with uncontrolled seizures may be on a special diet called the **ketogenic diet.** This diet is high in fat, low in carbohydrates, and low in protein. It is thought to achieve some seizure control through the ketosis that results from the metabolism of fat instead of glucose. These children should not be given any glucose solutions either orally or intravenously so as not to interfere with the ketosis so meticulously maintained by the child's family and caregivers.

In another example, many patients who have had organ transplantations must take antirejection drugs and are continually monitored by their physicians. This situation constitutes a chronic illness even though the transplanted organ(s) may be functioning well. These individuals are usually at a higher risk for infection due to the immunity suppression effects of their medications. Signs and symptoms of an infectious process may be the reason for a request for assistance.

Assistive Technology

Technology has made a tremendous difference in the lives of many children. This technology includes an array of medical equipment such as tracheostomies, gastrostomy tubes and buttons, central venous access devices, and so on. Families and caregivers usually receive education about caring for the specific equipment or device while in the hospital before discharge. However, they may experience a great deal of anxiety once the patient returns home.

Once at home, it can be very frightening if a malfunction occurs or the device does not operate as it did in the hospital. EMS may be called at the first sign of trouble, especially in the first few weeks during the adjustment phase. The EMT–I may be expected to "save the day" without having actual experience with the equipment in use.

It may be helpful to meet with personnel from the social services departments in the hospitals in your area. Encourage them to notify the ambulance service with whom the patient may be in contact regarding the presence of specialized equipment in the home. After these details are received, the EMT–I can visit the residence to gather more information from all parties involved. It may also be helpful to review what procedures should take place if a disaster (e.g., earthquake, tornado, flooding, and so on) or other event occurs that can cause a loss of power.

TRACHEOSTOMY

A tracheostomy is used as a temporary or permanent device. In some patients, it provides protection against secretions that may be aspirated. In other patients, it is necessary because of direct trauma to the airway or weakened respiratory muscles or after prolonged mechanical ventilation (Figure 34-25).

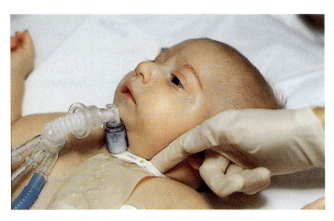

FIGURE 34-25 ▲ Some children may have a tracheostomy in place as a temporary or permanent device to aid in breathing.

Mucous plugs commonly obstruct the lumen of the tracheostomy tube because it is of such a small diameter. This obstruction may lead to cardiac arrest if the patency is not restored. Assessment should include a detailed inspection of the tracheostomy device and site. Is it patent? Are secretions present, and if so, what color and consistency are they? Is there any bleeding noted around the site?

Obstruction of the tracheostomy requires immediate action. Difficulty clearing secretions, improper positioning, or incorrect insertion of the tube during replacement may lead to obstruction. Place the patient in a sitting position as long as trauma is not suspected. Removal of the tube and direct suctioning of the stoma may be necessary to relieve the blockage.

The tracheostomy tube should be suctioned if it is occluded. Only approximately 4 to 5 seconds of suctioning are necessary because the tube is so short. If the EMT–I cannot remove the obstruction or cannot insert the suction catheter, he or she should remove the entire tube. He or she should suction the stoma, or opening in the neck, and insert a new tube if it is available and the EMT–I has

TABLE 34-12

Central Venous Access Devices

TYPE OF CATHETER	BENEFITS	MAINTENANCE CONSIDERATIONS
Peripherally inserted central catheter (PICC)	Used for therapy of short to moderate duration Lease costly	Antecubital vein is the most common site, but it may limit movement of arm Risk of infection May become dislodged easily (most are not sutured into place)
TUNNELED CATHETER Hickman Broviac	Used for long-term therapy Easy to use for self-administered infusions	Daily heparin flushes required Must be clamped or have clamp ready at all times Site must be kept dry Risk of infection Protrudes from body Susceptible to damage May be pulled out May alter body image of child
IMPLANTED PORTS Port-A-Cath Infus-A-Port Mediport	Used for long-term therapy Reduced risk of infection Only slight bulge on chest; completely under skin Increased safety (under skin and no maintenance care) Reduced cost for family Regular physical activity (including swimming) not restricted Heparinized monthly and after each infusion	Must pierce skin to access port Pain associated with needle insertion (may use local anesthetic like EMLA cream) Special needle (Huber) required to access port Must prepare skin before injection Catheter may dislodge from port especially if child "plays" with site Generally not allowed to engage in vigorous contact sports Difficult for self-administered infusions

Modified from Wong DL: *Whaley and Wong's nursing care of infants and children,* ed 6, St Louis, 1999, Mosby.

been trained to do so. If another tracheostomy tube is not available, a standard infant ET tube can be substituted.

If unable to ventilate through the stoma and the upper airway is patent, the EMT–I should manually occlude the stoma. Bag-valve-mask ventilation should be performed over the nose and face until orotracheal intubation can be done or a replacement tracheostomy tube becomes available.

In older children who are responsive, alternative methods of communication may be necessary. Some will use a communication board or simply write down their needs on a piece of paper. The EMT–I must be sure to ask what method is best for each particular patient.

CENTRAL VENOUS ACCESS DEVICES

Some patients who require frequent IV medications, repeated blood testing, administration of blood products, or administration of large quantities and/or concentrations of fluids may have a central venous access device inserted. Central venous access devices (VADs) provide extended access to a vein without the need for repeated venipunctures or infusions.

There are several types of devices (Table 34-12). All catheters end at the superior vena cava or the right atrium (Figure 34-26). Some of them may be used for fluid resuscitation or medication administration in an emergency. Follow local protocols or consult with the medical control physician. Medication and fluid may be given directly through the tubing for a peripherally inserted central catheter or through the injection cap for Hickman and Broviac catheters (Figure 34-27). The implanted devices (e.g., a Medi-Port) can only be accessed using a special needle called a *Huber needle* (Figure 34-28).

VAGUS NERVE STIMULATOR

Some patients with seizures that have not responded to medication may have a **vagus nerve stimulator (VNS)** in place. These devices are used in patients over 12 years of age and provide a pattern of stimulation to

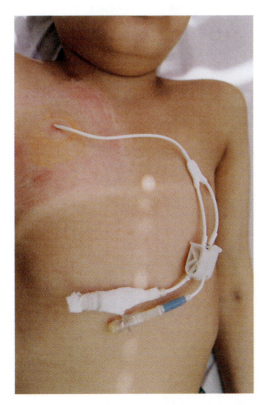

FIGURE 34-26 ▲ Central venous catheter insertion and exit site. (From Wong DL: *Whaley and Wong's nursing care for infants and children,* ed 6, St Louis, 1999, Mosby.)

FIGURE 34-27 ▲ External venous catheter (note redness from dressing site). (From Wong DL: *Whaley and Wong's nursing care of infants and children,* ed 6, St Louis, 1999, Mosby.)

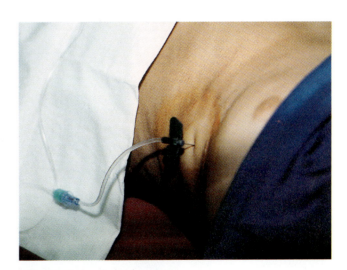

FIGURE 34-28 ▲ Implanted venous access device with Huber needle placement. (From Wong DL: *Whaley and Wong's nursing care of infants and children,* ed 6, St Louis, 1999, Mosby.)

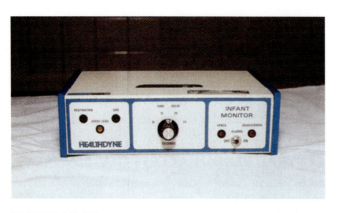

FIGURE 34-29 ▲ Apnea monitor. (From McSwain NE et al: *The basic EMT: comprehensive prehospital patient care,* ed 2, St Louis, 2001, Mosby.)

the vagus nerve to stop the progression of seizure activity. The generator is implanted under the skin and can also be activated by the patient if necessary. If the patient's heart rate is slow, consider a problem with this stimulator. Relay its presence to the medical control physician, and treat the patient for bradycardia.

APNEA MONITORS

Many premature infants are sent home with apnea monitors to warn parents and caregivers of any lapses in breathing (Figure 34-29). Some monitors also warn of bradycardia or tachycardia. An alarm sounds if the device does not detect a breath within a specific time interval or if there is a significant change in the infant's heart rate.

The EMT–I will most likely be called to the home to assist with CPR, to transport the infant back to the hospital, or simply to provide reassurance to frightened

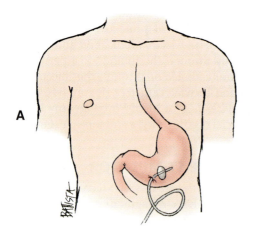

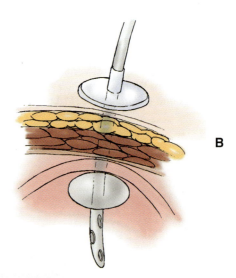

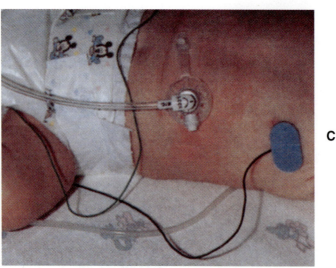

FIGURE 34-30 ▲ Some children have a gastrostomy tubes (**A and B**) or a button (**C**) for feeding. (**C** from McSwain NE et al: *The basic EMT: comprehensive prehospital patient care,* ed 2, St Louis, 2001, Mosby.)

parents. If the infant does not need to be transported, the EMT–I should let the family know that the EMS agency is available in the future if the infant's condition changes.

GASTROSTOMY TUBE OR BUTTON

A gastrostomy tube or button is used for children who cannot take food by mouth for an extended period of time. Various types of devices are used, and each is inserted and secured in a different way (Figure 34-30). The EMT–I should look at the insertion site for bleeding or to see if the tube has become dislodged. If the tube is secured within the stomach, he or she should be aware that more bleeding may occur internally. If there is any suspicion of internal bleeding, further evaluation is necessary at the hospital.

Medications

Some children take many medications for their particular disability. The EMT–I should obtain this information from the parents or examine medication bottles if necessary.

The EMT–I should determine when the child last took each medication. In someone with a gastrointestinal illness, nausea and vomiting may preclude the patient from taking or absorbing the drugs, which may in turn precipitate other serious consequences.

During assessment of the patient, obvious medication side effects may include drowsiness, irritability, or puffiness such as that seen with steroids. These side effects should be noted in the EMT–I's documentation.

Latex Allergies

In 1989, latex allergy was found to be a serious problem in children with spina bifida. Due to repeated exposure to products containing latex (e.g., catheters, gloves, and so on), children become sensitive to the latex and develop life-threatening allergic reactions. These allergies continue into adulthood.

It is important to know immediately if a pediatric patient is sensitive to latex. If a sensitivity or allergy is present, the child must not come into contact with any latex products or even be near equipment with latex (Box 34-7). Assemble a latex-free kit that can be stored in the ambulance for use when needed.

Family Issues

Dealing with a child with special health care needs can be stressful for the entire family. The family should be included during the EMT–I's assessment of the pediatric patient, because they have been forced to become experts regarding their child and his or her disability or special circumstance. The EMT–I should trust family members when they say there is a change in their

child's routine behavior. If the family is providing treatment on the EMT–I's arrival (e.g., suctioning their child or performing CPR), the EMT–I should either allow them to finish the procedure while he or she gathers more information or gently assume a primary role. The family should be allowed to assist in providing treatment if they prefer to do so. If the family is overwhelmed or significantly stressed, the EMT–I may need to be more assertive. However, the EMT–I should not simply take over as the medical professional and push the family aside.

Frequent hospitalizations may be a big part of these families' lives; and as part of the emergency response team, the EMT–I might see many different emotions at play. The child may be unusually fearful if past experiences with medical personnel have been painful or unpleasant. Parents may express frustration with yet another trip to the hospital, or they may be complacent about it.

It is also important to consider the siblings of the child with special needs. Their lives have been disrupted by the amount of care their brother or sister requires, frequent hospitalizations, and constant questions about why that child cannot do things other children are doing. If a sibling is at the scene, the EMT–I should include him or her in the treatment whenever possible and appropriate. He or she should listen to the sibling and let him or her help hold the patient's favorite blanket, doll, or toy as reassurance.

BOX 34-7

ITEMS THAT MAY CONTAIN LATEX

Adhesive bandage strips
Airways
Blood pressure cuff and tubing
Bulb syringe
Catheters
Dressings
Elastic bandages
Electrode pads
Endotracheal tubes
Gloves
Intravenous tubing and bags
Medication vials
Nasogastric tubes
Oxygen masks and cannulas
Spacer (from metered dose inhaler)
Stethoscope tubing
Suction tubing
Syringes (disposable)
Tape
Tourniquet

From Wertz E: *Emergency care for children,* Albany, NY, 2001, Delmar Thomson Learning.

If the EMT–I notices that the family is particularly anxious, he or she should pass this information on to the staff in the emergency department. This is a time when social service personnel, nutritionists, or other medical specialists may be able to provide some assistance or guidance.

General Considerations

Many children with special needs are at higher risk for medical complications or traumatic events. Some children will have an increased susceptibility to infection resulting from immunity-suppressing medications. Others may show signs of skin breakdown from the use of braces or splints. Yet another group may have physical impairments that can result in decreased reflexes, low muscle tone, altered sensation, or even paralysis, which can limit their protective mechanisms.

The EMT–I should look for a medical identification (such as Medic-Alert) bracelet or necklace on these patients but should not rely on this solely as an indication of a chronic problem. Many parents do not have them for their younger child for fear the child will pull it off or actually be hurt by it. It may, however, be present on an older child.

Ask the parent, caregiver, or school nurse if an *emergency information form* (EIF) is available. In October 1999, the AAP and the American College of Emergency Physicians (ACEP) finalized a document that provides standard information that would be helpful to emergency personnel (Figure 34-31). They authored a joint policy statement advocating the use of this form for children with special health care needs (Box 34-8). MedicAlert also participates in the project and stores the information if the child has a MedicAlert bracelet or necklace.

The document is completed and updated by the child's primary care physician. It then should be given to the parents, child care provider, school nurse, emergency department personnel, dispatch center, EMS provider, or to an individual at a place where the child spends a part of his or her day. During an emergency, this form relays pertinent information that may affect treatment.

If this form is not currently available, it can be seen on ACEP's website of the (http://www.acep.org/public/specialneeds/html). The form can be downloaded or printed from that site.

It is crucial to involve medical direction as soon as possible in situations involving children with special needs. Early communication will help ensure adequate treatment, as well as the proper patient destination. In addition, the staff at the receiving facility will be properly prepared for the EMT–I's arrival.

As the EMT–I gains more confidence in treating these types of patients, he or she should take part in educating other EMS personnel in the area by doing the following:
- Become more familiar with different types of disabilities.

- Incorporate the discussion of various disabilities into pediatric assessment and treatment modalities.
- Understand the importance of conveying information to the other members of the healthcare team.
- Use the parents as a resource for information and advocacy.

One way the EMT–I can take a proactive approach is to ask if the service area includes children at home with any type of disability, special education programs, special clinics, or seasonal residential camps (Figure 34-32). If any of these are within the EMT–I's jurisdiction, he or she should take an active role. The EMT–I can visit the child's home, the educational program, or camp and make sure adequate information is available to summon EMS assistance (e.g., the correct telephone number for dispatch). The EMT–I can meet the staff and educate them as to the skills he or she possesses and how he or she can work with them in an emergency. The EMT–I also can offer to provide CPR training as a community service and be available to work at the camp as an EMS provider or as part of a medical personnel team if qualified.

Most importantly, the EMT–I should interact with some of the children (e.g., giving them tours of the ambulance, demonstrating how different pieces of equipment are used). This interaction makes children feel more comfortable in the EMT–I's environment should an emergency require EMS services, and it will certainly give the EMT–I an opportunity to get to know a piece of the child's world.

Remember that the child for whom the EMT–I is caring is a person first and a person with a disability second. For many families, it takes quite a bit of time to adjust to a chronic illness. In many cases, the mixed emotions about this "change in plans" surface at different times throughout the child's life, one of which may be the emergency situation in which the EMT–I is involved. The EMT–I's sensitivity and compassion toward the child and the family during this time can help everyone involved appreciate the unique characteristics of these special children. See Box 34-9 for Guidelines for Disability Awareness.

SPECIAL CONSIDERATIONS

Pain Management

Many professionals tend to underestimate the existence of pain in children. One of the reasons for inadequate management of pain is a lack of understanding of what pain is—a personal phenomenon that *cannot* be experienced by any other individual. Essentially, pain is what the person says it is, existing when the person says it does. It includes both verbal and nonverbal expressions of pain.

Some children are unable to verbally express pain or are afraid to let someone know they are in pain. Box 34-10

Last name:

Emergency Information Form for Children With Special Needs

American College of
Emergency Physicians*

American Academy
of Pediatrics

| Date form completed By Whom | Revised | Initials |
| | Revised | Initials |

| **Name:** | Birth date: | Nickname: |

| Home Address: | Home/Work Phone: |

| Parent/Guardian: | Emergency Contact Names & Relationship: |

| Signature/Consent*: | |

| Primary Language: | Phone Number(s): |

Physicians:

| Primary care physician: | Emergency Phone: |
| | Fax: |

| Current Specialty physician: Specialty: | Emergency Phone: |
| | Fax: |

| Current Specialty physician: Specialty: | Emergency Phone: |
| | Fax: |

| Anticipated Primary ED: | Pharmacy: |

| Anticipated Tertiary Care Center: |

Diagnoses/Past Procedures/Physical Exam:

1.

2.

3.

4.

Synopsis:

Baseline physical findings:

Baseline vital signs:

Baseline neurological status:

*Consent for release of this form to health care providers

FIGURE 34-31 ▲ **Emergency Information Form (EIF) for Children with Special Health Care Needs.**

Continued

Last name:

Diagnoses/Past Procedures/Physical Exam continued:

Medications:

Significant baseline ancillary findings (lab, x-ray, ECG):

1.

2.

3.

4.

Prostheses/Appliances/Advanced Technology Devices:

5.

6.

Management Data:

Allergies: Medications/Foods to be avoided   **and why:**

1.

2.

3.

Procedures to be avoided   **and why:**

1.

2.

3.

Immunizations

Dates				
DPT				
OPV				
MMR				
HIB				

Dates				
Hep B				
Varicella				
TB status				
Other				

Antibiotic prophylaxis: Indication: Medication and dose:

Common Presenting Problems/Findings With Specific Suggested Managements

Problem	Suggested Diagnostic Studies	Treatment Considerations

Comments on child, family, or other specific medical issues:

Physician/Provider Signature: **Print Name:**

FIGURE 34-31, cont'd ▲ Emergency Information Form (EIF) for Children with Special Health Care Needs.

BOX 34-8

AMERICAN COLLEGE OF EMERGENCY PHYSICIANS POLICY STATEMENT

Emergency Information Form for Children with Special Health Care Needs

Emergency physicians and pediatricians provide medical care to many children with special needs because of chronic, complex medical illnesses. Care of these children may be complicated by the lack of patient history information, and unusual and uncommon disease processes.

To optimize emergency care of children with special needs, the American College of Emergency Physicians supports the following principles:

- A mechanism should be available to quickly identify the child with special health care needs when that child presents for emergency care.
- Records of each child's special needs should be maintained in an accessible and usable format.
- The exact form in which relevant information is stored may vary depending on individual physician and patient preference.
- A universally accepted form should be disseminated for use by prehospital providers, parents, physicians, and other child advocates.

Approved by the American College of Emergency Physicians Board of Directors and the American Academy of Pediatrics, December, 1998. Available at: http://www.acep.org/policy/po400267.html

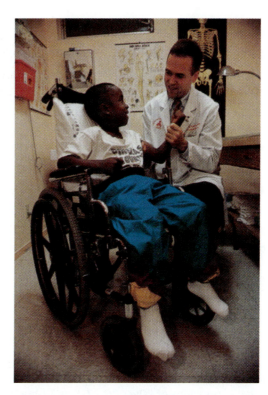

FIGURE 34-32 ▲ Visit a special clinic to learn more about children with special health care needs. (From McSwain NE et al: *The basic EMT: comprehensive prehospital patient care,* ed 2, St Louis, 2001, Mosby.)

outlines some of the more common expressions of pain according to the child's developmental level.

The EMT–I should make every attempt to make the infant or child as comfortable as possible. Strategies for relieving pain without medication include the following:

- *Always* be honest with the child.
- Express concern regarding the child's pain.
- Prepare the child before a potentially painful procedure but avoid "planting" the idea of pain. Instead of saying, "This is going to hurt," say, "Sometimes this feels like a stick or a pinch, and sometimes it doesn't bother people. Tell me what it feels like to you."
- Use "nonpain" descriptors whenever possible. Say, "It feels like intense heat," instead of "It is a burning pain."
- Encourage parents to stay with the child whenever possible.
- Have child take a deep breath and "blow the hurt away."
- Have child yell or say "ouch" by focusing on "yelling loud or soft as you feel it hurt. That way I know what you are feeling."
- Hold an infant or young child in a comfortable, well-supported position whenever possible (e.g., vertically against the chest and shoulder). Repeat one or two words softly such as "Mommy's here" or "Daddy's here."

BOX 34-9

GUIDELINES FOR DISABILITY AWARENESS

Use the word "disability" instead of handicapped.
Refer to the person first and the disability second, e.g., the child with mental retardation instead of the retarded child.
Use the child with a disability instead of the disabled child.
Never refer to someone as "wheelchair bound" or "confined to a wheelchair," because a wheelchair actually makes the person more mobile.
Avoid negative descriptions whenever possible. Do not use "invalid," "afflicted with," or "suffers from." Do not refer to children with Down syndrome as "mongoloids" or to children with epilepsy as "epileptics." Do not call seizures "fits."
Do not use "normal" to describe people who do not have disabilities. Use "typical" or "people without disabilities."
Do not refer to a person's disability unless it is relevant.

Modified from COALITION for Tennesseans with Disabilities: Talking about disability: a guide to using appropriate language, Nashville, Tenn, 1994, The COALITION.

BOX 34-10

DEVELOPMENTAL CHARACTERISTICS OF CHILDREN'S RESPONSES TO PAIN

YOUNG INFANTS

Generalized body response of rigidity or thrashing, possibly with local reflex withdrawal of stimulated area

Loud crying

Facial expression of pain (brows lowered and drawn together, eyes tightly closed, mouth open and squarish) (see Fig. 26-3)

Demonstrates no association between approaching stimulus and subsequent pain

OLDER INFANTS

Localized body response with deliberate withdrawal of stimulated area

Loud crying

Facial expression of pain and/or anger (same facial characteristics as pain but eyes may be open)

Physical resistance, especially pushing the stimulus away *after* it is applied

YOUNG CHILDREN

Loud crying, screaming

Verbal expressions of "Ow," "Ouch," or "It hurts"

Thrashing of arms and legs

Attempts to push stimulus away *before* it is applied

Uncooperative; needs physical restraint

Requests termination of procedure

Clings to parent or other significant person

Requests emotional support, such as hugs or other forms of physical comfort

May become restless and irritable with continuing pain

All these behaviors may be seen in anticipation of actual painful procedure

SCHOOL-AGE CHILDREN

May see all behaviors of young child, especially *during* painful procedure but less in anticipatory period

Stalling behavior, such as "Wait a minute" or "I'm not ready"

Muscular rigidity, such as clenched fists, white knuckles, gritted teeth, contracted limbs, body stiffness, closed eyes, wrinkled forehead

ADOLESCENTS

Less vocal protest

Less motor activity

More verbal expressions, such as "It hurts" or "You're hurting me"

Increased muscle tension and body control

Data from Craig KD and others: Developmental changes in infant pain expression during immunization injections. *Soc Sci Med* 19(12):1331-1337, 1984; and Katz E, Kellerman J, Siegel S: Behavioral distress in children with cancer undergoing medical procedures: developmental considerations, *J Consult Clin Psychol* 48(3):356-365, 1980.
From Wong DL: *Whaley and Wong's nursing care of infants and children,* ed 6, St Louis, 1999, Mosby.

The infant or child may need pharmacologic sedation for certain procedures. Follow local protocols, and consult with the medical control physician for appropriate medications and dosages.

Family Involvement

The EMT–I should remember to involve the parents, caregivers, or teachers throughout the call because it is often emotionally as well as physically traumatizing to the child and the family. In addition, if the illness or accident occurs in a crowded area such as a school or playground, other children or the patient's brothers or sisters may be in the area. They also may be frightened by the entire experience and may need some extra emotional support.

Transport Guidelines

When determining the destination for infants and children, evaluate the seriousness of the illness or injury
- Is the child critically ill?

- Is the child critically injured?
- Does the child have a chronic illness that is being treated at a specific hospital?
- Can the child go to the local community hospital only for initial evaluation before being transferred to a tertiary center?
- Is there a credentialed pediatric trauma center in the area?
- Is there a tertiary facility able to appropriately manage the child's critical illness?
- Is air transport needed to get the child to the appropriate receiving facility?

A critically injured child or one with a mechanism of injury in which a critical injury is suspected should go to a pediatric trauma center. If one is not available in the local community, air transport should be considered.

Controversy exists regarding transport to the local community hospital. If the child is in respiratory or cardiac arrest, some medical directors feel it is in the child's best interest to be initially stabilized at a local facility. Other medical directors feel that if the instability is caused by a major underlying traumatic or medical

CASE HISTORY FOLLOW-UP ■ ■ ■

En route to the emergency department, the crew performs an ongoing assessment of EMT–I Ward's child. Audible wheezes are still present, and he continues to use his neck muscles to breathe. The pulse oximeter indicates an oxygen saturation of 89%. The crew contacts medical direction to advise them of the patient's status, his medication history, and their 5-minute estimated time of arrival to the hospital. Because wheezes are still present, the on-line physician directs the crew to administer a second dose of albuterol by inhalation, but the drug has little effect on his respiratory status.

On arrival at the hospital, EMT–I Ward's son is quickly evaluated by the emergency department physician. An IV line is established, and a respiratory therapist begins to administer a bronchodilator via a nebulized updraft. Within minutes, the wheezes begin to clear and his color improves. Although he looks weary, EMT–I Ward knows her son is going to be fine.

EMT–I Ward is aware that an asthma attack can be life-threatening. She also knows that medications often are required to reverse reactive airway disease. She hopes her son will outgrow this illness. Until then, however, EMT–I Ward and her family must be prepared to manage this common childhood emergency.

event, the child's care will be unnecessarily delayed by the initial transport. If definitive care is needed, these physicians feel it is necessary to take the extra time to get the child to a location where the underlying cause can be adequately treated.

One goal of the Emergency Medical Services for Children program is to have a tiered transport system for pediatric patients that are critically ill or injured. The child is first transported by EMS (primary transport) to an Emergency Department Approved for Pediatrics (EDAP). This facility has minimum pediatric staffing, equipment, and supplies available for initial stabilization of the pediatric patient. The child is then transported (secondary transport) to an appropriate Pediatric Critical Care Center (PCCC) where a higher level of care can be given, including a pediatric intensive care unit (PICU) and other pediatric and trauma care specialists as necessary.

Remember that not all children need a tertiary level of care. It is appropriate to take the child with a broken ankle or the child that needs stitches in her arm after a sports injury to the local community hospital. Ideally, these local hospitals should have EDAPs so that appropriate staffing and equipment are available.

Regardless of the type of pediatric emergency, protocols should be developed and communicated to prehospital providers BEFORE an incident occurs in which they are needed. Many systems have pediatric triage guidelines that are followed based on certain criteria. Some of these guidelines are specific to trauma, and some of them are specific to medical emergencies. They are usually approved by the local, system, and/or regional medical director and updated on an annual basis. Again, work with the local medical director to review the guidelines for transport or establish some if they are not already present.

SUMMARY

- The EMT–I should try to speak to the child as much as possible to explain what is happening. If the patient is a young child, simple distraction from the activities at hand may be better than attempting to logically detail all of the actions. Diversionary tactics such as allowing the child to play with a toy or teddy bear can be quite helpful.

- When faced with a potential spinal injury in a child, the EMT–I must rule out life-threatening injuries before turning his or her attention to full-body immobilization. Initial manual stabilization of the head and cervical spine should begin immediately, as the EMT–I assesses the airway. Further immobilization should not occur until adequate assessment and treatment have been completed. When immobilization can be performed, the EMT–I should select the best equipment available.

- Pediatric illness or injury can be frightening to even the most experienced EMS provider. On those days when life is not too busy, the EMT–I should take the opportunity to review the equipment he or she would use to immobilize the pediatric patient. The EMT–I can practice pediatric assessment with his or her own children or children of other EMS or fire department members. This is great experience for the EMT–I as well as for the children. As they say, "Practice makes perfect." Once the EMT–I feels more confident with the process and the equipment, all of his or her concentration can be directed toward patient care.

- Children with special health care needs present another challenge. The EMT–I should become familiar with various disabilities and assistive technology used for children. Visits to local agencies, facilities, or camps in the service area will provide an opportunity to interact with these children before an emergency.

- The EMT–I must be adequately trained to deal with pediatric emergencies. He or she should concentrate on the differences between adults and infants or children. The assessment and treatment of these patients should be performed with those differences in mind. Special attention should be paid to the pediatric airway, because respiratory distress usually precedes cardiac dysrhythmias. Infants and children can compensate longer while in shock, yet deteriorate rapidly when their bodies can no longer maintain that compensation.

BIBLIOGRAPHY

American Academy of Pediatrics: *Emergency preparedness for children with special health care needs, Journal Title;* 104(4), 1999.

American Academy of Pediatrics: *Pediatric education for prehospital professionals,* Sudbury, MA, 2000, Jones and Bartlett Publishers.

American Academy of Pediatrics, Committee on Pediatric Emergency Medicine: Emergency Preparedness for Children with Special Health Care Needs, *Pediatrics* 104(4): e53; 1999.

American College of Emergency Physicians: *Emergency information form for children with special needs.* Available at: http://www.acep.org/public/specialneeds/html.

Anderson K, Anderson L, Glanze W: *Mosby's medical, nursing, and allied health dictionary,* St Louis, 1998, Mosby.

Foltin G, Tunik M, Cooper A: *Teaching resource for instructors in prehospital pediatrics,* New York, 1998, Center for Pediatric Emergency Medicine.

Jackson PL, Vessey JA: *Primary care of the child with a chronic condition,* St Louis, 1996, Mosby.

Krajicek MJ: *Instructor guide for the care of infants, toddlers, and young children with disabilities and chronic conditions,* Austin, Tex, 1998, Pro-Ed.

Maternal and Child Health Bureau, Health Resources and Services Administration: *National center established to improve care for children with special needs (press release),* US Department of Health and Human Services, 2000.

McPherson M: A new definition of children with special health care needs, *Pediatrics* 102(1):137-139, 1998.

McSwain N et al: *The basic EMT,* ed 2, St Louis, 2000, Mosby.

Mitchell NA: Innovative informations: latex allergy—accessing information on the Internet. *J Emerg Nurs* 32(1):51-52, 1997.

National Association of EMTs: *Prehospital trauma life support,* ed 4, St Louis, 1999, Mosby.

Wallace H et al: *Mosby's resource guide to children with disabilities and chronic illness,* St Louis, 1997, Mosby.

Wertz E: Children with special health care needs. In L Bernardo and D Thomas, editors: *Core curriculum for pediatric emergency nursing,* Des Plaines, Ill, 2000, Roadrunner Press.

Wertz E: *Emergency care of children,* Albany, NY, 2001, Delmar Thomson Learning.

Wong D: *Whaley and Wong's nursing care of infants and children,* ed 6, St Louis, 2001, Mosby.

WEBSITES WITH ADDITIONAL INFORMATION

American Academy of Pediatrics: http://www.aap.org.

American College of Emergency Physicians: http://www.acep.org

Center for Pediatric Emergency Medicine: http://www.cpem.org

Emergency Medical Services for Children: http://www.ems-c.org

Geriatrics

▪▪▪ CASE HISTORY

It is 4:00 AM when EMT–Is Valencia and Travis receive a call for a 78-year-old man complaining of shortness of breath. On arrival they locate the address in an apartment on the top floor of a three-story building without a functional elevator. After carrying their equipment up three flights of stairs, they discover an elderly male sitting in an armchair in an apartment living room. He appears pale, diaphoretic, and mildly tachypneic. He is only able to speak in three- or four-word sentences due to his dyspnea. While EMT–I Travis begins the patient assessment, EMT–I Valencia notices more than 30 prescription bottles sitting on the kitchen table, as well as another 20 bottles scattered throughout the bedroom and bathroom. As she collects the prescription bottles, she notes that there are prescriptions from numerous doctors and hospitals. A significant number of the bottles appear to be empty. EMT–I Travis' assessment of the patient reveals a frail, tachypneic male who continues to have respiratory difficulty. He is noted to have mild jugular venous distention in his neck veins, bilateral rales on auscultation of the lungs, and significant lower extremity edema. The patient gives a history that he has become too weak to even walk across the room to answer the door or to take his medications. He has been unable to get out of the apartment for the last 3 weeks due to his progressive dyspnea. He has also missed his last two appointments to see his physician due to his inability to navigate the three flights of stairs required to get to the parking lot and his car.

LEARNING OBJECTIVES

CHAPTER GOAL
Upon completion of this chapter, the EMT–Intermediate will be able to use assessment findings to formulate a management plan for the geriatric patient.

Cognitive Objectives
As an EMT-Intermediate you should be able to do the following:
- Describe dependent and independent living environments.
- Identify local resources available to assist the elderly and discuss strategies to refer the at-risk patient to appropriate community services.
- Discuss expected physiological changes associated with aging.
- Describe common physiological reactions associated with aging.

- Discuss problems with mobility in the elderly.
- Discuss problems with continence and elimination.
- Describe communication strategies used to provide psychological support.
- Discuss factors that may complicate the assessment of the elderly patient.
- Discuss common complaints, injuries, and illnesses of elderly patients.
- Discuss pathophysiological changes associated with the elderly in regards to drug distribution, metabolism and drug elimination.
- Discuss the impact of polypharmacy, dosing errors, medication non-compliance, and drug sensitivity in patient assessment and management.
- Discuss the impact that aging has on various body systems.
- Discuss the assessment and management of the elderly patient with complaints related to the following body systems:
  - Respiratory
  - Cardiovascular
  - Nervous
  - Endocrine
  - Gastrointestinal

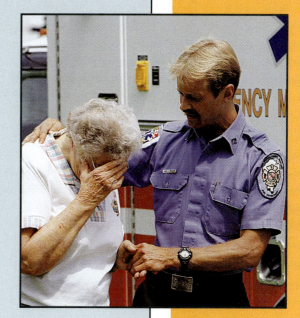

- Describe the assessment of central nervous system dysfunction in the elderly including cerebrovascular disease, dementia, Alzheimer's disease, and Parkinson's disease.
- Discuss the assessment of the elderly patient with gastrointestinal problems, including gastrointestinal bleeding and bowel obstruction.
- Discuss the normal and abnormal changes with age related to toxicology.
- Discuss the assessment and management of the elderly patient in response to environmental factors.
- Discuss the normal and abnormal changes of the musculoskeletal system with age.
- Discuss the unique assessment and management skills required to evaluate the elderly trauma patient.

Affective Objectives
As an EMT–Intermediate you should be able to do the following:
- Demonstrate and advocate appropriate interactions with the elderly.
- Recognize and appreciate the multiple impediments to physical and emotional well being in the elderly.

Psychomotor Objectives
As an EMT–Intermediate you should be able to do the following:
- Demonstrate the ability to assess a geriatric patient.
- Demonstrate the ability to apply assessment findings to the management plan for a geriatric patient.

INTRODUCTION

Although a significant proportion of medical resources is routinely applied to the geriatric population, some special needs are often overlooked or underserved. The percentage and size of the geriatric population in the United States continue to grow steadily (Table 35-1). This is largely due to improved access to health care, improved pharmacological tools for battling disease, and safer home and work environments.

The vast majority of the most critical patients that emergency medical services (EMS) typically encounters (those with cardiac disease, severe respiratory disease, or stroke) belong to the geriatric population (Figure 35-1). It is crucial that the EMT–Intermediate (EMT–I) recognize the unique influences that affect the elderly's (1) response to injury and disease, (2) psychosocial requirements and resources, and (3) physical barriers that inhibit maximum activity (Table 35-2).

Each culture in society is unique in their acceptance and treatment of the population that composes the geriatric age group. The social status and resources available and applied to the patient are derived from both societal and familial views of aging. The living environment can vary significantly. Many geriatric patients are able to function independently, residing in their own residence. It is not uncommon to encounter automobile drivers who are in their mid- to late nineties. There are numerous types of assisted living facilities that range from simply providing assistance with food or transportation to having multiple nursing, physical therapy, and pharmacy resources available to the patient 24 hours a day (Box 35-1).

As a patient requires additional assistance, options may include placement in a skilled nursing facility with

TABLE 35-1

Demographics of Aging

YEAR	POPULATION >65 YEARS (%)	POPULATION >85 YEARS (%)
1960	9.2	5.6
1990	12.5	9.7
2000(est.)	12.6	12.3
2020(est.)	16.5	12.1
2040(est.)	20.6	18.0

Day JC: Population projections in the United States, *Current Population Reports P25*, No 1130, Washington DC, US Government Printing Office, 1996.

constant nursing support or home health nursing services for either portions of the day or continuously.

COMMON PROBLEMS

Some of the most significant problems that members of our population face as they age involve difficulties with general mobility. Due to difficulties with ambulation, coordination, and strength, the incidence of falls is greatly increased. Although there can be many reasons for mobility difficulties, not being able to ambulate normally can have multiple consequences, including the following:

- Difficulty preparing or eating food with subsequent poor nutrition
- Difficulty with elimination
- Skin abrasions, injuries, and circulatory compromise from falling
- Additional orthopedic or intracranial injuries from falling
- Decreased medication compliance due to difficulties ambulating to where medications are stored

Aside from the physical effects on the patient who experiences decreased mobility, there are important psychological implications. The loss of independence may lead to episodes of depression, general loss of confidence in abilities, and concerns over feeling "old" in the eyes of society.

It is not uncommon for EMS providers to receive calls to assist an elderly member of their community who has fallen. After assisting these patients, they may desire no further EMS care and decline transportation to the hospital. It is important for the EMT–I to identify which patients have particular high risks for falls and subsequent additional injuries. Certainly any patient who has a history of falls should have the etiologic factors of the falls investigated. Geriatric patients who have central nervous system (CNS) disorders, including generalized weakness, impaired vision, dizziness, or cerebral vascular accidents, can also be at risk for falls.

Finally, never underestimate the potential side effects of medications the patient may be taking. There are

---

STREET WISE

The EMT–I will encounter patients that are living alone in homes or apartments. Some of these elderly patients may only be marginally getting by. The slightest challenge, either medically or socially, may incapacitate their "independence." They may require emergency social intervention in addition to medical care. Share any concerns with the hospital medical staff or local social service agencies.

HELPFUL HINT

- The vast majority of diseases that are experienced by the geriatric population are discussed in depth in other chapters. This chapter attempts to focus on the specific assessment and management skills needed to properly care for the elderly patient in general with or without specific medical problems.

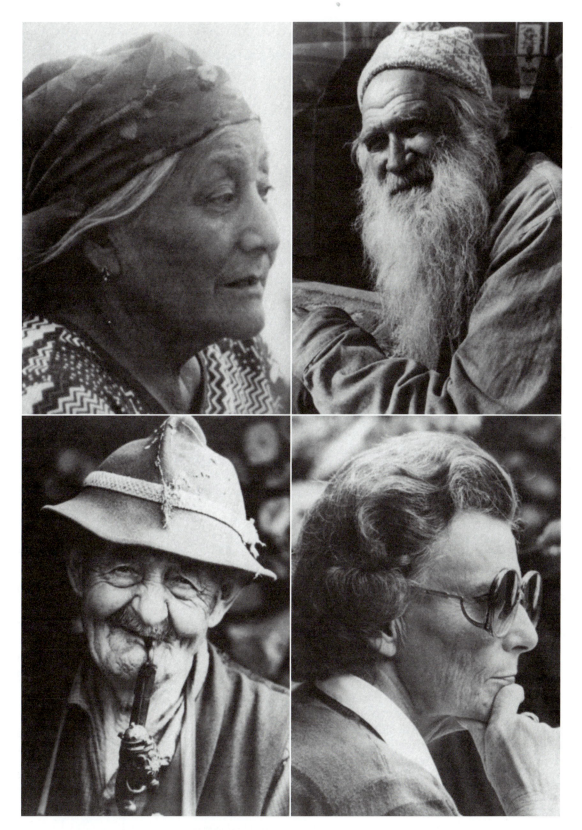

FIGURE 35-1 ▲ Faces of aging. (Rod Schmall from Ebersole P, Hess P: *Toward healthy aging: human needs and nursing response*, ed 5, St Louis, 1998, Mosby.)

TABLE 35-2

Leading Cause of Death among Persons Age 65 and Greater in 1995

CAUSE OF DEATH	NUMBER	ALL PERSONS >65 YEARS (%)
Heart disease	605,637	34.5
Neoplasm	384,186	21.9
CVA	139144	7.9
COPD	97,896	5.6
Pneumonia/infulenza	82,989	4.7
Diabetes mellitus	48,974	2.8
MVA	8,145	0.5
All other causes	386,249	22.0

Murphy S: Deaths: final for 1998, *National Vital Statistics Report* Vol 48, No 11, Hyattsville, Md, National Center for Health Statistics, 2000.
COPD, chronic obstructive pulmonary disease; *CVA,* cerebral vascular accident; *MVA,* motor vehicle accident (crash).

BOX 35-1

RESOURCES FOR ELDERS IN NEED

Emergency departments
Hospital social services
Government social service agencies
Local law enforcement
Local religious organizations
Community agencies (e.g., United Way)
Neighbors, local and distant family members

hundreds of over-the-counter and prescription medications that have effects on the CNS or may cause generalized weakness. Asking the patient if he or she has started any new medications or changed the dose or frequency of any medications may help clarify the cause of the fall.

Changes in Normal Sensation

VISION

As humans approach the age of 40 years, changes in vision become more common. The most significant changes include cataracts and glaucoma. **Cataracts** are opacities within the lens of the eyes, distorting and preventing light sensation. **Glaucoma** is the presence of an elevated intraocular pressure within the eye that can lead to vision loss. Many members of the older population also require the assistance of glasses which, if not present, can lead to impairment in their ability to recognize potential hazards, take medications, and prepare food.

HEARING

There is a measurable decay in hearing as the aging process progresses. Decreased hearing impairs the patient's ability to comprehend instructions and commands. It may also impair proper communications between the prehospital providers and the patient. Many patients experience extreme frustration when unable to adequately understand conversation directed to them.

The EMT–I should recognize that diminished hearing may be a significant barrier to proper communication.

SPEECH

Factors that can impair the patient's ability to properly conduct speech include CNS insults from strokes and anatomical derangements in the larynx or pharynx. Changes can occur in the quality of the patient's voice, rate of speech, fluency of speech, and even word retrieval. This may lead to impairment of the patient's ability to communicate past history, pain, physical complaints and questions (Figure 35-2).

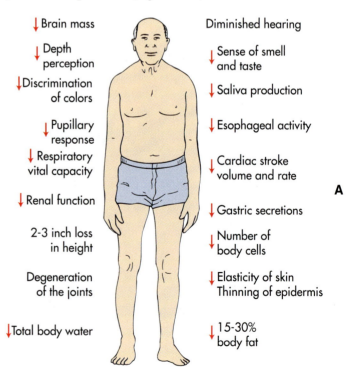

↓ Brain mass
↓ Depth perception
↓ Discrimination of colors
↓ Pupillary response
↓ Respiratory vital capacity
↓ Renal function
2-3 inch loss in height
Degeneration of the joints
↓ Total body water

Diminished hearing
↓ Sense of smell and taste
↓ Saliva production
↓ Esophageal activity
↓ Cardiac stroke volume and rate
↓ Gastric secretions
↓ Number of body cells
↓ Elasticity of skin Thinning of epidermis
↓ 15-30% body fat

A

FIGURE 35-2 ▲ **A, Changes related to aging.**
(A from National Association of Emergency Medical Technicians: *PHTLS: Basic and advanced prehospital trauma life support,* **ed 4, St Louis, 1999, Mosby.)**

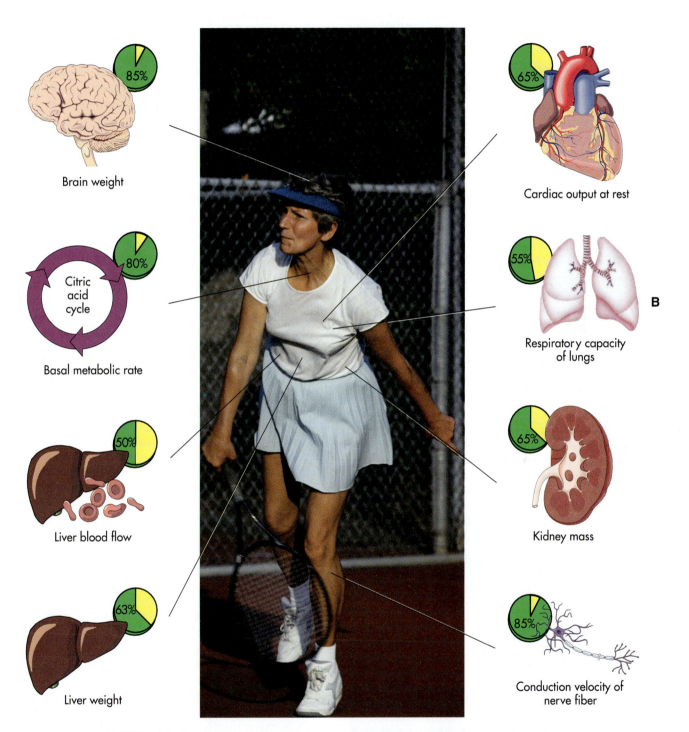

Brain weight

85%

Basal metabolic rate

Citric acid cycle

80%

Liver blood flow

50%

Liver weight

63%

Cardiac output at rest

65%

Respiratory capacity of lungs

55%

B

Kidney mass

65%

Conduction velocity of nerve fiber

85%

FIGURE 35-2, cont'd   ▲   **B,** Biological changes associated with maturity and aging. Insets show proportion of remaining function in the organs of a person in late adulthood compared to a 20-year-old person. (**B** from Thibodeau GA, Patton KT: *Structure and function of the body,* ed 11, St Louis, 2000, Mosby.)

PAIN PERCEPTION

Aside from the normal decline in pain perception with aging, a number of medical conditions, including **diabetes mellitus,** alter the patient's ability to perceive pain normally. This may lead patients to inadvertently injure themselves or not recognize the significance of an injury when it has occurred. The patient may not realize when a medical condition is worsening due to the decreased pain perception.

Problems With Continence and Elimination

Incontinence is the inability to prevent urination or bowel movements. In elderly patients, this can be a common source of embarrassment and may significantly reduce their ability to ambulate or have adequate social interactions. Incontinence can be due to a decrease in the typical bladder capacity or involuntary bladder contractions. Additionally, some medications can lead to changes in the patient's ability to control the bladder or bowels. Incontinence that is not cared for appropriately, leading to prolonged exposure to urinary or fecal matter on the skin, can lead to tissue irritation, excoriation, and even infection.

In contrast to incontinence problems, there are also significant complications from elimination difficulties in the elderly. Prostate gland enlargement can lead to urinary retention in men. In addition, urinary tract infections in men or women can lead to voiding difficulties. Acute or chronic renal failure will ultimately diminish the normal urine output over time.

Constipation in the elderly population can result from inadequate fluid intake, improper diet, or medications. Patients who are on chronic pain control medications typically are plagued with frequent bouts of constipation that even lead to bowel obstruction. Inflammatory disorders such as diverticulitis or malignancy such as colorectal cancer can lead to bowel elimination difficulties as well.

GENERAL ASSESSMENT

There are unique aspects in evaluating every geriatric patient. First of all, the EMT–I should display patience throughout all aspects of the examination. Changes in the patient's cognitive function may delay processing of questions or formulating a response to the EMT–I's inquires. The patient may take additional time performing measures such as removing clothing or ambulating.

A thorough psychosocial history should be obtained by the EMT–I. Often, elderly patients live alone, with little family or support network. The EMT–I's ability to properly gather this information is crucial because he or she may be the only health care provider who can objectively report the living conditions in the home environment for the patient. Factors that need to be assessed for every geriatric patient include the following:
- What is the patient's ability to provide for his or her own activities of daily living or self-care?
- What is the patient's support system? Does he or she live with family or other adults? Are there neighbors or other health care providers that are involved in providing assistance?
- What is the patient's normal level of activity each day?
- Is the patient compliant with medications? This includes whether the patient is able to get prescriptions filled.
- Does the patient have the physical dexterity to open prescription bottles or pick up small tablets?

Communicating With the Elderly Patient

The first step in effective communication with the elderly patient is recognizing that there may be barriers that can prohibit the patient from understanding the

EMT–I. Assist the patient with locating any hearing aids or eyeglasses, if needed. Ensuring adequate lighting during the assessment and treatment may help the patient feel more comfortable. As with any patient, ensure the person's dignity is preserved by respecting requests and making him a participant in his care.

> **STREET WISE** ✳
>
> It is not uncommon for the patient's chief complaint to be very different from the acute medical event that may be affecting him. Although it is important to understand the patient's expectations and desires, the EMT–I should not overlook any apparent difficulties the patient may be experiencing.

Physical Examination

The physical examination begins as the EMT–I approaches the patient. Visual clues as to the patient's respiratory status, overall mental status, and level of distress can be observed. After a rapid initial assessment ensures the airway is patent, ventilation and breathing are adequate, and the patient has adequate pulses, then a set of vital signs should be taken and recorded. A more focused and detailed examination should then be undertaken, which includes a head to toe examination.

1. *Neurologic*—The patient should be assessed for level of alertness, interactiveness, or the presence of confusion. General symmetric muscle strength should also be noted.
2. *Head, Eyes, Ears, Nose, Neck, and Throat (HEENNT)*
   - *Head*—Examination should include swelling (cephalohematoma), bleeding, bruising, and evidence of scars from recent cranial surgery. Also look for facial asymmetry.
   - *Eyes*—Evaluate pupillary response to light stimulation and gross visual acuity. This can be accomplished by asking the patient if objects appear blurry or normal.
   - *Ears*—Identify any bleeding or drainage. This may indicate a skull fracture.
   - *Nose*—It is important to note nasal obstruction or congestion, especially if oxygen is administered by nasal canula.
   - *Neck*—The patient should be evaluated for the presence or absence of jugular venous distention (JVD), which can indicate congestive heart failure and other cardiac problems.
   - *Throat*—Note the presence of foreign bodies in the patient's oropharynx, including dentures. Always utilize this step to further evaluation the integrity of the patient's airway.
3. *Pulmonary*—Lung sounds should be thoroughly assessed, listening throughout full respiratory cycles. The absence of rales, wheezes, or rhonchi does not necessarily imply clear breath sounds. It is critical that the EMT–I make the distinction between normal lung sounds and the absence of lung sounds (as is frequently encountered in patients with severe chronic obstructive pulmonary disease [COPD]).

> **STREET WISE** ✳
>
> Although asymmetric pupils immediately raise concern in patient evaluation, the cause may be very benign. A small percentage of the normal population typically has asymmetric pupils. Another cause of nonreactive pupils may be a prosthetic eye. Ocular diseases such as glaucoma or cataract surgery may cause the pupil to react in an unexpected fashion. The EMT–I should inquire if the patient had previously noticed or been told that their pupils were abnormal.

> **STREET WISE** ✳
>
> Many patients with COPD are very knowledgeable about the disease. These patients can provide helpful information on what types of therapies are beneficial.
>
> Key questions to ask the elderly patient in acute respiratory distress:
> - Do you have a history of asthma, COPD/ emphysema, congestive heart failure (CHF), or similar illnesses?
> - Are you normally on home oxygen? How many liters (L) per minute?
> - What therapies have you tried since becoming ill? Have they helped?
> - Have you been intubated before? How long ago?
>
> *Asking these questions will allow the EMT–I to gauge the severity of the patients illness, anticipated response to prehospital therapy, and plan for more advanced interventions if the patient declines rapidly.*

4. *Cardiac*—The cardiac evaluation in the geriatric patient in the prehospital setting consists of taking serial blood pressure and pulses. If there is any concern over aortic aneurysms, or dissection, the pulses and blood pressure should be taken in both upper and lower extremities.

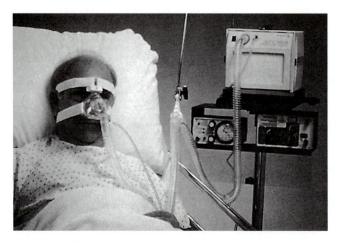

FIGURE 35-3 ▲ Patient wearing nose mask for noninvasive support with pressure support ventilation (BIPAP). (Respironics, Inc.)

CLINICAL NOTES

Some patients with advanced COPD or conditions such as severe sleep apnea may require more aggressive ventilatory therapy constantly or while sleeping (Figure 35-3). These machines function similar to a ventilatory by providing positive airway pressure throughout portions or all of ventilation. These devices fit tightly over the patient's nose alone or mouth and nose. They typically also provide supplemental oxygen and can be used by the patient during transport if the device is portable. Additional oxygen may be delivered by placing the patient on a nasal cannula before the mask if placed by the patient. If the patient is unable to participate in wearing the mask due to diminished neurological status, then the BIPAP/CPAP therapy should be abandoned, and more aggressive therapy with bag-valve-mask ventilation or endotracheal intubation should be initiated.

CLINICAL NOTES

Many patients who have hypertension or other heart disease may be placed on medications that limit the heart's ability to produce the typical physiological responses of tachycardia when illness, injury, or shock are present.

5. *Abdomen*—The abdomen should be assessed for generalized tenderness, pulsating masses, or distention. It may be difficult for prehospital providers to auscultate for bowel sounds due to high levels of ambient noise heard in the prehospital setting. The proper examination for bowel sounds can be time consuming and generally will not alter prehospital therapy.

6. *Extremities*—There should be a general assessment for any obvious deformity, fracture, bruising, or abrasions. It should be noted whether the patient has the ability to walk, or move all extremities.

Ideally, patients would present with the classic signs and symptoms of their medical illnesses. Although there are variances throughout the population, the EMT–I will often encounter elderly patients who have acute medical illnesses or injuries that may not display the expected signs or symptoms of their insult. The following factors may affect this:

- Other medical illnesses the patient may perceive as more crucial or worrisome
- Patient misinterpretation of the illness due to the absence of the classic signs and symptoms
- Changes in the patient's ability to properly sense pain or discomfort
- Medications that may affect the patient's response to pain, or normal physiological response to pain or injury

CLINICAL NOTES

Proper assessment is an ongoing, cyclical, process that continues to provide monitoring of the patient, including vital signs, ventilation, pain, and neurological status. Assessment should never be limited to a single "snapshot" of the patient. Acute neurological or cardiac events can cause the patient to deteriorate rapidly. Constant monitoring of the patient allows the EMT–I to anticipate critical changes and prepare the appropriate therapy.

GENERAL MANAGEMENT

Airway and Ventilation

Proper airway management in the elderly essentially follows typical adult airway management. Special considerations include the following:

- Foreign bodies in the oropharynx, dentures or partial dentures, may impair intubation attempts.
- Adequate bag-valve-mask ventilation of patients may be difficult in certain patients once dentures are removed. Consideration may be needed to replace the dentures to allow adequate ventilation.
- Patients experiencing acute neurological events may lose their ability to adequately protect their own airway. Aspiration can cause significant respiratory compromise.

Circulation

Special considerations in the geriatric population in regard to circulatory support include the following:

- *Intravenous (IV) access*—Many patients in the elderly population have small or friable veins. This may make venipuncture and IV access difficult.
- *IV fluid administration*—Caution should be used in the quantity of IV fluid administered to patients who have any history of cardiac disease, especially CHF. This may precipitate acute respiratory failure and require additional ventilatory support. Monitor the patient for increased rales, respiratory effort, tachypnea, and difficulty with speaking may assist the EMT–I in determining that additional IV fluids should be withheld.

STREET WISE

Closely monitor the flow (drip) rate of any intravenous fluids that a patient may be receiving. Flow control devices can be unexpectedly moved during patient care and transportation causing unintended administration of a fluid bolus. This can worsen conditions such as CHF.

Pharmacological Intervention

The following special considerations must be made any time an elderly patient is given medications:

- *Sensitivity*—The normal adult physiological process of drug metabolism slows as the body ages. In addition, there are other drugs that may compete with the normal metabolic process. Drugs that are typically broken down rapidly in a normal healthy adult may have significantly prolonged degradation and

---

CLINICAL NOTES

Lidocaine is a cardiac agent typically administered to patients experiencing ventricular irritability with ventricular tachycardia, ventricular fibrillation, or frequent premature ventricular contractions. The metabolism of lidocaine by the liver is significantly reduced in the elderly population, and a standard adult dose may have greater and potentially more toxic effects. This is the reason why lidocaine doses are typically reduced in the elderly.

---

therefore may exhibit prolonged length of action and effect (Table 35-3).

- *Side effects*—Elderly patients typically experience more adverse reactions to prescription medications than younger patients. This may result from physiological changes or interactions with other medications.

Transport Considerations

Moving the elderly patient may not be as simple as asking him or her to sit on the ambulance cot. The geriatric patient may have significant problems with joints or the spine. This may lead to difficulty sitting on a cot in a normal position. Every effort should be made to transport the patient in the position of most comfort. As the human body ages, bone density changes, and these patients are more prone to fracture, sometimes with only trivial force. In addition, changes in body mass and body fat composition may cause tissue injury by how the patient is positioned during transport.

TABLE 35-3

Drugs with Greater or Prolonged Effects due to Reduced Metabolism or Elimination in the Elderly

DRUG	CLASS
Ibuprofen	Analgesics/antiinflammatory
Morphine	Analgesics
Meperidine	Analgesics
Diltiazem	Cardiovascular agent
Lidocaine	Cardiovascular agent
Propranolol	Cardiovascular agent
Verapamil	Cardiovascular agent
Furosemide	Diuretic
Diazepam	Psychoactive

SPECIFIC SYSTEM ASSESSMENT AND INTERVENTION

Respiratory System

With the aging process, there are significant changes in the patient's respiratory status. There is decreased lung function due to chronic exposure to pollutants in the atmosphere, decreased efficiency in the alveolar capillary exchange, decreased tone of the respiratory muscles, and changes in the CNS's respiratory center. The common causes of pulmonary diseases in the elderly include pneumonia, pulmonary embolism, and obstructive lung disease.

PNEUMONIA

Pneumonia is a leading cause of death in the elderly population. Many of these patients have co-morbid diseases such as stroke, malignancy, or other metabolic derangements that inhibit the body's normal response to infection.

PULMONARY EMBOLISM

Classically pulmonary embolism (blood clot in the pulmonary vasculature) presents with acute onset of shortness of breath that may have associated chest pain and tachycardia. If the blood clot is large enough, occluding a significant portion of blood flow through the lungs back to the heart, then syncope, sudden hypotension, and even cardiac arrest can occur. Non-fatal pulmonary embolisms may be very difficult to diagnose due to the fact that tachypnea may be the only physical finding. This may be accompanied by anxiety and overt respiratory distress. Examination will reveal a patient who may be mild to moderately tachypneic and have an elevated pulse rate. Pulse oximetry may also reveal the patient to be hypoxic.

CLINICAL NOTES

Deep venous thrombosis (DVT) occurs when blood clots in larger veins. The most common site for DVTs are in the upper legs, but they can also occur in the upper arms. These blood clots can dislodge and travel through the vena cava to the right side of the heart and then become lodged in the pulmonary vasculature as a pulmonary embolism. Patients with symptoms of a pulmonary embolism may also complain of recent extremity pain or swelling.

OBSTRUCTIVE LUNG DISEASE

Patients who have a history of chronic bronchitis, emphysema, or COPD also have recurrent exacerbations requiring acute EMS intervention. Assessment of these patients typically reveals tachypnea, shallow respirations, and diffuse wheezing.

CLINICAL NOTES

Patients with advanced obstructive lung disease can have such severe disease that airflow is restricted to a significant degree, and wheezing may not be heard. It is important for the EMT–I to discriminate between normal breath sounds and the absence of breath sounds such as those associated with severe COPD. Management of these patients involves transporting in a position of comfort, providing IV line, bronchodilator therapy and oxygen support. If the patient is hypoxic, oxygen should be administered at high flow rates. Local medical control may have specific guidelines for the rate of oxygen administration in COPD patients.

ASSESSMENT OF PATIENTS WITH RESPIRATORY DISORDERS

In evaluating patients with respiratory difficulties, there are specific questions that should be asked:
- Does the patient have any history of prior respiratory difficulties, including pneumonia, chronic bronchitis, COPD, or pulmonary embolism? Is there home oxygen use, and has the patient been compliant?
- Does the patient take any medications for chronic lung disease, including metered dose inhalers or steroids?

Physical examination of these patients begins with observing the general respiratory effort as the EMT–I approaches the patient. Additional clinical indicators can be discovered by evaluating the respiratory rate, effort of respirations, retractions, or wheezing.

Breath sounds, by themselves, are not solely reliable for evaluating overall respiratory status. Evaluating the patient's whole respiratory effort, mental status, and pulse oximetry in combination will help the EMT–I properly estimate the patient's pulmonary status.

Cardiovascular System

Geriatric patients are at higher risk for cardiac disease. A high percentage of EMS calls relate to patients being evaluated for chest pain or palpitations. As individuals age, arteries tend to become more rigid. There is decreased peripheral resistance throughout the whole vascular system, which ultimately causes reduced blood flow to all organs. Patients with hypertension can further have cardiac and vascular damage due to the effects of the elevated blood pressure.

ASSESSMENT OF CARDIAC PATIENT

When evaluating elderly patients for acute illnesses it is important to place the acute events in a frame of reference compared to the normal level of activity. This can be accomplished by asking the following questions:

- What is the patient's general level of physical activity? Has the patient experienced any discomfort, dyspnea, or increasing fatigue in the recent past?
- Has there recently been any change in the patient's diet? The EMT–I should recognize that meals high in salt content may exacerbate CHF.
- What medication is the patient taking? This may help guide the EMT–I to recognize that the patient is taking medications for the treatment of angina or high blood pressure. Inquiries should also be made regarding any newly prescribed medications, any alterations in regular medication pattern, and compliance with prescribed medication regimen.
- Specific questions regarding any chest pain, length of chest pain, nature, and radiation of chest pain should be obtained.
- Does the patient experience any increased respiratory difficulties at nighttime? Patients with gradually

worsening CHF may experience orthopnea or shortness of breath when they lie flat, due to the redistribution of fluids in the lungs when the patient is no longer upright.
- Has the patient experienced any palpitations, rapid heartbeats, or skipped beats?

PHYSICAL EXAMINATION OF THE CARDIAC PATIENT

As with any patient, the geriatric cardiac patient should receive a full head-to-toe assessment. This includes a rapid initial assessment, followed by vital signs and then a more focused and detailed examination. Of particular note, the EMT–I should evaluate the following:

- Hypertension with assessment of orthostatic vital signs when indicated.
- Dependent edema in the patient's legs or sacral area.
- Examination for strength and regularity of pulses in all extremities.
- Signs of dehydration, including tachycardia, low blood pressure, tenting of the skin, poor skin turgor, dry lips and mucous membranes, or tachycardia.

MANAGEMENT OF THE CARDIAC PATIENT

Proper management of patients experiencing cardiovascular disorders include placing the patient in a position of comfort, establishing an IV life line, administering oxygen based on the patient's respiratory requirements, and performing ongoing cardiac monitoring en route to the hospital. Administration of oral nitroglycerin may be indicated in patients with chest pain and an acceptable blood pressure.

Patients who have irregular heartbeats, or cardiac dysrhythmias, must be continually monitored while being transported. An automated external defibrillator, or manual defibrillator with proper personnel, should be available to the patient at all times.

Nervous System

One of the most difficult organ systems to evaluate in any patient, and even more so in the elderly, is the CNS. Geriatric patients are at particular risk for suffering devastating events such as hemorrhagic stroke, embolic **stroke**, or metastatic brain disease. They may also suffer from head injuries from falls or trauma.

In general, cognitive functions decline in advancing years because of a combination of dysfunction of sensory organs, as well as decreased stimulus processing within the brain. These manifest as difficulties with recent memory, general psychomotor slowing of activities, increased forgetfulness, and a delayed reaction time.

Stroke • Sudden loss of neurological function due to intracranial hemorrhage or embolism.

STREET WISE

A new area that the EMT–I must investigate is the use of herbal medications. These preparations are typically purchased over the counter and do not require prescriptions. They have tremendous variability in their composition and physiological effects on the body. Patients may be reluctant to divulge that they are using herbal medications, as some patients feel they are attempting self-therapy without the guidance of their physician.

ASSESSMENT OF THE NERVOUS SYSTEM

Proper neurological assessment of the geriatric patient is best conducted in a systematic and unhurried fashion. Some key neurological findings are subtle and can be missed if the EMT–I rushes through the examination. Key components of the history of present illness include the following:

- Determine when the current neurological event started. If the patient is unable to verbalize the exact time of symptom onset, family members may be able to provide the time at which the patient was last seen acting with normal mentation. Also determine if the onset of the patient's symptoms was gradual (over days or weeks) or acute (over minutes or hours).
- Maintain a calm demeanor and do not appear rushed.
- Speak clearly and directly to the patient with very direct questions or commands.
- Allow the patient time to formulate answers and respond to questions.

HELPFUL HINT

- It is extremely important to try and establish the patient's normal pattern of activity and ability to care for himself. Family members can be very important in relaying information regarding these changes.

PHYSICAL EXAMINATION OF THE NEUROLOGICAL PATIENT

Patients who are the victims of an acute neurological event should have a rapid and thorough assessment. The neurological examination should consist of the following:

- Evaluation of general neurological level of consciousness (AVPU)
- Observation of general motor tone and ability to ambulate or move independently
- Observation for any improvement or deterioration and any abnormalities noted on initial assessment

The Cincinnati Prehospital Stroke Scale is another tool that is useful in the rapid evaluation of an acute stroke patient (Box 35-2).

MANAGEMENT OF THE NEUROLOGICAL PATIENT

Prehospital management of most acute neurological events is essentially limited to supportive care. Patients should be transported in a position of comfort, with the head elevated approximately 30 degrees on the cot. If the patient is a victim of trauma or there is a concern for cervical spine injury, the patient should be fully supine with cervical spine immobilization and a long backboard. The patient should be placed on oxygen and if available, cardiac monitoring should be performed.

BOX 35-2

CINCINNATI PREHOSPITAL STROKE SCALE

FACIAL DROOP
Ask patient to smile or show their teeth.
Normal: Both sides of face move equally well.
Abnormal: One side of face does not move as well as other.

ARM DRIFT
Ask patient to close eyes and hold both arms out.
Normal: Both arms move the same or both arms do not move at all.
Abnormal: One arm does not move or one arm drifts down compared to the other.

SPEECH
Ask patient to say, "You can't teach an old dog new tricks."
Normal: Patient uses correct words with no slurring.
Abnormal: Patient slurs words, uses inappropriate words, or is unable to speak.

CLINICAL NOTES

Newer therapies are available for the treatment of patients suffering from acute stroke. These therapies involve administration of thrombolytic, or clot-busting, medications to the patient within a specific time frame. The EMT–I should recognize patients who are suffering from acute stroke and provide rapid assessment and transportation to a hospital that can care for acute stroke victims. The critical information required when considering thrombolytic therapy for stroke patients require the EMT–Is' assistance in answering. These include the following:

- At what time, specifically, did the symptoms start? If the patient does not know what time the symptoms started, what time was the patient last observed acting normally?
- Has the patient been a victim of any recent falls or trauma?
- Does the patient have a history of hypertension or any known bleeding disorders?
- Has the patient had any recent surgery?

It is critical that the EMT–I provide constant reevaluation of the patient's neurological status. In general, acute neurological events such as hemorrhage, embolic stroke, or head injury from trauma, have a rapidly progressing course that may ultimately compromise the patient's airway or cardiovascular system.

Endocrine System

DIABETES

Approximately 20% of the geriatric population has diabetes mellitus. In addition, another 20%, or 40% have some derangement or impairment of normal glucose metabolism and glucose tolerance. It is important to recognize that some geriatric patients may have diabetes and experience hyperglycemia without being aware of the disease. In addition, patients with known diabetes who take insulin or other hypoglycemic agents may have episodes of hypoglycemia due to difficulty taking their medications or difficulties obtaining proper food intake after taking their medications.

Gastrointestinal System

Elderly patients frequently voice complaints that involve the gastrointestinal system. Nausea, vomiting, diarrhea, constipation, or abdominal pain can all originate within the gastrointestinal system but may also be secondary to other medical illnesses, physiological conditions, or medications.

Common gastrointestinal disorders in the elderly include the following:
- *Nausea*—This may be due to common gastrointestinal disorders that any adult can experience. Elderly patients have decreased gastric motility, which may lead to increased frequency of nausea. It is important to recognize that nausea may be a sign to a more serious medical condition such as acute myocardial infarction or early signs of diabetic ketoacidosis. Many elderly patients take numerous medications that produce a side effect of nausea.
- **Hiatal hernia**—Hiatal hernia is the protrusion of a portion of the stomach from its normal position in the abdomen through the diaphragm. Symptoms of a hiatal hernia typically include epigastric or lower thoracic discomfort and complaints of acid reflux or dyspepsia. It is estimated that approximately 40% of the population has hiatal hernias, but most people have no symptoms.
- **Gastrointestinal hemorrhage**—Gastrointestinal bleeding can come from a number of sources. Bleeding within the stomach itself can come from duodenal or peptic ulcers. Bleeding from the lower gastrointestinal system may be related to infection, polyps, vascular malformations, or malignancy. Patients who give any history of hematemesis (blood noted within the vomitus) or patients complaining of bright-red blood noted on bowel movements or dark, tarry bowel movements (melena) should receive a thorough examination at a hospital.
- **Bowel obstruction**—This can be caused by abdominal wall hernias, primary or metastatic tumors, constipation, postsurgical adhesions, and even infections. Symptoms typically include abdominal cramping that is initially intermittent but gradually

becomes constant and severe. Bowel obstructions are usually accompanied by vomiting and abdominal distention.

Patients can have gastrointestinal bleeding without any symptoms, which can lead to profound anemia. These patients should have orthostatic vital signs, a thorough assessment, and an IV line established. Risk factors for gastrointestinal bleeding include frequent alcohol consumption, tobacco use, and use of non-steroidal antiinflammatory medication. A particular bacterium, *H. pylori,* has been identified as also contributing to the development of peptic ulcer disease.

ASSESSMENT OF PATIENTS WITH GASTROINTESTINAL DISORDERS

Following the initial assessment and vital signs, the focused and detailed examination should be performed. Specific areas that should be assessed include the following:

- General hydration of the patient
- Abdominal examination consisting of identifying areas of tenderness and observing for abdominal distention
- Management primarily consists of supportive care, transporting in a position of comfort, and establishing an IV line. Oxygen therapy may be beneficial if there is any suspicion that the patient may be having a myocardial infarction or is in any distress.

Central Nervous System

STROKE

Strokes are also referred to as **cerebral vascular accidents (CVAs) or brain attacks.** Patients experiencing an acute stroke can exhibit a wide spectrum of neurological findings. These may include weakness or numbness in the extremities, acute mental status changes, difficulty swallowing, or difficulty speaking. The EMT–I should be patient while interacting with the stroke victim, since speech comprehension and speech processing may take longer than in healthy patients.

TRANSIENT ISCHEMIC ATTACKS

Transient ischemic attacks (TIAs) are acute neurological deficits that resolve over time. Both stroke and TIAs are discussed at length in Chapter 27.

✖ **Delirium** • Organic brain dysfunction resulting in confusion, abnormal behavior, or hallucinations.

✖ **Dementia** • Progressive loss of intellectual function.

DELIRIUM

Delirium consists primarily of organic brain dysfunction and will present with patients experiencing confusion, abnormal behavior, or hallucinations. It can be caused by many factors, including electrolyte derange-

ments, infections, fever, medications, and even tumors. Drugs of abuse and alcohol ingestion can also lead to delirium. Many causes of acute delirium are reversible but may be challenging to identify clearly. If uncorrected, the insulting factors in the acute delirium patient may lead to more permanent neurological changes.

ASSESSMENT OF THE DELIRIUM PATIENT

A thorough past medical history must be obtained to assist in identifying a chronic medical condition that may contribute to the acute delirium. The medical history evaluation should focus on the patient's general activity over the previous few days, food and fluid intake, changes in medication, and consumption of intoxicants. Family members should be asked about the patient's general affect and behavior over the previous 24 to 48 hours.

DEMENTIA

A significant portion of the aging population develops dementia with age. Up to 60% to 80% of the nursing home patients have some type of dementia in addition to other medical/physical conditions. **Dementia** is a progressive loss of intellectual function. Memory, reasoning, and orientation to time, location, and even self can all be affected. For the most part, dementia is considered irreversible and typically has a progressive course. The patient becomes more and more dependent on other caretakers for safety and general activities of daily living. Dementia can be caused by large strokes, multiple smaller strokes, genetic influences, infections, or Alzheimer's disease.

ASSESSMENT OF THE DEMENTIA PATIENT

The dementia patient is generally noted to be disoriented, have difficulty maintaining attention, and may exhibit aphasia or confused speech. It is not uncommon for these patients to be exhibiting auditory or visual hallucinations as well.

> ● **HELPFUL HINT**
> - Dementia is loss of memory and intellectual function and typically not reversible. Delerium is unusual behavior, hallucinations, or confusion that may be due to a reversible medical condition.

✖ **Alzheimer's Disease** • Form of dementia with progressive loss of memory

ALZHEIMER'S DISEASE

It is estimated that over four million Americans have **Alzheimer's disease,** which represents approximately 65% of all the dementias in the elderly population. Alzheimer's disease is a progressive loss of cognitive function and has been associated with anatomical changes within the cerebral cortex. The disease typically has a subtle onset, with patients noticing diminished performance in normal tasks. Memory loss, episodes of depression, fear and anxiety may occur. Although research into Alzheimer's disease is intense, the current therapy is fairly limited. EMS should provide supportive care, assessment for other acute medical or traumatic conditions, and transportation to the hospital.

Parkinson's Disease ● Degenerative nervous system disorder resulting in tremor and muscle rigidity.

PARKINSON'S DISEASE

Parkinson's disease is a slowly progressing degenerative disorder of the nervous system. It is typically dis-

tinguished by a tremor at rest, sluggish initiation of movements, and muscle rigidity. It affects 1 in 250 people over age 40 years and approximately 1 in 100 people over age 65 years. The primary site of insult is an area of the brain known as the basal ganglia, which helps to initiate actions such as lifting an arm and other movements. It also coordinates changes in posture. In Parkinson's disease, cells within the basal ganglia degenerate. In some cases the cause of Parkinson's disease may be infection or insults from drugs or toxins. Largely though, the cause of Parkinson's disease in most patients is never identified.

Prehospital treatment of the Parkinson's disease patient involves a general assessment and then supportive care. Specific assessment for other medical conditions or acute injury should be completed.

SPECIAL CONSIDERATIONS
Toxicology in the Elderly

On average, the elderly patient may take four to five prescription medications routinely, as well as numerous over-the-counter medications. Not only is the patient at risk from drug interactions, but there are physiological changes within the body that place the patient in jeopardy. These include decreased elimination due to decreased kidney function, decreased metabolism in the liver, or inhibition from other drugs.

There may be alterations in gastrointestinal absorption due to hypomotility within the bowel.

For any given drug, geriatric patients are typically more likely to have more significant side effects from the medication compared with the younger population. This is especially true with side effects involving the CNS.

Substance Abuse

Substance abuse in the elderly can occur. There are significant psychological changes and stresses that may contribute to this. Many older patients suffer from depression or anxiety and may turn to intoxicants for some form of comfort. It is important to note that smaller amounts of intoxicants may be responsible for significant levels of impairment in the geriatric patient.

Signs of substance abuse may be subtle and can include mood swings, bouts of depression, anger, episodes of confusion, hallucinations, or falls. The family should be questioned regarding changes in the patient's general affect and behavior, as well as access to medications. It should be noted that the EMT–I should briefly scan the patient's home to identify the number of medication bottles and types of substances the patient may be using. This information should be related to the hospital and may be very useful to the health care team.

Environmental Emergencies in the Elderly

The geriatric patient is very sensitive to changes in temperature. Many patients lack adequate financial resources to properly heat or cool their residences and can suffer from environmental insults. In addition, changes in CNS function place the patient at further risk. Patients with dementia or delirium may wander outside in the colder climates without adequate thermal protection. These patients may have difficulty remembering where they live and getting back into a warm environment. Hyperthermia can result from inadequate fluid intake and high ambient temperatures. The elderly population represents the vast majority of fatalities that occur during heat waves. Ensuring that elderly patients have adequate fluid access, ventilation, and access to climate-controlled temperatures can help avoid untoward consequences. There are additional causes of hyperthermia in the elderly that may be seen in response to infection, brain injury, or medication use. In general, strategies for preventing hyperthermia or hypothermia center on a proper social support structure. Patients should be in a safe environment and have proper supervision adequate to their level of neurological derangement and risk of injury.

Trauma

ORTHOPEDIC INJURIES

Osteoporosis, or a loss of calcium in the bone, contributes to a significant number of orthopedic fractures in the elderly. Patients can fracture a long bone, spinal bone, or pelvis with significantly less energy compared with a normal healthy adult. Hip fractures typically are the most common orthopedic condition encountered in the elderly population. It can happen simply from falling from a standing position. In some patients who have limited mobility, osteoporosis can be advanced, and fractures can occur with only trivial manipulation.

CARDIAC CONSIDERATIONS

In general, most elderly patient's cardiac function and cardiac output are reduced. This leads to a decreased compensatory mechanism when shock or other blood loss occurs. In addition, many elderly patients are on cardiac medications that may limit the heart's ability to mount the normal cardiac response to maintain adequate organ perfusion following a traumatic insult.

HEAD INJURIES

Generalized cerebral atrophy (loss of brain tissue) causes the brain to be more mobile within the skull (Figure 35-4). Bridging blood vessels between the brain and the skull can have additional tension during injury, leading to intracranial bleeding. In particular, subdural hematomas are common after blunt head injury. Physical signs and symptoms may be subtle and even absent initially but can gradually develop over time. Patients with a progressively deteriorating level of consciousness, agitation, confusion, or focal neurological findings after trauma should be considered to

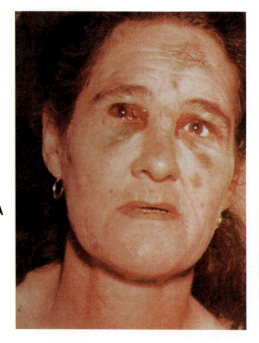

A

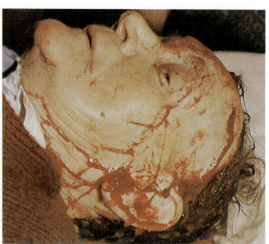

B

FIGURE 35-4 ▲ Scalp wounds can cause significant hemorrhage. (From London PS: *Colour atlas of diagnosis after recent injury*, London, 1990, Wolfe Publications Ltd.)

have an intracranial hemorrhage and be cared for appropriately.

BURNS

Serious burns can cause significant mortality in the elderly population. Preexisting diseases such as diabetes mellitus, lung disease, or malignancy can make it very difficult for the body to tolerate and ultimately heal from a severe burn. Elderly burn patients are at specific risk for infection from the burn and may have a prolonged hospitalization while attempting to recover. There are additional stresses placed on the patient's heart during an acute burn that may place the patient at additional risk for a myocardial infarction as a secondary component of the injury.

ASSESSMENT OF THE ELDERLY TRAUMA PATIENT

Any elderly patient who is "found down" should be assessed for the possibility of traumatic injury. The EMT–I should realize that falls from standing or even from a bed can produce significant trauma in this population. The initial assessment should be completed rapidly, followed by a set of vital signs and then a thorough head-to-toe trauma assessment and focused examination. Steps should be taken to maintain proper cervical spine stabilization throughout the assessment. Oxygen should be quickly applied to the patient and consideration for establishing an intravenous access should be made. The patient must have serial evaluations and repeat vital signs to assess for deterioration in condition. Additional management includes the following:

1. *Immobilization*—Although many of these patients will require cervical and long board immobilization, previous neurological injuries or orthopedic conditions may prohibit the patient from lying completely flat. Supporting the patient by placing pads, sheets or blankets in void areas between the patient and board may help provide some immobilization while also providing some comfort to the patient. These patients are at particular risk for early decubital ulcer formation from prolonged exposure to unpadded long spinal boards. Every attempt should be made to provide some padding before placing the patient on the board (Figure 35-5).

2. *Airway*—High-flow oxygen via nonrebreather mask should be placed on all geriatric trauma patients. Assessment of the airway for foreign bodies, particularly dentures or partial dentures, should be done early in the evaluation. If the patient has inadequate ventilatory effort, then the EMT–I should assist the ventilations with a bag-valve-mask device.

3. *IV access*—IV lines should be considered. It is critical to closely monitor the volume of IV fluids administered because certain cardiac conditions, especially CHF, can deteriorate with excess fluid administration.

4. *Geriatric abuse*—As mentioned earlier, it can be difficult for some family members or caretakers to provide 24-hour-per-day care for their elderly patients. This may invoke periods of rage, anger, or hostility that are directed at the elderly person. Every effort should be made while on scene to evaluate the social and physical conditions in which the patient lives. Additional clues that abuse may be occurring may include the following:
   - Frequent EMS calls for falls or injuries
   - Multiple orthopedic injuries from trivial falls
   - Multiple areas of bruising in various stages of healing
   - Evidence of burns or other scars in various stages of healing

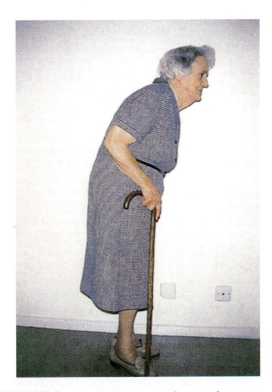

FIGURE 35-5 ▲ Kyphosis, an abnormal curvature of the spine, requires special padding and support during transport. (From National Association of Emergency Medical Technicians: *PHTLS: Basic and advanced prehospital trauma life support,* ed 4, St Louis, 1999, Mosby.)

5. *Neglect*—Aside from direct physical injury, abuse can also occur in the form of neglect:

- Lack of provision of necessary water, fluid, and food
- Lack of providing necessary medications
- Lack of proper hygiene, especially bathing the patient after episodes of incontinence.
- Failure to properly assist the patient with elimination

If the EMT–I suspects any neglect or physical abuse, he or she should inform the hospital staff on the patient's arrival. If for some reason, the patient is not transported to a hospital, then local law enforcement officials should be notified and proper social service agencies should be contacted. In some areas, there are specific laws addressing the mandatory reporting of elder abuse. The EMT–I should become familiar with any policies in their area that pertain to this important matter.

CASE HISTORY FOLLOW-UP ■■■

During their assessment of the patient EMT–Is Valencia and Travis determine there are many factors in the patient's physical environment that are acting as barriers to proper medical care. His current medical crisis limits his ability to walk. Physically moving around a room to take medications or prepare food is exhausting for him. It is nearly impossible for him to navigate the three flights of stairs required to get to the parking lot and his car.

EMT–I Valencia remembers being told by her instructor that she is the eyes and ears of the physician who will ultimately be responsible for the patient. She knows that valuable insight to the patient's ability to care for himself can be gathered by noticing the living conditions, general cleanliness, and access to medications. This patient's medications are essentially in a state of disarray, with many bottles empty and scattered. Also important is the fact that the patient has medications from many hospitals and physicians; this may indicate a lack of routine health care with a primary care provider.

Both EMT–Is recognize this patient is exhibiting the classic signs and symptoms of CHF: shortness of breath, tachypnea, rales, lower extremity edema, and JVD. They treat the patient by placing him placing into a position of comfort, applying oxygen by high-flow nonrebreather mask, establishing an IV line, and providing cardiac monitoring. The EMT–Is initiate diuretic therapy with furosemide and administer sublingual nitroglycerin to promote vasodilatation. They then promptly transport the patient to the hospital, recognizing that his condition may deteriorate rapidly, possibly ventilatory assistance by bag-valve-mask device.

SUMMARY

- The vast majority of critical patients encountered by EMS will be part of the geriatric population.
- Advanced heart disease, myocardial infarction, emphysema, and stroke all require the EMT–I to provide a thorough assessment and proper interventions.
- There are effects on all body systems as humans age.
- Normal changes in the body's physiology and CNS place the patient at risk from falls and dangerous side effects of medications.
- The EMT–I must recognize the potential for communication barriers due to hearing loss, speech recognition, and difficulties talking due to pulmonary or CNS insults.
- New therapies for the treatment of acute stroke require the accurate determination of onset of symptoms and rapid transportation to a hospital that can provide therapy.
- Elder abuse and neglect are growing problems that oblige the EMT–I to assume the role of patient advocate and report any concerns to the Emergency Department staff or local authorities.

ASSESSMENT-BASED MANAGEMENT

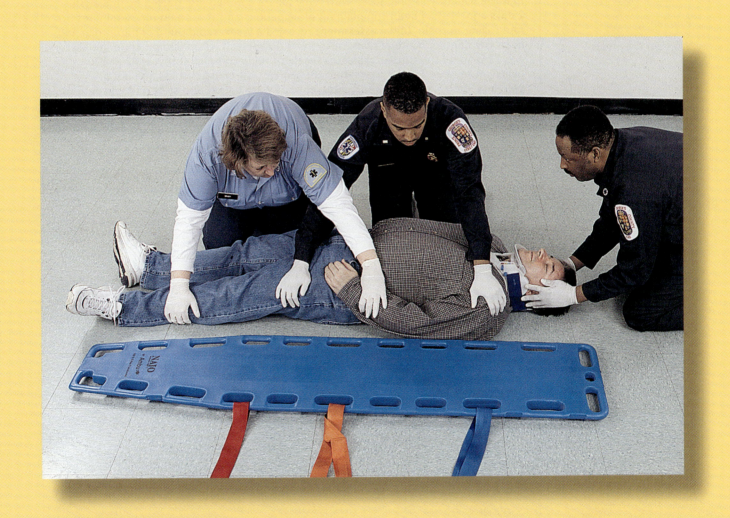

Assessment-Based Management

Key Terms

Field Impression

Multitasking

Pertinent Negatives

Preplan

Working Diagnosis

▪▪▪ CASE HISTORY

EMT–Is Anderson and Meehan return to their station after a call involving a 51-year-old male in full arrest. The call was initially received as "shortness of breath," but on arrival the EMT–Is discovered the patient to be severely dyspneic. The patient's wife reported that the patient was diagnosed with renal failure and had just started hemodialysis 2 days ago. He had been complaining of palpations and chest pain for 30 minutes before calling for help. Initial assessment revealed a weak, rapid pulse of more than 160 beats per minute, bilateral rales, pallor, and diaphoresis. His blood pressure initially was 72/34, and the cardiac monitor revealed a wide-complex tachycardia at 220 beats per minute. Shortly thereafter, the patient lost consciousness and became pulseless. Advanced life support interventions were begun and after multiple defibrillation attempts a perfusion rhythm of sinus tachycardia was restored.

At the station, they spend the next hour reviewing the call, discussing areas of improved efficiency in the assessment and treatment components of the patient's care, and preparing to present the call at the next run review session with the department's medical director.

LEARNING OBJECTIVES

CHAPTER GOAL

Upon completion of this chapter, the EMT–Intermediate will be able to integrate the principles of assessment-based management to perform an appropriate assessment and implement the management plan for patients with common complaints.

Cognitive Objectives

As an EMT–Intermediate you should be able to do the following:

- Explain how effective assessment is critical to clinical decision-making.
- Explain how the EMT–Intermediate's attitude affects assessment and decision making.
- Explain how uncooperative patients affect assessment and decision-making.
- Explain strategies to prevent labeling and tunnel vision.
- Develop strategies to decrease environmental distractions.

- Describe how manpower considerations and staffing configurations affect assessment and decision making.
- Synthesize concept of scene management and choreography to simulate emergency calls.
- Explain the rolls of the team leader and the patient care provider.
- List and explain the rationale for carrying the essential patient care items.
- Explain the general approach to the emergency patient.
- Describe how to effectively communicate patient information person to person, over the telephone, via radio communications, and in writing.
- Explain the general approach, patient assessment, and management priorities for patients who complain of the following:

▪ Chest pain	▪ Altered mental status
▪ Medical and traumatic cardiac arrest	▪ Shortness of breath
	▪ Trauma
▪ Acute abdominal pain	▪ Allergic reaction
▪ Gastrointestinal bleeding	▪ Pediatric emergencies

Affective Objectives
As an EMT–Intermediate you should be able to do the following:
- Appreciate the use of scenarios to develop high-level clinical decision-making skills.
- Advocate and practice the process of complete patient assessment on all patients.
- Value the importance of presenting the patient accurately and clearly.

Psychomotor Objectives
As an EMT–Intermediate you should be able to do the following:
- Acting as team leader, choreograph and organize the emergency medical services response team, perform a patient assessment, provide appropriate treatment, and present cases verbally and in writing using programmed patient scenarios.
- Acting as team leader, assess a programmed simulated patient and make decisions relative to interventions and transportation, provide the interventions, properly secure and transport the patient, encourage teamwork and integration, and practice various roles in patient care for the following common medical emergencies:

▪ Chest pain	▪ Spine injury
▪ Cardiac arrest (traumatic and medical)	▪ Blunt multiple trauma
	▪ Penetrating trauma
▪ Acute abdominal pain	▪ Elderly fall
▪ Gastrointestinal bleeding	▪ Athletic injury
▪ Altered mental status	▪ Head injury
▪ Shortness of breath	▪ Allergic reactions
▪ Syncope	▪ Pediatric emergencies including respiratory distress, fever and seizures
▪ Trauma	
▪ Isolated extremity fracture	
▪ Femur fracture	

INTRODUCTION

The most important skill that any medical practitioner can possess is the ability to effectively assess the patient (Figure 36-1). Failure to perform an adequate assessment leads the EMT–Intermediate (EMT–I) to potentially underestimate the severity of illness or injury, potentially not discovering acute life-threatening injuries or medical conditions. This may unfortunately lead to not initiating the proper treatment for the condition that is truly affecting the patient. Effective assessment skills involve the continuous gathering, evaluation, and ongoing synthesizing of the information that the EMT–I learns from the environment and the patient. This will allow the EMT–I to have a functional understanding of the patient's current medical crisis, make the appropriate determination of which actions are necessary, and initiate the appropriate treatment and transportation decisions.

THE NEED FOR INFORMATION

The right information is the key to making the right decisions regarding patient management. There is no single source of information that will typically lead the EMT–I to have a full understanding of the patient's needs. There are numerous sources of information that the EMT–I must rely on before conclusions are drawn regarding the nature, type, and severity of the medical, or traumatic emergency.

One of the most important and critical steps in gathering information regarding the patient is learned from the patient history. It is often said that more than 80% of medical diagnoses are based on history alone. The history is primarily and most often gained from the patient themselves but also can be gathered from friends, family members, or medical records at the patient's home. Obtaining the history of present illness does not simply involve asking the patient what is wrong and writing down the response verbatim. An effective history-taking process involves asking key and focused questions regarding certain components of the patient's signs and symptoms throughout the history taking. These key questions should be focused towards the chief complaint and associated problems that are learned during the history-taking process. It is crucial that the EMT–I possess knowledge of the disease or injury process to determine which key questions are needed. In addition, the EMT–I needs to be suspicious for different working diagnoses that may become apparent while obtaining the patient history.

The second key component of information gathering is the physical examination. The physical examination is used to support diagnostic clues gained during the history of present illness, as well as to ensure that basic life functions are occurring appropriately. Unfortunately, in the high-energy, fast-paced situations that involve most medical or traumatic emergencies, the physical examination is often hurried, only partially completed, or even completely overlooked. It is understandable that certain situations may limit the EMT–I's ability to perform a complete physical examination due to environmental conditions, bulky patient clothing, or the necessity to initiate treatment and transportation. Even in these situations, the focus physical examination should include the vital signs, as well as attention to the body systems associated with the chief complaint.

Development of a Working Diagnosis

As information is gathered through the history of present illness and physical examination, this information is cognitively compared with information already in the EMT–I's knowledge base. Patterns within the information learned will prompt the EMT–I to suspect certain medical conditions or injuries. As the EMT–I learns more about medical and traumatic conditions and cares for more patients in the field, their knowledge base increases. A solid foundation of medical knowledge, coupled with effective assessment skills increases the chances of the proper **working diagnosis** being determined in the field, appropriate interventions undertaken, and the best chances for the best patient care.

- ✖ **Field Impression** • Initial impression of current diagnosis based current presentation and past education and experiences.
- ✖ **Working Diagnosis** • Initial determination of the medical condition based on information available and subject to modification.

The Development of Field Impressions

As the EMT–I assesses the patient and gathers information for the history process, pattern recognition takes place, and a working differential diagnosis begins to formulate. Some EMT–I's refer to a "gut instinct" that helps them determine therapy. This is essentially using

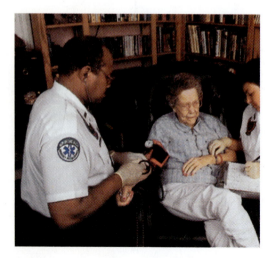

FIGURE 36-1 ▲ Assessment is an important skill for the EMT–I. (From Henry MC, Stapleton ER: *EMT prehospital care,* ed 2, Philadelphia, 1997, WB Saunders.)

pattern recognition that is learned from previous patient care experiences. After the formulation of a **field impression,** a plan of action must ensue. The severity of the patient's condition, as well as the nature of the environment where the patient is being cared for also affect the degree to which field interventions can occur.

Effective assessment also plays a significant role in protocol selection. The determination of the proper working diagnosis allows the EMT–I to select the appropriate treatment protocol. Proper assessment not only allows the EMT–I to know how to apply the protocols, but it also helps identify situations in which deviations from protocols are necessary.

Assessment and Decision Making

There are numerous factors that have gone into the process of patient assessment and decision making. These include the attitude of the EMT–I, the patient's demeanor, horrific or distracting injuries, environmental factors, and personnel resources.

The practiced approach to patient assessment includes the proper attitude at the beginning of the encounter. The proper attitude is developed with a knowledge base composed of understanding of traumatic injuries and medical emergencies, training and proper use of life-saving equipment, and understanding responsibilities to the patient that the EMT–I assumes. Although the emergency medical services (EMS) system is typically associated with public safety, the role that the prehospital medical provider assumes is better typified by considering it a public service. The EMT–I has a responsibility to be the advocate for the patient, caretaker for the patient, and uphold the desires of society in treating people in need.

Any patient assessment will be flawed if the EMT–I is judgmental at any time during the encounter. This may lead the EMT–I to ignore critical information, or neglect to ask important questions in the history gathering. Judging or labeling patients unfortunately makes the EMT–I assume certain aspects of the patient's overall condition that may easily be false. Additionally, patients, friends or family members are very quick to recognize when their trusted caregivers have assumed "an attitude." This may severely limit cooperation and information sharing, and it may lead to critical treatment not being undertaken.

> ### STREET WISE
>
> EMS is in the business of caring for sick and injured patients. Many patients with critical and complex medical conditions require the services of EMS routinely. Examples include patients with respiratory disorders such as COPD or asthma, and patients with metabolic disorders such as diabetes mellitus. Patients with these complex medical conditions may need EMS for their typical complaint but are not immune from developing other medical emergencies. The EMT–I should not minimize new complaints the patient possesses or only focus on the problems the patient has encountered before. Every "frequent flyer" should receive a through and complete assessment as if it was the first encounter for that EMT–I with that particular patient.

Another component of the EMT–I's attitude in patient assessment is the thoughtfulness put into each component of the decision-making process. "Locking on" to a specific working diagnosis early in the assessment process may make the EMT–I overlook crucial pieces of information from the history or physical examination that may reveal the more life-threatening condition. The EMT–I will best serve the patient with a practiced habit of a thorough history and assessment of each patient encounter.

Patient Demeanor

The vast majority of patients that the EMS provider encounters are genuinely thankful for the care being provided and are totally cooperative with the history and assessment process. This type of behavior by the patient facilitates exchange of information, assessment, and treatment.

There will be times, however, when the patient's attitude and behavior may create barriers to the flow of information. Patients that are belligerent, uncooperative, angry, or abusive, may be experiencing underlying medical or traumatic emergencies that are the root cause for their behavior. Such causes include the following:

- Hypoxia
- Hypovolemia/shock
- Hypoglycemia

> ### STREET WISE
>
> EMS professionals routinely encounter patients that are under the influence of alcohol. Many traumatic injuries are related to alcohol abuse, and many patients with chronic alcohol abuse have developed serious medical conditions. In a thorough assessment, the experienced EMT–I will recognize that belligerent or confused behavior that the intoxicated appearing patient is exhibiting may be due to alcohol intoxication, head injury, or other medical conditions. Simply attributing behavior to alcohol ingestion may cause the EMT–I to overlook a critical and life-threatening condition.

- Head injury
- Stroke
- Alcohol intoxication
- Drug intoxication
- Psychiatric conditions

The EMT–I should never assume that a patient's behavior is due to intoxication or the patient's personality until more life-threatening possibilities have been excluded.

Environmental Factors

Physicians and nurses enjoy the luxury of performing patient assessments in well-lit, temperature-controlled, relatively quite emergency departments. Unfortunately, this is not the case for most assessments the EMT–I will perform (Figure 36-2). Typically, lighting may be inadequate, noise levels from machinery or crowds may make communication and history taking difficult, obstacles may be present to limit EMT–I and patient movement, and even winds and temperatures may make proper assessment and therapy difficult.

Consideration should also be made to the dynamics that occur at mass casualty incidents. The resources of the first responding EMS units are typically overwhelmed by the multitude of patients and "helpful" bystanders. A mildly injured vocal patient may distract the EMT–I, whereas a much more seriously injured patient who is unable to call for help may receive no attention. Additionally, bystanders may be demanding that the EMT–I treat their particular friend or family member, even though other patients on the scene may require a higher degree of care.

There cannot be enough emphasis placed on the need for the EMT–I to consider the safety of the overall scene as they approach, assess, and treat the patient. This is not limited to dangers posed by aggressive bystanders or family members, but also dangers that can be encountered on the scenes of motor vehicle accidents, industrial accidents, water-related emergencies, and hazardous material situations.

Personnel Resources

The personnel composition of the responding EMS unit will directly affect the manner in which history is obtained, the patient is assessed, and therapy is initiated. In addition, the number of patients encountered may divide typically plentiful resources and only allow one EMT–I per patient. The components of history taking, assessment and therapy will then need to occur in a sequential, step-wise fashion.

If there are two EMT–Is available for patient care, this allows for history taking, assessment and even therapy to be initiated almost simultaneously. It is important to recognize the need for an organized team approach to patient assessment and interventions. Without this, a member of the team may overlook critical pieces of information regarding the patient's current medical emergency, injury, or pertinent medical history when that information is needed.

ORGANIZATION OF THE EVALUATION AND TREATMENT TEAM

One of the great challenges of prehospital care is preparing for the response to the tremendous variety and uniqueness of medical and traumatic emergencies. With any given 9-1-1 call, there can be many levels of responders providing assistance. These include bystanders that are providing some initial care, law enforcement first responders, Fire Department based first responders, EMT's, EMT–Is or paramedics and varying levels of basic and advanced life support providers. Although it may be useful having additional support in providing care, having an unorganized, piecemeal, segmented evaluation may not be providing the best patient care. Initial responders may relay a piece of information to the EMT–I that may not be entirely accurate. It is essential in every patient encounter to have one person that is ensuring that a thorough patient assessment is completed. In the rush to provide care at critical emergencies, many providers will be attempting to provide some therapy to the patient, while history-taking and overall scene assessment may not be occurring.

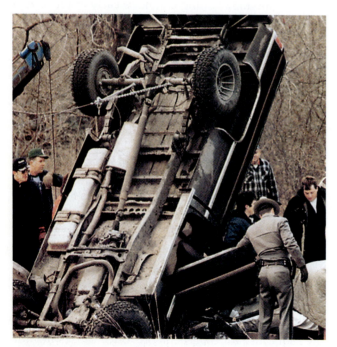

FIGURE 36-2 ▲ The EMT–I works in an uncontrolled environment. (From Henry MC, Stapleton ER: *EMT prehospital care*, ed 2, Philadelphia, 1997, Saunders.)

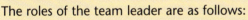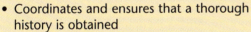 **Preplan** • An organized, predetermined approach to commonly encountered situations.

One way to ensure that each EMS response to a call for help results in a coordinated, seamless patient care assessment and intervention is to develop and practice a preplan. The EMT–I should be familiar with the capabilities of all other members of the EMS crew. Before the patient is even reached, team members should have roles assigned so that job responsibilities are clear and can be immediately undertaken. Recognizing the EMT–I may be the only advanced life support provider on scene, basic assessment duties and history taking can be undertaken by the EMT, while the EMT–I performs advanced life support interventions. The EMS crew should avoid always performing the same duties for each patient encounter. Rotating specific job duties, so that each team member gets exposed to history taking, assessment, and interventions will allow the whole crew to maintain critical skills that are needed for optimal patient care (Figure 36-3).

Patient Care Providers

The success of the prehospital patient care team not only depends on the strengths of the team leader but also the attributes of all of the patient care providers present. Job duties include the following:
• Gathering information from relatives and bystanders
• Obtaining vital signs
• Helping ensure overall scene safety
• Performing interventions, including attaching monitoring leads, oxygen, venous access, splinting and wound care

In addition, if other advanced life support scene providers are present, duties may include administering medications, placing endotracheal tubes or other airway maneuvers, and assisting as a triage officer during mass casualty incidents

Tools for the Trade

A tremendous amount of emphasis has been placed on the proper history taking and physical assessment, helping the EMT–I make the appropriate working diagnosis for the patients for which he or she cares. Although much of the success of selecting the correct working diagnosis is based on the intellectual preparedness and knowledge base, neither of these replace nor reduce the need for having the correct tools for facilitating assessment and interventions.

The EMT–I must assume with each patient encounter that they will be facing the worst situation possible. Typically, for critical patients, there is just not enough time to go back and retrieve the critical equipment from the ambulance. In these patients, certain essential lifesaving interventions may be initiated while the assessment process is still occurring. Neglecting to bring key equipment to the patient can seriously compromise

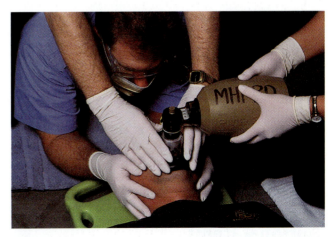

FIGURE 36-3 ▲ Coordination is the key to providing efficient care of the critical patient. (From National Association of Emergency Medical Technicians: *PHTLS: Basic and advanced prehospital trauma life support*, ed 4, St Louis, 1999, Mosby.)

overall patient care. The following several factors that influence bringing in the right equipment to the patient:

- *Portability*—Equipment that is essential to patient care needs to be sized and packaged in a manner that allows easy storage in the ambulance, rapid access, and easy transport to the patient. Large items and particularly heavy items can be difficult to move. This may lead the EMT–I to leave those items on the ambulance.
- *Critical need items*—The EMT–I must bring those items that are critical in providing airway and circulatory support to the high acuity patient. These items not only include oxygen delivery systems and pharmaceuticals but also the cardiac monitor and defibrillation devices.

Items of critical need include the following:
- Airway devices
- Oral and nasal airway adjuncts
- Suction devices, including rigid and flexible suction catheters
- Laryngoscope and a selection of laryngoscope blades
- A selection of endotracheal tube sizes, stylets, and endotracheal tube securing devices
- Manual ventilation bag-valve-mask device or pocket mask for manual mouth ventilation
- Oxygen tank and regulator
- Selection of oxygen delivery systems including a nonrebreather face mask, simple face mask, nasal cannulas, extension tubing, and aerosol delivery devices
- Cardiac monitors and either manual or automated defibrillators
- Basic assessment tools
  - Sphygmomanometer
  - Stethoscope
  - Flashlight
  - Scissors
- Inclusive dressings for thoracic injuries
- Large bore intravenous (IV) catheter for thoracic needle decompression of tension pneumothorax
- Gauze pads and dressings
- Bandages, tape, and compression dressings
- Splinting devices
- Cervical collars

In addition to assessment tools, always carry infection control supplies for all patient care providers. These include gloves, eye shields, and masks.

These are the critical items that should be brought in to every patient encounter. Neglecting any item will be going in unprepared and potentially leading to an unanticipated problem during patient care.

Optional Items

There are certain types of equipment that can be selected for different types of patient encounters (Figure 36-4). Certainly advanced cardiac life support medications may not be anticipated in patients with orthopedic

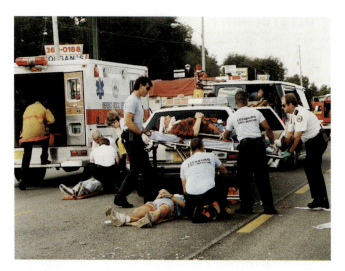

FIGURE 36-4 ▲ Each emergency situation calls for specific equipment to be used. (From McSwain NE Jr et al: *The basic EMT: comprehensive prehospital patient care*, St Louis, 1997, Mosby.)

injuries. Similarly, a long spinal board may not be needed in patients who are experiencing congestive heart failure (CHF). The equipment carried in to each patient encounter, outside of the essential items listed above, will depend on the reported patient problems, local medical protocols, personnel resources available on the responding unit, and accessibility to the patient.

Venous Access

Most medications delivered by the EMT–I are administered via IV. Even regarding those medications administered sublingually, subcutaneously, or intramuscularly, most patients are in critical enough condition that IV access is warranted. Venous access supplies should either be available with the essential response equipment or located with medications in the ambulance's drug box.

GENERAL APPROACH TO THE PATIENT

The EMT–I's initial approach to the patient will set the tone for all aspects of the patient encounter. The EMT–I should approach the patient, appearing calm and well organized. The patient places a tremendous amount of trust in the EMS system and in the EMT–I when picking up the telephone and calling 9-1-1 for help. The EMT–I must portray a high degree of confidence and skill to the patient to maintain that trust. The EMT–I will establish a provider-patient relationship immediately on making patient contact. The approach to establishing a relationship with the patient, or "bedside manner," will facilitate the ease at which the EMT–I gains information from the patient and undertakes interventions. Patients that have concern over the abilities of their caregiver often will comment on negative aspects of the encounter to providers once the patient is at the hospital and may therefore require a more significant amount of time when obtaining consent to begin therapies.

One way to ensure that the prehospital patient care team comes across as a strong, confident, highly skilled unit is to have preestablished preplans designating roles and assignments.

Identify one team member that will essentially function as team leader and carry on all dialogue with the patient. It can be quite distressing for patients to have two or three different caregivers bombarding the patient with questions or repeating the same question each time a new caregiver thinks of it. The team member that is obtaining history and interacting with the patient should maintain eye contact with the patient and speak at a level the patient can easily understand. Ask open-ended questions and listen thoroughly for the patient's answers. The key to a successful history-taking process is not only asking the right questions but also listening for the detailed answer.

Make sure that all necessary equipment is initially brought in. If the patient senses the members of the team are having to constantly go back to get equipment needed for initial care, this may jeopardize the trust the patient has in the caregivers.

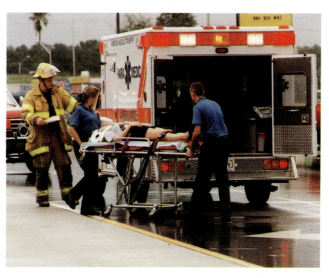

FIGURE 36-5 ▲ **There are situations that prompt the EMT–I to immediately transport the patient to the hospital.** (From McSwain NE Jr et al: *The basic EMT: comprehensive prehospital patient care,* St Louis, 1997, Mosby.)

- Observing the number of patients on the scene, in areas to which patients may have self-evacuated and determining total number of victims in mass casualty incidents.

> **STREET WISE**
>
> The EMT–I should recognize that tunnel vision could easily occur during scene size-up due to critical patients or serious hazards. Other patients and hazards may be neglected. The EMT–I must develop the habit of performing a complete and thorough scene size-up on each call.

The Initial Assessment

The initial assessment sets the tone for the entire patient encounter. Any information gleaned during the initial assessment guides the EMT–I not only in the interventions that are needed but also at the speed at which those should take place.

The different types of approaches based on the initial assessment can be categorized three ways:

1. *Evacuation approach*—With the initial assessment, the EMT–I determines that critical life-saving interventions are needed that cannot be provided by on-scene caregivers (Figure 36-5). This approach is most commonly encountered in trauma patients with penetrating injuries to the thorax or abdomen. Medical and pediatric patients who are developing airway obstructions may also fit into this category. Situations where hazards or threats on the scene may also fall into this category. It is best to immediately transport these patients to an

> **STREET WISE**
>
> One of the keys to being an excellent emergency care provider is not only providing patient assessment and determining what interventions are needed at the current moment, but also anticipating changes in the patient's condition that may require more aggressive resuscitative efforts. Anticipation of these changes will prompt the EMT–I to ensure the correct equipment is at hand if, in fact, those changes take place and the patient becomes more critical.

Scene Size-up

The EMT–I should begin to formulate the overall scene size-up immediately on approaching the scene. This includes the following:

- Observing ambient temperature and weather conditions that may affect the patient's medical condition, hinder EMS access to the patient, or transportation
- Identifying hazards in the environment, including weather, traffic, hostile bystanders, chemicals, fire, or animals
- Noting mechanism of injury information, including the patient's relative position, location of vehicles, or weapons

area where a more thorough assessment and intervention can occur.

2. *Resuscitative approach*—The initial assessment identifies patients in immediate need of intervention and can be initiated by the EMT–I. This typically involves patients that may have the following life-threatening situations:
   - Cardiac or respiratory arrest
   - Respiratory failure or distress
   - Unstable cardiac dysrhythmias
   - Seizures
   - Altered mental status
   - Coma
   - Hypotension and shock
   - Major trauma including patients with possible C-spine injuries

3. *Uncomplicated approach*—Patients are identified that can follow a more contemplative approach to additional assessment intervention. These patients typically do not need immediate intervention. In these cases, a more "relaxed" patient history, physical assessment, and interventions can be undertaken.

Identifying Problems

One of the hallmarks of an EMS system is the systematic approach to patient assessment. This is designed to help the EMT–I identify key life-threatening conditions that may require immediate intervention. The practice of assessing the ABCs on each patient encountered helps the EMT–I identify those rare occasions that a life threatening condition is actually present but not initially identified during scene size-up. A very systematic approach to patient evaluation should be undertaken with each patient encounter. This approach should be practiced and repeated on every patient for whom the EMT–I cares. This includes rapidly identifying the chief complaint, assessing the degree of distress the patient is currently experiencing, performing an initial assessment, taking a complete set of vital signs, compiling in a focused interview of the relevant history, and making a focused physical examination.

CLINICAL NOTES

The key to identifying an acute medical problem is having an adequate knowledge base to recognize when a pattern of patient complaints or physical findings fit with a specific disease pattern. If the EMT–I does not recognize a pattern when it does exist, the correct diagnosis may not be suspected and the appropriate treatment may not occur.

✖ **Multitasking** • The ability to process information to formulate multiple decisions and actions simultaneously.

Multitasking

Multitasking involves another characteristic of successful EMT–I practice; the ability to process multiple pieces of information, determine actions that need to be taken, and perform these actions while continuing to assess the patient. A simple example of multitasking is when the patient is interviewed while the EMT–I is performing the physical assessment. Until the EMT–I is comfortable doing both at the same time, the history should be obtained separately, with key findings of the history documented before the assessment is undertaken. In the rush to perform a thorough physical examination, the inexperienced EMT–I may not listen to key components of the patient history. This may lead the EMT–I to make the incorrect working diagnosis.

Patient Reliability

A significant amount of importance is placed on the patient's ability to describe the events of the illness or injury and any pain being experienced. Critical to the patient's description is the EMT–I's ability to properly listen and pick up on clues that would help support a working diagnosis. There is a tremendous amount of variability in individual's perception of pain. For example, a patient with an ankle sprain may be in a tremendous amount of discomfort and unable to carry on conversation due to the pain. Another patient may have a deformed thigh and obvious femur fracture but may be capable of carrying on complete conversations, appearing very comfortable. The EMT–I should also understand certain conditions will cause the sensation of pain in one particular area, but the offending etiologic factor of the pain is not in that area. For example, irritation of the subdiaphragmatic space either above the liver or the spleen from infection, injury, or blood may actually cause pain in the shoulder on that side. This is known as the Kerr's sign.

In summary, the EMT–I's primary function is to perform rapid, initial scene assessment, patient history, and patient assessment, as well as to begin interventions for the most likely working diagnosis, keeping in mind and anticipating what the worst case scenario might be.

COMMUNICATIONS

Communications is one of the most critical components of prehospital care. Not only is effective communications necessary among different members of the prehospital care team, but relating critical patient information over the radio to medical command authorities and the physician and nursing staffs is vitally important in the continuum of patient care. Failure to effectively communicate is often identified as one of the weakest links in the prehospital-to-hospital transition of patient care. Although the variety and nature of medical and traumatic emergencies that the EMT–I will encounter vary tremendously, one universal aspect of every patient encounter is that communications with other health care providers will be necessary. In almost every emergency run, the EMT–I will communicate with the hospital either for medical command orders or for patient report before transport. Additionally, effective communications are needed face to face at the hospital when patient care is being turned over to the nursing and physician staff. Communication skills are also important when writing in the patient care record. In all of the above aspects, the key components of the patient encounter are transmitted to the people that will be using the information.

Using effective and practice communication skills will help the EMT–I gain more trust and credibility within the health care system. A flawless patient presentation can only occur after the patient has had a thorough and adequate assessment by the EMT–I. If the assessment is only partially complete, and key pieces of information are not performed the receiving facility may have a difficult time understanding the condition of the patient.

> **STREET WISE**
>
> An organized and succinct patient report will demonstrate to the hospital staff that a patient has had an appropriate assessment and the EMT–I appears competent.

The emergency department staff will appreciate a report that is organized, including the key components of the history of present illness, past medical history, vital signs, and current patient assessment, as well as interventions (Figure 36-6). It is very difficult to understand what is wrong with a patient and what was done to the patient when patient reports are unorganized, rambling, include trivial pieces of information, or omit key pieces of information. In addition, these unorganized reports reflect poorly on the skills and overall credibility of the EMT–I.

It is the role of the EMT–I to communicate precisely with their medical command and emergency department staffs the exact condition and needs of the patient. This is crucial when calling for medical command orders. If the medical command physician or nurse has a poor understanding of exactly what the patient's current emergency or current needs are, then they are very unlikely to approve any interventions for the patient until a more thorough examination can take place at the hospital.

Highlights of Effective Communication

Effective communication can be practiced as follows:
- Concise reports typically last approximately one minute or less.
- Follow relatively standard reporting formats that are utilized by all EMS providers in the region. This may include the SOAP (subjective, objective, assessment plan) format.
- Reports pertinent pieces of the history of present illness, past medical history, and physical findings
- Reports pertinent negative findings. EXAMPLE: *A patient complaining of shortness of breath has a past medical history of congestive heart failure. He would be expected to have rales on auscultation of the lungs and may have edema of the lower extremities. If these physical findings were absent, they would be considered* **pertinent negatives** *and should be reported. This may lead the medical providers to consider other working diagnosis as the cause of the dyspnea.*

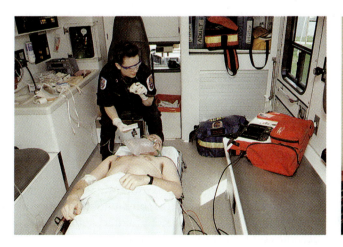
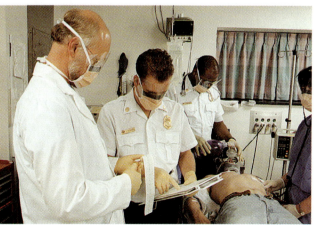

FIGURE 36-6 ▲ The EMT–I must be able to communicate precisely with their medical command and emergency department staffs. (From American College of Emergency Physicians; Pons PT, Cason D, chief editors: *Paramedic field care: a complaint-based approach,* St Louis, 1997, Mosby.)

The very first part of the medical report should include the working diagnosis. The remainder of the report should include basic health history, vital signs, and transmission of specific information to help support the working diagnosis.

It is inappropriate for the EMT–I to go through the patient report making the hospital staff "guess" what the working diagnosis is until the end of the report. The following sections detail a correctly conducted report, a poor presentation, and the key components of a good report.

GOOD REPORT

"Good morning Metro, this is Medic 4. We are en route to your facility with an 8-minute estimated time of arrival (ETA) with a 59-year-old male experiencing CHF. He has a history of CHF and ran out of his furosemide 3 days ago. He has been experiencing more shortness of breath for the last 2 days. He called 9-1-1 this morning because his breathing was getting much worse. Vital signs show a pulse of 120, blood pressure (BP) 180/105, respiratory rate of 32. Pulse oximetry is 84% on room air and 92% on nonrebreather mask. The patient is in mild-to-moderate respiratory distress with pale diaphoretic skin. Lungs have diffuse rales bilaterally, and there is significant edema noted in his lower extremities. Cardiac monitor shows sinus tachycardia, and an IV has been established. He feels more comfortable after oxygen administration. We have administered 40 mg of IV furosemide and one sublingual nitroglycerin. Repeat BP is 150/74. Do you have any questions or further orders?"

POOR PRESENTATION

"Uh, Metro. We got a guy here who called us for difficulty breathing. His pulse oximetry was 84% when we arrived on scene. Heart rate is 120; blood pressure is 180/105. He is kind of sweaty and looks a little pale. We'll be there in 5 minutes . . . out."

What is missing? Review the example of the good report above and notice how key elements of history, assessment, and therapy can easily be communicated and help facilitate the continuum of care at the emergency department.

A standardized approach to giving the patient care report can be facilitated by using information written on the run sheet or using a preprinted card that helps guide the EMT–I with a pattern at which to give the report. As the EMT–I gains more experience, he or she will rely less on a preprinted card and will be able to give the patient care report flawlessly as a matter of practice and habit.

KEY COMPONENTS

- The age, gender, and a general description of the degree of distress
- Chief complaint or reason the ambulance was called
- Nature of present emergency—medical or traumatic
- Pertinent findings from the history of present illness, including pertinent negatives
- Past medical history including allergies, medications, and pertinent medical history
- Assessment findings, working diagnosis, and treatment initiated or planned by EMS
- Physical examination, including vital signs, pertinent positive findings, and pertinent negative findings
- Field impression (What does the EMT–I think is wrong with the patient and what is the current working diagnosis?)
- Plan (What interventions have been undertaken already? What interventions are needed, including any interventions that require medical command approval?)

CLINICAL NOTES

EMS often encounters patients with a very wide and complex past medical history. It can be sometimes difficult to discriminate what components of the past medical history are pertinent to the current emergency. When communicating to the hospital, the EMT–I should only relay information that appears to be relevant to the patient's current medical crisis. Additional information can be given to the hospital once the ambulance has arrived.

The key to developing a flawless patient care report is to develop good habits in the reporting structure. Using small preprinted forms until the EMT–I is comfortable giving report without additional tools can be helpful. The EMT–I can help facilitate development of this practice by practicing presenting patients with other team members and observing more seasoned providers give patient care reports.

PREPARING FOR COMMON COMPLAINTS

It is impossible for EMT–Is to prepare for every type of patient they will encounter through the course of their career. There are common problems to be knowledgeable of regarding assessment and intervention skills. To become comfortable and efficient in caring for these patients, the EMT–I should practice scenario-based simulations to prepare. Results of practicing these types of scenarios include the following:

- Organization of the EMS response team
- Practicing assessment and identification of common physical findings for particular medical emergency or injury
- Practicing interventions based on the assessment and physical findings, in particular, those that vary with local medical control protocols
- Practice communicating information learned about the patient and interventions to simulated hospital and medical command staff.

In addition to practicing verbal patient scenarios, the EMT–I should also become involved in practicing laboratory-based simulations using EMS equipment and simulated patients (mannequins or patient actors). The goals for these simulations should include the following:

- Assessment of the mannequin or patient actor
- Verbalizing and discussing the formulation of the working diagnosis based on the assessment
- Verbalizing and discussing interventions that would be made based on the working diagnosis
- Verbalizing transportation issues involved with that particular patient
- Verbalizing and discuss various roles that other team members would assume during the simulated patient encounter

The EMT–I should practice scenarios based on the following types of common presentations:

- Chest pain
- Stable chest pain with cardiac arrhythmias
- Stable chest pain with bradycardia
- Bradycardia with worsening chest pain or hypertension
- Stable narrow-complex tachycardia
- Unstable narrow-complex tachycardia
- Stable wide-complex tachycardia
- Unstable wide-complex tachycardia
- Ventricular ectopy
- Cardiogenic shock and hypotension
- Cardiac arrest
- Traumatic cardiac arrest
- Medical cardiac arrest
- Ventricular fibrillation
- Ventricular tachycardia
- Asystole
- Pulseless electrical activity
- Termination of resuscitation in the field
- Determination of dead-on-arrival patients
- Abdominal pain

- Acute abdominal pain with normal vital signs
- Acute abdominal pain with hypotension
- Gastrointestinal bleeding
- Upper gastrointestinal bleeding with normal vital signs
- Upper gastrointestinal bleeding with hypotension and tachycardia
- Lower gastrointestinal bleeding
- Lower gastrointestinal bleeding with hypotension and tachycardia
- Altered mental status
- Alcohol overdose
- Drug overdose (street drugs, over-the-counter medications, and prescription pharmaceuticals)
- Seizure
- Hypoglycemia
- Stroke
- Closed head injury
- Dyspnea
- Acute asthma exacerbation
- Pulmonary edema/CHF
- Hyperventilation
- Smoke inhalation and toxic fume inhalation
- Trauma
- Multiple blunt trauma including motor vehicle accident and falls from height
- Penetrating trauma
- Head injury
- Spine injury
- Impaled objects
- Isolated extremity fractures
- Femur fracture
- Athletic injuries
- Elderly victims of falls
- Allergic reactions
- Medical reactions
- Insect stings
- Animal bites, including snake envenomations
- Local reactions versus systemic reactions
- Pediatric
- Difficulty breathing
- Respiratory arrest
- Cardiac arrest
- Dehydration
- Shock
- Major trauma
- Fever
- Seizures
- Extremity injuries

In reviewing the patient that EMT–Is Anderson and Meehan cared for, it is important to focus on the development of the working diagnosis based on the informational stimuli gathered during assessment. The "dispatch diagnosis" of shortness of breath should prompt responders to quickly review the common causes of shortness of breath in the adult and initial prehospital interventions. These can include asthma, pneumonia, chronic obstructive pulmonary disease, pulmonary edema, CHF, pulmonary embolism, pneumothorax, and dysrhythmias. The recent past medical history of renal failure and hemodialysis should raise concern over acute pulmonary edema or electrolyte disturbances that often plague this population of patients.

The current illness is characterized as beginning with palpitations and chest pain, which are both seen with tachydysrhythmias. This is confirmed with the ECG tracing of a wide-complex tachycardia. Physical examination confirms a rapid pulse. Rales also increase the concern for pulmonary edema secondary to the rapid heart rate.

Combining prearrival preparation, appropriate history-taking techniques, and a thorough examination will allow the EMT–I to properly weigh useful data and apply them to the development of the working diagnosis and subsequent treatment plan. Proper reflection on all aspects of the call will allow the EMT–Is to be better prepared for the next similar patient.

SUMMARY

- Preparation and development of a fund of knowledge allows the EMT–I to recognize disease and injury patterns.
- EMT–Is should have a clear understanding of each team member, including assignment of roles before beginning patient assessment.
- Formulation of the correct working diagnosis, using history-taking and physical-examination techniques is important.
- The proper equipment should be at hand to perform the patient assessment. Any additional equipment that may be needed should be anticipated early and made available when a change in patient condition develops.

- Effective communications with the patient, EMS team members, hospital personnel over the radio, and hospital personnel face-to-face should be conducted when turning over care at the emergency department.
- The skills described in this chapter can be strengthened not only through experience but also by simulating patient encounters and discussing assessment and intervention skills with more experienced providers.
- Each patient encounter will have its own level of uniqueness. The EMT–I will be well served by developing and practicing the habit of a systematic approach to patient history, physical examination, interventions and communications.

APPENDIXES

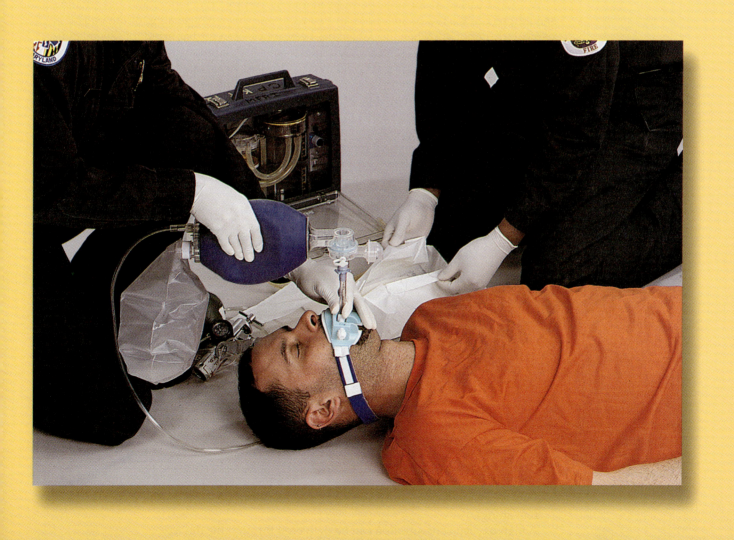

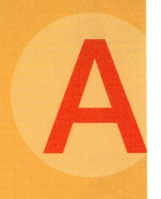

Alternative Airway Procedures

The following procedures, although not included in the current DOT curriculum for EMT–Intermediates (EMT–I), are used in some areas. For this reason, they are covered here, in the Appendix of this textbook. Follow local protocols for the indications and use of these procedures.

As stated earlier in most cases, manual airway control, ventilation, and oxygenation should precede the use of advanced airway adjuncts. This reoxygenating of the patient is particularly important when the patient has been apneic or in cardiac arrest for several minutes before help arrives. Prompt initiation of ventilatory support procedures allows the EMT–I to correct profound hypoxia and hypercarbia. However, due to the high pharyngeal pressures (leading to gastric insufflation) created by most ventilatory support procedures, an advanced airway adjunct should be in place as soon as possible to reduce the risk of regurgitation and possible aspiration. The following two adjuncts are advanced-level procedures:

- Esophageal obturator airway and esophageal gastric tube airway
- Endotracheal (ET) intubation performed digitally and with use of a lighted stylet

These procedures offer more benefits than basic airway adjuncts; however, they also carry more risks.

ESOPHAGEAL OBTURATOR AIRWAY

Description

The esophageal obturator airway (EOA) is a large-bore plastic tube that is open at the top end and closed at the other end (Figure A-1). The closed end has a rounded surface and a cuff. On insertion of the tube into the esophagus, the distal cuff is inflated with 30 to 35 mL of air. This inflation effectively occludes the esophagus and prevents regurgitation. Ventilations are delivered through the open end, which is housed in a removable clear plastic face mask. When a proper seal is maintained between the patient's face and the EOA mask, air exits the tube through 16 holes located along its side at the level of the hypopharynx.

Advantages

- It is easy to insert and does not require visualization of the upper airway.
- It prevents gastric distention and regurgitation.
- It delivers ventilations at the level of the hypopharynx.
- It makes it easier to insert an endotracheal tube (because there is only one passageway remaining).
- A high oxygen concentration can be delivered through the device.

Disadvantages

- It can be accidentally passed into the trachea, resulting in life-threatening airway obstruction.

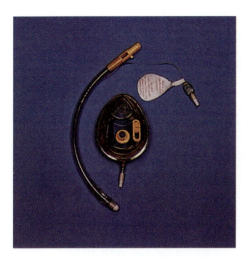

FIGURE A-1 ▲ Components of the esophageal obturator airway (EOA). (From Sanders MJ: *Mosby's paramedic textbook,* St Louis, 1994, Mosby.)

- It may tear or rupture the pharyngeal or esophageal walls during insertion.
- It requires the EMT–I to maintain an effective seal between the mask and the patient's face. Failure to do so results in inadequate tidal volumes being delivered to the patient.
- It does not keep the patient from aspirating foreign materials (e.g., blood or vomitus) present in the upper airway.

Contraindications

To reduce risks associated with its use, the EOA should not be employed in patients who are experiencing any of the following:
- Breathing on their own
- Under 16 years of age
- Under 5 or over 6 feet 7 inches tall.
- Have swallowed caustic substances.
- Have a history of esophageal disease or alcoholism
- Have a gag reflex

Because insertion of the EOA will stimulate the gag reflex, it should only be used in the unresponsive patient. If the patient's responsiveness improves and the gag reflex returns, the EOA must be removed. During insertion or removal of the device, a suction unit should be set up near the patient and checked to make sure it is working properly.

STREET WISE

The EOA should be used with caution in patients experiencing narcotic drug overdose or hypoglycemia because both conditions can be reversed with medication administration and the patient can regain a gag reflex.

Procedure

To insert an EOA the EMT–I should do the following:
1. Employ body substance isolation (BSI) precautions.
2. Open the airway manually using the head-tilt/chin-lift or jaw-thrust.
3. While maintaining ventilatory support, preoxygenate the patient with a bag-valve-mask device supplied with 100% oxygen.
4. Ask another EMT–I to take over ventilating the patient.
5. Select the proper equipment for EOA insertion and check it as follows:
   - Assemble the airway by connecting the tube to the mask. It will click into place when properly seated.
   - Pull back on the plunger of the syringe and draw in 30 to 35 mL of air. Attach the syringe to the one-way valve of the inflation tube and inflate and deflate the distal cuff of EOA to check for leaks. When inserting the tip of the syringe into the one-way inflation valve, use a twisting action to properly seal the syringe.
   - Inflate the mask through the one-way valve until the mask cushion is firm enough to provide a good seal against the patient's face.
   - Lubricate the EOA tube with a water-soluble lubricant if necessary.
6. Kneel at the top of patient's head, placing it into a neutral or slightly flexed position (if trauma is not suspected).
7. Elevate the tongue by grasping the jaw and tongue between the thumb and index finger of the left hand, lifting it anteriorly.
8. With the mask attached, hold the EOA tube at its midpoint, in a J-shaped position.
9. Insert the tip of EOA tube into patient's mouth and advance the tube, following the curvature of the pharynx.
10. Continue inserting the tube until the mask rests on the patient's face. If resistance is met, the tube should be withdrawn and another attempt made. Never use force to insert the tube because pharyngeal or esophageal trauma/laceration can occur. The patient should receive assisted breathing between insertion attempts.
11. Advance the tube until the mask is seated against the patient's face.
12. Seal the mask firmly over the patient's mouth and nose.
13. Attach a ventilatory device (e.g., bag-valve-mask device) to the 15-mm connector and deliver a breath. Look for chest rise and auscultate for breath sounds. If chest rise and lung sounds are absent with assisted breathing, placement of the EOA into the trachea should be suspected and the tube withdrawn.
14. If the chest rises and lung sounds are present, inflate the distal cuff with approximately 30 to 35 cubic centimeters of air (Figure A-2, *A*). The amount

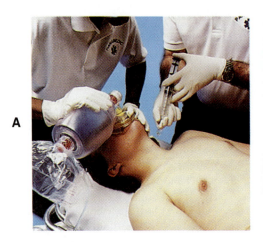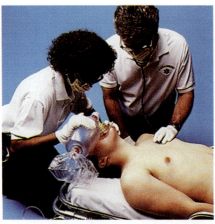

FIGURE A-2 ▲ **A,** Verify placement of the tube and inflate the cuff with 30 to 35 mL of air. **B,** Ventilate the patient, rechecking for proper tube placement, chest rise, and lung sounds. (From Sanders MJ: *Mosby's paramedic textbook,* St Louis, 1994, Mosby.)

of air used to inflate the distal cuff is considered patient-dependent (i.e., smaller patients need less). Check the pilot bulb to verify that air is inflating the distal cuff (a filled pilot balloon indicates that the distal cuff is inflated). The abdomen also should be auscultated to ensure proper placement of the EOA tube.

15. Keeping pressure on the plunger and using a reverse twisting action to prevent accidental loss of air, remove the syringe from the one-way valve.

16. Ventilate the patient with the head tilted backward (Figure A-2, *B*). This position helps to maintain an open airway. While ventilating the patient, recheck for proper placement, chest rise, auscultate over the stomach and listen for lung sounds. Make sure there is a good seal between the patient's face and the EOA mask and that the head is properly positioned.

17. If the patient begins to wake or display gag reflex, turn the patient's head to one side and prepare to suction while deflating the distal cuff and removing the EOA.

✖ **Carina** • Bifurcation of the trachea into the right and left mainstem bronchi.

Under normal circumstances the distal cuff of a fully inserted EOA lies below the level of the **carina.** However, in some patients the cuff may actually lie above the level of the carina. Subsequently, inflation of the distal cuff can obstruct the airway as the posterior membranous portion of trachea is compressed. It is recognized by lung sounds and chest rise that are present before inflation of the distal cuff but that disappear after the 30 to 35 mL of air is introduced. To correct this problem, air should be withdrawn from the distal cuff until effective air exchange is restored. It may be necessary to remove the EOA if there is any indication that the obstruction is still present.

Avoiding Incorrect Placement

Great care must be taken when inserting the EOA, because incorrect placement into the trachea will block air flow into the lungs. Before inserting the EOA, the EMT–I must make sure the head and neck are placed in a neutral or flexed forward position. A hyperextended position can cause the tip of the tube to be directed anteriorly into the trachea. When inserting the EOA, the tube should be grasped between its upper and middle thirds in the same way a pencil is grasped. This technique facilitates gentle maneuvering of the tube posteriorly and reduces the risk of pharyngeal trauma. Lastly, the tube must be stored in such a way as to prevent the tube from curling. A curled tube is more likely to drift upward into the trachea during insertion and thus should not be used.

Removal of the EOA

In some cases, it may be necessary to remove the EOA in the field. Given the potential for regurgitation during removal of the device, the patient should be placed on his or her side with suction immediately available. The distal cuff must then be deflated and the tube withdrawn in a steady and gentle manner. Ideally, an endotracheal tube should be in place to protect the airway from aspiration.

ESOPHAGEAL GASTRIC TUBE AIRWAY
Description

The esophageal gastric tube airway (EGTA) is an improved version of the EOA (Figure A-3). Its main advantage is that its tube is open all the way down. This design permits passage of a gastric tube for decompres-

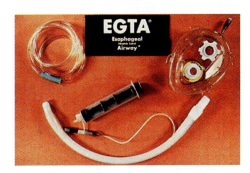

FIGURE A-3 ▲ Esophageal gastric tube airway. (Brunswick Biomedical Technologies, Inc.; Wareham, Mass., from Sanders MJ: *Mosby's paramedic textbook,* St Louis, 1994, Mosby.)

sion of the stomach, which alleviates gastric distention and allows suctioning of stomach contents prior to removal of the device. The face mask also is different. Instead of one port, like the EOA, the EGTA has two: one for attachment of the esophageal tube and one for connection to a ventilatory device. During assisted breathing, air is blown into the ventilation port of the mask. With the esophagus blocked, the air has nowhere to go but into the trachea and lungs. The technique for insertion and the complications of the EGTA are the same as those of the EOA.

Endotracheal Intubation With an EOA in Place

There may be situations when the EMT–I is required to place an ET tube in patients who have been intubated with an EOA. Although somewhat cumbersome, ET intubation can be accomplished with the EOA in place.

The steps for performing ET intubation with an EOA in place are basically the same as orotracheal intubation, but additionally, the EMT–I should do the following:

1. Remove the EOA mask by pinching the obturator tube where it extends through the plastic housing and lifting off the mask
2. Insert the laryngoscope blade into the right side of the patient's mouth. With a sweeping action, displace the tongue and EOA tube to the left. Proceed with intubation in the usual manner.
3. Under direct observation, insert the ET tube into the glottic opening and pass it until the distal cuff disappears past the vocal cords. Then advance the tube slightly (½ to 1 inch). The appropriate precautions should be used to ensure that the tube has passed into the glottic opening because the distensible esophagus can easily accommodate two tubes, the esophageal obturator and the ET tube.

4. Hold the tube in place with one hand to prevent displacement. Inflate the distal cuff with the appropriate amount of air and remove the syringe without releasing pressure on the plunger.
5. Attach a bag-valve-mask to the 15/22-mm adapter of the tube and deliver several breaths.
6. Check for proper tube placement (lung sounds, chest rise, absence of sounds in the epigastrium when ventilations are delivered).
7. Reoxygenate the patient with a bag-valve device supplied with 100% oxygen.
8. Secure the ET tube in place with umbilical tape while continuing to maintain ventilatory support.
9. With suction available, deflate the distal cuff of the EOA. Hold the ET tube firmly in place and remove the EOA tube in a steady manner. The EOA tube must be removed to prevent esophageal or tracheal damage that may result from having two distal cuffs in place at the same time.
10. Recheck for proper placement.
11. Maintain ventilatory support, checking periodically to ensure proper tube position.

DIGITAL INTUBATION

Several hundred years ago intubation was performed without the benefit of a laryngoscope and was known as digital (finger) or tactile (touch) intubation. Today, this procedure is useful for a number of prehospital care situations including when the patient is deeply comatose or in cardiac arrest and proper positioning is difficult to achieve (e.g., extrication situation). A primary benefit of the procedure is that it does not require manipulation of the head and neck. Additionally, because this technique does not necessitate visualization, it may be useful in patients who have facial injuries that destroy the anatomy or when copious amounts of blood, vomitus, or other secretions block the EMT–I's view despite adequate suctioning attempts. Two other uses for the procedure are when there is equipment failure or in disaster situations when intubation equipment is in short supply.

To perform digital intubation the EMT–I should do the following:

1. Employ BSI precautions. At a minimum, gloves and goggles should be worn. A face mask and gown also should be worn when splashing is likely.
2. While maintaining ventilatory support, preoxygenate the patient with a bag-valve-mask device supplied with 100% oxygen. If copious amounts of vomitus, blood, or secretions are present, the patient should be suctioned before intubation is attempted.
3. Direct a partner or first responder to provide ventilatory support of the patient.
4. Assemble and check the equipment as follows:
   - Appropriately sized ET tube
   - Malleable stylet
   - Water-soluble lubricant

- 5- to 10-mL syringe
- Bite block
- Tape or ET tube–securing device

5. Insert the stylet into the ET tube and bend the tube and stylet combination into a J-shaped or hockey-stick configuration.

6. With a fellow crew member or partner stabilizing the patient's head and neck in an in-line position, kneel at the patient's left shoulder, facing the patient. Place the bite block (or other such device) between the patient's teeth to prevent injury to the fingers.

7. Insert the middle and index fingers of the left hand into the patient's mouth. Alternating fingers, "walk" down the patient's tongue, pulling the tongue and epiglottis away from the glottic opening, within reach of the probing fingers (Figure A-4, *A*).

8. Palpate the epiglottis with the middle finger.

9. Press the epiglottis forward and insert the ET tube into the mouth anterior to the fingers.

10. Advance the tube with the right hand (Figure A-4, *B*). Use the index finger of the left hand to maintain the tip of the tube against the middle finger, guiding the tip to the epiglottis.

11. Use the middle and index fingers to manipulate the tube tip until it is between the epiglottis (in front) and the fingers (behind). Then advance the tube with the right hand through the cords as the index and middle fingers of the left hand press the tube forward to prevent it from falling back into the esophagus.

12. Once the tube is in the trachea, hold it in place with one hand to prevent displacement.

13. Inflate the distal cuff with the correct amount of air (approximately 5 to 10 mL of air). Immediately remove the syringe without releasing pressure on the plunger.

14. Attach a bag-valve-mask device to the 15- or 22-mm adapter of the tube and deliver several breaths. Check for proper placement of the tube by watching for chest rise and listening for the absence of sounds in the epigastrium and the presence of lung sounds while ventilations are delivered.

15. Reoxygenate the patient with a bag-valve-mask supplied with 100% oxygen.

16. Secure the ET tube in place with a commercial device or umbilical tape while maintaining assisted breathing.

17. Maintain ventilation, periodically checking to ensure proper tube position.

TRANSILLUMINATION (LIGHTED STYLET) METHOD

An alternative way of performing ET intubation is the transillumination method. With this method, a bright light, introduced into the larynx or trachea, shines through the soft tissues of the neck. This illumination allows the EMT–I to pass an ET tube through the glottic opening without having to directly visualize the structures. As with digital intubation, this procedure permits

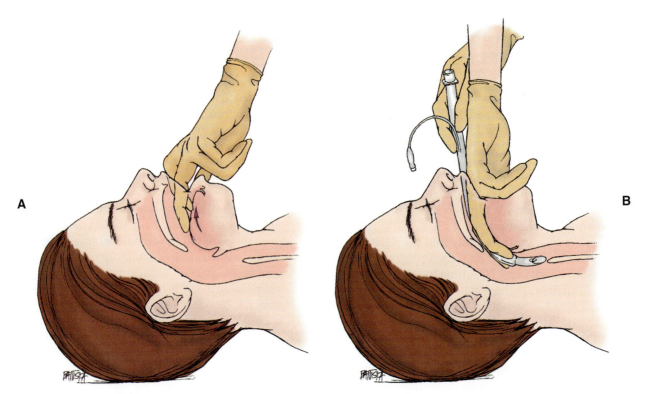

FIGURE A-4 ▲ Digital intubation. **A,** "Walk" down the patient's tongue. **B,** Insert the ET tube into the mouth anterior to the fingers.

ET intubation to be performed without manipulating the head and neck. To perform the transillumination technique, a bendable stylet is used. At its distal end is a small high-intensity bulb. A small battery supplies power for the device.

Contraindications

In nonemergency situations, this method is not recommended for patients who have epiglottitis or when a foreign body is in the airway.

The biggest problem associated with this technique is that outside light can make it difficult to see the light from the stylet. This method works best in a darkened room and with thin patients. In direct sun or bright daylight the patient's neck should be shielded.

To perform the transillumination technique the EMT–I should do the following:

1. Employ BSI precautions. At a minimum, gloves and goggles should be worn. A face mask and gown also should be worn when splashing is likely.
2. While maintaining ventilatory support, preoxygenate the patient with a bag-valve-mask device supplied with 100% oxygen.
3. Direct a partner or first responder to provide ventilatory support of the patient.
4. Assemble and check the equipment as follows:
   - Appropriately sized ET tube
   - Lighted stylet
   - Water-soluble lubricant
   - 5- to 10-mL syringe
   - Bite block
   - Tape or ET tube securing device

5. Insert the stylet into the ET tube and bend the tube and stylet combination to form a tight, 90-degree angle.
6. Placing the bend too proximal or making "too soft" a bend may make proper tube placement difficult.
7. Turn on the stylet light.
8. Grasp the lower jaw and lift it anteriorly. This elevates the tongue and the epiglottis.
9. Introduce the lightwand through the mouth, then use a gentler, rocking motion to place the tube in the glottic opening.
10. When the lightwand enters the glottis, a clearly defined glow transilluminates the cartilage.
11. Hold the tube in place with one hand to prevent displacement and remove the stylet.
12. Inflate the distal cuff with the correct amount of air (approximately 5 to 10 mL of air). Immediately remove the syringe without releasing pressure on the plunger.
13. Attach a bag-valve-mask device to the 15- or 22-mm adapter of the ET tube and deliver several breaths. Check for proper tube placement (chest rise, absence of sounds in the epigastrium, and presence of lung sounds when ventilations are delivered).
14. Recheck for proper tube placement and continue delivering ventilations while securing the tube in place.
15. For both alternative types of ET intubation, the esophageal detector device and end-tidal carbon dioxide detector should be used to verify correct placement of the tube. Also, the pulse oximeter should be attached to help determine the patient's oxygen saturation.

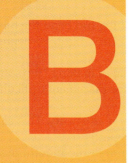

Administration of Thiamine in the Hypoglycemic Patient

Typically, when patients are hypoglycemic, 50% dextrose can be administered and the hypoglycemia reversed. However, in those who are malnourished or who are alcoholics, the administration of 50% dextrose may have little to no effect. The reason is that these patients are often thiamine deficient. Thiamine, or vitamin B-1, is necessary for the final conversion of glucose into adenosine triphosphate (ATP). A vitamin is a substance that the body cannot manufacture but is required for metabolism. Most vitamins needed by the body are acquired through diet. Chronic alcoholic intake hinders the absorption, intake, and use of thiamine, whereas malnutrition results in too little thiamine being brought into the body.

Thiamine deficiency can produce several significant neurological symptoms. These include Wernicke's syndrome and Korsakoff's psychosis. Wernicke's syndrome is an acute and reversible encephalopathy characterized by an unsteady gait, eye muscle weakness, and mental derangement. Korsakoff's psychosis is a significant memory disorder and may be irreversible.

In the thiamine-deficient patient, the administration of 50% dextrose will be ineffective in the overall reversal of hypoglycemia. For this reason thiamine administration should be considered in patients with suspected thiamine deficiency before or at the same time as dextrose is being administered. Thiamine is delivered either intravenously or intramuscularly at a dose of 100 mg.

THIAMINE

Generic name	Thiamine
Brand name	Betaxin
Class	Vitamin (B-1)
Mechanism of action	Thiamine joins with ATP to form thiamine pyrophosphate coenzyme, which is needed for carbohydrate metabolism. Most vitamins used by the body are acquired through diet; however, certain states such as alcoholism and malnourishment affect the intake, absorption, and use of thiamine.
Indications and field use	1. Coma of unknown origin (with administration of dextrose 50% or naloxone), especially if alcohol may be involved
2. Known or suspected thiamine deficiency
3. Delirium tremens
4. Beriberi (rare)
5. Wernicke's encephalopathy
6. Korsakoff's syndrome
Contraindications	There are no contraindications to the administration of thiamine in the emergency setting.
Adverse reactions	There are few side effects with thiamine use. However, the following have been reported:
● Dyspnea, and respiratory failure
● Hypotension (after rapid injection or large dose)
● Anxiety
● Diaphoresis
● Nausea and vomiting
● Allergic reaction (usually from intravenous [IV] injection; very rare); angioedema
Incompatabilities/ drug interactions	None significant
Adult dose	100 mg IV or intramuscular [IM] (IM is preferred)
Pediatric dose	Not recommended in the prehospital setting
Onset of action	Onset is rapid
Peak effects	Duration depends on degree of deficiency
Dosage forms/packaging	1000 mg in 10 mL vial (100 mg/mL)
100 mg in 1 mL vial (100 mg/mL)

NOTE: Pregnancy safety is Category A (Category C if dose exceeds Food and Drug Administration recommendations). Large IV doses may cause respiratory difficulties, and anaphylactic reactions have been reported.

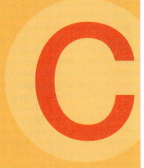

Glucagon Administration in the Hypoglycemic Patient

When an intravenous (IV) line cannot be established, hypoglycemic patients may benefit from subcutaneous (SQ) or intramuscular (IM) administration of glucagon. Glucagon can help raise serum glucose levels by stimulating the breakdown of liver glycogen. The return to consciousness after administration of glucagon typically takes from 5 to 20 minutes. This is a much slower process than is achieved through administration of 50% dextrose. Glucagon only works if there are adequate stores of glycogen available. It is ineffective in chronic alcoholics, those with liver disease, states of starvation, adrenal insufficiency or chronic hypoglycemia. Glucagon must be reconstituted immediately prior to its administration. A dose of 0.5 to 1.0 mg IV is usually adequate.

Glucagon exerts a positive inotropic action on the heart and decreases renal vascular resistance.

GLUCAGON

Generic name	Glucagon
Brand name	GlucaGen
Class	Hyperglycemic
Mechanism of action	Converts glycogen (stored in the liver) to glucose
Indication and field use	Use when unable to administer IV dextrose in cases such as the following: • Hypoglycemia • Patient with unknown cause of coma, seizure, or altered mental status
Contraindications	Patients with known pheochromocytoma (catecholamine producing tumor of the adrenal gland) or known hypersensitivity to glucagon
Adverse reactions	Nausea and vomiting (NOTE: These adverse reactions may also be seen in patients with hypoglycemia)
Incompatibilities/drug interactions	1. Potential diminished effect in patients taking propranolol 2. Potentially increases risk of bleeding in patients taking warfarin
Adult dose	1 mg
Pediatric dose	0.025 to 0.1 mg/kg with 1mg maximum dose
Routes of administration	Primarily IM, but also approved for SQ and IV
Onset of action	1 to 10 minutes
Peak effects	30 minutes
Duration of action	60 minutes
Dosage forms/packaging	1 mg ampules + 1 mL ampule of diluting solution

NOTE: Glucagon is effective in treating hypoglycemia only if sufficient liver glycogen is present. Because glucagon is of little or no help in states of starvation, adrenal insufficiency, or chronic hypoglycemia, hypoglycemia in these conditions should be treated with glucose.

Medical Terminology D

Medical terminology differs from "plain English" in that it is a special vocabulary used in the medical field. Whenever an unfamiliar word is used, you must learn its meaning, spelling, pronunciation, and proper usage. Learning medical terminology is an ongoing process of vocabulary building. Consistent use of a medical dictionary is essential. Understanding medical terms will help you communicate with members of the health care team, such as doctors, nurses, paramedics, and other EMS professionals.

Medical terms often can seem complex in their spelling and pronunciation. They can be confusing and overwhelming unless you know how they came into being and what they mean. It is much easier to remember the meaning of a medical term if you know where it came from. Most medical terms come from Greek or Latin words. The original words and their meanings are interesting (e.g., muscle comes from a Latin word for *mouse*). It was thought that the movement of a muscle under the skin resembled the scampering of a mouse. The coccyx, the lower end of the spine, is named for the cuckoo because it was thought to resemble the cuckoo's bill.

WORD BUILDING

Whenever you encounter a new word, try to break it up into its component parts. Some medical terms are very long, but they become less threatening when broken into smaller parts. If you can figure out the meaning of each part of a word and then combine the meanings, you will have the essential meaning of the word. Many medical words consist of two or three parts: the prefix (beginning), the word root (center), and the suffix (end) (Box D-1).

WORD ROOTS

The foundation of a word is the **word root.** The word root establishes the basic meaning of the word and is the part to which the prefixes (before) and suffixes (after) are added. Some word roots are complete words but not all. The same word root may have different meanings in different fields of study. You may have to consider the context of a word before assigning its meaning.

NOTE: Suffix, prefix, affix, and fixation all have fix as their word root.

Word Root • The foundation of a word; establishes the basic meaning of a word.

Some words contain more than one word root. Each word root retains its basic meaning in the word (Table D-1). These words are called *compounds*. Simple examples of compound words containing two word roots are *frostbite* and *bedpan*. A more complicated example is *osteoarthritis*. The combining form osteo comes from the word root *oste*, meaning bone. The word root *arthr* means joint or joints. The suffix *-itis* means inflammation. Therefore the combining word *osteoarthritis* means inflammation of the bone joints.

BOX D-1

WORD BUILDING

PERICARDIUM
peri- is a prefix meaning around.
-cardi is a word root meaning heart.
Pericardium is a membrane around the heart. (The pericardium is a sac that encloses the heart, holding in fluid.)

PERICARDITIS
peri- is a prefix meaning around.
-cardi is a word root meaning heart.
-itis is a suffix meaning inflammation.
Pericarditis means inflammation around the heart. (In pericarditis, the pericardium becomes inflamed due to a microorganism or a variety of other causes.)

MYOCARDIUM
my/o is a combining form meaning muscle.
-cardi is a word root meaning heart.
Myocardium means heart muscle.(The myocardium is the middle and thickest tissue of the heart, which is composed of cardiac muscle.)

ENDOTRACHEAL
endo- is a prefix meaning inside of.
trache/o is a combining form for trachea, or the windpipe.
trache/al means pertaining to the trachea.
Endotracheal means pertaining to the inside of the trachea. (In endotracheal intubation a tube is inserted through the mouth or nose into the trachea to open an airway.)

PYROMANIA
pyr/o- is a combining form meaning fire.
-mania is a suffix that means excessive preoccupation.
Pyromania is excessive preoccupation with fire. (A mania is a type of psychosis characterized by inappropriate overactivity.)

PYROPHOBIA
pyr/o- is a combining form meaning fire.
-phobia is a suffix meaning abnormal fear.
Pyrophobia is abnormal fear of fire.

TABLE D-1

Common Word Roots

WORD ROOT	MEANING	WORD ROOT	MEANING
arthr-	joint	later-	side
brachi-	arm	mel-	limb
bucc-	cheek	my-	muscle
cardi-	heart	nas-	nose
carp-	wrist	nephr-	kidney
cephal-	head	occipit-	back of head
chondr-	cartilage	ophthalm-	eye or eyes
cost-	rib	oss-	bone
cyst-	bladder	ot-	ear
cyt-	cell	phleb-	vein
encephal-	brain	pulm-	lungs
enter-	intestine	rhin-	nose
faci-	face	somat-	body
fibr-	fibers	splen-	spleen
gastr-	stomach	thorac-	chest
gloss-	tongue	ventr-	front
gnath-	jaw	viscer-	viscera
hist-	tissue		

PREFIXES

✖ **Prefix** • A sequence of letters that comes before the word root and often describes a variation of the norm.

A **prefix** introduces another thought or explains the word root (Table D-2). It is added before the word root and changes or adds to its meaning. For example, the prefix *sub-* in subcutaneous means below. The word *cutaneous* means skin; therefore subcutaneous is below the skin. Another word, *atypical*, which means not typical, can be easily understood when you know that it is formed by adding the prefix *a-*, meaning not, to typical, which is the word root.

TABLE D-2

Common Prefixes

PREFIXES	MEANINGS	EXAMPLES
a-, an-	without, from	apnea (without breath); asepsis (without infection)
ab-	away from	abnormal (away from the normal)
ad-	toward, to, near	adhesion (something stuck to)
aden-	pertaining to gland	adenitis (inflammation of gland)
ana-	up, toward, apart	anastomosis (joining of two parts)
ante-	before, in front of, forward	antenatal (occurring or formed before birth)
anti-	against, opposing	antiseptic (against or preventing sepsis)
bi-	two, double, twice	bilateral (both sides)
circum-	around, about	circumoral (around the mouth)
contra-	opposed, against	contraindication (indication opposing usually indicated treatment)
derma-	skin	dermatitis (inflammation of the skin)
dia-	through, completely	diagnosis (knowing completely)
dys-	difficult, bad, painful	dyspnea (difficulty breathing)
ecto-	outer, outside	ectopic (out of place)
edem-	swelling	edema (swelling)
endo-	within, inner	endometrium (within the uterus)
ep-, epi-	upon, on, over	epidermis (on the skin)
erythro-	red	erythrocyte (red blood cell)
hemi-	half	hemiplegia (paralysis of one side of the body)
hyper-	excessive, above	hyperplasia (excessive formation)
hypo-	under, deficient	hypotension (low blood pressure)
infra-	below, beneath	infrascapular (below the scapular bone)
inter-	between	intercostal (between ribs)
intra-	within	intralobar (within the lobe)
macro-	large	macroblast (abnormally large cell)
micro-	small	microdrip (small drop)
my-	pertaining to muscle	myoma (muscle tumor)
para-	beside, beyond, after	parathyroids (along side of thyroid)
per-	through, excessive	perforation (a breaking through)
peri-	around	periosteum (covering of bone)
post-	after, behind	postpartum (after childbirth)
pre-	before, in front of	prediastolic (before diastole)
retro-	backward, behind	retroflexion (bending backward)
semi-	half	semilunar (half moon)
sub-	under, beneath	subdiaphragmatic (under the diaphragm)
supra-	above, superior, excess	supraventricular (above the ventricles)

Examples of Prefixes

The word root *-pnea* means breath. If we add the prefix *a-*, meaning not, we have the new word *apnea*, meaning without breath. The word root *-logy* means study of. If we add the prefix *bio-*, we have the new word *biology*, meaning the study of life. The word root *-cardia* means heart. If we add the prefix *brady-*, meaning slow, we have the new word *bradycardia*, meaning slow heart.

SUFFIXES

Suffix • A sequence of letters that occurs at the end of the word, which often describes a condition of or act performed on the word root.

The **suffix** is added at the end of a word and changes or adds to its meaning (Table D-3). For example, the suffix

-ase indicates an enzyme. Lipase (*lip-*, meaning fat, plus *-ase*) is an enzyme that digests fats. Gastritis, meaning inflammation of the stomach, is a combination of the word root *gastr-*, meaning stomach, and the suffix, *-itis*, meaning inflammation.

Examples of Suffixes

The word root *neur-* means nerve. If we add the suffix *-algia*, meaning pain, we have the new word *neuralgia*, meaning pain along a nerve. The word root *psych-* means the mind. If we add the suffix *-osis*, meaning condition, we have the new word *psychosis*, meaning condition of the mind. The word root *hepato-* means liver. If we add the suffix *-megaly*, meaning enlargement, we have the new word *hepatomegaly*, meaning enlargement of the liver.

COMBINING FORMS AND VOWELS

✖ **Combining Form** • A word root followed by a vowel.

✖ **Combining Vowel** • A vowel that is added to a word root before a suffix.

Some word roots cannot combine with other word roots and/or suffixes without help (Table D-4). For example, *gastr-*, meaning stomach, cannot gracefully combine with *megaly*, meaning enlargement. The resulting term, *gastrmegaly,* is an impossible word. The hyphen at the end (or beginning) of a **combining form** indicates that it is not a completed word. A combining form is a word root with an added vowel, known as a **combining vowel.** We solve this problem by adding a vowel at the end of the word root, in this case, an *o* at the end of *gastr.* The result, *gastro-*, is referred to as a *combining form* because it is used when combining the root with other roots or suffixes. Gastr + o + megaly makes *gastromegaly,* or enlargement of the stomach. In this appendix, we will indicate word roots with combining vowels with a slash: gastr/o.

Examples of Combining Forms and Vowels

cardi + o + logy = cardiology (study of the heart)

neur + o + logy = neurology (study of the nervous system)

USING A MEDICAL DICTIONARY

A medical dictionary is very useful during the EMT–I course, and it is indispensable to the EMT–I. When choosing a medical dictionary, look for one that includes abbreviations, symbols, and pronunciations.

TABLE D-4

Common Combining Forms

COMBINING FORM	MEANING
brachi/o-	arm
carp/o-	wrist
cephal/o-	head
cervic/o-	neck
encephal/o-	brain
faci/o-	face
gloss/o-	tongue
nas/o-	nose
ot/o-	ear
pil/o-	hair
steth/o-	chest
thorac/o-	chest, thorax
thyr/o-	thyroid gland
trache/o-	trachea
ureter/o-	ureter
vas/o-	vessel
vesic/o-	bladder, blister
viscer/o-	viscera

TABLE D-3

Common Suffixes

SUFFIXES	MEANING	EXAMPLES
-algia	pain	neuralgia (pain along a nerve)
-cyte	cell	leukocyte (white blood cell)
-ectomy	cutting out	tonsillectomy (cutting out of tonsils)
-emia	blood	anemia (lack of blood)
-esthesia	sensation	anesthesia (without sensation)
-genic	causing	carcinogenic (cancer causing)
-gram	record	angiogram (record or graph of)
-itis	inflammation	tonsillitis (inflammation of the tonsils)
-logy	science, study of	biology (study of life)
-ostomy	creation of an opening	gastrostomy (artificial opening of)
-oma	tumor	neuroma (nerve tumor)
-osis	condition of	psychosis (condition of the mind)
-paresis	weakness	hemiparesis (one-sided weakness)
-phagia	eating	polyphagia (excessive eating)
-plegia	paralysis	hemiplegia (one-sided paralysis)
-pnea	breathing	apnea (no breathing)
-phasia	speech	aphasia (inability to speak)
-phobia	fear	hydrophobia (fear of water)
-rhythmia	rhythm	arrhythmia (variation from normal rhythm)
-rrhea	flow or discharge	pyorrhea (discharge of pus)
-taxia	order, arrangement of	ataxia (without muscle coordination)
-uria	to do with urine	polyuria (excessive secretion of urine)

Some medical dictionaries are generic to all medical specialties, whereas others are aimed at particular professions such as emergency medical services (EMS), nursing, or allied health. Check with your course instructor or a local bookstore to see which dictionary would be best for you.

PRONUNCIATION AND SPELLING

A useful way to familiarize yourself with each medical term is to say it aloud several times, learning to pronounce it correctly. Soon, it will become part of your vocabulary.

Spelling is especially critical since misspellings can cause confusion and even lead to misdiagnosis. If you are unsure of a word's spelling, you should consult a medical dictionary. It is also important to be aware that some medical terms sound alike but are spelled differently. For example, ileum (il'e-um) is a part of the small intestine, and ilium (il'e-um) is a part of the pelvic, or hip, bone.

A misspelled word may also completely alter the meaning of a term. For example, hyperglycemia (hi"per-gli-se'me-ah) is too much blood sugar, and hypoglycemia (hi"po-gli-se'me-ah) is too little blood

sugar. Words spelled correctly but pronounced incorrectly may be easily misunderstood. For example, urethra (ur-re'thrah) is the urinary bladder to the external surface, and ureter (u-re'ter) is one of two tubes that leads from the kidney to the urinary bladder.

The above examples illustrate the importance of learning correct pronunciation and spelling of medical terms.

ABBREVIATIONS

Abbreviation • A shorter way of writing something.

Some **abbreviations** are standard and used universally, such as OH for Ohio and Dr. for Doctor. Some abbreviations are specific to organizations or professions; outside the medical profession MCI (multicasuality incident) is a long-distance company. Some abbreviations have found their way into our spoken language, such as ASAP.

Abbreviations in the medical field are fairly universal, but you should check with your local EMS provider or hospital for their approved list of abbreviations. When in doubt about whether to use an abbreviation, you should write out the term in full. Table D-5 lists some of the most common medical abbreviations used by the EMT–I.

TABLE D-5

Common Medical Abbreviations and Symbols

ABBREVIATIONS

ABBREVIATION	MEANING	ABBREVIATION	MEANING
a̅	before	CO	carbon monoxide
abd	abdomen	c/o	complains of
ac	before meals	CO₂	carbon dioxide
ad lib	as much as needed, as desired	CSF	cerebrospinal fluid
AIDS	acquired immune deficiency syndrome	CVA	cerebrovascular accident
A & P	anatomy and physiology	CVD	cerebrovascular disease
AMI	acute myocardial infarction	CVP	central venous pressure
amp	ampule	D/C	discontinue
ant	anterior	drsg	dressing
ax	axillary	Dx	diagnosis
bid	twice a day	ECG or EKG	electrocardiogram
BM	bowel movement	EC	emergency center
BP	blood pressure	ED	emergency department
BSA	body surface area	EEG	electroencephalogram
c̄	with	EMS	Emergency Medical Services
C	centigrade, Celsius	ER	emergency room
Ca	cancer, calcium	ext	extract or external
CAD	coronary artery disease	F	Fahrenheit
caps	capsule	fx	fracture
CBC	complete blood count	GB	gallbladder
cc	cubic centimeter(s)	GI	gastrointestinal
CC	chief complaint	gm or g	gram(s)
CCU	cardiac care unit, coronary care unit, critical care unit	gr	grain(s)
		GSW	gunshot wound
cm	centimeter(s)	gtt	drop
CNS	central nervous system	gtts	drops
		GU	genitourinary

Continued

Common Medical Abbreviations and Symbols—cont'd

ABBREVIATIONS—cont'd

ABBREVIATION	MEANING
Gyn	gynecological
h	hour
hb, hgB	hemoglobin
HPI	history of present illness
hs	hours of sleep
hx	history
ICU	intensive care unit
IM	intramuscular
IV	intravenous
kg	kilogram(s)
KVO	keep vein open
L	liter(s)
lat	lateral
lb	pound
LLQ	left lower quadrant
LUQ	left upper quadrant
MAE	moves all extremities
mcg	microgram(s)
MCI	multicasualty incident
mg	milligram(s)
MI	myocardial infarction
mL	milliliter(s)
mm	millimeter(s)
mmHg	millimeters of mercury
NG	nasogastric
NKA	no known allergies
NPO	nothing by mouth
noc	night
NS	normal saline
O_2	oxygen
OB	obstetrics
OR	operating room
os	mouth
oz	ounce
P	pulse, phosphorus
$\bar{p}$	after
pc	after meals
PDR	Physician's Desk Reference
PE	physical examination, pulmonary embolus
PID	pelvic inflammatory disease
PMH	past medical history
po	orally
post	posterior
prep	preparation
prn	as needed, as desired, whenever necessary
pt	patient
$\bar{q}$	every
qd	every day
qh	every hour
q2h	every two hours
qid	four times a day
qm	every morning
qn	every night
qod	every other day
R	respiration, rectal
RLQ	right lower quadrant
R/O	rule out
ROM	range of motion
RUQ	right upper quadrant

ABBREVIATION	MEANING
Rx	drug, prescription, therapy
$\bar{s}$	without
SC, SQ	subcutaneously
SL	sublingual
SOB	shortness of breath
sol, soln	solution
stat	immediately
S & S	signs and symptoms
tab	tablet
T	temperature
tid	three times a day
TKO	to keep open
TPR	temperature, pulse, and respirations
tsp	teaspoon
ULQ	upper left quadrant
URQ	upper right quadrant
USP	US Pharmacopeia
VC	vital capacity
VS	vital signs
wt	weight
x-ray	roentgen ray

SYMBOLS

SYMBOL	MEANING
=	equal to
+	positive
−	negative
↑	increased
↓	decreased
°	degree
@	at
PO_2	partial pressure of oxygen
PCO_2	partial pressure of carbon dioxide
#	pound
>	greater than
<	lesser than
♀	female
♂	male

SELECTED ABBREVIATIONS USED FOR SPECIFIC DESCRIPTIONS

ABBREVIATION	MEANING
ASCVD	arteriosclerotic cardiovascular disease
ASHD	arteriosclerotic heart disease
ca	cancer
CNS	central nervous system
DJD	degenerative joint disease
DTs	delirium tremens
D_5W	5% dextrose in water
GI	gastrointestinal
GYN	gynecology
ICU	intensive care unit
LOC	level of consciousness
MI	myocardial infarction
NS	normal saline
PE	physical exam
RL	Ringer's lactate
Rx	prescription

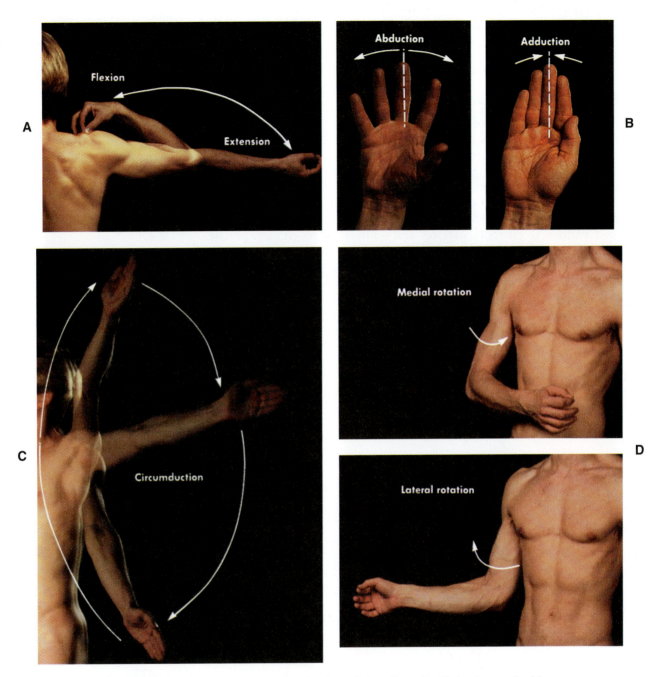

FIGURE D-1 ▲   **A,** Flexion and extension of the elbow. **B,** Abduction and adduction in the fingers. **C,** Circumduction of the shoulder. **D,** Medial and lateral rotation of the arm. (From Seeley R: *Anatomy and physiology,* ed 3, St Louis, 1995, Mosby.)

BODY MOVEMENTS

Terminology is also given to movements. Understanding these terms will help you in your description and documentation of patient complaints and injuries. It also will allow for better communication over the radio or cell phone to the receiving hospital.

Movements

Most movements have to do with some kind of motion at a joint (Figure D-1). Flexion decreases the angle at a joint

by bringing two parts closer together, whereas extension increases the angle by moving the parts further apart. For example, the movement of squatting causes flexion in the knees and hips, whereas standing up causes extension in the same joints. Abduction is the act of moving a part away from the midline of the body, whereas adduction means moving the part toward the midline.

Circumduction is the swinging of a body part in a circle. For example, drawing a circle in the sand with your foot would cause your leg to swing in a circle. Rotation means twisting or turning a part on its own axis. A lateral rotation of the arm twists the hand so that the thumb is turned outward, away from the midline of the body. A medial rotation turns the thumb inward, toward the midline.

SUMMARY

Medical terms are made up of combinations of word roots, prefixes, and suffixes. It is important to get into the habit of breaking down complex words into their separate parts when studying medical terminology. Because medical terms can sometimes be very long and complex, words are separated to help improve understanding of how they are put together.

As you various word roots, prefixes and suffixes, you will better understand, interpret, and define new medical terms. In addition, you should make a practice of looking up new terms in a glossary or dictionary when studying. Spelling and pronunciation are essential elements of effective communication with other health professionals; errors endanger the patient and the EMT–I's reputation. So much is involved in medical terminology that it can be regarded as a separate course of study in itself.

Understanding certain movements for orientation to the human body is essential for identifying and reporting location of injuries. A knowledge of medical terminology and body orientation will help make your communication and documentation of patient information much more precise.

GLOSSARY

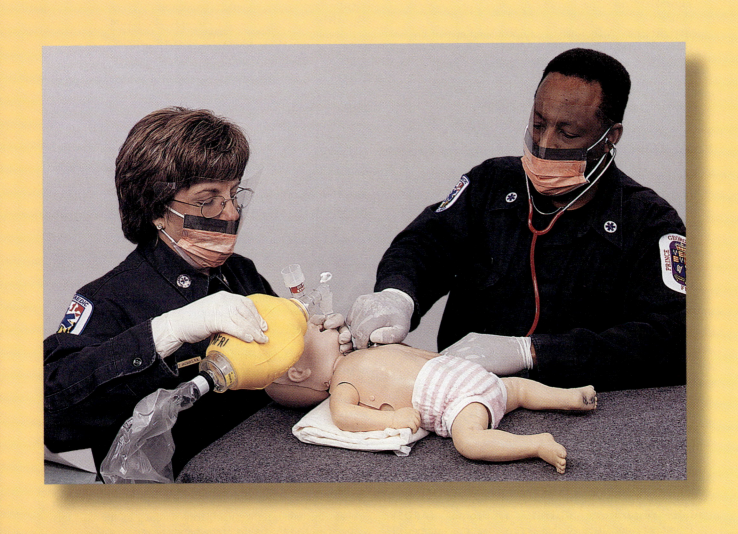

abandonment A form of negligence that occurs when the relationship between the EMT–I and the patient is terminated by the EMT–I without ensuring continuity of care for the patient.

abbreviation A shorter way of writing something.

abdominal aortic aneurysm The "outpouching" of the abdominal portion of the aorta due to atherosclerosis.

abdominal cavity The body cavity extending from below the diaphram to the pelvic bone.

abnormal behavior Any action that deviates from society's norms and expectations.

abruptio placenta The premature detachment of the placenta.

absolute refractory period The time during myocardial repolarization during which no stimuli will depolarize the myocyte.

absorption The process by which medications enter the body.

accessory muscles of respiration The muscles in the neck and intercostal space that assist the diaphragm with respirations.

acclimatization The body's adjustment to a new environment.

acetylcholine A cholinergic neurotransmitter that crosses the synapse to reach a postsynaptic neuron or effector organ; is also affected in organophosphate and nerve agent poisoning.

acetylcholinesterase The enzyme responsible for breakdown of the neurotransmitter acetylcholine.

acid A substance that increases the hydrogen ion concentration of water; a substance with a pH less than 7.0.

acrocyanosis Occurring in newborns, peripheral cyanosis involving bluish color to the hands and feet.

acronym Word that is formed by combining the first letter or letters of a name or a phrase. EXAMPLE: *SOAP*, Subjective, Objective, Assessment, and Plan.

action potential Electrical term for the process of depolarization and repolarization of a cell.

activated charcoal Medication administered orally that can be beneficial in certain overdoses and poisonings; acts by binding to the offending agent and preventing gastric absorption.

active transport The movement of a solute across a membrane from an area of lower concentration to an area of higher concentration.

acute abdomen Intense abdominal pain due to inflammation, infection, or hemorrhage.

acute mountain sickness Occurring after rapid ascent by an unacclimatized person to altitudes in excess of 8,000 feet; with symptoms including dizziness, headache, irritability, breathlessness, or euphoria.

acute pulmonary edema A quick, excessive backup of fluid in the lungs.

adenosine A cardiac medication that depresses the atrioventricular (AV) node and sinoatrial (SA) node activity; useful in terminating paroxysmal supraventricular tachycardia (PSVT).

adult respiratory distress syndrome (ARDS) Pulmonary insufficiency that occurs due to a number of bodily insults. Pathological findings include alveolar and interstitial edema due to leaking capillaries.

adventitious lung sounds Sounds heard during auscultation of the chest and are usually abnormal.

adverse reactions Undesirable side effects of a drug.

aerobic metabolism Metabolism that occurs with oxygen.

aerosol A gas under pressure that contains a drug that is breathed in.

affect A person's outward manifestations of emotion.

afterdrop phenomenon The reflex vasodilation that may occur after active external rewarming of patients experiencing hypothermia.

afterload The pressure the ventricular muscles must generate to overcome the higher pressure in the aorta.

agonist Drugs that interact with a receptor to stimulate a response.

air embolism The presence of air bubbles in the central circulation after inappropriate ascent while diving.

albuterol An inhaled beta-2 agonist used in treating bronchospasm.

alcohol abuse Excessive alcohol consumption that leads to medical, behavioral, or social changes in an individual.

alcohol withdrawal syndrome Physical reactions a person experiences when he or she abruptly stops consuming alcohol.

alcoholism A dependence on alcohol.

algorithms A defined standard medical care guidelines that follow a specific pattern.

allergen A stimulus that promotes an allergic response.

allergic reaction An exposure to any substance to which an individual is sensitive, resulting in skin, airway, or other bodily reactions.

alpha effects The stimulation of alpha-receptors that leads to vasoconstriction.

alternating current (AC) Electrical current that reverses direction.

Alzheimer's disease Central nervous system disorder characterized by progressively debilitating dementia.

ambient air Environmental or room air.

American Hospital Formulary Service A source of drug information that contains concise information arranged according to drug classifications.

American Medical Association Drug Evaluation A set of standards for evaluating drugs.

amiodarone A cardiac medication useful in treatment for both atrial and ventricular dysrhythmias.

amitriptyline A tricyclic antidepressant medication.

amniotic sac Protective membranous sac that insulates and protects the fetus during pregnancy.

amoxapine A tricyclic antidepressant medication.

ampule A glass container containing a drug; the bottle must be broken at the neck to retrieve the medication.

anaerobic metabolism Metabolism without oxygen.

anaphylactic reaction A severe allergic response to a foreign substance that the patient has had contact with before.

anaphylaxis Allergic reaction.

anatomic figure Diagram of a human body, with anterior and posterior views. Part of some run reports, it is used to mark and label patient's injuries or physical findings.

anatomic position Positioning of the body upright with eyes directed straight ahead, arms hanging by the side, feet together, and the palms of the hands facing forward.

anatomy The study of structures and organs of the body.

angina pectoris An intermittent attack of chest pain and related symptoms due to a reduction in blood flow to the heart muscle.

anoxia Lack of oxygen.

antagonist Drugs that attach to a receptor but do not stimulate a response or prevent a response.

antegrade amnesia Type of amnesia in which there is no recall of events immediately after recovery of consciousness.

anti-sludge An acronym used to describe anticholinergic poisoning.

antibody The part of the immune system that recognizes antigens and initiates an immune response.

antigen Any substance identified by antibodies as foreign and promotes an immune response.

antihistamines Class of medications used to treat insomnia and cold symptoms and is useful in treating allergic reactions.

antispasmodics Group of medications used to treat nausea, vomiting, and abdominal cramps; has anticholinergic properties.

antivenin Class of medications designed to treat patients who have sustained bites from specific snakes.

anxiety-hyperventilation syndrome Syndrome with tachypnea without physiological demand for increased oxygen, leading to respiratory alkalosis.

aortic valve The valve located between the aorta and the left ventricle and heard in the second heart sound.

aphasia An abnormal neurological condition in which language function is defective or absent due to an injury to the cerebral cortex.

apnea The absence of breathing.

apneustic breathing The pattern of respirations characterized by a prolonged inspiratory phase, followed by expiration apnea.

apothecary system A system for measuring medication dosage.

appendicitis The inflammation of the appendix.

arteries Vessels that carry blood away from the heart.

aspirate The taking of foreign material into the lungs during inhalation.

assault Threatening, attempting, or causing fear of offensive physical contact with a patient or other individual.

asthma A recurring condition of completely or partially reversible acute airflow obstruction in the lower airway.

asystole The absence of any cardiac activity.

ataxia A coordination dysfunction due to brain injury, intoxication, medications, or metabolic disorder.

ataxic (Biot's) breathing A type of breathing characterized by a series of several short inspirations and followed by long, irregular periods of apnea.

atelectasis Alveolar collapse.

atria The chambers in the heart that receive blood from other parts of the body.

atrioventricular node The electrical conduction node in the heart that separates atrial conduction and ventricular conduction.

atrophy The loss of tissue substance, typically brain or muscle, due to chronic conditions.

atropine Cardiac medication that blocks discharge from the parasympathetic nervous system, resulting in increased heart rate.

aura A warning sign that consists of seeing, hearing, or smelling something unusual before losing consciousness.

auscultation The act of listening for sounds within the body to evaluate the condition of the heart, lungs, abdomen; typically performed with a stethoscope.

automaticity The ability to self-generate electrical activity (action potential) without the need for extraneous nerve stimulation.

autonomic nervous system A specialized subdivision of the peripheral nervous system that regulates involuntary functions of the body.

AVPU scale A neurological response scale relating the patient's response to stimuli: Alert, Verbal, Painful, Unresponsive.

baroreceptors Sensory nerve endings that adjust blood pressure as a result of vasodilation or vasoconstriction.

barrel chest Thorax anatomy that suggests the presence of long-standing chronic obstructive lung disease (COPD).

base A substance that decreases the concentration of hydrogen ions; a substance with a pH greater than 7.0.

battery Criminal offense of attempting to inflict bodily injury on another.

Battle's sign Ecchymosis or bruising behind the ears present with a basilar skull fracture; may be a late sign.

behavioral emergency A situation in which the patient feels he or she has, in some way, lost control of his or her life.

behavioral seizures Seizures in adults that involve a brief "absence" spell or other abnormal behavior.

benzodiazepine A class of sedative agents useful for treating seizures.

beta receptors Receptors located on bronchial smooth muscle that initiate bronchodilation when stimulated.

biotelemetry The process of transmitting physiological data, such as an electrocardiogram over distance, usually by radio.

biotransformation Changes of a drug's free components into substances for elimination of the body.

bleb Air-filled sac within the lung that has been present since birth.

blood pressure A measurement of the force within the arteries created by the flow of blood.

blood pressure cuff A device used to measure blood pressure, also known as a *sphygmomanometer*.

blunt trauma A nonpenetrating force applied to the body, typically from vehicle crashes or falls.

board-like rigidity Spasms of the anterior abdominal wall muscles due to abdominal pain or inflammation.

body language Nonverbal gestures; posture; or evidence of rage, elation, hostility, depression, fear, anger, anxiety, or confusion.

body substance isolation Concept that regards all body tissues and fluids potentially infected; includes bloodborne, food-borne and air-borne pathogens.

body substance isolation precautions The use of protective equipment to minimize the chances of the EMT–I being exposed to contagious diseases.

bowel obstruction A blockage of the intestinal tract.

bowel sounds Sounds created by peristalsis of material and air through the intestines.

bradycardia Heart rate less than 60 beats per minute.

bradypnea Slower than normal breathing rate.

breath sounds Sound of air passing in and out of the respiratory passageways as heard with a stethoscope.

breech presentation In childbirth, a delivery in which the baby's buttocks or feet present before the head.

bronchial breath sounds Normal sounds heard over the anterior sternum, abnormal if heard elsewhere in the lungs, indicating consolidation of normal lung tissue.

bronchiolitis An infection of the lower respiratory tract, which is most often caused by a virus.

bronchorrhea Discharge of fluid in the bronchi.

bronchospasm The tiny muscle layers surrounding the bronchioles spasm and narrow the lumen of the airways.

bronchovesicular breath sounds Sounds intermediate between tracheal sounds and vesicular sounds, suggesting fluid in the lungs.

Broselow tape A reference guide containing pediatric resuscitation information.

bruits Moderate- to high-pitched "whooshing" sounds that represent turbulent blood flow in arteries.

buccal medication A drug dissolved between the cheek and the gum. It is absorbed across the mucous membrane of the mouth.

bullae Defects that are formed from the destruction of normal lung tissue in conditions such as chronic obstructive pulmonary disease.

Bundle of His Part of the cardiac conduction system in the ventricles.

capillaries Microscopic thin-walled vessels through which oxygen, carbon dioxide, and other nutrients and waste products are exchanged.

capnometer Electronic device that measures how much carbon dioxide is exhaled during breathing; end tidal CO_2.

carbon dioxide drive Stimulation of the normal respiratory reflex due to elevation of carbon dioxide in the blood.

carbon monoxide A colorless, odorless gas produced during combustion; binds to hemoglobin and prevents proper oxygen transportation.

carbonaceous Containing carbon.

carboxyhemoglobin Tightly bound carbon monoxide-hemoglobin molecule that prevents proper oxygen-hemoglobin binding and oxygen delivery.

cardiac arrest The absence of functional cardiac activity.

cardiac conduction system The pathway through which electrical impulses travel in the heart.

cardiac cycle The repetitive pumping process of blood that begins with the onset of cardiac muscle contraction and ends with the beginning of the next contraction.

cardiac dysrhythmia A disorder of cardiac rhythm.

cardiac monitor An electronic device for the continuous observation of cardiac function.

cardiac output The amount of blood pumped through the circulatory system in one minute.

cardiac tamponade The pericardial sac filling with sufficient blood or other fluid to prevent adequate ventricular movement.

cardiogenic pulmonary edema A type of pulmonary edema due to cardiac etiology, such as congestive heart failure, myocardial infarction, and valve disease.

cardiogenic shock Cardiac failure whereby the heart cannot sufficiently pump blood to the rest of the circulatory system.

cardiotoxicity A substance that produces a toxic effect on the heart.

carina Point at which the trachea divides (bifurcates, or separates into two sections) into the right and left mainstem bronchi.

carpopedal spasm Spasm of the fingers and toes typically seen during prolonged episodes of hyperventilation.

cartilage Connective tissue found primarily in the joints that allows for movement.

cataracts Opacities within the lens of the eyes distorting and preventing light sensation.

cation An ion with a positive charge.

caudal Near the lower end of the torso.

cavitation An opening produced by a force that pushes body tissues laterally away from the tract of a projectile.

cells The basic building blocks of all life.

centigrade scale A temperature scale, using 0 degrees as the freezing point and 100 degrees as the boiling point of water.

central cyanosis Particularly concerning in newborns, a bluish color to the trunk and face.

central nervous system The portion of the nervous system comprised of the brain and the spinal cord.

central neurogenic hyperventilation A pattern of breathing marked by rapid and regular respirations at a rate of about 25 per minute.

cephalopelvic disproportion A potentially difficult delivery due to the relative large size of the fetus in relation to the mother's pelvis.

cerebral autoregulation The adjustment of blood vessel capacity and resistance to maintain an optimal state of blood flow to the brain despite fluctuations in the mean arterial blood pressure.

cerebral homeostasis The maintenance of brain perfusion and oxygenation despite fluctuations in the mean arterial blood pressure.

cerebral ischemic syndromes Any process that disrupts blood flow to brain tissue.

cerebrospinal fluid Clear fluid surrounding the brain and spinal cord that acts as a cushion.

cerebrovascular accident (CVA) Also known as a *stroke*, this is a condition that results from a disruption of circulation to the brain, causing ischemia and damage to brain tissue.

certification Action by which an agency or association grants recognition to an individual who has met its qualifications.

cervix The interior, narrow portion of the uterus that opens into the vagina.

chemical name Drug name that gives the exact description of the chemical structure of the drug.

chemoreceptors Receptors in the blood vessels that detect changes in the chemical composition of the blood.

Cheyne-Stokes breathing An abnormal pattern of breathing, characterized by alternating period of apnea and deep, rapid breathing.

chief complaint Brief statement describing the reason for the patient's seeking medical attention.

child Individuals from age 1 to 8 years.

cholecystitis An occlusion of the gallbladder duct leading to inflammation and pain.

cholinergic agents A group of agents that lead to stimulation of the parasympathetic nervous system.

chronic bronchitis Also known as *chronic obstructive pulmonary disease* or *emphysema*; involving damage to the pulmonary alveoli typically due to long-term tobacco abuse.

chronic obstructive pulmonary disease (COPD) Progressive and irreversible disease of the airway marked by decreased inspiratory and expiratory capacity of the lungs.

chronotropic state Rate of cardiac muscle contraction.

cilia Fine, oscillating hairs on the cells that line the lungs.

circulatory system The body system composed of the heart, blood, and blood vessels that are responsible for the circulation of blood.

classic heat stroke Failure of the body's temperature regulation mechanisms over the course of time, leading to the inability to rid the body of excess heat.

closed injury or fracture An injury where there is a break in the bone but no disruption of the skin.

closed-ended question A question that is answered with a simple yes, no, or a few words.

codeine A narcotic agent used to treat painful conditions.

cognitive systems The part of the central nervous system that is involved in the maintenance of awareness and the "conscious" normal waking state.

coma A state of unresponsiveness characterized by the absence of spontaneous eye movements and response to painful stimuli and vocalization.

compartment syndrome Syndrome of ischemia and compromised circulation that can occur from a vascular and crush injury.

compendium of drug therapy A source of drug information distributed to practicing physicians.

compensated hypothermia A type of hypothermia in which the body's temperature is being maintained by the body's intrinsic thermogenesis.

complex-partial seizures Seizure that involves a brief "absence" spell or other abnormal behavior; also known as *behavior seizure* or *petit mal seizure.*

concept formation Pattern of understanding based on initial information gathered during patient assessment.

conduction The transmission of heat from warmer to cooler objects in direct contact.

conductivity The ability to transmit an appropriate electrical stimulus from cell to cell throughout the myocardium.

confrontation A direct but potentially disruptive communication with the patient.

congestive heart failure (CHF) An inability of the heart to pump blood caused by heart muscle damage.

conjugate gaze When both eyes move in the same direction.

connective tissue A type of tissue that binds other types of tissue together.

consensual pupillary reaction The constriction of the pupil in the eye opposite of the eye with the light stimulus.

consent Agreement or approval.

constricting band Used in the treatment of snakebites, a snug band placed 5 to 10 cm proximal to the bite that does not compromise arterial or venous flow.

contagious Any disease that can be spread from person to person.

continuous quality improvement An evaluation of services provided and the results achieved as compared with accepted standards.

contractility The extent and velocity (quickness) of muscle fiber shortening.

contracture Permanent condition of a joint characterized by flexion and fixation.

contraindications Conditions or instances for which a drug should not be used.

Controlled Substances Act An act passed in 1970 that regulates the manufacture and distribution of drugs whose use may result in dependency.

contusion Bruising below the dermis caused by blunt trauma.

convection The transfer of heat by circulation of heated particles.

cor pulmonale Right-sided heart failure due to difficulty pumping blood through lung tissue damaged in chronic obstructive pulmonary disease.

coral snakes Venomous snakes found in the United States that are brightly colored, with alternating black, white (or yellow), and red bands that encircle the entire body.

core body temperature The true body temperature typically measured by invasive means at the hospital.

coronary artery disease Plaque development resulting in narrowing of the coronary arteries.

coronary circulation The arterial system of blood supply from the aorta to the myocardium.

costovertebral angle Angle formed where the lowest rib meets the spinal column.

counter-regulatory hormones The hormones glucagon and epinephrine, which have the opposite effects of insulin, raising blood sugar.

crackles Crackling or bubbling sounds that represent fluid in the alveoli and are present in heart failure or pneumonia.

cranial In or near the head.

crepitus A palpable or audible crunching produced by movement of a body part.

cricoid cartilage The narrowest part of the child's upper airway.

cricothyroid membrane Membrane situated between the cricoid and thyroid cartilages of the larynx.

cross tolerance An increase in tolerance to other drugs in the same class.

croup A respiratory illness that occurs in children between 3 months and 3 years of age; also called *laryngotracheobronchitis.*

crowning Occurring during labor, when the newborn's head is easily visible on inspection of the perineal area.

cumulative effect Increasing by steps with an eventual total that may go past the expected result.

current health status Overall review of the patient's general health including use of alcohol, drugs, and smoking.

Cushing reflex When increased intracranial pressure causes a slowing pulse rate, deep or erratic respirations, and increasing blood pressure.

cyanosis A bluish discoloration of the skin due to inadequate oxygenation.

D50 A medication used to treat hypoglycemia, contains 25 grams of glucose in 50 mL of water.

data interpretation Comparing current information with past education and experience to draw conclusions.

decerebrate posturing The patient presents with stiff and extended extremities and retracted head.

decode Converting a message into understandable language.

decompression sickness An illness occurring during or after ascent secondary to rapid release of nitrogen bubbles.

decorticate posturing A sign of neurological compromise that presents with arms flexed, fists clenched, and legs extended.

dedicated land lines Telephone lines with continuous direct connection from one geographical location to another.

defibrillation An electrical shock delivered to the heart to restore an effective rhythm.

definitive care In-hospital care that resolves the patient's illness or injury after a definitive diagnosis has been established.

delirium An unusual behavior, delusion, or confusion that may be due to a reversible medical condition.

delirium tremens A severe state of alcohol withdrawal consisting of delirium, hallucinations, and nervous system hyperactivity.

dementia A loss of memory and intellectual function that is typically not reversible.

demographic information Documentation that includes patient's name, address, age, telephone number, and parent's name if the patient is a minor.

depolarization The cardiac myocyte activation resulting in electrical discharge and muscle contraction.

depressants Medication, toxins, or poisons that depress the central nervous system.

depression A psychiatric disorder marked by sadness, inactivity, difficulty in thinking and concentration, a significant increase or decrease in appetite and time spent sleeping, feelings of dejection and hopelessness, and sometimes suicidal tendencies.

detailed assessment A continuation of the patient assessment process in which in-depth information is obtained concerning the patient and his or her condition.

diabetes mellitus A chronic disease of the endocrine system caused by a decrease in the secretion or activity of the hormone insulin.

diabetic ketoacidosis A metabolic condition consisting of hyperglycemia, dehydration, and the accumulation of abnormal compounds, called *ketones* and *ketoacids*, in the body; also called *diabetic coma.*

diaphoresis Profuse sweating.

diaphragm A wide muscular partition separating the thoracic, or chest, cavity from the abdominal cavity.

diastole The relaxation of the heart.

diazepam A benzodiazepene medication used for sedation and treatment of active seizures.

diffusion A passive process of molecules moving from an area of higher concentration to an area of lesser concentration.

digital comunications Data or sounds that are converted into digital code for transmission.

digital intubation The placement of an endotracheal tube using guidance by fingers.

diphenhydramine (Benadryl) An antihistamine medication used to treat allergic reactions and anaphylaxis.

direct current (DC) Electrical current that flows only in one direction.

direct pupillary reaction The constriction of the pupil when exposed to a light stimulus.

dislocations A separation of two bones at the joint.

distal Farthest from a reference point.

distribution Moves the drug from the bloodstream into the tissues and fluids of the body.

diuretic A medication used to promote kidney production of urine.

diverticulitis The inflammation of small intestinal "outpouchings" (diverticuli).

diverticulosis The "outpouching" of the weakened wall of the colon, forming small pouches that may lead to inflammation, abscess, infection, or rupture.

do not resuscitate order (DNR) A physician's order indicating that a patient is not to be resuscitated in the event of a cardiac arrest.

documentation Process used to record patient information.

dorsalis pedis pulse The pulse of the dosalis pedis artery, found on the foot lateral to the extensor tendon of the great toe.

dorsum In reference to anatomic position—back of.

dosage errors An unintentional mistake in calculating or administering a medication.

doxepin A tricyclic antidepressant medication.

dromotropic state The rate of cardiac electrical conduction.

drowning Death within 24 hours after a submersion accident.

drowsiness Diminished level of consciousness due to fatigue, intoxication, medications, hypoxemia, head injury, or metabolic disorder.

drug A substance taken into the body to affect change to one or more body functions, often to prevent or treat a disease or condition.

drug action The cellular change produced by a drug.

drug allergy Allergy to a drug shown by reactions ranging from a mild rash to severe allergic reaction and shock.

drug dependence A physical state where withdrawal symptoms occur when a person discontinues the use of drugs.

drug effect Degree of a drug's physiological change.

Drug Enforcement Agency (DEA) Established in 1970, the DEA deals with controlled substances only and enforces laws against manufacture, sale, and use of illegal drugs.

drug inserts Literature found in all drug packages; supplies detailed information about the drug.

drug tolerance When the body becomes accustomed to a particular drug over a period.

drug toxicity Results from overdosage, ingestion of a drug intended for external use, or buildup of the drug in the blood due to impaired metabolism or excretion.

drug withdrawal A set of signs and symptoms that develop in a person after abrupt cessation of taking a drug.

dry drowning Hypoxemia due to prolonged water immersion with minimal water insult to the lungs due to laryngeal spasm.

dullness Medium-pitched sound normally heard over solid organs during palpation.

duplex Communication system that uses two frequencies for each channel to transmit and receive messages, thus allowing simultaneous two-way communications.

duty to act The medical care provider has an obligation to provide care.

dysarthria Impaired speech due to dysfunction of the tongue or other muscles essential to speech.

dysphonia Difficulty in speaking.

dyspnea Shortness of breath or difficulty in breathing.

dysrhythmia An abnormal cardiac rhythm.

ecchymosis Bruises; discoloration of the skin or mucous membranes due to leakage of blood in the subcutaneous tissue.

ECG Abbreviation for electrocardiogram.

echoed Immediately repeating back each radio transmission received.

eclampsia A condition whereby a pregnant female experiences seizures in addition to preeclampsia; usually occurs during the third trimester of pregnancy.

ectopic pregnancy The implantation of a fertilized egg outside of the uterus; usually occurs in the fallopian tube.

edema Swelling due to accumulation of fluid in the tissues.

ejection fraction The percentage of blood that is ejected in during ventricular contraction.

electrocardiogram A record of the electrical activity within the heart.

electrolytes Salts that when dissolved in a solvent break up into ions that are capable of conducting an electrical current.

elixir Drug dissolved in alcohol with flavoring added.

Emergency Medical Dispatcher (EMD) A specially trained person who receives calls for emergency assistance and ensures proper emergency medical services response.

emergency medical services (EMS) system An organized approach to providing emergency care to the sick and injured.

Emergency Medical Technician (EMT) A person trained according to criteria established by the Department of Transportation in the care of the acutely sick or injured person.

empathetic responses Identifying with the patient's feelings or symptoms.

emphysema A form of chronic obstructive pulmonary disease; lung tissue damage with loss of elastic recoil of the lungs.

EMS System An organized approach to providing emergency care to the sick and injured.

EMT–Basic The primary level of EMT–Basic training; requires completion of a minimum 110-hour EMT–Basic training program meeting Department of Transportation standards.

EMT–Intermediate EMT who has completed training beyond the EMT–Basic level; the degree of training and skills practiced varies widely between states and EMS systems.

EMT–Paramedic EMT who has advanced training in patient assessment, medical emergencies, pharmacology, trauma, obstetrics, rescue, behavioral emergencies, and other EMS activities.

emulsion Drug combined with water and oil; must be thoroughly shaken to disperse the medication evenly.

encephalitis The inflammation of the brain tissue due to infection.

encode Putting an idea or message into a language or code.

encoder A device that blocks out radio traffic that is not directed at the specific base station.

encrypting The scrambling of a message in order to prevent illicit access to the information.

endocrine system The body system comprised of ductless glands that are responsible for hormone production.

endotracheal Within or through the trachea.

endotracheal intubation The insertion of an open-ended tube into the trachea.

enhanced 9-1-1 Emergency phone number that includes a visual system that displays the caller's phone number and address.

enteral Administration of a drug along any portion of the gastrointestinal tract.

enteric-coated tablet A compressed dry form of a drug coated to withstand the stomach acidity and dissolve in the intestines.

entrance wound The site on the body where a missile or electricity first strikes it.

envenomation Snakebites that involve the transfer to venom into the patient.

environmental emergency A medical condition caused or exacerbated by weather, terrain, atmospheric pressure, or other local factors.

environmental exposures Injuries or effects to the body due to the environment; such as lightning, excessive heat, or cold.

epicardium The surface layer of cardiac muscle that is covered by the pericardium.

epiglottitis An inflammation of the epiglottis, which most often occurs in children from 3 to 7 years of age.

epilepsy Seizures spontaneously recurring over a span of years.

epinephrine A drug that stimulates the adrenal glands and narrows the blood vessels; also called *adrenalin*.

erythrocytes Red blood cells.

eschar A tough, nonelastic coagulated collagen of the dermis; scab or dry crust resulting from a thermal or chemical burn.

escharotomy A surgical incision made into necrotic tissue of a burn; expands the tissue and decreases ischemia from a circumferential burn.

esophageal varices Distended, friable esophageal veins prone to spontaneous hemorrhage.

esophagitis Inflammation of the esophagus from infection, alcohol, or medication.

ethics The discipline dealing with what is good and bad.

eupnea Normal inhalation and exhalation.

evaporation The loss of heat at the surface from vaporization of liquid.

evisceration The protrusion of an internal organ or peritoneal contents through a wound or surgical incision, particularly in the abdominal wall.

excitability The ability to respond to an appropriate electrical stimulus.

excretion The elimination of waste products from the body.

exertional heat stroke The failure of the body's temperature regulation mechanisms rapidly during periods of heavy exertion, leading to the inability to rid the body of excess heat.

exit wound The site on the body where a missile or electricity leaves it.

expressed consent Given when the patient provides verbal or written consent for the EMT–I to examine, care for, and transport the patient to an appropriate medical facility.

extracellular fluid Fluid found outside of the cell membranes.

extrinsic asthma Occurs when some specific outside substance such as pollen causes the bronchioles to narrow.

facial droop Asymmetry on one side of the face that may indicate an acute stroke.

facilitated diffusion Transports molecules of a substance across a cell membrane that would otherwise be impermeable to the substance.

facilitating behaviors Patterns of behaviors and actions that promote efficient and appropriate patient care.

facilitation A combination of verbal and nonverbal actions that encourage the patient to say more.

Fahrenheit Scale Temperature scale, using 32 degrees as the freezing point and 212 degrees as the boiling point of water.

fallopian tubes   A pair of muscular tubes that extend from the uterus into the pelvic cavity.

false imprisonment   Intentional and unjustifiable detention of a person against his will.

Federal Communications Commission (FCC)   The federal agency established to control and regulate all radio communications in the United States.

Federal Food, Drug, and Cosmetic Act   An amended act requiring that the safety of a drug must be proven before it can be distributed to the public; also requires that labels be used to list the possible habit-forming properties and side effects of drugs.

Federal Trade Commission (FTC)   An agency of the federal government that regulates drug advertising.

feedback   Confirmation from the receiver that a message has been received and understood.

femoral pulse   The pulse of the femoral artery palpated near the inguinal crease.

fentanyl   A narcotic medication.

fetus   An unborn child.

fibrosis   Abnormal formation of scar tissue in the connective tissue framework of the lungs following inflammation or pneumonia and in pulmonary tuberculosis.

fight or flight response   A sympathetic stimulation to prepare the body when in a dangerous situation.

fingerstick blood glucose (sugar) test   A process by which a drop of blood is obtained from the finger to determine blood glucose (sugar) level.

FiO$_2$ Percentage of oxygen in inspired air.

first heart sound   The first heart sound heard over the parasternal area largely due to closure of the mitral valve.

First Responder   Trained person who provides initial care until other EMS providers arrive on the scene.

flail chest   Injury that occurs when two or more ribs are broken in two or more places, resulting in paradoxical motion of the flail segment.

flat affect   Limited emotional components of a patient's demeanor.

flexion   The act of bending or being bent.

fluid extract   An alcohol solution of a drug from a vegetable source. The most concentrated of all fluid preparations.

focal motor seizures   Seizure activity involving only parts of the body, not generalized.

focused history and physical examination   An in-depth examination to determine the severity and cause of the patient's condition; includes both a hands-on examination and a gathering of the patient's history.

fontanelles   Soft spots on the top of an infant's head.

Food and Drug Administration (FDA)   Established to review drug applications and petitions for food additives; inspect factories where drugs, cosmetics, and foods are made; and to remove unsafe drugs from the market.

formable splint   A splint that accommodates the shape of the injured extremity.

fourth-degree burn   Full-thickness injury that penetrates the subcutaneous tissue, muscle, fascia, periosteum or bone.

fractures   A break in the continuity of bone or cartilage.

frontal   Vertical line dividing the body into a front and back portion.

frostbite   The formation of ice crystals within the tissues.

full-thickness burn   A burn that extends through all layers of the epidermis and dermis.

furosemide   A potent diuretic used in treatment of congestive heart failure.

gag reflex   Retching or striving to vomit; it is a normal reflex triggered by touching of the soft palate or the throat.

gastritis   Inflammation of the lining of the stomach.

gastrointestinal bleeding   Refers to *hemorrhage* anywhere in the gastrointestinal tract.

gastrointestinal (GI) system   The body system responsible for digestion.

general survey   A universal overview of the patient's general condition.

generalized major motor seizures   Seizure activity involving the entire body; also known as *tonic-clonic seizures.*

generic name   The nonproprietary designation of a drug.

geriatric abuse   Situations in which periods of rage, anger, or hostility are directed at an elderly person.

GI hemorrhage   Any bleeding from the upper or lower gastrointestinal tract.

Glasgow Coma Scale   A numerical scale used for neurological assessment in a critical patient.

glaucoma   The presence of an elevated intraocular pressure within the eye that can lead to vision loss.

glottis   The slitlike opening between the vocal cords.

glucose   Sugar used as fuel by the cells of the body.

goblet cells   Cells that line the respiratory tract and normally produce a layer of mucus that is continuously swept out of the lungs by cilia.

good samaritan laws   Laws that may provide immunity from prosecution or civil suit for people who render care at the scene of an emergency.

grand mal seizure   Generalized major motor seizure.

gravida   The total number of times a woman has been pregnant.

gross negligence   The willful and reckless giving of care that causes injury to the patient.

grunting   Abnormal, short, and loud breaks during exhalation.

guarding   The intentional avoidance of pain caused by abdominal palpation by tensing abdominal muscles.

gurgling   A bubbling sound from fluid in the airways, common in pneumonia, congestive heart failure, or excess oral secretions.

half-life   Time required by the body, tissue, or organ to metabolize or inactivate half the substance taken in.

hallucinogens   Induce a sense of euphoria and hallucinations.

Harrison Narcotic Act of 1914   The first federal legislation designed to stop drug addiction or dependence.

HBV   Abbreviation for hepatitis B virus.

headache   Head pain due to any etiology.

heat cramps   Cramps or pains in the muscles that occur due to heat exposure.

heat exhaustion   More severe loss of fluid and salt than occurs in heat cramps, usually following exertion in a hot, humid environment.

heat stroke   A failure of the body's temperature regulation mechanisms; also called sunstroke.

hematochezia   The presence of bright red blood in the stool.

hematocrit   The volume percentage of red blood cells in whole blood.

hematoma   Swelling caused by leaking blood vessels below the dermis.

hematuria   Blood in the urine.

hemiplegia   Weakness on one side of the body typically due to stroke.

hemoglobin   A protein that bonds oxygen to red blood cells.

hemoglobinuria   A burn that extends through all layers of the epidermis and dermis.

hemolysis   Breakdown of red blood cells.

hemopericardium   Blood in the pericardium.

hemoperitoneum   Blood in the peritoneum.

hemopneumothorax   Air and blood accumulation in the pleural cavity.

hemoptysis   Blood in sputum produced when coughing.

hemorrhagic stroke   A stroke caused by nontraumatic intracranial bleeding.

hemothorax   Blood collects in the pleural space.

hemotoxicity   Damage or insult affecting the blood.

hepatitis B virus (HBV)   A virus that causes an inflammation of the liver.

heroin   A narcotic agent typically abused intravenously.

hiatal hernia   The protrusion of a portion of the stomach from its normal position in the abdomen through the diaphragm, resulting in epigastric or lower thoracic discomfort and complaints of acid reflux or dyspepsia.

high permeability pulmonary edema   Pulmonary edema due to leakage or increased capillary permeability due to systemic or pulmonary insult.

high pressure pulmonary edema   Cardiogenic pulmonary edema.

high-altitude cerebral edema   A type of high-altitude illness causing increased intracranial pressure.

high-altitude illness   A group of syndromes that are the result of decreased atmospheric pressure due to increased elevations, resulting in hypoxia.

high-altitude pulmonary edema   A type of high-altitude illness that leads to increased pulmonary artery pressures and pulmonary edema that develop in response to hypoxia.

histamine   A cellular substance released into the body during anaphylactic shock; may cause airway compromise and vasodilation.

history of present illness/injury   Events or complaints associated with the patient's complaint.

HIV   Abbreviation for human immunodeficiency virus.

homeostasis   The normal state of balance between all of the body's systems.

hydrocodone   A narcotic medication.

hypercarbia   Excessive partial pressure of carbon dioxide in the blood.

hypercholesterolemia   Elevated levels on cholesterol in the blood.

hyperglycemia   The elevation of the blood sugar level above normal.

hyperglycemic hyperosmolar nonketotic coma   A state where the blood sugar is markedly elevated but no acidosis or accumulation of ketones is present.

hyperkalemia   Elevated levels of potassium in the blood.

hyperresonant   Low-pitched, loud tone that is heard in conditions of excess air such as pneumothorax or abdominal obstruction.

hypersensitivity   Allergy to a drug shown by reactions ranging from a mild rash to severe allergic reaction and shock; also called *drug allergy*.

hypertension   Consistently elevated blood pressures above the normal range.

hypertensive   The condition of having high blood pressure.

hypertensive emergency   A sudden increase in blood pressure that leads to problems with in the nervous system, the kidneys, or the heart.

hypertonic solution   A solution that has an osmotic pressure greater than that of normal body fluid.

hyperventilation   A respiratory rate greater than the required for normal body function.

hyperventilation syndrome   Tachypnea without physiological demand for increased oxygen leading to respiratory alkalosis.

hypoglycemia   An abnormally low blood sugar level.

hypokalemia   Low level of potassium in the blood.

hypoperfusion   Fluid passing through an organ or part of the body that does not have properly oxygenated blood.

hypoperfusion syndrome   Shock.

hypotension   Continuous blood pressure below normal, typically below 100 mm Hg systolic.

hypotensive   The condition of having low blood pressure.

hypothermia   A condition in which the core (or internal) body temperature (CBT) is less than 95° F due to either decreased production of heat or increased heat loss from the body.

hypotonic solution   A solution that has an osmotic pressure less than that of normal body fluid.

hypoventilation   A reduced rate or depth of breathing, often resulting in an abnormal rise of carbon dioxide.

hypovolemic shock   A form of shock caused by the loss of blood or fluid volume from the body.

hypoxemia   Insufficient oxygenation of the blood.

hypoxia   Reduced oxygen supply to the cells.

hypoxic drive   A secondary respiratory mechanism that stimulates breathing due decreasing levels of oxygen in the blood.

idea   The intended meaning of the communication.

idiopathic seizure   Seizures with no known cause.

idiosyncratic reactions   An abnormal or unexpected reaction to a drug peculiar to a certain patient. This is not technically an allergy.

IgE   Abbreviation for immunoglobulin E, a type of antibody unique in that it is the only type of antibody involved in an anaphylactic reaction.

imipramine   A tricyclic antidepressant medication.

immune system   The body system that protects the body from foreign materials.

immunization   Process of rendering a person immune or of becoming immune.

implied consent   The EMT–I assumes that a patient who is severely ill or injured would want care if he or she were able to respond.

incontinence   The inability of the patient to control urination or bowel movements.

indications   Disease states or instances for which a drug is prescribed.

inert gases   Gases that generally cause no direct tissue toxicity but can be harmful by displacing oxygen.

infant   Children under the age of one year.

inferior   Below or lower, on the body.

information stimuli   Data that the EMT–I is exposed to from multiple sources: patient, environment, assessment, family.

informed consent   The patient consents to care only after receiving all the information necessary to understand his or her condition and the risks and benefits of care and refusal of care.

ingestion   A medication or poison that enters the body through the gastrointestinal track.

inhalation   Administration of drugs, water vapors, or gases by inspiration of the substance(s) into the lungs.

inhalation injury   An upper and/or lower airway injury that results from thermal and/or chemical exposure.

initial assessment   A quick evaluation of the patient to determine immediate life-threatening emergencies.

injection   The process by which a medication or substance enters the body by penetration through the skin, typically using a needle.

inotropic state   The strength of cardiac contraction.

inspection   The act of visually evaluating the patient.

insulin   An endocrine hormone responsible for moving glucose (sugar) molecules from the blood into the cells.

integumentary system   The body system comprised of the skin and its appendixes.

intercostal retractions   The increased use on intercostal muscles due to respiratory difficulty.

interference   Preventing or inhibiting clear reception.

interpretation   The synthesizing of information learned from multiple sources to draw a conclusion.

interstitial fluid   Fluid found outside of the blood vessels in the spaces between the body's cells.

intracellular fluid   Fluid found within individual cells.

intracerebral hematoma   Accumulation of blood within the tissue of the brain.

intracranial pressure   Pressure within the skull.

intradermal   Injection of a drug within the dermis.

intralingual   Injection of a drug within the tongue.

intramuscular   Injection of a drug within the muscle.

intraosseous   Administration of medication directly into the bone marrow of a long bone.

intrapulmonary shunting   The circulation of blood to nonventilated alveoli. This results in the blood having the same oxygen content as systemic venous blood.

intrathecal   Injection of a drug through the theca of the spinal cord into the subarachnoid space.

intravascular fluid   Fluid found within the vascular system; comprises the fluid portion of blood; plasma.

intravenous cannulation   The placement of a catheter into a vein.

intrinsic asthma   Asthma defined as no specific substance can be identified as causing bronchospasm.

intubation   Passing a tube into an opening of the body.

involuntary guarding   The tensing of the abdominal wall muscles due to abdominal pain or peritoneal irritation.

ipecac   Medication that stimulates the central nervous system to induce vomiting.

ipratropium   A bronchodilating agent used in the treatment of asthma and chronic obstructive pulmonary disease with anticholinergic affects.

ipsilateral   On the same side of the body.

irritant gases   Gases that produce irritation to the skin, eyes, oropharynx, lungs, or skin.

ischemia   A lack of oxygen to an organ.

ischemic heart disease   The general phrase that includes coronary artery disease, myocardial infarction, angina pectoris, and ischemia related congestive heart failure.

isotonic solution   A solution that has the same osmotic pressure as bodily fluids.

jaundice   The yellowish discoloration of the skin, mucous membranes, and sclera of the eyes caused by greater than normal amounts of bilirubin (a breakdown product of hemoglobin) in the blood.

joints   Occur where two or more bones meet or articulate.

jugular venous pressure   The abnormal distention of the jugular veins seen in conditions such as congestive heart failure and cardiac tamponade.

Kehr's Sign   The complaint of pain in the left shoulder that might be caused secondary to irritation of the adjacent diaphragm from splenic hematoma or hemoperitoneum.

ketoacids   Compounds containing the carbonyl and carboxyl groups.

ketones   Substances formed during the breakdown of fatty acids in periods of faulty carbohydrate metabolism.

kilogram   A metric measurement of weight.

kinematics   The process of predicting injury patterns that may result from the forces and motions of energy.

Kussmaul respirations   Rapid and deep respirations usually found in patients with diabetes or others with imbalances of the acid content in their bodies.

kyphoscoliosis   Lateral curvature of the spine; can interfere with normal breathing.

large-bore catheter   Catheter with a large interior diameter (14 to 16 gauge).

lateral   To the side.

lead   Summation of cardiac voltage changes between electrodes that are placed in different places on the body.

Lefort fracture   Fracture pattern produced in the mid-face region.

lethargy   A diminished level of consciousness or activity.

leukocytes   White blood cells.

level of consciousness (LOC)   The degree of awareness a patient has regarding their immediate surroundings.

libel   The injury of a person's character, name, or reputation by false and malicious writings.

licensure   Process by which a governmental agency grants permission to an individual to engage in a given occupation on finding that the applicant has attained the minimal degree of competency necessary.

lidocaine   An antidysrhythmic drug.

liniment   An oily liquid used on the skin.

lip pursing   Exhaling through puckered-out lips, typical in states of respiratory difficulty.

local effect   Limited to the area where it is administered.

lorazepam   A benzodiazepene sedative agent useful in the treatment of active seizures.

lower gastrointestinal (GI) bleeding   Bleeding due to a lesion of the GI tract below the level of the duodenum.

lymphatic system   The body system comprised of capillaries, thin vessels, valves, ducts, nodes, and organs that allows for the transport of lymph through the body.

major trauma   Injuries involving multiple organ systems or significant injury to one organ system.

maladaptive behavior   Behavior indicating that a person is unable to properly adapt to various challenging circumstances.

mandible   The large bone forming the lower jaw.

mast cell   A specialized type of white blood cell.

maxilla   One of a pair of large bones that form the upper jaw.

mean arterial pressure (MAP) Diastolic pressure plus one-third of the pulse pressure.

meconium A thick, greenish-black material that is normally expelled from the intestine shortly after birth and provides evidence of patency of the gastrointestinal tract.

meconium aspiration syndrome Occurs when the fetus or newborn inhales the thick, sticky meconium, causing airway obstruction and respiratory difficulty.

medial A plane that passes near the midline of the body.

medical ambiguity Vagueness in symptoms or complaints that limit the ability to determine a specific diagnosis.

medical asepsis The practices used to prevent the transfer of pathogenic organisms from person to person, place to place, or person to place.

medical communications Communication between the EMT–I and medical direction or the receiving hospital.

medical control Supervision and management of an EMS system and the field performance of EMTs.

medical direction Medical supervision of an EMS system and the field performance of EMTs.

megahertz (MHz) Radio frequencies designated by cycles per second.

melena Black, tarry stool indicative of gastrointestinal bleeding.

meningitis An inflammation of the membranes that surround the brain and spinal cord.

menstrual cycle The hormone-controlled cycle of altering the uterine lining each month in preparation for egg implantation.

meperidine (Demerol) A narcotic medication.

metabolic acidosis A condition in which the level of bicarbonate is low in relation to the levels of carbonic acid.

metabolic alkalosis A condition in which the level of bicarbonate is high in relation to the level of carbonic acid.

metabolism The sum of all chemical processes that take place in the body as they relate to the movement of nutrients in the blood after digestion, resulting in growth, energy, release of wastes, and other body functions.

metric system A decimal system of weights and measures based on the meter and the kilogram.

midsagittal A vertical line dividing the body into right and left halves.

mild hypothermia Hypothermia with a core body temperature of greater than 90° F.

milliequivalent The concentration of electrolytes in a certain volume of solution based on the number of available ionic charges.

minute volume The volume of air exchanged in one minute.

miscarriage A sudden and unexpected loss of pregnancy; also called spontaneous abortion.

mitral valve The valve between the left atrium and left ventricle.

morphine Narcotic medication used for painful conditions, congestive heart failure, and chest pain.

motor tics Spasmodic muscular contraction most commonly involving the face, head, mouth, eyes, and neck.

mucous membrane A thin layer of connective tissue lining many of the body cavities through which air passes via small, mucus-secreting glands. The mucus is a thick, slippery secretion that functions as a lubricant and protects various surfaces.

multiple sclerosis A disease resulting from spotty destruction of the myelin coat of CNS tissue.

multiplex Duplex system that allows transmission of voice and data simultaneously.

multi-system trauma Serious injury occurring in two or more major systems of the body.

muscle coordination The ability of muscles to move as a whole.

muscle strength The amount of force generated on testing of muscle groups.

muscle tone The tension created by normal muscle with normal nerve innervation.

muscular rigidity Hardness, or stiffness of the extremities, typically due to neurologic disease.

muscular system The body system composed of contractile tissue that allows for movement.

myocardial infarction (MI) The death of heart muscle caused by a lack of oxygen.

myocardium The heart muscle.

myoglobinuria Molecular complex responsible for the red color of muscle and for its ability to store oxygen.

naloxone (narcan) A narcotic antagonist agent used to reverse the effects of narcotics.

narcotic act The act that made the possession of heroin and marijuana illegal.

narcotics A substance that dulls senses and relieves pain in moderate doses.

narrative Portion of the run report that is written out longhand.

nasal administration Injection of a drug or substance into the nasal mucosa.

nasal flaring Widening of the nostrils during inspiration, seen more often in children with respiratory distress.

nasal septum In the nose, the wall dividing the nostrils. It is made up of bone and cartilage covered by mucous membrane.

near drowning The patient survives at least 24 hours after a submersion accident, although death may eventually occur.

nebulizer Device that propels liquid medication into a fine mist for inhalation.

neck vein distention A bulging outward of the veins in the neck.

needle Sharp stainless steel hollow tube that is used to penetrate the skin and blood vessel.

negligence Professional conduct that falls below the standard of care.

neonate A baby during the first 28 days of life.

nervous system The body system that controls the body's functions.

neurogenic shock A form of shock in which the nervous system is no longer able to control the diameter of the blood vessels.

neuroprotective agents General classification of medications being developed to protect brain tissue during acute stroke or trauma.

neurosis An anxious reaction to a perceived fear.

neurotoxicity A toxic effect on the CNS.

nitrogen narcosis The development of an apathetic, slightly euphoric mental state due to the narcotic effect of dissolved nitrogen that occurs during diving.

nitroglycerin A tablet or spray commonly prescribed to cardiac patients; acts to dilate blood vessels to increase oxygen flow to the myocardium.

noise Anything that interferes with receiving a message.

norepinephrine A naturally occurring hormone also used as an exogenous cardiac medication that stimulates the heart.

normal percussion note The sound typically heard during percussion of the chest.

normal sinus rhythm The normal electrical activity and rate of the heart.

normotension The condition of having normal blood pressure.

nortriptyline A tricyclic antidepressant medication.

nuchal rigidity Pain and stiffness encountered when attempting to move the neck; typically due to irritation of the meningeal lining of the brain.

obstructive airway disease A generic term for a spectrum of diseases, the most common being asthma and chronic obstructive lung disease.

obtundation A reduced level of consciousness resulting in insensitivity to unpleasant or painful stimuli.

occiput The back portion of the head.

occupational exposures Exposure to gas, chemicals, or other harmful substances that occurs at the workplace.

official name The drug name that is listed in one of the official publications.

open injury or fracture A break in the bone and disruption of the skin.

open-ended question Questions that require more than a simple, often one-word answer.

opisthotonic posturing Acute arching of the back with the head bent back on the neck, the heels bent back on the legs, and the arms and hands flexed rigidly at the joints.

OPQRST Acronym for assessing the complaint, signs, and symptoms of a patient: Onset, Provocation, Quality, Radiation, Severity, Time.

oral medication A drug that is swallowed and absorbed from the stomach or small intestine.

oral report Description of the case given by the EMT–I to medical direction or the receiving hospital.

ordinary negligence Acts or omissions that occur in the attempt to deliver proper care.

organelles Components of cells that carry out the processes necessary for life within each cell.

orotracheal Through the mouth.

orthopnea Worsening of shortness of breath when lying down.

orthostatic hypotension A condition in which a patient's blood pressure suddenly drops on standing up.

oscilloscope Television-like screen that displays an electrical current such as the impulse that travels through the heart's conduction system.

osmosis The movement of water across a semipermeable membrane.

ovaries A walnut-sized pair of glands located on each side of the uterus in the upper pelvic cavity.

overdose Excessive exposure to a substance that has normal treatment uses.

oxygenation The delivery of oxygen to the hemoglobin in the bloodstream.

P wave The first component of the electrical cardiac cycle that represents atrial depolarization.

pallor An unnatural paleness or absence of color in the skin.

palpitation A sensation of pounding or racing of the heart.

pancreatitis Inflammation of the pancreas typically due to alcohol abuse or gallstones.

para The total number of times a woman has given birth.

paradoxical chest movements When part of the chest wall moves in a direction opposite to the rest of the chest.

paraplegia A condition in which the lower extremities become paralyzed.

parasympathetic division Part of the nervous system that originates in the brain and sends messages to affect organs by the cranial nerves. It affects the heart, stomach, and gastrointestinal tract; also called the cholinergic division.

parasympathetic nervous system Division of the autonomic nervous system responsible for slowing the heart rate, intestinal activity, respiratory rate, and pupillary responses.

parenteral drugs Drugs administered into the body by subcutaneous, intramuscular, or intravenous routes.

paresthesia A condition in which the patient complains of tingling or numbness in the arms or legs.

Parkinson's Disease A central nervous system disorder characterized by tremor, progressive loss of motor control and speech difficulty.

paroxysmal nocturnal dyspnea Awakening at night with severe shortness of breath.

partial agonist Drugs that interact with a receptor to stimulate a response but inhibit other responses.

partial-thickness burn A burn that involves the epidermis and dermis but no underlying tissue; also called a *second-degree burn.*

past medical history Significant past medical illnesses or traumatic injury that the patient has experienced.

patent Wide open.

patent airway An open, unblocked airway.

pathogens Microorganisms capable of causing disease in a suitable host.

pathophysiology The study of disease mechanisms.

PCO_2 Abbreviation for partial pressure of carbon dioxide.

Peak Expiratory Flow Rate The measure of the peak rate of air movement during forced exhalation; useful in evaluation respiratory capacity in patients with conditions such as asthma and chronic obstructive pulmonary disease.

peak flow meter Device used to measure peak expiratory flow rates.

pelvic inflammatory disease Inflammation of the female internal genitalia usually due to sexually transmitted disease.

penetrating trauma Any type of invasive injury to the body in which an opening is created.

peptic ulcer disease Illness due to erosions in the lining of the gastrointestinal tract.

percussion A physical examination technique involving tapping a finger over body structures to elicit a sound.

perfusion The process by which oxygenated blood is delivered to the body's tissue and wastes are removed from the tissue.

pericardium The protective layer of membranes covering the heart.

perineum The external female genital region between the urinary opening (urethra) and the anus or rectal opening.

peripheral cyanosis In newborns, peripheral cyanosis involving bluish color to the hands and feet.

peripheral nervous system The portion of the nervous system comprised of cranial nerves, the spinal nerves, and the autonomic nervous system.

peristalsis Propulsive, muscular movements of the intestines.

peritonitis Inflammation of the lining of the abdominal cavity, typically due to hemorrhage or infection.

permeability The degree to which a substance is allowed to pass through a cell membrane.

personal protective equipment Equipment used to protect providers from communicable disease or hazardous chemicals.

pertinent negative The absence of a sign or symptom or lack of a response to treatment that helps substantiate or identify a patient's condition.

pertinent positive The presence of a sign or symptom or response to treatment that helps substantiate or identify a patient's condition.

petit mal seizures A seizure manifesting as a brief absence spell or other abnormal behavior.

pH Potential of hydrogen and is measurement of hydrogen ion concentration.

pharmacodynamics The study of the effects of drugs on the body.

pharmacokinetics The movement of the drugs through the body, including absorption, distribution, metabolism, and excretion.

pharmacology The study of drugs and their effects and actions on the body.

phonation Process of generating sounds or speech with the vocal cords.

photophobia Pain or increased sensitivity to bright light.

Physicians' Desk Reference (PDR) Widely used reference for drug information.

physiology The study of the functions and processes undertaken by the body.

pitting edema Pressure over an edematous area results in a depression in the skin.

placenta A disk-shaped spongy organ that develops in the uterus during pregnancy. The placenta exchanges oxygen and nourishment from the mother to fetus and transfers waste products from the fetus to the mother's bloodstream via blood vessels in the umbilical cord.

placenta previa An abnormal positioning of the placenta in the uterus.

plasma The fluid or water portion of the blood.

platelets Formed elements suspended in plasma that are essential to blood clotting.

pleuritic chest pain Chest pain that varies in quality with respiration, cough, or chest movement.

pneumatic antishock garment (PASG) An inflatable garment sometimes used on patients with severely low blood pressure or serious pelvic instability.

pneumonia Inflammation of the lungs, commonly caused by bacteria.

pneumothorax A condition in which air is present in the pleural space.

po$_2$ Abbreviation for partial pressure of oxygen.

point of maximum impulse (PMI) The area of apical heartbeat, found in the midclavicular fifth intercostal space.

poisoning An exposure to a substance that is generally only harmful and has no usual beneficial effects.

polarized Myocardial cell potential to contract and transmit electrical wave.

popliteal pulse The pulse of the popliteal artery palpated behind the knee.

position of function Immobilizing the injured hand with wrist dorsiflexion and finger flexion.

posterior Toward the back of the body.

posterior tibial pulse Pulse located posterior to the medial malleolus of the ankle.

postictal state The period of a decreased level of consciousness after a seizure that is followed by a gradual return to normal consciousness.

potentiation One drug prolongs or multiplies the effect of another drug.

PR segment The component of cardiac electrical cycle before the QRS complex that represents a pause at the atrioventricular node.

pralidoxime (2-PAM) An antidote used in organophosphate and nerve agent exposure that acts by reactivating cholinesterase.

prearrival medical instructions Instructions for initial care of the patient, often provided by the emergency medical dispatcher, to a person who calls for EMS assistance.

preeclampsia Hypertension and excess fluid retention occurring during pregnancy.

preexcitation syndromes The presence of abnormal conduction pathways between the atria and ventricles.

prefilled syringe A syringe and drug solution packaged together to be used to deliver a single dose.

prefix A sequence of letters that comes before the word root and often describes a variation of the norm.

preinfarction angina Chest pain at rest, considered a type of unstable angina.

preload The passive stretching force exerted on the ventricular muscle at the end of diastole.

premature or preterm infant Infant born before completion of 37 weeks gestation.

premature ventricular contractions Extra cardiac beats originating from the ventricle, interrupting the normal sinus rhythm.

primary apnea Apnea of the newborn that can be reversed by touching and stimulating the baby.

procainamide A cardiac medication that can suppress both atrial and ventricular dysrhythmias.

professional A person who has certain special skills and knowledge in a specific area and conforms to the standards of conduct and performance in that area.

progressive angina Chest pain that is accelerating in frequency and duration.

prolapsed cord During childbirth, a delivery in which the umbilical cord presents during delivery.

propoxyphene (Darvon) A narcotic medication.

protocols Written instructions listing guidelines for the care of patients with specific conditions, illnesses, or injuries.

proximal Nearest the origin of a structure.

psychogenic shock Simple fainting, occurs when blood vessels dilate, allowing blood to pool.

psychosis A mental condition, whereby the patient has lost his or her sense of reality.

pulmonary circulation Vascular system that transports unoxygenated blood from the right ventricle, through the lung-alveolar complex, returning oxygenated blood to the left atrium.

pulmonary edema An excessive backup of fluids in the lungs.

pulmonary embolism The blockage of a pulmonary artery by foreign matter.

pulmonary thromboembolism The blockage of a pulmonary artery by a blood clot.

pulmonary valve A cardiac valve between the right ventricle and the pulmonary circulation.

pulse oximeter A device used to determine the percent of hemoglobin bound to oxygen in the blood.

pulse pressure Measurement of pressure obtained by subtracting the diastolic pressure from the systolic pressure.

pulse rate The number of heartbeats in a minute.

pulseless electrical activity (PEA) A condition in which there is electrical activity in the heart, but no muscle contraction and no pulse.

pupillary reactivity The reactivity of a patient's pupils to light.

Pure Food and Drug Act A law enacted in 1906 to prevent the manufacture and trafficking of mislabeled, poisonous, or harmful food and drugs.

Purkinje fibers Specialized cardiac cells that conduct current from the bundle branches to the individual myocardial cells.

pyelonephritis An infection of the kidney(s) causing flank pain, dysuria, nausea, vomiting, and abdominal pain.

QRS complex A component of cardiac electrical complex that represents ventricular depolarization.

quadriplegia A condition in which all four extremities become paralyzed.

quality improvement An evaluation of services provided and the results achieved as compared with accepted standards.

raccoon eyes Bilateral ecchymosis or bruising around the eye present with a basilar skull fracture.

radiation The transmission of heat through space.

radio frequency The number of times per minute a radio wave oscillates.

rales A crackling or bubbling sound in the lungs.

rapid transport Delivering the patient with multi-system trauma to definitive care without unnecessary delay.

rapid trauma assessment A quick and thorough hands-on examination of the trauma patient to evaluate his or her condition.

rapture of the depths Nitrogen narcosis that occurs during diving.

rebound tenderness An intense pain elicited on withdrawal of direct pressure on a point in the abdomen, signifying intraabdominal irritation or inflammation.

reciprocity Mutual exchange of privileges or licenses by two certifying agencies.

rectal medication A drug is inserted into the rectum.

red blood cells Cells in the blood that contain hemoglobin and are responsible for oxygen transport.

reevaluation Ongoing assessment of the patient to determine change in condition or response to therapy.

reflection Repeating the patient's words (or your summary of them) back to make certain you both are communicating.

registration Act of enrolling one's name in a "register" or book of record.

regurgitation A passive, backward flow of gastric contents from the stomach into the oropharynx.

relative refractory period The period during the myocardial repolarization in which a sufficiently stronger than normal stimulus will initiate depolarization of the myocyte.

repeater system Devices that receive transmissions from relatively low-wattage transmitters on one frequency and retransmit them at a higher power on another frequency, increasing the range of the transmissions.

repolarization The period after depolarization in which the myocyte returns to the resting state.

reproductive system The body system responsible for sexual reproduction.

research The scientific study, investigation, and experimentation in order to establish facts and determine their significance.

respiration The mechanism of inspiring air and expiring carbon dioxide.

respiratory acidosis An abnormal condition with high blood levels of carbon dioxide.

respiratory alkalosis An abnormal condition with low levels of carbon dioxide and large amounts of alkali in the blood.

respiratory rate The number of breaths that occur in one minute.

respiratory system The body system that allows for the exchange of oxygen and carbon dioxide in blood.

response to treatment The patient's response or lack of response to the care that was rendered.

restoration of spontaneous circulation Condition that occurs when the patient is resuscitated to the point of having a pulse without cardiopulmonary resuscitation.

resuscitation To provide efforts to return spontaneous pulse and breathing to the patient in a full cardiac arrest.

retractions The inward movement of the soft tissues of the chest, commonly the suprasternal notch and the intercostal spaces; typically associated with respiratory compromise or airway obstruction.

retrograde amnesia The lack of recall of events before an injury.

retroperitoneal space Potential space behind the "true" abdominal cavity.

rewarming shock Reflex vasodilation that may occur after active external rewarming of patients suffering from hypothermia.

Rh factor An antigen factor considered during blood typing.

rhabdomyolysis Breakdown of striated or skeletal muscle.

rhonchi A coarse gurgling sound in the lungs during the process of breathing.

rigid splint A splint that requires positioning of the body part to fit the splint's shape.

rigidity A condition characterized by hardness and stiffness.

Rule of Nines A system used to estimate the percentage of body surface involved in a burn injury.

Rule of Palms A method to estimate burn size by visualizing the patient's palm as an indicator of 1% of the total body surface area.

run critiques Sessions where providers and medical control physicians review run reports and/or case histories to identify positive and negative aspects of care.

ruptured ovarian cyst A painful condition that occurs when a large ovarian cyst on an ovary ruptures.

ruptured viscus A rupture of a hollow organ within the abdomen, typically the duodenum due to peptic ulcer disease.

sagittal A vertical line dividing the body into right and left portions.

SAMPLE history acronym   An acronym for obtaining a patient's history (signs and symptoms, allergies, medications, past medical history, last oral intake, and events leading to present event).

scaphoid   An abdominal wall that is markedly concave or hollowed.

scene size-up   The immediate evaluation of an emergency scene for the safety of the crew, patient, and bystanders.

sclera   The white aspect of the eyes.

sclerotic   Hardening or thickening of tissues.

scope of practice   Description of what assessment and treatment skills an EMT–I may legally perform.

second heart sound   S2, the heart sound that follows S1, large due to the aortic valve closure.

secondary apnea   Apnea of the newborn that will not reverse with simple stimulation techniques and requires assisted ventilation.

secondary drowning   The recurrence of respiratory distress (usually in the form of pulmonary edema or aspiration pneumonia) after successful recovery from the initial incident.

seizure   A sudden, intense episode of heightened electrical activity in the brain.

semipermeable   Cell membranes that allow only certain substances to pass through them.

septic shock   A form of shock caused by an infection resulting in a massive vasodilation of the circulatory system.

serous membrane   A two-layer epithelial membrane that lines body cavities and covers the surfaces of organs.

severe hypothermia   Hypothermia with a core body temperature of less than 90° F.

shakes   Group of symptoms that occur during alcohol withdrawal including tremor, restlessness, and difficulty sleeping.

shock   A state of inadequate tissue perfusion along with the body's attempt to compensate for the lack of adequate tissue perfusion.

side effect   Any effect of a drug that is unintended.

simple partial seizures   Seizure activity involving only parts of the body, not generalized.

simplex   Radio communication that can occur in only one direction at a time.

sinoatrial node   Point of origin of a cardiac electrical impulse, located high in the right atrium.

sinus arrhythmia   Slight irregularities in rhythm that vary with a person's breathing.

situational awareness   Process by which all facets of the scene and patient are integrated to create an overall picture of the current event.

skeletal system   The framework of the body comprised of bones that allows for protection and movement of the body.

skin   The tough, supple membrane that covers the entire surface of the body.

slander   The utterance of false statements that defame and damage another's reputation.

SLUDGE   An acronym used to describe effects of cholinergic poisoning.

snoring respirations   Noisy, raspy breathing, usually with the mouth open.

sodium bicarbonate   A medication used in the treatment of some overdoses and for correcting severe acidosis.

solutes   A substance dissolved in a solution.

solvent   A dissolving substance, usually a liquid.

special sensory system   The system of the body responsible for the five senses.

spectrum of acuity   The wide range of patient presentations, illnesses, or injuries.

spinal shock   A complete transection of the spinal cord that causes the patient to lose sensation and voluntary movement below the injury.

spontaneous abortion   A sudden and unexpected loss of pregnancy; also called *miscarriage.*

spontaneous pneumothorax   A sudden accumulation of air in the pleural space.

ST segment   The period during the cardiac cycle after ventricular depolarization (QRS) and ventricular repolarization (T-wave).

stable angina   Chest pain that the patient historically feels, which starts with exertion and is relieved with rest and is not worsening in nature.

standard of care   The degree of medical care and skill that is expected of a reasonably competent EMT–I acting in the same or similar circumstance.

standing orders   EMT–I field interventions that are completed before contacting medical control.

Starling's Law of the Heart   Increased return to the heart stretches the ventricles, leading to increased cardiac contractility.

status asthmaticus   A severe prolonged asthma attack that does not respond to standard medications.

status epilepticus   A series of seizures without an interval of wakefulness between them.

sterilization   The process of cleaning equipment that results in complete destruction of all living organisms, including bacterial spores and viruses.

stethoscope   An instrument consisting of two earpieces connected by means of flexible tubing to a diaphragm used to auscultate various body sounds.

stimulants   Medications or drugs that stimulate the central nervous system.

straddle injuries   Trauma to the perineal area, typically from falls with legs abducted.

striae   Stretch marks.

stridor   A high-pitched noise heard on inspiration.

stroke   A condition that results from a disruption of circulation to the brain, causing ischemia and damage to brain tissue; also called *cardiovascular accident.*

stroke volume   The amount of blood pumped into the cardiovascular system as a result of one heart contraction.

stupor   A state of lethargy and unresponsiveness where a person seems unaware of the surroundings.

stylet   A bendable plastic-coated wire useful in facilitating endotracheal intubation.

subarachnoid hematoma   A collection of blood or fluid in the subarachnoid space.

subcutaneous   Under the skin.

subcutaneous emphysema   Presence of air beneath the skin (in the subcutaneous tissues), giving it a characteristic crackling sensation on palpation.

subcutaneous injections   Injections that are given into the fatty layer of tissue below the skin.

sublingual   Under the tongue.

substance abuse   The habitual utilization of medications, street drugs, alcohol, or other intoxifying products.

suicide   The intentional taking of one's life.

suicide attempt A planned event in which the patient has a true intent to die.

suicide gesture Something done by a person intended to ask for help, rather than to die.

superficial burn A burn that only involves the epidermis; also called a *first-degree burn.*

superior Above or in a higher position.

supine hypotensive syndrome Occurs during late pregnancy when the enlarged uterus places pressure on the inferior vena cava, reducing blood flow back to the heart.

suppository One or more drugs mixed in a firm base that dissolves gradually at body temperature.

supraclavicular retractions The use of supraclavicular muscles to aid with ventilation during periods of respiratory distress.

surfactant Material in the lungs that line the alveoli and respiratory passages, reducing surface tension and allowing for easier respiration.

suspension Finely ground drugs that are dissolved in a liquid, such as water.

sympathetic division A part of the nervous system whose primary effect is to increase the heart rate, bronchiole dilation, and increased metabolism and strength; also called the adrenergic division.

sympathetic nervous system Division of the autonomic nervous system that is responsible for constriction of blood vessels, elevation of blood pressure and heart rate, and a feeling of nervousness in a stressful situation.

syncope A transient state of unresponsiveness due to inadequate perfusion of the brain from which the patient has recovered.

synergism Two drugs working together.

systemic circulation The vascular system that delivers oxygenated blood from the left ventricle to the body through arteries and returns to the right atrium through the venous system.

systemic effect Pertaining to the whole body rather than one of its parts.

systemic lupus erythematosis An autoimmune disease that can cause inflammation of brain tissue.

systemic toxins Toxins that have a broad effect on multiple systems of the body.

systole Each contraction of the heart.

tachycardia An elevated heart rate above 100 beats per minute.

tachyphylaxis Rapid development of tolerance.

tachypnea A rapid breathing rate.

tenderness Pain with movement or palpation of an area of the body.

tendons White fibrous tissue that attaches muscles to bones.

tension pneumothorax Condition that occurs when air in the pleural space under pressure, effects the opposite lung, causing inadequate ventilation, and proper cardiac functioning.

tenting A sign of dehydration, the skin remains up when gently pinched.

tetany A condition characterized by cramps, seizures, twitching of the muscles, and sharp flexion of the wrist and ankle joints; sometimes accompanied by attacks of stridor.

the bends Decompression sickness.

The White Paper A 1966 report published by the National Academy of Sciences entitled Accidental Death and Disability.

therapeutic effect A drug's desired effect and the reason the drug is prescribed.

thermolysis The normal bodily means of heat loss and gain.

threshold The critical level at which myocyte depolarization occurs.

thromboembolus An aggregation of clumped RBCs and platelets that travel through the circulation.

thrombolytics "Clot-busting drugs" that chemically dissolve the blockage in blood vessels.

thrombophlebitis An inflammation of the veins typically associated with a superficial blood clot.

thrombotic stroke An acute stroke due to a blood clot in the cerebral circulation.

tissue Groups of similar cells working together to accomplish a common function.

TKO rate "To keep open" rate of infusing the intravenous solution; it is also referred to as *KVO* (keep vein open) and is equal to approximately 8 to 15 gtts (drops) per minute.

tolerance An individual's capacity to endure medications.

tonic-clonic seizure movements Alternating, jerking movements, typically seen in generalized seizures.

Torsade de Pointes A unique variant of polymorphic ventricular tachycardia, meaning "twisting about the points," characterized by QRS complexes that alternate (usually gradually) between upright deflections and downward deflections.

tort The breach of a legal duty or obligation resulting in an injury, either physical, mental, or financial.

tort law Law that covers a private or public wrong or injury that occurs due to a breach, or break, of a legal duty or obligation.

toxidromes Patterns of toxicity seen in groups of drugs, poisons, or toxins.

tracheal lumen Cavity or channel within the trachea.

tracheal tugging Situation in which the Adam's apple appears to be pulled upward on inspiration; occurs in the presence of airway obstruction.

traction splint A splint designed to maintain mechanical in-line traction to help realign fractures, commonly used with femur fractures.

trade name The brand of the drug that is registered by the United States Patent Office.

transceivers The radio component that serves as both a transmitter and receiver.

transcutaneous pacing The process by which regular electrical stimulation is supplied to the myocardium through an external pacemaker with leads positioned on the thorax.

transdermal Through the skin.

transient ischemic attack (TIA) A strokelike neurological deficit that completely resolves within minutes to hours; also called a *mini-stroke.*

transverse A horizontal line dividing the body into an upper and lower portion.

trauma center Specially recognized hospitals providing emergency and specialized intensive care to critically ill and injured patients.

traumatic asphyxia A severe crushing injury to the chest and abdomen.

treatment orders Treatment directive given to the EMT–I by medical direction.

tremor The rhythmic, purposeless, quivering movements resulting from the involuntary alternating contraction and relaxation of opposing groups of skeletal muscles.

trench foot A condition resembling frostbite that historically affected the feet of soldiers who kept their feet in wet socks and shoes for long periods

tricuspid valve The cardiac valve between the right atria and the right ventricle.

tricyclic antidepressant drugs A class of antidepressant medications; in overdose situations, it can have diverse effects on the autonomic nervous system and cardiac conduction system.

tripod position Bodily position taken by patients with severe respiratory distress; involves leaning forward on the hands.

trunking Communication equipment that allows multiple agencies or systems to share frequencies.

turgor The elasticity of the skin.

type I diabetes (insulin-dependent) A disease in which patients typically have disease onset at a younger age, are prone to diabetic ketoacidosis, and require insulin injections to live.

type II diabetes (non–insulin-dependent) The type of diabetes in which the onset is after the teenage years and may be controlled with diet or noninsulin medications.

U-wave Typically not present in the cardiac cycle, these waves follow the T-wave and represent myocardial damage of electrolyte disorders (hypokalemia).

umbilical The attachment between the fetus and the placenta.

unintentional poisoning Poisoning where there is no intent by any individual to poison or hurt someone.

United States Pharmacopeia A reference for drug information.

unstable angina Angina that either is new in onset or differs from a patient's typical stable angina pattern.

upper gastrointestinal (GI) bleeding Bleeding that originates anywhere in the GI tract from the mouth to the duodenum.

urban hypothermia Cold stress among the aged, intoxicated, or debilitated that can cause fatal hypothermia.

urinary system The body system responsible for the removal of waste products from the body in the form of urine.

uterine rupture Rupture of the uterus during pregnancy; has a high mortality rate for both mother and fetus and occurs most commonly after the onset of labor.

uterus A hollow, muscular organ shaped like an inverted pear located in the pelvic cavity between the urinary bladder and the rectum.

vagal maneuvers Techniques that stimulate the parasympathetic nervous system and may be tried to terminate PSVT in hemodynamically stable patients.

vagina The birth canal or passageway between the uterus and the external genitalia or perineum.

vagolytic Anticholinergic drugs that block the parasympathetic nervous system.

vasopressin A naturally occurring antidiuretic hormone, which, in high doses, acts as a powerful vasoconstrictor.

veins Blood vessels that transport blood back to the heart.

ventilation The process by which air and oxygen is inspired and carbon dioxide is expired.

ventricles The lower chambers of the heart muscle that are responsible for the majority of blood movement.

ventricular conduction disturbances Delays in cardiac electrical conduction through either the bundle branches (right or left) or the fascicles (anterior or posterior).

ventricular fibrillation Erratic, uncoordinated firing of multiple sites in the ventricle, resulting in no cardiac output.

ventricular tachycardia Wide-complex tachycardia with a focus in the ventricles and varying degrees of cardiac output.

verapamil A calcium channel blocker that slows conduction and increases refractoriness in the atrioventricular node.

vesicular breath sounds A normal sound of rustling or swishing heard with the stethoscope over the lung periphery, these sounds are usually higher pitched during inspiration and fade rapidly during expiration.

vials Glass or plastic medication containers that have a self-sealing rubber stopper on the top, from which multiple doses may be drawn.

vipers A class of poisonous snakes found in the United States.

visual acuity examination A brief examination to determine how accurately the patient is seeing.

vital signs The measurement of key bodily functions including pulse, blood pressure, and respiratory rate.

volatile chemicals A group of agents of abuse including aerosols, glues, and gasoline.

wet drowning Hypoxemia due to prolonged water immersion with significant water insult to the lungs.

wheezes A high-pitched squeal in the lungs during the process of breathing.

wide open rate No restrictions of fluid flow from the intravenous bag to the patient.

working diagnosis Perceived medical illness or injury that is affecting the patient based on current information.

zone of coagulation The central area of the burn wound that has sustained the most intense contact with the thermal source.

zone of hyperemia The periphery of the zone of stasis and has increased blood flow as a result of the normal inflammatory response.

zone of stasis Stasis surrounds the critically injured area and consists of potentially viable tissue, despite the serious thermal injury.

INDEX

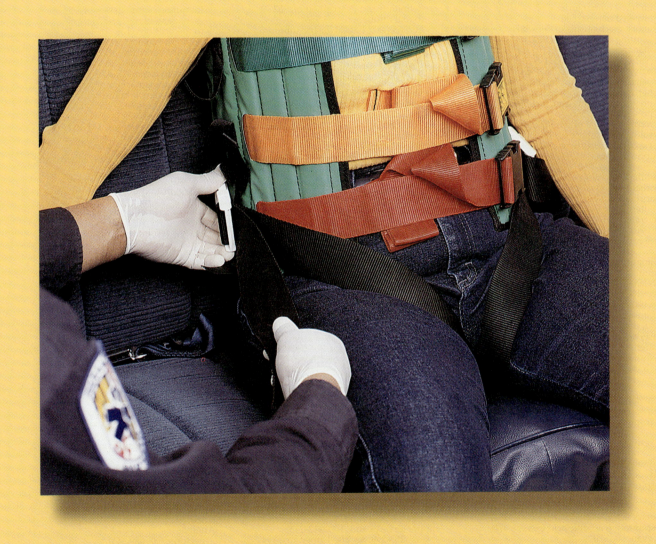